LOW BACK SYNDROMES

Integrated Clinical Management

NOTICE

LOW BACK SYNDROMES

Integrated Clinical Management

Edited by:

Craig E. Morris, DC, DACRB, FAFICC, CSCS

Adjunct Associate Professor, Cleveland Chiropractic College, Los Angeles
Post-Graduate Faculty, Southern California University of Health Sciences
Post-Graduate Faculty, Rehabilitation, Canadian Memorial Chiropractic College, Palmer Chiropractic College
Chairman, Manipulation and Manual Medicine Committee, American Back Society
Chiropractic and Rehabilitation Consultant, National Hockey League Players' Association (NHLPA)
Torrance, California

McGraw-Hill
Medical Publishing Division

New York Chicago San Francisco Lisbon London Madrid Mexico City
Milan New Delhi San Juan Seoul Singapore Sydney Toronto

The McGraw-Hill Companies

Low Back Syndromes: Integrated Clinical Management

2 3 4 5 6 7 8 9 0 QPD/QPD 0 9 8 7

ISBN 0-07-137472-8

This book was set in Palatino by TechBooks, Inc.
The editors were Michael Brown and Christie Naglieri.
The production supervisor was Catherine Saggese.
Project management was provided by TechBooks, Inc.
Quebecor World was printer and binder.

This book is printed on acid-free paper

Cataloging in Publication Data for this book is on file at the Library of Congress.

This book is dedicated to:

Jana and our four—

Andrei H., Jana A., Christopher L., and Cameron S.

and

Those patients who ultimately benefit from the

instruction contained within these pages

and

Vlad

Contents

PART V. REHABILITATION OF THE LOW BACK/707

PART VI. CLINICAL MANAGEMENT/819

Contributors

Andrew R. Block, PhD
The WellBeing Group, Plano, Texas
Chapter 19: Biopsychosocial Factors in Low Back Syndromes
Chapter 33: Presurgical Psychological Screening for Low Back Syndromes

Nikolai Bogduk, BSc (Med), MBBS, PhD, MD, DSc, Dip Anat, Dip Pain Med, FAFRM, FAFMM, FFPM (ANZCA)
Professor of Pain Medicine, University of Newcastle, and Head, Department of Clinical Research, Royal Newcastle Hospital Newcastle, New South Wales, Australia
Chapter 31: Evidence-Based Treatment of Back Pain

Alan Breen, DC, PhD, MIPEM
Director, Institute for Musculoskeletal Research and Clinical Implementation—AECC, Bournemouth, Dorset, United Kingdom
Chapter 14: Subjective and Objective Outcomes Assessment of Low Back Syndromes

David C. Byfield, BSc Hons, DC, MPhil, FCC (Ortho)
Head of Subject—Chiropractic, Principal Lecturer, Welsh Institute of Chiropractic, University of Glamorgan, Pontypridd, Wales, United Kingdom
Chapter 8: The Posterior Joint Syndromes: Zygapophyseal and Sacroiliac Joints

V. Cascioli, M: Tech Chiropractic
Senior Lecturer, University of Glamorgan; Doctor of Chiropractic Pontypridd, Wales, United Kingdom
Chapter 8: The Posterior Joint Syndromes: Zygapophyseal and Sacroiliac Joints

J. David Cassidy, DC, PhD, DrMedSc
Professor of Epidemiology, Department of Public Health Sciences, University of Toronto; Senior Scientist, Division of Outcomes and Population Health, Toronto Western Hospital Research Institute, Toronto, Ontario, Canada
Chapter 11: Nonspecific Low Back Pain and Chronic Low Back Syndromes

Leon Chaitow, ND, DO
Honorary Fellow, School of Integrated Health, University of Westminster, London, United Kingdom
Chapter 13: Functional Examination for Low Back Syndromes

David A. Chapman-Smith, LLB (Hons)
Attorney at Law, The Chiropractic Report, Toronto, Ontario, Canada
Chapter 36: Risk Management for Low Back Syndromes

Alan L. Colledge, PT, MD, FAADEP
Medical Director, Labor Commission of Utah; Associate Clinical Professor, Department of Family and Preventative Medicine, Rocky Mountain Center for Occupational & Environmental Health, University of Utah; Medical Chair, International Association of Workers Compensation Boards and Commissions Impairment and Pain Committees, Provo, Utah
Chapter 34: Management of Occupational Low Back Injuries

Michael Scott DeBerard, PhD
Associate Professor of Psychology, Utah State University, Logan, Utah
Chapter 34: Management of Occupational Low Back Injuries

Rick B. Delamarter, MD
Associate Clinical Professor, Department of Orthopaedic Surgery, University of California, Los Angeles School of Medicine; Medical Director, The Spine Institute at Saint John's Health Center, Santa Monica, California
Chapter 32: Clinical Decision Making: When to Recommend Back Surgery

Anthony DeLitto, PT, PhD, FAPTA
Associate Professor and Chair, Department of Physical Therapy, University of Pittsburgh; Director of Research, Comprehensive Spine Center, Vice-President for Education and Research, Centers for Rehab Services/University of Pittsburgh Medical Center, Pittsburgh, Pennsylvania
Chapter 29: Clinical Management of Athletes with Low Back Syndromes

Ronald Donelson, MD, MS
President, SelfCare First, LLC, Hanover, New Hampshire
Chapter 15: McKenzie Protocols for Mechanical Assessment of the Low Back

Mark S. Edinger, DC, DABCO
Post-graduate faculty, National University of Health Sciences; Co-Director of Yeomans-Edinger Chiropractic Center, SC, Ripon, Wisconsin
Chapter 14: Subjective and Objective Outcomes Assessment of Low Back Syndromes

Jake Epker, PhD
Private Practice, Mobile, Alabama
Chapter 19: Biopsychosocial Factors in Low Back Syndromes

Leonard J. Faye, DC, FCCSS (Canada) Hon
Private practice, Post-Graduate Lecturer, Los Angeles, California
Chapter 25: Manual Therapeutic Techniques for Low Back Syndromes: An Overview

Steven Z. George, PT, PhD

Assistant Professor, Department of Physical Therapy, Brooks Center for Rehabilitation Studies, Center for Pain Research and Behavioral Health; University of Florida, Gainseville, Florida

Chapter 29: Clinical Management of Athletes with Low Back Syndromes

Philip E. Greenman, DO, FAAO

Emeritus Professor, Department of Osteopathic Manipulative Medicine, Emeritus Professor, Department of Physical Medicine & Rehabilitation, Michigan State University College of Osteopathic Medicine, East Lansing, Michigan

Chapter 25: Manual Therapeutic Techniques for Low Back Syndromes: An Overview

Jaroslaw P. Grod, DC, FCCS (C)

Professor and Director, Continuing Education, Canadian Memorial Chiropractic College, Toronto, Ontario, Canada

Chapter 2: Functional Anatomy of the Lumbar Spine

Kambiz Hannani, MD

Director, Spine Specialty Institute, West Covina, California

Chapter 32: Clinical Decision Making: When to Recommend Back Surgery

Steven L. Heffner, DC, Diplomate MDT

Faculty Member, Canadian Memorial Chiropractic College, Southern California, University of Health Sciences; Mechanical Diagnosis and Therapy Specialist of the Spine and Extremities, Laurel Health System, Wellsboro, Pennsylvania

Chapter 15: McKenzie Protocols for Mechanical Assessment of the Low Back

Chapter 22: McKenzie Protocols for Mechanical Treatment of the Low Back

Walter Herzog, PhD

Professor, Faculties of Kinesiology, Medicine and Engineering, Canada Research Chair for Molecular and Cellular Biomechanics, Associate Dean for Research (Kinesiology), University of Calgary, Calgary, Alberta, Canada

Chapter 3: Low Back Biomechanics: Structure and Function of the Low Back

Chapter 21: The Biomechanics of Spinal Manipulation

Drew Heusch, PhD

Senior Lecturer, Welsh Institute of Chiropractic, University of Glamorgan, Pontypridd, Wales, United Kingdom

Chapter 8: The Posterior Joint Syndromes: Zygapophyseal & Sacroiliac Joints

Paul Hodges, PT, PhD, MedDr

Professor and NHMRC Senior Research Fellow, Division of Physiotherapy, The University of Queensland, St. Lucia, Queensland, Australia

Chapter 5: Functional Control of the Low Back

Edward B. Holmes, MD, MPH

Assistant Professor, Occupational Medicine, University of Utah; Chief Medical Consultant, Disability Determination Services for Social Security, Salt Lake City, Utah

Chapter 34: Management of Occupational Low Back Injuries

Paul D. Hooper, DC, MPH, MSc

Professor, Southern California University of Health Sciences, Whittier, California

Chapter 11: Nonspecific Low Back Pain and Chronic Low Back Syndromes

Chapter 20: Manipulation Techniques for Low Back Syndromes

Eric L. Hurwitz, DC, PhD

Associate Professor in-Residence, University of California, Los Angeles School of Public Health, Department of Epidemiology, Los Angeles, California

Chapter 4: Epidemiology of Low Back Syndromes

Gary Jacob, DC, LAc, MPH, CHES, DipMDT

Associate Faculty, Clinical Sciences, Southern California University of Health Sciences, Private Practice, Los Angeles, California

Chapter 22: McKenzie Protocols for Mechanical Treatment of the Low Back

Vladimir Janda, MD, DSc (1928–2002)

Professor Emeritus, Department of Rehabilitation Medicine, Postgraduate Institute of Medicine, Charles University Hospital, Prague, Czech Republic

Chapter 5: Functional Control of the Low Back

Chapter 23: Mobilization Methods for Low Back Syndromes

Chapter 25: Manual Therapeutic Techniques for Low Back Syndromes: An Overview

Muffit L. Jensen, DC

Associate Professor, Cleveland Chiropractic College, Los Angeles, Burbank, California

Chapter 23: Mobilization Methods for Low Back Syndromes

Hugh I. Johnson, MPA

Regional General Manager, Utah Transit Authority, Orem, Utah

Chapter 34: Management of Occupational Low Back Injuries

Kendall M. Jones, MD, DABR

Medical Director, Plano Radiology Center, Plano, Texas

Chapter 16: Diagnostic Imaging Approaches to the Evaluation of Low Back Syndromes

Matthew H. Kowalski, DC, DABCO

President, New England Spine Institute, PC, Holbrook, Massachusetts

Chapter 6: The Intervertebral Disc and its Syndromes

Chapter 7: The Stenotic Syndromes

James Kutz, BS, JD

Partner, Post & Schell Law Firm, Harrisburg, Pennsylvania; Adjunct Professor, Dickenson School of Law, Penn State University, Harrisburg, Pennsylvania

Chapter 36: Risk Management for Low Back Syndromes

Andre Labbe, PT, MOMT

Clinical Instructor—Louisiana State University Medical Center Department of Physical Therapy, Louisiana State University; Owner/Director of Clinical Operations—Advantage Physical Therapy, Harahan, Louisiana

Chapter 27: Rehabilitation of the Surgical Lumbar Spine Patients

Richard C. Lehman, MD

Medical Director, US Center for Sports Medicine; Medical Director, Florida Panthers, Hockey Team, National Hockey League; Consulting Orthopedic Surgeon, University of California, Los Angeles Track and Field Team, St. Louis, Missouri

Chapter 29: Clinical Management of Athletes with Low Back Syndromes

Chapter 30: Clinical Management of Elite Athletes with Low Back Syndromes

Gideon Letz, MD, PMH

Assistant Clinical Professor, University of California, San Francisco; Medical Director, State Compensation Insurance Fund; Occupational Medicine Physician, Kaiser Permanente, San Francisco, California

Chapter 10: Red Flags for Serious Disease in Low Back Syndromes

Peter W. McCarthy, BSc, PhD

Head of Chiropractic Research Unit, Welsh Institute of Chiropractic, University of Glamorgan, Pontypridd, Wales, United Kingdom

Chapter 8: The Posterior Joint Syndromes: Zygapophyseal and Sacroiliac Joints

Robin McKenzie, MNZSP, MNZMTA, RPT

McKenzie Institute International, Waikauae, New Zealand

Chapter 15: McKenzie Protocols for Mechanical Assessment of the Low Back

Chapter 22: McKenzie Protocols for Mechanical Treatment of the Low Back

Vert Mooney, MD

Clinical Professor of Orthopaedics, University of California, San Diego; President, US Spine and Sport Foundation, San Diego, California

Chapter 35: Clinical Management of Chronic, Disabling Low Back Syndromes

Craig E. Morris, DC, DACRB, FAFICC, CSCS

Adjunct Associate Professor, Cleveland Chiropractic College, Los Angeles; Post-Graduate Faculty, Southern California University of Health Sciences; Post-Graduate Faculty, Rehabilitation, Canadian Memorial Chiropractic College, Palmer Chiropractic College; Chairman, Manipulation and Manual Medicine Committee, American Back Society, Chiropractic and Rehabilitation Consultant, National Hockey League Players' Association (NHLPA); Torrance, California

Chapter 1: The Clinical Evolution of Low Back Syndromes

Chapter 9: Myofascial Pain in Low Back Syndromes

Chapter 10: Red Flags for Serious Disease in Low Back Syndromes

Chapter 11: Nonspecific Low Back Pain and Chronic Low Back Syndromes

Chapter 12: History and Physical Examination for Low Back Syndromes

Chapter 13: Functional Examination for Low Back Syndromes

Chapter 20: Manipulation Techniques for Low Back Syndromes

Chapter 23: Mobilization Methods for Low Back Syndromes

Chapter 25: Manual Therapeutic Techniques for Low Back Syndromes: An Overview

Chapter 26: Rehabilitation Strategies in Low Back Syndromes

Chapter 27: Rehabilitation of the Surgical Lumbar Spine Patients

Chapter 28: Lumbopelvic Sensorimotor Training and Functional Stabilization

Chapter 30: Clinical Management of Elite Athletes with Low Back Syndromes

Chapter 36: Risk Management for Low Back Syndromes

Chapter 37: Low Back Syndromes: A Final Perspective

Donald R. Murphy, DC, DACAN

Clinical Assistant Professor, Brown University School of Medicine; Clinical Director, Rhode Island Spine Center, Providence, Rhode Island

Chapter 10: Red Flags for Serious Disease in Low Back Syndromes

Chapter 25: Manual Therapeutic Techniques for Low Back Syndromes: An Overview

Chapter 26: Rehabilitation Strategies in Low Back Syndromes

Chapter 28: Lumbopelvic Sensorimotor Training and Functional Stabilization

Srdjan S. Nedeljkovic, MD

Assistant Professor of Anaesthesia, Harvard Medical School; Fellowship Education, Director, Pain Management Center, Brigham and Women's Hospital, Boston, Massachusetts

Chapter 17: Minimally Invasive Approaches to the Evaluation of Low Back Syndromes

Chapter 24: Minimally Invasive Procedures for the Treatment of Low Back Syndromes

Niels Grunnet-Nilsson DC, MD, PhD

Director of Studies, Institute of Sports Science and Clinical Biomechanics; Faculty of Health Science, University of Southern Denmark, Odense, Denmark

Chapter 11: Nonspecific Low Back Pain and Chronic Low Back Syndromes

Roger E. Pack, MPT, OCS

Clinical Supervisor, Physical Therapy, Spine and Sports Center, Provo, Utah

Chapter 34: Management of Occupational Low Back Injuries

Phil Page, PT, ATC, MS, CSCS

Manager of Clinical Education & Research, The Hygenic Corporation, Baton Rouge, Louisiana

Chapter 27: Rehabilitation of the Surgical Lumbar Spine Patients

Diane N. Resnick, DC

Assistant Professor, Southern California University of Health Sciences; Clinical Education Coordinator, University Health Center, Pasadena, Pasadena, California

Chapter 12: History and Physical Examination for Low Back Syndromes

Scott Rose, PT

Certified Manual Physical Therapist Candidate through the NAIOMT; Clinical Director Advanced Training and Rehabilitation, Chesterfield, Missouri

Chapter 30: Clinical Management of Elite Athletes with Low Back Syndromes

Greg Roskopf, MA

Owner/Founder, Muscle Activation Techniques, Denver, Colorado

Chapter 30: Clinical Management of Elite Athletes with Low Back Syndromes

Kim Ross, DC, PhD

Associate Professor, Chairperson for the Department of Applied Chiropractic, Canadian Memorial Chiropractic College, Toronto, Ontario, Canada

Chapter 3: Low Back Biomechanics: Structure and Function of the Low Back

Michael J. Schneider, DC, PhD (cand.)

PhD candidate in Rehabilitation Science, University of Pittsburgh; Doctor of Chiropractic, Private Practice, Pittsburgh, Pennsylvania

Chapter 9: Myofascial Pain in Low Back Syndromes

Paul G. Shekelle, MD, PhD

Professor of Medicine, University of California, Los Angeles School of Medicine; Staff Physician, West Los Angeles, Veterans Affairs Medical Center, Los Angeles, California

Chapter 4: Epidemiology of Low Back Syndromes

Dennis R. Skogsbergh, DC, DABCO, DACBR

Texas Back Institute, Plano, Texas; Quantum Diagnostic Imaging, Richardson Texas

Chapter 6: The Intervertebral Disc and its Syndromes

Chapter 7: The Stenotic Syndromes

Chapter 16: Diagnostic Imaging Approaches to the Evaluation of Low Back Syndromes

Rand S. Swenson, DC, MD, PhD

Associate Professor of Medicine (Neurology) and Anatomy Dartmouth Medical School, Hanover, New Hampshire

Chapter 18: Neurodiagnostic Approaches to the Evaluation of Low Back Syndromes

Bruce P. Symons, MSc, DC

Research Associate, Human Performance Laboratory, Faculty of Kinesiology, University of Calgary; Village Square Chiropractic & Rehabilitation Clinic, Calgary, Alberta, Canada

Chapter 3: Low Back Biomechanics: Structure and Function of the Low Back

Joe L. Verna, DC

San Diego, California

Chapter 35: Clinical Management of Chronic, Disabling Low Back Syndromes

Robert A. Walker, PhD

Professor and Head, Department of Basic Sciences, New York Chiropractic College, Seneca Falls, New York

Chapter 2: Functional Anatomy of the Lumbar Spine

Mark Webster, BSc, DC, MSc, FCC (Ortho)

Award Leader and Senior Lecturer, Welsh Institute of Chiropractic, University of Glamorgan, Pontypridd, Wales, United Kingdom

Chapter 8: The Posterior Joint Syndromes: Zygapophyseal and Sacroiliac Joints

Steven G. Yeomans, DC, DABCO, FACO

Post-graduate Faculty, National University Health Sciences, Northwestern University Health Sciences, Palmer College of Chiropractic, Los Angeles College of Chiropractic; Doctor of Chiropractic; Co-Director and President of the Yeomans-Edinger Chiropractic Center, SC, Ripon, Wisconsin

Chapter 14: Subjective and Objective Outcomes Assessment of Low Back Syndromes

Introduction

Dr. Craig Morris has asked me to write a brief Introduction for the upcoming textbook on low back syndromes. During the past 30–40 years this writer has become more and more convinced of the value of using a book like this as a reference on frequent occasions in his or her daily work.

In an intriguing novel, *The Torch*, the well known neurosurgeon Dr. Wilder Penfield gives the reader fascinating insight into the life and times of Hippocrates who taught and practiced medicine on the Aegean island of Cos more than 2,000 years ago. He is recognized today as one of the founders of modern medicine. His home and clinic were adjacent to the harbor. Every evening after a hard day's work he and his students and assistants foregathered under the famous Plane Tree for a glass of wine and for serious discussion of that day's work. Many erudite physicians and therapists throughout the world have accepted Hippocrates' approach over the centuries as the basis for learning and teaching in many of the best universities in the world. Fellows at Oxford and Cambridge Colleges have since the 14th century followed the Hippocratic practice, developing what they have called the Combination Room. In college halls the fellows have met evening by evening in such a room for dinner and afterwards for the drinking of very carefully prepared and selected College Port of the highest possible standard. This was combined with both light and serious discussion of an infinite variety of topics. Through such an informal activity many important discoveries have been made over the years in scientific and other fields.

For *Low Back Syndromes: Integrated Clinical Management*, we can recognize two main approaches: (1) that of cooperation in which we are careful not to tread on one another's toes, and (2) that of combination in which we aim to synthesize two or more approaches to form an entirely new one. I believe that one very important aim of the participants in this present volume is to stimulate the formation of a great many Combination Rooms all over the world in which well recognized teachers and practitioners meet together to wine and dine and "sip their port" and in such an informal setting lay the foundations for an entirely new approach to the topic.

A brief account of a personal approach made by two of us to the "Combination Room" idea serves to further clarify my point. In 1944 after 3 years as physician and surgeon at an Anglican Mission Hospital near Mombasa, I was offered a job by the Kenya government as doctor in charge of a Rehabilitation Centre in Nairobi for African soldiers discharged from the Kenyan army, to improve their health before discharge from the forces. My colleague, Mr. Frank Keer, was trained as a British army radiographer (i.e. radiological technician) in China. Neither of us had any formal training in Rehabilitation Medicine. As we set about this task, a completely different field of medical practice soon presented itself, the treatment of African patients with tuberculosis of the spine and other joints. We decided to tackle this urgent problem with but little approval from the medical authorities, using three different approaches to treatment for lesions of the spine: (1) to put the spine at rest with the patient in a plaster of Paris shell; (2) when the general condition of the patient was satisfactory, to undertake a bone grafting operation to immobilize the affected part of the spine to prevent increasing deformity and promote healing of the affected bone and joints; and (3) Frank's idea, to give each patient several periods of exercises to arms and legs each day to stimulate the overall health and well being of the patient. This threefold regime usually lasted about three months. It seemed good to add to this the pleasant environment of a garden with bougainvilleas, roses and jacaranda trees. In retrospect we realized that this regime was in fact a combination of traditional and complementary medicine. The results were effective in 80% of patients who would otherwise be crippled. This exciting and accidental discovery demonstrated to us that much better results could be obtained by combining orthodox traditional and complementary methods and that the overall general health of the patient was almost as important as the local treatment of disease in the spine. We later added the benefits of occupational therapy, arranging for each patient to spend time each day, while still in a plaster shell, making sisal doormats for which he or she was paid a small amount of money. Years later in Canada, this first Kenyan ad hoc experiment was put into practice in a more elaborate way in other fields of medicine and surgery. In fact it was the beginning of a new approach that incorporated several different disciplines. For those of us so engaged, this type of experiment led to what proved to be the development of a form of complementary medicine. Chiropractors such as Drs. Gordon Potter, David Cassidy, and Dale Mierau had a very important role in this.

Tools such as this book help us to remain abreast of the varied clinical options available. The relentless pursuit of friendly relations with colleagues in other branches of health care is highly desirable, allowing us the opportunity to learn and work together as described in the Hippocratic approach and in the development of the Combination Room. In so doing, our patients become the ultimate beneficiaries.

It is the combination of varying schools of clinical thought and scholarly traditionalism that leads me to invite the reader to explore the combined knowledge contained within the ensuing pages of this text.

W. H. Kirkaldy-Willis, MA, MD, LLD (Hons), FRCS, (E and C), FACS, FICC (Hons)
Emeritus Professor of Orthopaedics, University of Saskatchewan, Canada
Past President, Canadian Orthopaedic Research Society
Past President, International Society for the Study of the Lumbar Spine
Past President, North American Spine Society
Past President, American Back Society

Foreword

One year ago, Craig Morris asked if I would write a Foreword for his new multidisciplinary book, *Low Back Syndromes* (LBS). I considered the request and said something like "I'd like to have a look at it before I can agree to do this." The first to arrive was the table of contents. At first glance, it appeared to be principally authored by one discipline (chiropractors) and the topics did not appear to connect or convey how this story was going to flow. My first impression was that this is a blind attempt to understand "the elephant" from a chiropractic perspective. How wrong I was.

Some of you may be familiar with the Hindu fable by John Godfrey Saxe that begins:

It was six men of Indostan
To learning much inclined
Who went to see the Elephant
(Though all of them were blind)
That each by observation
Might satisfy his mind

The first approached the Elephant
And happening to fall
Against his broad and sturdy side
At once began to bawl
"God bless me!-but the Elephant
Is very like a wall!"

And so each of the men explored a single, yet different, part of the elephant, proclaiming after much inspection and palpation that the elephant was either like a wall, a tree trunk, a snake, a dagger, or a rope. And yet, since the beast they were investigating was much bigger than they could feel (and they were blind), none of them fully understood the elephant.

And so these men of Indostan
Disputed loud and long
Each in his own opinion
Exceeding stiff and strong,
Though each was partly in the right,
And all were in the wrong!

The Moral
So, oft in theologic wars
The disputants, I ween,
Rail on in utter ignorance
Of what each other mean,
And prate about an Elephant
Not one of them has seen!

This, in my opinion, has been the history of the diagnosis and treatment of low back and pelvic girdle pain.

The proofs arrived and I began to read Chapter 1—The Clinical Evolution of Low Back Syndromes, by Craig Morris. This is an excellent review of the scope of the problem and discusses the economic impact of LBS in both industrialized and less developed countries as well as the natural history of low back pain (LBP). Morris goes on to describe the evolution of the various paradigms (views of "the elephant") including the arrival of the "disc paradigm" through to the current focus on a "biopsychosocial paradigm." He explains how and why the Cochrane review was done (and who Cochrane was) as well as the origins of the current push for evidence-based health care. This is indeed a well-written overview and introduction to the complex problem of syndromes involving the low back.

I was excited and very interested in what was to come. After reading six or seven more chapters, I realized that the material truly represented a multidisciplinary perspective, and not just a singular approach. I felt that I had been exposed to the structure and function of the intervertebral discs, the zygapophyseal joints, the muscles (core and others), and the emotional state of "the elephant"; however, I still had no consensual framework or paradigm for how all this structure, neurophysiology and mind set helped me as a clinician treat "the elephant." What is the best way to get him moving or at least feeling better? What is exposed through reading the various chapters is that we not only have what Janda called "terminological chaos" but also assessment and treatment chaos with relatively little consistent evidence yet to guide us in clinical practice.

Then I read Chapter 37—Low Back Syndromes: A Final Perspective, by Morris. "The lack of a universally accepted classification system that subdivides nonspecific back pain remains one of the key links to gaining control of disabling LBS".

This is only one of many "pearls" in this chapter that demonstrate that Morris has a clear view of the elephant and has taken on this mammoth task to encourage each of us to remove our blinders, to focus on something less familiar and to consider how we can go forward from here to resolve the current dilemma of LBS. We cannot yet be evidence-based, there isn't enough evidence or understanding of the whole elephant, some parts are better than others but are still isolated from the whole problem.

Another pearl from Chapter 37: "Each clinician must realize that today's research or guidelines are not final products, but rather the latest in an ongoing production. In order for clinicians to provide the optimal treatment of their specific patient's needs, a dynamic balance between clinical experience, clinical research, and clinical guidelines must be continually reestablished."

Yes, indeed and this will require:

1. Standardized terminology regarding the classification of low back impairment vs. pain.
2. Clinical reasoning with respect to the volume of assessment tests/procedures that are possible, yet not always applicable.
3. The development of treatment protocols specific to the impairment and not to non-specific low back pain.
4. Greater interprofessional communication and collaboration than is currently the global standard.

Only then will we have the ability to develop more sound studies (randomized and controlled) to test the efficacy of treatment programs that are specific to each subgroup of impairment leading to low back pain. Until then, the best evidence-based treatment will be to use a multimodal approach that considers the biomechanical, neuromuscular, and emotional needs of the patient. It is time to remove the blindfolds, to question our own paradigms, and to grow towards a clearer view of this big picture.

So my recommendation would be to start with Chapter 1, then read Chapter 37, and then explore the journey into the varying views of the elephant (all the other chapters), recognizing that each can only consider a part of the whole problem. This text, together with the sharing of ideas and research through multidisciplinary conferences, is a huge step towards finally getting the big elephant moving. Congratulations Craig, I'm looking forward to the second edition!

DIANE LEE (PHYSIOTHERAPIST)
White Rock, British Columbia

Foreword

For a social problem that crosses many cultures, Dr. Morris has provided a volume of work addressing the problem by engaging the expertise of multiple disciplines. A pain in the back has probably been in existence ever since humans decided to stand on two feet. Back problems have been prevalent in the work place ever since someone started to pay attention and keep records. In fact, it seems the more attention we give to this social disease (my personal label for the malady), the more ubiquitous it becomes.

This social disease provides justification (to varying degrees depending on the group) for the existence of spinal surgeons (orthopedic and neurological), doctors of chiropractic, physical therapists, osteopaths, naturopaths, acupuncturists, biomechanists, psychologists, massage therapists, exercise physiologists, athletic trainers, personal trainers, exercise gurus, etc. and etc. International and national scientific and academic bodies bow allegiance to this social phenomenon to the point that they publish expensive journals and host annual meetings in exotic places, focused on this single subject.

Over the years, a single cause linked to a single cure has plagued the industry with expensive care heaped on those beleaguered with a wide range of manifestations of this once-thought-to-be unique phenomenon. The varied outcomes associated with the methods of treating and managing back problems have brought relief to some but have also failed many, leading to mental if not physical invalidism, unproductive citizenry, reluctant third-party payers, distraught patients and family, and individual providers making a handsome living off the backs of others.

Governments of industrialized countries have poured millions on millions of dollars into research seeking an understanding of the cause of this social phenomenon. Progress has produced many new theories and elaborate diagnostic schemes relating to the cause, multiple techniques and procedures relating to the care and clinical guidelines, and protocols emanating from the "evidence." Yet, the problem and the business related to the problem continue to grow.

Since this social disease has impact across multiple disciplines, I recommend this book for all who have any interest in back related syndromes. There is more than a morsel for all who are feeding at the table of resolving back problems. Perhaps this is even an insight, a guidepost to the future solution of the back pain dilemma. If specialists and generalists in multiple disciplines can read each others' works, learn from each others' experiences and carve out space for the benefit of each others' procedures, perhaps, just perhaps, the patient, the person suffering from this malady, will receive care that may speed recovery, reduce residual complications, cut costs, eliminate drug and physician dependence, and put John and Jane Q. Public back into the work force. Perhaps the dilemma of back related syndromes would begin to diminish.

Dr. Morris is to be applauded for his success in herding a group of professionals into a common corral, obtaining their vision and wisdom, creating a coherent collection of commentary and providing all of this in a publishable product worthy of digestion. I applaud all the contributors for the immensity and completeness of their work. I hope that each will be diligent in reading and assimilating the work of their colleagues.

Reed Phillips, DC, PhD
President, Southern California University of Health Sciences
Whittier, California

Preface

The main motivation for this book was impatience, an example that good things can indeed arise from less-than-admirable qualities. After growing tired of trying to search out the various methods and updated rationales of differing schools of thought regarding the assessment and treatment of low back conditions, I felt that a text published encapsulating these strategies was only a matter of time. Because it was not forthcoming, I ultimately decided to invite leading authorities of these approaches to explain their methods as contributors of chapters. So here it is. . . .

The day of isolated approaches for low back syndromes is past. Multidisciplinary approaches have arrived and this now requires an updated, broad, clinical perspective. New demands are being placed on health care providers like never before. Patients and third-party groups now expect opinions regarding procedures from providers who do not perform those procedures. Surgeons are asked to opine regarding non-surgical measures in which they have no training and, conversely, non-surgeons are invited to comment on surgical measures. Regardless of one's specialty, he or she is now expected to have sufficient current knowledge of the other disciplines' approaches to either comment on or co-manage specific cases.

Some explanation and clarification regarding this book is appropriate. It is important to understand why I used the term of "low back syndromes" instead of other options such as "low back pain" in the title. Professor Nikolai Bogduk stated on many occasions that low back pain and sciatica are separate disorders, a statement with which I am in agreement. The same can be said for the so-called "pseudo-sciatic" conditions such as pain referred to the lower extremities via myofascial or posterior joint origin. Nevertheless, they all have a common point in that they arise from the same anatomic region. Therefore, I decided to describe this collage of disorders as low back syndromes. For the sake of organization of this text, it provides a relatively convenient generic umbrella beneath which subtopics can be placed.

Second, there is the issue of multiple professional disciplines, and specialties within those disciplines, being integrated as contributors throughout the book. I attribute this approach to those individuals who have heavily influenced me with their tutelage and by their example. They helped to teach me that relieving spinal pain, or any other type of human ailment, far exceeds the boundaries of any single discipline. Instead, they demonstrated that clinical excellence, professional pragmatism and personal service must set the real standard. For this guidance, I must thank Toby Friedman, MD, Bob Morris, DC, Donald Sage, MD, Richard Vincent, DC, Karel Lewit, MD, DSc, Scott Haldeman, DC, MD, PhD, Aubrey Swartz, MD, Pharm D,and D Allan MacKenzie, MD

Third, you will notice that there are at times contrasting perspectives when comparing opinions of various contributors of the book. This is not meant to be confusing, but it is by design an attempt to demonstrate that respected opinions in this field of healthcare can vary significantly. I feel that the real answers to todayís questions regarding low back disorders will become clarified when those leaders who are involved in the solutions clearly understand and respect all of the perspectives and then apply scientific rigor and the clinical arts to the mix. This text is designed to be a tool in that regard.

I would like to thank my high school journalism teacher, Ms. Konnie Krislock, for inspiring me to continue writing. Despite the fact that I did not pursue journalism as a profession as she hoped, she strongly felt I should write in professional journals should I become a doctor. One never knows the impact that such suggestions might have in the future.

Without the assistance and support of three key individuals, this book would never have been initiated or completed. These include my wife, Jana, and my friend and colleague, Donald Murphy, DC. It was Don's book, *Conservative Management of Cervical Spine Syndromes* (McGraw-Hill, 1999), that inspired me to move forward with this project. In addition he contributed three chapters to this text and provided wise counsel on a variety of issues.

The third key person, who helped me to organize this book and provide invaluable and sage advise, was my dearly departed friend and mentor, the late Professor Vladimir Janda (MD, DSc). Even in failing health and a half-a-world away, he was always available for me. His insights and enthusiasm for this project helped to bolster me in the early stages, and his memory inspired me in the later stages when he was no longer with us. Revered around the world by allopaths, chiropractors, osteopaths, and physical therapists, he along with those previously mentioned reinforced the value of interprofessional respect and cooperation. His fingerprints of brilliance are evident throughout the pages of this text.

There are a host of contributors who provided additional assistance beyond what should have been reasonably asked of them. These include Dennis Skogsbergh, DC, Matthew Kowalski, DC, Philip Greenman, DO, Kim Ross, DC, PhD, Paul Hooper, DC, MS., Srdjan Nedeljkovic, MD, Leon Chaitow, ND, DO, and Steven Heffner, DC.

I would like to also thank the library facilities and staff at the Southern California University of Health Sciences, Cleveland Chiropractic College, Los Angeles, and the University of California, Los Angeles Medical Library.

Finally, I would like to thank the staff at McGraw-Hill Publishers for their support and patience. Special thanks goes to Mr. Michael Brown, my publisher, and also to Ms. Christie Naglieri, Ms. Maya Barahona, Ms. Seema Koul, and John Hannon, DC for their editorial assistance.

PART

I

OVERVIEW

CHAPTER

1

THE CLINICAL EVOLUTION OF LOW BACK SYNDROMES

Craig E. Morris

OUTLINE

OBJECTIVES

1. Provide a brief insight into the problem of low back syndromes.
2. Present a brief explanation of the factors that led to this problem.
3. Discuss key leaders who influenced the clinical evalution in low back disorders.
4. Discuss the advent of Evidence Based Health Care.
5. Introduce the biopsychosocietal model of chronic, disabling pain.

INTRODUCTION

Low back disorders are as old as man. Whether the malady is confined to the spine or referred to the pelvis and periphery, these manifestations nevertheless share a common lumbopelvic origin. These local and referred conditions are collectively called the *low back syndromes* (LBS), a group that continues to impact the human race in a variety of ways.

Over the past century, LBS have become increasingly problematic, receiving an escalating amount of attention and concern in the medical, industrial, and political world because of the burdens placed on health-care and social care systems.[1,2]

Because of the health-care world's failure to bring LBS under control, Waddell[3] labeled back pain "a twentieth century medical disaster." If this is so, then continuing spiraling economic and social costs would present a crippling burden to national economies, making LBS a twenty-first-century societal catastrophe.

In an era of dramatic and widespread societal advances, why would an archaic issue like LBS be such a problem? The answer to this question is complex and indeed requires explanation. This chapter will attempt to provide a brief account of various factors that led to this increased interest. In so doing, it is intended to lay the groundwork for a deeper understanding of the issues presented in the subsequent chapters of this textbook.

THE SCOPE OF THE PROBLEM

Low back pain is the most prevalent of all musculoskeletal conditions, afflicting nearly everyone at some time in their life.[1] LBS are the most important disorders associated with absence from work in the welfare states.[4] Waddell noted lifetime prevalence of back pain between 59% and 84%.[3] The 1-year prevalence rate has been estimated between 15% and 40%,[3,5,6] while between 4% and 33% of the population will experience back pain at any one point.[1,3] It should be noted that most of the statistics usually involve low back pain rather than all LBS. Therefore, the prevalence of this group of disorders is not known, except to say that it is greater than local back pain alone, of which it is a subset.

Industrialized countries have experienced a dramatic increase in the utilization and costs associated with LBS in recent decades.[2,7] There is evidence that LBS patients utilize more overall medical care proportionally for non-LBS conditions than those without LBS.[8,9]

However, wide variations in cost estimates among different studies make it difficult to clearly determine the real direct and indirect costs of this malady.[10] For example, Figure 1–1 demonstrates cost estimates for low back disorders among two large studies[8,10] that reached far different conclusions.

Although the direct costs of LBS (i.e. the cost of care from providers, hospitals, diagnostics, pharmaceuticals, etc.) are enormous, the indirect costs (i.e. costs for disability, administrative activities, lost productivity, etc.) are several times greater.[7,11] Figure 1–2 demonstrates two studies[7,11] that found indirect costs for LBS to be seven to eight times greater than the direct costs.

Although the problem of LBS afflicts all industrialized countries.[12] There is recent evidence that the costs were lower in Great Britain than in Germany.[13] Perhaps these lower costs are associated with sociocultural and pesion program changes, which led to a measurable decline in British LBS-associated disability.[14]

Non-industrialized countries demonstrate interesting trends in LBS, despite a real paucity of research. A South West Nigerian population demonstrated back pain rates similar to industrialized countries, although there was much less associated lost time from work.[15] A second study found that back pain rates were significantly lower in developing countries than in wealthier countries.[16] That paper also found that heavy physical laborers in developing countries demonstrated lower back pain rates than urban workers in both affluent and low-income countries, bringing into question the notion that back pain is associated with hard physical labor.[16]

THE "NATURAL" HISTORY OF BACK PAIN

Acute low back pain appears to be a relatively benign problem, often described as "self-limiting." Nachemson stated that only 10% suffer disabling back pain after 6 weeks[17] and later noted that the natural history studies show an excellent prognosis for low back pain and a good prognosis for those with sciatica.[18] Coste et al. found that 90% of the patients with acute low back pain recovered within 2 weeks.[19] In an extremely positive summary, van den Hoogen et al. found that "All aspects of suffering caused by low back pain tend to diminish over time."[20]

However, statistics may be deceiving, since these numbers may not take into account the issue of recurrence, where patients whose back pain abates

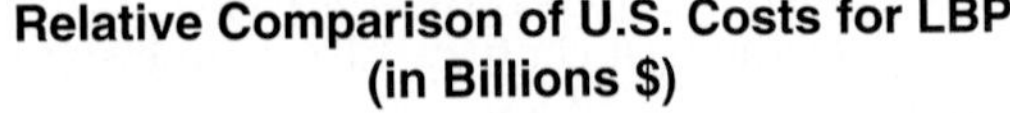

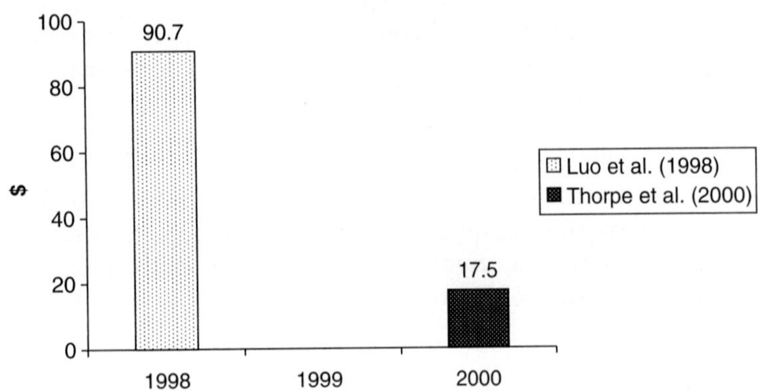

FIGURE 1–1. Graphic comparison of estimated costs for treatment of back problems in the United States. The significant variation provides a clear picture of the difficulties of accurately determining the true financial burden of LBS.

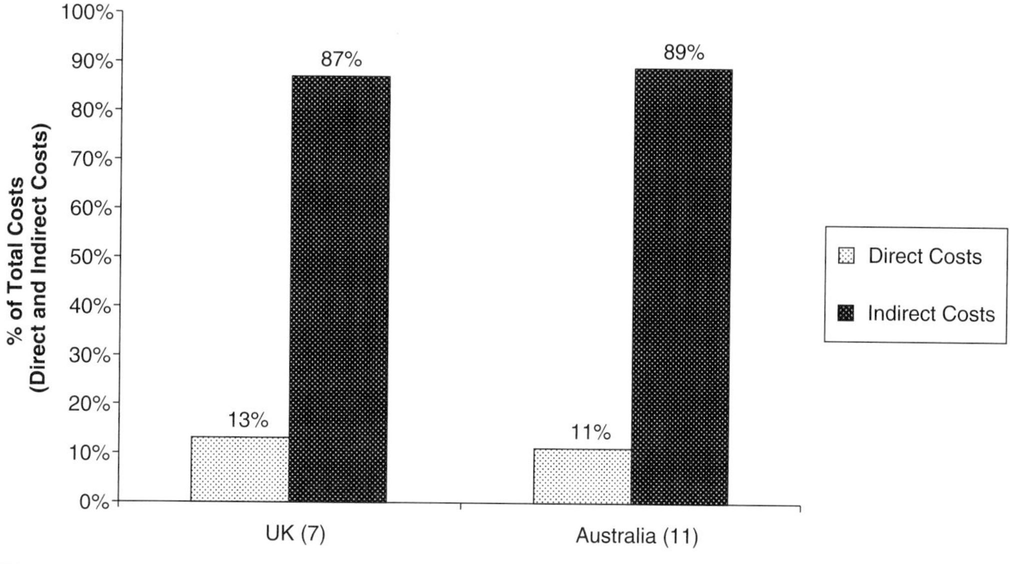

FIGURE 1–2. Comparison of direct and indirect costs of low back problems, demonstrating that the direct costs are dwarfed by the indirect costs.

only to later return. For example, Carey et al. found that, from 208 randomly selected clinics, patients with low back pain who were pain-free for 3 months following the initial visit were again monitored at 6 and 22 months.[21] The recurrence rates of this patient population were significant. Between 8% and 14% of the patients experienced a recurrence during the period 3–6 months following the initial visit. The numbers worsened among those between 6 and 22 months, with recurrence rates varying from 20% to 35%. It was noted that recurrence rates were higher for HMO (i.e., Health Maintenance Organization—a comprehensive, private-sector, American-managed care program that includes inpatient and outpatient treatment) patients than for non-HMO patients. The numbers are yet worse for another study, in which about two thirds demonstrated recurrences over a 1-year period and some one third of those who previously lost work-time were again disabled due to a back pain relapse.[22]

Like many aspects of LBS, the statistics regarding recurrence rates are quite variable, leading one to avoid overreliance on any one study and perhaps reminding all to remember Mark Twain's famous warning, "There are lies, damned lies, and statistics!" One recent study demonstrated such statistical variation by using three separate measures of back pain recurrence for the same group of patients. Wasiak et al.[23] demonstrated such statistical variability by comparing a claims-based recurrence rate of 7.1%, a care-based recurrence rate of 12%–49%, and a disability-based recurrence rate of 6%–17%.

The reason for these recurrence rates is not known; however, research has demonstrated that there may be far more involved than simply pain. Indeed, it is now clear that reduced or alleviated back pain does not necessarily mean that the back condition is fully resolved. Hides et al. demonstrated that patients who experienced their initial onset of back pain that quickly improved subsequently demonstrated atrophy and fatty infiltration of the local multifidus musculature 10 weeks later.[24] The same authors later reported that patients who received traditional medical treatment *and* exercise avoided multifidus fatty infiltration and atrophy, while those who received only traditional medical treatment (i.e., no exercise) sustained it.[25]

These findings suggest that the seemingly contradictory notion that acute back conditions are self-limiting with an excellent natural history, but that there is a high liklihood of a significant residual remains. It must be understood that the pain recedes, but other factors may indeed persist that lead to recurrences. What these factors are and how relevent each one may be remains uncertain. Therefore, an approach that focuses upon the presence or amelioration of pain in the short-term appears to be somewhat simplistic, although concrete evidence directly tying additional complicating factors to chronicity and recurrence remains elusive.

COSTS OF CHRONICITY

It stands to reason that, because of escalating overall costs, the incidence of back pain must have skyrocketed over the past several decades. Astonishingly, the overall incidence of back pain itself appears to be relatively stable, according to one noted Finnish study.[26]

Four years later, another Finnish paper demonstrated that the prevalence of back pain remained essentially unchanged, but also added that the rates among individual subgroups varied significantly. Those individuals with lower education, lower income, blue-collar jobs, and jobs that required laborious work were at highest risk.[27]

The problem of LBS does not lie in the increasing incidence of these disorders, but rather in the incidence of *disabling* low back conditions, the *chronicity* of those problems, and the *associated societal sequelae.*

Nachemson et al. found that 50% of workdays lost is attributable to 15% of the working population. They also stated that 80% of the social and health-care costs were directed toward only 10% of patients with chronic pain and disability.[28]

Sick leave costs are a major cost driver of chronic LBS. Indeed, a recent German study observing the economic consequences of low back pain for 1 year following a rehabilitation program found that the greatest costs were associated with sick leave.[29]

To make matters worse, these statistics may not properly address a component that has until recently been all but ignored: *presenteeism*. Presenteeism is lost industrial productivity caused by workers who perform their work at a decreased capacity. Prior estimates of lost productivity measured individuals who did not work, but ignored those who were present, yet less productive due to illness.

There is no currently accepted measure to realistically quantify the lost productivity yield associated with presenteeism, although it is believed to be monumental. For example, one third of the employed persons polled in a recent study stated that they had gone to work two or more times during the past year when they should have taken sick leave.[30] Stewart et al. stated that 76% of lost productive time, defined as absence or reduced performance due to common pain conditions (headache, backache, etc.), was due to reduced productivity while at work.[31] They estimated the lost productive time in the United States for a 1-year period between August 2001 and July 2002 at $61.2 billion. Perhaps these statistics are reliable, as they represent approximately a sixfold increase compared to the estimates of the British study above (£10.67 billion in 1998)[7], when accounting for the US-UK population ratio.[32]

Recent studies have demonstrated increasing evidence that the subacute stage post-injury (4–12 weeks) is a critical period in preventing disability.[33] If one accepts this notion, then early and effective treatment avoids costs of prolonged care and the majority of resources should be used during the initial 3 months of treatment. Figure 1–3 demonstrates the chronological annual costs of claims in the California workers' compensation system. This defines an example of a problem where costs have spiraled out of control, with a small portion of the resources (less than 10% of the costs, in fact) being attributed to the first year of care. The overall costs are unknown due to time limitations of the study, and in reality may be limited only by the patients' life span.

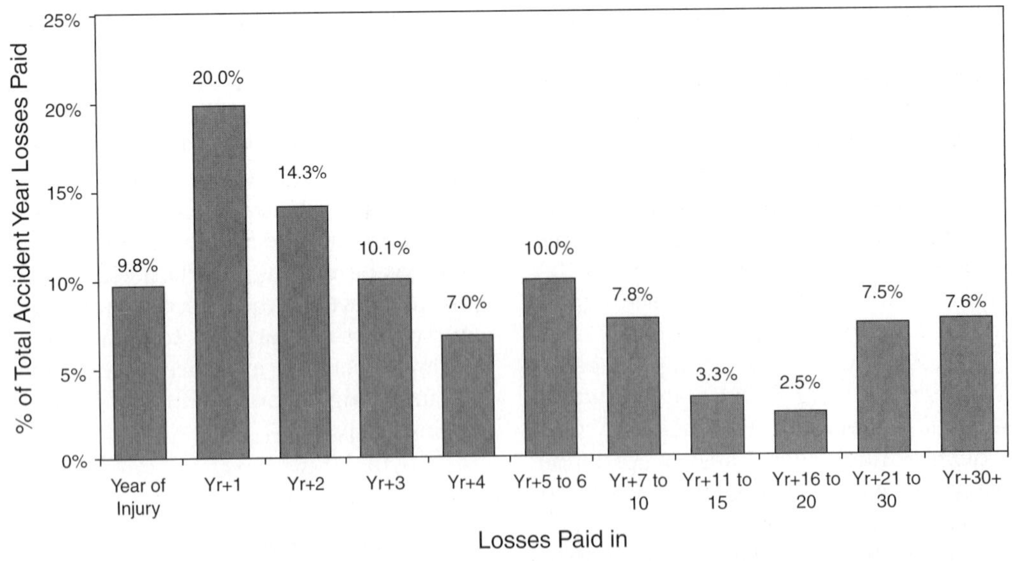

FIGURE 1–3. California workers' compensation costs. This 2003 graphic demonstrates that a relatively small percentage of financial resources are expended during the initial period of treatment. Instead, vast resources are dispersed over the next decade, providing a classic example of the burden of chronicity. *(Modified with permission from the Workers' Compensation Research Institute Rating Bureau of California.)*

In an age where statistical/analytical summaries can be produced to provide comprehensive economic landscapes, it becomes quite easy to overlook the individual and familial toll of disabling back syndromes. While the cultural architecture of the twenty-first century continues to evolve, the family unit nevertheless remains the building block of societies. As such, the stress that disability brings to the individual and his or her family must not be ignored. For example, Strunin and Boden described significant changes that occur when family members become disabled with chronic back pain, causing restructuring of family responsibilities, alterations in the performance of household and parenting duties, and compromised leisure activities with family and spouse. Increases in depression and anger led to mounting strains on family relationships.[34] In another study, Eriksen et al. demonstrated a strong correlation between long-term disability and separation or divorce.[35]

In summary, the national costs of LBS are staggering, while the toll on individuals can be devastating.

SOCIETAL PARADOX

In a time of advancing technologies, scientific research, mass communication, and organized healthcare standards, it would seem incongruous that such an aged, nagging issue as low back disorders would continue to plague today's advanced societies. The reasons for this paradox are indeed complex and may be associated less with the degree of back pain itself. Rather, the relative societal issues and costs associated with the condition appear to be where the true burden to industrialized nations occurs. Understanding the societal issues and measuring the losses associated with this condition is no simple matter, since it moves far beyond economic issues and includes a human toll on an individual, familial, social, and societal level. A brief explanation will be provided in the ensuing pages.

To appreciate the series of events that led to the current situation requires a little reminiscense from a multifactorial perspective.

SPINAL CONDITIONS OF ANTIQUITY AND PIVOTAL CLINICIANS OF HISTORY

Spinal disorders have been documented in the studies of ancient cadaveric specimens. For example, spinal problems consisting of infectious diseases, degeneration, malformation, cancer, in addition to understandable posttraumatic events, were found in a group of 700 South Americans dating back more than 8000 years.[36]

A Colombian pre-Hispanic mummy, belonging to the ancient Guane society, was found to have spinal tuberculosis, or Pott's disease, with the stereotypical angular kyphosis present.[37]

Egyptian mummies have demonstrated such conditions as Sheuermann's disease, scoliosis, and spondyloarthropathy.[38]

Ramesses II ("The Great"), one of the most famous of all mummies, demonstrated clear signs of spinal pathology. Indeed, it demonstrates significant diffuse osteophytic changes that are dèbat due to either ankylosing spondylitis or diffuse idiopathic skeletal hyperostosis.[39,40]

Hippocrates the Koan (fifth to fourth century BC), the great Greek physician who is considered the father of modern medicine, wrote extensively about orthopedics, including the spine. Two of his most important treatises on the subject were entitled "On Joints" and "On Nature of Bones." He organized diseases of the spine into five categories:

1. Kyphosis as a result of (a) disease or (b) spinal injury
2. Scoliosis
3. Concussion
4. Dislocations of the vertebrae
5. Fractures of the spinous processes

Hippocrates devised treatment for scoliosis in the fifth century BC, and for traumatic fractures. He designed two traction devices, namely, the Hippocratic Ladder, generally used for dislocations of joints, and the Hippocratic Board or Bench, generally used for spinal curvature, and established treatment protocols that endured for centuries. He was the first to give an account of spinal diseases and describe tuberculous spondylitis.[41] His work set the stage for future approaches to LBS.

Galen of Pargamum (second century AD) was another Greek physician who supported and expanded many of Hippocrates' theories and methods. He was the unquestioned authority on medicine from the second century until the sixteenth century AD. He broke new ground on spinal anatomy and on physiology, established standards in research, and developed theories that covered many of the medical specialties. Perhaps his greatest contributions were concerned with injuries of the spinal cord.[42,43]

Rheumatism, a colloquial term for painful musculoskeletal conditions, has afflicted famous and influential humans throughout history. Ceccarelli noted that numerous kings, queens, and popes were plagued by gout for centuries.[44] Those with low back pain and sciatica, considered a rheumatic condition until the mid-nineteenth century,[45] included Jacob of biblical times and also Thomas Jefferson.[46] Chronic polyarthropathy afflicted King Constantine of Greece and Mary Queen of Scots.[47] While these events occurred prior to the days of uniform medical records or statistical analysis, these historically famous individuals who suffered from various LBS might present a glimpse of what was occurring among the masses.

SETTING THE STAGE

Back Disability Prior to and during the Nineteenth Century

Prior to the nineteenth century, low back conditions seemed to have had little, if any, impact on human society as a whole.[47] Disabled individuals consisted of the blind, deaf, dumb, epileptics, and the insane rather than those with back problems. Musculoskeletal disabilities were an issue, however, that invariably covered amputees, such as soldiers following the American Civil War of the mid-nineteenth century. However, the amputees of that period were typically placed into jobs with minimal physical demands which allowed them to earn a living, such as making brooms or tools. The lack of societal support programs meant that the established social system, typically the family or religious institutions, provided support for the disabled.

Allan and Waddell noted that disability from back pain began to appear only in the late nineteenth century.[45] They also stated that this was preceded by two seminal ideas—back pain came from the spine and was caused by injury. Boni added that the herniated intervertebral disc was also recognized during this time period,[48] although its relationship to sciatica was discovered later. Thereafter, backache and sciatica were treated together.

Too Much Information and Too Little Knowledge

Although some consider the information age to have started with Alexander Graham Bell's invention of the telegraph, Dewar stated that it actually began with Gutenberg and his printing press in 1492 Germany.[49] This allowed mass distribution of the printed media, and everything relating to mass transportation of information then ensued. The information age provided impetus for the industrial age, the nuclear age, the space age, and the digital age. The information age was then catapulted further with the transmission of information over lines and then over "airwaves."[49] A third generation has now evolved with the advent of the computer and the internet. The impact of each event on society has been, and remains, profound. In the relative chronology of the human experience, the transmission of information has advanced at near-light speed over a relatively brief period.

The profound impact of increasing amounts of information has been as great in the field of health care as any other aspect of society. The number of medical articles and journals grew exponentially between 1750 and the early 1990s, at which point more than 34,000 references from 4000 journals were added monthly to the US National Library of Medicine's database.[48] Organized medicine, confronted with a growing body of information that more than one person could possibly absorb, divided the load by establishing a variety of specialties of practice and research. This was a successful remedy, although temporary. In the last decade of the twentieth century, the topic of *information overload* was brought forward by Arndt,[50] Faber,[51] and Hunt and Newman.[52] The number of journals leveled off in the early 1990s,[53] so there are currently over 400,000 biomedical articles produced annually.[54]

Ironically, the failure to control disabling back syndromes among countries that employ the most advanced health-care systems demonstrates that a plethora of information does not guarantee sufficient knowledge to resolve the problem.

Urbanization, Industrialization, and the Human Response

In order to provide a brief summary of the etiology of the epidemic of disabling LBS, one must travel beyond the parameters of the classic clinical texts and explore the causative societal factors.

The nineteenth century brought dramatic changes in the Western world, with a transition from a rural, agrarian-based population to an urban, industrially based society.[55,56] The transition in the human social and physical experience was dramatic. Machines were gradually introduced to perform physically demanding chores previously done by humans and animals. Whereas individuals previously performed a variety of physical demands in the fields, for example, throughout the day, city workers became gradually more confined to repetitive tasks that required less physical demands performed through a more limited range of motion. Although sitting at the workplace was less common in the past, productivity-driven industry necessitated a gradual transition to this less physically demanding, relatively static strategy. This strategy was exemplified by the introduction of the assembly line, a model designed to allow workers to remain in place with the target product being assembled passed by. By and large, this transition to a less physically demanding means of making a living was considered a significant societal advance because of increased productivity, it progressively may have increased the risk of physical deconditioning. In addition to remaining in prolonged, constrained postures at work, increased interaction within the burgeoning urban population logically created increased risks of emotional stresses amid mounting productivity demands and interpersonal interactions. Instead of earning a living, a broad-based strategy that required individuals to manufacture all of their needs, urbanization and industrialization brought forth the new concept of "earning an income."[55]

In summary, the industrial revolution brought forth advances in productivity while paradoxical changes occurred to the individual in terms of limited physical demands and increased emotional stresses.

The Disaster

The nineteenth and twentieth centuries brought the most dramatic changes to date in human history in terms of population, technology, sociology, and economy. History records monumental advances in travel, manufacturing, communications, and quality of life. Ironically, the benefits have proven to be a "double edged sword," in that there have been, and continue to be, unanticipated prices paid for these advances. This is certainly so with the following topics providing examples of these unanticipated complications:

- *Mass transit evolution:* There were relatively few trains and motorcars at the turn of the 20th century. The ensuing decades brought forth an explosion in the numbers of mass-produced motorized ground, water, and air transportation devices. As the numbers and utilization of these high-speed mechanical wonders increased, so did the number of acceleration/deceleration-type injuries. This brought about a new complication to the societal mix: financial compensation claims for such injuries. Indeed, clinics were established to provide treatment for this new type of trauma that was initially related to trains, which were called the Railway Institutes.[57,58] Finally, emerging transportation technologies provided new opportunities for large-scale relocation of varying nationalities to form new urban intercultural melting pots.
- *Social engineering and the welfare state:* The key issue for most individuals of the nineteenth century Western world was survival. For those who were fortunate enough to be free from enslavement, they had the opportunity to independently fend for themselves and their families. If they were unable to accomplish this, then there were few options for their survival. As countries gained wealth, a framework to establish more complex strategies to protect the needy few was engineered. This led to the beginning of the welfare state in a growing number of industrialized countries.[55] This focus has evolved in many modern day countries so that quality of life issues, rather than survival issues, are now at the forefront. This includes continuing income in case of a significant illness or injury. Insurance from disabling conditions is based on the simple notion that many members of a society can take up the slack for the few who are unable to perform their share of the work. With time, these assurances became less appreciated, as they became routinely expected entitlements. These expectations gradually transitioned within the population and become a birthright. It has been suggested that LBS are a "culture driven disorder."[59] While this approach appears to be the only fair way to take care of the disabled population, one question must be asked: What happens if the number of disabled individuals swell to the point that the workers can no longer support them?[2,60]
- *Workers' compensation:* The idea for national protection of the worker injured on the job was the brainchild of "The Iron Chancellor", Otto von Bismarck, in the nineteenth century.[61] This was largely a political plan designed to unify the disparate Germanic principalities into one nation. Workers' compensation insurance is now a commonly accepted strategy in various formats among many nations around the world. While this should be considered a social triumph, research has consistently proven that workers who are injured on the job fare far worse in their recoveries and subsequent ability to compete in the open labor market compared to individuals who are not injured at work. Because of the added complexity of the management of industrially related LBS, Chapter 34 is dedicated to this challenging topic.
- *Clinician profiles:* Humans are a compilation of their respective experiences, the expression of which carries into their professional lives. Clinicians, therefore, are prone to beliefs that can facilitate or interfere with their patients' recovery. On the basis of years of experience of teaching family care medical residents, Williamson et al. noted three barriers among residents regarding teaching their patients' psychosocial factors of chronicity.[62] These issues include their beliefs regarding their role as physicians in primarily ruling out organic disease; believing that the patient also primarily requests ruling out organic disease; and physician concerns about approaching patients as people, who may indeed suffer from many of the same psychosocial problems as the physician himself or herself. Like any other group, physicians vary in their communication skills and it has been demonstrated that they often have very different opinions compared to those of their patients regarding the quality of information transmitted regarding musculoskeletal conditions during clinical interaction.[63]
- *Health-care advances:* Improvements in technologies, communication, and research led to dramatic progress in a variety of human maladies. These

advances are credited with expanding the understanding of etiological aspects of disease, of diagnostics and treatment methods, many of which are explained in the ensuing chapters of this textbook. With these evolving standards, increased societal confidence led to increasing dependence on, and expectations of, treatment of conditions previously managed independently, such as many mild to moderate back pain. Unfortunately, it has been estimated that the etiology of up to 85% of all back problems cannot be determined, a cautious reminder regarding overconfidence in the diagnosis and treatment of LBS.[28,64]

- *Racial/cultural variations:* A variety of races and cultures combined to form new national social and societal complications. These groups had different values, mores, and perspectives regarding work ethic, gender, and health-care issues, requiring a broader understanding of the psychosocial aspects of LBS in order to properly mange these conditions. Indeed, a great deal of research has shown that cultural issues affect perceptions about pain and disease including issues related to chronic disabling LBS.[65–68] In an era where one must be careful to be sensitive to respect variations among ethnicities, genders, and cultures, it becomes rather easy for the health-care community to simply avoid these potentially uncomfortable topics instead of confronting and establishing strategies designed to address the individual needs of each.

While these changes were not evenly distributed to all of humanity globally, the majority of the residents of the more industrialized countries benefited from the advances. In so doing, the role of government gradually changed. Instead of being designed to provide personal safety, from invasion for example, and an opportunity for prosperity if one worked diligently, populations came to expect that they were "entitled" to prosperity and to protection from loss of prosperity, regardless of the diligence of their work.

These factors were not independent of each other, but were synergistically intermingled to establish a ripe environment barriers to recovery from LBS: the growth of a *disability mindset*.

CLINICAL ASSESSMENT, PERSPECTIVE, AND TREATMENT OPTIONS: A BRIEF HISTORICAL REVIEW

Although an in-depth review of the key clinical contributors to the advancement of the current understanding of LBS is beyond the scope of this chapter, tribute is paid to a select few in order to gain an appreciation of this clinical evolution.

General Anesthesia

The discovery of general anesthesia brought dramatic changes in surgery, allowing procedures to be painlessly performed on motionless, unconscious patients. Several people are credited with bringing general anesthesia forward to become a mainstay for surgical procedures, such as spinal surgery; however, there is evidence that Crawford Williamson Long, was the first to use ether during surgery on March 30, 1842.[69,70] Whereas spinal surgery was previously left for the few cases where patients would either agree to, or were incapable of stopping, such a painfully invasive procedure, the advent of general anesthesia allowed surgery to be utilized to a far broader range of cases and conditions.

Antiseptic Techniques

Joseph Lister, brought antiseptic surgical methods and wound management to the medical world. His teaching and 1867 classic text *Antiseptic Principles of the Practice of Surgery* brought about dramatic decreases in postoperative fatality, allowing this branch of medicine to be used among a broader spectrum of conditions with less risk.[71,72]

Manual/Physical Methods

Although manual healing methods such as massage and manipulation have been utilized throughout history, a few noted individuals brought various schools of thought to the modern age. Andrew Still introduced a new clinical paradigm he termed osteopathy in 1855.[73,74] D. D. Palmer brought forth his model of chiropractic in 1895.[75–77] Two leaders in manual medicine emerged in England around the turn of the twentieth century, James B. Mennell and John Cyriax, whose work was continued by their respective sons, John Mennell and James Cyriax, that heavily influenced the direction of orthopedic medicine, physical medicine, and physical therapy.[78–81]

Diagnostic Imaging

Wilhelm Roentgen was the first to use radiation to produce radiographic images.[82–84] Indeed, his observations regarding the use of x-ray for clinical assessment spawned what later became the specialty of radiology. It was Roentgen's work that allowed for later advances in diagnostic imaging such as scintigraphy, computerized tomography (CT), and magnetic resonance imaging (MRI).[82]

Neurology

Sir Charles Sherrington played a pivotal role in establishing the groundwork for the clinical understanding and expansion of neurophysiological principles for the twentieth century. His contributions earned him the 1932 Nobel Prize for Physiology or Medicine. Just like the other leaders presented here, other clinical pioneers heavily influenced him. In Sherrington's case, Pavlov, Bell, Cajal, and Jackson[85] were key influential figures. Sherrington is credited with bringing forth the concept of the synapse,[86] clarifying the physiological mechanism of the stretch reflex (also known as Liddell–Sherrington reflex), helping to organize dermatomal mapping,[85] coining the term *proprioception*[87] and his most renowned achievement "Sherrington's law of reflex inhibition."[87] His classic text *The Integrative Action of the Nervous System*, first published in 1906, provided insights and brilliant deductive reasoning to explain complexity of the nervous system while presenting the material in an organized and readable manner.[87]

Medication

While chemical treatments for infirmities have been used throughout history, one compound stands above the others in history for its utilization in, among other things, LBS: aspirin. Aspirin, an extract of willow tree bark, was first sold by Bayer Laboratories on March 6, 1899. The Assyrians and Egyptians were aware of the analgesic effects of willow tree bark and Hippocrates recommended women in labor to chew on willow leaves. After Frenchman Charles Gerhardt developed a crude form of aspirin, it was apparently forgotten until Felix Hoffmann later rediscovered it. Sir John Vane received the 1982 Nobel Prize in Medicine for his discovery of aspirin's mechanism as an inhibitor of prostaglandin synthetase,[88] emphasizing the societal importance of this "wonder drug." The success of aspirin, with its analgesic, antipyretic, and anti-inflammatory properties, contributed to societal acceptance of pharmacological and allopathic methods of health care.

SURGERY AND THE "DYNASTY OF THE DISC"

Although the idea of disc material compressing on the spinal cord was previously introduced by Walter Dandy in 1929,[89] the importance of this concept was emphasized with case studies 5 years later. The year of 1934 was an especially important year in the historical evolution of LBS. This was when two New England spine surgeons named William Mixter and Joseph Barr proved that sciatica could be caused by a herniation of the nucleus pulposus compressing on the spinal nerve root. These results were published in 1934,[90] spawning an increased focus on pathoanatomical etiology of back syndromes that was facilitated by new technologies in identifying and surgically correcting them.

The significance of this event cannot be overemphasized in the assessment and treatment of LBS. A recent review of German spine-related literature in the twentieth century noted a heterogeneous group of conditions that were considered and discussed in the first part of the century.[91] It was later noted that the focus was almost exclusively devoted to the diagnosis and treatment of the degenerative disc. Interestingly, it was only in the last decade of the century that interest returned to non-disc-related spinal issues. In retrospect, two factors were identified as causes of the disc paradigm:

1. A tendency to prefer organic, visible abnormalities as etiologies.
2. An inclination to trust technical diagnostic results more than clinical judgment.

These preferences led to overreliance on diagnostic studies such as CT and MRI. In fact, it was not until 1984 that Wiesel et al. performed the first quality normative study for low back by utilizing CT technology,[92] finding 35.4% of asymptomatic controls with no back history to have positive findings (disc herniation, disc degeneration, or spinal stenosis). Boden et al. found similar results on lumbar assessment of individuals with no history of back pain and found a 36% rate of disc herniation.[93] Subsequent normative studies found even higher rates of positive findings,[94,95] leading to the gradual acceptance of the *benign disc lesion* and requiring clinicians to look beyond the imaging studies and correlate additional clinical factors into their assessment.

Despite the evidence of increasing recent interest in non-disc-related conditions,[91] spinal surgery rates have risen since the 1930s. Cherkin et al. found that the international rates varied significantly among 11 developed countries and found that the United States had a 40% higher rate than any other country and more than five times higher than in England and Scotland.[96] Indeed, the number of lumbar spine surgeries performed in the United States increased from 1990 to 2000 by one third, from over 300,000 to nearly 400,000. The number of lumbar spine fusion surgeries increased by 179% during that period, with the highest percentage occurring in the age group 60 and over.[97] For further information on this topic, Chapter 32 of this text provides an in-depth explanation of spinal surgical procedures.

THE BIOPSYCHOSOCIAL MODEL

George Engel, a psychiatrist, brought forth the biopsychosocial model of disease in the middle of the twentieth century.[98–101] This broadened the biomedical model of disease that focused heavily on infectious and organic pathology on which medicine had been based. With this addition, human interactions and emotions were added to the mix of infirmities, overcoming the Cartesian model that separated body from soul centuries earlier.

Of course, transitions, albeit important ones, rarely happen overnight. The biopsychosocial model was not immediately integrated into all forms of treatment. This was true with treatment for low back conditions, and so the organic model persisted for some time. Waddell, in his epic 1987 Volvo Award winning paper, introduced this model to the spine world, changing the way in which back syndromes were addressed.[102]

With the biopsychosocial model, a variety of factors in patients' lives influence the risk of chronic pain syndromes. These factors are addressed in detail in Chapter 19, while being covered in varying degrees in a number of other later chapters.

Although Engel's strategy for LBS added new levels of complexity to a comparatively simple and comfortable biological model, *bringing it to light at least allowed for the possibility of understanding and clinically integrating these principles*. Indeed, it may be such academic provocation that is necessary for progress to occur.

THE SPORTS MEDICINE MODEL

The modern integration into the sports medicine model for the treatment of disabling spinal conditions occurred in the final decades of the twentieth century and is attributed to Tom Mayer.[103] He noted that athletes tended to regain their functional capacity very effectively despite frequent severe injuries that would not resolve as successfully with patients from the general public. He stated that the athlete, passionately focused on returning to his or her sport as quickly as possible, usually returned when they were able to play at a competitive level rather than when they were free of pain and their injuries completely "healed." This concept helped to expose the difference between "hurt versus harm," in which health-care providers could counsel their patients that a return to increasing activities were not necessarily injurious despite the pain, but were instead often beneficial.

The sports medicine model helped to overcome the long-standing passive strategy of bed rest for back problems that had been popular throughout the twentieth century by orthopedists. Indeed, Professor Joel Goldthwait, the man credited by Lewin as making "the medical profession scientifically 'back-conscious,'"[104] stated the following in 1937:

> Since it is almost impossible to use any form of support that will satisfactorily protect the joints when patients are ambulatory, it is best to put these patients to bed for a week or ten days, with local applications to the low back in order to stimulate circulation. This management affords the expectation of a rapid recovery and early return to work.[105]

The sports medicine model helped to overcome the era passive of back healing utilizing bed rest. It also promoted the notion that patients who focused on resumption of their lives instead of dwelling on their pain tended to have better outcomes.

THE CONTRIBUTION OF PROFESSOR ARCHIBALD COCHRANE

Archibald Cochrane was a British physician who, in the later twentieth century, indelibly altered the course of health care. Outspokenly pragmatic, he promoted reasonable principles regarding how health care should be organized for society. He stated that health-care resources would always be limited and that such resources should therefore be provided utilizing methods that have been scientifically proven to be the most effective.[106,107]

Professor Cochrane also stated that much of medicine was based on poor research standards. In 1979, he wrote, "It is surely a great criticism of our profession that we have not organized a critical summary, by specialty or subspecialty, adapted periodically, of all relevant randomized controlled trials."[107]

It was Cochrane's influence that ultimately led to the 1993 formation of the international organization named in his honor. "The Cochrane Collaboration" established strict methodological criteria by which research is qualified and integrated within an organized framework. The Cochrane Library subsequently provides an updated list of quarterly papers that pass the methodological muster.

Finally, Professor Cochrane is given credit for providing influential impetus for the development of a new paradigm for the teaching and organization of global health care, what has become known as evidence-based Health Care.[108]

EVIDENCE-BASED HEALTH CARE

Evidence-based health care (EBHC) is something of an enigma due to a variety of associated paradoxical scenarios. Also known as evidence based medicine (EBM), EBHC is essentially a new approach to the organization and practice of health care despite the fact that its roots date back to the mid-nineteenth century Paris.[109] Also, the practice of EBHC appears to be widely interpreted despite a rather circumscript definition. Finally, a variety of governmental and provider groups are increasingly utilizing EBHC strategies to more effectively control clinical practice standards and torein in costs. However, others have raised concerns about this trend because of patient and provider treatment freedoms.[110] Such ambivalence exemplifies the current state of EBHC.

The term "evidence-based medicine" is a clinical learning strategy that was coined and developed by instructors at McMaster Medical School in Canada in the 1980s.[111] The first published description of this new paradigm was by Guyatt in 1991.[108] As such, the clinical world has been exposed to this relative neophyte for little more than a decade.

EBM has been defined by Rosenberg and Donald as "the process of systematically finding, appraising, and using contemporaneous research findings as the basis for clinical decisions."[111] Sackett, described as another leader in the EBM movement,[108] was the lead author of another paper that subsequently provided a second, excellent definition, explaining it as "the conscienscious, explicit, and judicious use of current best evidence in making decisions about the care of individuals."[109]

In a relatively short period, EBHC is setting a standard on which national and international health-care bodies, teaching institutions, individual providers, and those who oversee and pay for such methods to be provided are coming to rely.

Interestingly, one of those credited with bringing EBHC forward presented potential flaws in the strategy.[109] Alvan Feinstein was the lead author in a 1997 paper that expressed concerns that EBM is almost exclusively based on randomized trials and meta-analyses and does not include a number of treatments or patients seen in clinical practice.[112] It was noted that the type of information on which EBM is based is rarely available for important clinical issues such as etiology, prognosis, diagnosis, or conditions that depend on pathophysiological changes. The paper went on to state that:

> The laudable goal of making clinical decisions based on evidence can be impaired by the restrictive quality and scope of what is collected as "best available evidence." That authoritative aura given to the collection, however, may lead to major abuses that produce inappropriate guidelines or doctrinaire dogmas for clinical practice.[112]

With this warning, one of the acknowledged leaders in bringing this paradigm forward provides a succinct warning that EBHC has the capacity for significant benefit or abuse. Perhaps the difference between the two is subject to one's interpretation, biases, or even prejudices. Of course, there is no place for prejudice in EBM, as it is the very antithesis of the scientific theory on which the model is based.

EBHC is quickly becoming the "gold standard" for determination of appropriate methods for assessment and treatment of health care. If the above-noted concerns are heeded, then this may help to provide needed organization in the nebulous area of LBS.

Because of the emerging importance of EBM at this point in the history of LBS, Chapter 31 provides an in-depth summary of this topic, including a practical example of case management utilizing many of these principles.

CONCLUSION

At the dawn of the twenty-first century, chronic disabling LBS appears to be the cataclysmic result of a series of factors: a predisposition of symptomatic risk to the majority of the population; difficulty in objectifying its cause or even its presence; psychological, industrial, and cultural factors; high expectations from health-care systems and from accessible social pensions. In the end, LBS appear to be more than a biopsychosocial issue, but rather a *societogenic complex* in which the populace moves, acts, or thinks as a group. Instead of the individual being influenced by the social environment, the societal current may instead pull him or her along as disabling LBS and pensions become more commonly accepted. If this is so then one of the abherant results of societal evolution is that of a new biopsychosocietal model (see Figure 1–4), where accepted societal standards regarding available disability options can impact the individual's future vocational decision making. In other

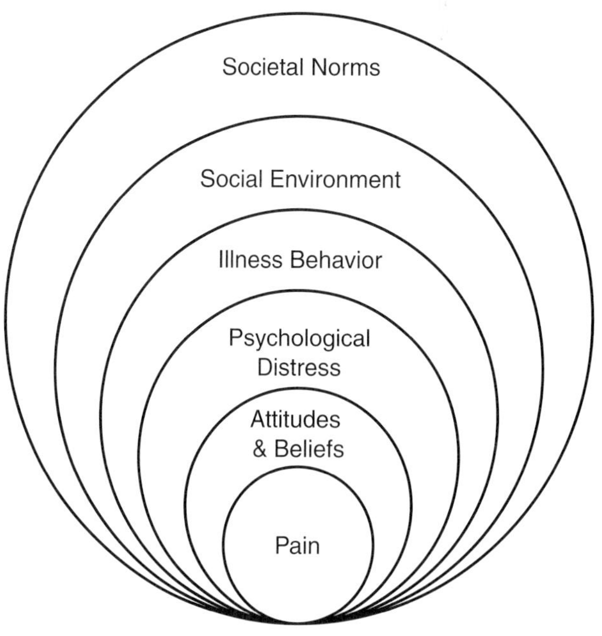

FIGURE 1–4. The biopsychosocietal model of disabling pain. (after Waddell[3] and Loeser[110])

words, should one work for an income or be disabled for an income?

SUMMARY

1. The multifactorial nature of LBS is briefly sketched here.
2. The complexity of the etiological aspects of LBS is indeed daunting.
3. An historical perspective of low back syndromes was presented.
4. A biopsychosocietal model of disapling pain was introduced, describing how evolving societal norms influence on an individual's response, both emotionally and physically, to painful conditions such as low back syndromes.
5. Perhaps the greatest irony of all is that despite the burden to society, the truly devastating consequences of chronic, disabling LBS occur to the individual, that person for whom society was designed to protect.
6. The ensuing chapters of this textbook are designed to provide such understanding.

REFERENCES

1. Woolf A, Pfleger B. Burden of major musculoskeletal conditions. *Bull World Health Organ* 2003;81(9):646–656.
2. Nachemson A. Chronic pain—The end of the welfare state. *Qual Life Res* December 1994;3(Suppl 1): S11–S17.
3. Waddell G. *The back pain revolution*, 2nd ed. Edinburgh: Churchill Livingstone, 2004:74.
4. Reiso H, Nygard JF, Jorgensen GS, Holanger R, Soldal D, Bruusgaard D. Back to work: Predictors of return to work among patients with back disorders certified as sick. A two-year follow-up study. *Spine* July 1, 2003;28(13):1468–1473; discussion 1473–1474.
5. Frymoyer J, Cats-Baril W. An overview of the incidence and costs of low back pain. *Orthop Clin North Am* 1991;22:263–271.
6. Papageorgiou A, Croft P, Ferry S, Jayson M, Sillman A. Estimating the prevalence of low back pain in the general population. *Spine* September 1, 1995;20(17): 1889–1894.
7. Maniadakis N, Gray A, The economic burden of back pain in the UK. *Pain* January 2000;84(1):95–103.
8. Luo X, Pietrobon R, Sun S, Liu G, Hey L. Estimates and patterns of direct health care expenditures among individuals with back pain in the United States. *Spine* January 1, 2004;29(1):79–86.
9. Mapel D, Shainline M, Paez K, Gunter M. Hospital, pharmacy, and outpatient costs for osteoarthritis and chronic back pain. *J Rheum* 2004;31(3):573–583.
10. Thorpe K, Florence C, Joski P. Which medical conditions account for the rise in health care spending? *Health Aff* August 5, 2004;W4:437–445.
11. Walker BF, Muller R, Grant WD. Low back pain in Australian adults: he economic burden. *Asia Pac J Public Health* 2003;15(2):7987.
12. Mikheev M. *Ceremonial address to the World Chiropractic Congress*, London, United Kingdom, May 27, 1993.
13. Raspe H, Matthis C, Croft P, O'Neill T. Variation in back pain between countries: The example of Britain and Germany. *Spine* April 23, 2004;29(9):1017–1021.
14. Waddell G, Aylward M. *Low back pain, disability and social security benefits: A literature review and analysis.* Dept of Social Security Research Report. London: Department of Social Security, 2001.
15. Omokhodion F. Low back pain in an urban population in Southwest Nigeria. *Trop Doct* January 2004;34(1): 17–20.
16. Volinn E. The epidemiology of low back pain in the rest of the world. A review of surveys in low- and middle-income countries. *Spine* August 1, 1997;22(15): 1747–1754.
17. Nachemson A. Advances in low-back pain. *Clin Orthop* November 1985;(200):266–278.
18. Nachemson A. Newest knowledge of low back pain. A critical look. *Clin Orthop* June 1992;(279):8–20.
19. Coste J, Delecouillerie G, Cohen de Lara A, Le Parc J, Pailaggi J. Clinical course and prognostic factors in acute low back pain: An inception cohort study in primary care practice. *BMJ* February 26, 1994; 308(6928):577–580.
20. van den Hoogen H, Koes B, van Eijk J, Bouter L, Deville QW. Pain and health status of primary care patients with low back pain. *J Fam Pract* February 1997; 44(2):187–192.
21. Carey T, Garrett J, Jackman A, Hadler N. Recurrence and care seeking after acute back pain: Results of a long-term follow-up study. North Carolina Pain Project. *Med Care* February 1999;37(2):157–164.
22. Hestbaek L, Leboeuf-Yde C, Manniche C. Low back pain: What is the long-term course? A review of studies of general patient populations. *Eur Spine J* 2003;12:149–165.
23. Wasiak R, Pransky G, Verma S, Webster B. Recurrence of low back pain: Definition–sensitivity analysis using administrative data. *Spine* October 1, 2003; 28(19):2283–2291.
24. Hides J, Richardson C, Jull G. Multifidus muscle recovery is not automatic after resolution of acute, first-episode low back pain. *Spine* December 1, 1996; 21(23):2763–2769.
25. Hides J, Jull G, Richardson C. Long-term effects of specific stabilizing exercises for first-episode low back pain. *Spine* June 1, 2001;26(11):E243–E248.
26. Leino P, Berg M, Puska P. Is back pain increasing? Results from national surveys in Finland during 1978/9–1992. *Scand J Rheumatol* 1994;23(5):269–276.
27. Heistaro S, Vartiainen E, Heliovaara M, Puska P. Trends of back pain in eastern Finland, 1972–1992, in relation to socioeconomic status and behavioral risk factors. *Am J Epidemiol* October 1, 1998;148(7): 671–682.
28. Nachemson AL, Waddell G, Norlund AI. Epidemiology of neck and low back pain. In: Nachemson AL,

Jonsson E, eds. *Neck and back pain: The scientific evidence of causes, diagnosis and treatment*. Philadelphia: Lippincott Williams & Wilkins, 2000:165–188.
29. Merkesdal S, Bernitt K, Busche T, Bauer J, Mau W. Comparison of costs-of-illness in patients with low back pain 12 months prior and after orthopedic inpatient and outpatient rehabilitation. *Rehabilitation (Stuttg)* April 2004;43(2):83–89.
30. Aronsson G, Gustafson K, Dallner M. Sick but yet at work. An empirical study of sickness presenteeism. *J Epidemiol Community Health* 2000;54(7):502–507.
31. Stewart W, Ricci J, Chee E, Morganstein D, Lipton R. Lost productive time and cost due to common pain conditions in the US workforce. *JAMA* November 12, 2003;290(18):2443–2454.
32. The world factbook. www.cia.gov/cia/publications/factbook/fields/2119.html.
33. Feldman JB. The prevention of occupational low back pain disability: Evidence-based reviews point in a new direction. *J Surg Orthop Adv* Spring 2004;13(1):1–14.
34. Strunin L, Boden LI. Family consequences of chronic back pain. *Soc Sci Med* April 2004;58(7):1385–1393.
35. Eriksen W, Natvig B, Bruusgaard D. Marital disruption and long-term work disability. A four-year prospective study. *Scand J Public Health* September 1999;27(3):196–202.
36. Gerszten P, Gerszten E, Allison M. Diseases of the spine in South American mummies. *Neurosurgery* January 2001;48(1):208–213.
37. Sotomayor H, Burgos J, Arango M. Demonstration of tuberculosis by DNA ribotyping of *Mycobacterium tuberculosis* in a Colombian prehispanic mummy. *Biomedica* June 2004;24(Suppl 1):18–26.
38. Schermuly W, Eggebrecht A. The radiology of Egyptian mummies. *Rofo* November 1976;125(5):389–396.
39. Chhem R, Schmit P, Faure C. Did Ramesses II really have ankylosing spondylitis? A reappraisal. *Can Assoc Radiol J* October 2004;55(4):211–217.
40. Feldkeller E, Lemmel E, Russell A. Ankylosing spondylitis in the Pharaohs of ancient Egypt. *Rheumatol Int* January 2003;23(1):1–5.
41. Marketos S, Skiadis P. Hippocrates: The father of spine surgery. *Spine* July 1, 1999;24(13):1381–1387.
42. Marketos K, Skiadas P. Galen: A pioneer of spine research. *Spine* November 15, 1999;24(22):1358–1362.
43. Xarchas K, Bourandas J. Injuries and diseases of the spine in the ancient times. *Spine* July 1, 2003; 28(13):1481–1484.
44. Ceccarelli G. Archeology in medicine: Digging up into the tophi of Popes, Dukes and Kings. *Reumatismo* 2003;55(2):123–130.
45. Allan B, Waddell G. An historical perspective on low back pain and disability. *Acta Orthop Scand Suppl* 1989;234:1–23.
46. Appelboom T. The past: A gallery of arthritics. *Clin Rheumatol* December 1989;8(4):442–452.
47. *Disability history*. Washington State University, 2004. www.ccer.org/Dis_Hist/disability/index.htm.
48. Boni T. From sciatica to intervertebral disc replacement. On the history of a disease concept. *Orthopade* December 2000;29(12):1033–1043.
49. Dewar J. *The information age and the printing press: Looking backward to see ahead*. Rand Publication President's Award Paper, 1997.
50. Arndt K. Information excess in medicine. Overview, relevance to dermatology, and strategies for coping. *Arch Dermatol* September 1992;128(9):1249–1256.
51. Faber R. Information overload. *BMJ* 1993;307:383.
52. Hunt R, Newman R. Medical knowledge overload: A disturbing trend for physicians. *Health Care Manage Rev* Winter 1997;22(1):70–75.
53. Moorman P, van der Lei J. An inventory of publications on computer-based records: An update. *Methods Inf Med* 2003;42(3):199–202.
54. Davis D, Ciurea I, Flanagan T, Perrier L. Solving the information overload problem: A letter from Canada. *Med J Aust* 2004;180(6, Suppl):S68–S71.
55. Degler C, Cochran T, SeSantis V, et al. *The democratic experience*, 3rd ed. Glenview, IL: Scott, Foresman & Co., 1973.
56. Shola Orloff A. *The politics of pensions. A comparative analysis of Britain, Canada, and the United States, 1880–1940*. Wisconsin: University of Wisconsin Press, 1993.
57. Siemerink-Hermans H. The "railway spine": alleged spinal injury caused by railway concussions as a basis for financial claims in 19th century England. *Ned Tijdschr Geneeskd* April 11, 1998;142(15):864–868.
58. Harrington R. On the tracks of trauma: Railway spine reconsidered. *Soc Hist Med* August 2003;16(2):209–223.
59. Aceves-Avila F, Ferrari R, Ramos-Remus C. New insights into culture driven disorders. *Best Pract Res Clin Rheumatol* April 2004;18(2):155–171.
60. Nachemson A. Backache—The bane of the welfare state? *Nord Med* 1994;109(3):70–71.
61. Sigerist H. From Bismark to Beveridge: Developments and trends in social security legislation 1943. *J Public Health Policy* 1999;20(4):474–496.
62. Williamson P, Beitman B, Katon W. Beliefs that foster physician avoidance of psychosocial aspects of health care. *J Fam Pract* December 1981;13(7):999–1003.
63. Woolf A, Zeidler H, Haglund U, et al. Musculoskeletal pain in Europe: Its impact and a comparison of population and medical perceptions of treatment in eight European countries. *Ann Rheum Dis* 2004;63: 342–347.
64. Deyo R. Measuring the functional status of patients with low back pain. *Arch Phys Med Rehabil* December 1988;69(12):1044–1053.
65. Kposowa A, Tsunokai G. Searching for relief: Racial differences in treatment of patients with back pain. *Race Soc* 2004;5:193–223.
66. Cassisi J, Umeda M, Deisinger J, Sheffer C, Lofland K, Jackson C. Patterns of pain descriptor usage in African Americans and European Americans with chronic back pain. *Cultur Divers Ethnic Minor Psychol* February 2004;1(1):81–89.
67. McCracken L, Matthews A, Tang T, Cuba S. A comparison of blacks and whites seeking treatment for

chronic pain. *Clin J Pain* September 2001;17(3):249–255.

68. Bates M, Rankin-Hill L, Sanchez-Ayandez M, Mendez-Bryan R. A cross-cultural comparison of adaptation to chronic pain among Anglo-Americans and native Puerto Ricans. *Med Anthropol* February 1995;16(2):141–173.
69. Agris J. Stamps commemorating medicine. "Dr. Crawford Williamson Long" the Father of Anesthesia. *J Dermatol Surg Oncol* May 1980;6(5):415.
70. Carmichael E. Crawford Williamson Long—Discoverer of surgical anesthesia. *J Med Assoc State Ala* January 1967;36(7):843–857.
71. Newsom S. Pioneers in infection control—Joseph Lister. *Hosp Infect* December 2003;55(4):246–253.
72. Watson-Jones R. The debt of orthopedic surgery to Joseph Lister. *J Bone Joint Surg Br* February 1967;49(1):1–2.
73. Hamonet C. Andrew Taylor Still and the birth of osteopathy (Baldwin, Kansas, USA, 1855). *Joint Bone Spine* February 2003;70(1):80–84.
74. Burns S, Burns J. Andrew Taylor Still, M.D.: Founder of osteopathy. *J Altern Complement Med* Fall 1997;3(3):213–214.
75. Donahue J. The man, the book, the lessons: The chiropractor's adjuster, 1910. *Chiropr Hist* December 1990;10(2):35–43.
76. Tutashinda K. D.D. Palmer: A new look at an old visionary. *Chiropr Hist* December 1995;15(2):103–104.
77. Terrett AJ. The genius of D.D. Palmer: An exploration of the origin of chiropractic in his time. *Chiropr Hist* June 1991;11(1):31–38.
78. Kent H. James Beaver Mennell (1880–1957). *Arch Phys Med Rehabil* December 1957;38(12):785.
79. Mennell JB. *Massage—Its principles and practice*, 2nd ed. London: J & A Churchill, 1920.
80. Cookson J. Orthopedic manual therapy—An overview. Part II. The spine. *Phys Ther* March 1979;59(3):259–267.
81. Cyriax J. *Cyriax's illustrated manual of orthopaedic medicine*, 2nd ed. London: Butterworth-Heinemann, 1993.
82. Riesz P. The life of Wilhelm Conrad Roentgen. *AJR Am J Roentgenol* December 1995;165(6):1533–1537.
83. Yochum T. 1895–1995: Diagnostic imaging in its first century. *J Manipulative Physiol Ther* November–December 1995;18(9):618–625.
84. Elke M. One century of diagnostic imaging in medicine. *Experientia* July 14, 1995;51(7):665–680.
85. Greenblatt S. John Hughlings Jackson and the conceptual foundations of the neurosciences. *Physis Riv Int Stor Sci* 1999;36(2):367–386.
86. Tansey E. Not committing barbarisms: Sherrington and the synapse, 1897. *Brain Res Bull* 1997;44(3):211–212.
87. Sherrington C. *The integrative action of the nervous system*, 1st ed. London: Archibald Constable and Co. Ltd., 1906.
88. Levesque H, Lafont O. Aspirin throughout the ages: A historical review. *Rev Med Interne* March 2000;21(Suppl 1):8s–17s.
89. Dandy WJ. Loose cartilage from intervertebral disc simulating tumor of the spinal cord. *Arch Surg* 1929;19:660–672.
90. Mixter W, Barr J. Rupture of the intervertebral disc with involvement of the spinal canal. *NEJM* 1934;211:210–211.
91. Lutz G, Butzlaff M, Schultz-Venrath U. Looking back on back pain: Trial and error of diagnoses in the 20th century. *Spine* August 15, 2003;28(16):1899–1905.
92. Wiesel S, Tsourmas N, Feffer H, Citrin C, Patronas N. A study of computer-assisted tomography. I. The incidence of positive CAT scans in an asymptomatic group of patients. *Spine* September 1984;9(6):549–551.
93. Boden S, Davis D, Dina T, Patronas N, Weisel S. Abnormal magetic resonance scans of the lumbar spine in asymptomatic subjects. A prospective investigation. *J Bone Joint Surg Am* March 1990;72(3):403–408.
94. Jenson M, Brant-Zawadzki M, Obuchowski N, Modic M, Malkasian D, Ross J. Magnetic resonance imaging of the lumbar spine in people without back pain. *N Engl J Med* July 14, 1994;331(2):69–73.
95. Boos N, Rieder R, Schade V, Spratt K, Semmer N, Aebi M. The diagnostic accuracy of magnetic resonance imaging, work perception, and psychosocial factors in identifying symptomatic disc herniations. *Spine* December 15, 1995;20(24):2613–2625.
96. Cherkin D, Deyo R, Loeser J, Bush T, Waddell G. An international comparison of back surgery rates. *Spine* June 1, 1994;19(11):1201–1206.
97. Deyo R, U.S. national trends for lumbar spine surgery for degenerative conditions, 1990–2000.
98. Engel G. A unified concept of health and disease. *Perspect Biol Med* 1960;3:459–485.
99. Engel G, Reichsman F, Segal H. A study of an infant with gastric fistula. Behavior and the rate of total hydrochloric acid secretion. *Psychosom Med* September–October 1956;18(5):859–871.
100. Engel G. The need for a new medical model: A challenge to biomedicine. *Science* 1977;196:129–136.
101. Engel G. The biopsychosocial model and the education of health professionals. *Ann N Y Acad Sci* 1978;310:169–181.
102. Waddell G. A new clinical model for the treatment of low-back pain. *Spine* September 1987;12(7):632–644.
103. Mayer T. Functional restoration: The sports approach to the chronically disabled worker. Presented at Chronic Pain and the Primary Physician, Houston, TX, December 2, 1989.
104. Lewin P. *The back and its disk syndromes*. Philadelphia: Lea & Febiger, 1955.
105. Goldthwait J. Low-back lesions. *J Bone Joint Surg* July 1937;19(3):810–812.
106. Cochrane A. *Effectiveness and efficiency. Random reflections on health services*. London: Nuffield Provincial Hospitals Trust, 1972.
107. Cochrane A. 1931–1971: A critical review, with particular reference to the medical profession. In: *Medicine*

for the year 2000. London: Office of Health Economics, 1979:1–11.

108. Guyatt G, Cook D, Haynes B. Evidence based medicine has come a long way. *BMJ* October 30, 2004;329:990–991.
109. Sackett D, Rosenberg W, Muir Gray J, Haynes R, Richardson W. Evidence based medicine: What it is and what it isn't. *BMJ* January 13, 1996; 312:71–72.
110. Loeser JD. Concepts of Pain. In: Stanton-Hicks M, Boas R, eds. *Chronic Low Back Pain*. New York, Raven Press, 1982.
111. Rosenberg W, Donald A. Evidence based medicine: An approach to clinical problem-solving. *BMJ* April 29, 1995;310:1122–1126.
112. Feinstein A, Horwitz R. Problems in the "evidence" of "evidence-based medicine." *Am J Med* December 1997;103(6):529–535.

CHAPTER

2

FUNCTIONAL ANATOMY OF THE LUMBAR SPINE

Robert A. Walker and Jaroslaw P. Grod

OUTLINE

OBJECTIVES

1. To provide an overview of the anatomy of the lumbar spine.
2. To provide a morphological overview of additional regional anatomy.
3. To present the reader with a variety of functional insights as they correlate with lumbopelvic anatomy.

INTRODUCTION

Pain syndromes emanating from the low back have been a human nemesis throughout history. In keeping with human nature, mankind confronted this challenge by striving to better understand and resolve this age-old adversary. Of course, uncovering the anatomical makeup of this troublesome region formed the basis of increased understanding and therapeutic strategies. As will be discussed in later chapters, recent gains in understanding of low back physiology, along with the ensuing array of pathological conditions that can be called low back syndromes, have spawned alterations in the perspective in which anatomy is appreciated in a rapidly changing academic and clinical environment. In the past, anatomy and physiology were considered relatively disparate subjects. Recently, increased interest in the physiological aspects of anatomy and, conversely, the anatomical aspects of physiology has blurred their distinction.

One of the challenges in writing a textbook that focuses on one region, such as the low back, is that one must establish topical parameters with which to abide when, practically speaking, such borders do not really exist. With this seeming contradiction in mind, the authors will focus their attention on lumbopelvic regional anatomy. However, this chapter will also explore a functional model of anatomy. In so doing, topics will be initiated that will allow for greater depth in subsequent chapters.

This chapter presents a basic outline of the soft tissue and osseous anatomy of the anatomical regions germane to the understanding of low back syndromes. Hence, the so-called neuromusculoskeletal aspects of the lumbopelvic region will be emphasized. However, adjacent regions will at times be addressed in order to clarify the topic, cover material for later chapters, or to provide comparison with the region of focus. This chapter begins with an overview of the cutaneous innervation of blood supply of the back, and then proceeds to the fascia and musculature, and then examines the neural anatomy and regional osteology.

INNERVATION AND BLOOD SUPPLY OF THE BACK

Cutaneous nerves and vessels in the back pierce the muscles and deep fascia covering the musculature and then continue inferolaterally to reach the skin. It is important to note that the superficial and intermediate back muscles, which function during upper limb movement and respiratory activity respectively, are both innervated by ventral rami of spinal nerves. The deep or true back muscles receive their motor innervation from the dorsal rami of spinal nerves.

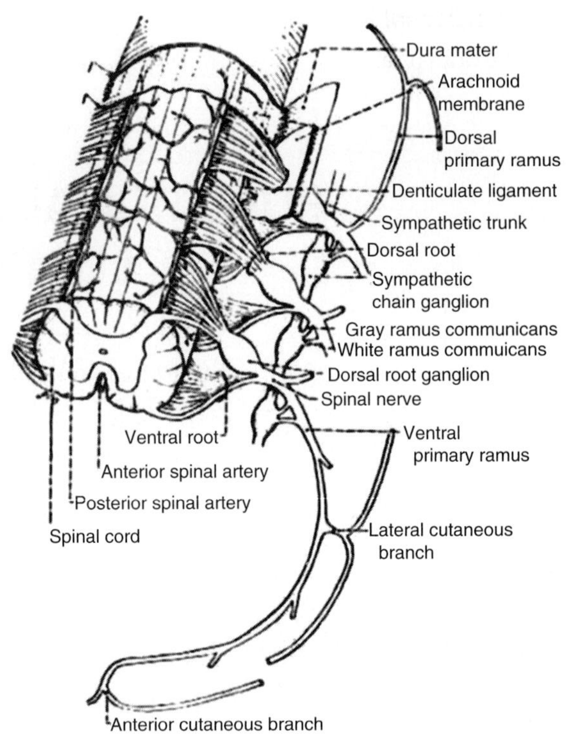

FIGURE 2–1. Branches of a typical spinal nerve. (*After Woodburne.*)

The dorsal rami of spinal nerves are generally smaller than the ventral rami. As a rule, each dorsal ramus divides into a medial and a lateral branch (Fig. 2–1) The dorsal rami of the first cervical nerve (C1), the fourth and fifth sacral nerves (S4 and S5), and the coccygeal nerve (C×1) are exceptions to this rule. These dorsal rami *do not* split into medial and lateral branches. Both the medial and lateral branches of the remaining spinal nerves will supply muscles, but only one branch of each dorsal ramus will become cutaneous. Which branch becomes cutaneous depends upon the spinal level of the nerve. In the *upper half of the back,* the *lateral branch* remains in the deep back muscles that it supplies, whereas the medial branch supplies the muscles and then continues to the skin. In the *lower half of the back* and most of the buttock, the *medial branch* remains in the muscles it supplies, and the lateral branch innervates muscles and then continues to become a cutaneous branch. *Therefore, the cutaneous nerves found in the upper part of the back are the medial branches of dorsal rami, whereas those in the lower part of the back are the lateral branches.* This is the general pattern, but there are some exceptions, as noted below.

Clinical Pearl: The dorsal rami of spinal nerves are generally smaller than the ventral rami. As a rule, each dorsal ramus divides into a medial and a lateral branch.

Thoracic Dorsal Rami

Thoracic dorsal rami all divide into medial and lateral branches. Cutaneous branches may descend as many as four rib spaces before becoming cutaneous. Thus lower thoracic dorsal rami may innervate areas of skin inferiorly to the level just above the iliac crests. As with the cervical dorsal rami, one branch will become cutaneous after innervating muscles, while the other branch will remain purely muscular. This change occurs between T6 and T7.

T1–T6: The situation is as in the cervical region. The *medial branch becomes cutaneous* after innervating intrinsic muscles, while the lateral branch remains purely muscular. Medial branches supply and pass between semispinalis and multifidus, and then pierce the rhomboids and trapezius (without innervating them) to become cutaneous. Lateral branches increase in size from superior to inferior, passing between longissimus and iliocostalis, and supplying the remaining intrinsic muscles.

T7–T12: The situation is reversed. The *lateral branch becomes cutaneous* after innervating intrinsic muscles, while the medial branch remains purely muscular.

Lumbar Dorsal Rami

Lumbar dorsal rami also divide into medial and lateral branches and follow the pattern of the lower six thoracic dorsal rami. *Medial branches* are short and end in the multifidi, which they supply. They remain purely muscular. *Lateral branches* supply the erector spinae. In addition, the lateral branches of L1, L2, and L3 become cutaneous by piercing the aponeurosis of latissimus dorsi and supply skin of the gluteal region, reaching as far inferior as the level of the greater trochanter. *Intermediate branches* have only muscular distribution, to the lumbar fibers of the longissimus muscle. Within this muscle they form an intersegmental plexus. The intermediate branch of the L5 dorsal ramus supplies the lowest fibers of the longissimus, which arise from the L5 transverse process and attach to the medial aspect of the iliac crest.

Sacral Dorsal Rami

Medial branches: Small and innervate the multifidus.

Lateral branches: Lateral branches of S1, S2, and S3 join with one another and the lateral branch of the dorsal ramus of L5 and with S4 in a series of loops dorsal to the sacrum. From these loops run a series of filaments to form another series of loops dorsal to the sacrotuberous ligament deep to the gluteus maximus. The rami of this region form a type of neural meshwork over the sacrum, which makes neurotomy procedures and the like impossible as stated in Chapter 24. From these, two or three *gluteal branches* arise, which pierce the gluteus maximus to become cutaneous along a line from the posterior superior iliac spine to the apex of the coccyx.

Dorsal rami of S4 and S5 do not divide into medial and lateral branches. They unite with each other and the coccygeal dorsal ramus (C×1) to form loops dorsal to the sacrum. Filaments from these loops supply the skin over the coccyx.

Coccygeal Dorsal Ramus

The coccygeal dorsal ramus (C×1) does not divide into medial and lateral branches. It forms loops with the dorsal rami of S4 and S5 as noted above.

BLOOD SUPPLY

Small arteries and veins accompany the dorsal rami forming segmentally arranged neurovascular bundles. The blood vessels in the thoracic region are dorsal branches of the posterior intercostal arteries that accompany the dorsal rami of thoracic spinal nerves. In the lumbar region the arteries are dorsal branches of the four, paired lumbar arteries. The posterior intercostal arteries and lumbar arteries are branches of the descending aorta. The accompanying veins are named similarly.

MUSCLES AND FASCIA

General Plan of the Back Musculature

The muscles of the back consist of two large groups: the intrinsic back musculature and the extrinsic back musculature. The extrinsic back musculature consists of those muscles with attachments to the dorsal portion of the ribs or to the vertebral column but which are of hypaxial (i.e., beneath the axis of the skeleton, subvertebral, hyposkeletal) origin embryologically, and are therefore innervated by ventral rami of spinal nerves. With a few exceptions, these muscles are concerned principally with movements of the upper limbs, but can act secondarily on the vertebral column. These include the trapezius, latissimus dorsi, levator scapulae, rhomboideus major, rhomboideus minor (Fig. 2–2), serratus posterior superior and inferior (Fig. 2–3), anterior and posterior cervical intertransversarii, and lateral lumbar intertransversarii.

Clinical Pearl: The extrinsic back musculature consists of those muscles with attachments to the dorsal portion of the ribs or to the vertebral column but which are of hypaxial origin embryologically, and

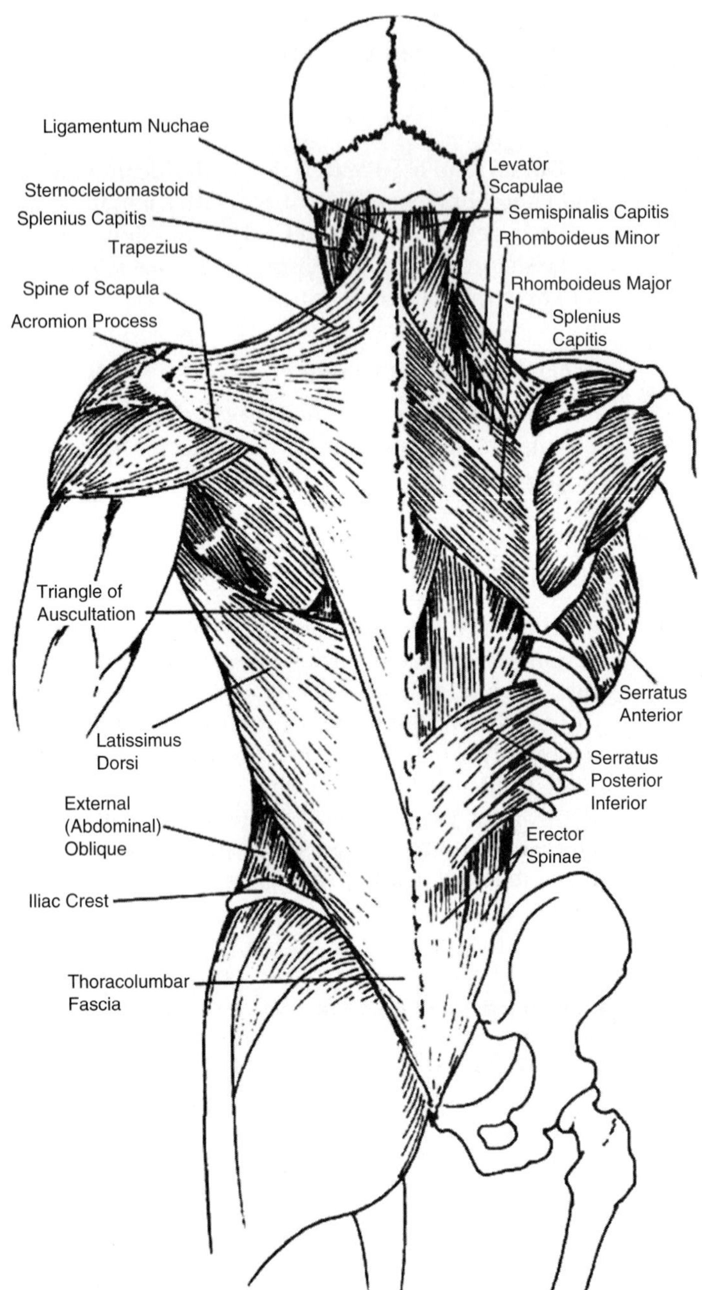

FIGURE 2–2. The superficial back muscles: trapezius, latissimus dorsi, levator scapulae, rhomboideus major, rhomboideus minor. (*Courtsey of William Yee, Anatomy Department, New York Chiropractic College, New York.*)

are therefore innervated by ventral rami of spinal nerves.

The intrinsic back musculature consists of the "true" back muscles: those that are of epaxial (i.e., at or above the level of the axis of the skeleton, supravertebral) origin embryologically are innervated by dorsal rami of spinal nerves, including the splenius muscles, the erector spinae group, the transversospinalis group, the interspinales, the thoracic and medial lumbar intertransversarii, and the four suboccipital muscles—obliquus capitis superior and inferior and rectus capitis posterior major and minor. Each will be described in turn below.

The Thoracolumbar Fascia

The *thoracolumbar fascia* is the fascial sheath that encloses the erector spinae muscle group. It has been a region of increased focus over the past few years as new insights into the functional aspects of this tissue have come to light (see Chapters 4 and 9). It is a subdivision of the vertebral fascia surrounding the intrinsic muscles of the back and neck (Fig. 2–4). It is continuous with the *fascia nuchae* which surrounds the splenius group of intrinsic muscles. In the thoracic region, it is relatively thin and transparent. In the lumbar region it is much thicker and is composed of three layers that attach to the lumbar spinous and transverse processes. The anterior and middle sheets

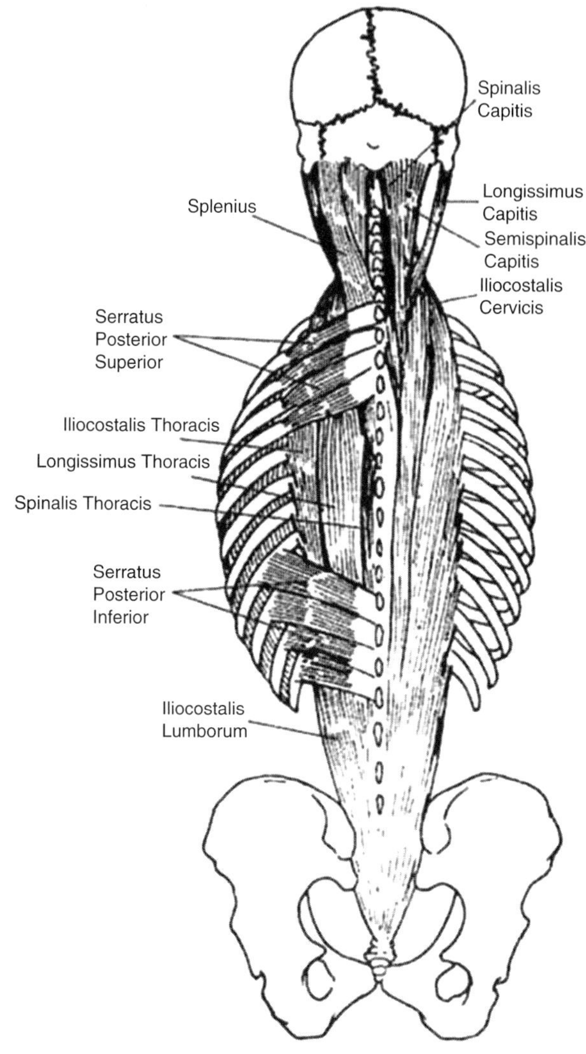

FIGURE 2–3. Serratus posterior superior and inferior and the erector spinae muscle group. (*Courtsey of William Yee, Anatomy Department, New York Chiropractic College, New York.*)

enclose the quadratus lumborum muscle. The middle and posterior sheets enclose the erector spinae muscle group. All threesheets fuse lateral to the quadratus lumborum to form the *lateral raphe* and provide attachment for the transversus abdominis, internal oblique, external oblique, and latissimus dorsi muscles. Additionally, it gives origin to some of the superficial and intermediate muscles of the back.

The anterior layer of the thoracolumbar fascia lies anterior to the quadratus lumborum muscle in lumbar region, and ventral to the intrinsic muscles of back above the lumbar region. It ends medially in the transverse processes of lumbar vertebrae. Laterally, it combines with the aponeurosis of the transversus abdominis muscle.

The *posterior lumbocostal ligament* is a thickening of the anterior layer between the twelfth rib and the transverse process of L1.

The middle layer is formed when the anterior layer splits to surround the quadratus lumborum muscle. The middle layer lies posterior to the quadratus lumborum and anterior to the intrinsic muscles of the back in the lumbar region. It is not present in the thoracic region.

The posterior layer covers the erector spinae posteriorly. It is composed of superficial and deep laminae. It ends laterally in the lumbar region by blending with the aponeurosis of the transversus abdominis muscle. In the thoracic region it blends with the fascia of the intercostal muscles. Superiorly, it blends with the nuchal fascia.

The posterior layer of the thoracolumbar fascia has received a significant amount of attention in recent years because of its importance in load transfer from trunk to legs. Vleeming et al. found that a variety of individual muscles cause displacement of the posterior layer during traction in 10 human specimens. The superficial lamina was displaced by latisimus dorsi, gluteus maximus, and erector spinae. The deep lamina was displaced by traction of the biceps femoris. Finally, tension was found to be transmitted to the contralateral posterior fascial layer caudal to the L4 level. These findings contributed significant insights into the functional anatomy of the thoracolumbar fascia as a key link in effective transference of loading from spine to legs during gait.[3]

Clinical Pearl: The posterior layer of the thoracolumbar fascia has received a significant amount of attention in recent years because of its importance in load transfer from trunk to legs.

The thoracolumbar fascia exhibits a wide area of attachments:

1. Medially
   (a) Ligamentum nuchae
   (b) Tips of the spinous processes
   (c) Supraspinous ligament
   (d) Thoracic and lumbar transverse processes
   (e) Median sacral crest
2. Laterally
   (a) Angles of the ribs lateral to the insertions of the iliocostalis muscle
   (b) Blends with the intercostal fascia
   (c) Blends with fascia of the transversus abdominis

The nuchal fascia covers the splenius muscles in the neck. It forms from the posterior portion of the prevertebral fascia. It attaches superiorly to the skull below the superior nuchal line. Inferiorly it is continuous with the thoracolumbar fascia.

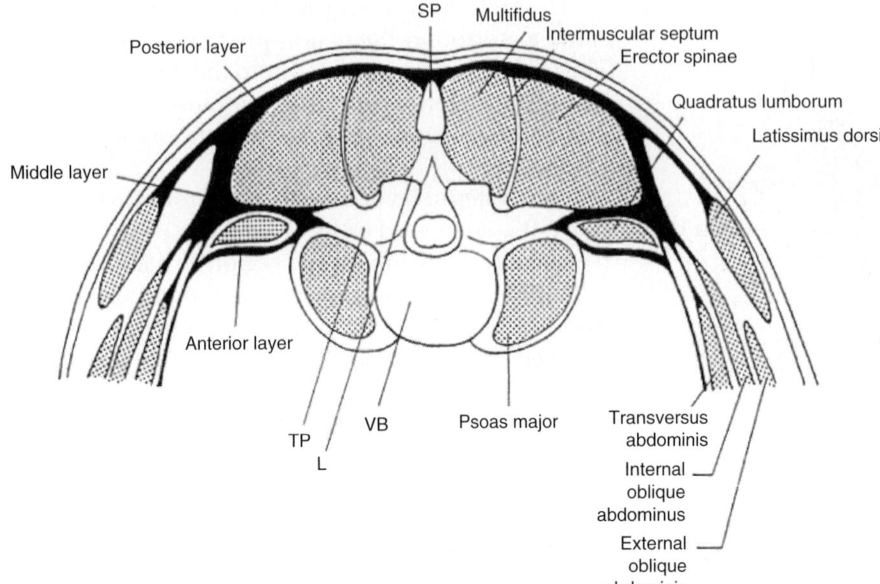

FIGURE 2–4. The musculature and thoracolumbar fascia (TLF) in graphic cross-section of the lumbar spine. Note the TLF posterior layer lying dorsal to the erector spinae and multifidus musculature, its middle layer between the erector spinae and the quadratus lumborum muscle, and its anterior layer ventral to the quadratus lumborum. Laterally the thoracolumbar fascia blends with the aponeurosis of the transversus abdominis muscle. Key: L, lamina; SP, spinous process; TP, transverse process; VB, vertebral body. (*After Porterfield and DeRosa.*[2])

Details of the Back Muscles

The muscles of the back are arranged into three layers[4]: superficial layer, intermediate layer, and deep or intrinsic layer.

1. The *superficial layer* (Fig. 2–2) of muscles all act on the upper limb and are innervated by ventral rami of spinal nerves. They consist of
   (a) Trapezius
   (b) Latissimus dorsi
   (c) Levator scapulae
   (d) Rhomboideus major
   (e) Rhomboideus minor
2. The, *intermediate layer* (Fig. 2–3) of muscles serves respiratory functions. They are also innervated by ventral rami. They consist of
   (a) Serratus posterior superior
   (b) Serratus posterior inferior
3. The *deep layer* of muscles are the true or *intrinsic* back muscles (including the segmental and suboccipital muscles) and are innervated by the dorsal rami of spinal nerves (with the exception of some of the intertransversarii). These intrinsic back muscles can be further subdivided into superficial, intermediate, and deep layers. These layers consist of the following:
   (a) The superficial layer includes the splenius capitis and splenius cervicis. These muscles will not be discussed, as they exceed the parameters of the chapter.
   (b) The intermediate layer includes the erector spinae muscle group (Fig. 2–3), composed of
   - Iliocostalis lateral column
     –lumborum
     –thoracis
     –cervicis
   - Longissimus (intermediate column)
     –thoracis
     –cervicis
     –capitis
   - Spinalis (medial column)
     –thoracis
     –cervicis
     –capitis

   (c) The deep layer includes the following:
   - Transversospinalis group (Fig. 2–5), composed of
     –semispinalis
     –multifidus
     –rotatores longus
     –rotatores brevis
   - Segmental muscles (Fig. 2–6), composed of
     –intertransverse muscles (intertransversarii)
     –interspinous muscles (interspinales)
     –levator costarum

Of the superficial and intermediate extrinsic muscles, only the latissimus dorsi and serratus posterior inferior are of concern with reference to the low back.

Contraction of a muscle can occur concentrically, eccentrically, or isometrically. Actions will, for this chapter, be defined as concentric contractions unless otherwise explained.

Latissimus Dorsi (Fig. 2–2) The muscle arises from the spinous processes of the lower six thoracic, all lumbar, and upper sacral vertebrae. It arises from the lumbar and sacral vertebrae by way of the vast *thoracolumbar fascia*. This fascia covers the deep (intrinsic) muscles

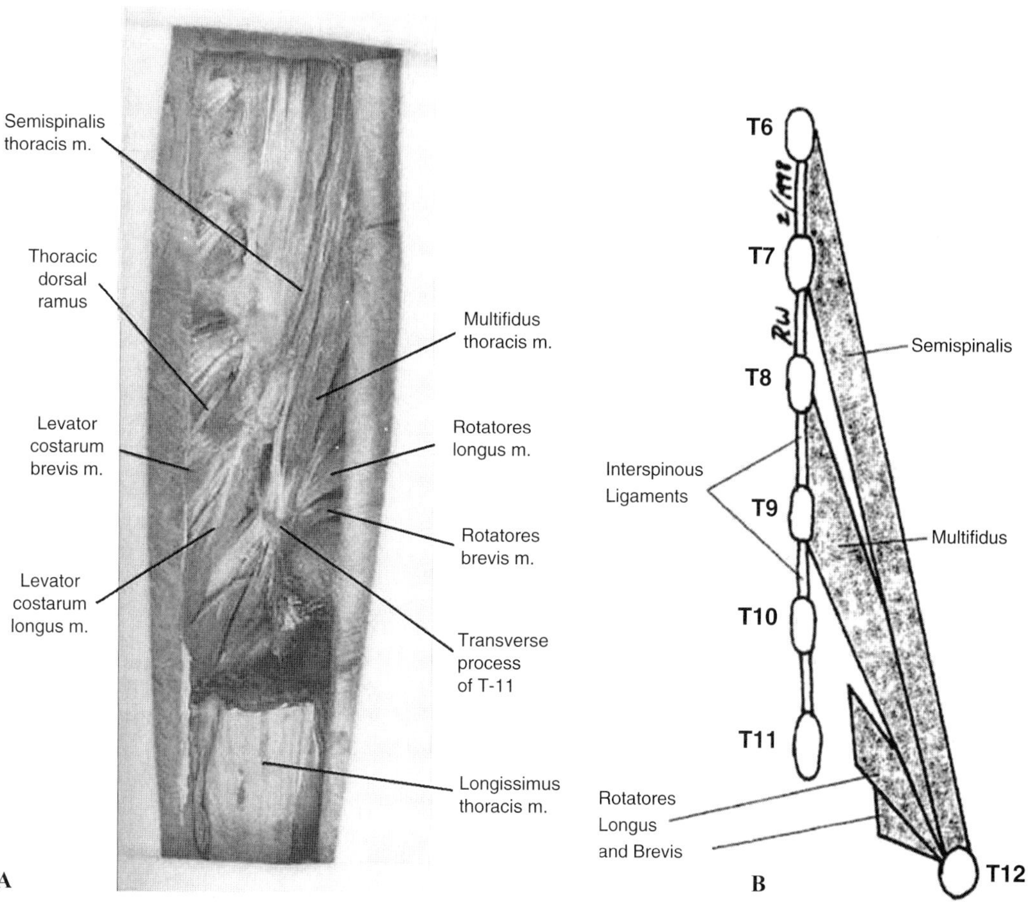

FIGURE 2–5. Transversospinalis muscle group. Note the four parts: semispinalis, multifidus, rotatores longus, and rotatores brevis. *A*. Photograph of a cadaveric specimen. *After Cramer and Darby.*[5] *B*. Diagrammatic representation. (*By Robert A. Walker.*)

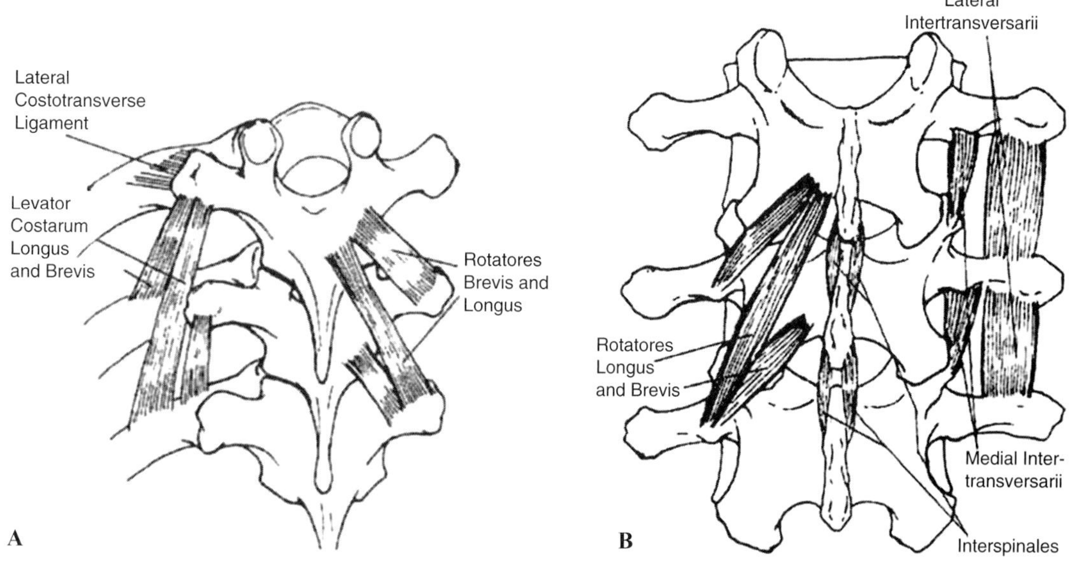

FIGURE 2–6. Segmental muscles of the thoracic (*A*) and lumbar (*B*) regions. (*Courtsey of William Yee, Anatomy Department, New York Chiropractic College, New York.*)

of the back, from the posterior part of the iliac crest, and from muscular slips from the lower three or four ribs. These muscular slips also interdigitate with the external oblique muscle. Its superior border extends laterally from the spinous processes of T6 and T7. Its most lateral fibers interdigitate with those of the *external oblique* below the origin of the *serratus anterior*. Superiorly, the muscle fibers converge into a broad tendon that is inserted into the humerus. Close to the tendon, the muscle receives its nerve supply from the *thoracodorsal nerve*, a branch of the brachial plexus of the upper limb. The *thoracodorsal artery* accompanies the nerve.

Origin: Spinous processes of the lower six thoracic, all lumbar, and the upper sacral vertebrae, from the posterior part of the iliac crest, and from the lower three or four ribs by muscular slips which interdigitate with the external oblique.
Insertion: Crest of the lesser tubercle and floor of the bicipital groove of the humerus.
Innervation: Thoracodorsal nerve (C6–C8).
Blood supply: The thoracodorsal artery.
Action: Extension, medial rotation, and adduction of the arm. With the shoulder girdle and humerus fixed, the latissimus dorsi elevates the ipsilateral innominate bone.

Serratus Posterior Inferior (Figs. 2–2 and 2–3)

Origin: Spinous processes of T10 or T11 to L2.
Insertion: Lower three of four ribs lateral to their angles.
Innervation: Ventral rami of lowest four thoracic nerves (T9–T12).
Blood supply: Posterior intercostal arteries.
Concentric action: Depresses lower ribs, draws them down and back. The serratus posterior inferior has historically been considered as muscle of expiration, although there is no evidence of a respiratory role. In fact, some electromyographic studies have refuted this, while a greater proprioceptive role than previously thought may exist for this muscle.[6]

Clinical Pearl: The serratus posterior inferior has historically been considered as muscle of expiration, although there is no evidence of a respiratory role. In fact, some electromyographic studies have refuted this, while a greater proprioceptive role than previously thought may exist for this muscle.

Erector Spinae (Fig. 2–3) The *erector spinae* group is the largest muscle mass in the back. It extends from the pelvis to the skull and from the midline laterally to approximately the angles of the ribs or one hand breadth to either side of the vertebral spines. Its tendinous origin is from the sacrum, the iliac crest, and the spinous processes of the lumbar and of the last two thoracic vertebrae. The fibrous tissue becomes largely muscular in the upper lumbar region and becomes divisible into three distinct columns: *iliocostalis, longissimus,* and *spinalis*. The details of only the lumbar and thoracic portions of the erector spinae will be discussed here.

The *iliocostalis* is the most lateral portion and is divided into the *iliocostalis lumborum, iliocostalis thoracis*, and *iliocostalis cervicis*. The *iliocostalis lumborum* is the lowest part of the muscle and divides into six or seven slips that insert into the lower borders of the lower six or seven ribs at about the level of the angles. The *iliocostalis thoracis* arises from the upper borders of the lower six ribs medial to the insertions of the *iliocostalis lumborum*, which partially overlaps it. The *iliocostalis thoracis* runs vertically and inserts by separate slips into the upper six ribs and sometimes the transverse process of the seventh cervical vertebra. The *iliocostalis cervicis* arises medial to the *iliocostalis thoracis* near the angles of the upper six ribs and inserts into the transverse processes of the fourth, fifth, and sixth cervical vertebrae.

The middle column of erector spinae is the *longissimus group* composed of the *longissimus thoracis, longissimus cervicis*, and *longissimus capitis*. The *longissimus thoracis* arises from the thoracolumbar fascia and accessory processes of the lumbar vertebrae. It inserts into the tips of the transverse processes of the lower nine thoracic vertebrae and lower nine ribs.

The most medial portions of the erector spinae superior to the lumbar region are the *spinalis muscles*, which include the *spinalis thoracis, spinalis cervicis*, and *spinalis capitis*. This group is not present in lumbar region, but is covered here to be complete. The spinalis group are the smallest and most poorly defined of the erector spinae muscles. The *spinalis thoracis* is relatively easy to identify and most constant. However, the *spinalis cervicis* may or may not be demonstrable. The *spinalis thoracis* lies medial to the *longissimus thoracis*. The two are partially blended at their origins. It also arises from the spinous processes of the eleventh thoracic through the second lumbar vertebrae and inserts into the spinous processes of the upper four to eight thoracic vertebrae.

1. Iliocostalis (lateral column of erector spinae)
   (a) Iliocostalis lumborum
      Origin: Thoracolumbar fascia.
      Insertion: Lower borders of the lower six or seven ribs near the angles.
      Innervation: Dorsal rami of lumbar spinal nerves.

Blood supply: Posterior intercostal arteries, lumbar arteries.
Action: Extension and lateral flexion of vertebral column.

(b) Iliocostalis thoracis
Origin: Upper borders of lower six ribs medial to insertions of iliocostalis lumborum.
Insertion: Upper six ribs and sometimes the transverse process of C7.
Innervation: Dorsal rami of thoracic spinal nerves.
Blood supply: Posterior intercostal arteries.
Action: Extension of vertebral column.

2. Longissimus (middle column of erector spinae)

(a) Longissimus thoracis
Origin: Thoracolumbar fascia and accessory processes of the lumbar vertebrae.
Insertion: Transverse processes of the lower nine thoracic vertebrae and the lower nine ribs.
Innervation: Dorsal rami of thoracic spinal nerves (T1–T12).
Blood supply: Posterior intercostal and lumbar arteries.
Action: Extension and lateral flexion of the vertebral column.

(b) Longissimus lumborum (longissimus thoracis pars lumborum)

Although not traditionally described, a number of workers now recognize a lumbar portion of the longissimus, inserting into the transverse processes of lumbar vertebrae.[7,8]

3. Spinalis (medial column of erector spinae)

(a) Spinalis thoracis
Origin: Blends with longissimus thoracis and arises from spinous processes of T11–L2.
Insertion: Spinous processes of upper four to eight thoracic vertebrae.
Innervation: Dorsal rami of thoracic spinal nerves (T1–T12).
Blood supply: Posterior intercostal arteries.
Action: Extension and lateral flexion of the vertebral column.

Transversospinalis (Fig. 2–5) The *transversospinalis muscles* lie deep to the erector spinae and occupy the space between the transverse and spinous processes of the vertebral column. As a muscle group, their fibers tend to run from transverse processes below to spinous processes above. Hence, their collective name, *transversospinalis*. The muscle group consists of three subdivisions: the *semispinalis*, *multifidus*, and *rotatores*. The details of only the lumbar and thoracic portions of the transversospinalis muscle group will be discussed here.

The *semispinalis* consists of three groups of muscle: the *semispinalis thoracis*, *semispinalis cervicis*, and *semispinalis capitis*. The *semispinalis* muscles are the longest, and most superficial fibers of the transversospinalis muscles, usually crossing from four to six vertebral levels from origin to insertion. The *semispinalis thoracis* arises from the transverse processes of the lower six thoracic vertebrae and inserts into the spines of the upper thoracic and lower cervical vertebrae.

The *multifidus* lies deep to the *semispinalis in the cervical and thoracic spine*. In the lumbar region, however, the multifidus is the most medial of the lumbar musculature. Although it is considered a deep layer muscle, it has no other overlying muscle in this region (Fig. 2–4) It is thickest in the lumbar region and extends upward into the cervical region. There are no clear cut distinctions between regional attachments. By convention, the layer is described as one entire muscle, the *multifidus*, with plural appropriately being *multifidi*. The *multifidus* is covered by the *semispinalis* in the cervical and thoracic regions. It is covered posteriorly by posterior layer of the thoracolumbar fascia and then loosely by the the erector spinae aponeurosis (ESA) in the lumbar. The ESA is a broad fibrous sheet of connective tissue that originates with fibers from the longissimus thoracis medially and iliocostalis lumborum laterally, with an additional minimal contribution of superficial multifidus fibers from upper lumbar segments. The ESA inserts into the ilium, sacrum, and the lumbar and sacral spinous processes.[9]

Multifidus fibers cross from two to four vertebral levels between their attachments of origin and insertion. The lumbar part of the muscle arises from the dorsal sacrum, the posterior superior iliac spine, the deep surface of the tendon of origin of the erector spinae muscle, and the lumbar mamillary processes. The thinner thoracic bundles arise from all of the thoracic vertebrae. The still thinner cervical bundles arise from the articular processes of the lower four cervical vertebrae. The fiber bundles pass upward and medially to insert into all the spinous processes from the fifth lumbar to the axis.

The *rotatores* lie deep to the *multifidus* and are the deepest muscles of the *transversospinalis* group with the shortest fibers extending only one or two vertebral levels. Each muscle has a single origin and single insertion. The *rotatores* are present in the cervical, thoracic, and lumbar regions of the back and are divided into *rotatores longus* and *rotatores brevis*. Each *rotatores longus* arises from the transverse process of one vertebra, crosses the vertebra immediately above and inserts into the spinous process of the vertebra two levels above the vertebra of origin.

1. Semispinalis thoracis
   Origin: From the transverse processes of the lower six thoracic vertebrae.
   Insertion: Spinous processes of upper thoracic and lower cervical vertebrae.
   Innervation: Dorsal rami of thoracic spinal nerves (T1–T6).
   Blood supply: Posterior intercostal arteries.
   Actions:
   Bilaterally: Extension of the vertebral column.
   Unilaterally: Rotation of the vertebral column toward the opposite side.
2. Multifidus
   Multifidus (lumborum, thoracis, and cervicis portions)
   Origin: Posterior surface of sacrum, posterior sacroiliac ligament, mamillary processes of lumbar vertebrae, transverse processes of thoracic vertebrae, and articular processes of cervical vertebrae 4 through 7.
   Insertion: Spines of the vertebrae 2 to 4 segments superior to the vertebra of origin.
   Innervation: Dorsal rami of all spinal nerves.
   Blood supply: Posterior intercostal and lumbar arteries, deep cervical branch of the costocervical trunk.
   Action: Extension, lateral flexion, trunk stabilizer during rotation, extension, and lateral motions of the pelvis. There appears to be a division of function between the deep and superficial aspects of this muscle, as noted below. Also, the multifidus, in concert with several other muscles, has been shown to be integrally involved with intrinsic stability of the lumbopelvic spine, which is briefly discussed later.

The lumbar muscles produce different forces on the spinal motion segments. Each muscle produces shear forces and compressive forces and also acts as a moment-producer. These muscles provide segmental stability to the spine while also ensuring mobility.[10]

Clinical Pearl: The superficial multifidus contributes to the control of spine orientation and the deep multifidus has a role in controlling intersegmental motion.

The multifidus has become the center of a great deal of attention in recent years. The reason for such interest will be touched upon in this chapter and will be covered in more depth in Chapter 5. The key feature of the lumbar multifidus muscles is the repeating series of fascicles originating from the laminae and spinous processes of the lumbar vertebrae. They are the longest and most medial of the lumbar transversospinalis muscles. The L1–L5 slips of the multifidus muscle spread out laterally to their insertions. Multifidus fascicle insertions are attached directly to the posterior sacrum, and indirectly to the sacroiliac joint and the ilium via the posterior sacroiliac ligament.

Clinical Pearl: Multifidus fascicle insertions are attached directly to the posterior sacrum, and indirectly to the sacroiliac joint and the ilium via the posterior sacroiliac ligament.

The activity of the deep and superficial fibers of the lumbar multifidus during voluntary arm movement has been studied. The deep and superficial fibers of the multifidus are differentially active during single and repetitive movements of the arm. The superficial multifidus contributes to the control of spine orinetation and the deep multifidus has a role in controlling intersegmental motion.[11]

When investigating acute low back pain, remission of painful low back symptoms in acute subjects seem to indicate that there is no spontaneous multifidus muscle recovery. Perhaps one reason for the high recurrence rate of low back pain following the initial episode is lack of localized muscle support.[12] In another study 80% of the patients with low back pain showed the presence of multifidus muscle atrophy and leg pain.[13]

3. Rotatores longus and Rotatores brevis
   Origin: From the transverse processes of vertebrae.
   Insertion: Lamina of the vertebra immediately superior (rotatores brevis), or into the lamina of the second vertebra above the vertebra of origin (rotatores longus).
   Innervation: Dorsal rami of spinal nerves.
   Blood supply: Posterior intercostal arteries, lumbar arteries.
   Action: Rotation of the vertebral column.

The small cross-sectional design of the rotatores makes it a poor generator of force and as a result a poor contributor to rotation and twisting. The rotatores have four to seven times more muscle spindles than the multifidus.[14] Perhaps the rotatores behave as length transducers or vertebral location sensors at the lumbar joint. And perhaps they are affected by manual therapies especially with the joint at end range.[15] These are but a few thoughts to consider while pondering the anatomy of the lumbar spine. The rotatores may have more a proprioceptive function than a rotatory function. Although they appear to lack the mechanical advantage to be primary rotators, they may be accessory muscles of rotation. According to McIntosh et al.,[16] none of the lumbar back muscles can be considered rotators. The oblique abdominal muscles are the principal rotators of the trunk. It has been demonstrated[14,17,18] that muscles such as the rotatores longus and rotatores brevis are placed in locations of such poor mechanical advantage that they are unlikely to produce the movements to which they have historically been ascribed. Generally, such small muscles are synergistic at best to other larger, more effective muscles. Additionally, they generally have much higher proportions of muscle spindles than larger muscles. Therefore, it is suggested[14,17,18] that such small, redundant muscles act as "kinesiological monitors," in other words, proprioceptive organs. In the back, the rotatores would serve such a function, while the oblique abdominal muscles produce the functional rotation.

Segmental Muscles of the Back (Fig. 2–6) The segmental muscles extend from one vertebra to the next without skipping any levels. This group includes the interspinales and intertransversarii. The levatores costarum brevis and the rotatores brevis may also be considered with this group.

The interspinales are well developed in the cervical and lumbar regions, but poorly developed or lacking in the thoracic region. In the lumbar region they take the form of well-developed single muscle bellies connecting the tips of the spinous processes to one another.

The intertransversarii run vertically between adjacent transverse processes. Like the interspinales, these muscles are generally well developed in the cervical and lumbar regions, but poorly developed or absent from the thoracic region. The lumbar region contains two intertransversarii on each side: a medial and a lateral muscle. The lateral muscles pass between adjacent transverse processes. The medial muscles pass from the mamillary process of the vertebra below to the accessory process of the vertebra above.

The levatores costarum muscles consist of 12 pairs of muscles, which arise from thoracic transverse processes and insert between the tubercle and the angle of the rib below. They function to elevate the ribs and aid in inspiration. They are located deep to the erector spinae muscles. Each has a brevis portion, which reaches the rib immediately inferior, and a longus portion, which inserts two ribs below the transverse process of origin.

1. Levatores costarum
   Origin: Twelve pairs, from transverse processes of seventh cervical and first through eleventh thoracic vertebrae.
   Insertion: On external surface of rib below vertebra of origin between the tubercle and the angle.
   Innervation: Dorsal rami of lowest cervical and thoracic spinal nerves (C8, T1– T11).
   Blood supply: Posterior intercostal arteries.
   Action: Elevate ribs, assist in inspiration, rotates, and laterally flexes vertebral column.
2. Thoracic and lumbar interspinales
   Origin: Superiorly on spine of vertebra.
   Insertion: Inferiorly on spine of vertebra immediately superior to vertebra of origin; not always present in thoracic region.
   Innervation: Dorsal rami of spinal nerves.
   Blood supply: Muscular branches of the posterior intercostal arteries, lumbar arteries, deep cervical branches of the costocervical trunk.
   Action: Extension of vertebral column.
3. Thoracic and lumbar intertransversarii
   Origin: Superiorly on transverse processes of vertebrae.
   Insertion: Inferiorly on transverse processes of vertebrae immediately superior to vertebra of origin; most highly developed in cervical and lumbar regions.
   Innervation: Dorsal rami of spinal nerves, except lateral intertransversarii in lumbar and lower thoracic; these exceptions are innervated by ventral rami.
   Blood supply: Muscular branches of posterior intercostal and lumbar arteries.
   Action: Lateral flexion of vertebral column.

Abdominal Muscles

Muscles of the abdominal wall exert their effects on the lower back as well as maintaining the body wall, including the quadratus lumborum and the three flat muscles of the abdominal wall.

1. Quadratus lumborum (Fig. 2–7)
   Origin: Iliolumbar ligament and posterior part of the iliac crest.
   Insertion: Inferior border of the twelfth rib, transverse processes of lumbar vertebrae 1 to 4.
   Innervation: Subcostal nerve (ventral ramus of twelfth thoracic spinal nerve); ventral rami of lumbar spinal nerves 1, 2, and 3 (T12, L1–L3).
   Blood supply: Lumbar branch of the iliolumbar artery.
   Action: Depresses and fixes the twelfth rib. Acts as a muscle of expiration by fixing the twelfth rib and thereby stabilizing the inferior attachments of the diaphragm. Laterally flexes the vertebral column when concentrically contracting unilaterally. With the pelvis fixed and

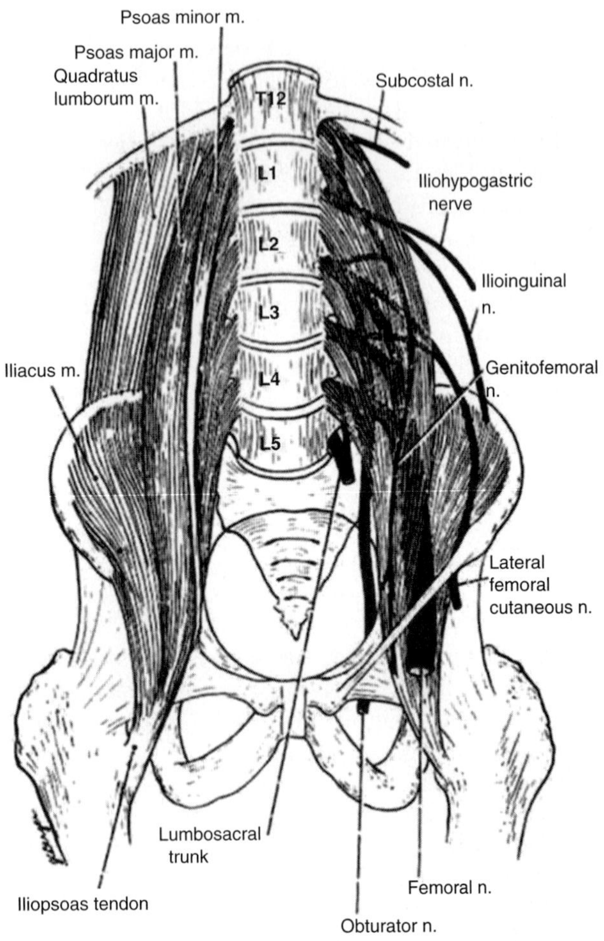

FIGURE 2–7. Quadratus lumborum, iliacus, psoas major, and psoas minor. Anterior view. (*After Woodburne.*)

contracting bilaterally, it probably helps extend the lumbar vertebral column. Unilateral, concentric contraction of the quadratus lumborum leads to ipsilateral flexion, with concurrent stabilizing eccentric contraction of the contralateral quadratus lumborum. Also, the quadratus lumborum concentrically lowers the lower ribs, so it eccentrically aids in stable inspiration and concentrically assists expiration. This is important because the strategies for the so-called respiratory "synkinesis" techniques of muscle energy are reversed with the quadratus lumborum (compared with almost all other skeletal muscle) in the mobilization chapter.

2. Obliquus externus abdominis (Fig. 2–8)
   Origin: Eight fleshy strips that arise from the external and inferior borders of the lower eight ribs, interdigitating with serratus anterior and latissimus dorsi.
   Insertion: Ventral half of the external aspect of the iliac crest, remainder via a wide aponeurosis that helps constitute the rectus abdominis sheath, and via the sheath into the linea alba. The lower border of its aponeurosis forms the inguinal ligament.
   Innervation: Ventral rami of lower six thoracic and first two lumbar spinal nerves (T7–T12, L1, L2).
   Blood supply: Superior and inferior epigastric arteries.
   Action: Compresses abdomen, supports abdominal viscera, active in forced expiration. Via actions on the ribs rotates the vertebral column to the contralateral side. Bilateral contraction helps flex lumbar vertebral column.
3. Obliquus internus abdominis: (Fig. 2–8)
   Origin: Thoracolumbar fascia, anterior two thirds of the iliac crest deep to obliquus externus abdominis, lateral two thirds of the inguinal ligament.
   Insertion: Costal cartilages of the last three ribs, and then via its aponeurosis into the rectus sheath and thus into the linea alba.
   Innervation: Ventral rami of lower six thoracic and first two lumbar spinal nerves (T7–T12, L1, L2).
   Blood supply: Superior and inferior epigastric arteries, deep circumflex iliac artery.
   Action: Compresses abdomen, supports abdominal viscera, active in forced expiration. Via actions on the ribs rotates the vertebral column to the ipsilateral side. Bilateral contraction helps flex lumbar vertebral column.
4. Transversus abdominis (Fig. 2–8)
   Origin: Deep surfaces of the lower six costal cartilages, middle layer of the thoracolumbar fascia, anterior two-thirds of the iliac crest, deep to the obliquus internus abdominis.
   Insertion: Via the rectus sheath into the linea alba with the oblique abdominal muscles.
   Innervation: Ventral rami of the lower 6 thoracic ventral rami, iliohypogastric nerve and ilioinguinal nerve (T7–T12, L1, L2).
   Blood supply: Deep circumflex iliac artery; inferior epigastric artery.
   Action: Compresses abdomen, supports abdominal viscera, active in forced expiration. Key muscle for intrinsic (core) stability, which will be discussed later.

Pelvic Diaphragm (Fig. 2–9) The pelvic diaphragm forms the lowest portion of the body wall and encloses the pelvic viscera, giving them support and restraining the abdominal contents. It consists of the levator ani muscle, the coccygeus muscle, and the fascia covering their internal and external surfaces. The levator ani muscle is described as having two portions based upon their origins: the pubococcygeus and iliococcygeus. The coccygeus muscle is also referred to

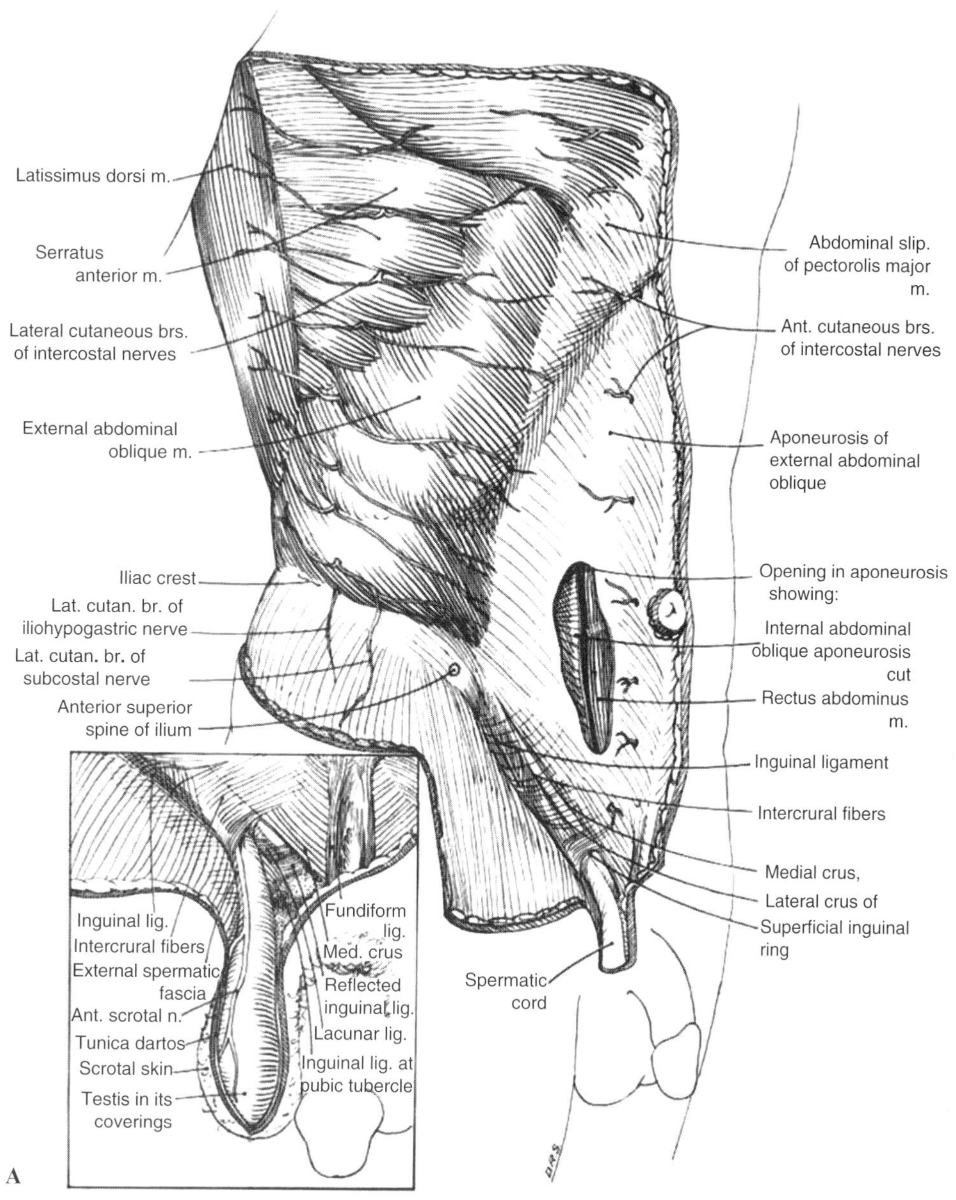

FIGURE 2–8. Obliquus abdominis externus, obliquus abdominis internus, transversus abdominis. *A.* Obliquus abdominis externus.

as the ischiococcygeus muscle. It is posterior to the levator ani but is contiguous with it and in the same plane.

1. Levator ani (pubococcygeus and iliococcygeus)
   Origin: Body of the pubis, tenindous arch of the obturator fascia, and the ischial spine.
   Insertion: Perineal body, coccyx, anococcygeal ligament, walls of prostate, vagina, rectum and anal canal.
   Innervation: nerve to levator ani (S4, sometimes contributions from S3 and/or S5) via the pudendal plexus.
   Blood supply: Branches of the internal pudendal, inferior rectal, and inferior gluteal arteries.
   Action: Supports pelvic viscera; raises the pelvic floor, resists increased abdominal pressure. Pubococcygeus portion the inferior end of the rectum toward the pubis, constricting the rectum and vagina. Key muscle for intrinsic (core) stability, which will be discussed later.
2. Coccygeus (ischiococcygeus)
   Origin: Ischial spine and sacrospinous ligament.
   Insertion: Coccyx and last segment of sacrum.
   Innervation: Branches of the ventral rami of fourth and fifth sacral nerves via the pudendal plexus.
   Blood supply: Branches of the internal pudendal and inferior gluteal arteries.
   Action: Draws the coccyx anteriorly, supports the coccyx, forms the pelvic diaphragm with the

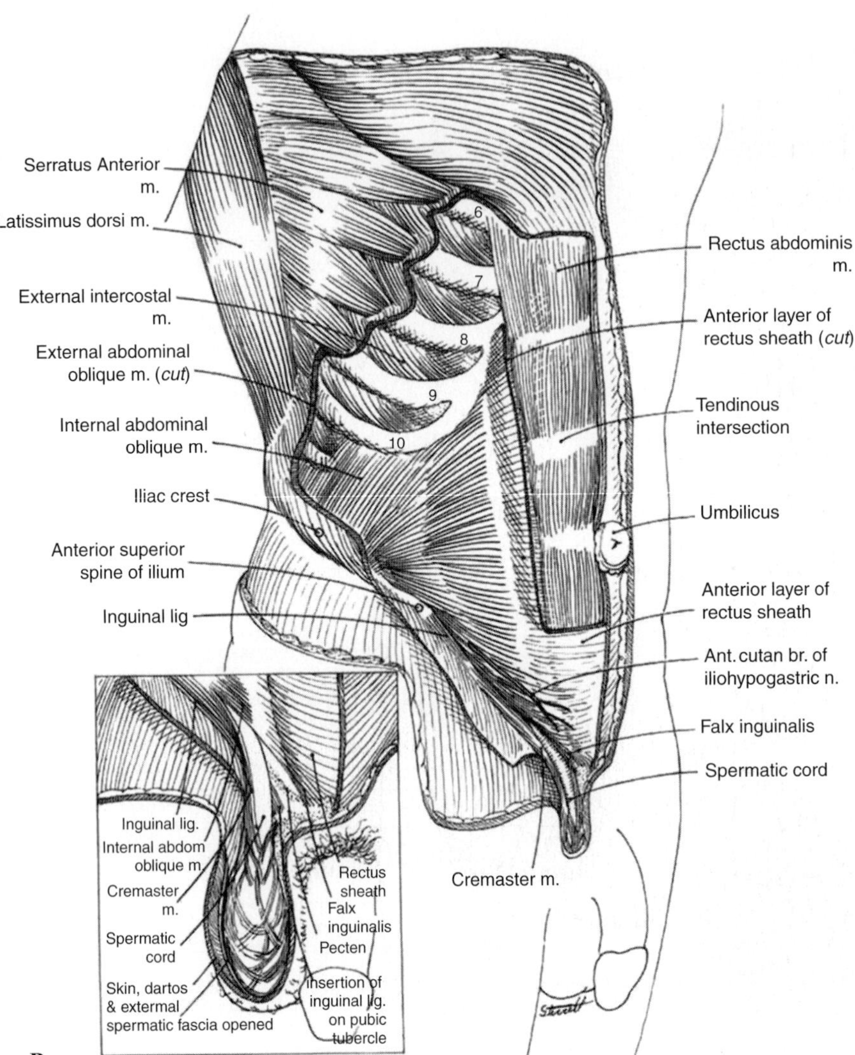

FIGURE 2–8. *B.* Obliquus abdominis internus. (Continued)

levator ani. Key muscle for intrinsic (core) stability, which will be discussed later.

3. Iliacus and psoas major and minor (Fig. 2–7)
   (a) Iliopsoas: The iliopsoas is the term applied to the iliacus and psoas major muscles collectively, as they insert into the lesser trochanter of the femur by a common tendon.
   (b) Iliacus:
   Origin: Superior two thirds of the iliac fossa; iliac crest; anterior sacroiliac, lumbosacral, and iliolumbar ligaments; ala of sacrum.
   Insertion: With the tendon of the psoas major into the lesser trochanter of the femur, capsule of the hip joint, and the shaft of the femur.
   Innervation: Femoral nerve (L2, L3).
   Blood supply: Iliac branch of the iliolumbar artery and the superior gluteal artery.
   Action: Flexes the thigh, flexes the pelvis when the thigh is fixed.
   (c) Psoas major:
   Origin: Anterior and inferior surfaces of the transverse processes, bodies, and intervertebral discs of all five lumbar vertebrae. Interestingly, the muscle bundles of each upper lumbar segment are not longer than the lower ones, as one might expect. Instead, the tendonous slips are longer at each successive rostral vertebral level. This design allows for a more uniform load along the length of the lumbar spine. In addition, the vertical orientation of the muscle increases axial loading and also isolates its capacity as a hip flexor.[9]
   Insertion: After passing beneath the inguinal ligament and anterior to the capsule of the hip joint, inserts with the iliacus (as the iliopsoas muscle) into the lesser trochanter of the femur.

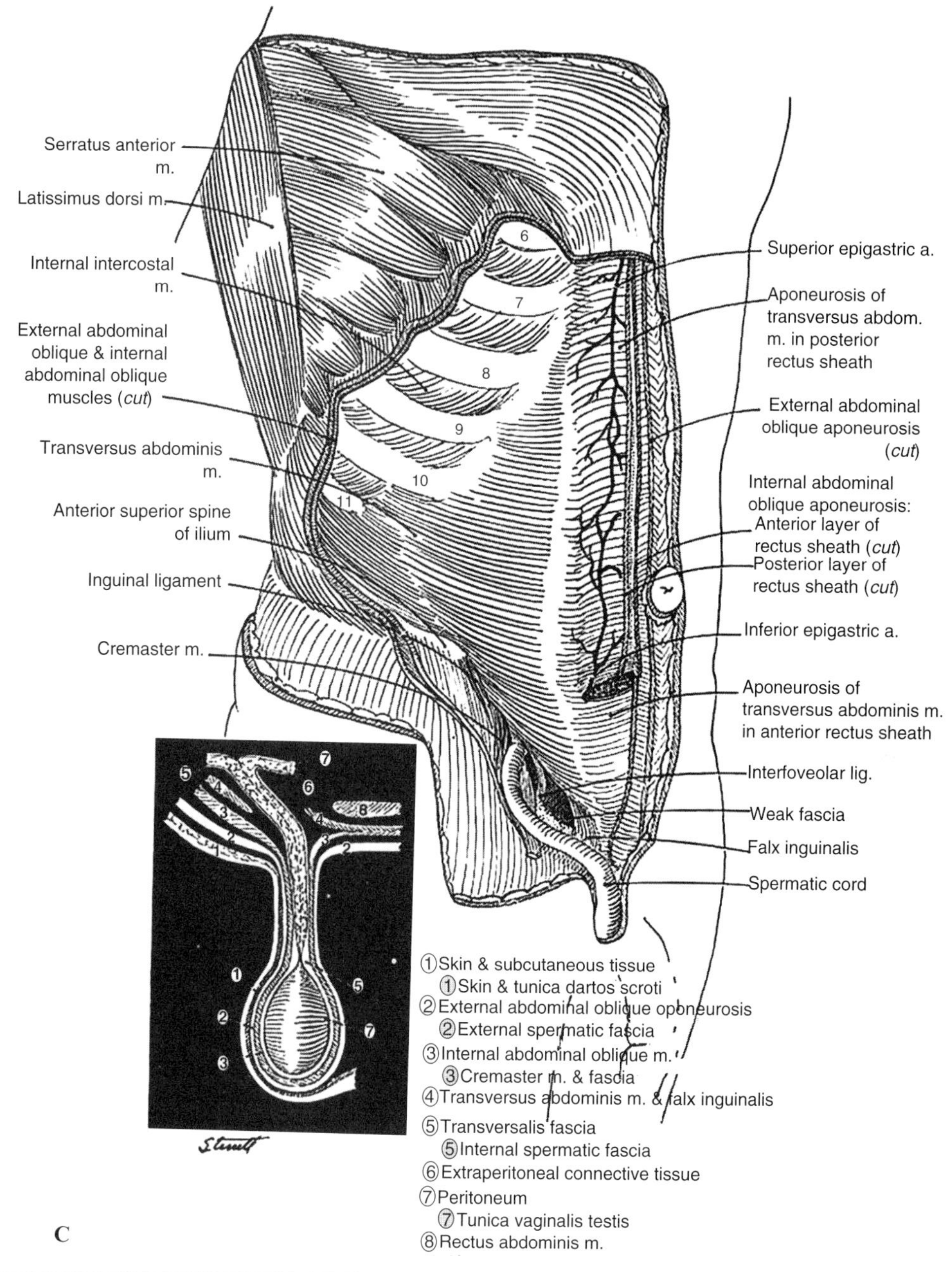

FIGURE 2–8. (Continued) *C.* Transversus abdominis. (*After Woodburne.*)

Innervation: Branches of the lumbar plexus including contributions from the ventral rami of lumbar spinal nerves 2, 3, and 4 (L2, L3, L4).

Blood supply: Lumbar branch of the iliolumbar artery.

Action: Flexes the thigh at the hip joint.

While mechanically it appears to be a medial rotator of the thigh, electromyographic studies show it to be active during lateral rotation. The psoas may have minimal ability to produce any significant range of motion at the lumbar spine.[9] It attaches anteriorly to every lumbar vertebra and disc (except L5/S1). According to Bogduk, the psoas acts on the lumbar spine to generate a longitudinal force to enhance spinal stability via axial compression. However, contrary to common belief, it has a minimal effect on the lumbar lordosis.[9]

(d) Psoas minor: The psoas minor is often absent, and is absent bilaterally in half of subjects.

Origin: Sides of the bodies of the twelfth thoracic and first lumbar vertebrae and the intervertebral disc between them.

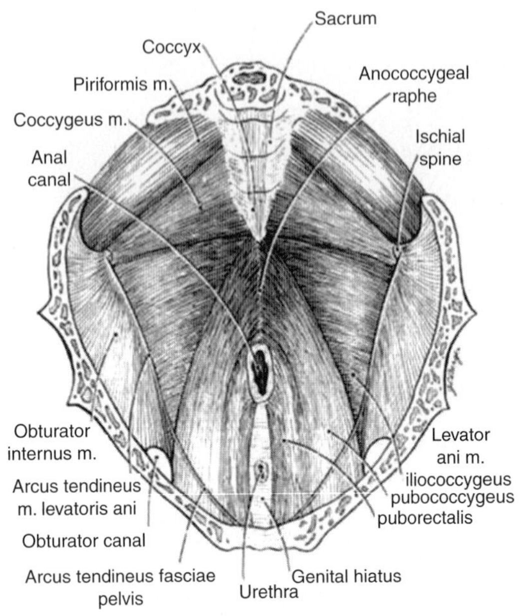

FIGURE 2–9. Pelvic diaphragm. Superior view. Posterior is at top of the illustration. (*After Woodburne.*[1])

Insertion: Pectineal line and iliopectineal eminence of the innominate bone.
Innervation: Ventral ramus of the first (and sometimes second) lumbar spinal nerve (L1, L2).
Blood supply: Lumbar branch of the iliolumbar artery.
Action: Flexes pelvis on the vertebral column.

4. Diaphragm (Fig. 2–10)

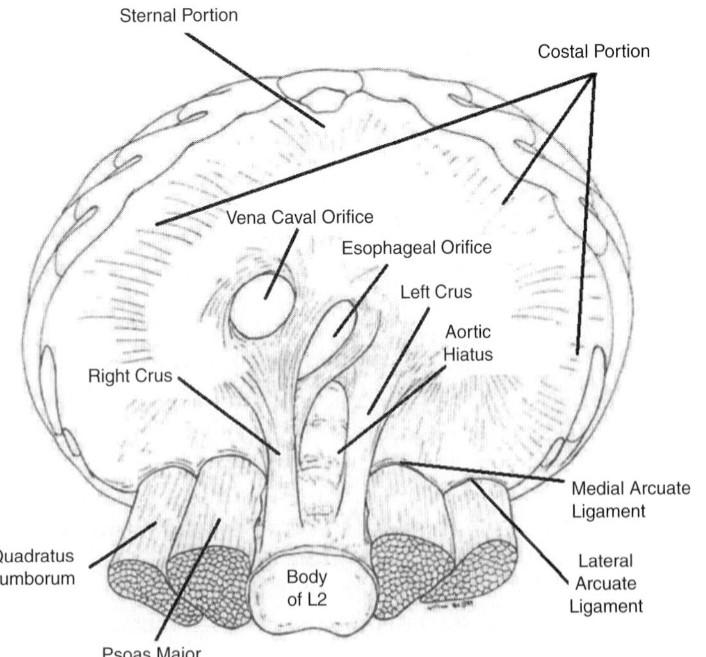

FIGURE 2–10. Diaphragm and associated structures. Inferior view. (*Courtsey of William Yee, Anatomy Department, New York Chiropractic College, New York.*)

Origin: Sites of attachment of the diaphragm.
Sternal part: Attaches by two slips to posterior part of xiphoid process.
Costal part: Attaches to internal surfaces of lower six ribs and costal cartilages. Interdigitates with transversus abdominis muscle.
Lumbar part: Attaches to medial and lateral arcuate ligaments by two crura (singular: crus), in addition to the anterior bodies of the upper three lumbar vertabrae.

- *Right crus*: Broader and longer than left. Attaches to anterolateral aspect of bodies and intervertebral discs of vertebrae L1–L3.
- *Left crus:* Attaches to corresponding parts of L1 and L2, shorter than right.
- Medial tendinous arches of both crura converge over aorta at level of thoracolumbar disc (intervertebral disc T12/L1). This constitutes the *median arcuate ligament.*

Lateral arcuate ligament: Thickening of fascia where diaphragm overlies the quadratus lumborum muscle. Fibers run from the ligament to the central tendon of the diaphragm.
Medial arcuate ligament: Thickening of fascia where the diaphragm overlies the psoas major muscle. Fibers run from the ligament to the central tendon of the diaphragm.
Insertion: Central tendon of diaphragm, an aponeurosis of interwoven collagenous fibers. It is located nearer the front of the thorax than the rear, so muscle fibers are longer posteriorly.

Innervation: Principal motor innervation is from the phrenic nerve (C3–C5), with some peripheral innervation from intercostal nerves.

Blood supply: Superior and inferior phrenic arteries, musculophrenic artery, and pericardiacophrenic artery.

Action: The essential muscle of respiration. Contraction of the diaphragm results in a lengthening of the thoracic cavity, thereby increasing the volume of the thoracic cavity, increasing negative pressure and thereby drawing air into the lungs. Contraction of the diaphragm is responsible for about two thirds of the volume of inspired air. Key muscle for intrinsic (core) stability, which will be discussed next.

Functional Aspects of the Diaphragm, Pelvic and Abdominal Musculature, the Psoas Major, and Lumbar Stability

As previously noted, recent interest in understanding lumbopelvic function and dynamic stability has led to a renewed interest in the regional anatomy. Lumbar stability is dependent upon an interrelationship among the thoracoabdominal diaphragm, the pelvic diaphragm, the muscles of the abdominal wall, and the psoas major.[23,24] Through its segmental attachments, and links to the diaphragm and pelvic floor, psoas can axially compress the lumbar spine and thus play a role in spinal stability. It is therefore an important stabilizer of the lumbar spine. Gibbons and coworkers[25–27] report significant fascial relations of the psoas major muscle.

The medial actuate ligament is a continuation of the superior psoas fascia that continues superiorly to the diaphragm. The right and left crura of the diaphragm attach to the anterolateral parts of the bodies of vertebrae L1–L3. On both sides of the body, the crura and their fascia blend with the psoas major and its fascia until they pass more anteriorly to blend with the anterior longitudinal ligament.[25] As the psoas major passes inferiorly, its inferomedial fascia becomes thicker at its most inferior portion and becomes continuous with the fascia of the pelvic floor. The psoas fascia also forms links with the conjoint tendon, transversus abdominis, and the internal oblique. As psoas passes over the pelvic brim, the fascia of the posterior fascicles attaches firmly to the pelvic brim.[25–29]

The musculature of the body wall, thoracoabdominal diaphragm, and pelvic diaphragm, form a cylinder. The roof of the cylinder is the diaphragm, while the pelvic diaphragm forms the floor. The wall of the cylinder is formed by the abdominal and posterior spinal musculature, especially transversus abdominis and the segmental fibers of lumbar multifidus.[19–21] Psoas major is connected to the diaphragm and the pelvic floor through fascial attachments and interdigitations of the diaphragm and psoas major. This arrangement allows psoas to act as a link between the diaphragm and the pelvic floor that helps to maintain stability of the lumbar cylinder mechanism. Fascial tension, created by the contraction of the diaphragm, pelvic floor, psoas major, and abdominal musculature, results in an increase in intra-abdominal pressure (IAP), which results in further stiffening, and thus increasing the stability of the spine. Increased fascial tension may directly restrict intervertebral motion or provide gentle segmental compression. Transversus abdominis influences the stability of the spine via modulation of IAP or increased tension in the thoracolumbar fascia. Hodges and Richardson[22] stated that their study shows that contraction of the transversus abdominis was significantly delayed in patients with low back pain with all movements. This model is discussed in greater detail in Chapter 5.

Clinical Pearl: Fascial tension, created by the contraction of the diaphragm, pelvic floor, psoas major, and abdominal musculature results in an increase in IAP, which results in further stiffening, and thus increasing the stability of the spine.

During inspiration, tension within the diaphragm increases. Thus the cylinder becomes more stable. During expiration, the diaphragm relaxes, and the result is that the cylinder becomes less stable. Transversus abdominis contracts earlier in expiration,[23] presumably to compensate for this decrease in stability of the pressurized cylinder.[21] Coactivation of the diaphragm and abdominal muscles causes a sustained increase in IAP, whereas inspiration and expiration are controlled by opposing activity of the diaphragm and abdominal muscles to vary the shape of the pressurized abdominal cavity.[30] One study indicated that changes in trunk muscle activity and IAP with respiratory efforts modulate spinal stiffness. Also, the diaphragm may magnify spinal stiffness via attachment of its crural fibers to the lumbar vertebrae.[31]

OSSEOUS ANATOMY

The adult human skeleton is composed of 206 bones, which can be divided into an *appendicular* and an *axial skeleton*. The *appendicular skeleton* consists of the bones of the upper and lower limbs and their associated girdles. The *axial skeleton* consists of the *cranium* (or *skull*), the *vertebrae*, and *associated structures*.[4]

This chapter will consider the osteology and articulations of the vertebral column.

BONES OF THE VERTEBRAL COLUMN

The Vertebral Column in General

The human *vertebral column* is composed of 33 segments or *vertebrae*. Some are fused in adult life, so that the total number of individual bones is only 26. Between each vertebral segment is a fibrocartilaginous *intervertebral disc*.

The vertebrae may be broken into five groups, cranially to caudally:

Cervical	7 bones
Thoracic	12 bones
Lumbar	5 bones
Sacral	5 segments fused into one bone
Coccyx	4 segments typically fused into one bone

It should be noted that these are the most typical numbers of vertebrae in each segment, but that there can be some variation. There is rarely (in fact, virtually never) any variation in the number of cervical vertebrae, but it is fairly common to find one more or one less segment in the lumbar, sacral, and coccygeal segments of the vertebral column. The probability that an atypical number of vertebrae will be encountered increases caudally.

The vertebral column serves three primary functions: (i) to support the trunk and transmit its weight to the pelvis and lower limb; (ii) to house and protect the spinal cord and its membranes; (iii) to provide a central axis for the thorax (each rib articulates with a vertebra and coordinated motion of the ribs is a critical aspect of normal breathing) and protect its contents. (The thorax also serves as the attachment point of the forelimb.) All vertebrae are formed along a common plan, but vary according to their positions and functions in the spinal column. These parts may be examined in a typical vertebra.

Regions of the Vertebral Column

As mentioned above, the vertebral column can be divided into five groups or regions: cervical, thoracic, lumbar, sacral, and coccygeal. Vertebrae of each region demonstrate specific characteristics that are diagnostic for that region. All 33 vertebral segments and their associated intervertebral discs taken together constitute the *vertebral column*.

In the human being, the vertebral column demonstrates a series of *curvatures* associated with these different regions (Fig. 2–11). There are *four curvatures* in the human vertebral column: the *cervical curvature*, the *thoracic curvature*, the *lumbar curvature*, and the *sacral curvature* (the curve of the coccyx continues along the sacral curvature). In most terrestrial vertebrates, the vertebral column demonstrates a single horizontal arc that is convex dorsally, and is supported cranial and caudally by the pectoral and pelvic limbs. Human beings, however, are unique in our *bipedal* form of walking and in that humans habitually balance all of the weight of the trunk over the pelvic limb and girdle alone, with the vertebral column held more or less vertically over the sacrum.

Embryologically, there is present a single dorsoconvex arc in the human vertebral column, just as is true of other terrestrial vertebrates. The *thoracic* and *sacral curvatures* of the human adult vertebral column are convex dorsally, and are called *primary curvatures*, as they were present embryologically and are the adult remnants of this embryological curvature. The *cervical and lumbar curvatures* begin to appear before birth, but are not really obvious until later. They are referred to as *secondary curvatures*. The *cervical curvature* becomes apparent when the infant begins to hold its head up. It can be obliterated by flexing the neck, but it is present in normal standing, sitting, and walking. The *thoracic curvature* is formed by the articulation of the 12 thoracic vertebrae. It is permanent. The *lumbar curvature*, which becomes pronounced as a child begins to walk, is generally greater in women and less in men, while the *sacral curvature* is generally slightly greater in men than in women, though the sexes overlap a great deal in this feature.

Osteological Features of Vertebrae in General

The most anterior portion of a typical vertebra is the *body*. The *body* is the largest portion of a vertebra and is approximately cylindrical in shape. Its *cranial (superior)* and *caudal (inferior) surfaces* are roughened and give attachment to the *intervertebral discs*. Located around the circumferences of the cranial and caudal surfaces of the body are slightly elevated rims. The diameters of the cranial and caudal surfaces of the vertebral bodies are somewhat greater than the diameter of the center portion of the body so that it appears constricted or "waisted." The posterior surface of the body faces the vertebral foramen, and contains one or more large, irregular openings, the *foramina vasculare (basivertebral foramina)*, for the passage of the basivertebral veins (Fig. 2–12).

The bodies of the vertebrae transmit the weight of a person's body, and muscular and other compressive forces (i.e., reaction forces from walking, running, jumping, etc.). The vertebrae are separated from one another by fibrocartilaginous intervertebral discs, which transmit forces from one vertebra to the next. Posterior to the vertebral body is the *vertebral arch*, formed by the *pedicles* and *laminae*. (The *neural arch* is the developmental structure that contributes both to the vertebral arch and to part of the vertebral body. It is sometimes used, incorrectly, as a synonym for vertebral arch.) The vertebral arch, along with the posterior surface of the vertebral body, encloses an opening, the

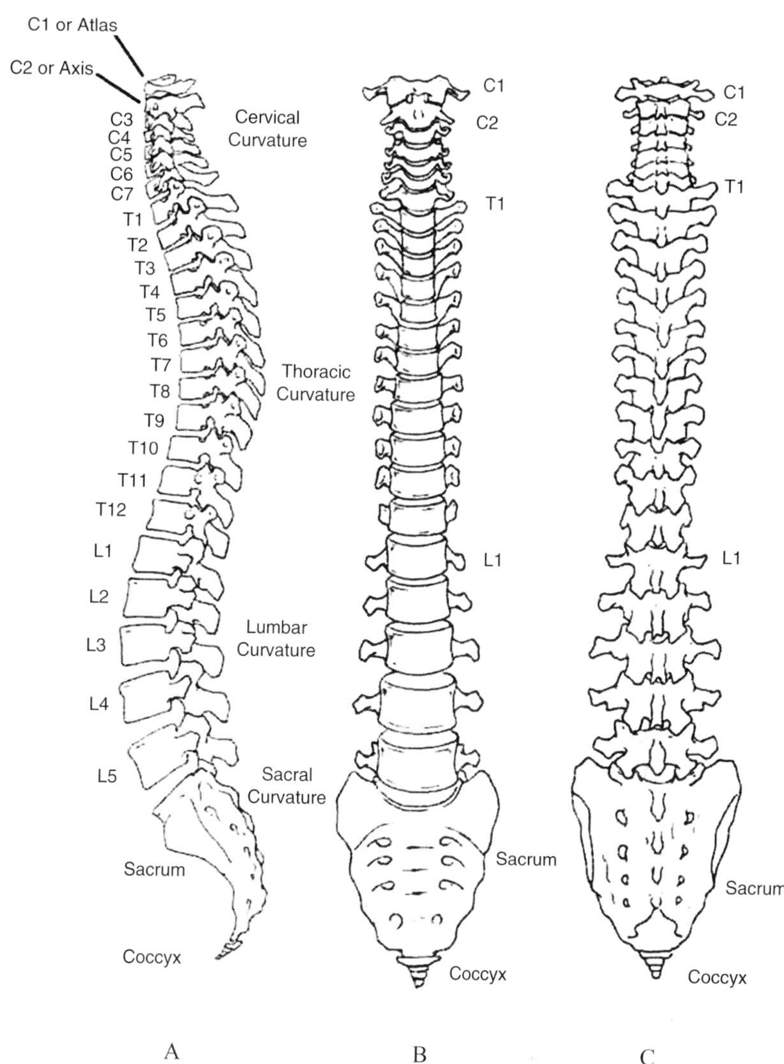

FIGURE 2–11. Bony vertebral column and curvatures. *A.* Left lateral view. *B.* Anterior view. *C.* Posterior view. (*After Walker et al.*[32])

vertebral foramen. The spinal cord and its associated membranes pass through the *vertebral canal*, formed by the vertebral foramina of all the vertebrae. The vertebral arches do not bear weight, but rather protect the spinal column, and are connected to one another by strong ligaments.

The vertebral arch consists of a pair of *pedicles* and a pair of *laminae*. These two portions of the arch together support seven processes: four *articular processes*, two *transverse processes*, and one *spinous process*. Each vertebral arch can be divided into right and left halves posteriorly by the spinous process. Laterally, each half can be divided into anterior and posterior portions by the transverse process. The portion of the arch between the body anteriorly and the transverse process posteriorly is the *pedicle*. It is by the pedicle that the vertebral arch is attached to the vertebral body. It is short, strong, and rounded. The portion of the vertebral arch between the transverse process and the spinous process is the *lamina* (plural *laminae*). The lamina is flat and platelike. Arches of adjacent vertebrae articulate with one another by means of *superior and inferior articular processes*. The articular processes are also known as *zygapophyses* (singular: *zygapophysis*). On each side of the vertebral arch, the superior articular process is located superior to the transverse process, while the inferior articular process is located inferior to the transverse process. Each inferior articular process articulates with the superior articular process of the vertebra below it. These form small synovial joints, and each articular process bears a small smooth *articular facet*.

Because the craniocaudal height of the pedicles is less than the height of the bodies of the vertebrae to which they are attached, there exist "notches" or depressions on the superior and inferior surfaces of the pedicles. These are the *superior vertebral notches* above the pedicles and the *inferior vertebral notches* below them. The inferior vertebral notch is much deeper than the superior because the pedicle attaches nearer the superior surface of the vertebral body than the inferior surface of the body. The superior and inferior

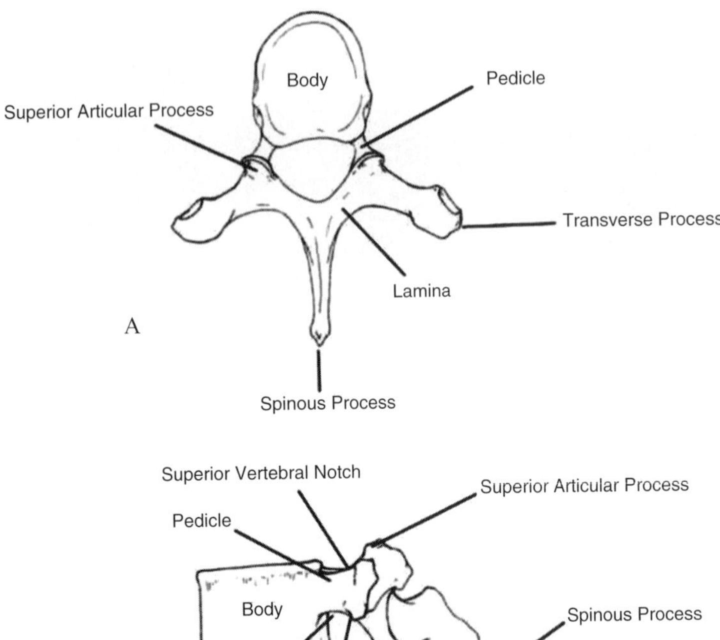

FIGURE 2–12. Osteological features of vertebrae in general. *A.* Superior view. *B.* Left lateral view. (*After Walker et al.*[32])

vertebral notches of adjacent vertebrae form the *intervertebral foramen*. It is through these intervertebral foramina that the spinal nerves exit the spinal column to reach their peripheral distributions.

In addition to the body, the pedicles, the laminae, the transverse processes, the spinous process, and the articular processes, associated with each vertebra is a *costal element*. The costal element takes a different form in different regions of the spinal column. *Costal* means "rib." In the thoracic region, the costal element is not a part of the *thoracic vertebra*, but is present as a separate bone, the *rib* (Latin: "costa"). In *cervical, lumbar,* and *sacral vertebrae*, the costal element is incorporated into the vertebrae. In *cervical vertebrae,* the costal element is present as the *anterior and posterior costal tubercles*, the *anterior costal bar*, and the *costal lamella*, all parts of the transverse process.These define the anterior and lateral borders of the characteristic *transverse foramen* of cervical vertebrae. In *lumbar vertebrae*, the costal element also forms the bulk of the transverse process (the "true" transverse process being represented by the *accessory processes*). In the *sacral vertebrae* the costal elements become incorporated into the *lateral masses* of the sacrum. The *coccygeal vertebrae* consist primarily of degenerate bodies and lack costal elements. The specific details of thoracic and lumbar vertebrae are discussed in the following sections.

Regional Osteology of the Thoracic and Lumbar Vertebral Column

Thoracic Vertebrae There are 12 *thoracic vertebrae* (Fig. 2–13). They are intermediate in size between the cervical and lumbar vertebrae. They are unique in that they articulate with the *ribs*. They are easily distinguished by the presence of *costal facets* on the sides of the bodies for articulation with the heads of the ribs, and facets on their transverse processes for articulation with the tubercles of the ribs. Some of the thoracic vertebrae bear complete, rounded *costal facets* (T1, T10–T12) by which a rib articulates with a single vertebral body. In most of the thoracic vertebrae (inferior portion of T1, T2–T8, superior portion of T9) each side of the body bears both a superior and inferior semicircular-shaped costal facet, called a *demifacet*. The *inferior demifacets* of the more cranial vertebrae combine with the *superior demifacets* of the adjacent caudal vertebrae to form a cuplike cavity that receives the head of the rib. The articulations between the heads of the ribs and the costal facets form the *costovertebral joints*. The *costotransverse joints* are formed by the articulation of the tubercles of the ribs with the transverse processes of the thoracic vertebrae.

The *bodies* of the thoracic vertebrae, in the midthoracic region, are heart shaped, and as broad anteroposteriorly as mediolaterally. The body is slightly thicker

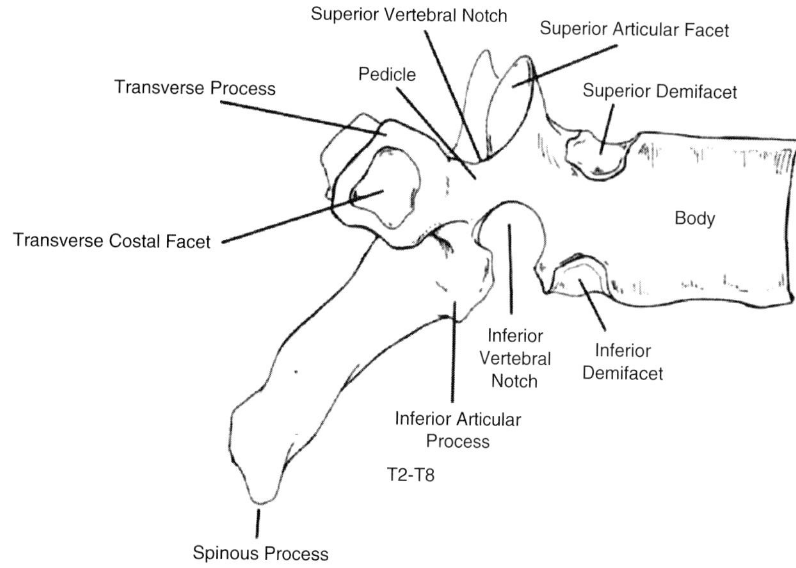

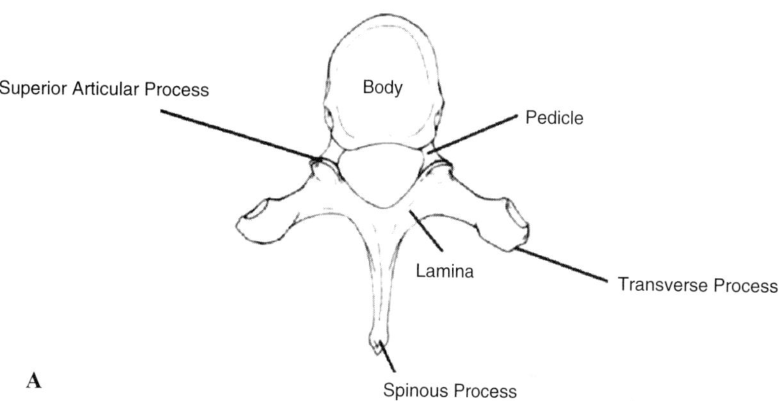

FIGURE 2–13. Thoracic vertebrae. *A.* Typical thoracic vertebrae (T2–T8), right lateral and superior views.

dorsally than ventrally, contributing to the thoracic curvature of the spine. *Superior demifacets* are located just anterior to the pedicles, while the *inferior demifacets* are located just anterior to the inferior vertebral notch. The *pedicles* are directed slightly cranially. The *superior vertebral notches* are very shallow and scarcely recognizable. The *inferior vertebral notches* are large, and deeper than in other regions of the spine. The *laminae* are broad and thick and, unlike other regions of the column, overlap those of the vertebrae below. The *vertebral foramen* is small and circular.

The *spinous processes* of thoracic vertebrae are long, and directed obliquely inferior. The thoracic spinous process ends in a single tubercle. In T1 and T2, the process is more horizontal, and the interspinous spaces are large. In T3 and T4, they are more oblique but the interspinous spaces are still large. The spinous processes of T5–T8 are very oblique and overlap to a greater extent than do the spinous processes of more cranial vertebrae and the interspinous spaces become smaller. The processes of T9 and T10 are oblique with small interspinous spaces, while those of T11 and T12, like those of the lumbar vertebrae, are horizontal.

The *superior articular processes* are thin and platelike, and project up from the junctions of the pedicles and laminae. The articular facets are practically flat and face dorsally and laterally. The *inferior articular processes* are fused to a considerable extent with the laminae, and project only slightly beyond the inferior border of the laminae. The articular facets are directed ventrally and medially, and are nearly vertical.

The *transverse processes* arise from the vertebral arch just posterior to the superior articular processes and pedicles. They are long, thick, and strong with an obliquely posterior and lateral direction. On the ventral surface of the lateral extremity of the transverse process is the *transverse costal facet*, which is the facet for articulation with the tubercle of the rib.

In general, the body of *first thoracic vertebra* will bear an entire costal facet for the first rib, and an inferior demifacet for the superior portion of the head of the second rib. The body of the first thoracic vertebra

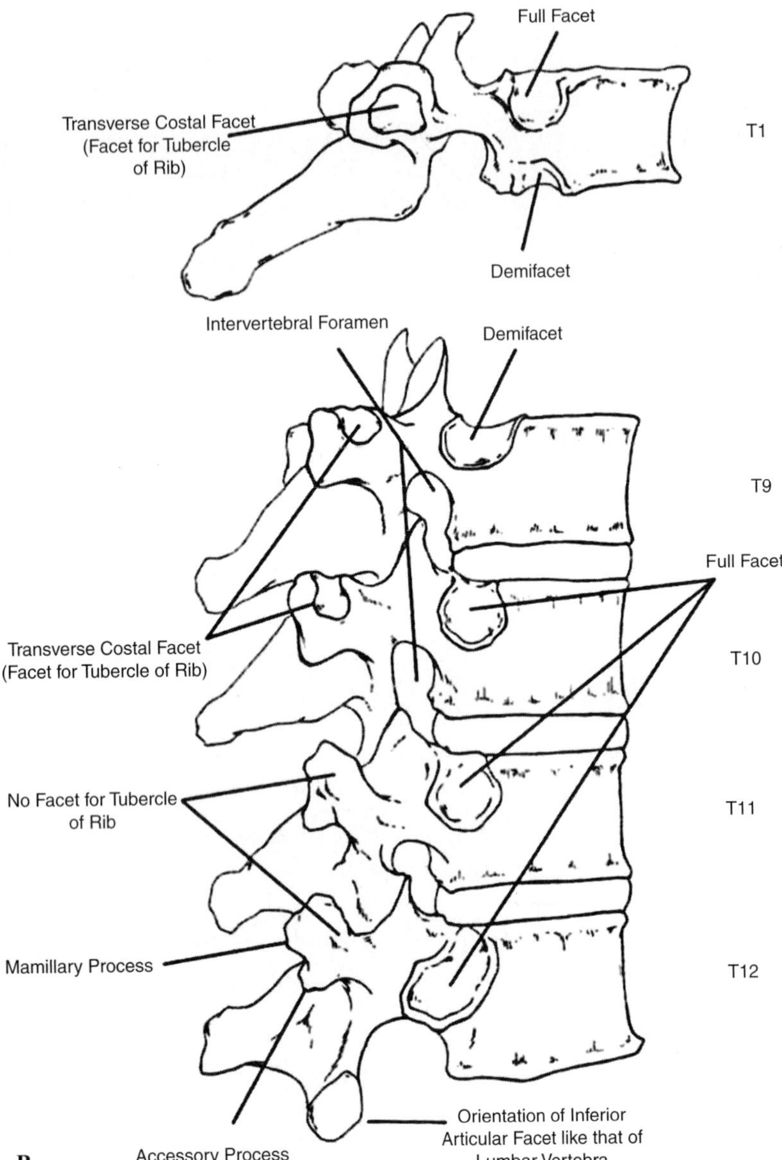

FIGURE 2–13. (Continued) *B.* Thoracic vertebrae with distinguishing characteristics (T1, T9–T12), right lateral view. (*After Walker et al.*[32])

is transversely broad, like a cervical vertebra. The spinous process is long, thick, and almost horizontal.

The *second through eighth thoracic vertebrae* are the most typical. They bear two demifacets on each side, a superior and an inferior.

The *ninth thoracic vertebra* usually bears only a superior demifacet and no inferior demifacet. In some persons, however, it may bear both a superior and a small inferior demifacet.

The *tenth thoracic vertebra* usually bears one large circular articular facet on each side, placed partly on the pedicle and partly on the body. In the case of the ninth thoracic vertebra bearing a small inferior demifacet, the tenth then bears one large demifacet on each side.

The *eleventh thoracic vertebra* approaches the lumbar vertebrae in size and form. It bears only a single costal facet on each side, which is large and placed upon the lateral aspect of the pedicle. The pedicles are thicker and stronger in the eleventh and twelfth thoracic vertebrae than in any other part of the column. In both the eleventh and twelfth thoracic vertebrae, *transverse processes* are short and *bear no transverse costal facets*.

The *twelfth thoracic vertebra* is very similar to the eleventh. It may be distinguished, however, by its inferior articular facets. They are convex and directed laterally like those of the lumbar vertebrae. As noted above, it bears no transverse costal facets on its transverse processes. In many ways, the twelfth thoracic vertebra is a transitional vertebra between the thoracic and lumbar regions, just as the first represented a transition between the cervical and thoracic regions. T12 will exhibit *accessory processes*, which are very

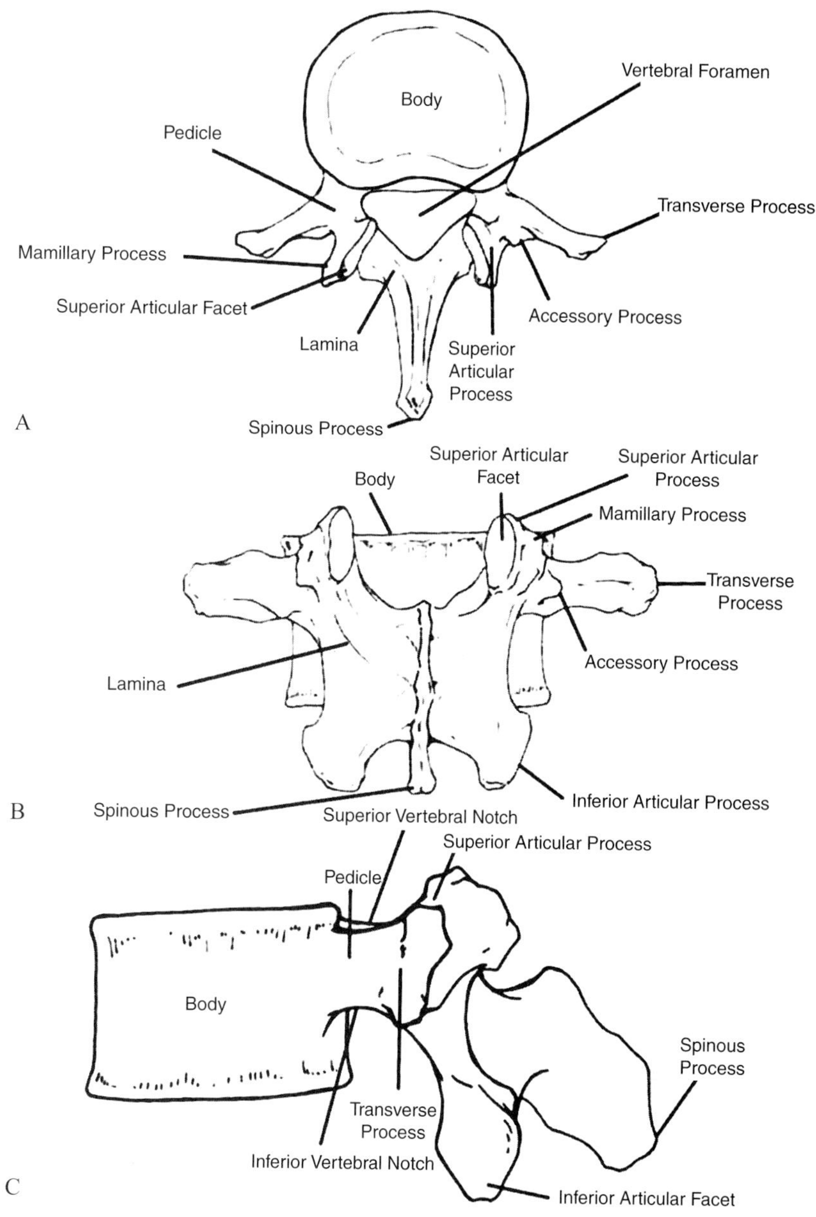

FIGURE 2–14. Lumbar vertebrae. *A.* Superior view. *B.* Posterior view. *C.* Left lateral view. (*After Walker et al.*[32])

small rough elevations on the inferolateral surfaces of the transverse processes. They are also found occasionally on T11 and T10. The *mamillary processes* are small round enlargements on the superior aspect of the transverse processes of T12 and possibly T11 and T10. Both accessory and mamillary processes are characteristic of lumbar vertebrae, though their locations are slightly different (probably because of the developmental origins of thoracic and lumbar transverse processes from transverse and costal elements, respectively).

The *intervertebral foramina* in the thoracic region have the following borders:

superior—inferior vertebral notch of cranial vertebra
inferior—superior vertebral notch of caudal vertebra
posterior—joint capsule of zygapophyseal joint
anterior—body of cranial vertebra, articular capsule of costovertebral joint

Lumbar Vertebrae (Fig. 2–14) There are normally five *lumbar vertebrae*. Aside from the fused upper sacral segments, the *lumbar vertebrae* are the largest vertebrae. They are characterized by *large bodies*, the presence of *mamillary processes* and *accessory processes*, and a *lack of transverse costal facets or transverse foramina*.

The *body* is large, wider transversely, and a little thicker ventrally. It is flattened or slightly concave superiorly and inferiorly. The sides of the body are concave. The *vertebral foramen* is triangular, but smaller than in the cervical region. The *transverse processes* are anterior to the articular processes (instead of posterior

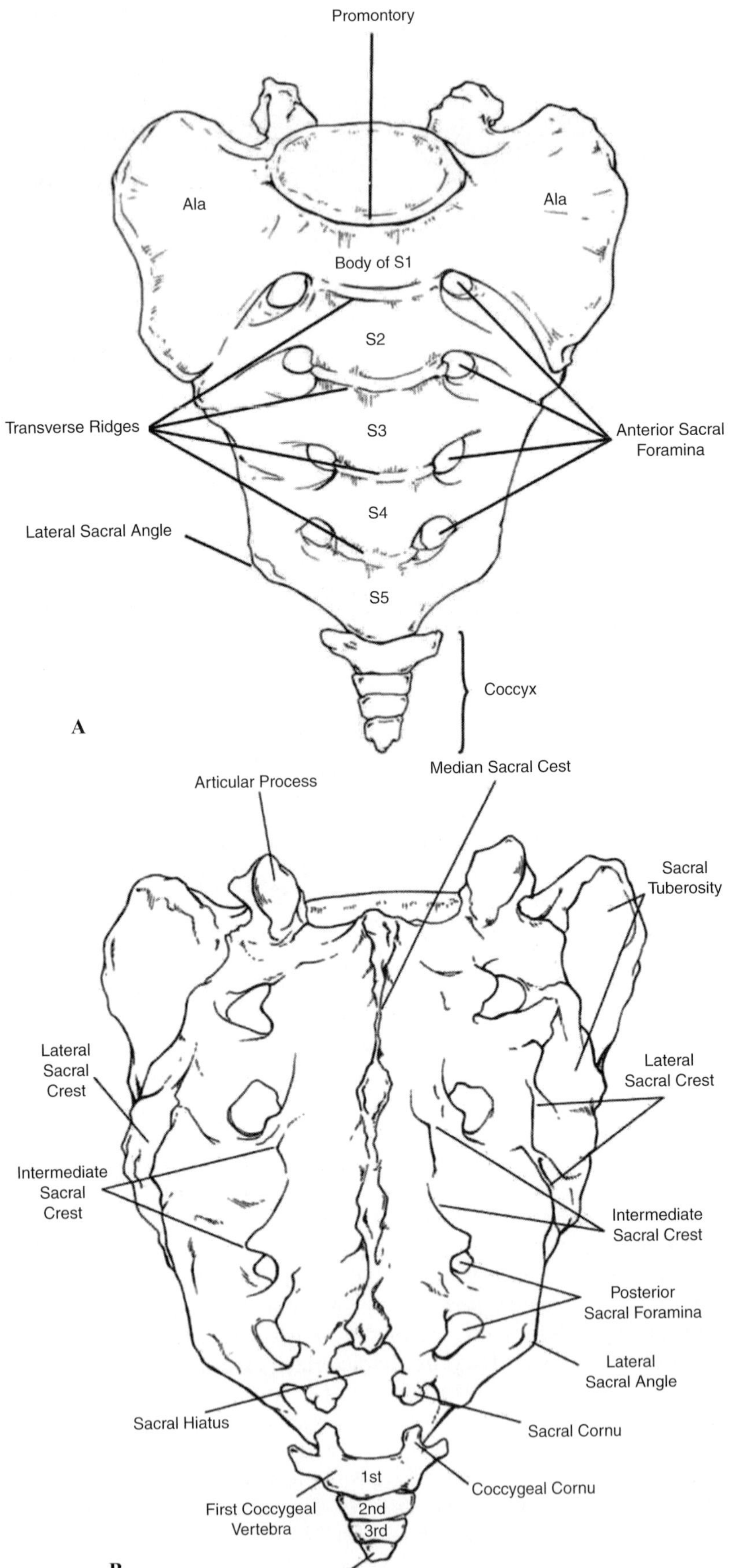

FIGURE 2–15. Sacrum and coccyx. *A.* Anterior view. *B.* Posterior view.

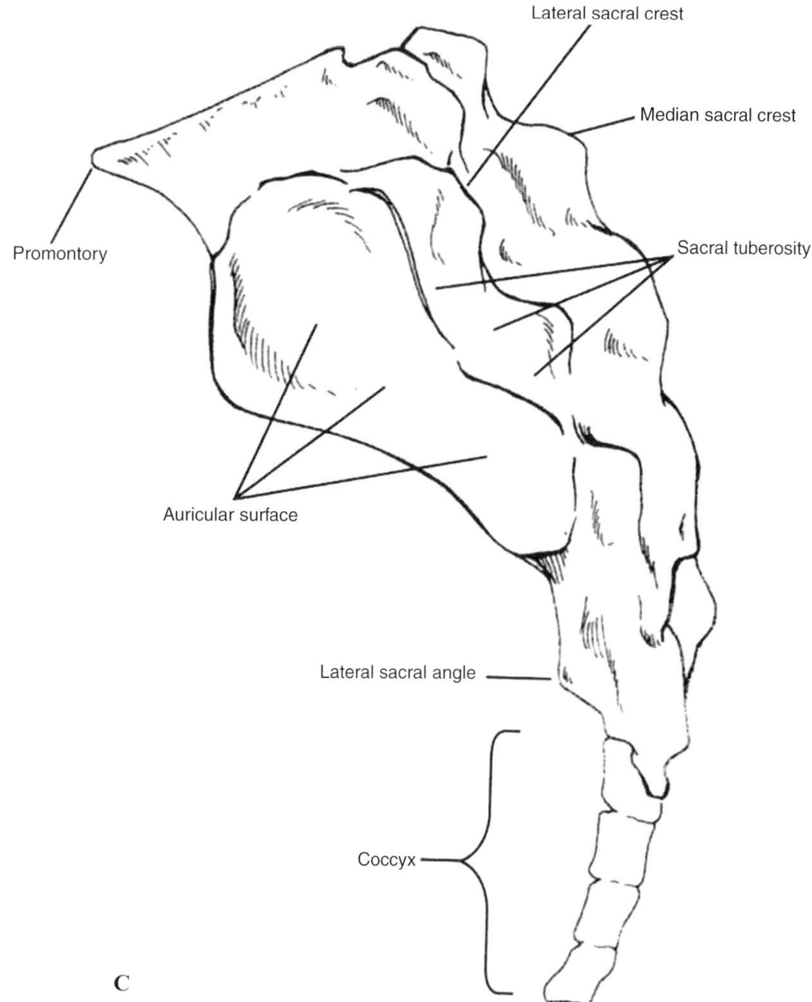

FIGURE 2–15. (Continued) *C*. Left lateral view.

to them as in the thoracic vertebrae) and posterior to the inferior vertebral notch. They are long, slender, and horizontal in the cranial three lumbars, while they incline a little caudally in the caudal two lumbars. The *accessory processes* are small, rough elevations on the dorsal surfaces at the bases of the transverse processes.

The *spinous process* is thick, broad, and quadrilateral in shape. It is thickest caudally. The spinous process of the *fifth* lumbar vertebrae is small for the lumbosacral angle.

The *superior articular processes* possess slightly concave, vertical facets which face medially and dorsally. On the posterolateral borders of the superior articular processes are found round enlargements, the *mamillary processes*. The *inferior articular processes* possess convex, vertical facets which face laterally and ventrally.

The *pedicles* unite with the cranial part of the body. As a result, the *inferior vertebral notches* are very deep, while the *superior vertebral notches* are shallow. The *laminae* are tall superoinferiorly, narrow mediolaterally, and robust.

The *intervertebral foramina* allow the passage of lumbar spinal nerves to exit the vertebral canal. In the lumbar region, the borders of the foramina are the following:

superior—inferior vertebral notch of cranial vertebrae
inferior—superior vertebral notch of caudal vertebrae
posterior—zygapophyseal joint capsule
anterior—bodies of cranial and caudal vertebrae and their intervertebral disc

Sacrum (Fig. 2–15) The *sacrum* is a large triangular mass formed by the fusion of five vertebrae. It forms the posterosuperior wall of the pelvic cavity, being wedged between the auricular surfaces of the two os coxae. It presents for examination of a *base*, a *pelvic* (ventral) *surface*, a *dorsal surface*, two *lateral surfaces*, and an *apex*. The base of the sacrum is superior and articulates with the fifth lumbar vertebrae, while its apex is inferior and articulates with the coccyx. Because the sacrum is formed by the fusion of five (on average) separate vertebrae, all the typical features of

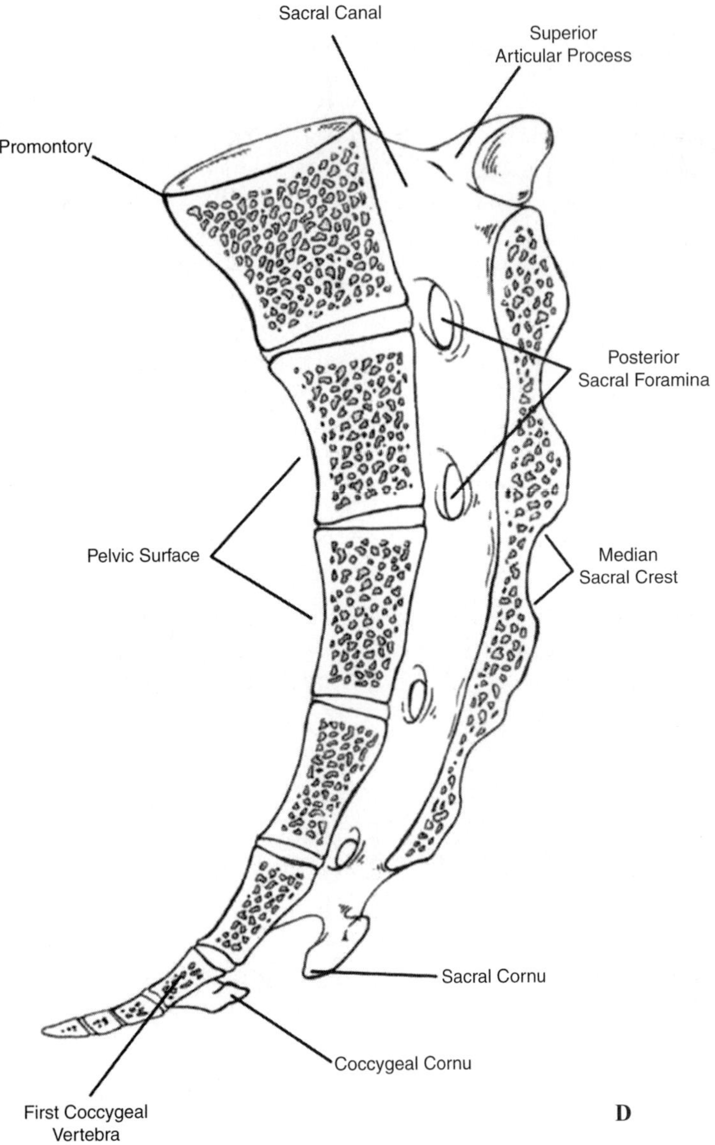

FIGURE 2–15. (Continued) *D.* Coronal section viewed from the left. (*After Walker et al.*[32])

a vertebra are present in the sacrum, though in modified form.

The *base* is the superior surface of the body of the first sacral vertebral segment. The base projects ventrally to form the lumbosacral angle. The *promontory* is the ventral border of superior surface of the body of S1. It is the most ventral portion of the sacrum and helps define the border of the pelvic inlet. The *sacral canal* is formed by the five vertebral foramina of the sacral vertebrae. The *ala* (Latin: "wings") are the lateral processes extending from the bodies of S1 and S2. They are formed by the fusion of the costal elements of the sacral vertebrae. They support the auricular surfaces. The *superior articular processes* of the sacrum articulate with the inferior articular facets of the fifth lumbar vertebra. The articular facets face dorsomedially.

The *pelvic surface* is concave in shape. It is characterized by four *transverse ridges*, which indicate the site of fusion of the five sacral vertebrae. Also on the pelvic surface are four pairs of *anterior sacral foramina*. They communicate with the sacral canal by means of the intervertebral foramina and allow the passage of the ventral rami of the first four sacral nerves, and the lateral sacral arteries and veins.

The *posterior (dorsal) surface* is convex and narrower than the pelvic surface. In the midline, the *median sacral crest* is surmounted by three or four tubercles, the rudimentary spinous processes of the first three or four sacral segments. The *sacral groove* is a shallow groove on either side of the median sacral crest. It is formed by the union of the laminae of the sacral vertebrae. The *sacral hiatus* is a defect in the floor of the sacral groove inferiorly. It is due to the nonfusion of the laminae of S5 with those of S4. On either side of the dorsal surface, on the lateral aspect of the sacral groove, is the *intermediate sacral crest*. It is a linear series of tubercles produced by the fusion of the articular processes of the sacral vertebrae. At the distal ends of the intermediate crests are the two *sacral cornu*. These are the inferior articular processes of S5 and articulate via ligaments with the coccyx. The *lateral sacral crest* is formed by the fusion of three or four transverse tubercles, which are rudimentary transverse processes of the sacral vertebrae. There are four *posterior sacral foramina* between the intermediate and lateral sacral crests. These allow the exit of the dorsal rami of the sacral spinal nerves from the sacral canal.

The *lateral surface* of the sacrum is dominated by the *auricular surface*. This surface articulates with the similarly shaped auricular surface of the ilium. The *sacral tuberosity* is the rough area between the auricular surface and the lateral sacral crest. It has deep impressions for the attachments of the interosseous sacroiliac ligaments. Caudal to the auricular surface the lateral surface is nonarticular. More caudally the lateral surface curves medially to the body of the fifth sacral vertebra at the *lateral sacral angle*.

The *apex* of the sacrum is its caudal end. It presents a *facet* for articulation with the coccyx. This is the inferior surface of the body of the fifth sacral vertebra.

In order to increase the size of the pelvic cavity for childbirth, the female sacrum is wider, relatively shorter, and its pelvic surface faces more caudally than in the male because of the specialized growth of the ilium that decreases the acuity of the greater sciatic notch.

Coccyx (Fig. 2–15) The *coccyx* is the most caudal portion of the vertebral column. It is formed by the fusion of (usually) four rudimentary vertebral bodies. As a rule, only the first coccygeal vertebra possesses rudiments of transverse processes and superior articular processes. These articular processes are termed the *cornu* of the coccyx. The coccyx is as a site of muscle attachment for the pelvic floor.

Ribs (Fig. 2–16) The *ribs* are elastic arches of bone, which, together with the thoracic vertebrae, the sternum, and the costal cartilages, form the skeleton of

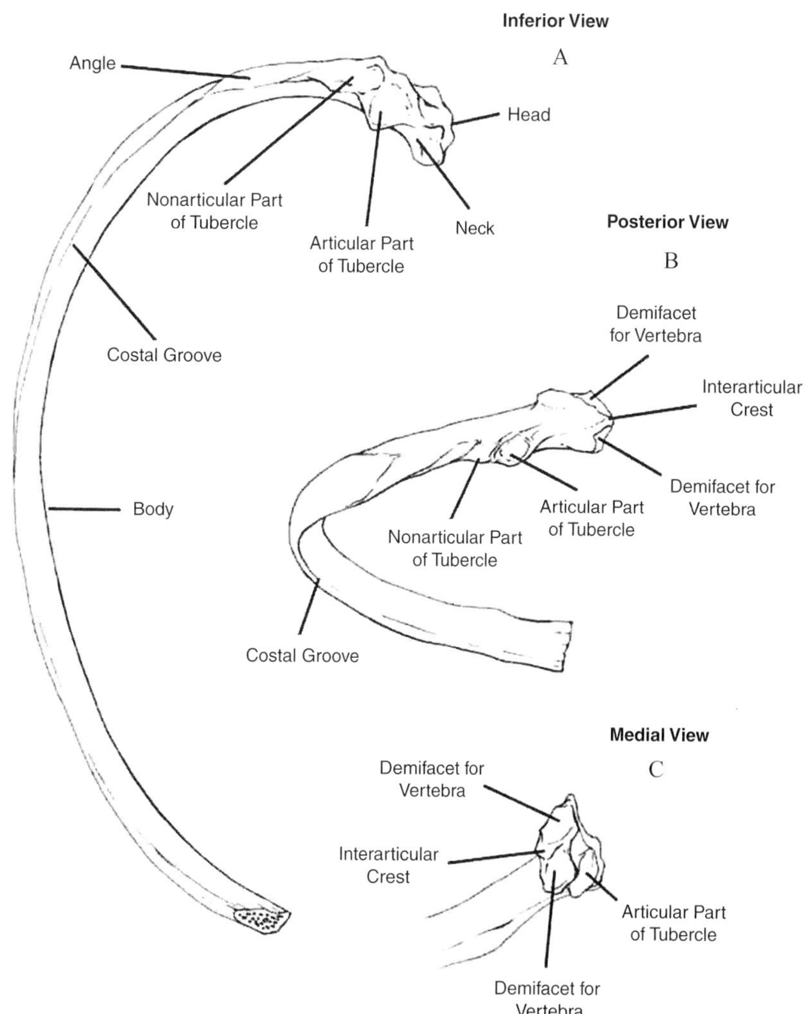

FIGURE 2–16. Osteology of a typical rib. *A.* Inferior view. *B.* Posterior view. *C.* Medial view. (*After Walker et al.*[32])

the thorax. There are 12 pairs of ribs. The first 7 pairs articulate posteriorly with the bodies and transverse processes of the thoracic vertebrae, and anteriorly, via their *costal cartilages*, with the sternum. The costal cartilages are composed of hyaline cartilage. Their dorsal ends articulate with the ventral extremities of ribs 1–10. Their ventral ends articulate either with the sternum (ribs 1–7), or with the costal cartilage of the rib above them (ribs 8–10). Ribs 1–7 are referred to as the *true* or *vertebrosternal ribs*. The remaining five pair are referred to as the *false ribs*. Pairs 8, 9, and 10 have their costal cartilages attaching to the costal cartilage of the rib above, and are also known as the *vertebrochondral ribs*. Pairs 11 and 12 are also known as the *floating ribs*. Their extremities are embedded in the musculature of the posterior thoracic wall. They are tipped with hyaline cartilage, but do not articulate with the sternum or other costal cartilages. Furthermore, unlike the cranial 10 pairs of ribs, the eleventh and twelfth pairs do not articulate with the transverse processes of their corresponding vertebrae.

The description that follows applies to the more typical *third through tenth ribs*. The first and second ribs and eleventh and twelfth ribs present features unique to them, which diverge from this common pattern.

Each rib has two extremities, a *dorsal or vertebral extremity* and a *ventral or sternal extremity*. The intervening portion of the rib is the *body or shaft*. The dorsal extremity bears a *head*, a *neck*, and a *tubercle*.

The *head* bears a kidney-shaped *articular facet* divided into superior and inferior *demifacets* by a horizontal *interarticular crest* (crest of the head). The superior portion of this articular facet is for articulation with the inferior demifacet of a thoracic vertebra, while the inferior portion is for articulation with the superior demifacet of the vertebra below. These *demifacets* on the heads of the ribs vary in their configurations in the same manner as the costal facets and demifacets of the thoracic vertebrae.

The *neck* is a flattened portion of the rib extending laterally from the head. The ventral surface of the neck is flat and smooth, while the dorsal surface is roughened for attachments of various ligaments. It has a cranial and a caudal border. The cranial border bears a rough *crest of the neck* for the attachment of the anterior layer of the superior costotransverse ligament. The caudal border is rounded.

The *tubercle* of the rib is a raised area on the posterior surface of the dorsal extremity at the junction of the neck and the body. It consists of an *articular portion* and a *nonarticular portion*. The *articular portion* is more caudal and medial, and bears a small oval facet for articulation with the transverse process of the more caudal of the two vertebrae with which the head articulates. The lateral *nonarticular portion* is roughened and receives the attachment of the lateral costotransverse ligament.

The *body* of the rib is thin and flat, and has two surfaces, an *external surface* and an *internal surface*. The body has a rounded *superior border* and a sharp *inferior border*. A little beyond the tubercle, the body is marked by a prominent line which gives attachment to a tendon of the iliocostalis muscle. This is the *angle* of the rib. At the angle of the rib, the shaft turns anteromedially. The distance between the tubercle and the angle progressively increases from the second to the tenth rib. Along the inferior margin of the internal surface of the rib is the *costal groove*. This groove is on the inferior border of the rib dorsally, but just ventral to the angle it comes to lie on the internal surface of the rib. The superior edge of the groove is rounded and gives attachment to the internal intercostal muscle. The inferior border of the groove, which is also the *inferior border of the body* of the rib, is sharp. The groove houses the intercostal nerve, artery, and vein. The *sternal extremity* of the body is flattened and presents a hollow oval which receives the rounded end of the costal cartilage.

The *first rib* is the most curved and the shortest. It has no angle and the body is flattened horizontally. Its cranial surface is marked by two grooves and the *scalene tubercle*. The *scalene tubercle* is toward the sternal extremity near the internal edge of the rib and is the site of attachment of the scalenus anterior muscle. It separates two grooves. The ventral groove is the *groove for the subclavian vein*, while the more dorsal groove is the *groove for the subclavian artery*. The head bears no interarticular crest, and so has only a single articular facet.

Near the middle of the external surface of the *second rib* is a rough *tuberosity for the serratus anterior*. While the serratus anterior attaches along the external surface of the first eight or nine ribs, its attachment to the second rib is particularly well-marked.

The *eleventh and twelfth ribs* are the floating ribs. Each has a single, large articular facet on the head, and no interarticular crest. They also have no neck or tubercle. The eleventh has a slight angle and a shallow costal groove, while the twelfth demonstrates neither.

The Sternum (Fig. 2–17) The *sternum* is composed of three parts: the *manubrium*, the *body* (or *gladiolus*), and the *xiphoid process*.

The *manubrium* is the most superior part of the sternum. At the center of its superior border is the *jugular (suprasternal) notch*. On either side of the jugular notches are the *clavicular notches*, which bear articular facets for articulations with the sternal ends of the clavicles.

The *body* is the largest portion of the sternum, and is composed of four sternebrae or segments that become fused in adulthood. The manubrium joins the body of the sternum at the *sternal angle* (Angle of

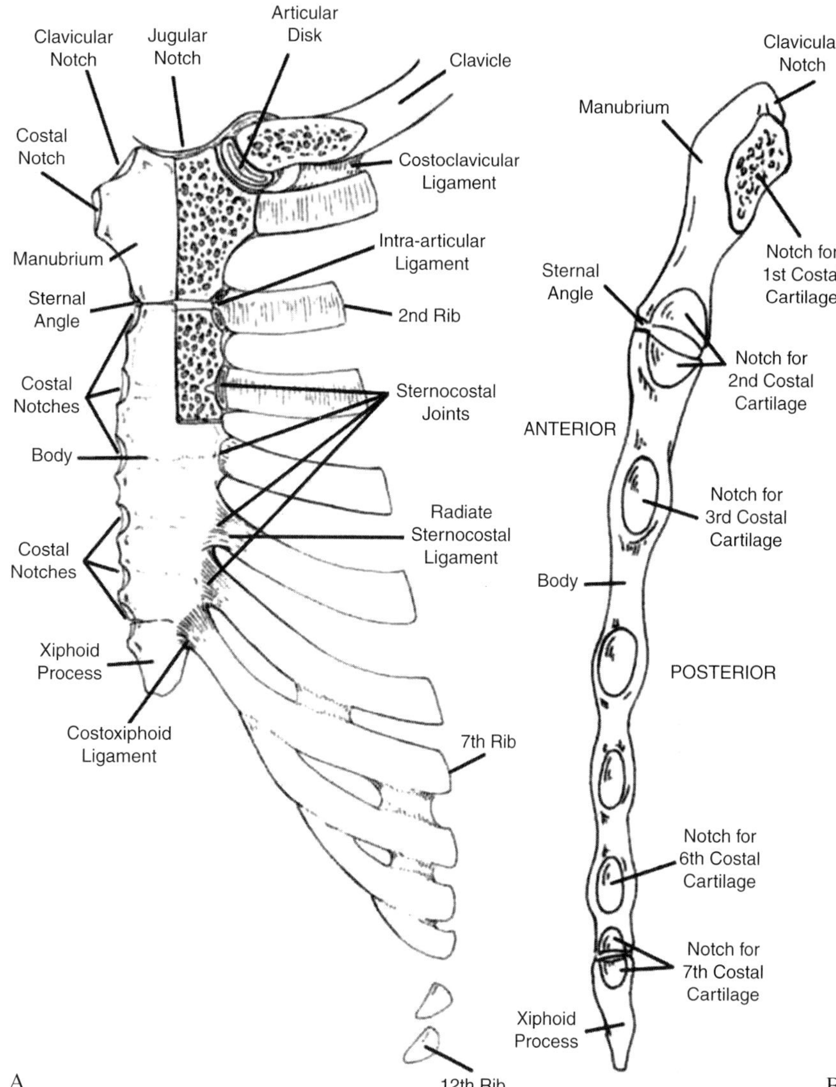

FIGURE 2–17. The sternum. *A.* Anterior view. *B.* Left lateral view. (*After Walker et al.*[32])

Louis), which is an important anatomical landmark. At the sternal angle, the *second costal cartilages* articulate with both the manubrium and the body. The costal cartilages are composed of hyaline cartilage and run between the sternum and the ventral extremities of the ribs. Since the second ribs lie at the level of the easily palpable sternal angle, the ribs can be counted with accuracy in the living subject. On either side of the sternum are seven *costal notches* for articulations with the costal cartilages. There is one complete notch and one half costal notch on either side of the manubrium. There are four complete notches and two half-notches on each side of the body. The xiphoid process also possesses a half-notch for the costal cartilage of the seventh rib on each side.

The most inferior and smallest segment of the sternum is the *xiphoid process*. It is thin and elongated. It is cartilaginous throughout youth, and progressively ossifies with age. It may remain partly cartilaginous, however, throughout life. It articulates with the body of the sternum at the *xiphisternal junction*. The costal cartilages of the seventh ribs articulate with the xiphoid process.

Os Coxae (Innominate or Hip Bone) (Fig. 2–18) The pelvic girdle attaches the lower limb to the axial skeleton. The pelvic girdle consists of the two *os coxae* and the *sacrum*. (The *os coxae* is better known by its trivial names *hip bone* or *innominate bone*. Its official name in the *Terminologica Anatomica* is *os coxae*, but innominate is commonly used.) The innominates articulate with the sacrum at the sacroiliac joint, and together they form the bony *pelvis*. Each innominate articulates with the lower limb at the hip joint.

In the adult, the *innominate* is present as a single, irregularly shaped bone. In the child, however, it consists of three separate bones, the *ischium*, the *ilium* and the *pubis*, which are united by a Y-shaped hyaline growth cartilage in a central depression called the *acetabulum* (the hemispherical socket for the femur). These three bones fuse to one another at adolescence. The upper bladelike bone is the *ilium*. At the

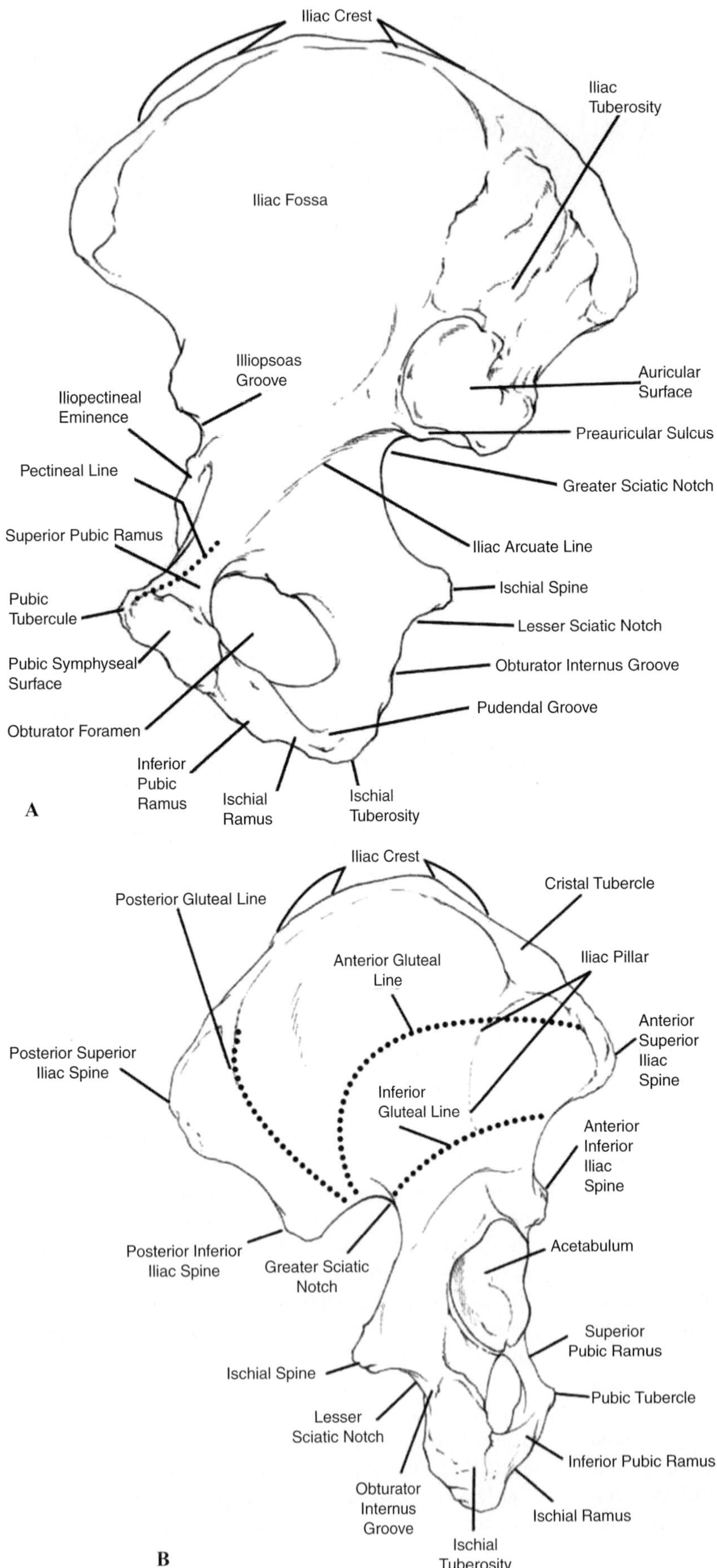

FIGURE 2–18. Os coxae (innominate or hip bone). *A.* Medial view of right innominate. *B.* Lateral view of right innominate.

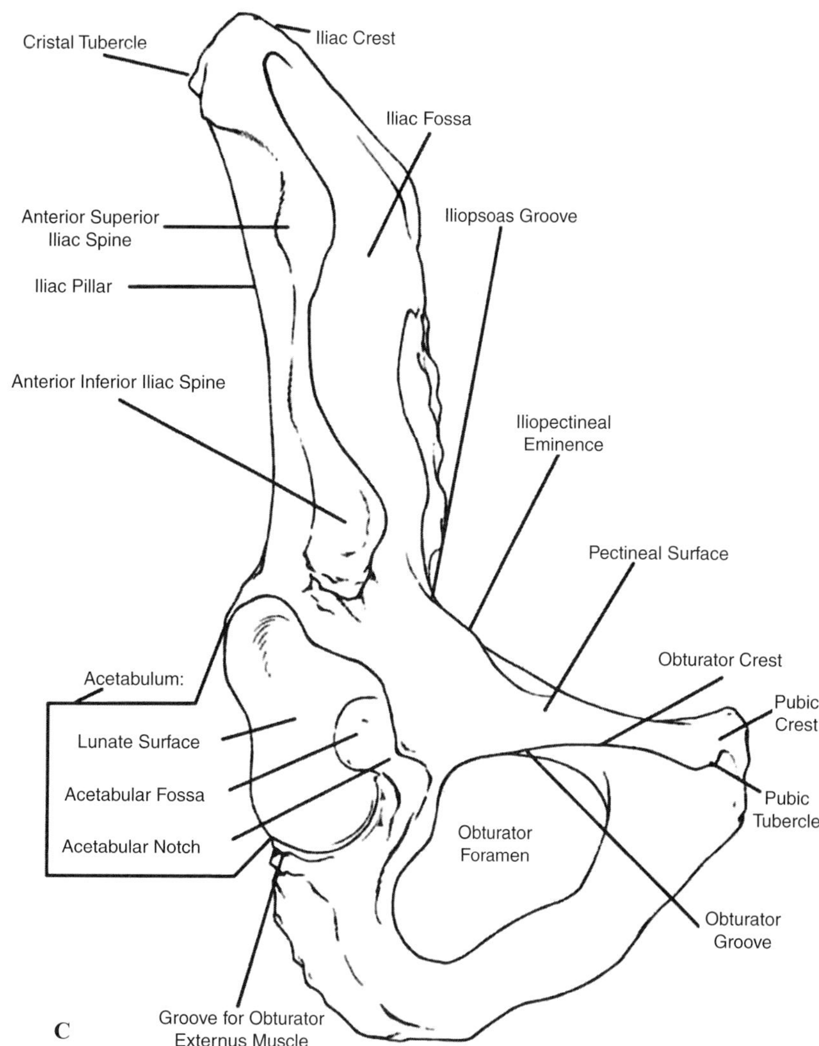

FIGURE 2–18. (Continued) *C*. Anterior view of right innominate. (*After Walker et al.*[32])

acetabulum (Latin: "vinegar cup"; the hemispherical socket for the femur) it is fused to the *pubis* anteriorly and the *ischium* inferiorly. The two innominates are joined to the sacrum at the bilateral *sacroiliac joints,* and to each other at the anterior *pubic symphysis*.

Much of the internal surface of the ilium is taken up by the *iliac fossa,* from which the iliacus muscle originates. The blade itself is surmounted by the *iliac crest,* which is formed by a separate *apophysis* during development. (An *apophysis* is a secondary center of ossification forming under a muscle attachment, also known as a *traction epiphysis*.) The iliac crest serves as attachment for the internal and external oblique and transversus abdominis muscles of the abdominal wall. Its anteriormost projection is the *anterior superior iliac spine,* which provides attachment for the sartorius muscle. Inferior to this is the *anterior inferior iliac spine,* which is also formed from a separate apophysis. The upper portion of the anterior inferior iliac spine gives origin to the straight head of the rectus femoris muscle. A teardrop-shaped lower portion (with the point of the teardrop pointed posteriorward) gives origin to the iliofemoral ligament and directly abuts the rim of the acetabulum. The second head of the rectus femoris muscle arises from a small depression a few millimeters above the acetabular rim more posteriorly. Just anteromedial and inferior to the anterior inferior iliac spine is the *iliopsoas groove,* which provides passage for the iliopsoas muscle as it passes over the femoral head to its insertion on the lesser trochanter of the femur. The medial wall of this groove is sometimes formed by the bossing (swelling), which results from the fusion point of the ilium and the pubis. This is called the *iliopectineal (iliopubic) eminence*. There is a sharp border between the iliac blade bearing the origin of the iliacus and its more inferior portion which forms the true pelvis. This sharp border is called the *iliac arcuate line*. It junctures the *auricular surface* at its apex. Just inferior to the auricular surface is the *preauricular sulcus* (also known as the *paraglenoid sulcus*). This groove is more common and better developed in females than in males. Its origin and function are controversial, but may be related to changes in adjacent ligaments induced by hormones associated with pregnancy and/or childbirth. Between the auricular surface and the iliac crest is a very rugose (roughened) region called the *iliac tuberosity*. This tuberosity is for the attachment of the *interosseous sacroiliac ligament*.

The *exterior surface of the ilium* gives rise to two important muscles of gait, the gluteus medius and the minimus. The minimus occupies the anterior portion, with its attachment outlined by the anteriormost extent of the ilium, the anterior iliac crest, and a line that originates from the iliac crest and passes posteroinferiorly toward the greater sciatic notch (see below). This is the *anterior gluteal line*. The medius is attached posterior to the anterior gluteal line from an almost circular area outlined by the crest and a second line, the posterior gluteal line. The *posterior gluteal line* is a short continuation of the iliac crest toward the *greater sciatic notch*. The posterior terminus of the iliac crest is the *posterior superior iliac spine*. Note that the posterior gluteal line and posterior part of the crest (anterior from the posterior superior spine for a distance about 1–2 in) forms a rugose triangular area. To this area is attached a portion of the gluteus maximus muscle (the bulk of its origin is from the sacrum). A vague line may run from the *anterior inferior iliac spine* to the greater sciatic notch delineating the inferior extent of the gluteus minimus origin. This is the *inferior gluteal line*. Also note that the iliac blade is bent back relative to the massive portion of the innominate which houses the acetabulum. The ilium's inferior surface thus forms the *greater sciatic notch*, which is shaped in males very much like an inverted fishhook, and in females very much like a boomerang. That is, the walls of the notch are much more divergent from one another in females than in males. The posterior terminus of this notch is the *posterior inferior iliac spine*. The anterior terminus of the notch is actually located on the ischium and is called the *ischial spine*.

In external view the ilium will display a distinct thickening of its body about one third the distance from the anterior superior iliac spine to the posterior superior iliac spine. This thickened region runs from the iliac crest to the acetabular lip. It is called the *iliac pillar*. At the juncture of the pillar with the crest, there is a thickening of the latter called the *cristal tubercle*. The pillar is crossed by the anterior gluteal line.

The lower portion of the acetabulum is formed by the *corpus* or *body* of the *ischium*. From this a large *ischial ramus* projects anteriorly and joins the inferior ramus of the pubis. The inferior portion of the corpus is surmounted by a large rugose region, called the *ischial tuberosity*. The tuberosity is formed by the posterior terminus of a separate apophysis which surmounts the length of the ischiopubic ramus. The ischial tuberosity's surface is highly rugose and faceted. These facets are for the origin of the so-called hamstring muscles. The superiormost facet gives origin to the semimembranosus muscle. The next facet is for the biceps femoris muscle, and the most inferior is for the origin of the semitendinosus muscle. These three muscles arise from the more vertical portion of the tuberosity, before it becomes sharply angled to provide a horizontal surface for the attachment of the adductor magnus muscle. There is a distinct groove between the ischial tuberosity and the remaining surface of the ischium on its internal surface. This is the *pudendal groove* for the pudendal nerve and the internal pudendal vessels. Between the ischial tuberosity and the *ischial spine* is a second involution of the lesser pelvis, called the *lesser sciatic notch*. A groove may be occasionally palpated just inferior to the ischial spine for the obturator internus muscle: the *obturator internus groove*. A second groove is formed by the anterosuperior edge of the ischial tuberosity and the lower lip of the acetabulum. This is the *obturator externus groove*. The pubis and ischium together surround a large opening called the *obturator foramen*. It is closed by a membrane during life. Its outer surface gives attachment to the obturator externus muscle, while its internal surface gives attachment to the obturator internus muscle.

The *pubis* is formed of two separate portions called *rami* (the *superior and inferior rami*) and a central portion which provides the attachment to the two rami and to the pubic symphysis called the *corpus* or *body*. The arcuate line of the ilium is continuous onto the superior ramus of the pubis, and may be followed anteriorly to a large anterior projection called the *pubic tubercle*. The continuation of the *iliac arcuate line* on the pubis is called the *pectineal line* (or the *pecten*). The *iliac arcuate line* and the *pectineal line* together form the *linea terminalis*. The *pectineal line* together with the *iliac arcuate line* and the *sacral promontory* form the brim of the lesser or "true" pelvis, which is the area inferior to this brim. Medial to the pubic tubercle is the *pubic crest*. The surface of the superior ramus just anterior to the pectineal line is called the *pectineal surface*. A second ridge or line runs from the pubic tubercle to the acetabular rim. This is the *obturator crest*. It gives attachment to the pubofemoral ligament. The *inferior ramus of the pubis* joins the *ramus of the ischium*. It gives origin to the three adductor muscles of the thigh. At the apex of the obturator foramen on the inferior and posterior aspect of the superior ramus of the pubis is the *obturator groove* for the passage of the obturator nerve and vessels. In life this is converted into the obturator canal by the obturator membrane.

The *acetabulum* bears a *lunate* (*articular*) *surface*, an *acetabular notch*, a *rim*, and a central nonarticular portion, the *acetabular fossa*. The acetabulum is traditionally described as being composed of 2/5 ilium, 2/5 ischium, and 1/5 pubis. In life, a fibrocartilaginous labrum attaches to and deepens the acetabular rim. The acetabular notch is a gap in the acetabular rim and is actually closed in life by the *transverse acetabular ligament*. Additionally, a small ligament of the head of the femur runs from this transverse acetabular ligament to the fovea capitis, a small depression in the center of the head of the femur.

JOINTS/LIGAMENTS, BARRIER CONCEPT, END-FEEL

The Anterior Longitudinal Ligament (Fig. 2–19)

The *anterior longitudinal ligament* is a strong band of fibers forming a syndesmosis which extends along the anterior surface of the bodies of the vertebrae from the occiput to the sacrum. This ligament is specialized in the region of the atlas and axis. From its lateral aspects, fibers spread out to form the anterior atlantoaxial ligament between the atlas and axis and anterior atlantooccipital membrane between the atlas and occipital. Its morphology is more typical in lower cervical vertebrae and the rest of the column. It is thicker in the thoracic than in the lumbar or cervical regions. It is somewhat thicker as well over the vertebral bodies than over the intervertebral discs. It attaches to the basilar portion of the occipital bone, the anterior tubercle of the atlas, the body of the axis, the prominent margins of the vertebral bodies and intervertebral discs of the vertebrae down to the superior part of the anterior surface of the sacrum. In the cervical area it is thin and narrow, and in general it is *narrow cranially and wider caudally*.

The anterior longitudinal ligament is composed of superficial, intermediate, and deep fibers. The superficial fibers are the longest and extend over four to five vertebrae. Intermediate fibers extend two to three vertebral levels, while the deep fibers are shorter, crossing only between adjacent vertebrae. In addition to its mechanical function, morphological studies have found nerve supply to confirm proprioceptive function assisting in posture, movement, muscle tone and reflexes.[33,34,35] The anterior longitudinal ligament in summary functions to limit extension of the spinal column, in addition to providing important proprioceptive information.

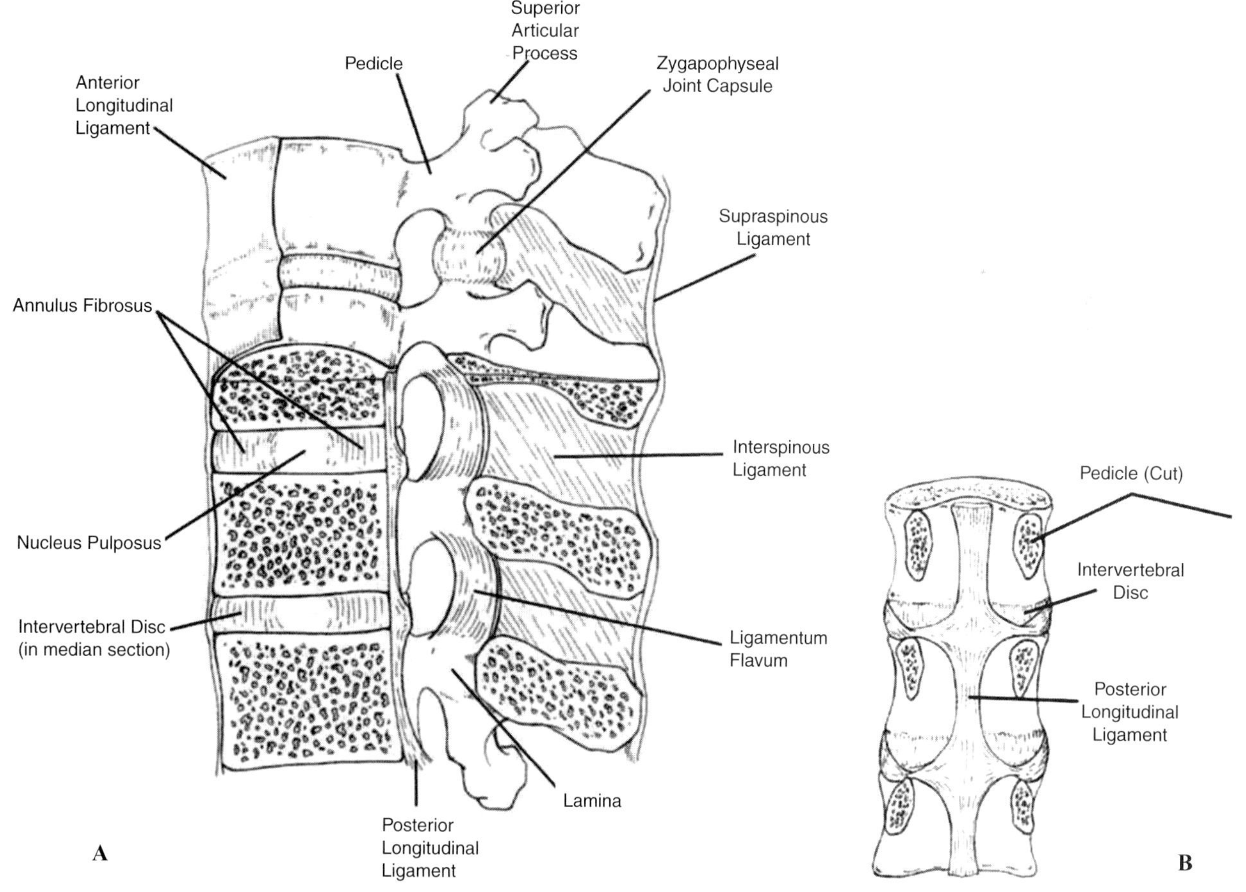

FIGURE 2–19. Anterior and posterior longitudinal ligaments, intervertebral syndesmoses, supraspinous ligament. *A.* Left lateral view in partial coronal section, lumbar region. *B.* Posterior view of lumbar column demonstrating the posterior longitudinal ligament. (*After Walker et al.*[32])

Clinical Pearl: The anterior longitudinal ligament, in summary, functions to *limit extension* of the vertebral column, in addition to providing important proprioceptive information.

The Posterior Longitudinal Ligament

The *posterior longitudinal ligament* forms another vertebral syndesmosis and attaches to the dorsal surfaces of the bodies of the vertebrae within the vertebral canal. The portion of the posterior longitudinal ligament superior to the axis is specialized as the *tectorial membrane*. The posterior longitudinal ligament extends from the axis to the sacrum and lies within the sacral canal. It consists of superficial and deep layers of fibers. The superficial fibers cross three to four vertebrae, while the deep fibers run between adjacent vertebral bodies. This ligament is not firmly attached to vertebral bodies, because the basivertebral veins and the vertebral venous plexus are situated between it and the vertebral bodies. The posterior longitudinal ligament is *broad cranially and narrow caudally*. In the lower thoracic region and lumbar region it is denticulated, being broad over the intervertebral discs and narrow over the vertebral bodies and to provide important propriceptive information.[33,34,35]

Clinical Pearl: The posterior longitudinal ligament, in summary, functions to limit flexion of the vertebral column and to provide vital proprioceptive input.

The synovial joints between articular processes of the vertebrae are of the plane synovial type, and are known as *zygapophyseal joints*. They are also referred to as *posterior joints, facet joints, apophyseal joints*, and most recently *z-joints* as a short form to zygapophyseal joints. The term *zygapohpyseal* has is roots from two Greek words—*zygos*, meaning bridge or yoke, and *apophysis*, which means outgrowth. The *articular capsules* of the zygapophyseal joints surround the margins of the articular processes. The fibrous articular capsules are thin and loose, and longer and looser in the cervical region than elsewhere. The size, shape, and movements of the zygapophyseal joints vary from vertebral level to vertebral level. These joints may contain fat pads or fibroadipose menisci (articular discs), especially in the lumbar region. They are innervated by medial branches of dorsal rami of spinal nerves, both the ascending branch of the dorsal ramus below and the descending branch of the dorsal ramus above the joint.

Clinical Pearl: The synovial joints between articular processes of the vertebrae are of the plane synovial type, and are known as *zygapophyseal joints*. They are also referred to as *posterior joints, facet joints, apophyseal joints*, and most recently *z-joints* as a short form to zygapophyseal joints.

An important clinical element that continues to be questioned and debated by both researchers and clinicians is whether the *zygapophyseal joint* and capsule may be a source of idiopathic low back pain. Berven and his group underscore the importance of the *zygapophyseal joints* as important structural components that contribute to the stability of the lumbar motion segments. They allude to the *zygapophyseal joints* as a significant cause of low back pain.[36] A Japanese study looked at the distribution of referred pain from lumbar *zygapophyseal joints* (L1/L2 to L5/S1) and the medial branches of the lumbar dorsal rami (Th 12 to L5) in patients with chronic low back pain. The study group included patients with chronic low back pain undergoing either *zygapophyseal joints* joint injection or radiofrequency facet denervation. A total of 71 joints and 91 medial branches were studied in 48 subjects. The distribution of referred pain from the L1/L2 to L5/S1 *zygapophyseal joints*, and the medial branches of the dorsal rami from L1 to L5 were similar for each level stimulated. The overlap of referred pain between each level was considerable.[37]

A study done on white rabbits showed that *zygapophyseal joints* contain group-III and group-IV mechanosensitive units with low to high thresholds. Several units responded to movement of the joint. Units with high threshold and slow conduction velocity may serve as nociceptors. Units with lower thresholds may serve as proprioceptors (more on propioception at the end of this chapter). The high-threshold group-III units neurophysiological charactersitics suggest that the *zygapophyseal joints* may be a source of low back pain.[38]

The vertebral arches are also connected to one another by the following ligaments:

Supraspinous ligament
Ligamentum nuchae
Interspinous ligament
Intertransverse ligament
Ligamentum flavum (plural: ligamenta flava)

The latter three ligaments (interspinous ligament, intertransverse ligament, and ligamentum flavum) constitute the *intervertebral syndesmosis*.

Intervertebral (Segmental) Syndesmoses (Fig. 2–19)

Ligamenta Flava: Segmental Syndesmosis The *ligamenta flava* (Singular: *ligamentum flavum*) connect the laminae of adjacent vertebrae from the axis to the first segment of the sacrum. It is specialized as the *posterior atlantoaxial ligament or membrane* between the posterior arch of the atlas and the laminae of the axis, and the *posterior atlantooccipital membrane* between the posterior arch of the atlas and the posterior margin of the foramen magnum. They consist of two lateral portions which begin posterior to the articular processes and extend posteriorly to the point where the laminae meet to form the spinous process. They are composed primarily of yellow elastic tissue (flavum; Latin: "yellow"). In the *cervical region* the ligamenta flava are thin, but broad and long. They are thickest in the *lumbar region*, and of intermediate thickness in the *thoracic region*. There is one pair between adjacent vertebrae, and they run from the anterior and inferior surface of the more superior lamina to the posterior and superior surface of the more inferior lamina. They function to brake the separation of the laminae in flexion of the vertebral column. Elastin fibers permit them to stretch and regain their shapes.

Interspinous Ligaments: Segmental Syndesmoses The *interspinous ligaments* are thin and membranous and connect adjoining spinous processes and extend from the root to the apex of each process. The interspinous ligaments function to limit flexion of the vertebral column. They meet the *ligamenta flava* ventrally and the supraspinous ligament dorsally. They are narrow and elongated in the thoracic region and thicker and quadrilateral in the lumbar region. In the cervical region, they are incorporated into the ligamentum nuchae.

Intertransverse Ligaments: Segmental Syndesmoses The *intertransverse ligaments* connect the transverse processes of adjacent vertebrae, and function to limit lateral flexion of the vertebral column. In the cervical region they are represented by only a few irregular fibers, and are largely replaced by the intertransverse muscles. In the thoracic region they are well-developed cords that are blended intimately with adjacent muscles, while in the lumbar region they are thin and membranous.

Supraspinous Ligament (Fig. 2–19) Continuous sydesmoses of the lumbar and thoracic spine include the anterior and posterior longitudinal ligaments (previously described) and the supraspinous ligament. The *supraspinous ligament* is a strong fibrous cord that connects the apices of the spinous processes from the seventh cervical vertebra to the sacrum. It has superficial, intermediate, and deep fibers. The superficial fibers span three to four vertebrae, the intermediate span two to three, and the deep run between adjacent vertebrae. It is thicker and broader in the lumbar region than in the thoracic, where it is relatively thin. In the cervical region above C7 the supraspinous and interspinous ligaments are specialized as the *ligamentum nuchae.*

Iliolumbar Ligament (Fig. 2–20) There are certain ligaments that have been implicated in the cause of low

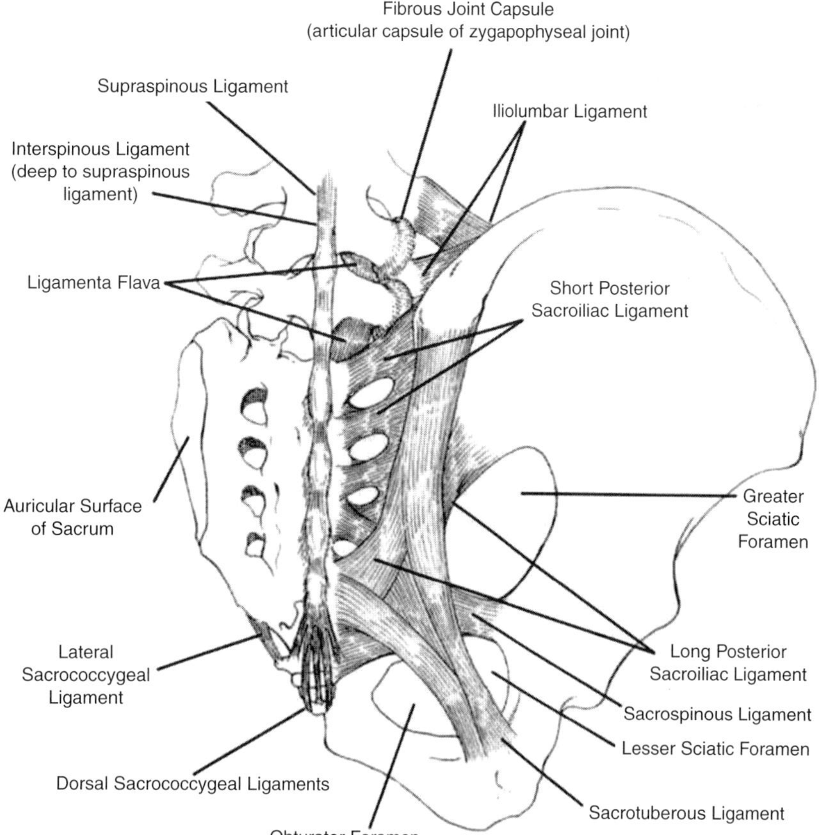

FIGURE 2–20. Iliolumbar ligament, long dorsal sacroiliac ligament, lumbosacral joint, sacroiliac joint, sacrococcygeal joint, ligaments connecting the sacrum and ischium, posterior view. (*After Walker et al.*[32])

back pain. The *iliolumbar ligament* is referred to as the most important ligament for restraining movement at the lumbosacral junction. Some authors state that it may play a key role in restraining movement in the sacroiliac joints. This ligament is oriented in the coronal plane, perpendicular to the sacroiliac joint.[39] One study assessed whether the *iliolumbar ligament* is able to restrict sacroiliac joint mobility in embalmed cadavers. Cutting both iliolumbar ligaments produced significantly increased sacroiliac joint mobility.[40]

Questions arise regarding whether low back pain is at times due to injury to the iliolumbar ligaments. As one of three pelvic-lumbar ligaments (including *sacrotuberous* and *sacrospinous ligaments*), it develops about the twelfth week of gestation. What is apparent is that this ligament is a major stabilizing factor between the vertebral spine and the pelvis and that its innervation is similar to the posterior lumbar ligaments. One interesting observation is that this ligament is present only in animals that assume an erect posture.[41] One theory espouses that microtrauma to the iliolumbar ligaments is the primary cause of chronic low back pain[41] because of the following:

- The iliolumbar ligament as a stabilizer is the weakest component of the "multifidus triangle." The multifidus triangle (now an outdated term) is created by the ilium and its articulations with the pelvis, the sacrum and its articulations with the fifth lumbar vertebra, and the attachment of the fifth lumbar vertebra back to this ilium via the iliolumbar ligament.
- The iliolumbar ligament increases susceptibility to injury due to angulated attachments.
- The iliolumbar ligament being a primary inhibitor of excess sacral flexion.
- The iliolumbar ligament being a highly innervated nociceptive tissue.
- The iliolumbar ligament plays an increased role in disc degeneration.

Clinical Pearl: One interesting observation is that the iliolumbar ligament is present only in animals that assume an erect posture.

The Long Dorsal Sacroiliac Ligament (Fig. 2–20) The *long dorsal sacroiliac ligament* is easily palpated in the area caudal to the posterior superior iliac spine. One dissection study of the sacral and lumbar regions showed that the long dorsal sacroiliac ligament is closely related anatomically with the erector spinae muscle, the posterior layer of the thoracolumbar fascia, and a specific part of the sacrotuberous ligament. The sacrotuberous ligament was also found to be contiguous with fibers of the ipsilateral biceps femoris. It appears to be an important link between legs, spine, and arms. The long dorsal sacroiliac ligament should not be neglected when diagnosing patients with low back pain or peripartum pelvic pain.[42]

Intervertebral Disc (Fig. 2–21) The *intervertebral discs* constitute a specific type of synarthrodial joint, a *symphysis*. They adhere to the superior and inferior surfaces of the adjacent vertebrae by thin layers of hyaline cartilage called *vertebral end plates*, which are considered to be an integral part of the disc. Each disc consists of *the vertebral end plates*, an outer laminated *annulus fibrosus*, and an inner *nucleus pulposus*. The annulus fibrosus is fibrocartilage, while the nucleus pulposus (better developed in cervical and lumbar regions) is made up, at birth, of soft, gelatinous mucoid material and a few multinucleated notochordal cells. Notochordal cells disappear in the first decade of life, and the substance of the nucleus pulposus is replaced gradually by fibrocartilage. Thus with maturity the nucleus pulposus becomes less distinct from the rest of the disc.

Intervertebral discs are present between vertebral bodies from C2 to the sacrum, and a rudimentary disc is present between S5 and C×1. They are generally thicker anteriorly than posteriorly in the cervical and lumbar regions, which creates the *spinal curvatures* in these regions. The intervertebral discs are nearly flat in the thoracic spine. They are thinnest in the upper thoracic spine, and thickest in the lumbar spine. The outer *annulus fibrosus* has a narrow outer collagenous zone, and a wider, inner fibrocartilaginous zone. The annulus fibrosus consists of a number of laminae, with fibers of adjacent laminae set obliquely to one another, and at a 30 degree angle relative to the horizontal (see Fig. 6–1). The oblique arrangement of fibers in adjacent laminae in the lumbar region imparts great torsional strength to disc. Additionally, the outer laminae bulge externally, while the inner laminae bulge internally toward the nucleus pulposus. The annulus fibrosus is thickest anteriorly and thinnest posteriorly. The functions of the annulus fibrosus are to enclose and retain the nucleus pulposus, absorb compressive shocks, form a structural unit between vertebral bodies, and allow restricted motion between adjacent vertebral segments.

The inner *nucleus pulposus* accounts for 40% of the bulk of the disc. The nucleus pulposus contains the remains of the notochord and has a high water content. Notochordal cells disappear during the first decade of life, and are replaced eventually by fibrocartilage. The nucleus pulposus is relatively larger at birth, but decreases in relative size as they dehydrate with age. The nucleus pulposus is better developed in the cervical and lumbar regions than in the thoracic region, and lies nearer the posterior part of the disc than the anterior. Functions of the nucleus pulposus are to provide a resilient spacer allowing motion between

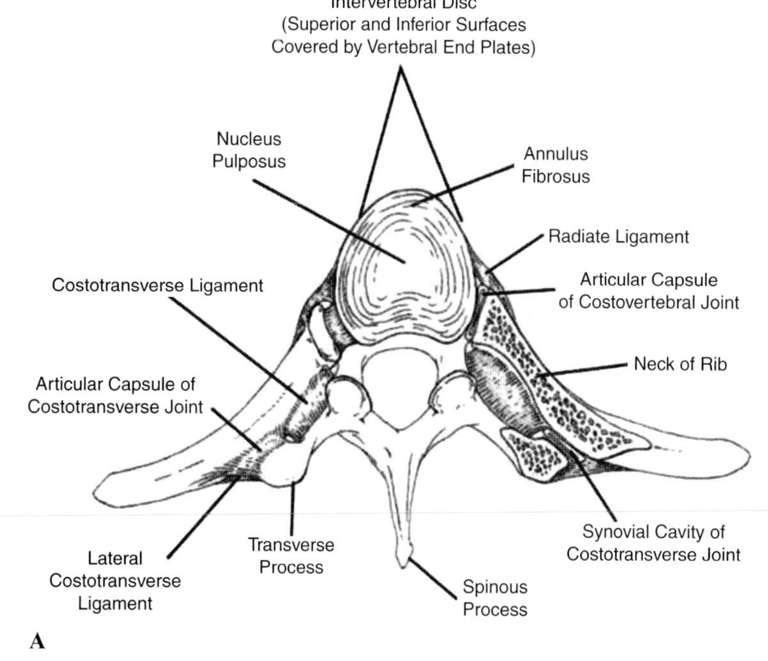

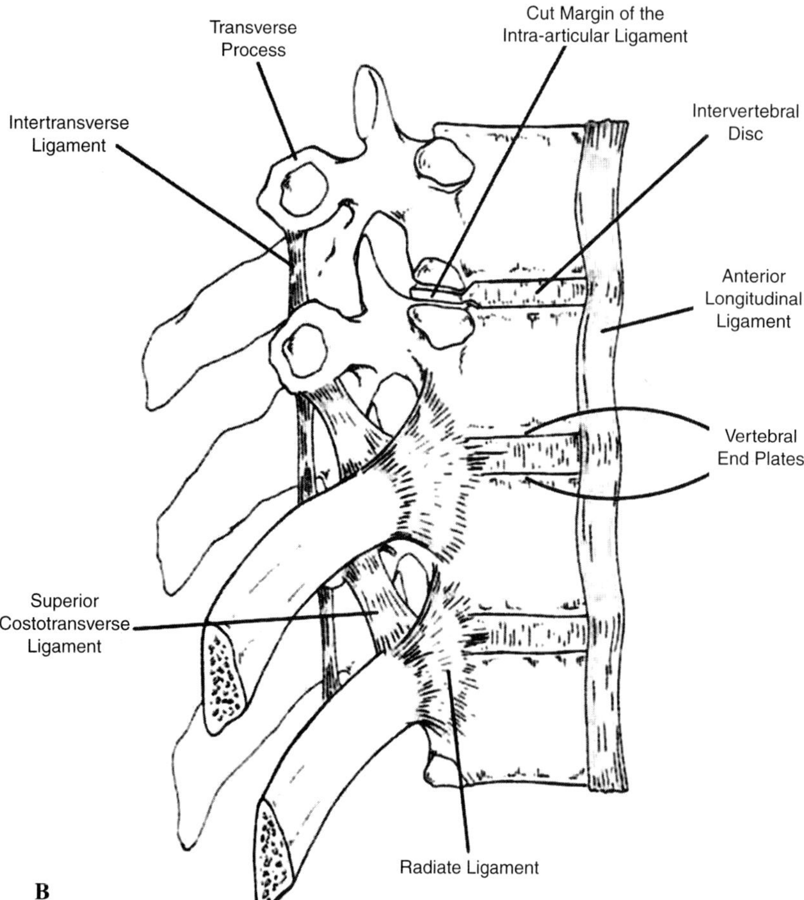

FIGURE 2–21. Intervertebral disc. *A.* Superior view of the intervertebral disc and associated structures in the thoracic region. *B.* Right lateral view of the intervertebral discs in the thoracic region. (*After Walker et at.*[32])

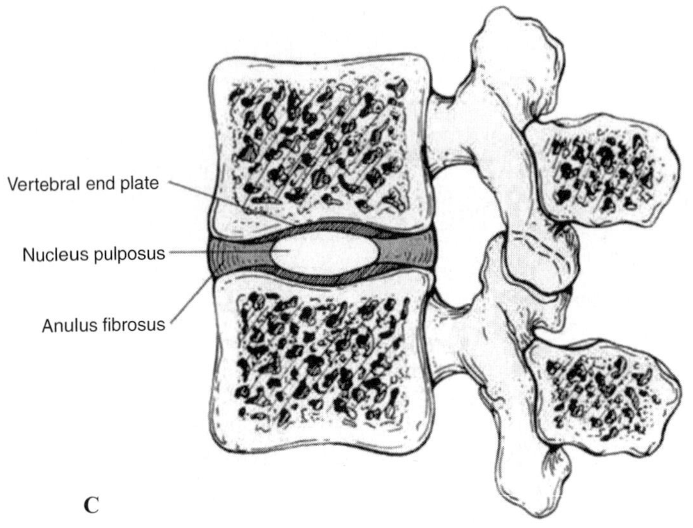

FIGURE 2–21. (Continued) *C.* Left lateral view of a coronal section of an intervertebral disc in the lumbar region. (*After Cramer and Darby.*[5])

vertebral segments, and to distribute compressive forces (but they are noncompressible, although deformable, themselves).

The *vertebral end plates* help prevent the vertebral body from suffering damage from pressure and contain the annulus fibrosus and nucleus pulposus within their normal borders. A rupture of the nucleus pulposus through the end plate is known as a *Schmorl's node*.

Intervertebral discs are avascular structures, but do have vasculature that surrounds their peripheries. They are attached to the anterior and posterior longitudinal ligaments, and to the heads of the ribs by the intra-articular ligaments. They contribute about one fifth of the total height of the vertebral column, and are relatively thicker in the lumbar and cervical regions, and thus contribute to greater mobility in these regions. They are thinnest, and essentially flat anteroposteriorly, in the thoracic region. Also, the discs are thicker anteriorly than posteriorly in the lumbar and cervical regions, thus helping to create the lumbar and cervical curvatures.

The functions of the intervertebral disc are to bear weight (with bodies of vertebrae), distribute loads, and to dissipate shock (acting as "shock absorbers"). High water content aids this function. They become less capable of holding water with age as nucleus becomes progressively replaced by fibrocartilage. They also have a higher water content in the morning than later in the day. The intervertebral discs also act as a flexible buffer between rigid vertebrae, and permit adequate motion at low loads while providing stability at higher loads.

Many issues regarding the intervertebral disc remain enigmatic. A few of these issues will be discussed here with more precise information in the chapters ahead. The natural history of extruded lumbar intervertebral discs were studied using magnetic resonance imaging (MRI). Forty-nine patients ranging in age from 19 to 57 were included in this study. The signal intensity ratio (SIR) was measured. The size of the herniated nucleus pulposus (HNP) with a SIR value of 1.2 and higher on T2-weighted MRI images decreased with time. The HNP with a SIR below 1.2 did not show any size reduction. The SIR of 1.2 and higher is a good indicator predicting spontaneous reduction of the HNP. The reduction of the lumbar disc herniation may be due to dehydration in the HNP.[43]

Clinical Pearl: The production of proinflammatory mediators within the nucleus pulposus may be a major factor in the genesis of painful lumbar disc.

Lumbar facet joint asymmetry has been targetted in the past as a culprit in intervertebral disc herniation. Few studies have addressed this issue, but one study that included 136 patients with intervertebral disc herniation used computed tomography to study this problem. In the end there was no difference in the distribution of the more coronally or sagitally facing facet joints with respect to the side of herniation. These results did not support the hypothesis that facet asymmetry is associated with lumber intervertebral disc herniation.[44]

Videman and his group studied the associations between back pain and lumbar MRI findings. This was a retrospective monozygotic twin cohort study involving 115 monozygotic male twin pairs between 35 and 69 years of age. The findings of this study raised more questions about the underlying cause of low back pain. The sensitivities of the only three significant MRI parameters, *disc height*, *disc narrowing*, and *annular tears*, are poor.[45]

The intervertebral disc may be a source of inherent pain due to mechanical or chemical irritation. It

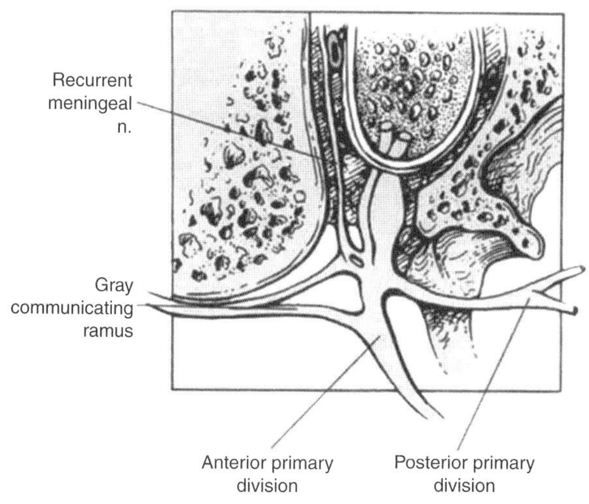

FIGURE 2–22. Innervation of the intervertebral disc. Anterior is to the left, and lateral toward the bottom of the illustration. (*After Cramer and Darby.*[5])

is innervated with the outer portion of the annulus fibrosus (Fig. 2–22). Most of the innervation in adults occurs in the lateral part of the disc and less innervation occurs in the posterior region. The anterior part has the least amount of nerve supply.[46] The lumbar sinu-vertebral nerves (SVNs), branches of the lumbar ventral rami, and the gray rami communicantes are the sources of nerve supply for the lumbar discs.[47] Because the gray rami communicantes innervates the discs at various levels, there is a possibility that discogenic pain from a single level may affect more than one recurrent branch of the spinal nerves. When there is a free nerve ending in proximity to blood vessels in the disc there may be a motor or vasosensory action. The anulus fibrosus contains very few blood vessels, which makes it unlikely be the action for the majority of nerve fibers in the anulus fibrosus. Unequivocal proof that disc pain is caused by a particular nerve is still lacking. There is some indication that the disc can be associated with pain.[48]

Clinical Pearl: Because the gray rami communicantes innervates the discs at various levels, there is a possibility that discogenic pain from a single level may affect more than one recurrent branch of the spinal nerves.

Mechanoreceptors were found in the outer two to three lamellae of the human intervertebral disc and anterior longitudinal ligament. Their presence may have clinical and physiological implications.[49]

Clinical Pearl: Mechanoreceptors were found in the outer two to three lamellae of the human intervertebral disc and anterior longitudinal ligament. Their presence may have clinical and physiological implications.

Nerve ingrowth deeper into diseased intervertebral disc has been studied as it relates to chronic pain. Samples of human intervertebral discs were analyzed using immunohistochemical techniques. Nerve fibers in the outer third of the annulus fibrosus in 48 (60%) of the 80 samples of intervertebral discs were identified. Among patients with chronic low back pain, nerves have been found to extend into the inner third of the annulus fibrosus and even into the nucleus pulposus in 21 (46%) and 10 (22%) samples, respectively. These isolated nerve fibers within diseased intervertebral discs and their association with pain allude to an important function for nerve growth into the intervertebral disc in the pathogenesis of chronic low back pain.[50]

Clinical Pearl: Among patients with chronic low back pain, nerves have been found to extend into the inner third of the annulus fibrosus and even into the nucleus pulposus.

Herniated intervertebral disc tissue has been implicated in production of a number of proinflammatory mediators and cytokines. In a recent study high levels of proinflammatory mediator was found in disc tissue from patients undergoing fusion. The production of these proinflammatory mediators within the nucleus pulposus may be a major factor in the genesis of painful lumbar disc.[51]

Innervation of the Lumbar Spine The intervertebral disc is innervated by the SVN (also known as the recurrent meningeal nerve) posteriorly, the ventral rami and gray rami communicantes posterolaterally, and the gray rami communicantes and branches of the sympathetic trunk anterolaterally (Fig. 2–22).

The SVN was first described in 1850 by von Luschka.[52] The SVN innervates the ventral portion of the lumbar spine including structures such as the dural sac, anulus fibrosis, posterior longitudinal ligament, blood vessels of the ventral region, and vertebral bodies.[53] The ventral rami and gray rami communicans innervate the lateral and anterior annuli fibrosi. They are not innervated by the SVN. Discogenic pain is mediated by the SVNs and this hypothesis is reinforced by the anatomical and clinical features.[54]

Clincal Pearl: The sinu-vertebral nerve was first described in 1850 by von Luschka.

In a study of 25 adult cadavers various patterns of rami communicantes were investigated. The posterior aspect of the intervertebral disc and the posterior longitudinal ligament were found to receive sinu-vertebral nerves originating from the deep transverse rami. This suggests two types of innervation, one originating directly from the spinal nerve segmentally and one reaching the vertebral structures via the sympathetic nerves nonsegmentally. This may indicate that these nerves are potentially involved in the proprioception of the spinal column.[55]

Clinical Pearl: The posterior aspect of the intervertebral disc and the posterior longitudinal ligament were found to receive sinu-vertebral nerves originating from the deep transverse rami. This suggests two types of innervation, one originating directly from the spinal nerve segmentally and one reaching the vertebral structures via the sympathetic nerves nonsegmentally.

Lumbosacral Joint (Fig. 2–20) Lumbar vertebrae are joined with the sacrum and pelvis via the *anterior and posterior longitudinal ligaments*, the *intervertebral disc* between L5 and S1, the *ligamenta flava*, the *interspinous and supraspinous ligaments*, and *articular capsules of the zygapophyseal joints*. Additionally, the fifth lumbar vertebra (and occasionally the fourth) is joined with the pelvis via one additional ligament on each side, the *iliolumbar ligaments*. The *iliolumbar ligament* consists of a *superior band* and an *inferior band* (also known as the *lumbosacral ligament*). Both bands attach medially to the transverse process of L5. The *superior band* runs from the transverse process of L5 to crest of the ilium immediately ventral to the sacroiliac articulation. The *inferior band* runs from the transverse process of L5 to the base of the sacrum, where it blends with the *anterior sacroiliac ligament*. These two bands limit lateral flexion of the lumbar spine.

Sacroiliac Joint (Fig. 2–20) The *sacroiliac articulation* occurs between the *auricular surface of the ilium* and the matching *auricular surface of the sacrum*. This joint is a synchondrosis. The joint has a very special character because the sacral portion develops from somitic mesoderm while the innominate portion develops from lateral plate mesoderm. The sacral portion presents a typical chondral surface (and is also a growth center [epiphysis]). The surface of the innominate portion has a different texture and includes a significant amount of fibrocartilage. The two parts of the joint are united by patches of softer fibrocartilage. Over a considerable extent of the joint, especially in later life, there may be a synovial cavity, so that it exhibits some characteristics of a plane synovial joint. There are three ligaments of this joint: the anterior sacroiliac ligament, the posterior sacroiliac ligament, and the interosseous sacroiliac ligament.

The *anterior sacroiliac ligament* extends from the base and lateral parts of the ventral surface of the sacrum to the margins of the auricular surface of the ilium. The *posterior sacroiliac ligament* consists of both long and short fibers. The *short posterior sacroiliac ligament* runs from intermediate and lateral sacral crests to the posterior superior iliac spine and internal lip of the iliac crest at its dorsal end. The *long posterior sacroiliac ligament* runs from the lower part of the lateral sacral crest to the posterior superior iliac spine, where some of its fibers merge with the fibers of the *sacrotuberous ligament* (described below). The *interosseous sacroiliac ligament* is located between the sacroiliac joint and the posterior sacroiliac ligaments, uniting the tuberosities of the ilium and the sacrum. It is a large syndesmosis lying deep to the posterior sacroiliac ligament.

Clinical Pearl: The long dorsal sacroiliac ligament has intimate anatomical connections with the erector spinae muscles, the posterior layer of the thoracolumbar fascia, and a particular part of the sacrotuberous ligament. Here lies another source of myofascial pain.

During flexion and extension of the trunk, some rotation may occur at the sacroiliac articulation.[56] The axis of rotation is located 5–10 cm inferior to the sacral promontory. The greatest amount of motion of the sacrum relative to the innominate bones occurs in rising from a sitting position. The sacral promontory moves forward (a movement called *nutation*) as much as 5 or 6 mm as body weight pushes down on the top of the sacrum. In contrast, anterior rotation of the sacral apex is termed *counternutation*. Less posterior motion occurs at the sacral apex. The range of motion is the same in males and nonpregnant females, but *nutation* and *counternutation* increase in pregnancy.

Clinical Pearl: The sacral promontory moves forward (a movement called *nutation*) as much as 5 or 6 mm as body weight pushes down on the top of the sacrum.

Ligaments Connecting the Sacrum and Ischium (Fig. 2–20) Two ligaments connect the sacrum and the ischium. These are the sacrotuberous ligament and the sacrospinous ligament.

The *sacrotuberous ligament* extends from the posterior inferior iliac spine, the fourth and fifth transverse tubercles and caudal part of the lateral margin of the sacrum and coccyx to the inner margin of the tuberosity of the ischium. Its more proximal fibers fuse with the long posterior sacroiliac ligament. The sacrotuberous ligament has been found to provide an important functional chain between the biceps femoris, the sacroiliac joint, the posterior thoracolumbar fascia, and the trunk, in the transference of loading from the spine to the leg. It is found that some of the biceps femoris fibers do not terminate at the ischium, but continue with the sacrotuberous ligament.[3]

The *sacrospinous ligament* is a thin triangular sheet attached by its broad base to the lateral margins of the sacrum and coccyx. Its apex is attached to the ischial spine. The sacrotuberous and sacrospinous ligaments close the *greater and lesser sciatic notches* of the ilium to create the *greater and lesser sciatic foramina.*

Sacrococcygeal Joint (Fig. 2–20) This is a slightly moveable joint between the first coccygeal vertebra and the fifth sacral vertebra. A small intervertebral disc is present between these two vertebral bodies. The following ligaments strengthen this joint: the ventral sacrococcygeal ligament, the superficial dorsal sacrococcygeal ligament, the deep dorsal sacrococcygeal ligament, the lateral sacrococcygeal ligaments, and the intercornual (interarticular) ligaments.

The *ventral sacrococcygeal ligament* consists of a few irregular fibers running from the ventral surface of the sacrum to the ventral surface of the coccyx which blend with the periosteum. The *superficial dorsal sacrococcygeal ligament* runs from the free margin of the sacral hiatus and attaches to the dorsal surface of the coccyx. It closes the posterior aspect of the most distal part of the sacral canal and corresponds to the ligamenta flava. The *deep dorsal sacrococcygeal ligament* corresponds to the posterior longitudinal ligament and is a flat band which arises from the posterior aspect of the fifth sacral segment inside the sacral canal and attaches to the dorsal surface of the coccyx deep to the superficial dorsal sacrococcygeal ligament. The *lateral sacrococcygeal ligaments* are present on either side of the coccyx. They run from the rudimentary transverse processes of the first coccygeal vertebra to the lower lateral angle of the sacrum. They complete the foramina for the fifth sacral nerve. The *intercornual ligaments* connect the cornua of the sacrum and coccyx.

THE CONCEPT OF SPINAL JOINT DYSFUNCTION

Theories on joint dysfunction include entrapped or pathological meniscus, abnormal paraspinal muscle function, and abnormal biomechanical processes within the synovial joint.[57] This anatomy chapter has provided a plethora of potential anatomical consequence that may result in joint/segmental dysfunction leading to pain and disability. Consider the following anatomical scenarios as potentiators of joint/segmental dysfunction:

- Contraction of the multifidus muscle may cause lesions in the zygapohyseal joints and disc.
- The iliolumbar ligament is a major stabilizer of L5 on the sacrum and has a direct restraining effect on the movement in the sacroiliac joints. This may have consequences in the etiology of sacroiliac joint pain.
- The long dorsal sacroiliac ligament has intimate anatomical connections with the erector spinae muscles, the posterior layer of the thoracolumbar fascia, and a particular part of the sacrotuberous ligament. Here lies another source of myofascial pain.
- There is some evidence that the diaphragm may be involved in postural control of postural stability during sudden voluntary movements of the limbs.
- Intra-abdominal pressure partly contributes to spinal stability.
- The presence of mechanoreceptors in the outer portion of the intervertebral disc may have clinical and physiological implications.

Ponder these preceding factors while reading further chapters. They will provide more data for demystifying these anatomical scenarios.

PROPRIOCEPTION

Proprioception is a term that is used in injury evaluation, rehabilitation, and posture/balance assessment. It has been defined as the neurological ability of the body to assess information or inputs coming from muscles, joints, tendons, and various other mechanoreceptors. These inputs are modulated via three different motor control centers of the central nervous system (CNS):

1. spinal level
2. lower brain (brainstem, cerebellum) level
3. cortical level

Proprioceptive inputs are analyzed at a subconscious level by the first two CNS centers and consciously at the cerebral cortex.[58]

Proprioception is a subconscious means of providing afferent input from the periphery to the CNS. While much anatomical focus has been directed to the segmental aspects of the muscular and skeletal systems, perhaps in order to organize such a complex topic, relatively little has been discussed regarding the contiguity of the fascial system and the interdigitations of adjoining tendinous insertions. Fascia surrounds, interweaves, and connects the neuromusculoskeletal system into one continuous sheet of tissue, so that the slightest change in tension in one region stimulates receptors in adjoining regions.

As such, proprioceptors provide a vital and uninterrupted continuum of sensory input from which the CNS can organize a coordinated efferent response, optimizing locomotion along countless kinetic chains.

Clinical Pearl: Fascia surrounds, interweaves, and connects the neuromusculoskeletal system into one continuous sheet of tissue, so that the slightest change in tension in one region stimulates receptors in adjoining regions.

Proprioception is measured by two general methods. One method is designed to assess position sense, which requires subjects to reproduce previous positions or ranges of movement. The second method is designed to assess movement sense, which is assessed by determining thresholds to the perception of movement and its direction.[59] Cutaneous receptors in the hand seem to play an important role in hand proprioception. Spinal afferent nerves may appear to convey proprioceptive data from structures such as the interspinous, supraspinous, and flaval ligaments, lumbar discs, and paraspinal muscles.

The effects of proprioception on lumbar muscle function and stability of the lumbar spine remain uncertain.[60] Inadequate or aberrant proprioception has been theorized as a significant factor contributing to chronic low back pain. However, a recent study found that in a group of patients with chronic low back pain no proprioceptive deficits could be clearly identified. This agrees with other studies that intimate that patients with low back pain experience no proprioceptive deficits.[50] Yet other studies indicate that there may be a direct connection between the structures that provide internal cues for the body's ability to sense nociceptive influence affecting the afference of these structures. Differences in proprioception do exist between individuals with back pain and those without back pain.[61,62]

A study measuring repositioning error (RE) in 20 subjects with low back pain with 20 control subjects showed that RE in patients with low back pain was significantly higher than that of control subjects in flexion, and significantly lower than that of control subjects in extension. The increase in RE of patients with low back pain during flexion implicates loss of proprioception.[63] This is why Janda developed a sensory stimulation program with a focus on proprioceptive retraining. This appears to be an effective rehabilitation tool.[64] Another study investigated the role of paraspinal muscle spindles in lumbosacral positioning sense in low back pain subjects and asymptomatic subjects. The findings of this study indicated that low back pain patients have a less refined position sense than normal subjects. This may be due to altered paraspinal muscle spindle afferent and central processing of the sensory input. In addition, muscle vibration can be an interesting expedient for improving proprioception and enhancing muscle control.[65]

Anatomy provides the foundation for comprehending physiology, neurology, and pathology as well as forming new engrams in developing and integrating clinical strategies. This chapter has attempted to set the stage for the following chapters by painting the portrait of the embryological end-stage known as the human lumbar spine. It will hopefully lead to a better understanding of the challenge of managing the problem of low back pain.

ACKNOWLEDGMENTS

Original artwork for this chapter (Figs. 2–2, 2–3, 2–6, and 2–10) was prepared by William Yee, DC, LAc, Flushing, New York. Drawings commissioned by the Anatomy Department of New York Chiropractic College (NYCC) while he was a work study student at NYCC. For all other illustrations, see credit as given.

SUMMARY

1. This chapter provided an overview of lumbopelvic region anatomy.
2. Because of the increasing understanding of low back function, an expanded morphological explanation has been provided.
3. This chapter described various aspects of functional anatomy which combines morphological explanation with functional correlates.
4. A special emphasis was placed on the contiquity of the fascial system in contrast with the classically taught segmented muscular system. The uninterupted fascia with its mechanoreceptors.
5. The information provided in this chapter is designed to assist the reader by providing an anatomical cornerstone for ensuing chapters of this text.

REFERENCES

1. Woodburne RT. *Essentials of human anatomy*, 6th ed. Oxford, London, 1978.
2. Porterfield JA, DeRosa C. *Mechanical low back pain: Perspectives in functional anatomy*. Philadelphia: W. B. Saunders, 1991.
3. Vleeming A, Pool-Goudzwaard AL, Stoeckart R, van Wingerden JP, Snijders CJ. The posterior layer of the thoracolumbar fascia. Its function in load transfer from spine to legs. *Spine* April 1, 1995;20(7):753–758.
4. Walker RA, Lovejoy CO, Bedford ME, Yee W. *Skeletal and developmental anatomy for students of chiropractic*. Philadelphia: F.A. Davis, 2002:81–137.

5. Cramer GD, Darby SA, eds. *Basic and clinical anatomy of the spine, spinal cord, and ANS*. St. Louis: Mosby, 1995.
6. Bogduk, N. A reappraisal of the anatomy of the human erector spinae. *J Anat* 1980;131:525–540.
7. Vilensky JA, Baltes M, Weikel L, Fortin JD, Fourie LJ. Serratus posterior muscles: Anatomy, clinical relevance, and function. *Clin Anat* July 2001;14(4):237–241.
8. Bustami, Faraj MF. A new description of the lumbar erector spinae muscle in man. *J Anat* 1986;144: 81–91.
9. Bogduk N. *Clinical anatomy of the lumbar spine and sacrum*, 3rd ed. New York: Churchill Livingstone, 1997:101–117.
10. Kaigle AM, Holm S, Hansson T. Experimental instability in the lumbar spine. *Spine* 1995;20:421–430.
11. Moseley GL, Hodges PW, Gandevia SC. Deep and superficial fibers of the lumbar multifidus muscle are differentially active during voluntary arm movements. *Spine* 2002; 27(2):E29–E36.
12. Hides JA, Richardson CA, Jull GA. Multifidus muscle recovery is not automatic after resolution of acute, first-episode low back pain. *Spine* 1996;21(23):2763-2769.
13. Kader DF, Wardlaw D, Smith FW. Correlation between the MRI changes in the lumbar multifidus muscles and leg pain. *Clin Radiol* 2000;55(2):145–149.
14. Nitz AJ, Peck D. Comparison of muscle spindle concentrations in large and small human epaxial muscles acting in parallel combinations. *Am Surg* 1986;52:273–277.
15. McGill S. *Low back disorders: Evidence-based prevention and rehabilitation*. Champaign: Human Kinetics, 2002: 60–61.
16. Macintosh JE, Pearcy MJ, Bogduk N. The axial torque of the lumbar back muscles: Torsion strength of the back muscles. *Aust N Z J Surg* March 1993; 63(3):205–212.
17. Buxton DF, Peck D. Density of muscle spindle profiles in the intrinsic forelimb muscles of the dog. *J Morphol* March 1990;203(3):345–359.
18. Peck D, Buxton DF, Nitz A. A comparison of spindle concentrations in large and small muscles acting in parallel combinations. *J Morphol* June 1984;180(3):243–252.
19. Morris JM, Lucas DB, Bresler B. Role of the trunk in stability of the spine. *J Bone Joint Surg* 1961;43A: 327–351.
20. Bartlink DL. The role of intra-abdominal pressure in relieving the pressure on the lumbar vertebral discs. *J Bone Joint Surg* 1957;39B: 718–725.
21. Richardson C, Jull G, Hides J, Hodges P. *Therapeu tic exercise for spinal stabilisation: Scientific basis and practical techniques*. Edinburgh: Churchill Livingstone, 1999:41–59.
22. Hodges, P, Richardson C. Inefficient muscular stabilization of the lumbar spine associated with low back pain. A motor control evaluation of transverses abdominis. *Spine* 1996;21 (22):2640–2650.
23. Hodges PW, Richardson CA, Gandevia SC. Contractions of specific abdominal muscles in postural tasks are affected by respiratory maneuvers. *J Appl Phys* 1997;83(3): 753–760.
24. Hodges, PW. Functional control of the low back. In: Morris, CE, ed. *Conservative management of low back syndromes*. New York. McGraw-Hill, 2005: xxx–xxx.
25. Gibbons SGT. A review of the anatomy, physiology and function of psoas major: a new model of stability. In: *Proceedings of the tragic hip: Trouble in the lower quadrant. 11th Annual National Orthopaedic Symposium*, Halifax, 1999. Cited in: Gibbons SGT, Comerford MJ, Emerson PL. Rehabilitation of the stability function of psoas major. Available at: http://www.kineticcontrol.com/pages/references/Publications/Psaos.htm.
26. Gibbons SGT. The model of psoas major stability function. In: *Proceedings of 1st International Conference on movement dysfunction*, Edinburgh, Scotland, 2001. Cited in: Gibbons SGT, Comerford MJ, Emerson PL. Rehabilitation of the stability function of psoas major. Available at: http://www.kineticcontrol.com/pages/references/Publications/Psoas.htm.
27. Gibbons SGT, Pelley B, Molgaard J. Biomechanics and stability mechanisms of psoas major. In: *Proceedings of 4th Interdisciplinary World Congress on low back pain*, Montreal, Canada, 2001. Cited in: Gibbons SGT, Comerford MJ, Emerson PL. Rehabilitation of the stability function of psoas major. Available at: http://www.kineticcontrol.com/pages/references/Publications/Psoas.htm.
28. McVay CB, Anson BJ. Aponeurotic and fascial continuities in the abdomen, pelvis and thigh. *Anat Rec* 1940:76 (2): 213–232.
29. Williams PL, Bannister LH, Berry MM, et al. *Gray's anatomy*, 38th ed. Edinburgh: Churchill Livingstone, 1995:868–870.
30. Hodges PW, Gandevia SC. Changes in intra-abdominal pressure during postural and respiratory activation of the human diaphragm. *J Appl Physiol* 2000;89:967–976.
31. Shirley D, Hodges PW, Eriksson AE, Gandevia SC. Spinal stiffness changes throughout the respiratory cycle. *J Appl Physiol* October 2003;95(4):1467–1475.
32. Walker RA, Lovejoy CO, Bedford ME, Yee W. *Skeletal and developmental anatomy for students of chiropractic*. Philadelphia: FA Davis, 2002,86.
33. Higuchi K, Sato T. Anatomical study of lumbar spine innervation. *Folia morphol (warsz.)* 2002;61(2):71–79.
34. Roberts S, Eisenstein S, Menage J, Evans E, Ashton I. Mechanoreceptors in intervertebral discs. Morphology, distribution, and neuro peptides. *Spine* December 1995;20(24):2645–2651.
35. Pionchon H, Tommasi M, Pialat J, et al. Study of the innervation of the spinal ligaments at the lumbar level. *Bull Assoc Anat (Nancy)*. September 1986;70(210):63–67.
36. Berven S, Tay BB, Colman W, Hsu SS. The lumbar zygapophyseal (facet) joints: A role in the pathogenesis of spinal pain syndromes and degenerative spondylolisthesis. *Semin Neurol* 2002;22(2):187–196.

37. Fukui S, Ohseto K, Shiotani M, Ohno K, Karasawa H, Naganuma Y. Distribution of referred pain from the lumbar zygapohyseal joints and dorsal rami. *Clin J Pain* 1997;13(4):303–307.
38. Yamashita T, Cavanaugh JM, el-Bohy AA, Getchell TV, King AI. Mechanosensitive afferent units in the lumbar facet joint. *J Bone Joint Surg Am* 1990;72(6):865–870.
39. Pool-Goudzwaard AL, Kleinrensink GJ, Snijders CJ, Entius C, Stoeckart R. The sacroiliac part of the iliolumbar ligament. *J Anat* 2001;199(Pt 4):457–463.
40. Pool-Goodzwaard A, Hock van Dijke G, Mulder P, Spoor C, Snijders C, Stoeckart R. The iliolumbar ligament: Its influence on stability of the sacroiliac joint. *Clin Biomech (Bristol, Avon)* 2003;18(2):99–105.
41. Sims JA, Moorman SJ. The role of the iliolumbar ligament in low back pain. *Med Hypotheses* 1996;46:511–515.
42. Vleeming A, Pool-Goudzwaard AL, Hammudoghlu D, Stoeckart R, Snijders CJ, Mens JM. The function of the long dorsal sacroiliac ligament: Its implication for understanding low back pain. *Spine* 1996;21(5):556–562.
43. Henmi T, Sairyo K, Kanematsu Y, Kajikawa T, Katoh S, Goel VK. Natural history of extruded lumbar intervertebral disc herniation. *J Med Invest* 2002;49 (1–2):40–43.
44. Cassidy JD, Loback D, Yong-Hing K, Tchang S. Lumbar facet joint asymmetry. *Spine* 1992;17(5):570–574.
45. Videman T, Battie MC, Gibbons LE, Maravilla K, Manninen H, Kaprio J. Associations between back pain history and lumbar MRI findings. *Spine* 2003; 28(6):582–588.
46. Holm, Indahl A, Solomonow M. Sensorimotor control of the spine, *J Electromyogr Kinesiol* 2002;12(3):219–234.
47. Bogduk N, Twomey L. Nerves of the lumbar spine. In: *Clinical anatomy of the lumbar spine.* New York: Churchill Livingstone, 1992:116–117.
48. Yamashita T, Minaki Y, Oota I, Yokogushi K, Ishii S. Mechanosensitive afferent units in the lumbar intervertebral disc and adjacent muscle. *Spine* 1993; 18(15):2252–2256.
49. Roberts S, Eisenstein SM, Menage J, Evans EH, Ashton IK. Mechanoreceptors in the intervertebral disc. Morphology, distribution, and neuropeptides. *Spine* 1995;20(24):2645–2651.
50. Freemont AJ, Peacock TE, Goupille P, Hoyland JA, O'Brien UJ, Jayson MI. Nerve ingrowth into diseased intervertebral disc in chronic back pain. *Lancet* 1997;19;350(9072):178–181.
51. Burke JG, Watson RW, McCormack D, Dowling FE, Walsh MG, Fitzpatrick JM. Intervertebral discs which cause low back pain secrete high levels of proinflammatory mediators. *J Bone Joint Surg Br* 2002;84(2):196–201.
52. von Luschka H: *Die nerven des menschlichen wirbelkanales.* Tubingen, Germany: Laupp and Siebeck, 1850.
53. Bogduk N. The innervation of the lumbar spine. *Spine* 1983;8(3):286–293.
54. Raoul S, Faure A, Robert R, et al. Role of the sinuvertebral nerve in low back pain and anatomical basis of therapeutic implications. *Surg Radiol Anat* 2002;24: 366–370.
55. Higuchi K, Sato T. Anatomical study of the lumbar spine innervation. *Folia Morphol (Warsz)* 2002; 61(2):71–79.
56. Soames RW, Atha J. The role of the antigravity musculature during quiet standing in man. *Eur J Appl Physiol Occup Physiol* 1981;47(2):159–167.
57. Leach R. *The chiropractic theories*, 3rd ed. Baltimore: Williams & Wilkins, 1994:121.
58. Koumantakis GA, Winstanley J, Oldham JA. Thoracolumbar proprioception in individuals with and without low back pain: Intratester reliability, clinical applicability, and validity. *J Orthop Sports Phys Ther* 2002;32(7):327–335.
59. Swinkels A, Dolan P. Regional assessment of joint position sense in the spine. *Spine* 1998;23(5):590–597.
60. Brumagne S, Lysens R, Spaepen A. Lumbosacral repositioning accuracy in standing posture: A combined electrogoniometric and videographic evaluation. *Clin Biomech* 1999;14:361–363.
61. Grod J, Diakow P. Effect of neck pain on verticality perception: A cohort study. *Arch Phys Med Rehabil* 2002;83:412–415.
62. Gill KP, Callaghan MJ. The measurement of lumbar proprioception in individuals with and without low back pain. *Spine* 1998;23(3):371–377.
63. Newcomer KL, Laskowski ER, Yu B, Johnson JC, An K. Differences in repositioning error among patients with low back pain compared with control subjects. *Spine* 2000;25(19):2488–2493.
64. Bullock-Saxton JE, Janda V, Bullock MI. Reflex activation of gluteal muscles in walking: An approach to restoration of muscle function for patients with low back pain. *Spine* 1993;18:704–708.
65. Brumagne S, Cordo P, Lysens R, Verschueren S, Swinnen S. The role of paraspinal muscle spindles in lumbosacral position sense in individuals with and without low back pain. *Spine* 2000;25(8):989–994.

CHAPTER

3

BIOMECHANICS OF THE LOW BACK

Kim Ross, Walter Herzog, and Bruce P. Symons

OUTLINE

OBJECTIVES

1. Introduce the reader to biomechanical principles of the low back.
2. Provide definitions for key concepts upon which principles of low back biomechanics are based.
3. Integrate biomechanical concepts with low back functional anatomy.
4. Explain various spinal loads associated with injury and rehabilitation.
5. Describe loads associated with different spinal positions and activities.

INTRODUCTION

The demand for conservative care practitioners and their treatments is due to the fact that 70% of the population will suffer from low back pain (LBP) at some point in their life,[1] with a yearly prevalence rate of 50%.[2] This prevalence rate also appears to be true historically: Conservative low back treatment has been practiced in one form or another for thousands of years.[3] Therefore, suffering from LBP appears to be a normal part of life, and only the exceptional individual escapes unafflicted. Why are humans, as a species, so susceptible to LBP?

The authors will describe a circuitous route to demonstrate the value in mastering the biomechanics and anatomy of the human spine, a relatively onerous task, but it is important to reinforce the scientific and clinical merit of doing so. The answer to why humans are so prone to LBP lies primarily in the structure and function of the human spine. In most terrestrial vertebrates, the spine serves as a horizontal scaffold from which the appendicular skeleton articulates. In contrast, human bipedalism has forced this scaffold into a vertical column: the spine, particularly the lumbar spine, which serves as a support to balance the upper body over the pelvis. Obviously, this configuration is not stable—if a craftsman were to build a solid dining table, one would probably choose four legs over two. The inherent biomechanical instability of adapting to bipedalism, and the inevitable forces that impact the vertebral column, has resulted in *Homo sapiens* groaning over their backs for millennia.

BASIC BIOMECHANICS

The key question to be answered in this chapter is "What is biomechanics and how does it relate to LBP?" Before attempting to answer the second half of that question, the first half must be addressed. Biomechanics is the science that deals with the external and internal forces acting on a biological system, and the effects these forces have on the system. Biomechanics is commonly divided into the two subsets: kinematics and kinetics. Kinematics describes the motion of an object, without consideration of the forces that cause the motion. Kinetics is concerned with the forces producing motion. This discussion will begin with kinetics, as forces are required to produce accelerated motion.

Kinetics

To understand injury and rehabilitation of the lower back, it is important for the reader to understand some basic kinetic concepts such as forces. These concepts entail different types of loads to which tissues may be subjected: Newton's laws of motion, and moments.

What Are Forces? Force is something that cannot be directly described, but instead is typically defined by the action it produces. For example, a frictional force shows its action by slowing down an object. The frictional forces of brakes on wheels allow for a deceleration of a bike. Similarly, frictional forces between ice and a rock cause a rock to stop in the sport of curling. Force is measured in Newtons, where 1 Newton is the force required to accelerate a mass of 1 kilogram by 1 meter per square second. Forces cause motion, but a stationary system may also be subjected to forces. As a man sits motionlessly and reads this text, the force of gravity pushes him into his chair. However, there is no motion because the chair is pushing up on the buttocks with an equal magnitude of force, but in the opposite direction, and along a line coincident with the resultant gravitational force. The stationary, seated reader is, in this instance, in a state of *static equilibrium*.

Static equilibrium is a motion state in which all particles of a system (in this case, the seated man) move with a constant velocity (constant speed and constant direction) relative to an inertial reference frame. For a special *reference frame* (the one that moves at the same constant velocity as the system of interest), the system appears motionless. The sum of all the external forces acting on the system (reader) is zero. For a system in *static equilibrium*, it is always true that the sum of all the external forces, and the sum of all the external moments acting on the system, is zero. However, note that the reverse is not correct in general. That is, if the sum of all external forces and the sum of all external moments acting on a system is zero, the system is not necessarily in static equilibrium. However, if now another person pushes the same reader from the side, the stationary reader will move because of the additional unbalanced force. At this point, the sum of all external forces acting on the reader's body does not add up to zero, and as a result, the reader is thrown off his static equilibrium, and is accelerated in the direction of the resultant force.

The reader interested in a greater understanding of these biomechanical principles, in addition to the ensuing principles, briefly covered in this chapter is directed to the text by Herzog, which provides far greater explanation into this challenging topic.[4]

Internal and External Forces Before addressing internal and external forces, it is necessary to define the notion of a *mechanical system*. A mechanical system is a system of points that is defined by the engineer. For example, if a woman is interested in the way the human body moves, her system of interest may be the entire human body. But if her interest is in a herniated disc, then the system of interest is the herniated disc. Therefore, in the first system, the forces acting on the herniated disc by muscles, ligaments, vertebral bodies, etc., are internal forces. Conversely, the forces from these same muscles, ligaments, vertebral segments, etc., would be considered external forces in the second example because the reference point has been altered to focus on the disc. Newton's laws of motion relate only to the external forces acting on a body; therefore, it is important to know what forces one is interested in before defining the system of interest.

Internal forces are defined as all the forces acting *within* the system of interest. For example, if the system of interest is the entire human body, then the components of the body such as ligaments, muscles, bones, tendons and fascia exert internal forces, and these forces cannot be obtained using Newton's laws for the defined system.

External forces, on the other hand, are all the forces acting externally on, or *outside*, the system of interest. These forces are typically divided into *contact forces* and *remote forces*. Contact forces are all the forces that occur because of the contact of the target system with its environment. The person sitting in the chair and reading this text will experience forces from the chair on his buttocks and back, forces from the floor on his feet, and the pushing force from the other person, mentioned above. Remote forces are all the forces that

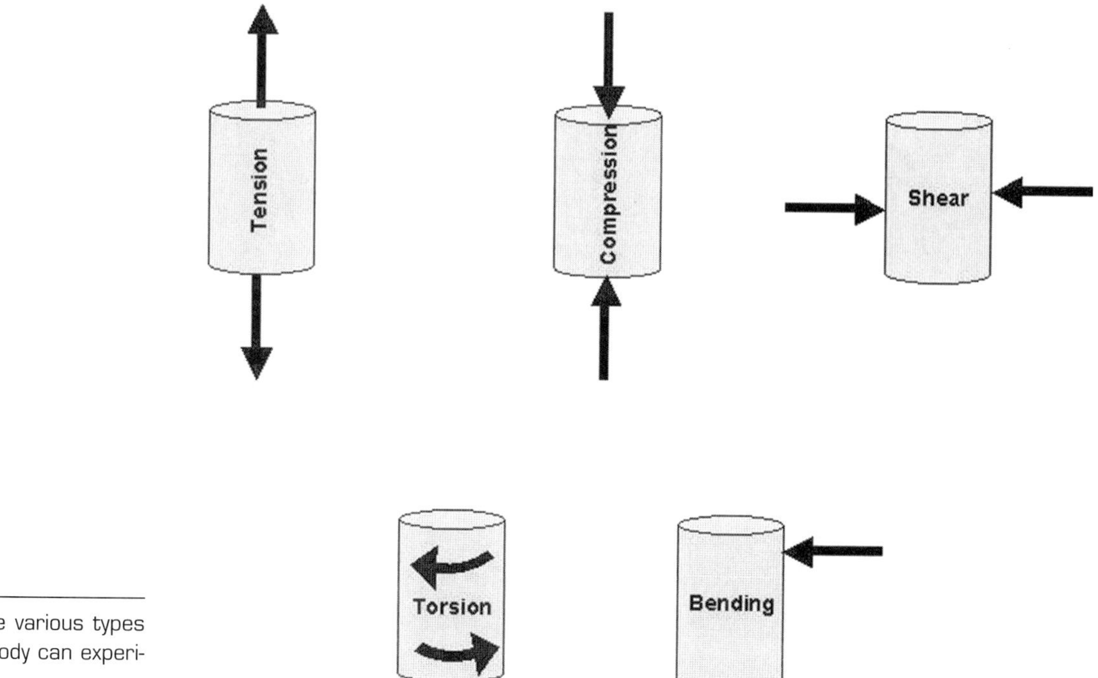

FIGURE 3–1. The various types of loads which a body can experience.

act on the system but are not caused by contact with the environment. These include electrostatic forces, magnetic forces, and the most important of these in the biomechanics context, the force of gravity. Counteracting the force of gravity may be in large part responsible for injuries of tissues in the low back, which is a topic that will be discussed later in this chapter.

Types of Mechanical Loads Forces acting on a system create mechanical *stresses*. Depending on the loading produced by a force, different types of stresses are created inside the system of interest.

Tensile force, the first principle, is sometimes simply referred to as *tension*. Tensioncreates a so-called *axial stress*, which tends to pull apart the molecules of the system. As a result the object tends to stretch in the direction of the tensile force (Fig. 3–1). Hanging from a chin-up bar creates tension in the intervertebral discs because the gravitational force exerts an axial load on the back.

Compression, i.e., the second principle, in contrast, is caused by forces pressing the system of interest together along the longitudinal axis. It results in *axial stress* that tends to push the molecules of the system together (Fig. 3–1). The intervertebral discs and zygapophyseal and sacroiliac joints are exposed to compression in a standing person. The force of gravity acting on the torso pushes down on the disc, while the reaction force from the ground pushes up on the disc, thereby creating a compressive stress.

Shear is the third principle of stress (next to tensile and compressive stress) (Fig. 3–1). For example, a force that tends to slide one vertebra in the anterior direction relative to the one below would create a shear stress between the two vertebrae.

The loads discussed above are termed *simple loads*. In other words, they produce only one type of stress. However, there are a number of loading conditions that will create different types of stresses on the system of interest simultaneously. For example, a *bending load* (Fig. 3–1) produces different types of stresses at different locations of the system. Flexion of the spinal column, for example, produces a compressive stress on the anterior portion of the vertebrae, and a tensile stress on the posterior part of the vertebrae. Lateral bending will cause compression on the side of bending (i.e., the concave side) and tension on the contralateral side (i.e., the convex side). In the middle of the vertebral column, there exists an axis that experiences neither compression nor tension and this axis is referred to as the *neutral axis*.

Torsional loading (Fig. 3–1) also causes different portions of the object to undergo different stresses. Torsional loading involves twisting of an object about its longitudinal axis. Torsion produces shear stresses in the system, and these shear stresses increase as one moves from a neutral torsion axis in the center of a symmetric system to its outside. Twisting one's body to the right or left creates a torsional load in the discs of the spine, and hence would produce a shear stress.

Addition of Forces To properly understand how forces affect the lower back, it is important to understand how forces add together. For example, suppose the system of interest is a single vertebra, and the

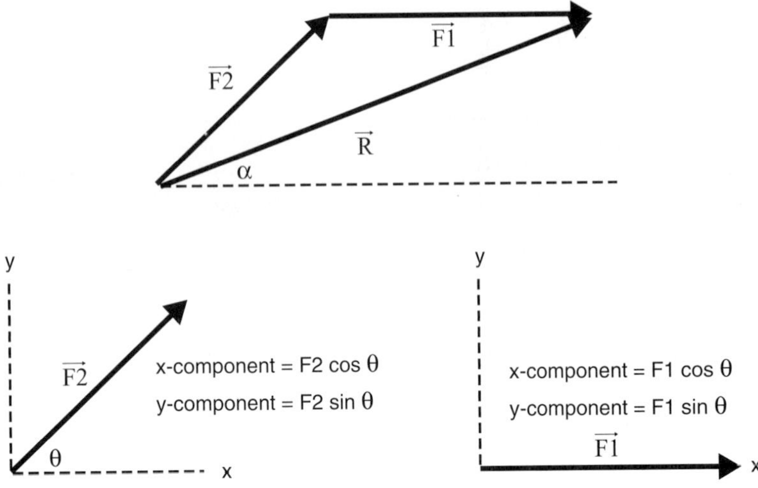

$$R = \sqrt{(F2 \cos\theta + F1 \cos\theta)^2 + (F2 \sin\theta + F1 \sin\theta)^2}$$

$$\alpha = \tan^{-1} (F2 \sin\theta + F1 \sin\theta) / (F2 \cos\theta + F1 \cos\theta)$$

FIGURE 3–2. Determining the resultant magnitude *R* and direction (α) of two forces.

question is how it behaves mechanically when subjected to a series of external forces. The vertebra is subjected to the force of gravity acting on each particle of the system but this distributed gravitational force can be replaced by a single force (the weight of the vertebra) acting through the system's center of mass. Contact forces acting on the vertebra include the forces of the adjacent vertebrae acting through contacts with the zygapophyseal joints and the discs, the attached ligaments and muscles, and other surrounding tissues. Each of these forces acts in a particular direction and possesses a particular magnitude. However, even though many forces may act upon the vertebra simultaneously, it is possible to determine the resultant effect of all these forces on the system. This single force obtained by vector addition of all the individual forces is known as the *resultant force*. If the system of interest is in a state of static equilibrium, the resultant force acting on the vertebra will be zero.

So how are forces added together to obtain the resultant force? First, it must be understood that a force is a *vector*, meaning that every force has a magnitude and a direction. In mechanics, vectors can be represented graphically with arrows. The length of the arrow shows its magnitude, and the direction is indicated by the direction of the arrow, positive being defined from the tail to the tip of the arrow. Mathematically, vectors are represented in inertial reference frames by a combination of unit vectors multiplied by the appropriate constants. Graphically, forces are added by attaching the tail end of one vector to the head of the other vector while maintaining their original orientation. This process is continued until all force vectors have been arranged tail to tip. Figure 3–2 shows a simple version of how this is done where two forces, described as $\vec{F1}$ and $\vec{F2}$, have been added by adding the tail of $\vec{F1}$ to the head of $\vec{F2}$. The resultant force is determined by drawing a line from the tail of $\vec{F2}$ to the head of $\vec{F1}$ (Fig. 3–2). When adding force vectors algebraically, the resultant force of two forces is obtained by adding the corresponding components of the two force vectors. For example, assume that vector $\vec{F1}$ is 3 units in the x direction and 0 units in the y direction; then $\vec{F1} = 3x + 0y$. If the force vector $\vec{F2}$ is 2.5 units in the x and y directions, then $\vec{F2} = 2.5x + 2.5y$. The resultant force of these two forces, the resultant force vector $\vec{R}$, is then given by $\vec{R} = (3 + 2.5)x + (0 + 2.5)y$, or $\vec{R} = 5.5x + 2.5y$ (Fig. 3–3).

Free Body Diagrams For some situations, a *free body diagram* is a good way to determine resultant forces

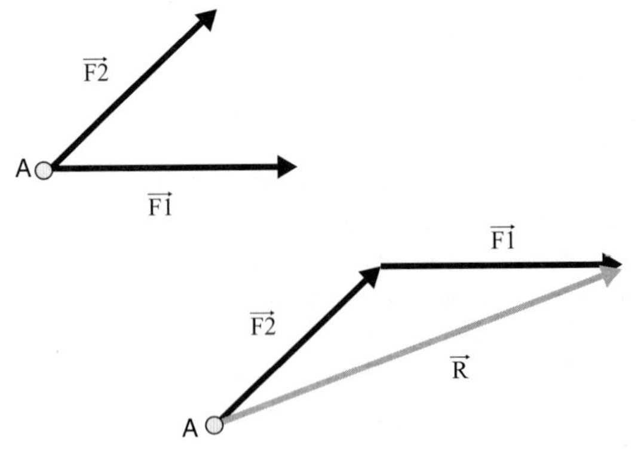

FIGURE 3–3. Two forces shown in vector form acting on point A. The magnitude of the forces is represented by the length and the direction of the force is represented by the direction of the arrow head. The net effect of these two forces produces a single force (the resultant or $\vec{R}$).

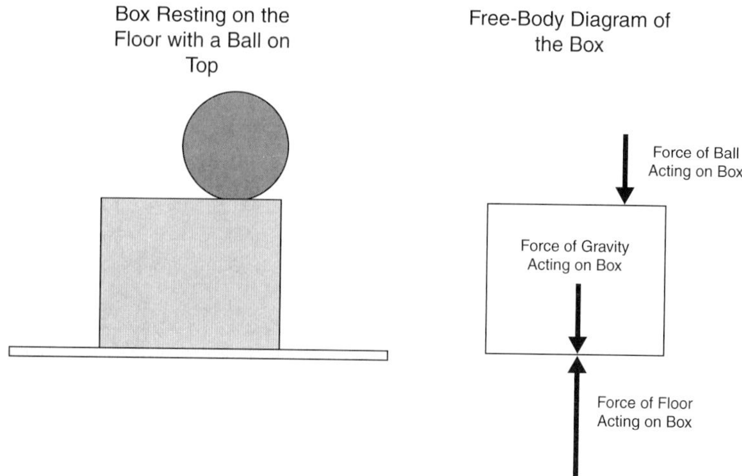

FIGURE 3–4. Building a free body diagram. The ball, the floor, and gravity are replaced by their force effect on the box.

acting on an object. However, it is important to warn the reader that the concept of a free body diagram is not always a feasible way to approach a mechanical problem. For example, in situations in which kinematic constraints have to be satisfied by external forces, the principle of virtual work is typically the preferred choice of solution. When using the free body diagram approach to calculate an external force acting on a system, the following steps should be performed: first, identify the system of interest (e.g., a vertebral body) and isolate it from all its surroundings; second, draw all the external contact and remote forces acting on the system of interest. For example, imagine a box placed on the floor with a ball on its top. A force vector representing the contact force of the ball acting on the box replaces the ball. Another force vector representing the force of the floor acting on the box replaces the floor. In addition, the force of gravity is shown to be acting through the center of mass of the box (i.e., this is the weight of the box) (Fig. 3–4).

Newton's First Law (The Law of Inertia) Newton's first law states, "A system continues in its state of rest, or uniform motion, unless it is acted upon by a resultant external force." In other words, if there is no external resultant force acting on the system, it will travel in uniform motion relative to any inertial reference frame. Uniform motion is defined as a translation of the system in which the velocity (vector) of each particle of the system is the same and constant.

Newton's Second Law (F = ma) Newton's second law states, "The rate of change in momentum of a particle is proportional to the resultant external force acting on the particle." Stated simply, the second law says that if a particle is acted upon by a resultant force, it will be accelerated in the direction of the applied force, and its acceleration will be directly proportional to the force and inversely proportional to the object's mass. From Newton's second law, it is clear that resultant forces cause accelerations.

Newton's Third Law (Action–Reaction) Newton's third law states,"For every action, there is an equal but opposite reaction." Simply stated, for every force acting from one system onto another, there is an equal and opposite force from the second system onto the first. Recalling the previous example of the man sitting in the chair, his weight exerts a force on the chair. If he does not move (i.e., he is in a state of static equilibrium), the chair will exert a force against him of equal magnitude, *but in the opposite direction*. Or, as another example, if in the lumbar spine the L5 vertebra is exerting a force on the L5–S1 disc, then the disc exerts a force of equal magnitude, but opposite direction, on the L5 vertebra.

What Are Moments? When a force applied to an object of interest produces an angular acceleration, then that force is said to have produced a moment on that object. For example, when opening a door by the handle, the door rotates around the hinges. The force applied to the handle produces a moment about the hinges, thereby causing rotation. The magnitude of the moment is dependent on two variables: the magnitude of the force, and the perpendicular distance of the line of action of the force from the turning axis. A moment ($\vec{M}$) is mathematically defined as $\vec{M} = \vec{r} \times \vec{F}$, where $\vec{r}$ is a location vector from any point of the line of action of the force to the turning axis, and $\vec{F}$ is the force producing the moment. "$\times$" is the symbol for the cross or vector product of two vectors. Note that the vector product is not commutative; therefore, the order of the vector notation is crucial. Note further that the above vector equation can be replaced by the scalar notation $M = d \cdot F$, where now M refers to the magnitude of the moment, d is the perpendicular distance from the line of action of the force to the axis of rotation, and F is the force magnitude. The "·" (i.e., the period between the d and the F in the equation above) now symbolizes a normal scalar multiplication.

The unit of measure for moments is Newton meters or Nm. Returning to the above example of the door, one notes that doorknobs are typically located far from the hinges. This design is not by accident, because on placing the doorknobs in this location, the distance (d) from the line of action of force application to the hinges is large. As a result, the magnitude of force required to open the door is small. If the handle were located close to the hinge, the force magnitude would have to be increased to open the door. A second example may clarify just how important moments are to everyday life. Imagine trying to loosen a nut from a bolt using only the head of a wrench. In most cases, this would be an impossible task because the forces required to loosen the bolt would be too great. However, wrenches are designed with long handles attached to the head. Since the *moment arm*, afforded by the handle, is greatly increased compared to the above situation, a small force would produce the required moment to loosen the nut.

Moments Affecting Human Tissue So how do moments impact the tissues of the human body? An example is provided in Figure 3–5, demonstrating a schematic representation of an arm (vertical segment) and forearm and hand (represented by one horizontal segment). When the biceps muscle, which inserts into the radius of the forearm, contracts concentrically, the elbow will flex provided the biceps force is greater than any external forces acting on the forearm–hand. The biceps force vector is shown as $\vec{F}_{ms}$. Assuming that the arm (vertical segment) is fixed, the biceps is going to

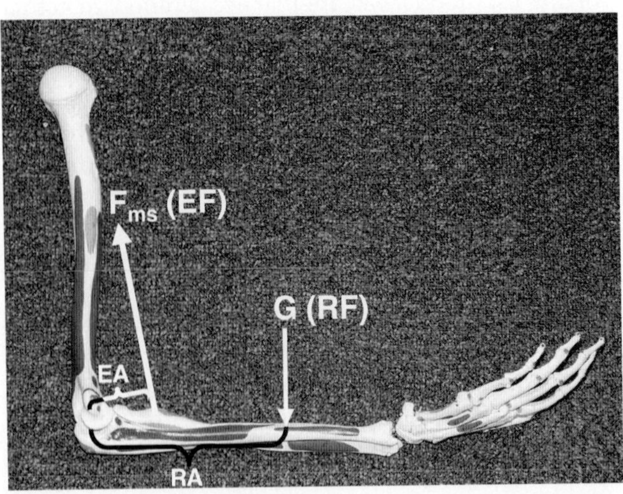

FIGURE 3–5. The moment acting on the forearm and hand about the elbow is equal to (EF × EA) + (RA × RF).

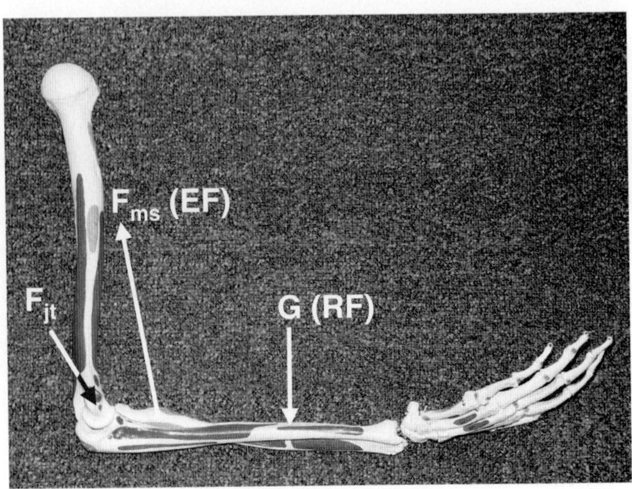

FIGURE 3–6. Arm being held at 90 degrees (the joint reaction force $\vec{F}_{jt}$ is also shown).

move the horizontal segment. Please note that the moment arm for the biceps is quite short. The weight of the forearm–hand segment ($\vec{G}$)acts through the center of mass of the forearm–hand and it opposes the intended motion. Note that the moment arm for the gravitational force is quite long. If one wishes to keep the arm in a 90-degree orientation as shown in Figure 3 5, the sum of the moments acting about an axis through the elbow joint needs to be zero. For this to occur, $\vec{F}_{ms}$ needs to be considerably greater than $\vec{G}$ because of the difference in the moment arms of the two forces. In fact, if $\vec{F}_{ms}$ and $\vec{G}$ are the only forces acting on the forearm–hand segment, a zero moment at the elbow would imply that $\vec{F}_{ms} \times EA = \vec{G} \times RA$, or $\vec{F}_{ms}/\vec{G} = RA/EA$. However, for that static equilibrium to be established, not only does the sum of all moments about an axis through the elbow joint have to be zero, but the sum of all forces acting on the horizontal segment must be zero as well. Given the magnitudes and directions of the two forces shown in Figure 3–5, there must be at least one additional force acting on the horizontal segment so that a zero resultant force can be obtained. Figure 3–6 shows that this force is applied by the humerus on the radius in the form of a *joint reaction force* ($\vec{F}_{jt}$).

The concept of moments is important in understanding the loads imposed on the spinal column.[5] If a person is standing and bends forward at the hip (hip flexion), the weight of the upper body, arms, and head have a particularly long moment arm relative to sagittal plane axes through the centers of rotation in the lumbar spine, producing a sizable moment. For the tissues of the spine (muscular, fascial, tendinous, and ligamentous) to oppose that moment, great forces are required, because of the relatively short moment arm of these tissues relative to the lumbar spine rotation centers. Like the joint reaction force described above for the elbow, there will be compressive forces acting on the lumbar vertebrae because of muscular, ligamentous, and other forces resisting the external moments created by the weight force during the forward bending action described above. The choice of which tissues resist the gravitational moment is the key to protecting the discs and vertebrae from excessive compression. *The greater the moment arm of the tissue providing the resistance moment, the smaller the force required to provide that resistance, and consequently the smaller the joint reaction forces and the compressive forces acting on the intervertebral discs.* A simple example may facilitate the understanding of this concept, using a man ("Person A") and a woman ("Person B") for two-person clarity. Take a long broom handle and place it in an anterior–posterior direction on the man's shoulder across the upper trapezius muscle (which will represent a lumbar disc). Place a 10-lb free weight on the anterior end of the handle (representing the flexion moment produced by gravity) while the woman holds the posterior end of the broom handle. The woman represents the resistance moment provided by the tissues of the lower back. Now have her slide her hands in an anterior direction along the broom handle until the hands are directly behind his upper trapezius. It should be noted that the compression on his upper trapezius becomes greater as her hands come closer. Eventually, if her hand contact is close enough to the upper trapezius, he may not be able to stand the pain of the load from the handle.

Kinematics

Most people can relate more easily to kinematics than kinetics because motion can usually be seen while forces cannot. However, the motions of lumbar vertebrae are very complex, and certainly not seen with the naked eye. For this prerequisite review some of the basic concepts in kinematics are provided.

Three coordinates can describe any point in space. These are typically designated along the x, y, and z axes of a Cartesian, right-handed coordinate system. However, the position of a rigid body in space cannot be described by the same system. Although the center of mass of that body can be located, its orientation is not quantified. For example, a vertebra sitting in space can have its center of mass described by x, y, and z coordinates, but it may be sitting upright, tilted by 45 degrees, lying on its side, upside down, etc. Therefore, along each x, y, and z axis, there is also a corresponding axis of rotation around that direction (see Fig. 3–7*B*). Thus, any body in space can be described as having 6 degrees of freedom of motion: 3 degrees of freedom can be used to describe the location of any point on the rigid body (e.g., the center of mass) along the x, y, and z directions, plus 3 degrees of freedom to describe the orientation of the rigid body around the axes of the coordinate system. These degrees of freedom will become important later as vertebral motion and the facet joints are discussed. In general, movement of the spine is not reported by x, y, and z coordinates, but rather by the anatomic planes. These anatomic planes are typically designated in reference to the x–y (coronal), x–z (transverse), and y–z (sagittal) planes of the coordinate system (see Fig. 3–7*A*).

Anatomic Planes and Motion Figure 3–8 shows a person in the "anatomic position." This figure is important, because physiologic motion will be discussed relative to this mannequin and the corresponding anatomic planes. For example, note that the palms of the hands face forward in the anatomic position. Therefore, if one stands in the anatomic position, curling the fingers into a fist would be described as "flexion" of the fingers. Subsequent wrist rotation of 180 degrees so that the palms face backwards and knuckles face forward, curling of the fingers into a fist is still "flexion" rather than extension, because this motion is *referenced* against the anatomic neutral position.

Based on the discussion above, the lumbar spine as a whole has 6 degrees of freedom of motion. While this following discussion would seem quite elementary, a clear explanation of the following movements provides a cornerstone for a variety of pertinent topics throughout this text. Imagine a man standing upright in the anatomic neutral position. Flexion is bending forward from the neutral position into a bow, with him looking "down" at the floor. Extension is leaning backwards from the neutral position, with him up looking "up" at the ceiling. Right lateral bending is bending over toward the right; imagine him standing with his hands by his sides, and sliding his right hand down his right thigh toward the knee. Left lateral bending is the same motion toward the left. Right rotation is spinning around his waist toward the right from the neutral position. Looking down from a "bird's-eye" view from above, he is spinning clockwise, and he should end up looking at the wall beside or behind him, depending on his degree of flexibility. Collectively, these movements are termed the ranges of motion of the lumbar spine.

Motion of the lumbar spine can be described as noted above, but in the scientific literature, motion is typically described for individual vertebrae or pairs of vertebrae. Table 3–1 summarizes the currently acknowledged ranges of motion for the lumbar spine and specific vertebrae. The numbers given represent the mean motion in degrees, followed by the lower and upper ranges in parentheses.

It can be observed clinically that most people have asymmetric ranges of motion—they can usually bend more to one side than the other. The values in Table 3–1

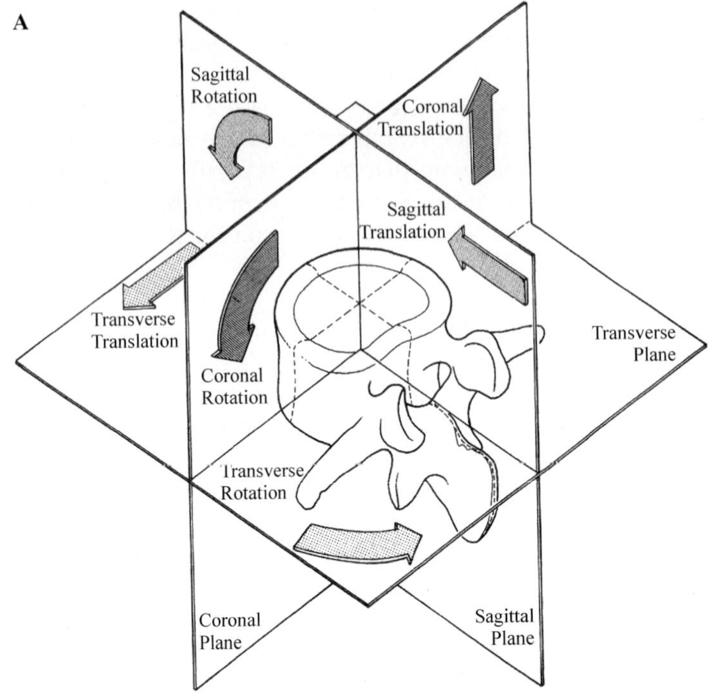

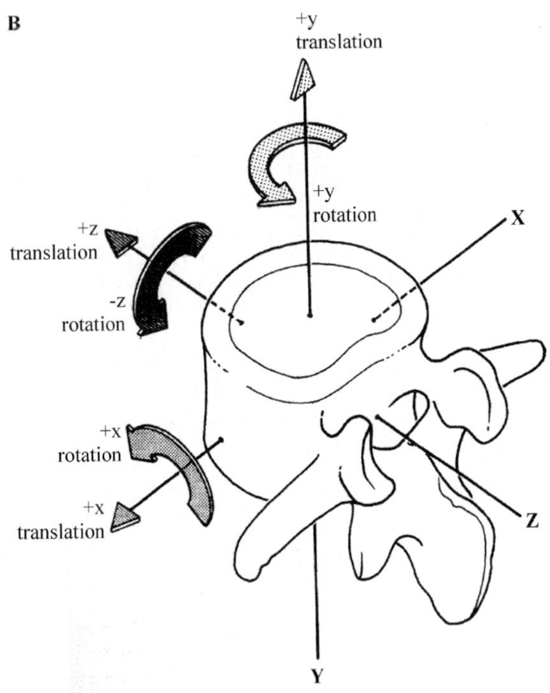

FIGURE 3–7. Principal planes (*A*) and principal axes (*B*) that are used to determine the linear and angular motion of a vertebra in space.

were obtained as an average over the general population. One point that needs emphasizing is the great range of values reported in Table 3–1. This range reflects the clinical observation that people vastly differ in their flexibility and stiffness values for lumbar motion segments.[7] Combined with the natural intrasubject asymmetries, it becomes extremely difficult for a conservative care practitioner to determine whether or not an observed asymmetry in range of motion, a vastly increased joint stiffness from normal, or an overall small range of motion represents a pathological finding, or is perfectly normal for the specific patient. So, why is it that motion segment L1–L2 has only 12 degrees of flexion while L5–S1 has 20 degrees? The

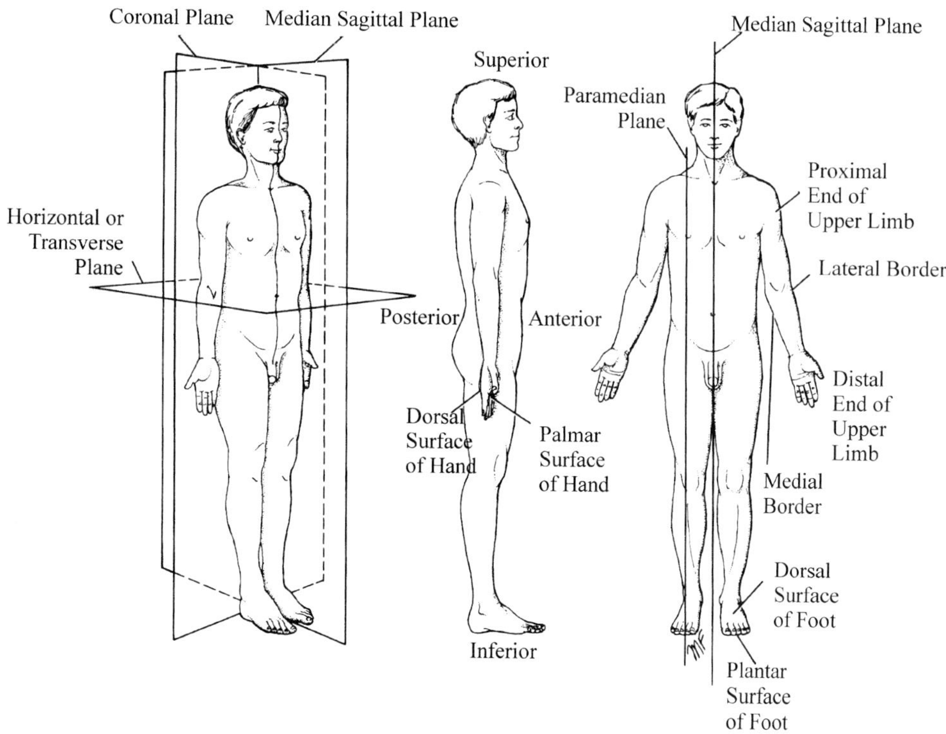

FIGURE 3–8. Principal planes of the human body.

answer lies partially in the orientation of the lumbar zygapophyseal or facet joints.

THE BIOMECHANICS OF THE LUMBAR SPINE

Now that the basic concepts in general biomechanics have been covered, it is appropriate to initiate a more specific discussion on the biomechanics of the spine itself. The human vertebral column is a complex structure of tissues that includes bones, joints, ligaments, muscles, connective tissues, nerves, blood vessels, and lymphatics. It functions as a whole; in isolation, any single structure cannot be understood in terms of the global physiologic functions of the spine. However, this same spinal complexity necessitates a reductionist approach to better understand its structure and function. Therefore, the following discussion will examine the lumbar spine by distilling it down to its components and systems. However, the reader is encouraged to bear in mind that lumbar and pelvic function and biomechanics cannot be adequately described by arithmetically adding all of its structural subunits. The understanding of how each structural subunit integrates into the whole lumbopelvic structure, and consequently affects the global biomechanics of the spine, is an area of growing research.

The topic of interest is the low back, which can be broadly described as the lumbar spine, the pelvis, the sacral spine plus the coccyx. Since the objective of this chapter is to review the biomechanics of the lumbosacral spine, the focus of this discussion will be those anatomic structures that have a direct effect on the physical mechanics and movement of the lumbar spine. Therefore, the innervation, blood supply, and lymphatic drainage will not be described.

TABLE 3–1. Range of Motion of Lumbar Motion Segments

Lumbar Motion Segment	Flexion plus Extension (degrees)	Lateral Bend (One Direction) (degrees)	Rotation (One Direction) (degrees)
L1–L2	12 (9–16)	6 (3–8)	2 (1–3)
L2–L3	14 (11–18)	6 (3–9)	2 (1–3)
L3–L4	15 (12–18)	8 (5–10)	2 (1–3)
L4–L5	17 (14–21)	6 (5–7)	2 (1–3)
L5–S1	20 (18–21)	3 (2–3)	5 (3–6)

Source: Adapted from White and Panjabi.[6]

FUNCTIONAL ANATOMY OF THE LUMBAR SPINE

From an engineering perspective, the lumbar spine represents a balance between the need for flexibility and the need for stability. These driving forces in the evolution of the lumbar spine are clearly reflected by its structure. The zygapophyseal joints, the ligaments, and the muscles that affect this region of the spine will be specifically addressed.

The Lumbar Zygapophyseal Joints

The zygapophyseal joints of the lumbar spine serve two main functions: First, they are weight-bearing structures; it has been reported that lumbar facets can carry up to 33% of the compressive load of the body, depending on the posture.[6] Furthermore, surgical resection of one or both facet joints of a vertebra generally leads to clinical instability. Second, since they are articulations, they allow for specific motions (and restrict other motions) of the lumbar spine. The heavy innervation of the lumbar facet joints with mechanosensitive and proprioceptive afferents also supports the notion of their key role in lumbosacral motion.[8]

The angulation of the facet joints varies throughout the lumbar spine; the upper lumbar facet joints tend to be longitudinal (~15 degrees from the coronal plane) and limit the amount of flexion–extension, whereas the facet joints of the lower lumbar spine tend to be diagonally oriented (~45 degrees from the coronal plane) and limit axial rotation while enabling flexion–extension. In general, the inclination of the facet joints increases sagittally as one moves inferiorly from L1 to L5. However, it must be kept in mind that the facets are curved rather than parallel. In any case, as a whole, the lumbar spine generally serves to resist torsion or rotation.

Clinical evidence suggests that facet joints may lose movement and become extremely stiff. The precise sequela leading to restricted motion in a stiff facet joint is not well understood. However, during conservative manipulative treatment of the involved motion segment, movement is thought to be reestablished, at least in part, through cavitation of the involved facet joint.

Research on finger joints demonstrates that application of a longitudinal force increases the corresponding metacarpophalangeal joint space. The amount of joint distraction is initially small, but upon cavitation of the joint, joint space increases, the joint becomes less stiff, and the range of motion is increased. Scientific evidence suggests that the articular noises associated with joint manipulation (i.e., high-velocity, low-amplitude thrust maneuvers) of the low back represent cavitation events of lumbar facet joints. The clinical interpretation of hearing (and feeling) this articular release is typically that of a successful treatment, and it is associated with increasing the range of motion and decreasing the stiffness of the affected motion segment. Whether this interpretation is correct remains a topic of scientific debate. However, it has been shown convincingly that "cavitation" does not produce a muscular reflex response,[9] as had been proposed in the literature.[10]

Although it is well acknowledged, and universally accepted, that spinal segments move relative to one another during everyday movements, an important question in conservative back care was whether relative movements of adjacent vertebrae could be achieved in the so-called "paraphysiological" zone, and if so, how much that movement might be. The paraphysiological zone of movement is defined here as the range of motion beyond that achieved by passive guidance with an appropriate force. When practitioners move a motion segment to the end range of passive motion, and then exert a thrust-like (high-speed, low-amplitude) force, the perception is that of motion. However, it is impossible to say whether that "perceived" motion was caused by neighboring motion segments that were not at the end range of passive motion, or if it was actual motion of the target segment beyond the passive range of motion. In a series of studies, Gál et al.[11,12] demonstrated on fresh unembalmed cadaveric specimens, using high-speed cinematography and three-dimensional kinematic analysis procedures, that movements in the paraphysiological zone indeed occurred with treatment. The relative movements were measured to be in the range of 1 mm in linear and 1 degree in angular displacement. These are relative movements that could cause facet joint cavitation, and may cause the increased range of motion and decreased joint stiffness following the thrust-like manipulative procedures.

Often, it is assumed that the vertebrae move freely in all 6 degrees of freedom. However, this is not the case in the intact spine. Owing to the orientation of the facets, ligamentous restraints, and muscular force, motions are generally *coupled* in the lumbar spine. For example, lateral bending of the lumbar spine in vivo is accompanied by axial rotation of the vertebrae toward the concavity created by the bending, and vice versa—rotation is accompanied by lateral bending.[13] In theory, any one particular motion (e.g., flexion) may be coupled to all five other degrees of freedom. However, in reality, motions are typically coupled to only one or two more motions to a varying extent, and the coupled motions are generally less than one-half the magnitude of the primary motion. The magnitude of the various coupled motions also depends on the specific lumbar vertebra involved. Flexion of the lumbar vertebra is accompanied by forward translation of the vertebrae in the sagittal plane, which helps to approximate the facet joint surfaces. Essentially, the vertebra tips forward as it bends forward. Extension is the reverse of flexion—there is a rotation of the vertebra backwards accompanied by a posterior translation of the vertebra.

The Lumbar Spinal Ligaments

In general, the lumbosacral spine derives most of its mechanical stability from its ligamentous and muscular support. In the living spine, the ligaments serve several functions, the most important of which is giving physical stability to the spine while allowing physiologic movement. Although the muscles can accomplish the same task, they require an active expenditure of energy. In contrast, ligaments provide passive support without energy cost.

In addition to their structural role in lumbopelvic biomechanics, ligaments also serve a functional role in that they provide afferent sensory feedback to the central nervous system to aid in performing the constant, second-by-second, balancing trick required to maintain bipedalism. Proprioceptors found in these ligaments, such as stretch receptors, constantly inform the spinal cord and higher centers of the instantaneous position, orientation, and alignment of the spine. In this section, the mechanically most important ligaments from posterior or dorsal to anterior will be described.

From an engineering perspective, ligaments are strongest in tension along the direction parallel to their fibers. Ligaments cannot support compressive loads and merely buckle if loaded. There is some similarity between ligaments and the steel cables that support a suspension bridge. Both structures are slightly elastic and can stretch, but are susceptible to fatigue failure if heavy loads are imposed over a long period. If one extends the suspension bridge analogy to the structure and functions of ligaments, then it becomes apparent why there are so many ligaments. For each degree of freedom of movement that the vertebral column has, there must be a corresponding ligament to stabilize the spine in that direction and restrict the motion beyond its physiologic end range. Naturally, there are large, strong ligaments that function along the major axes of motion, but there is also a vast array of small ligaments that are either vestigial or serve to restrict motion in some small but specific way. The physiologic strains tolerated by the major lumbar ligaments are summarized graphically in Figure 3–9.

Ligaments of the spine can fail. Rissanen[14] found that 20% of human cadaveric spines contained partially ruptured interspinous ligaments. Ligaments are virtually impossible to tear during normal everyday movements because of the small strains and strain rates produced in these activities. It appears that failure of ligaments at slow rates of stretching results in avulsion injuries, while high rates of loading produces mid-substance failures. Therefore, one might speculate that the large number of back ligament injuries observed on autopsy may be the results of trauma (e.g., from falling and contact sports) rather than from daily labor in physically demanding job situations.

The Muscles of the Lumbar Spine

The muscles of the low back serve two primary roles: (1) to move the lumbar spine through its range of motion while restricting unwanted movements, and (2) to increase the stiffness and stability of the lumbar

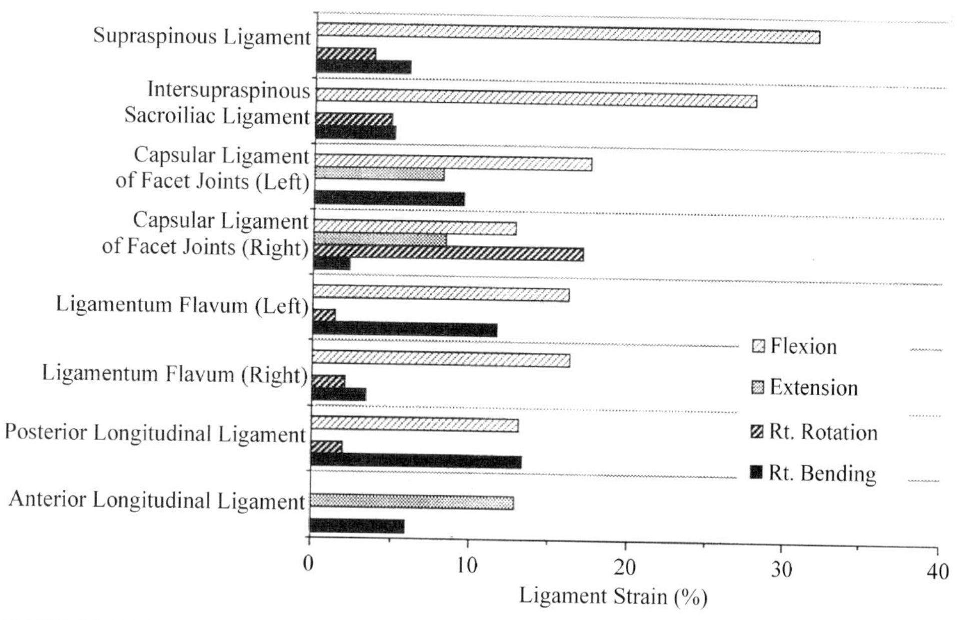

FIGURE 3–9. Physiologic strains that are tolerated by the major lumbar ligaments.

spine, for example to provide stability for controlled movement of the extremities. The properties of a muscle will vary depending on whether it is active or passive. The passive, inactivated muscle has physical characteristics similar to those of other soft tissues in the spine, whereas actively contracting muscle is the only tissue that can produce controlled force. If the muscles are fatigued because of repetitive cycles of loading, they may lose their protective functions in vivo. This potentially exposes individuals to injuries under circumstances where external loads could normally be tolerated safely.[15]

The spine is a highly unstable structure. Its shape (an essentially long, thin rod) makes the spine vulnerable to buckling failure. Buckling is the type of failure that occurs when a drinking straw is compressed longitudinally. Initially, the drinking straw will flex slightly under very little load, and then, all of a sudden will buckle (collapse) and no load can be supported anymore. Similarly, the unsupported human spine can merely withstand axial compression of about 20 N before it buckles.[16] Obviously, under physiologic, in vivo conditions this does not occur, otherwise human spines would fail just under the weight of the upper body.

Buckling of the spine in real life is prevented by a continuous and well-controlled activation of the back muscles. Specifically, co-contraction of pair (left and right) muscles provides the stiffness and stability that is required by the spine to withstand everyday loading, including the continuous support of body weight.

Researchers have attempted for a long time to determine the exact control of forces in back muscles during static weight bearing tasks and dynamic tasks of everyday living. Unfortunately, such attempts, although often excellently performed, have not had the desired success for two reasons: first, direct muscle force measurements in the back musculature are virtually impossible and, to the authors' knowledge, have never been performed in living humans; and second, theoretical approaches aimed at calculating the forces from measured external forces and electromyogram (EMG) are prone to large errors, because of the inherent redundancy of the musculoskeletal system "low back," and the grave uncertainties in relating electromyographic measurements to the corresponding muscle forces.

Let us consider these points. Direct, in vivo muscle force measurements are standard in a variety of experimental animal models.[17–19] However, such measurements can only be easily performed in muscles with long, free running tendons, a rarity in the low back. In addition, human ethics protocols are very strict; therefore, in vivo muscle force measurements in humans have been the exception, and have typically just been performed in very special circumstances. And, when such measurements have been made, calibration of the force transducers was done using a theoretical inverse dynamics approach,[20] thereby rendering the absolute force results unreliable.

Regarding the theoretical calculation of individual muscle forces, one has to deal with the redundancy of the musculoskeletal system.[21] Mathematically, a redundant system is a set of equations that contains more unknown variables than there are equations. Such a system of equations cannot be solved in a unique way. Consider the system below, consisting of one equation and two unknowns (x, y).

$$x + y = 10$$

This system has an infinite number of solutions; for example, $x = 10$, $y = 0$; or $x = 5$, $y = 5$; or $x = 0.3$, $y = 9.7$; or $x = 20$, $y = -10$; etc.

Musculoskeletal redundancy is characterized by the fact that the spine (and most other human and animal joints) has more muscles than there are degrees of freedom. For example, knee extension (1 degree of freedom) can be accomplished with any combination of forces from the four principal knee extensor muscles. The same is true for the spine, its joints, and its degrees of freedom. Reviews on the musculoskeletal redundancy problem, or the "general distribution problem," as it is typically called in biomechanics, are widely available.[21,22]

The most frequently used approach to solve the general distribution problem in biomechanics is optimization theory. This approach is based on two premises: First, it is known from direct, in vivo muscle force, and indirect, in vivo electromyographic measurements that a given task is typically performed in a stereotypical way. This means when a person walks, the coordination patterns of the muscles and the force contributions of the muscles to the required joint moments are similar from step to step. This occurs despite the musculoskeletal redundancy that, in theory, would allow for each consecutive step to be executed with a variety of different muscle force patterns. Second, it has been assumed that the stereotypic patterns of muscle force coordination are the result of optimizing a physiologic function, for example, the maximization of endurance,[21] the minimization of the metabolic cost of movement,[23,24] or, for the spine, the optimization of stability or stiffness. Although none of these optimization functions has been shown to be correct to date, the idea that muscles may be recruited and activated according to some overriding optimization rule has been proposed for centuries,[25] and, if the publication of scientific literature in this area is any indication, remains an appealing solution still today.

A special problem with the muscles of the back and their biomechanical function is the fact that many muscles span multiple joints (motion segments), that they have a broad range of geometries, and that their moment arms relative to the instantaneous joint axes remain unknown, as the instantaneous joint axes of vertebral motion segments in dynamic tasks remain ill described. McGill[26] describes the nonintuitive case of the quadratus lumborum and psoas. Psoas has often been identified as a stabilizer of the lumbar spine because of its anatomical position. However, its activation profile[27] suggests that psoas is very much a hip flexor rather than a lumbar spine stabilizer. On the basis of further electromyographic evidence, McGill[26] argues that likely quadratus lumborum exercises the spinal stabilization function often associated with psoas. Although the electromyographic evidence appears quite clear on this issue, the reader should be reminded that electromyographic activity should not be equated with muscle force. It is quite possible, although unlikely in the above case, that a high level of EMG is associated with no force (e.g., because of the length of the muscle[28]) while an electrically silent muscle may provide force, very much like a passive structure, such as a ligament. Therefore, inferring biomechanical function from electromyographic activity alone must always be considered with some caution.

So far, muscles have been discussed only as force generators that stabilize the spine, produce movements, and are capable of producing great torques for heavy lifting. However, there exist a number of small muscles in the back with minimal moment arms about the spinal axes of rotation. These muscles seem ill suited to produce forces and torques, especially when compared to some of the powerful muscles that exist in the low back region. The rotators are such small muscles that connect adjacent vertebrae and have been implicated to assist rotation of the spine. Similarly, the intertransversarii also attach to adjacent vertebrae in a fashion that contraction would create lateral flexion. Interestingly, it has been found that the rotators and intertransversarii have a 5–7 times greater density of muscle spindles[29] than other, larger muscles of the back. Muscle spindles are highly effective proprioceptors of muscle length and muscle rate of stretch. The anatomic placement of the rotators and intertransversarii between adjacent vertebrae, thus, could provide an intricate system of detection of relative location and position, as well as the rate of change of location and position, of adjacent vertebral bodies. Although not proven directly, such proprioceptive function of these muscles seems quite possible, and has been suggested previously, based on anecdotal evidence.[26]

Interestingly, when giving a high-speed, low-amplitude spinal manipulative treatment, reflex responses are observed consistently,[30] and some of these reflex responses have been directly associated with the reflex arc of the muscle spindles. It would be of interest to investigate if these spindle reflex responses originate in the rotators and intertransversarii, and therefore, might provide direct evidence of relative vertebral movement during spinal manipulative treatment.

HISTORY DEPENDENCE OF BACK PROPERTIES

The last piece of background information needed to understand low back injury and rehabilitation is how the tissues of the back respond to loading over time. The human spine is a viscoelastic structure. Although the bony part of the spine may be considered elastic without introducing great error, the associated soft tissue structures (tendon, muscles, ligaments, discs, and cartilage) are clearly viscoelastic and dominate the overall mechanical properties of the spine. Mechanically, the term *elastic* means that the force of a material (e.g., during compression) is always given as a function of its deformation, whereas the term *viscoelastic* means that not only deformation, but also the speed of deformation determines a material's instantaneous force. Therefore, the force response of a viscoelastic material depends on its deformation history. Some of the rate constants of the viscoelastic behavior of the spine are low, and the mechanical response of the spine depends exquisitely on the history of spine loading and deformation for the past few minutes, rather than seconds.

This long-lasting viscoelasticity of the human spine has potential implications for clinical practice. For example, one would expect the range of motion of the spine to be smaller, and stiffness to be greater in the fully hydrated spine (just after getting out of bed) compared to a less hydrated spine (at the end of the day). Similarly, if one wants to lift a heavy load, the chances of getting injured are greater when attempting to do so while sitting for the past 2 hours compared to having lifted similar weights just previously. Often, understanding a back injury has more to do with what a person did before the injury occurred, rather than what the person did at the time of injury occurrence.

THE SIGNIFICANCE OF LOADS ON THE LUMBAR SPINE TO INJURY AND REHABILITATION

The lumbar spine is continuously exposed to mechanical loading through the forces of gravity, muscular contraction, ligamentous tension, and disc compression. This section will discuss how everyday activities impose mechanical loads on the spine. It is hoped that these considerations might provide some insight into how low back injuries may occur. Advice will be provided that might help prevent injury or may improve the rehabilitation process.

Flexion–Extension Loads

The majority of work on range of motion and spinal loading has been done on sagittal plane motion (flexion–extension). The relevant question here is "Does sagittal plane motion cause low back injury?" It was commonly believed in the past that disc herniations resulted from a single excessive load.[31] However, it would appear that the production of a disc herniation is a process rather than a single event.[31] In one study, it was found that disc herniations occur with some regularity from repetitive flexion–extension cycles.[31] When axial compression was increased during these flexion–extension cycles, disc injuries appeared to occur with greater frequency and severity. What are the biomechanical reasons for such an observation? It has been determined that bending to full flexion changes the line of action of longissimus thoracis and iliocostalis lumborum, compromising their role to support anterior shear forces on the spine.[32] Macintosh et al.[33] found that there was a major change in shear forces in flexed postures as compared to upright standing. In that particular study they determined that flexion resulted in a net posterior shear force at the L5–S1 segment. McGill[34] states that the interspinous ligament is the dominant component in resistance to flexion. This ligament also creates large shear components that must be resisted by the zygapophyseal joint complex.

Adams and Dolan[35] found that repeated flexion in vitro over a period of minutes reduced the peak bending moment of the lumbar spine by 17%. In other words, the spines ability to resist a flexion load is decreasing as a result of the repeated load imposed upon it. A sustained 5-minute flexed posture reduced the bending moment by 42%. Adams[35] makes the point that if ligaments are stretched during prolonged flexed postures, such as might occur during sitting and gardening, then it is probably not wise to follow that activity with vigorous exercise, because the intervertebral discs would be lacking some ligamentous protection. Kong et al.[36] found that intradiscal pressures, forces in ligaments, and the load across facet joints increase with increased trunk flexion. These forces are increased when subjects held a load in their hands. Increasing the handheld loads, or increasing trunk flexion, resulted in an increase in the load-bearing role of the musculature compared to passive structures. The study by Kong et al.[36] provides some rationale to avoid activities that require repetitive flexion–extension cycles, especially when there is insufficient time for tissues to recover from the load imposed upon them.

Clinical Pearl: If the spinal ligaments are stretched during prolonged flexed postures, such as might occur during sitting and gardening, then it is probably not wise to follow that activity with an immediate bout of vigorous exercise, because the intervertebral discs may be lacking some ligamentous protection.

Lateral Bending Loads

Studies have revealed that lateral bending results in a considerable amount of coactivation of the muscles of the trunk.[37,38] Muscles on both sides of the trunk are activated to satisfy a lateral bending reaction torque, and to provide for spinal stabilization.[37] Without coactivation, the stability of the spine would be compromised during lateral flexion motions. As a consequence of the coactivation, spinal loads increase by as much as 25%, as compared to the situation with no coactivation.[38] The type of loading that is most likely affected by the coactivation of muscles in lateral bending is compression, anterior–posterior shear, and lateral shear. This type of loading has been implicated as a possible mechanism for increased risk of injury in the workplace.

Clinical Pearl: When people bend laterally, muscles on both sides of the trunk are activated, presumably to provide stability to the trunk during such movements. Without coactivation, the spine might be more likely to buckle during lateral flexion, and so become injured.

Axial Twisting Loads

Trunk twisting appears to load the spine and trunk muscles less than trunk flexion or holding weights in front of the body.[39] Nevertheless, axial twisting may represent a significant risk for spinal injury. Spinal compression, flexion–extension, and lateral bending moments are all generated during twisting movements.[40] According to McGill,[41] nonmuscular, passive tissues contribute significantly to axial torque, and the flexed and twisted spine is less able to resist applied torques than the straight and untwisted spine, thereby increasing the risk for injury.

Clinical Pearl: Trunk twisting appears to load the spine and trunk muscles less than trunk flexion or holding weights in front of the body. Nevertheless, axial twisting may represent a significant risk for spinal injury. Spinal compression, flexion–extension, and lateral bending moments are all generated during twisting movements.

Loads on the Spine Resulting from Lifting

Low back injury is a common occurrence during lifting activities. As a result, considerable research has been focused on the loads imposed on the low back during lifting tasks. A dramatic example of loading during lifting occurs in the sport of power lifting. It has been determined that compressive loads at L4–L5 of up to 17,000 N are not uncommon in power lifting.[42] In other words, the lumbar vertebrae of these athletes experience compressive loads of nearly 20 times their own body weight.

Flexion–extension moments of the spine tend to increase with increasing loads that must be lifted during a given task.[43,44] Also, the distance of the load in front of the person performing the task affects the load on the spine. It has been determined that the greater the distance from load to person, the greater the moment produced at L4–L5. When this distance exceeded 40 cm, the effect of the load on the L4–L5 moment was greatly amplified. This result was attributed to a change in the lifting technique that had to be adopted under these circumstances.[45]

Another factor that affects loading of the low back during lifting is the speed of lifting. Fast lifts have been shown to increase the peak low back extensor moment by 60%, as compared to slow lifts.[46] In addition, fast lifts have been shown to increase the torsion, and lateral-bending moments compared to slow lifts.[44,47] These results are to be expected as fast lifting will involve greater accelerations than slow lifting, and therefore, in accordance with Newton's second law of motion, the forces must be increased as well.

Another significant factor affecting injuries in lifting is fatigue. Marras and Granata[48] determined the spinal loading of workers during lifting tasks over a 5-hour period. It was observed that the workers changed their lifting technique and movement patterns significantly during the 5-hour test period. Spinal compressive loads decreased while anterior–posterior shear loads increased over time. These changed loading conditions at the end of the test period are typically associated with an increased risk for low back injury. Dolan and Adams[49] asked subjects to lift and lower a weight from the floor to their waist 100 times. By the end of the 100 lifts, the lumbar spine was being flexed an additional 7%, the bending moment acting on the lumbar spine increased and fatigue (as measured by electromyography) was apparent in the erector spinae musculature. When the spine is substantially flexed, even small increases in flexion cause relatively large increases in bending moment because the spine's resistance to bending increases rapidly as full flexion is approached. This increase in spinal bending was accompanied by a small decrease in peak extensor moment and spinal compression. The authors suggested that this reduction in peak extensor moment might reflect a change to a more stooped (bent back) posture as the muscles fatigued. They state that lifting with a bent back reduces extensor moments as it allows the subject to lean directly over the weight and bring it closer to the center of rotation in the intervertebral discs. However, even though the peak extensor moment decreased with fatigue, that part of it which was due to passive tension in noncontractile tissues would have increased because of the increase in lumbar flexion.

Finally, it has been shown that asymmetrical lifts produce a unique spinal loading pattern. Typically, lifts that are asymmetrical (i.e., not purely in the sagittal plane) increase the lateral bending and twisting moments.[50] In some studies, it has also been found that spine compression and lateral shear forces increased as lifting became more asymmetric.

What conclusions can be drawn about safe lifting? First, avoid flexion of the lumbar spine because it produces anterior shear on the vertebral bodies. Second, reduce the speed of lifting. Third, provide adequate rest periods between lifting tasks to avoid excessive muscular fatigue. Fourth, lift balanced loads in the sagittal plane to avoid asymmetric loading of the spine. Finally, hold objects as close to the body as possible during lifting to minimize the resultant extensor moment in the low back needed to counter the flexion moment caused by the object that is lifted.

Clinical Pearl: What conclusions can be drawn about safe lifting? First, avoid flexion of the lumbar spine because it produces anterior shear on the vertebral bodies. Second, reduce the speed of lifting. Third, provide adequate rest periods between lifting tasks to avoid excessive muscular fatigue. Fourth, lift balanced loads in the sagittal plane to avoid asymmetric loading of the spine. Finally, hold objects as close to the body as possible during lifting to minimize the resultant extensor moment in the low back needed to counter the flexion moment caused by the object that is lifted.

Does pain act as a warning of ill-advised lifting postures? One study would suggest that it does. Patients with chronic LBP were asked to lift in various postures, and it was determined that the peak L4–L5 reaction moments were less for a lifting posture that produced lower levels of self-reported back pain.[51] When interpreting the clinical significance of this study, it must be kept in mind that in addition to the L4–L5 reaction moments, there are many other things that may have changed when the subjects changed their posture. The study only suggests a correlation between the reaction moments and pain rather than a causal relationship.

Another point of interest may be the use of lifting belts. It has been suggested that lifting belts restrict motion of the torso and stiffen the spine, thereby protecting the tissues of the back. It has been determined that lifting belts indeed increased the stiffness about the frontal (lateral bending) and longitudinal axis (axial rotation) of the spine.[52] However, stiffness about a transverse axis (flexion–extension) seemed unaffected by the lifting belt. In another study, it was found that lifting belts reduced peak trunk angles, velocities, and accelerations of the trunk during a lift to upright posture. On average, there was a statistically significant reduction in spinal load associated with the use of an elastic lifting belt. However, it should be noted that despite this result being statistically significant, the data were so variable that some subjects actually experienced an increase in spinal loading while wearing the belt.[53] In a third study, subjects were asked to lift a box to a height of 79 cm and 60 degrees to the right. It was found that lifting belts reduced maximum spine flexion, spine flexion–extension angular velocities, and torso lateral bending angular velocity during the assigned task. On the other hand, the lifting belts increased hip and knee flexion. Subjects with belts lifted more slowly and used a squat lift technique rather than a stooping technique in which the lumbar spine is flexed.[54]

What is the effect of wearing a lifting belt on muscle activity in the low back? Thomas et al.[55] determined that the lifting belt reduced the peak-normalized EMG of the erector spinae group by an average of 3% during asymmetric lifts, but increased it by 2% in symmetric lifts. Others studied the effect of lifting belts on trunk muscle activity and intra-abdominal pressure (IAP).[56] An increase in IAP was found when subjects were wearing a belt compared to the no-belt condition. If the belt relieved the direct compressive load on the spine or assisted IAP to produce an extensor moment, then this would be reflected in diminished extensor muscle activity. As expected, holding the breath reduced extensor muscle activity, but wearing a belt did not augment this effect. From these results, it was concluded that prescription of abdominal belts to workers is not justified. Lavender et al.[57] suggested that lifting belts appear to alter the muscular response strategy in an unexpected manner. They concluded that the belt's effect might be less biomechanical and more psychological.

Clinical Pearl: Should workers wear a lifting belt to protect their lumbar spines? Studies regarding lifting belts have failed to show that they protect the low back.

Loads on the Lumbar Spine while Sitting

With a significant portion of the population of the industrialized world sitting in front of computers for large portions of their day, loading of the lumbar spine caused by sitting must be understood. Long periods of sitting may cause LBP.[58] So, is sitting worse for the lumbar spine than standing? In one study, it was found that people who rarely or never sit on their jobs had the highest incidence of LBP. Workers who sit frequently for short periods of time typically have a low incidence of LBP. [59] This finding is supported by the results of a study in which spinal shrinkage was measured for standing and sitting over a 6.5-hour work period.[60] Spinal shrinkage has been used as an indirect indicator of the compressive loading on the lumbar spine. It was found that standing produced 4.16 mm and sitting 1.73 mm of shrinkage. This result might be interpreted as an indication of greater compressive loading for standing compared to sitting. But other biomechanical variables should also be considered. Callaghan and McGill[61] determined differences in muscle activation between standing and unsupported sitting. They found that the erector spinae group had greater activation for sitting than standing. In fact, standing appeared to provide a rest for the erector spinae muscles, possibly because some of the loading was taken up by passive tissues.

What may be some of the strategies that can be used to reduce loading of the lumbar spine during sitting? It is assumed that loading is shared by many vertebral components when maintaining a lordotic posture, whereas flexed postures produce an increase in tensile forces in the region of the posterior annulus.[62] Callaghan and Dunk[63] found that electromyographic activity of the thoracic erector spinae decreases with a slumped sitting posture. According to the authors, since the thoracic erector spinae muscles have been shown to cross the lumbar spine and generate moments about the L4–L5 joint, the response of the thoracic erector spinae would be affected by the lumbar spine angle adopted in seated postures. Slumped sitting would likely increase the moment at the lumbar spine, as the center of gravity of the upper body would be displaced anterior to the L4–L5 joint. Since there is no increase in lumbar muscle activity and a decrease in thoracic activation levels during slumped sitting, it is likely that the passive tissues (ligaments, lumbodorsal fascia, etc.) of the spine would support the load moment. What strategy could possibly be used to produce a lumbar lordosis? It has been found that a posterior tilt of a seat combined with a reclined backrest produces lordosis of the low back.[64] In another study, the seat was modified to unload the ischial tuberosities and shift some of the loading to the thighs. This resulted in increased lumbar lordosis, sacral inclination, and lumbar spine disc height, and decreased muscular activity.[65] Furthermore, backrests with an anterior curvature produce the greatest lordosis.[66] However, a lordotic seat posture was also associated with a great amount of shrinkage, and hence, presumably, great lumbar spine loading.

Scientific evidence is confusing in this area of research, and the best sitting posture in terms of low back loading has not been identified. Researchers are coming to the conclusion that an important strategy to avoid LBP during sitting is to vary the posture.[61,67]. Prolonged posture leads to static loading of the soft tissues, and eventually may cause discomfort. Sitting still is also associated with an accumulation of metabolites, accelerating disc degeneration leading to disc herniation.[67] Therefore, static positions should be avoided, and the seated workers are advised to alter their position frequently, and include periods of standing and walking as part of their work routine. The constant change of posture causes loading of different tissues, thereby ensuring that no single tissue is subjected to long periods of static loading.

Clinical Pearl: Researchers are coming to the conclusion that an important strategy to avoid LBP during sitting is to vary the posture. Prolonged posture leads to static loading of the soft tissues, and eventually may cause discomfort.

Loads on the Lumbar Spine while Walking

Many clinicians suggest walking as a form of rehabilitation from low back injury. To determine if this is a wise choice of therapy, it is important to examine the loads imposed on the lumbar spine while walking. The peak disc compressive loads of the lumbar spine during walking vary between approximately 1.5 and 3 times body weight.[68,69]. In general, spinal loading increased as walking velocity increases. In addition, zygapophyseal joint forces generally increased with the cadence of walking. Peak *z*-joint forces were found to occur right after heel strike and toe-off.

Muscle activity in the low back during walking is concentrated in the extensors, which show a burst of activity at the time of ipsilateral toe-off.[70] Callaghan et al.[71] suggested that tissue loading during walking is below the levels caused by other rehabilitation tasks, suggesting that walking is a wise choice for general exercise and rehabilitation programs. One might assume that slow walking is better than fast walking, as the peak loads are lower. However, Callaghan et al.[71] noted that slow walking with restricted arm swinging produces a more static load, which may be more detrimental to certain tissues and may cause injuries at a greater rate than the more dynamic loading observed while walking fast.

If walking fast is a wise choice for general exercise,[71] then what are the effects of running on low back loading? Increased running speed has been associated with greater spinal shrinkage, and therefore, presumably, greater compressive loading of the spine.[72] The greatest shrinkage appears to occur in the first 15 minutes of the run, suggesting that shrinkage is a viscoelastic phenomenon, and thus presumably not a very good indicator of compressive spinal loading over time. Shrinkage in subjects with chronic LBP and asymptomatic individuals was found to be the same for a given running protocol.[72] The risk of LBP associated with jogging has been found to be low.[73] It has been suggested that jogging may protect from LBP. However, poor running technique, including excessive forward bending of the trunk, must be avoided.[74]

Clinical Pearl: Are the levels of spinal loading during walking considered safe for a rehabilitation program? Tissue loading during walking appears to be below the levels caused by other rehabilitation tasks, suggesting that walking is a wise choice for general exercise and rehabilitation programs.

Loads on the Lumbar Spine while Exercising

Clinicians frequently recommend abdominal exercises for rehabilitation of low back problems, or for preventing them to occur in the first place. An in-depth explanation of rehabilitative exercises and their clinical strategic utilization is covered in the rehabilitation section of this textbook (see Chapters 26–30), but a few relevant activities will be briefly covered here from a biomechanical perspective.

Sit-ups with bent knees has been said to stop psoas activation, but this idea has been disputed.[27] A flexed knee position was believed to realign psoas, and, as a consequence, it had been argued anecdotally that spinal compression might be reduced. However, psoas' line of action was found to not to change with flexed knees, and its activity for bent knee sit-ups appeared to be greater than during straight knee sit-ups. Of course, it is virtually impossible to determine the line of action of any muscle in vivo, and increased electromyographic activity does not necessarily translate to greater muscle force; thus, these results must be considered with caution. Nevertheless, McGill[5] recommends that most people should not perform sit-ups, but suggests a side bridge exercise for safer and more effective rehabilitation and prevention of low back injury. For lack of measurement of any disc pressures, or any internal forces, during these exercises, this recommendation that is based on the electromyographic levels of a single muscle must be taken as anecdotal. The side bridge exercise is practically demonstrated in Chapter 30.

Other clinicians have suggested that back extensor exercises are an important rehabilitation and prevention strategy. Exercises involving active trunk extension produced high joint forces and muscle activity levels.[75] Exercises with the spine held isometrically with leg extension demonstrated asymmetrical activity in the trunk muscles, thereby decreasing the load on the spine. In such an exercise, the patient starts in a position on their hands and knees. They then simply lift one leg and thigh in the direction of extension so that the lower limb becomes nearly parallel to the floor. They then reassume the hands and knee position and then lift the opposite leg and thigh. They concluded that single-leg extension tasks constitute a low risk exercise for initial extensor strengthening given the low spine load and mild extensor challenge. When combined with contralateral arm extensions, the challenge and demand of the exercise can be increased as the rehabilitation progresses. So in this case, the patient does exactly the same thing as with the leg extensions, except that in addition they lift the opposite arm and forearm until they are nearly parallel to the floor.

Another exercise that is frequently prescribed for low back rehabilitation is bicycling. Bicycling is said to prevent the ground reaction forces associated with running and walking. However, it has been stated that 30%–70% of cyclists suffer from cervical, thoracic, or lumbar back pain.[76] It has been suggested that one of the main problems causing these back problems was the seat angle. When the seat was adjusted so that there was an anterior inclination, there was a decrease in the hyperextension of the pelvic–spine angle, and 70% of cyclists with LBP reported a major improvement in the incidence and magnitude of their back pain. In another study, it has been suggested that cyclists' incidence of LBP can be reduced by placing the crank and pedals behind the saddle axis.[77] This position was said to produce more physiologic spine angles, resulting from a change in pelvis position. Finally, it has been determined that mechanical loading of the spine can be reduced by shifting weight onto the upper limbs, a position which is adopted by triathletes and competitive cyclists during time trials.[78] Therefore, cycling can be a beneficial exercise provided that the time is taken to ensure proper positioning on the bicycle.

Clinical Pearl: Sit-ups are said to impose large compressive loads on the spine, although direct load measurements have not been performed to date.

SUMMARY

Having reviewed some of the basic anatomy and biomechanics of the lumbar spine, it is now important to add all of the individual constituents to construct a dynamic, three-dimensional spine. This is a challenging mental exercise for most. Plastic models of the spine are useful for this purpose, but lack ligaments and muscles to simulate the biomechanics of the in vivo spine. Mathematical modeling is a promising avenue of investigation, but has inherently limited application to the in vivo lumbar spine.[79] To further confound this, the human spine is a living, growing structure that heals itself and adapts in a physiologically meaningful way to external stimuli. The bones can grow and deform, the discs can imbibe water or degenerate, the ligaments can change length, and the muscles vary in size and shape tremendously. Perhaps the clearest example of this point is the existence of coupled motions. Therefore, despite the static presentation of its biomechanics, the lumbar spine is a dynamic structure that defies current approaches to its complete description and understanding.

Despite these limitations, researchers endeavor to understand the loading characteristics of the lumbar spine during various activities, so that injury, from both a causative and preventative perspective, can be better understood and rehabilitation protocols can be based on increasingly sound scientific evidence for more effective recovery.

REFERENCES

1. Zdeblick TA. The treatment of degenerative lumbar disorders—A critical review of the literature. *Spine* 1995;20:126S–137S.
2. Bigos SJ, Bowyer O, Braeen G. *Acute low back problems in adults.* AHCPR Clinical Practice Guideline No. 14. Rockville, MD: Agency for Health Care Policy and Research, 1994. AHCPR Publication No. 95–0643.
3. Evans D. Mechanisms and effects of spinal high-velocity, low-amplitude thrust manipulation: Previous theories. *J Manipulative Physiol Ther* 2002;25:251–262.
4. Herzog, W. Basic mechanics. In: Herzog W, ed. *Clinical biomechanics of spinal manipulation.* New York: Churchill Livingstone, 1998:1–25.
5. McGill SM. *Low back disorders: Evidence-based prevention and rehabilitation.* Champaign, IL: Human Kinetics, 2002.
6. Panjabi MM, White AA. Physical properties and functional biomechanics of the spine. In: Panjabi M and White A, eds. Clinical biomechanics of the Spine, 2nd ed. Philadelphia, PA: Lippincott Williams & Wilkins 1990.
7. Ashton-Miller JA, Schultz AB. Biomechanics of the human spine and trunk. In: Pandolf KB ed. *Exercise and sports science reviews*, Vol. 16. American College of Sports Medicine Series. New York: MacMillan, 1988.
8. McLain RE, Pickar JG: Mechanoreceptor endings in human thoracic and lumbar facet joints. *Spine* 1998;23:168–173.
9. Herzog W: On sounds and reflexes. *J Manipulative Physiol Ther* 1996;19:216–218.
10. Brodeur R: The audible release associated with joint manipulation. *J Manipulative Physiol Ther* 1995;18:155–164.
11. Gál J, Herzog W, Kawchuk G, et al. Biomechanical studies of spinal manipulative therapy (SMT): Quantifying the movements of vertebral bodies during SMT. *JCCA* 1994;38:11–24.

12. Gál J, Herzog W, Kawchuk G, et al. Movements of vertebrae during manipulative thrusts to unembalmed human cadavers. *J Manipulative Physiol Ther* 1997;20:30–40.
13. Triano JJ. The mechanics of spinal manipulation. In: Herzog W, ed. *Clinical biomechanics of spinal manipulation*. Philadelphia, PA: Churchill Livingstone, 2000:92–190.
14. Rissanen PM: The surgical anatomy and pathology of the supraspinous and interspinous ligaments of the lumbar spine with special reference to ligament ruptures. *Acta Orthop Scand Suppl* 1960;46:1516–1521.
15. Solomonow M, Zhou BH, Lu Y, et al. Biomechanics of increased exposure to lumbar injury caused by cyclic loading. Part 1. Loss of reflexive muscular stabilization. *Spine* 1999;24:2426–2434.
16. Lucas D, Bresler B. *Stability of the ligamentous spine*, Vol. 40. California: Biomechanics Laboratory, University of California, 1961.
17. Walmsley B, Hodgson JA, Burke RE: Forces produced by medial gastrocnemius and soleus muscles during locomotion in freely moving cats. *J Neurophysiol* 1978; 41:1203–1215.
18. Hodgson JA: The relationship between soleus and gastrocnemius muscle activity in conscious cats—A model for motor unit recruitment? *J Physiol* 1983;337:553–562.
19. Herzog W, Leonard TR: Validation of optimization models that estimate the forces exerted by synergistic muscles. *J Biomech* 1991;24S:31–39.
20. Andrews JG: Biomechanical analysis of human motion. *Kinesiology* 1974;4:32–42.
21. Crowninshield RD, Brand RA: A physiologically based criterion of muscle force prediction in locomotion. *J Biomech* 1981;14:793–801.
22. Herzog W. Force-sharing among synergistic muscles: Theoretical considerations and experimental approaches. In: Holloszy JO, ed. *Exercise and sport sciences reviews*, 24th ed. Baltimore, MD: Williams & Wilkins, 1996:173–202.
23. Dul J, Johnson GE, Shiavi R, et al. Muscular synergism. II. A minimum-fatigue criterion for load sharing between synergistic muscles. *J Biomech* 1984;17:675–684.
24. Dul J, Townsend MA, Shiavi R, et al. Muscular synergism. I. On criteria for load sharing between synergistic muscles. *J Biomech* 1984;17:663–673.
25. Weber W, Weber E. *Mechanik der menschlichen Gehwerkzeuge*. Göttingen: W. Fischer-Verlag, 1836.
26. McGill SM. Functional anatomy of the lumbar and thoracic spine. In: Herzog W, ed. *Clinical biomechanics of spinal manipulation*. Philadelphia, PA: Churchill Livingstone, 2000:26–49.
27. Juker D, McGill SM, Kropf P, et al. Quantitative intramuscular myoelectric activity of lumbar portions of psoas and the abdominal wall during a wide variety of tasks. *Med Sci Sports Exerc* 1998;30:301–310.
28. Gordon AM, Huxley AF, Julian FJ: The variation in isometric tension with sarcomere length in vertebrate muscle fibres. *J Physiol* 1966;184:170–192.
29. Nitz AJ, Peck D: Comparisons of muscle spindle concentrations in large and small human epaxial muscles acting in parallel combinations. *Am Surg* 1986;52:273–277.
30. Herzog W, Scheele D, Conway PJW: Electromyographic responses of back and limb muscles associated with spinal manipulative therapy. *Spine* 1999;24:146–152.
31. Callaghan JP, McGill SM. Intervertebral disc herniation: Studies on a porcine model exposed to highly repetitive flexion/extension motion with compressive force. *Clin Biomech* 2001;16:28–37.
32. McGill SM, Hughson RL, Parks K. Changes in lumbar lordosis modify the role of the extensor muscles *Clin Biomech* 2000;15:777–780.
33. Macintosh JE, Bogduk N, Pearcey MJ. The effects of flexion on the geometry and actions of the lumbar erector spinae. *Spine* 1993;18:884–893.
34. McGill SM. Estimation of force and extensor moment contributions of the disc and ligaments at L4–L5. *Spine* 1988;13:1395–1402.
35. Adams MA, Dolan P. Time-dependent changes in the lumbar spine's resistance to bending. *Clin Biomech* 1996;11:194–200.
36. Kong WZ, Goel VK, Gilbertson LG, Weinstein JN. Effects of muscle dysfunction on lumbar spine mechanics. A finite element study based on a two motion segments model. *Spine* 1996;21:2197–2206.
37. McGill SM. A myoelectrically based dynamic three-dimensional model to predict loads on lumbar spine tissues during lateral bending. *J Biomech* 1992;25:395–414.
38. Marras WS, Granata KP. Spine loading during trunk lateral bending motions. *J Biomech* 1997;30:697–703.
39. Schultz AB, Andersson GB, Haderspeck K, Ortengren R, Nordin M, Bjork R. Analysis and measurement of lumbar trunk loads in tasks involving bends and twists. *J Biomech* 1982;15:669–675.
40. Marras WS, Granata KP. A biomechanical assessment and model of axial twisting in the thoracolumbar spine. *Spine* 1995;20:1440–1451.
41. McGill SM. The influence of lordosis on axial trunk torque and trunk muscle myoelectric activity. *Spine* 1992;17:1187–1193.
42. Cholewicki J, McGill SM, Norman RW. Lumbar spine loads during the lifting of extremely heavy weights. *Med Sci Sports Exerc* 1991;23:1179–1186.
43. Buseck M, Shilipplein OD, Andersson GB, Andriacchi TP. Influence of dynamic factors and external loads on the moment at the lumbar spine in lifting. *Spine* 1988;13:918–921.
44. Lavender SA, Li YC, Andersson GB, Natarajan RN. The effects of lifting speed on the peak external forward bending, lateral bending and twisting spine moments. *Ergonomics* 1999;42:111–125.
45. Schipplein OD, Reinsel TE, Andersson GB, Lavender SA. The influence of initial horizontal weight placement on the loads at the lumbar spine while lifting. *Spine* 1995;20:1895–1898.
46. Dolan P, Earley M, Adams MA. Bending and compressive stresses acting on the lumbar spine during lifting activities. *J Biomech* 1994;27:1237–1248.

47. Gagnon D, Gagnon M. The influence of dynamic factors on triaxial net muscular moments at the L5/S1 joint during asymmetrical lifting and lowering. *J Biomech* 1992;25:891–901.
48. Marras WS, Granata KP. Changes in trunk dynamics and spine loading during repeated trunk extensions. *Spine* 1997;22:2564–2570.
49. Dolan P, Adams MA. Repetitive lifting tasks fatigue the back muscles and increase the bending moment acting on the lumbar spine. *J Biomech* 1998;31:713–721.
50. Hooper DM, Goel VK, Aleksiev A, Spratt K, Bolte KM, Pope M. Three dimensional moments in the lumbar spine during asymmetric lifting. *Clin Biomech* 1998;13:386–393.
51. Wilson DJ, Hickey KM, Gorham JL, Childers MK. Lumbar spinal moments in chronic back pain patients during supported lifting: A dynamic analysis. *Arch Phys Med Rehabil* 1997;78:967–972.
52. McGill S, Seguin J, Bennett G. Passive stiffness of the lumbar torso in flexion, extension, lateral bending and axial rotation. Effect of belt wearing and breath holding. *Spine* 1994;19:696–704.
53. Granata KP, Marras WS, Davis KG. Biomechanical assessment of lifting dynamics, muscle activity and spinal loads while using three different styles of lifting belt. *Clin Biomech* 1997;12:107–115.
54. Giorcelli RJ, Hughes RE, Wassell JT, Hsiao H. The effect of wearing a back belt on spine kinematics during asymmetric lifting of large and small boxes. *Spine* 2001;26:1794–1798.
55. Thomas JS, Lavender SA Corcos DM, Andersson GB. Effect of lifting belts on trunk muscle activation during suddenly applied load. *Hum Factors* 1999;41:670–676.
56. McGill SM, Norman RW, Sharratt MT. The effect of an abdominal belt on trunk muscle activity and intra-abdominal pressure during squat lifts. *Ergonomics* 1990;33:147–160.
57. Lavender SA, Shakeel K, Andersson GB, Thomas JS. Effects of a lifting belt on spine moments and muscle recruitments after unexpected sudden loading. *Spine* 2000;25:1569–1578.
58. Rohlmann A, Wilke HJ, Graichen F, Bergmann G. Spinal load bearing during sitting in an office chair with a tilting back. *Biomed Tech* 2002;47:91–96.
59. Magora A. Investigation of the relation between low back pain and occupation. 3. Physical requirements: Sitting, standing and weight lifting. *Ind Med Surg* 1972;41:4–9.
60. Leivseth G, Drerup B. Spinal shrinkage during work in a sitting posture compared to work in a standing posture. *Clin Biomech* 1997;12:409–418.
61. Callaghan JP, McGill SM. Low back joint loading and kinematics during standing and unsupported sitting. *Ergonomics* 2001;4:280–294.
62. Hedman TP, Fernie GR. Mechanical response of the lumbar spine to seated postural loads. *Spine* 1997;22:734–743.
63. Callaghan JP, Dunk NM. Examination of the flexion relaxation phenomenon in erector spinae muscles during short duration slumped sitting. *Clin Biomech* 2002;17:353–360.
64. Lengsfeld M, van Deursen DL, Rohlmann A, van Deursen L.L, Griss P. Spinal load changes during rotatory dynamic sitting. *Clin Biomech* 2000;15:295–297.
65. Makhsous M, Lin F, Hendrix RW, Hepler M, Zhang LQ. Sitting with adjustable ischial and back supports: Biomechanical changes. *Spine* 2003;28:1113–1121.
66. Bendix T, Poulsen V, Klausen K, Jensen CV. What does a backrest actually do to the lumbar spine? *Ergonomics* 1996;39:533–542.
67. Pope MH, Goh KL, Magnusson ML. Spine ergonomics. *Annu Rev Biomed Eng* 2002;4:49–68.
68. Khoo BC, Goh JC, Bose K. A biomechanical model to determine lumbosacral loads during single stance phase in normal gait. *Med Eng Phys* 1995;17:27–35.
69. Cheng CK, Chen HH, Chen CS, Lee SJ. Influences of walking speed change on the lumbosacral joint force distribution. *Biomed Mater Eng.* 1998;8:155–165.
70. Cappozzo A. Compressive loads in the lumbar vertebral column during normal level walking. *J Orthop Res* 1984;1:292–301.
71. Callaghan JP, Patla AE, McGill SM. Low back three-dimensional joint forces, kinematics, and kinetics during walking. *Clin Biomech* 1999;14:203–216.
72. Garbutt G, Boocock MG, Reilly T, Troup JD. Running speed and spinal shrinkage in runners with and without low back pain. *Med Sci Sports Exerc* 1990;22:769–772.
73. Mundt DJ, Kelsey JL, Golden AL, et al, for the Northeast Collaborative Group on Low Back Pain. An epidemiologic study of sports and weight lifting as possible risk factors for herniated lumbar and cervical discs. *Am J Sports Med* 1993;21:854–860.
74. Liemohn W. Exercise and arthritis. Exercise and the back. *Rheum Dis Clin North Am* 1990;16:945–970.
75. Callaghan JP, Gunning JL, McGill SM. The relationship between lumbar spine load and muscle activity during extension exercises. *Phys Ther* 1998;78:8–18.
76. Salai M, Brosh T, Blankstein A, Oran A, Chechik A. Effect of changing the saddle angle on the incidence of low back pain in recreational bicyclists. *Br J Sports Med* 1999;33:398–400.
77. Fanucci E, Masala S, Fasoli F, Cammarata R, Squillaci E, Simonetti G. Cineradiographic study of spine during cycling: Effects of changing the pedal unit position on the dorso-lumbar spine angle. *Radiol Med* 2002;104:472–476.
78. Usabiaga J, Crespo R, Iza I, Aramendi J, Terrados N, Poza JJ. Adaptation of the lumbar spine to different positions in bicycle racing. *Spine* 1997;22:1965–1969.
79. Solomonow M, Zhou BH, Baratta RV, et al. Bioexponential recovery model of lumbar viscoelastic laxity and reflexive muscular activity after prolonged cyclic loading. *Clin Biomech* 2000;15:167–175.

CHAPTER

4

EPIDEMIOLOGY OF LOW BACK SYNDROMES

Eric L. Hurwitz and Paul G. Shekelle

OUTLINE

OBJECTIVES

1. To understand basic epidemiologic principles necessary for the critical evaluation of literature on lumbar spine disorders.
2. To become familiar with the epidemiologic measures used to describe the frequency and impact of lumbar spine disorders.
3. To become familiar with the epidemiologic measures used to describe associations of potential risk and prognostic factors with lumbar disease outcomes.
4. To become familiar with the prevalence, incidence, and economic impact of lumbar spine disorders.
5. To identify factors associated with the risk, prognosis, and consequences of lumbar spine disorders.
6. To understand the natural course of low back disorders and how this course may be influenced by other diseases and factors.
7. To become familiar with the multifactorial nature of low back pain and its consequences.
8. To describe the frequency and impact of low back disorders in the workplace.

9. To identify occupational factors associated with lumbar spine disorders in the workplace.
10. To become familiar with the evidence for and against low back pain prevention strategies in the workplace.

INTRODUCTION

Disorders affecting the low back are the most widespread and disabling musculoskeletal conditions in the United States and around the world. The primary purpose of this chapter is fourfold: (1) to introduce epidemiologic concepts necessary for the understanding of the low back literature; (2) to describe the frequency and impact of the most common low back disorders in society and in the workplace; (3) to discuss factors that may increase (or decrease) the risk of low back pain and associated syndromes; and (4) to review the evidence for and against strategies for the prevention of low back disorders in the workplace and elsewhere.

Given that epidemiology is perceived as daunting to many students, interns, and clinicians, it would be easy to simply bypass this chapter and move to other more academically comfortable topics. However, with an understanding of some basic terminology and practical applications, you will come to realize that epidemiology is not as threatening as the name may suggest. In fact, clinicians use epidemiology (possibly without realizing it) every time they take a patient's history and examination findings to make a differential diagnosis. For example, the history may include personal behaviors, occupational exposures, and comorbidities. The clinician integrates his knowledge of these factors and how they may be associated with certain conditions (e.g., smoking and lung cancer, high-fat diet and cardiovascular disease) with results from diagnostic tests to come up with possible diagnoses. This is clinical epidemiology. You will soon gain an appreciation for the relevance of epidemiology not only to clinical decision making, but also to patient communication, intra- and interprofessional dialogue, and reporting medical–legal and reimbursement issues.

EPIDEMIOLOGIC CONCEPTS

Before embarking on a tour of lumbar spine disorders, it is important to have a basic understanding of the terms, study designs, and definitions used in describing lumbar spine disorders and in the assessment of factors associated with these conditions. Epidemiology is the study of the distribution and determinants of health and disease in human populations.[1] Distribution refers to the frequency of disease according to time, place, and person, whereas determinants refers to those agents or factors that increase or decrease the probability of becoming ill or, if already ill, of recovering. Although the study of distribution of disease is often called descriptive epidemiology and the study of determinants is called analytic epidemiology, there are descriptive and analytic components to both types of study.

Measures of Disease Frequency and Association

Table 4–1 shows the most commonly used epidemiologic measures of frequency and association. A variety of statistical measures are used to describe disease frequency. Point prevalence, or simply prevalence, is the proportion of a defined population having the disease at a point in time. For example, if a survey is conducted today among 1000 residents of Los Angeles and 50 report having low back pain, then the prevalence of low back pain in this population is 50/1000, or 5%. Period prevalence, in contrast to point prevalence, is the number of existing cases plus the number of new cases occurring in a population over a specific period of time. For example, if the above survey asked respondents about their low back pain status during the past 2 weeks instead of today, and 80 reported having pain in the past 2 weeks, then the 2-week period prevalence would be 80/1000, or 8%. Cumulative incidence, or risk, is the proportion of a defined population "at risk" that develops disease over a specified period of time. "At risk" means that everyone in the population is free of the disease under study when follow-up begins. For example, in order to know the proportion of a population that develops low back pain during a 1-year period, one would follow a population initially free of low back pain and count those that develop pain during the year. If 1000 people are followed and 20 develop low back pain according to this definition, then the 1-year cumulative incidence, or 1-year risk of low back pain is 0.02 or 2%. Another incidence measure is incidence density. In contrast to cumulative incidence, which is a proportion, incidence density is a rate. In order to compute incidence density, it is necessary to know the time that each person in the population spent at risk of developing the disease. Once a person develops the disease, he is no longer at risk and thus he would no longer accumulate time at risk. If a population of 1000 people contributed 1000 person-years at risk of developing low back pain, and 100 people developed low back pain, then the incidence density would be 100/1000 person-years, or 0.1 low back pain cases per year.

Epidemiologic measures of association are used to assess the direction and magnitude of association of potential risk and prognostic factors with the disease or health outcome of interest. The specific measure

TABLE 4–1. Epidemiologic Measures of Frequency and Association, by Type of Measure

Type of Measure	Measure	Definition	Design
Frequency	Lifetime prevalence	Proportion of persons in population known to have had the disease for at least part of their lives	Cross-sectional
	Point prevalence	Proportion of persons in population with the disease at a specified point in time	Cohort, cross-sectional
	Period prevalence	Proportion of persons in population known to have had the disease at any time during a specified interval	Cohort, cross-sectional
	Cumulative incidence (CI; risk)	Proportion of population that experiences onset of health-related event during a specified time interval	Cohort
	Incidence density (ID; rate)	Number of events occurring during specified time interval divided by number of person-time units at risk during the interval	Cohort
Association	Prevalence ratio	Prevalence in one group ("exposed") divided by prevalence in another group ("unexposed")	Cross-sectional
	Cumulative incidence ratio (CIR; risk ratio)	Risk in one group ("exposed") divided by risk in another group ("unexposed")	Cohort
	Incidence density ratio (IDR; rate ratio)	Rate in one group ("exposed") divided by rate in another group ("unexposed")	Cohort
	Odds ratio (OR)	Odds of disease in one group ("exposed") divided by odds of disease in another group ("unexposed")	Cohort, cross-sectional, case-control

used is typically dependent upon the type of study and on the method of outcome assessment. The prevalence ratio is simply the ratio of two prevalence measures. For example, if the prevalence of low back pain in the United States is 10% and the prevalence in the United Kingdom is 8%, then the prevalence ratio, comparing the United States with the United Kingdom, is 0.10/0.08, or 1.25, meaning the prevalence of low back pain is 25% higher in the United States than in the United Kingdom. The cumulative incidence ratio, or risk ratio, is the ratio of the risk of disease in one group to the risk of disease in another group. For example, if a population of 1000 workers is followed for incident low back pain disability over a 5-year period, where half of the workers are females and half males, and 75 males and 75 females become low back disabled, then the 5-year risk ratio comparing males to females is 75/500 / 75/500 = 1.0. A ratio measure of 1.0, called the null value, means there is no association between the factor (e.g., sex) and the outcome (e.g., low back disability). Ratio measures greater than 1 indicate positive associations between the factor and the outcome, while ratio measures less than 1 indicate negative associations. If incidence densities rather than risks are measured, then the appropriate measure of association is the incidence density ratio, or simply the rate ratio. Alternatively, differences between risks or rates may be computed. These measures are called risk or rate differences, where the null value is 0 rather than 1. A measure of association often used in cross-sectional and case-control studies is the odds ratio, which is the ratio of 2 odds: the odds of disease in one group divided by the odds of disease in another group. The odds ratio is typically used when risk or rate ratios cannot be calculated, or because of its useful statistical properties in certain multivariable analyses.

Basic Research Strategies

A number of strategies and designs are used in epidemiologic research. The specific strategy or design depends primarily on the research objective, but also on time, budget, and other issues. The most common designs encountered in the epidemiology of lumbar spine and other musculoskeletal diseases are cross-sectional, cohort, and case-control studies. All designs involve some type of sampling from a larger population. It is this larger population to which the investigator would like to make inferences.

Clinical Pearl: Sampling is a key element of epidemiologic study design. The population from

TABLE 4–2. **Strengths and Limitations of Epidemiologic Research Strategies, by Type of Design**

Type of Design	Major Strengths	Major Limitations
Cross-sectional	Can examine multiple outcomes and exposures	Temporal relationship between exposure and outcome may not be clear
	Is relatively inexpensive and quick	Exposure information collected retrospectively may not be accurate
	Describes disease frequency (prevalence) in the population	Outcome status can influence the selection of subjects differentially by exposure status
		Cannot generally distinguish between predictors of disease occurrence and disease progression
Cohort	Can examine multiple outcomes for a specific exposure	Is inefficient for studying rare diseases
		Can be costly and time-consuming
	Can elucidate the temporal relationship between exposure and outcome	Validity and precision (accuracy) of results can be affected by loss to follow-up
	Outcome status is not likely to affect measurement of exposure	
	Outcome status is not likely to affect selection of subjects	
Case-control	Is relatively quick and inexpensive	Cannot estimate disease rates in the population (unless population-based)
	Is efficient for studying rare diseases and diseases with long incubation/latent periods	Exposure status can influence the selection of subjects differentially by outcome status
	Can examine multiple exposures for a single outcome	Retrospective exposure information may not be accurate
		Temporal relationship between exposure and outcome may not be clear
Experiment	Randomization achieves comparability between groups (if the sample size is large enough)	Is expensive and time-consuming
		Generalizability may be limited
		May be unethical or impractical to randomize

which the sample is drawn is the target population to which the investigator would like to draw conclusions.

Table 4–2 shows the major types of epidemiologic research designs and their strengths and limitations. Cross-sectional studies involve a sample of population on which exposures and outcomes are measured simultaneously. A survey is a type of cross-sectional study. These studies are often small but may include thousands of subjects, such as the National Health Interview Survey (NHIS) or the National Health and Nutrition Examination Survey (NHANES). Cross-sectional studies do not follow populations at risk, as do cohort studies. Prevalence ratios and prevalence odds ratios are the measures of association typically computed from cross-sectional data. Cohort studies start with a population at risk of the outcome, and thus prevalent cases are excluded; then this population is followed over time and assessed for outcome events. If the investigator is interested in assessment of prognostic factors rather than risk factors for the outcome, say low back pain, then the population at baseline would include only those subjects with low back pain, since people without current low back pain are not "at risk" of improvement. Risk and rate ratios are the measures of association most often used with cohort data. Case-control studies compare a group of cases (subjects with the outcome of interest) with a group of noncases (subjects without the outcome of interest) with respect to potential risk or prognostic factors. The odds ratio is the most common measure of association used with case-control data, though depending on how the cases are sampled, risk or rate ratios may also be used. If all the cases in a defined population are selected, then the study is a population-based case-control study. A recently developed variant of the case-control design is the case-crossover design, where control data are collected from the cases rather than from separate subjects.[2,3] Although this design has not been used in epidemiologic studies of low back syndromes, the case-crossover design may be appropriate for estimating the effects of transient exposures on acute onset events, such as certain occupational exposures and acute low back injury.

The studies described above are called observational designs because the investigator observes disease occurrence without having anything to do with who is and is not "exposed" to putative risk or prognostic factors. If the research question relates to the effect of an intervention or other factor amenable to being assigned, then an experiment or quasi-experiment is the design option. The intervention is randomized in an experiment, whereas it is assigned but through a nonrandomized process in a quasi-experiment. Randomization means that the probabilities of being assigned to each intervention group are the same from one person to the next. If the sample size is large, then comparability between groups is likely, thus bias from confounding (discussed below) is minimized.

Validity of Epidemiologic Data

Systematic error, or bias from sampling, data, and other sources may affect the validity of epidemiologic data. The major types of bias in epidemiologic studies are selection bias, information bias, and confounding. Random error does not result in bias per se, but causes measures of frequency and association to be relatively less precise. Systematic error can be reduced by ensuring unbiased sampling and measurement and by randomization or controlling for the effects of confounders in the analysis. Random error can be reduced by having a large study population and by using reliable instruments for assessing exposures and outcomes.

Clinical Pearl: Validity of epidemiologic data is adversely affected by systematic error, which may be reduced by ensuring unbiased sampling and measurement, and by randomization in clinical trials or controlling for the effects of confounders in observational studies.

Loss to follow-up in cohort studies and biased sampling in case-control studies are the major sources of selection bias in epidemiologic studies. Misclassification of exposures and outcomes in all types of studies are the major sources of information bias. Confounding is a potential source of bias in all observational studies and in small randomized studies. Effect estimates may be adjusted, or controlled, for the effects of confounding factors in the analysis. However, unlike randomized studies, which ensure comparability across exposure groups with respect to both known and unknown confounders, adjusting for confounders in the analysis only deals with variables that are measured in the study.

The amount of random error is reflected by the width of the confidence interval (CI) around the estimate of frequency or effect. Typically the 95% CI is computed. If the study were to be repeated again and again using the same methods (but with different samples of subjects), then 95 out of 100 of the calculated 95% CIs would include the true population parameter. It is this "truth" that is sought after but which cannot actually be observed in the study sample.

Internal validity refers to lack of bias in the effect estimates, whereas external validity refers to the extent to which the results may be generalizable to other populations and other circumstances. Many randomized clinical trials are conducted using strict inclusion/exclusion criteria that may not be reflective of primary care patient populations, for example. Although effect estimates from such studies may be internally valid (unbiased), they may not be applicable to other patient groups. The extent to which estimates are generalizable depends primarily on whether there are differences between the study population and the population to which results are to be generalized with respect to factors that modify the effect of the exposure on the outcome. For example, if a study population includes only males, then the results may not be generalizable to a population that includes males and females if the exposure effect is not the same for both sexes. Study samples may be stratified by potential effect modifiers, such as sex, in order to generate category-specific (e.g., male and female) estimates for the exposure effect.

NONSPECIFIC MECHANICAL LOW BACK AND LEG PAIN

Prevalence, Incidence, and Economic Impact

Table 4–3 shows the frequencies of low back pain and leg pain. The lifetime prevalence of low back pain in community-based populations has been estimated to be between 50% and 85%,[4–6,9–15] though Deyo, using data from the National Health and Nutrition Examination Survey (NHANES I) reported 13.8%.[8] Low back pain is defined in this latter study as pain lasting for at least 2 weeks. The point prevalence has been estimated to be between 6% and 35%,[9,13,17–19,21] while 10%–50% have reported low-back pain in the past year,[8,11,14,21] and 21%–39% in the past month.[10,12] Prevalence appears to peak in males around age 40 and in females between 50 and 60 years.[27,28] The notably wide variation in estimates is due primarily to inter-study differences in the definition of low back pain,[29] but also to differences in populations that may vary in how they perceive and evaluate pain.

Clinical Pearl: Low back pain is the third most commonly reported symptom, the second most frequent cause of worker absenteeism, and the most costly ailment of working-age adults in the United States.

TABLE 4–3. **Prevalence and Incidence of Low Back Pain in Adults, by Type of Frequency Measure**

Frequency Measure	Population	Frequency	Reference
Lifetime prevalence	Adult females, Sweden	70%	4
	Males, age 40–47, Sweden	61%	5
	Adults, age 18–64, Denmark	60%–80%	6
	Adults, United States	17.2%	7
	Adults, United States	13.8%	8
	Females, age 38–64, Sweden	66%	9
	Adults, age >30, Finland	75%	10
	Adults, United Kingdom	58%	11
	Adults, United Kingdom	59%	12
	Adults, age 20–69, Canada	84.9%	13
	Adults, age 30–50, Norway	66%	14
	Adults, Belgium	59%	15
	Adults, age 18–55, United States	70%	16
Point prevalence	Community sample, United Kingdom	15%	17
	Adults, age 18–64, United States	18%	18
	Adults, Sweden	6%	19
	Females, age 18–64, Sweden	35%	9
	Adults, Sweden	31%	20
	Adults, age 20–69, Canada	28.4%	13
	Adults, age 25–64, United Kingdom	19%	21
	Adults, age <60, United States	8.5%	22
	Adults, age >60, United States	5%	22
	Adults, Belgium	33%	15
1-year prevalence	Adults, United Kingdom	36%	11
	Adults, age >25, United States	18%	23
	Adults, United States	56%	24
	Adults, age >25, United States	10.3%	8
	Females, age 35–45, Sweden	69.5%	25
	Males, age 35–45, Sweden	63.2%	25
	Adults, age 25–64, United Kingdom	39%	21
	Adults, age 30–50, Norway	44%–54%	14
	Adults, age 18+, United States	56%	24
6-month prevalence	Adults, age 20–69, Canada	48.9%	13
1-month prevalence	Adults, age >30, Finland	21%	10
	Adults, United Kingdom	39%	12
	Adult males, United Kingdom	35%	12
	Adult females, United Kingdom	42%	12
2-week prevalence	Adults, Denmark	23%	26
1-year cumulative incidence	Adults, age 30, Denmark	11%	6
	Adults, age 25–64, United Kingdom	4.7%	21

Few studies have assessed the incidence of low back pain in general populations. Biering-Sörensen reported the 1-year incidence of low back pain among 30-year-olds at 11%,[6] while Hillman et al. reported a 1-year incidence of 4.7% among 25- to 64-year-olds in the United Kingdom.[21] Abenhaim reported a 1-year incidence of back-related compensated absence from work in Quebec at 1.4%.[30]

Low back pain is the third most commonly reported symptom, trailing only tiredness and headache.[24] Low back pain is the most costly ailment of working-age adults and is one of the most frequent complaints reported by patients seeking medical care.[31,32] Low back pain resulting in disability claims, which had been on the rise during most of the 1990s,[33] but which now may be leveling off,[34] is largely responsible for the estimated $33 billion spent annually in direct health care costs associated with low back pain care.[33] Back pain is the second most frequent cause of worker absenteeism,[35] resulting in $8.8 billion in work-related low back claims in 1995.[36] There is little evidence that the prevalence of low

TABLE 4–4. **Putative Sociodemographic, Behavioral, and Physical Risk/Prognostic Factors for Low Back Pain, by Type of Factor**

Type of Factor	Factor	Finding	References
Sociodemographic	Age	Increasing age	8,10,15,39–42
		Decreasing age	43
		No association	6,44,45
	Sex	M > F (disabling pain)	42
		M > F	46
		F > M (nondisabling pain)	42
		M = F	10,44,45,47
	Education	Less education	6,8,10,48–50
		Less education (disabling pain)	42,51
		No association	46,52,53
		No association (nondisabling pain)	42
	Marital status	Unmarried	23
		Living alone (males)	54
		Div/wid. (disability)	55
	Race/ethnicity	White vs. non-white	8,10,42
Sociodemographic	Employment	Unemployed	42,56,57
Behavioral	Smoking	Smokers	39,58–64
		No association	42,65,66
	Alcohol use	Drinkers	39,67
	Activity	Sedentary vs. active	40,64,65,68–70
		No association	46,53,58,71–75
Physical	Height	Increasing height	39,44,76
		No association	45,46,74,77–79
	BMI	High vs. low	39,44,75,80
		High vs. low (disabling pain)	42
		No association	45,46,71,77,81–84
	Strength	Increased strength	85–87
		No association	6,65,73,74,79,88–91
	Flexibility	Increased flexibility	88,92,93
		No association	74,78,79,94–96
	Leg length	Unequal vs. equal	97–100
		No association	74,82,93,101–104
Spinal deformity	Scoliosis/other	No association	45,48,71,105
	Spondylolisth.	Spondylolisthesis	52
		Spondylolisthesis (females)	106
		No association	10,71

back pain has increased appreciably over the past few decades.[14,37,38]

Risk and Prognostic Factors for Low Back Pain

Sociodemographic Factors Table 4–4 shows putative sociodemographic risk/prognostic factors for low back pain. Numerous studies have addressed the associations of factors such as age, sex, level of education, marital status, race/ethnicity, and employment status with low back pain. Most of the studies are cross-sectional, including persons with acute and chronic episodes, and thus cannot differentiate risk of developing a new episode of low back pain from prognosis. Age has been identified as a possible risk factor in many reports,[8,10,15,40–42] but has been discounted as a risk factor in others.[6,44,45] The highest prevalence of low back pain appears to occur between the ages of 55 and 64 years,[8] while disabling low back pain is most common in 35- to 54-year-olds.[42]

Low back pain has been found to affect males and females in similar proportions,[10,44–47] though males may be more likely to have disabling episodes while females may be more likely to have nondisabling back pain.[42] Females were almost 30% less likely to have incident low back pain in the recent British birth cohort study.[46]

Low level of education has been identified as a possible risk factor in a few studies,[6,10,42,48–51] but not in others.[46,52,53] In the 1958 British birth cohort study, low level of education and social class were predictive of incident low back pain in univariate analyses, but not in multivariable analyses, suggesting that other factors are responsible.[46] Hurwitz and Morgenstern[42] found that those with at least some college education were less likely to have a disabling back problem but equally likely as less educated persons to have a nondisabling back problem. This cross-sectional study also found back problems to be less prevalent among non-whites, as have other studies[8,10] and not surprisingly, disabling back problems were found to be less prevalent among employed persons.[42] The relatively better health status of people in the workforce ("healthy worker effect") is a plausible explanation for this finding. Other studies in the United States have reported similar findings.[56,57]

Behavioral Factors Table 4–4 shows putative behavioral risk/prognostic factors for low back pain. Personal behaviors such as smoking, alcohol use, and physical activity have been hypothesized as potential risk or prognostic factors for low back pain. Smoking in particular has been the focus of a multitude of cross-sectional, case-control, and cohort studies,[10,16,39,46,54,58–60,66,75,107–109] as well as systematic reviews.[14,111] The evidence suggests that smokers may be somewhat more likely than non-smokers to report low back pain, but the association between smoking and low back pain may not be causal. Alcohol use has also been shown to be associated with low back pain,[39,67] but like for smoking, the association may not be causal.

Clinical Pearl: Exercise and physical fitness have been shown to prevent low back pain; however, not all physical activities are created equal. The magnitude of risk reduction, if any, appears to be modified by the type of activity.

Exercise and physical fitness, including leisure-time physical activity, have been suggested as possible protective factors for low back pain in some studies,[40,64,68–70] but not in others.[40,46,58,71–74] Some physical activities may lead to low back pain while others may be protective; thus, the risk may be modified by type of activity. Similarly, prognosis may vary according to type of activity.[112] A recent review of 39 studies showed little association of leisure-time physical activity with musculoskeletal disorders, including low back pain, among workers, though sedentary leisure activity was found to be associated with an increased prevalence of low back pain and related sick leave.[113]

Physical Factors Table 4–4 shows putative physical risk/prognostic factors for low back pain. Height, weight or relative weight (body mass index [BMI]), strength, flexibility, posture, and other physical factors have been addressed in a number of studies. Standing height has been identified as a possible risk factor in a few studies,[44,39,76] though not in others,[45,77] including most prospective studies.[46,74,78,79] Obesity or BMI has also been identified as a predictor in a few studies,[39,42,49,75,80] but has been ruled out in many more.[45,46,71,77,81–84] Findings from a recent systematic review suggest that obesity may be a risk and prognostic factor for low back pain, but that the shape of the relationship is unclear.[114] Most prospective studies show no or negative associations between weight and low back pain.[65,74,78,79]

Clinical Pearl: Although most prospective studies have failed to demonstrate positive associations between body mass index or obesity and risk of low back pain, being overweight is associated with other adverse health outcomes that may influence prognosis.

Physical strength has been shown to be protective in some[85–87] but not all studies,[6,73,88–90] including many prospective cohort studies.[65,74,79,91] Similarly, inconsistent findings have been observed for associations between flexibility and low back pain.[88,92–96] Prospective studies tend not to show appreciable associations.[74,78,79,95] One prospective study found relatively longer hamstrings to be protective of recurrent low back in women,[74] though another prospective study failed to confirm this finding.[79]

Posture and leg-length inequality have been the focus of a few studies. The literature is inconsistent regarding these factors as possible determinants of low back pain. Regarding leg-length inequality of 2.5 cm or more, fewer studies suggest an association[97–100] than do not.[74,82,93,101–104] Large prospective studies have failed to find associations between leg-length inequality and low back pain.[74,103] Scoliosis and postural abnormalities have generally been shown not to be associated with low back pain.[45,48,71,105] whereas for spondylolisthesis, some investigators have detected associations[52] and others not.[10,71] A case-control study showed spondylolisthesis increased the odds of pain in women but not in men.[106]

Clinical Pearl: Leg-length inequality, scoliosis, and other postural abnormalities have generally been found not to increase the risk of low back pain and related disability.

Psychological and Psychosocial Factors Table 4–5 shows putative psychological and psychosocial risk/prognostic factors for low back pain. Psychological and psychosocial factors have been the subject of numerous investigations and recent review articles. Burton

TABLE 4–5. Putative Psychological and Psychosocial Risk/Prognostic Factors for Low Back Pain, by Type of Factor

Risk/Prognostic Factor	Factor	Finding	References
Risk factor	Psychological distress	Incident pain episodes	115
		Musculoskeletal pain	116
		Incident back pain	117
		Incident back consultation	117
	Catastrophizing	Incident pain episodes	118
	Fear avoidance	Incident pain episodes	118
	Depression	Incident back pain	117
		Incident back consultation	117
		No association with pain onset	119
Prognostic factor	Psychological distress	↑ Disability	120
		↑ Pain and disability	121
		↑ Sick leave	121
	Somatization	↑ Pain and disability	121
		↑ Sick leave	121
		↑ Disability	122,123
	Catastrophizing	↑ disability	120
	Fear avoidance	↑ Pain duration	124–126
		No association with pain duration	127,128
		↑ Pain and disability	121
		↑ Sick leave	121,126
		↑ Pain recurrence	129
		↑ Pain intensity	129
		Early retirement	129
	Pain intensity	↑ Disability	120
		↑ Pain intensity	124
		↑ Costs	130
		↑ Sick leave	131
		No association with sick leave	132
	Praying/hoping	↑ Disability	120
	Maladaptive coping	↑ Pain duration	120,133–135
	Depression/depressive symptoms	↑ Pain duration	116,119,129,134,136–138
		No association with pain duration	127,128,139
		↑ Disability	122,123
		↑ Pain and disability	121
		↑ Sick leave	121
		↑ Costs	130
		↑ Satisfaction	140
	Perceived stress/anxiety	↑ Pain duration	67,121,133,141
		↑ Pain intensity	124
		↑ Disability	126
		↑ Sick leave	126
	Psychopathology	↑ Sick leave (6 months)	127
		No association with sick leave (1 year)	128
	History of depression/anxiety	↑ Pain duration	16,67,116,141,142
		No association with pain duration	Leavitt, 1990 (336); Leino and Magni, 1993 (178)
	Alcohol/drug abuse history	↑ Pain duration	67,143

et al.[120] found that among patients with acute and subacute low back pain, history of low back trouble and psychosocial variables, especially passive coping strategies, were among the best predictors of disability at 1 year. The authors of another study that sought to identify predictors of chronicity among patients with acute low back pain found fear-avoidance variables to be the best predictors of continued pain and disability after 1 year.[121] Fear-avoidance variables include stressful life events, personality, previous pain history, and pain-coping strategies.[121] These and other studies[125,144–146] have found pain severity and other clinical examination findings to be only minimally associated with disability. Among workers with low back pain, dissatisfaction with work was found to be the strongest predictor of future medical care.[136] Scale 3 (hysteria) of the MMPI (Minnesota Multiphasic Personality Inventory Depression scale; and no measures of physical functioning) was predictive of low back pain among uninjured workers.[136] Mannion et al.[117] found that somatic anxiety and depression, as measured by the Modified Somatic Perception Questionnaire (MSPQ) and the Zung Depression Scale, respectively, predicted new episodes of low back pain among a population of health care workers without a history of low back pain.

A number of cross-sectional[23,42,48,55,57,147–151] and longitudinal studies.[46,54,133,136,139,152] and a case-control study[135] have addressed the influence of marital status and social support on low back pain and related disability. No clear patterns of increased or decreased risk associated with social support emerge from these data.

Two recent reviews of psychological factors and back pain are worth noting.[153,154] Linton[153] reviewed 37 prospective studies of risk and prognostic factors for back and neck pain and concluded, in part, that (1) psychological factors are associated with the onset of back and neck pain; (2) psychosocial factors may be predictive of back-related disability; and (3) depression and anxiety are associated with pain and disability. Future studies that consider more fully the associations of psychosocial factors, pain, and depression over time, and within a theoretical framework, were suggested. Hoogendoorn et al.[154] performed a systematic review of 11 cohort and 2 case-control studies of work- related and personal psychosocial risk factors for back pain, concluding that low social support, low job satisfaction, and low decision latitude may be predictive of back pain. The authors detailed the many methodologic problems of the studies included in their review, including failure to properly control for physical work exposures, and recommended that future studies consider these and other factors in order to better estimate the effects of psychosocial factors on back pain. Not included in the above reviews is the recent 1958 British birth cohort study, which found low control over one's life (also known as locus of control) predictive of incident low back pain at age 32–33 years in univariate and multivariate analyses.[46]

Clinical Pearl: Evidence from numerous prospective studies indicate that psychological factors are associated with the onset of low back pain, and in general, psychosocial factors are better than physical or clinical factors in predicting chronicity.

Turk[155] reviewed studies addressing psychosocial predictors of transitioning from acute to chronic pain. He concluded that in general, psychosocial factors are better than physical or clinical factors in predicting chronicity, and that pain chronicity has a multifactorial etiology, with many variables playing roles over time, which may itself interact with psychosocial variables, such as psychosocial distress, substance abuse, anxiety, depression, social support, coping, and job satisfaction. More recently, Pincus et al.[156] conducted a systematic review of prospective cohort studies that addressed psychosocial factors in the transition from acute to chronic low back pain. They concluded from the 6 studies (of 25 articles) that met their criteria for methodology, psychological measurement, and statistical analysis that "strong evidence" exists for distress and depressive mood and "moderate evidence" exists for somatization as relevant predictors of chronicity, and that further studies need to be conducted on the roles of coping strategies, fear avoidance, and other psychological factors.

Clinical and Other Factors The most consistent predictor of low back pain is past low back pain. This finding has been reported from numerous cross-sectional,[39] case-control,[43,157,158] and cohort[44,62,136,117,159,160–163] studies. Additional clinical factors that may be associated with low back pain include having a history of allergies,[164] hormone-replacement therapy among postmenopausal women,[165] family history of low back pain and certain genetic factors,[166] and pregnancy.[10,39,141,167–169] History of physical and sexual abuse has recently been linked to chronic back pain among women.[170,171]

Sciatica

The lifetime prevalence of sciatica (true radicular pain) has been estimated to be 5% in men and 4% in women.[76] Back pain with associated leg pain, which may be referred or radicular, has been shown to be much more common: 35% in men vs. 45% in women.[76] The 3-year incidence of sciatic pain among 25- to 49-year-old Finnish men was estimated to be 22% in machine operators, 24% in carpenters, and 14% in office workers.[172]

Possible risk factors for sciatica include male sex, age 30–50 years, height, obesity, and multiple pregnancies.[10,76,108] History of back pain has been shown to be an important predictor of sciatic pain as well as low back pain[53] Low back pain with associated sciatic pain has been shown to have a worse prognosis than back pain without sciatic pain.[173,174] As with low back pain, psychological factors may be important risk and/or prognostic variables.[172] A recent 1-year cohort study conducted among Finnish workers found increasing age, mental stress, long-term smoking, and work-related twisting to increase the risk of sciatic pain, while increasing age, mental stress, history of smoking, jogging, and poor job satisfaction to increase the risk of persistent pain.[175]

Natural Course of Low Back and Leg Pain There is a dearth of literature on the natural course of low back and leg pain. For classification purposes, back pain is often divided into rather arbitrary categories of acute, subacute, and chronic pain. Acute episodes are characterized by episodes of less than 1 month, subacute episodes lasting from 1 to 3 months, and chronic pain lasting more than 3 months.[176] This classification scheme fails to characterize the often recurrent nature of back pain in many individuals. For example, 25% of patients in primary care had appreciable low back pain 1 year after their initial episodes had resolved.[177] Other prospective studies of 1 year or longer duration have reported frequent recurrences.[178–181] Carey et al. reported recurrence rates of between 20% and 35% between 6 and 22 months among patients who were free of back pain 3 months after a health care visit for acute low back pain.[181] Carey et al. also reported from an inception cohort that 67% of patients with chronic low back pain at 3 months were functionally disabled at 22 months.[174] With the exception of prior history of back pain,[39,43,44,46,62,70,117,136,157,159,160–162,181,182] there are few factors predictive of prognosis or recurrence. Factors found to have some prognostic value in recent prospective studies are pain-related disability,[119,181,183] number of days in pain,[119] low level of education,[119] psychological distress[122,123,182] female sex,[119] and doctor-diagnosed disc disease.[181]

Comorbidity is common with low back pain. Low back pain sufferers have been shown to be more likely than nonsufferers to have other musculoskeletal pain,[71,184] to have other disabling health conditions,[42] and to go on sick leave from other conditions.[185] As discussed elsewhere in the chapter, psychological distress and depression have been shown to be highly correlated with low back and leg pain,[33,172,186,187] as are psychosomatic symptoms.[188] It is likely that psychological factors play roles in both the cause and consequence of low back pain and disability.[115,117,189]

Clinical Pearl: Persons with low back pain are much more likely than persons without pain to have comorbidities such as rheumatological ailments and other disabling conditions, and are more likely to use coping strategies that reinforce their pain and disability.

Coping with Chronic Low Back Pain and Disability

The types of strategies used by persons with acute or chronic pain to deal with their pain may affect their level of psychological disability and physical functioning.[190,191] Cross-sectional studies of persons with chronic pain have demonstrated that relatively more active coping strategies, such as increasing activities and purposely ignoring the pain are related to less psychological disability,[192–194] while diverting attention from the pain and ignoring the pain are related to greater levels of physical functioning.[193] Many studies of patients with chronic pain have shown benefits of cognitive therapy and other interventions that promote more effective coping strategies.[192,195] In a study of patients with chronic low back pain, those with comorbid depression were more likely to report passive coping strategies (e.g., praying, hoping) compared to patients without depression.[134] The temporal relationship between depression, coping style, and pain is unclear. It is not known if coping strategies are stable or if they change over time as pain persists, attenuates, or recurs. The psychophysiological mechanism by which coping, which may be viewed as a stress moderator[196] and pain interact also remains elusive.

Psychological Distress and Depression

Although many investigators have found cross-sectional and longitudinal associations between back pain and depression in clinic-based,[122,123,140,143,197] occupational,[48,116,136] and population-based[117,137,138,198,199] studies, the biological and psychosocial mechanisms responsible for the apparent link remain unclear,[115,119,200] and not all findings are consistent. Inter-study differences in populations and in the definitions of low back pain, as recently suggested,[29] may be responsible for some of the variability across studies.

Dionne et al.[122] demonstrated that in addition to initial functional limitations and number of pain days, measures of somatization and depression were the strongest predictors of low back pain related functional limitations at 2 years among primary care low back pain patients. At 1 year, those patients with continued low back pain and related disability also tended to have higher levels of depression.[119] Baseline depression was also among the major predictors of patient's self-report of poor outcome (patient felt "mixed," "mostly dissatisfied," "unhappy," or "terrible" about low back symptoms in the past 24 hours) at 7 weeks and 1 year among primary care low back pain patients in a health maintenance organization.[140] Other investigators have found cross-sectional associations between depression and low back pain.[137,143,198,201]

Measures of psychological distress predicted the onset of low back pain episodes during a 1-year follow-up period in a recent prospective cohort study.[115] A recent analysis of a subset of the 1958 British birth cohort found that psychological distress at 23 years of age predicted incident low back pain (adjusted OR = 2.52, 95% CI = 1.65, 3.86) at 32–33 years of age.[46] Other investigators found no association between depression and subsequent episodes of back pain during a 3-year period among enrollees of a health maintenance organization.[202] This apparent inconsistency may be due to differences in the populations, length of follow-up, or to differences in how depression and back pain were defined and measured. The importance of psychological variables in back and other musculoskeletal pain outcomes have been demonstrated in many studies.[48,116,123,136,138,143] Leino and Magni[116] found in their longitudinal study that depression predicted the onset of musculoskeletal pain. Polatin et al.[143] concluded that substance abuse and anxiety disorders precede chronic low back pain, while major depression precedes it in some cases and is a consequence of chronic low back pain in other patients. Magni et al.,[138] using data from the National Health and Nutrition Examination Survey I (NHANES I) and the National Health and Nutrition Epidemiologic Follow-Up Survey (NHEFS), found that depression was a predictor of development of chronic musculoskeletal pain 8 years later, and among nondepressed subjects of NHANES I, chronic neck and back pain predicted depression at follow-up 8 years later. Other investigators have also shown low back pain to precede psychological distress and depressive symptoms.[197] Among patients with low back pain enrolled in a recent randomized clinical trial, current pain and disability appreciably increased the odds of subsequent psychological distress, and current distress increased the odds of subsequent pain and disability, suggesting that pain/disability and psychological distress may be causes and consequences of each other.[203]

Clinical Pearl: Recent studies have shown that low back pain and disability increase the risk of psychological distress and depression, and that distress and depression increase the risk of subsequent pain, suggesting a possible bidirectional causal pathway between physical and psychological pain.

Self-reported pain and disability, scores on Scale 3 (hysteria) of the MMPI, and workers' compensation and personal injury status were the strongest predictors of return to work after 1 year among patients with acute pain (<6 weeks) in a prospective cohort study, while physical factors, such as injury severity and physical job demands, and psychopathology, such as major depression and substance and alcohol abuse, were not predictive.[127,128] Gatchel et al.[127,128] concluded that major psychopathology does not precede the onset of chronic low back disability. These and other investigators have shown that improvement in pain outcomes parallel improvement in psychological symptoms.[204,205] Among patients receiving care for lumbar disc prolapse or protrusion, psychological and social variables, including depression, pain coping strategies, and social support, were found to be among the most important predictors of persistent pain 6 months after initial treatment.[129] Depression and stressful work were the major predictors of applying for early retirement.[129]

The authors of a recent comprehensive review of chronic pain and depression concluded that depression is more prevalent among persons with chronic pain; however, based on the available evidence, they could not determine the temporal relationship between depression and chronic pain.[200] The authors identified many problems with studies of depression and chronic pain, including diagnostic criteria used for assessing depression (e.g., *DSM-IV* criteria for major depression vs. the use of scales such as the Beck Depression Inventory, Zung Depression Scale, and the Center for Epidemiologic Studies Depression [CES-D] Scale), issues of assessment of depression in persons with chronic pain (because persons with chronic pain may exhibit similar symptoms as depressed persons without pain), and the existence of many different pain syndromes (the existence or strength of the pain–depression relationship may vary according to the type, severity, and duration of the pain syndrome).

Prevention of Low Back Pain and Related Disability

Numerous randomized[206–219] and nonrandomized[220–225] studies of interventions designed to prevent low back pain or related disability have been published in the scientific literature. These interventions include lumbar supports,[206,207,220] back schools and related educational interventions,[208–214,219,221–224] exercises,[210,215–217] information,[218] and multidisciplinary programs.[225] Reviews of back schools,[226,227] lumbar supports,[226,227] and exercise[226–228] have been published. With the exception of certain exercise interventions, there is little evidence that lumbar supports and back schools and other education programs prevent initial or recurrent episodes of low back pain, or prevent acute pain from becoming chronic. There is also little empirical evidence suggesting that modification of risk factors, such as obesity, smoking, and psychosocial factors, prevents incident or recurrent low back pain episodes.[176,226] However, there is some evidence that cognitive-behavioral therapy may be helpful in preventing chronicity in certain cases.[229,230]

Clinical Pearl: With the exception of certain exercise interventions, there is little scientific evidence that lumbar supports and back schools and other educational programs prevent initial or recurrent episodes of low back pain, or prevent acute pain from becoming chronic.

LUMBAR INTERVERTEBRAL DISC AND ZYGAPOPHYSEAL JOINT DISEASE

Disc Herniation

The incidence of prolapsed lumbar intervertebral disc herniation (a noncontained disc, with nuclear material extending to the neural canal) among 20- to 64-year-olds is estimated to be between 0.1% and 0.5% per year.[231] Men are about 1.6 times more likely than women to be hospitalized for disc herniation.[76] Blue-collar workers and motor-vehicle drivers are the most likely occupational groups to be hospitalized, whereas professional workers are the least likely.[232] Weight and height were risk factors for disc-related hospitalizations among male US World War II military recruits.[233] Heliövaara[76] also showed that obesity and body height were predictive of sciatica due to lumbar disc herniation. Smoking has been shown to be associated with disc prolapse.[107] Psychological factors, including depression, avoidance behavior, nonverbal pain behavior, and lack of social support, were predictive of worse prognosis among patients with acute disc prolapse.[129]

One percent of lumbar disc herniations result in cauda equina syndrome.[234] A study of the natural history of disc herniation demonstrated reductions on follow-up in 63% of patients with magnetic resonance imaging (MRI)-verified disc herniations who did not undergo surgery.[235] However, disc herniation was recently shown to be a strong predictor of disc degeneration after 5 years in a study of 41 initially asymptomatic subjects.[236]

Disc and Zygapophyseal Joint Degeneration

The primary risk factor for lumbar disc degeneration is age.[237,238] Autopsy studies have revealed that little disc degeneration occurs up to the age of 30, after which the risk of degeneration increases linearly in both males and females, though males experience a greater increase in risk with age than females. At age 80–95 years, only 14% of men and 26% of women lack any intervertebral disc degeneration.[237] A more recent study of 600 autopsies reported no grade II or III disc degeneration at 20 years and about 90% at 70 years.[238] Finally, a study of 86 autopsies showed that by age 64 the likelihood of at least one disc herniation is close to 100%, as are signs of disc and zygapophyseal joint degeneration, including osteophytes, zygapophyseal joint osteoarthritis, and endplate irregularities.[239] This latter study also demonstrated that heavy physical loading was most strongly associated with annular ruptures, whereas occupations involving the least loading were associated with the least amount of degeneration.[239] Compared with house painters, concrete reinforcement workers were found to be more likely (OR = 1.8) to have disc space narrowing and more likely to have spondylophytes (OR = 1.6), again suggesting that physical loading is associated with degeneration.[240] Nerve-root involvement has been found in about 10% of patients with lumbar disc degeneration.[17] It should be noted that many investigators have found little correlation between the presence of disc or zygapophyseal joint degeneration and back or leg pain,[241,242] though one longitudinal study of 1167 45- to 64-year-old women showed that radiographically verified disc degeneration is almost 50% more common in those with subsequent back pain than without. Not surprisingly, the best predictor of disc degeneration was pre-existing degeneration at another spinal level.[243] Also, disc degeneration at age 15 was recently found to be a very strong risk factor for recurrent low back pain up to age 23 among those with recurrent low back pain at age 15.[244]

A population-based MRI study of 232 men (mean age = 49 years) revealed that disc height narrowing is most common at L4–L5, followed by L5–S1, L3–L4, and L2–L3.[245] This study also showed that endplate changes and osteophytes are somewhat more common in the lower thoracic spine than the lumbar spine. Degeneration has been shown to be relatively more common among certain athletes, including weight lifters, wrestlers, soccer and tennis players, and gymnasts,[246–248] though no association was found between long-distance running and disc degeneration.[249] A study of identical twins recently revealed that there may be a genetic influence with disc degeneration, finding high concordance with MRI signal intensity, disc narrowing and bulging, and endplate changes.[250] Similarly, a twin study with 172 monozygotic and 154 dizygotic twins showed heritability for lumbar disc degeneration (74%), 64% for severe disease, and 63% for extent of disease.[251] Predictors of lumbar disc degeneration in a recent longitudinal study of 41 asymptomatic subjects included disc herniation, lack of sports activities, and night shift work.[236]

LUMBAR SPINAL STENOSIS

Lumbar spinal stenosis is the reduction in the diameter of the vertebral canal (central stenosis), the lateral recesses, or the intervertebral foramina. Spinal stenosis may be developmental (congenital) or acquired. Acquired stenosis may be subdivided into degenerative, combined congenital and degenerative, spondylotic and spondylolisthetic, iatrogenic posttraumatic, and metabolic (e.g., Paget's disease).[252,253] Although the prevalence and incidence of the specific types of lumbar spinal stenosis are unknown, degenerative stenosis is the most common type of spinal stenosis. The primary risk factor for both congenital and degenerative spinal stenosis is age. Congenital stenosis typically becomes symptomatic in persons 20–30 years old, while degenerative stenosis becomes symptomatic in 50- to 60-year-olds, with females somewhat more likely to be affected than males.[253] Among asymptomatic persons older than 60 years of age, 21% were found to have central canal narrowing.[254] The most common segments affected are L3–L4 and L4–L5.[255] Leg pain and back pain are present in about 80% and 65%, respectively, of persons with degenerative spinal stenosis.[255] Maternal malnutrition and other factors in utero may influence the development of congenital stenosis, but no definitive data are available to confirm or refute this hypothesis.[254]

Few studies have addressed the natural history of spinal stenosis.[256–258] In general, these small studies show that in patients with stenosis of moderate severity, symptoms typically remain unchanged or improve slightly over time, while patients with more severe stenosis are more likely to get worse without conservative treatment or surgical intervention.

FIBROMYALGIA AND MYOFASCIAL PAIN

The low back is a common site for symptoms associated with fibromyalgia and myofascial pain syndrome.[259,260] According to the American College of Rheumatology (ACR) criteria for fibromyalgia, which require at least 11 of 18 anatomical sites to be tender upon 4 kg of pressure, the prevalence of fibromyalgia was recently estimated to be 2%,[261] with a higher prevalence among females. In 18- to 29-year-old females, the prevalence was 1%, whereas among 70- to 79-year-old females, the prevalence was 7%. The prevalence among males did not appreciably change with age, the peak being 1% among 70- to 79-year-olds. In addition to sex,[261–264] factors that have been shown in cross-sectional studies to be associated with fibromyalgia or chronic widespread pain include low educational level,[261,262] physical trauma,[265] and sexual abuse.[266] Comorbid medical illness,[266] irritable bowel syndrome,[267] physical stress,[262] sleep disturbance,[263] and depression[261,263,268,269] have also been reported to be associated with fibromyalgia. Given the cross-sectional nature of these studies, nothing definitive can be stated regarding the influence of these factors on causing or affecting the development of fibromyalgia.

There have been no large studies addressing the natural history of fibromyalgia or chronic widespread pain. Small studies of fibromyalgia patients followed up for 2–4 years show that the majority of patients continue to experience symptoms.[270–272] However, a prospective community-based study of chronic widespread pain showed that after 2 years, only 35% fulfilled the criteria for chronic widespread pain.[273]

LOW BACK DISORDERS IN THE WORKPLACE

Impact of Work-Related Pain and Disability

Low back pain is the most common musculoskeletal disorder in the workplace.[27] The 1-year prevalence of lost work time in the United Kingdom has been estimated to be 11% in men and 7% in women.[11] In the United States in 1988, 17.6% of the workforce (22.4 million people; 56% male) lost 149 million days of work.[35] Back pain is the second most frequent cause of worker absenteeism,[35] resulting in 5.6 million work-related back-pain cases and $8.8 billion in work-related low back claims in 1995.[36] The rate and duration of back-related disability claims appear to have decreased in recent years, however, in the United States and elsewhere.[36,274] The small proportion of workers absent for more than 6 months account for a much greater proportion of compensation and related disability costs.[275] The estimated overall prevalence of cases of work-related back pain with at least one lost workday was 4.6% of the working population.[35] The industry with the most lost workdays was construction for men (1.76 million days) and elementary and secondary schools for women (760,000 days).

The prevalence of low back pain in specific occupations has been addressed in a few cross- sectional studies. For example, among Australian helicopter pilots, the lifetime prevalence of low back pain was an estimated 64%[276]; Canadian Mounted policeman, 54.9%[277]; and nurses in the United Kingdom, 60%[278].

Among workers in four occupational sectors, point prevalence varied from 8% to 45% depending on how low back pain was defined (e.g., according to pain duration, pain intensity, health care use, sick leave).[29] The 1-year incidence of low back pain was an estimated 4.9% among nurses in Canada,[84] whereas the 4-year cumulative incidence was 9.2% among aircraft manufacturing workers in Washington.[279] The leading industries in which workers' compensation claims are awarded for gradual-onset back disorders in Washington State are nursing homes, roofing, wood-frame building construction, landscaping, and wallboard installation.[280]

Occupational Risk and Prognostic Factors

Occupation and Industry Comparing specific occupations to all workers using National Health Interview Survey data, among males the occupations at highest risk for back pain were construction laborers, carpenters, and industrial truck and tractor equipment operators. Among females, the highest risk occupations were nursing aides/orderlies/attendants, licensed practical nurses, maids, and janitors/cleaners.[281] The highest risk industries for work-related back pain among males were lumber and building material retailing, crude petroleum and natural gas extraction, and sawmills/planing mills/millwork. Among females, the highest risk industries were nursing and personal care facilities, beauty shops, and motor vehicle equipment manufacturing.[35]

Sociodemographic Factors Few studies of occupational groups have identified sex, age, or other sociodemographic factors as meaningful predictors of low back pain.[58,160,282] However, one recent cross-sectional study in Germany found high income to be protective for severe low back pain after controlling for work tasks (OR = 0.37),[283] while a study of utility workers in Ontario found being married to be a risk factor.[284] Being divorced or widowed has been shown to be associated with longer work-loss time.[147] Married men were shown to return to work sooner than unmarried men after work injury, while married women returned to work later.[151] The Panel on Musculoskeletal Disorders and the Workplace found increasing age and male gender as factors contributing to the development of pain and disability and to the acute-to-chronic pain transition.[285]

Behavioral Factors Smoking has been shown to predict the reporting of low back symptoms in numerous longitudinal studies[58,62,160,] and cross-sectional studies.[59] Leisure-time physical activity did not appear as an important predictor of low back pain in one 1-year cohort study of Canadian manufacturing employees,[160] though physical activity was slightly inversely associated with the development of low back pain over a 5-year period in another cohort study.[65] The authors of a recent review of 39 studies concluded little overall association between leisure-time physical activity and low back pain, though sedentary leisure activity was found to be associated with an increased prevalence of low back pain and related sick leave.[113]

Physical Factors Of the anthropometric factors studies in occupational populations, weight has been shown to increase the risk of low back pain in women,[44,62] though low BMI was predictive (OR = 2.0) in a recent case-control study in Ontario.[158] Fransen et al.[286] recently showed that obesity was predictive of transitioning from acute to chronic pain after 3 months of an initial workers' compensation claim. The Panel on Musculoskeletal Disorders and the Workplace found BMI as a factor contributing to the development of pain and disability and to the acute-to-chronic pain transition.[285] Height increased the risk of back symptoms among men in one 4-year-long cohort study,[44] but not in other shorter cohort studies.[62,282] One longitudinal study of firefighters demonstrated that aerobic capacity and fitness were protective for subsequent low back injury claims,[287] though these findings are not supported by other longitudinal studies.[58,62] Trunk and lifting strength were not found to be predictive in cohort studies of manual laborers[288] and nurses,[289] respectively. Abdominal muscle weakness was predictive of low back pain among utility workers in one cross-sectional study.[284] Flexibility among nurses was not shown to be a protective factor.[62]

Biomechanical Factors Table 4–6 shows putative occupational biomechanical risk/prognostic factors for low back pain. Specific physical work exposures that have been found to increase the risk of low back pain in working populations are lifting,[41,47,77,82–84,167,170,278,282,286,293,295,296,298–305,313–319] twisting,[53,320] lifting while twisting,[107,320] sitting,[232,290,321,322] standing,[41,61] driving,[16,54,61,80,107,141,232,316] pulling,[313–316] pushing,[313–316] carrying[313–316,323] and lowering,[313–316] bending,[41,71,282,320] bent or twisted posture,[53,77,283,298,301,306,309,310] and stretching and reaching.[316] Other exposures or conditions that have been linked to low back pain are heavy manual labor or physically demanding work,[41,48,76,158,282,283,315] physically stressful work,[39] repetitious work,[67,77,178,324] and jobs requiring the worker to stay in one position for long periods.[325] Work-related twisting was recently shown to increase the risk of incidental sciatic pain in a cohort study of Finnish workers.[175]

TABLE 4–6. Putative Occupational Biomechanical Risk/Prognostic Factors for Low Back Pain, by Factor

Factor	Population	Finding	Reference
Manual material handling	Selected occupations	Lifting → ↑ LBP	290
	Swedish cohort	Heavy lifting → ↑lifetime LBP	291
	US postal workers	Letter carriers → ↑back problems	292
	Australian nurses	Frequent lifting → ↑LBP past month	293
	Israeli miners	Lifting → ↑severe LBP	294
	US nurses	Lifts → ↑back injury	84
	US nurses	Lifts → ↑LBP (past 12 months)	295
	US nurses	Lifts → ↑self-reported back injury	296
	French hospital workers	↑material handling → ↑LBP (12 months)	297
	US firemen	Lifting → ↑LBP with sick days	83
	English nurses	Moving patients → ↑LBP (12 months)	278
	US/Swedish drivers, others	Frequent lifting → ↑LBP (12 months)	82
	Ontario survey	Frequent lifting → ↑severe back problems	47
	Workers	Lifting → ↑LBP (12 months)	298
	Tannery workers	Lifting → ↑LBP (12 months)	299
	Industrial workers	Lifting → ↑LBP (12 months)	300
	Steelworkers	Lifting → ↑LBP (12 months)	301
	Swedish workers	Heavy lifting → ↑LBP (12 months)	77
	Retail material handlers	Material handling → ↑back claim	302
	Retail employees	Lifting → ↑back claim	303
	English nurses	Lifting/transfer → ↑LBP	304
	Assembly workers	Lifting → ↑LBP claim	305
	US workers	Lifting → ↑herniated disc	107
Frequent bending and twisting/awkward postures	Finnish workers	Bending/twisting → ↑sciatica (12 months)	53
	Netherlands concrete workers	Twisted posture→ ↑LBP (12 months)	306
	US assembly workers	Flexing/twist./bending → ↑LBP claim	305
	Swedish construction workers	Bending → ↑LBP (12 months)	71
	Italian bus drivers, others	Awkward posture → ↑LBP (12 months)	81
	Netherlands crane/ office workers	Nonneutral trunk → ↑LBP (12 months)	307
	Italian tractor drivers, others	↑postural load → ↑LBP (12 months)	308
	Canadian blue collar workers	Awkward posture → ↑severe problems	47
	Workers	Awkward postures → ↑LBP (12 months)	298
	Swedish workers	Awkward postures → ↑LBP (12 months)	309
	Swedish workers	Bending/twisting → ↑LBP	77
	Nurses	Flexion → ↑LBP care	310
	Finnish workers	Twisting → ↑sciatica (12 months)	175
Heavy physical load	Dutch workers	Heavy load → ↑back complaints	311
	US workers	Heavy load → ↑LBP (12 months)	312
	Swedish workers	Heavy load → ↑LBP (12 months)	309
	40–47-year-old Swedes	Heavy load → ↑LBP past month	291
	Finnish nurses	Heavy load → ↑lifetime LBP	167
Repetitive motion	Swedish workers	Repetitive work → ↑LBP	77

Note: LBP = low back pain.

A critical National Institute for Occupational Safety and Health (NIOSH) review of 42 epidemiologic studies (30 cross-sectional, 8 cohort, and 4 case-control) of physical workplace factors and low back disorders concluded that there is "strong evidence" for a causal relationship between lifting/forceful movement and low back pain; "evidence" for a causal relationship of awkward posture and heavy physical work with low back pain; and "insufficient evidence" for a causal relationship between static work posture

TABLE 4–7. **Number of Prospective Epidemiologic Studies of Putative Work-Related Risk/Prognostic Factors for Low Back Pain Reviewed by the Panel on Musculoskeletal Disorders and the Workplace,[285] by Type of Factor and Type of Association**

Type of Factor	Factor	Type of Association		
		Null	Positive	Total
Biomechanical*	Manual material handling	4	24	28
	Frequent bending and twisting	2	15	17
	Heavy physical load	0	8	8
	Static work posture	3	3	6
	Repetitive movements	2	1	3
	Whole-body vibration	1	16	17
Work-related psychosocial†	High job demands	1	5	6
	Low decision latitude/control	0	2	2
	Low stimulus from work (monotony)	2	4	6
	Low social support at work	0	7	7
	Low job satisfaction	1	13	14
	High perceived stress	0	3	3
	High perceived emotional effort	0	3	3
	Perceived ability to return to work	0	3	3
	Work perceived dangerous to back	0	2	2
Personal psychosocial‡	Depression of anxiety	5	17	22
	Psychological distress	0	11	11
	Personality factors	3	4	7
	Fear-avoidance coping	1	8	9
	Pain behavior/function	1	6	7

* 43 separate studies.
† 21 separate studies.
‡ 38 separate studies.

and low back pain.[326] The Panel on Musculoskeletal Disorders and the Workplace concluded that "there is a clear relationship between back disorders and physical load" (e.g., manual material handling, load moment, frequent bending and twisting, and heavy physical work).[285] Table 4–7 shows the number of prospective epidemiologic studies of putative work-related risk/prognostic factors for low back pain reviewed by the Panel on Musculoskeletal Disorders and the Workplace.

A wealth of literature supports the hypothesis that whole-body vibration contributes to the development of low back pain.[39,47,61,76,77,81,82,107,298,306,308,309,327–330] A critical review published by NIOSH concluded that there is "strong evidence" favoring a causal relationship between whole-body vibration and low back pain.[326] The National Research Council and the Institute of Medicine (NRC/IOM) also concluded in their recently released report that whole-body vibration is clearly linked to back disorders in the workplace.[285] However, a recent review of studies published from 1986 through 1997 concluded that evidence was insufficient to establish a causal relation between whole-body vibration and low back pain.[331]

Clinical Pearl: Two expert panels convened by the National Institute for Occupational Safety and Health (NIOSH) and the Institute of Medicine (IOM) recently reviewed the literature on musculoskeletal disorders in the workplace and concluded that high physical load and whole-body vibration are linked to an increased risk of occupational low back pain.

A recent case-control study of automobile company employees showed that peak lumbar shear force, peak load handled, and cumulative lumbar disc compression were predictive of low back pain after controlling for the effects of psychosocial risk factors and other potential confounding variables.[158] Physical ergonomic stress was predictive of incident low back pain in the 1958 British birth cohort study.[166] Using strict criteria (e.g., measurement of risk not based solely on self-reports, outcome measures quantifiable on a continuous measurement, design either cohort, case-control, or randomized controlled trial [RCT]), the IOM panel identified 9 studies (5 cohort[28,282,300,332,333] and 4 case-control[305,318,319,334,335] studies) that addressed biomechanical risk factors for back pain. Risk factors identified from these studies include capacity/demand ratio (4 studies), load location (7 studies), load moment (5 studies), frequency (7 studies), kinematics (5 studies), spinal load (2 studies), 3-dimensional loading (5 studies), and multiple factors (7 studies). However, as noted by Davis and Heaney[336] and others, no studies to date have been able to adequately assess both biomechanical and psychosocial exposures in occupational settings.

Psychological and Workplace Psychosocial Factors Table 4–8 shows putative occupational psychosocial risk/prognostic factors for low back pain. Many psychological factors and psychosocial factors in the workplace have been linked to low back pain. These include monotony at work,[39,41,309] poor rating by a supervisor,[52] low job satisfaction,[5,15,41,48,62,67,78,89,136,178,316,320,324,346–348,352] emotionally stressful or anxiety-provoking work,[16,278,291] high psychological job demands,[339] low control,[339,341] poor workplace social environment,[158,309,337,338,340,343,345,346,353] and physical stress.[354] Poor job satisfaction was shown to increase the risk of persistent sciatic pain in a recent cohort study of Finnish workers.[175]

A number of reviews published in the past decade point to a few consistent risk factors. Bongers et al.[355] reviewed 49 cross-sectional studies and 15 longitudinal studies of psychosocial workplace factors on musculoskeletal pain, concluding that job demands, job control, monotonous work, perceived workload time pressure, and lack of social support were risk factors for pain. NIOSH reviewed 13 studies (10 cross-sectional and 3 cohort) of workplace psychosocial factors and back disorders, concluding that perceptions of intensified workload, low job control, and job dissatisfaction were associated with back disorders.[326] The Panel on Musculoskeletal Disorders and the Workplace examined studies addressing psychosocial factors and low back disorders.[285] They concluded that there is strong evidence for low job satisfaction, monotonous work, poor social support at work, high perceived stress, high perceived job demands (work pace), and perceived ability to return to work; and moderate evidence for low job control, emotionally demanding job, and perception that work could be dangerous to back. A recent systematic review of psychosocial factors that included 11 cohort studies and 2 case-control studies concluded that there is "strong evidence" supporting a link between low social support in the workplace and low job satisfaction and back pain; and "insufficient evidence" linking fast work pace, high qualitative demands (e.g., conflicting demands, interruption of tasks, intense concentration), low job content and low job control with back pain.[356]

Clinical Pearl: The Institute of Medicine's 2001 Panel on Musculoskeletal Disorders and the Workplace concluded that there is strong evidence for links between low back disorders and low job satisfaction, monotonous work, poor workplace social support, high perceived stress, and high perceived job demands.

Although negative psychosocial work characteristics (monotony, lack of control, lack of learning opportunities) and job dissatisfaction were predictive of incident low back pain in the univariate analyses of the 1958 British birth cohort study, these factors were not predictive after taking into account other back pain risk factors.[46] Acute psychological distress was predictive of new episodes of low back pain among nursing students in a recent prospective cohort study,[182] and psychological distress, defined as a General Health Questionnaire score of 6 or greater, was one of the predictors of transitioning from acute to chronic pain after 3 months of an initial workers' compensation claim.[286]

Workers' Compensation and Other Societal Factors Economic incentives, workplace organizational policies, litigation, cultural factors, and other societal factors have been shown to influence the reporting of pain, though findings from the literature are not entirely consistent. Furthermore, interpreting the relevant studies in this area is particularly problematic because of the general low quality of the studies and investigators' failure to account for confounding factors.[357,358] For example, back injuries occurring at work have been shown to result in more work-loss days than injuries occurring away from work[142,359]; however, the specific effect of workers' compensation or disability benefits contributing to these differences is not clear. Hadler et al. found no difference in work-loss time or time to return to work in his study comparing patients receiving workers' compensation for acute low back injury with patients who were not receiving compensation.[360] Other investigators have found differences in time to return to work between patients under different compensation schemes; however, uncontrolled differences between groups preclude meaningful interpretations of the studies' findings.[361,362] Several studies have shown compensation to be associated with factors such as heavy physical load, injury severity, income, education, and other variables that may confound the association between compensation and work-related injury outcomes.[363–366] Claims for work-related low back

TABLE 4–8. Putative Occupational Psychosocial Risk/Prognostic Factors for Low Back Pain, by Type of Factor

Type of Factor	Factor	Population	Finding	Reference
Risk factor	High psychological job demands	Swedish nursing aides	↑Psychological demands → ↑lifetime LBP	337
		Netherlands population cohort	↑Work pace → ↑LBP	311
		Swedish nurses	↑Demands → ↑LBP past month	338
		Swedish cohort	↑Demands → ↑intermittent chronic LBP	339
		Swiss workers	↑Demands → ↑LBP past month, male only	150
		Swedish nurses	↑Work demands → ↓LBP (no association)	340
	Low decision latitude/control	Netherlands population cohort	↓Intellectual discretion → ↑LBP	311
		Finnish cohort	Low control → ↑LBP	38
		Swedish nurses	↓Latitude → ↑LBP past month	338
		Swedish cohort	Low control → ↑intermittent chronic LBP	339
		Swiss workers	↓Discretion → ↑LBP past month, male only	150
		UK office workers	↓Job satisfaction → ↑LBP sick leave	341
		Construction workers	↓Latitude → ↓LBP (no association)	71
		Swedish nurses	Low control → ↓LBP (no association)	340
	Low stimulus/monotony	Female Swedes (40–47 years)	Monotonous work → ↑lifetime LBP	291
		Swedish cohort	Monotonous work → ↑LBP (past year)	342
		Population cohort	Monotony → ↑LBP (past year)	309
		Finnish cohort	Monotonous work → ↑sciatic incidence	108
		Swedish nurses	↓Stimulation → ↑LBP (no association)	340
		Aircraft assemblyman	Boredom → ↑LBP (no association)	160
	Low workplace social support	Finnish cohort	Coworker problems → ↑sciatic incidence	108
		Swedish nurses	↓Support from bosses → ↑LBP	347
		Danish salespersons	↓Social contact → ↑LBP (past year)	343
		US ironworkers	↓Social support → ↑work-related LBP	344
		Swedish workers	↓Social support → ↑1-year LBP previously	345
		Construction workers	Social support → ↓LBP (no association)	71
		Swedish cohort	Social support → ↓LBP (no association)	339
		US transit workers	↓Support from boss → ↑neck/LBP	346
	High perceived stress/emotional effort	Finnish workers	Frequent job stress → ↑sciatic pain	53
		Finnish cohort	Mental stress → ↑LBP and sciatic pain	39
		Construction workers	Mental stress → ↑LBP (past year)	71
		UK nurses	Frequent stress → ↑LBP (past year)	278
		Swedish workers	↑Job strain → ↑1-year LBP previously	345
		US transit workers	↑Job strain → ↑neck/LBP	346
		Israeli workers	↑Concentration → ↑LBP	320
		Israeli workers	↑Fatigue → ↑LBP	320
		UK nurses	↑Fatigue → ↑LBP (past year)	278
		NZ nursing students	↑Distress → ↑incident LBP (6 months)	182

(Continued)

TABLE 4–8. (cont.)

Type of factor	Factor	Population	Finding	Reference
	Low job satisfaction	Israeli workers	Not satisfied → ↑LBP	320
		Swedish nursing aides	↓Satisfaction → ↑lifetime LBP	337
		US aircraft workers	Job enjoyment→ ↓LBP	136
		Construction workers	Job satisfaction→ ↓LBP (past year)	71
		Belgium workers	Job satisfaction → ↓LBP (lifetime, 1 year)	15
		Swiss workers	↓Satisfaction → ↑LBP past month, male only	150
		UK workers	Job dissatisfaction → ↑incident LBP	347
		UK office workers	↑Satisfaction → ↑LBP-related sick leave	341
		US transit workers	↓Job dissatisfaction → ↑neck/LBP	346
		Netherlands physical workers	↓Satisfaction → ↑incident LBP, sick leave	348
		55-year-old Swedes	Job satisfaction → ↓LBP	48
		Population cohort	Job satisfaction → ↓LBP (past year)	80
		US nurses	↓Satisfaction → ↑LBP claims (18 months)	62
		Aircraft assemblymen	↓Satisfaction → ↑LBP (1 year)	160
		Australian nurses	Job satisfaction → ↓LBP (no association)	349
		Swedish cohort	Job satisfaction → ↓LBP (no association)	342
Prognostic factor	High psychological job demands	Cohort, 3 months	↑Demands → ↑return to work	131
	Low stimulus/ monotony	Acute LBP sufferers	Monotonous work → ↑sick leave (1 year)	132
		Acute spinal pain	Monotonous work → ↑sick leave (6 months)	126
		Workers on sick leave	Lack of variation → ↑LBP disability	350
	Low workplace social support	Acute disc prolapse	Daily hassles → ↑LBP intensity	129
		Cohort, 3 months	↓Relations at work → ↓return to work	131
		Workers on sick leave	Social isolation → ↑LBP disability	350
	High perceived stress/ emotional effort	Back pain <6 months	↑Job stress → ↓employment (30 months)	200
		Workers' compensation cases	↓Job stress → ↓return to work	133
		Workers on sick leave	↓Emotional effort→ ↑LBP disability	350
	Low Job satisfaction	Workers w/new LBP	Job satisfaction → ↑return to work	55
		Acute LBP patients	Job dissatisfaction→ ↑return to work (3 months)	183
		Female LBP patients <1 year	Job dissatisfaction→ ↑return to work (6 months)	351
		Acute spinal pain patients	Job dissatisfaction→ ↑sick-leave days (6 months)	126
		Workers on sick leave	Job dissatisfaction→ ↑LBP disability	350
		Workers w/acute LBP	↑Satisfaction→ ↑return to work (no association)	139
		Workers' compensation cases	↑Satisfaction → ↑return (no association @6 months)	133

injuries increased during the 1980s and through the mid-1990s, though again the effect of benefits on increasing claim rates is not clear-cut. Contributing to the ambiguity of cause and effect is evidence suggesting that providers may alter their clinical behavior according to whether patients are compensated or not.[367,368]

Litigation has been shown to negatively affect low back outcomes,[369,370] but like the workers' compensation literature, meaningful interpretations of the data are made difficult by the presence of bias in most of the relevant studies, and not all studies show a litigation effect.[371,372] Furthermore, the patient populations are highly selective, limiting the studies' external validity, and the association between litigation and pain may be bidirectional. For example, some low back sufferers may decide to seek attorney representation only after prolonged pain, while others may decide to seek attorney representation immediately following an acute injury. The interpretation of any "litigation" effect in studies composed of these two types of individuals would vary.

Clinical Pearl: Workers' compensation and litigation have been reported to negatively affect low back prognosis. However, interpretation of the studies is complicated by the presence of uncontrolled confounding, changes in provider behavior because of litigation or compensation status, and highly selective patient populations.

A few studies have looked at the effects of organizational policies on time lost from work, time to return to work, and other occupational outcomes.[373–376] In general, findings from these studies show that employers who are actively involved in their employees' health care, offer modified work when indicated, and are concerned about workers' career development are rewarded with fewer claims and fewer and shorter injury-related absences from work.

Prevention of Work-Related Low Back Disorders

Prevention strategies may be used in primary, secondary, or tertiary prevention. The goal of primary prevention is to prevent the onset of the condition, whereas the goal of secondary prevention is to improve the prognosis once the condition is present. Tertiary prevention seeks to maintain the function and activities of daily living of persons who are permanently disabled or impaired. Lumbar supports, back schools and education, and exercise are the preventive interventions that have received the most attention in the literature (see *Prevention of Low Back Pain and Related Disability* above). Ergonomics and risk factor modification have not been subjected to controlled clinical trials. A recent review of controlled clinical trials in industry identified 11 studies for inclusion.[227] The authors concluded from their analysis of 6 studies (including 4 RCTs) of education interventions that given the poor quality of the studies and that 5 of the 6 studies showed no effect on back pain incidence of absenteeism, these interventions are not effective for back pain prevention. They also found no evidence favoring lumbar supports from their analysis of 3 RCTs and 2 controlled clinical trials. All 3 RCTs of exercise interventions demonstrated effects on preventing back pain and/or work-loss days. Thus, the authors concluded that there is limited evidence for the effectiveness of exercise. However, all the studies were of low quality. Two recent studies, one a cohort study of back-belt use among material handlers[377] and another an RCT of an educational pamphlet to prevent disability following work-related low back injury,[378] add to the evidence that lumbar supports and educational interventions are ineffective. Back-belt use or its requirement did not reduce claim rates or self-reported low back pain,[377] and the pamphlet did not prevent or reduce low back pain, health care use, or work absenteeism.[378]

Clinical Pearl: Findings from randomized clinical trials of preventive strategies in the workplace indicate that educational interventions, lumbar supports, and back belts have little effect on worker absenteeism or self-reported pain. Exercise interventions have been shown to prevent low back pain and related work-loss days, though the evidence is limited to few studies of relatively low quality.

The Panel on Musculoskeletal Disorders and the Workplace noted that "there is a very large body of published literature about workplace interventions for the primary and secondary prevention" of back disorders, but that few of the studies meet strict validity criteria.[285] The panel concluded, in part that (1) interventions must mediate physical stressors, largely through the application of principles of ergonomics; (2) employee involvement is essential to successful implementation; (3) employee commitment demonstrated by an integrated program and supported by best practices review is important for success; (4) because of limitations in the scientific literature, a comprehensive and systematic research program supported by an infrastructure linking industry, labor, government, and academic efforts is needed to further clarify and distinguish the features that make interventions effective for specific musculoskeletal disorders; and (5) although generic guidelines have been developed and successfully applied in intervention programs, no single specific design, restriction, or practice for universal application is supported by the existing scientific literature.[285]

LOW BACK DISORDERS IN CHILDREN AND ADOLESCENTS

Back pain is the most common musculoskeletal disorder in youngsters.[110,379–387] Table 4–9 shows the

TABLE 4–9. Prevalence and Incidence of Low Back Pain in Children and Adolescents, by Type of Frequency Measure

Frequency Measure	Population (Country)	Frequency	Reference
Lifetime prevalence	6- to 13-year-olds (Canada)	23%	379
	14- to 18-year-olds (Canada)	33%	379
	11- to 12-year-olds (United Kingdom)	11.6%	380
	15-year-olds (United Kingdom)	50.4%	380
	13- to 16-year-olds (Denmark)	58.9%	381
	14-year-olds (Finland)	30%	382
	High schoolers (Australia)	57%	383
	9-year-olds (Belgium)	36%	384
Point prevalence	High schoolers (Australia)	17%	383
1-year prevalence	7-year-olds (Finland)	1%	385
	10-year-olds (Finland)	6%	385
	13- to 18-year-olds (Finland)	18%	385
	11- to 12-year-olds (United Kingdom)	11.8%	380
	15-year-olds (United Kingdom)	21.5%	380
	13- to 16-year-olds (Denmark)	50.8%	381
2-year cumulative incidence	Children (Sweden)	20%	386
1-year cumulative incidence	Mean age = 12.8 years (Finland)	17.6%	387
	Mean age = 13.8 years (Canada)	17.2%	110

prevalence and incidence of low back pain in children and adolescents. Estimates of lifetime prevalence range from about 10% to 60%, depending on the definition of the pain and the age range of the population studied. Estimates of 1-year prevalence are similarly variable, ranging from 1% among 7-year-olds in Finland[385] to 50.8% among 13- to 16-year-olds in Denmark.[381] Two cohort studies, one conducted in Finland[387] and one recently published from Canada,[110] each estimated the 1-year cumulative incidence of low back pain at about 17%.

Clinical Pearl: Although back pain is the most common musculoskeletal disorder in children, few factors have been shown to consistently increase their risk of pain. As with low back disorders in adults, the causes are likely multifactorial, involving the interplay of genetic, physical, psychological, and behavioral variables.

Table 4–10 shows putative sociodemographic, physical, psychosocial, and behavioral risk/prognostic factors for low back pain among children and adolescents. Increasing age[379,380,385,388–392] and female sex[49,101,381,386,389,390,393–395] have been shown to increase the risk of low back pain, though the latter finding has not been consistently demonstrated.[110,380,384,388,392] Genetic predisposition for low back pain,[94,384] sciatica,[396] intervertebral disc prolapse,[397–399] and disc degeneration[250–400] have been shown in recent observational studies. Few physical factors have been shown to consistently increase the risk of low back disorders among children, though specific competitive sports, including volleyball, bodybuilding, and gymnastics, have been found to be associated with low back pain.[246,380,389,390,395] Other behavioral factors, including smoking[110,381,386,387,395] and time spent in sedentary activities,[382,384,387,389,390,393,395] have been linked with low back pain in kids. Early childhood trauma and psychological distress have been found to increase the risk of low back pain in adolescents.[94,110,386,403]

SUMMARY

1. Principles of study design, analysis, and data interpretation are important in the understanding of estimates of frequency of low back disorders and estimates of association of putative risk and prognostic factors with the occurrence of these disorders. Cohort, cross-sectional, and case-control studies are the major observational designs used to investigate the epidemiology of low back disorders. Experimental (randomized) designs are appropriate for the evaluation of preventive interventions.

TABLE 4–10. Putative Sociodemographic, Physical, Psychosocial, and Behavioral Risk/Prognostic Factors for Low Back Pain among Children and Adolescents, by Type of Factor

Type of Factor	Factor	Finding	References
Sociodemographic	Age	Increasing age	379,380,385,388–392
	Sex	F > M	49,101,381,386,389,390,393–395
		M > F	110,380,384,388,392
		M = F	
	Education	Family education level	393
	History/genetic	Low back pain	94,384,390
		Sciatica	396
		IVD prolapse/herniation	397–399
		Disc degeneration	250,400
Physical	Height	Increasing height	70
		Sitting height	387
	Weight/BMI	Increasing weight	101
		↑ Weight (LBP prevalence)	70,381
		No association with LBP prevalence	382
		No association with LBP onset	70,387
			110
	Flexibility	↓Hip/knee mobility	101
		↓Extension/posterior thigh flexion	382
		↓Posterior thigh flexion	110,379
		No association with flexion–extension	380
		No association with mobility	393
	Strength	Weak abdominals	393
		↓Trunk flexor strength	392
		No association with isometric strength	110
		No association with isokinetic strength	401
	Endurance	↓Isometric (LBP prevalence)	70
		No association with LBP prevalence	402
		No association with LBP onset	70
	Fitness	Poor vs. not poor	381
	Posture	Hyperlordosis	393
		No association with lordosis	387
		No association with backpack	384
		Tight hamstrings	393
	Leg length	Unequal vs. equal	393
	Spinal history	Trauma history	382,389
		Early disc degeneration	70,244
		High growth spurt	110
Psychosocial	Psychological factors	Childhood trauma	403
		"Negative" factors	94
		Emotional factors	386
	Psychological distress	Low Mental Health (MHI)-5 score	110
Behavioral	Activity	≤2 day/week (LBP prevalence)	404
		No association with LBP onset	404
		No association with ↑activity	386,392,393
		↑Activity (LBP prevalence)	385,392
		No association with ↑activity	389
		↑Workout intensity	404
		Competitive sports	380,390,395,405
		Volleyball	389,390,395
		Bodybuilding	390,395
		Aerobics/tennis/cycling	390,395

(Continued)

TABLE 4–10. (cont.)

Type of Factor	Factor	Finding	References
		Gymnasts (LBP prevalence)	246,406
		Gymnasts (disc degeneration)	246,407,408
		No association with sports	110
	Smoking	↑Smoking (LBP prevalence)	381,386,389,395
		↑Smoking (LBP onset)	110
	TV watching	↑TV watching	389,390,395
		No association with TV watching	384
		↑Video game playing	384
	Sitting	Increased sitting	382,387,389,393,395
	Working	Leisure-time job	381
		School-year job	110

2. Prevalence and incidence measures are used to estimate the frequency of low back disorders in various populations and settings.
3. Associations of putative risk and prognostic factors with low back outcomes are most commonly estimated with ratio measures of effect, including prevalence, incidence (risk), and odds ratios.
4. Although the prevalence and incidence of nonspecific mechanical low back pain and other low back disorders depend on the population studied and on specific definitions used, the overall impact of disorders affecting the low back is large, with millions of persons affected and economic costs in the tens of billions of dollars.
5. A number of sociodemographic, behavioral, and physical factors have been identified as risk factors for low back disorders, though with the exceptions of age and history of low back problems, the literature is not consistent. Psychosocial factors, such as psychological distress and depression, have been shown to adversely affect prognosis in many studies.
6. The natural course of low back disorders depends on the specific disorder; however, a history of pain episodes has been shown to be one of the most consistent predictors of subsequent pain. Low back disorders have also been shown to be affected by the presence of comorbidities.
7. The causes and consequences of low back disorders are inherently multifactorial, with genetic, environmental, behavioral, and other factors influencing their onset, duration, and recurrence.
8. Low back pain is the most common and costly musculoskeletal ailment in the workplace, with consequences including disability, lost productivity, sick leave, and large workers' compensation expenses.
9. Many biomechanical and personal and workplace psychosocial factors have been found to affect the risk and prognosis of lumbar spine disorders in the workplace. Workers' compensation and other societal factors may also play important roles, though their specific influence is difficult to determine.
10. There are few valid data showing the effectiveness of low back pain and disability prevention interventions in the workplace.

REFERENCES

1. Last JM. *A dictionary of epidemiology*, 4th ed. New York, NY: Oxford University Press, 2001.
2. Maclure M, Mittleman MA. Should we use a case-crossover design? *Ann Rev Public Health* 2000;21:193–221.
3. Mittleman MA, Maldonado G, Gerberich SG, Smith GS, Sorock GS. Alternative approaches to analytical designs in occupational injury epidemiology. *Am J Ind Med* 1997;32:129–141.
4. Hirsch C, Jonsson B, Lewin T. Low back symptoms in a Swedish female population. *Clin Orthop* 1969;63:171–176.
5. Svensson HO. Low back pain in forty to forty-seven year old men. II. Socio-economic factors and previous sickness absence. *Scand J Rehabil Med* 1982;14:55–60.
6. Biering-Sörensen F. A prospective study of low back pain in a general population. I. Occurrence, recurrence and aetiology. *Scand J Rehabil Med* 1983; 15:77–79.
7. Cunningham LS, Kelsey JL. Epidemiology of musculoskeletal impairments and associated disability. *Am J Public Health* 1984; 74:574–579.
8. Deyo RA, Tsui-Wu YJ. Descriptive epidemiology of low back pain and its related medical care in the United States. *Spine* 1987; 12:264–268.
9. Svensson HO, Andersson GBJ, Johansson S, et al. A retrospective study of low back pain in 38- to 64-year old women: Frequency and occurrence and impact on medical services. *Spine* 1988; 13:548–552.
10. Heliövaara M. Risk Factors for low back pain and sciatica. *Ann Med* 1989; 21:257–264.

11. Walsh K, Cruddas M, Coggon D. Low back pain in eight areas of Britain. *J Epidemiol Commun Health* 1992; 46:227–230.
12. Papageorgiou AC, Croft PR, Ferry S, et al. Estimating the prevalence of low back pain in the general population: Evidence from the South Manchester back pain survey. *Spine* 1995; 20:1889–1894.
13. Cassidy JD, Carroll L, Cote P. The Saskatchewan health and back pain survey: The prevalence of low back pain and related disability in Saskatchewan adults. *Spine* 1998; 23:1860–1866.
14. Leboeuf-Yde C, Lauritsen JM. The prevalence of low back pain in the literature: A structured review of 26 Nordic studies from 1954 to 1993. *Spine* 1995; 20:2112–2118.
15. Skovron ML, Szpalski M, Nordin M, et al. Sociocultural factors in back pain: A population based study in Belgian adults. *Spine* 1994; 19:129–137.
16. Frymoyer JW, Pope MH, Clements JH, Wilder DG, MacPherson B, Ashikaga T. Risk factors in low back pain. *J Bone Joint Surg Am* 1983; 65:213–218.
17. Lawrence JS. Disc degeneration: Its frequency and relationship to symptoms. *Ann Rheum Dis* 1969; 28:121–137.
18. Nagi SZ, Riley LE, Newby LG. A social epidemiology of back pain in a general population. *J Chron Dis* 1973; 26:769–779.
19. Bjelle A, Allander E, Lundguist B. Geographic distribution of rheumatic disorders and working conditions in Sweden.*Scand J Soc Med* 1981; 91:119–126.
20. Brattberg G, Thorslund M, Wikman A. The prevalence of pain in a general population: The results of a postal survey in a county of Sweden. *Pain* 1989; 37:215–222.
21. Hillman M, Wright A, Rajaratnam G, et al. Prevalence of low back pain in the community: Implications for service provision in Bradford, U.K. *J Epidemiol Commun Health* 1996; 50:347–352.
22. Carey TS, Evans AT, Hadler NM, et al. Acute severe low back pain: A population-based study of prevalence and care-seeking. *Spine* 1996; 21:339–344.
23. Reisbord LS, Greenland S. Factors associated with self-reported back-pain prevalence: A population-based study. *J Chron Dis* 1985; 38:691–702.
24. Taylor H, Curran NM. *The Nuprin pain report*. New York: Louis Harris and Associates, 1985:1–233.
25. Linton SJ, Hellsing AL, Hallden K. A population-based study of spinal pain among 35–45 year old individuals: Prevalence, sick leave, and health care use. *Spine* 1998; 23:1457–1463.
26. Bredkjaer SR. Musculoskeletal disease in Denmark: The Danish Health and Morbidity Survey 1986–87. *Acta Orthop Scand* 1991; 62(Suppl 241):10–12.
27. Marras WS. Occupational low back disorder causation and control. *Ergonomics* 2000; 43:880–902.
28. Marras WS, Davis KG, Heaney CA, Maronitis AB, Allread WG. The influence of psychosocial stress, gender, and personality and mechanical loading of the lumbar spine. *Spine* 2000b; 25:3045–3054.
29. Ozguler A, Leclerc A, Landre MF, Pietri-Taleb F, Niedhammer I. Individual and occupational determinants of low back pain according to various definitions of low back pain. *J Epidemiol Community Health* 2000; 54:215–220.
30. Abenhaim L, Suissa S. Importance and economic burden of occupational back pain: A study of 2,500 cases representative of Quebec. *J Occup Med* 1987; 29:670–674.
31. Hart LG, Deyo RA, Cherkin DC. Physician office visits for low back pain. *Spine* 1995; 20:11–19.
32. Woodwell DA. National Ambulatory Medical Care Survey: 1997 summary. *Adv Data* 1999; 20:1–28.
33. Waddell G. Low back pain: A twentieth century health care enigma. *Spine* 1996; 15:2820–2825.
34. Hashemi L, Webster BS, Clancy EA. Trends in disability duration and cost of workers compensation low back pain claims (1988–1996).*J Occup Environ Med* 1998; 40:1110–1119.
35. Guo HR, Tanaka S, Halperin WE, Cameron LL. Back pain prevalence in U.S. industry and estimates of lost workdays. *Am J Public Health* 1999; 89:1029–1035.
36. Murphy PL, Volinn E. Is occupational low back pain on the rise? *Spine* 1999; 24:691–697.
37. Allan DB, Waddell G. An historical perspective on low back pain and disability. *Orthop Scand* 1989; 60(Suppl 234):10–23.
38. Leino P, Hänninen V. Psychosocial factors at work in relation to back and limb disorders. *Scand J Work Environ Health* 1995; 21:134–142.
39. Heliövaara M, Mäkelä M, Knekt P, Impivaara O, Aroma A. Determinants of sciatica and low-back pain. *Spine* 1991; 16:608–614.
40. Riihimaki H. Low-back pain: Its origin and risk indicators. *Scand J Work Environ Health* 1991; 17:81–90.
41. Svensson HO, Andersson GB. The relationship of low-back pain, work history, work environment, and stress: A retrospective cross-sectional study of 38- to 64-year old women. *Spine* 1989; 14:517–522.
42. Hurwitz EL, Morgenstern H. Correlates of back problems and back-related disability in the United States. *J Clin Epidemiol* 1997; 50:669–681.
43. Daltroy LH, Larson MG, Wright EA, et al. A case-control study of risk factors for industrial low back injury: Implications for primary and secondary prevention programs. *Am J Ind Med* 1991; 20:505–515.
44. Battie MC, Bigos SJ, Fisher LD, et al. Anthropometric and clinical measures as predictors of back pain complaints in industry: A prospective study. *J Spinal Disord* 1990; 3:195–204.
45. Burdorf A, Sorock G. Positive and negative evidence of risk factors for back disorders. *Scand J Work Environ Health* 1997; 23:243–256.
46. Power C, Frank J, Hertzman C, Schierhout G, Li L. Predictors of low back pain onset in a prospective British study. *Am J Public Health* 2001; 91:1671–1678.
47. Liira JP, Shannon HS, Chambers IW, et al. Long-term back problems and physical work exposures in the 1990 Ontario Health Survey. *Am J Public Health* 1996; 86:382–387.
48. Bergenudd H, Nilsson B. Back pain in middle age: Occupational workload and psychologic factors: An epidemiologic survey. *Spine* 1988; 13:58–60.

49. Viikari-Juntura E, Vuori J, Silverstein B, et al. A life-long prospective study on the role of psychosocial factors in neck–shoulder and low-back pain. *Spine* 1991; 16:1056–1061.
50. Dionne C, Koepsell TD, Von Korff M, Deyo RA, Barlow WI, Checkoway H. Formal education and back-related disability. In search of an explanation. *Spine* 1995; 20:2721–2730.
51. Deyo RA, Tsui-Wu YJ. Functional disability due to back pain. *Arthritis Rheum* 1987; 30:1247–1253.
52. Bigos SJ, Spengler DM, Martin NA, et al. Back injuries in industry: A retrospective study. III. Employee-related factors. *Spine* 1986; 11:252–256.
53. Riihimaki H, Tola S, Videman T, et al. Low-back pain and occupation. *Spine* 1989; 14:204–209.
54. Biering-Sörensen F, Thomsen C. Medical, social and occupational history as risk indicators for low-back trouble in a general population. *Spine* 1986; 11:720–723.
55. Cats-Baril WL, Frymoyer JW. Demographic factors associated with the prevalence of disability in the general population. *Spine* 1991; 16:671–674.
56. Volinn E, Lai D, McKinney S, et al. When back pain becomes disabling: A regional analysis. *Pain* 1988; 33:33–39.
57. Cheadle A, Franklin G, Wolfhagen C, et al. Factors influencing the duration of work-related disability: A population-based study in Washington State Workers Compensation. *Am J Public Health* 1994; 84:190–196.
58. Battie MC, Bigos SJ, Fisher LD, et al. A prospective study of the role of cardiovascular risk factors and fitness in industrial back pain complaints. *Spine* 1989; 14:141–147.
59. Boshuizen HC, Verbeek JH, Broersen J, et al. Do smokers get more back pain? *Spine* 1993; 18:35–40.
60. Deyo RA, Bass JE. Lifestyle and low-back pain. *Spine* 1989; 14:501–506.
61. Pietri F, Leclerc A, Boitel L, et al. Low-back pain in commercial travelers. *Scand J Work Environ Health* 1992; 18:52–58.
62. Ready AE, Boreskie SL, Law SA, et al. Fitness and lifestyle parameters fail to predict back injuries in nurses. *Can J Appl Phys* 1993; 18:80–90.
63. Toroptsova NT, Benevolenskaya LI, Karyakin AN, et al. "Cross sectional" study of low back pain among workers at an industrial enterprise in Russia. *Spine* 1995; 20:328–332.
64. Harreby M, Kjer J, Hesselsöe G, et al. Epidemiological aspects and risk factors for low back pain in 38 year-old men and women: A 25-year prospective cohort study of 640 school children. *Eur Spine J* 1996; 5:312–318.
65. Leino P. Does leisure time physical activity prevent low back disorders: A prospective study of metal industry employees. *Spine* 1993; 18:863–871.
66. Manninen P, Riihimaki H, Heliövaara M. Incidence and risk factors of low back pain in middle-aged farmers. *Occup Med* 1995; 45:141–146.
67. Vallfors B. Acute, subacute and chronic low back pain: Clinical symptoms, absenteeism and working environment. *Scand J Rehabil Med Suppl* 1985; 11:1–98.
68. Cady LD, Thomas PC, Karwasky RJ. Program for increasing health and physical fitness of firefighters. *J Occup Med* 1985; 2:111–114.
69. Heistaro S, Vartiainen E, Heliövaara M, Puska P. Trends of back pain in eastern Finland, 1972–1992, in relation to socioeconomic status and behavioral risk factors. *Am J Epidemiol* 1998; 148:671–682.
70. Salminen JJ, Erkintalo M, Laine M, et al. Low back pain in the young: A prospective three-year follow-up study of subjects with and without low back pain. *Spine* 1995; 20:2101–2108.
71. Holmstrom EB, Lindell L, Mortitz U. Low back and neck/shoulder pain in construction workers: Occupational workload and psychosocial risk factors. *Spine* 1992; 17:663–671.
72. Magnusson M, Almqvist M, Broman H, Pope M, Hansson T. Measurement of height loss during whole body vibrations. *J Spinal Disord* 1992; 5:198–203.
73. Troup JDG, Martin JW, Lloyd DCEF. Back pain in industry: A prospective study. *Spine* 1981; 6:61–69.
74. Biering-Sörensen F. Physical measurements as risk indicators for low-back trouble over a one-year period. *Spine* 1984; 9:106–119.
75. Mortimer M, Wiktorin C, Pernol G, Svensson H, Vingard E. Sports activities, body weight and smoking in relation to low-back pain: A population-based case-referent study. *Scand J Med Sci Sports* 2001; 11:178–184.
76. Heliövaara M. Body height, obesity, and risk of herniated lumbar intervertebral disc. *Spine* 1987; 12:469–472.
77. Saraste H, Hultman G. Life conditions of persons with and without low-back pain. *Scand J Rehabil Med* 1987; 19:109–113.
78. Troup JDG, Foreman TK, Baxter CE, Brown D. 1987 Volvo award winner in clinical sciences. The perception of back pain and the role of psychophysical tests of lifting capacity. *Spine* 1987; 12:645–657.
79. Videman T, Rauhala H, Asp S, et al. Patient-handling skill, back injuries, and back pain. An intervention study in nursing. *Spine* 1989; 14:148–156.
80. Biering-Sörensen F, Thomsen CE, Hilden J. Risk indicators for low back trouble. *Scand J Rehabil Med* 1989; 21:151–157.
81. Bovenzi M, Zadini A. Self-reported low back syndromes in urban bus drivers exposed to whole-body vibration. *Spine* 1992; 17:1048–1059.
82. Magnusson MI., Pope MH, Wilder DG, et al. Are occupational drivers at an increased risk for developing musculoskeletal disorders? *Spine* 1996; 21:710–717.
83. Nuwayhid IA, Stewart W, Johnson JV. Work activities and the onset of first-time low back pain among New York City fire fighters. *Am J Epidemiol* 1993; 137:539–548.
84. Venning PJ, Walter SD, Sitt LW. Personal and job-related factors as determinants of incidence of back injuries among nursing personnel. *J Occup Med* 1987; 29:820–825.
85. Chaffin DB, Herrin GD, Keyserling WM. Preemployment strength testing: An updated position. *J Occup Med* 1978; 20:403–408.

86. Leino P, Aro S, Hasan J. Trunk muscle function and low back disorders: A ten-year follow-up study. *J Chron Dis* 1987; 40:289–296.
87. McNeill T, Warwick D, Andersson G, et al. Trunk strengths in attempted flexion, extension, and lateral bending in healthy subjects and patients with low-back disorders. *Spine* 1980; 5:529–538.
88. Kujala U, Taimela S, Viljanen T, et al. Physical loading and performance as predictors of back pain in healthy adults: A 5-year prospective study. *Eur J Appl Physiol* 1996; 73:452–458.
89. Mostardi RA, Noe DA, Kovacic MW, et al. Isokinetic lifting strength and occupational injury: A prospective study. *Spine* 1991; 17:189–193.
90. Pedersen OF, Petersen R, Staffeldt ES. Back pain and isometric back muscle strength of workers in a Danish factory. *Scand J Rehabil Med* 1975; 7:125–128.
91. Battie MC, Bigos SJ, Fisher LD, et al. Isometric lifting strength as a predictor of industrial back pain reports. *Spine* 1989; 14:851–856.
92. Howell DW. Musculoskeletal profile and incidence of musculoskeletal injuries in lightweight women rowers. *Am J Sports Med* 1984; 12:278–282.
93. Pope M, Bevins T, Wilder DG, et al. The relationship between anthropometric, postural, muscular, and mobility characteristics of males, ages 18–55. *Spine* 1985; 10:644–648.
94. Balagué F, Skovron MI, Nordin M, et al. Low back pain in schoolchildren: A study of familial and psychological factors. *Spine* 1995; 20:1265–1270.
95. Battie MC, Bigos SJ, Fisher LD, et al. The role of spinal flexibility in back pain complaints within industry: A prospective study. *Spine* 1990; 15:768–773.
96. Sweetman BJ, Anderson JAD, Dalton ER. The relationships between little-finger mobility, lumbar mobility, straight-leg raising, and low-back pain. *Rheumatol Rehabil* 1974; 13:161–166.
97. Friberg O. Clinical symptoms and biomechanics of lumbar spine and hip joint in leg length inequality. *Spine* 1983; 8:643–651.
98. Friberg O. Results of radiologic measurements of leg-length inequality. *Spine* 1992; 17:458–460.
99. Giles LGF, Taylor JR. Low-back pain associated with leg length inequality. *Spine* 1981; 6:510–521.
100. Rowe ML. Low back disability in industry: Updated position. *J Occup Med* 1971; 13:476–478.
101. Fairbank JC, Pynsent PB, Van Poortvliet JA, et al. Influence of anthropometric factors and joint laxity in the incidence of adolescent back pain. *Spine* 1984; 9:461–464.
102. Grundy PF, Roberts CJ. Does unequal leg length cause back pain? *J Manipulative Physiol Ther* 1984; 2:256–258.
103. Hellsing AL. Leg length inequality: A prospective study of young men during their military service. *Upps J Med Sci* 1988; 93:245–253.
104. Soukka A, Alaranta H, Tallroth K, et al. Leg-length inequality in people of working age: The association between mild inequality and low-back pain is questionable. *Spine* 1991; 16:429–431.
105. Magora A. Investigation of the relation between low back pain and occupation: Neurologic and orthopaedic conditions. *Scand J Rehabil Med* 1975; 7:146–151.
106. Virta L, Ronnemaa T. The association of mild-moderate isthmic lumbar spondylolisthesis and low back pain in middle-aged patients is weak and it only occurs in women. *Spine* 1993; 18:1496–1503.
107. Kelsey JL, Githens PB, O'Connor T, et al. Acute prolapsed lumbar intervertebral disc: An epidemiological study with special references to driving automobiles and cigarette smoking. *Spine* 1984; 9:608–613.
108. Riihimaki H, Viikari-Juntura E, Moneta G, et al. Incidence of sciatic pain among men in machine operating, dynamic physical work, and sedentary work: A three-year follow-up. *Spine* 1994; 19:138–142.
109. Leboeuf-Yde C, Kyvik KO, Bruun NH. Low back pain and lifestyle. Part I. Smoking. Information from a population based sample of 29,424 twins. *Spine* 1998; 23:2207–2213.
110. Feldman DE, Shrier I, Rossignol M, Abenhaim L. Risk factors for the development of low back pain in adolescence. *Am J Epidemiol* 2001; 154:30–36.
111. Leboeuf-Yde C. Smoking and low back pain. A systematic literature review of 41 journal articles reporting 47 epidemiologic studies. *Spine* 1999; 24:1463–1470.
112. Vuori IM. Dose–response of physical activity and low back pain, osteoarthritis, and osteoporosis. *Med Sci Sports Exerc* 2001; 33(6, Suppl):S551–S586.
113. Hildebrandt VH, Bongers PM, Gul J, van Dijk FJ, Kemper HC. The relationship between leisure time, physical activities and musculoskeletal symptoms and disability in worker populations. *Int Arch Occup Environ Health* 2000; 73:507–518.
114. Leboeuf-Yde C, Kyvik KO. Is it possible to differentiate people with or without low-back pain on the basis of test of lumbopelvic dysfunction? *J Manipulative Physiol Ther* 2000; 23:160–167.
115. Croft PR, Papageorgiou AC, Ferry S, Thomas E, Jayson MI, Silman AJ. Psychologic distress and low back pain: Evidence from a prospective study in the general population. *Spine* 1995; 20:2731–2737.
116. Leino P, Magni G. Depressive and distress symptoms as predictors of low back pain, neck–shoulder pain, and other musculoskeletal morbidity: A 10-year follow-up of metal industry employees. *Pain* 1993; 53:89–94.
117. Mannion AF, Dolan P, Adams MA. Psychological questionnaires: Do abnormal scores precede or follow first-time low back pain? *Spine* 1996; 21:2603–2611.
118. Linton SJ, Buer N, Vlaeyen J, Hellsing AL. Are fear-avoidance beliefs related to a new episode of back pain? A prospective study. *Psychol Health* 1999; 14:1051–1059.
119. Von Korff M, LeResce L, Dworkin SF. First onset of common pain syndromes: A prospective study of depression as a risk factor. *Pain* 1993; 55:251–258.
120. Burton AK, Tillotson KM, Main CJ, et al. Psychosocial predictors of outcome in acute and subchronic low back trouble. *Spine* 1995; 20:722–728.
121. Klenerman L, Slade PD, Stanley IM, et al. The prediction of chronicity in patients with an acute attack of

low back pain in a general practice setting. *Spine* 1995; 20:478–484.

122. Dionne CE, Koepsell TD, Von Korff M, Deyo RA, Barlow WE, Checkoway H. Predicting long-term functional limitations among back pain patients in primary care settings. *J Clin Epidemiol* 1997; 50:31–43.
123. Main CJ, Wood PLR, Hollis S, et al. The distress and risk assessment method: A simple patient classification to identify distress and evaluate the risk of poor outcome. *Spine* 1992; 17:42–52.
124. Philips HC, Grant L. The evolution of chronic back problems. *Behav Res Ther* 1991; 29:435–441.
125. Waddell G, Newton M, Henderson I, et al. A fear-avoidance beliefs questionnaire (FABQ) and the role of fear-avoidance beliefs in chronic low back pain and disability. *Pain* 1993; 52:157–168.
126. Linton SJ, Hallden K. Can we screen for problematic back pain? A screening questionnaire for predicting outcome in acute and subacute back pain. *Clin J Pain* 1998; 14:209–215.
127. Gatchel RJ, Polatin PB, Kinney RK. Predicting outcome of chronic back pain using clinical predictors of psychopathology: A prospective analysis. *Health Psychol* 1995; 14:415–420.
128. Gatchel RJ, Polatin PB, Mayer TG. The dominant role of psychosocial risk factors in the development of chronic low back pain disability. *Spine* 1995; 20:2702–2709.
129. Hasenbring M, Marienfeld G, Kuhlendahl D, et al. Risk factors of chronicity in lumbar disc patients: A prospective investigation of biologic, psychologic, and social predictors of therapy outcome. *Spine* 1994; 19:2759–2765.
130. Engel CC, Von Korff M, Katon WJ. Back pain in primary care: Predictors of high health-care costs. *Pain* 1996; 65:197–204.
131. Hazard RG, Haugh LD, Reid S, Preble JB, MacDonald L. Early prediction of chronic disability after occupational low back injury. *Spine* 1996; 21:945–951.
132. Hellsing AL, Linton SJ, Kalvemark M. A prospective study of patients with acute back and neck pain in Sweden. *Phys Ther* 1994; 74:116–124; discussion 25–28.
133. Lancourt J, Kettelhut M. Predicting return to work for lower back pain patients receiving worker's compensation. *Spine* 1992; 17:629–640.
134. Weickgenant AL, Slater MA, Patterson TL, Atkinson JH, Grant I, Garfin SR. Coping activities in chronic low back pain: Relationship with depression. *Pain* 1993; 53:95–103.
135. Linton SJ, Buer N. Working despite pain: Factors associated with work attendance versus dysfunction. *Int J Behav Med* 1995; 2:252–262.
136. Bigos SJ, Battie MC, Spengler DM, et al. A prospective study of work perceptions and psychosocial factors affecting the report of back injury. *Spine* 1991; 16:1–6.
137. Magni G, Marchitti M, Moreschi C, et al. Chronic musculoskeletal pain and depressive symptoms in the National Health and Nutrition Examination. I. Epidemiological follow-up study. *Pain* 1993; 53:161–168.
138. Magni G, Moreschi C, Rigatti-Luchini S, et al. Prospective study on the relationship between depressive symptoms and chronic musculoskeletal pain. *Pain* 1994; 56:289–297.
139. Lehmann TR, Spratt KF, Lehmann KK. Predicting long term disability in low back injured workers presenting to a spine consultant. *Spine* 1993; 18:1103–1112.
140. Cherkin DC, Deyo RA, Street JH, Barlow W. Predicting poor outcome for back pain seen in primary care using patients own criteria. *Spine* 1996; 21:2900–2907.
141. Frymoyer JW, Pope MH, Costanza MC, et al. Epidemiologic studies of low-back pain. *Spine* 1980; 5:419–423.
142. Leavitt F. The role of psychological disturbance in extending disability time among compensable back injured industrial workers. *J Psychosom Res* 1990; 34:447–453.
143. Polatin PB, Kinney RK, Gatchel RJ, Lillo E, Mayer TG. Psychiatric illness and chronic low-back pain. The mind and the spine: Which goes first? *Spine* 1993; 18:66–71.
144. Linton SJ. The relationship between activity and chronic back pain. *Pain* 1985; 21:289–294.
145. Waddell G. A new clinical model for the treatment of low back pain. *Spine* 1987; 12:632.
146. Waddell G. Biopsychosocial analysis of low back pain. *Baillieres Clin Rheumatol* 1992; 6:523–557.
147. Volinn E, Koevering DV, Loeser JD. Back sprain in industry: The role of socioeconomic factors in chronicity. *Spine* 1991; 16:542–548.
148. Isacsson A, Hanson BS, Ranstam J, et al. Social network, social support and the prevalence of neck and low back pain after retirement: A population study of men born in 1914 in Malmo, Sweden. *Scand J Soc Med* 1995; 23:17–22.
149. Klapow JC, Slater MA, Patterson TL, et al. Psychosocial factors discriminate multidimensional clinical groups of chronic low back pain patients. *Pain* 1995; 62:349–355.
150. Foppa I, Noack RH. The relation of self-reported back pain to psychosocial, behavioral, and health-related factors in a working population in Switzerland. *Soc Sci Med* 1996; 43:1119–1126.
151. Baldwin ML, Johnson WG, Butler RJ. The error of using returns-to-work to measure the outcomes of health care. *Am J Ind Med* 1996; 29:632–641.
152. Muramatsu N, Liang J, Sugisawa H. Transitions in chronic low back pain in Japanese older adults: A sociomedical perspective. *J Gerontol B Psychol Sci Soc Sci* 1997; 52:S222–S234.
153. Linton SJ. A review of psychological risk factors in back and neck pain. *Spine* 2000; 25:1148–1156.
154. Hoogendoorn WE, Bongers PM, de Vet HC, et al. Flexion and rotation of the trunk and lifting at work are risk factors for low back pain: Results of a prospective cohort study. *Spine* 2000; 25:3087–3092.
155. Turk DC. The role of demographic and psychosocial factors in transition from acute to chronic pain. In: Jensen TS, Turner JA, Wiesenfeld-Hallin Z, eds. *Proceedings of the 8th World Congress on Pain*, Vol. 8. Seattle: IASP Press, 1997:185–213.
156. Pincus T, Burton AK, Vogel S, Field AP. A systematic review of psychological factors as predictors of

chronicity/disability in prospective cohorts of low back pain. *Spine* 2002; 27:E109–E120.
157. Ryden LA, Molgaard CA, Bobbitt S, et al. Occupational low-back injury in a hospital employee population: An epidemiologic analysis of multiple risk factors of a high-risk occupational group. *Spine* 1989; 14:315–320.
158. Kerr MS, Frank JW, Shannon HS, et al. Biomechanical and psychosocial risk factors for low back pain at work. *Am J Public Health* 2001; 91:1069–1075.
159. Harber P, Pena L, Hsu P, et al. Personal history, training, and worksite as predictors of back pain of nurses. *Am J Ind Med* 1994; 25:519–526.
160. Rossignol M, Lortie M, Ledoux E. Comparison of spinal health indicators in predicting spinal status in a 1-year longitudinal study. *Spine* 1993; 18:54–60.
161. Papageorgiou AC, Croft PR, Thomas E, et al. Influence of previous pain experience on the episode incidence of low back pain: Results from the South Manchester Back Pain Study. *Pain* 1996; 66:181–185.
162. Adams MA, Mannion AF, Dolan P. Personal risk factors for first-time low back pain. *Spine* 1999; 24:2497–2505.
163. Hellsing AL, Bryngelsson IL. Predictors of musculoskeletal pain in men: A twenty-year follow-up from examination at enlistment. *Spine* 2000;25:3080–3086
164. Hurwitz EL, Morgenstern H. Cross-sectional associations of asthma, hay fever, and other allergies with major depression and low-back pain among adults aged 20–39 years in the United States. *Am J Epidemiol* 1999; 150:1107–1116.
165. Brynhildsen JO, Bjors E, Skarsgard C, Hammar ML. Is hormone replacement therapy a risk factor for low back pain among postmenopausal women? *Spine* 1998; 23:809–813.
166. Harreby M, Neergaard K, Hesselsoe G, Kjer J. Are radiologic changes in the thoracic and lumbar spine of adolescents risk factors for low back pain in adults? A 25-year prospective cohort study of 640 school children. *Spine* 1995; 20:2298–2302.
167. Videman T, Nurminen T, et al. Low-back pain in nurses and some loading factors of work. *Spine* 1984; 9:400–404.
168. Mantle MJ, Greenwood RM, Currey HL. Backache in pregnancy. *Rheumatol Rehabil* 1977; 16:95–101.
169. Fast A, Shapiro D, Ducommon EJ, et al. Low-back pain in pregnancy. *Spine* 1987; 12:368–371.
170. Linton SJ, Lardén M, Gillow AM. Sexual abuse and chronic musculoskeletal pain: Prevalence and psychological factors. *Clin J Pain* 1996; 12:215–221.
171. Linton SJ. A population-based study of the relationship between sexual abuse and back pain: Establishing a link. *Pain* 1997; 73:47–53.
172. Pietri-Taleb F, Riihimaki H, Viikari-Juntura E, Lindstrom K, Moneta GB. The role of psychological distress and personality in the incidence of sciatic pain among working men. *Am J Public Health* 1995; 85:541–545.
173. Smedley J, Inskip H, Cooper C, Coggon D. Natural history of low back pain. A longitudinal study in nurses. *Spine* 1998; 23:2422–2426.
174. Carey TS, Garrett JM, Jackman AM. Beyond the good prognosis. Examination of an inception cohort of patients with chronic low back pain. *Spine* 2000; 25:115–120.
175. Miranda H, Viikari-Juntura E, Martikainen R, Takala EP, Riihimaki H. Individual factors, occupational loading, and physical exercise as predictors of sciatic pain. *Spine* 2002; 27:1102–1109.
176. Frank JW, Kerr MS, Brooker AS, et al. Disability resulting from occupational low back pain. I. What do we know about primary prevention? *Spine* 1996; 21:2908–2917.
177. Von Korff M, Saunders K. The course of back pain in primary care. *Spine* 1996; 21:2833–2837; discussion 2838–2839.
178. Bergquist-Ullman M, Larsson U. Acute low back pain in industry. A controlled prospective study with special reference to therapy and confounding factors. *Acta Orthop Scand* 1977; 170:1–117.
179. Abenhaim L, Suissa S, Rossignol M. Risk of recurrence of occupational back pain over three year follow up. *Br J Ind Med* 1988; 45:829–833.
180. Rossignol M, Suissa S, Abenhaim L. The evolution of compensated occupational spinal injuries. A three-year follow-up study. *Spine* 1992; 17:1043–1047.
181. Carey TS, Garrett JM, Jackman A, et al. Recurrence and care seeking after acute back pain: Results of a long-term follow-up study. North Carolina Back Pain Project. *Med Care* 1999; 37:157–164.
182. Feyer AM, Herbison P, Williamson AM, et al. The role of physical and psychological factors in occupational low back pain: A prospective cohort study. *Occup Environ Med* 2000; 57:116–120.
183. Coste J, Delecoeuillerie G, Cohen de Lara A, Le parc JM, Paolaggi JB. Clinical course and prognostic factors in acute low back pain: An inception cohort study in primary care practice. *BMJ* 1994; 308:577–580.
184. Skargren EI, Oberg BE. Predictive factors for 1-year outcome of low-back and neck pain in patients treated in primary care: Comparison between the treatment strategies chiropractic and physiotherapy. *Pain* 1998; 77:201–207.
185. Seferlis T, Nemeth G, Carlsson AM, Gillstrom P. Acute low-back-pain patients exhibit a fourfold increase in sick leave for other disorders: A case-control study. *J Spinal Disord* 1999; 12:280–286.
186. Von Korff M, Dworkin SF, Resche LL, et al. An epidemiologic comparison of pain complaints. *Pain* 1988; 32:173-183.
187. Akerlind I, Hornquist JO, Bjurulf P. Psychological factors in the long-term prognosis of chronic low back pain patients. *J Clin Psychol* 1992; 48:596–605.
188. Vikat A, Rimpela M, Salminen JJ, Rimpela A, Savolainen A, Virtanen SM. Neck or shoulder pain and low back pain in Finnish adolescents. *Scand J Public Health* 2000; 28:164–173.
189. Leino P. Symptoms of stress predict musculoskeletal disorders. *J Epidemiol Community Health* 1989; 43:293–300.
190. Rosenstiel AK, Keefe FJ. The use of coping strategies in chronic low back pain patients: Relationship

to patient characteristics and current adjustment. *Pain* 1983; 17:33–44.
191. Turner JA, Clancy S. Strategies for coping with chronic low back pain: Relationship to pain and disability. *Pain* 1986; 24:355–364.
192. Keefe FJ, Williams DA. A comparison of coping strategies in chronic pain patients in different age groups. *J Gerontol* 1990; 45:161–165.
193. Jensen MP, Karoly P. Control beliefs, coping efforts, and adjustment to chronic pain. *J Consult Clin Psychol* 1991;59:431–438.
194. Jensen MP, Karoly P. Pain-specific beliefs, perceived symptom severity, and adjustment to chronic pain. *Clin J Pain* 1992; 8:123–130.
195. Nicholas MK, Wilson PH, Goyen J. Operant-behavioural and cognitive-behavioural treatment for chronic low back pain. *Behav Res Ther* 1991; 29:225–238.
196. Lazarus RS, Folkman S. *Stress, appraisal, and coping.* New York: Springer, 1984.
197. Krishnan KR, France RD, Pelton S, McCann UD, Davidson J, Urban BJ. Chronic pain and depression. II. Classification of depression in chronic low back pain patients. *Pain* 1985; 22:279–287.
198. Magni G, Caldieron C, Rigatti-Luchini S, Merskey H. Chronic musculoskeletal pain and depressive symptoms in the general population. An analysis of the 1st National Health and Nutrition Examination Survey data. *Pain* 1990; 43:299–307.
199. Hansen FR, Biering-Sörensen F, Schroll M. Minnesota Multiphasic Personality Inventory profiles in persons with or without low back pain. A 20-year follow-up study. *Spine* 1995; 20:2716–2720.
200. Fishbain DA, Cutler RB, Rosomoff HL, Khalil T, Steele-Rosomoff R. Impact of chronic pain patients' job perception variables on actual return to work. *Spine* 1997; 13:197–206.
201. Croft P, Rigby AS. Socioeconomic influences on back problems in the community in Britain. *J Epidemiol Community Health* 1994; 48:166–170.
202. Von Korff M, Deyo RA, Barlow WE, Checkoway H. Predicting long-term functional limitations among back pain patients in primary care settings. *J Clin Epidemiol* 1997; 50:31–43.
203. Hurwitz EL, Morgenstern H, Yu F. Cross-sectional and longitudinal associations of low-back pain and related disability with psychological distress among patients enrolled in the UCLA Low-Back Pain Study. *J Clin Epidemiol* 2003; 56:463–471.
204. Gatchel RJ, Mayer TG, Capra P, Barnett J, Diamond P. Million Behavioral Health Inventory: Its utility in predicting physical function in patients with low back pain. *Arch Phys Med Rehabil* 1986; 67:878–882.
205. Naliboff BD, McCreary CP, McArthur DL, Cohen MJ, Gottlieb HJ. MMPI changes following behavioral treatment of chronic low back pain. *Pain* 1988; 35:271–277.
206. Van Poppel MNM, Koes BW, van der Ploeg T, et al. Lumbar supports and education for the prevention of low back pain in industry: A randomized controlled trial. *JAMA* 1998; 279:1789–1794.
207. Walsh NE, Schwartz RK. The influence of prophylactic orthoses on abdominal strength and low back injury in the workplace. *Am J Phys Med Rehabil* 1990; 69:245–250.
208. Bergquist-Ullmann M, Larsson U. Acute low back pain in industry. *Acta Orthop Scand Suppl* 1977; 170: 1–117.
209. Berwick DM, Budman S, Feldstein M. No clinical effect of back schools in an HMO. A randomized prospective trial. *Spine* 1989; 14:338–344.
210. Donchin M, Woolf O, Kaplan L, Floman Y. Secondary prevention of low-back pain. A clinical trial. *Spine* 1990; 15:1317–1320.
211. Leclaire R, Esdaile JM, Suissa S, Rossignol M, Roulx R, Dupiuis M. Back to school in a first episode of compensated acute low back pain: Clinical trial to assess efficacy and prevent relapse. *Arch Phys Med Rehabil* 1996; 77:673–679.
212. Lindequist S, Lundberg B, Wikmark R, Bergstad B, Loof G, Ottermark AC. Information and regime at low back pain. *Scand J Rehabil Med* 1984; 16:113–116.
213. Sirles AT, Brown K, Hilyer JC. Effects of back school education and exercise in back injured municipal workers. *AAOHN J* 1991; 39:7–12.
214. Stankovic R, Johnell O. Conservative treatment of acute low back pain. A 5-year follow-up study of two methods of treatment. *Spine* 1995; 20:469–472.
215. Gundewall B, Liljeqvist M, Hansson T. Primary prevention of back symptoms and absence from work. A prospective randomized study among hospital employees. *Spine* 1993: 18:587–594.
216. Kellett KM, Kellett DA, Nordholm LA. Effects of an exercise program on sick leave due to back pain. *Phys Ther* 1991; 71:283–291; discussion 291–293.
217. Linton SJ, Hellsing AL, Bergstrom G. Exercise for workers with musculoskeletal pain: Does enhancing compliance decrease pain? *J Occup Rehabil* 1996b; 6:177–190.
218. Symonds TL, Burton AK, Tillotson KM, Main CJ. Absence resulting from low back trouble can be reduced by psychosocial intervention at the workplace. *Spine* 1995; 20:2738–2745.
219. Daltroy LH, Iversen MD, Larson MG, et al. Controlled trial of an educational program to prevent low back injuries. *N Engl J Med* 1997; 337:322–328.
220. Anderson ST, Charlesworth RW. Rheumatologic disease among Air Force recruits: A multimillion-dollar epidemic. *Semin Arthritis Rheum* 1993; 22:275–279.
221. Feldstein A, Valanis B, Vollmer W, Stevens N, Overton C. The Back Injury Prevention Project pilot study. Assessing the effectiveness of attack, an injury prevention program among nurses, aides, and orderlies. *J Occup Med* 1993; 35:114–120.
222. Morrison GE, Chase W, Young V, Roberts WL. Back pain: Treatment and prevention in a community hospital. *Arch Phys Med Rehabil* 1988; 69:605–609.
223. Versloot JM, Rozeman A, van Son AM, van Akkerveeken PF. The cost-effectiveness of a back school program in industry. A longitudinal controlled field study. *Spine* 1992; 17:22–27.

224. Weber M, Cedraschi C, Roux E, Kissling RO, Von Kanel S, Dalvit G. A prospective controlled study of low back school in the general population. *Br J Rheumatol* 1996; 35:178–183.

225. Yassi A, Khokhar J, Tate R, Cooper J, Snow C, Vallentyne S. The epidemiology of back injuries in nurses at a large Canadian tertiary care hospital: Implications for prevention. *Occup Med (Lond)* 1995; 45:215–220.

226. Lahad A, Malter AD, Berg, AO, et al. The effectiveness of four interventions for the prevention of low back pain. *J Am Med Assoc* 1994; 272:1286–1291.

227. van Poppel MNM, Koes BW, Smid T, et al. A systematic review of controlled clinical trials on the prevention of back pain in industry. *Occup Environ Med* 1997; 54:841–847.

228. Gebhardt WA. Effectiveness of training to prevent job-related back pain: A meta-analysis. *Br J Clin Psychol* 1994; 33:571–574.

229. Hasenbring M, Ulrich HW, Hartmann M, Soyka D. The efficacy of a risk factor-based cognitive behavioral intervention and electromyographic biofeedback in patients with acute sciatic pain. An attempt to prevent chronicity. *Spine* 1999; 24:2525–2535.

230. Morley S, Eccleston C, Williams A. Systematic review and meta-analysis of randomized controlled trials of cognitive behaviour therapy and behaviour therapy for chronic pain in adults, excluding headache. *Pain* 1999; 80:1–13.

231. Gyntelberg F. One year incidence of low back pain among male residents of Copenhagen aged 40–59. *Dan Med Bull* 1974; 21:30–36.

232. Kelsey JL, Hardy RL. Driving of motor vehicles as a risk factors for acute herniated lumbar intervertebral disc. *Am J Epidemiol* 1975; 102:63–73.

233. Hrubec Z, Nashold BS Jr. Epidemiology of lumbar disc lesions in the military in World War II. *Am J Epidemiol* 1975; 102:367–76.

234. Shapiro S. Medical realities of cauda equina syndrome secondary to lumbar disc herniation. *Spine* 2000; 225:348–351.

235. Bozzao A, Gallucci M, Masciocchi C, Aprile I, Barile A, Passariello R. Lumbar disk herniation: MR imaging assessment of natural history in patients treated without surgery. *Radiology* 1992; 185:135–141.

236. Elfering A, Semmer N, Birkhofer D, Zanetti M, Hodler J, Boos N. Risk factors for lumbar disc degeneration: A 5-year prospective MRI study in asymptomatic individuals. *Spine* 2002; 27:125–134.

237. Heine J. Uber die Arthritis deformans. *Virchows Arch Pathol Anat* 1926; 260:521–663.

238. Miller JAA, Schmatz C, Schultz AB. Lumbar disc degeneration: Correlation with age, sex, and spine level in 600 autopsy specimens. *Spine* 1988; 13:173–178.

239. Videman T, Nurminen M, Troup JD. 1990 Volvo Award in clinical sciences. Lumbar spinal pathology in cadaveric material in relation to history of back pain, occupation, and physical loading. *Spine* 1990; 15:728–740.

240. Riihimaki H, Mattsson T, Zitting A, Wickstrom G, Hanninen K, Waris P. Radiographically detectable degenerative changes of the lumbar spine among concrete reinforcement workers and house painters. *Spine* 1990; 15:114–119.

241. Magora A, Schwartz A. Relation between the low back pain syndrome and x-ray findings. 2. Transitional vertebra (mainly sacralization). *Scand J Rehabil Med* 1978; 10:135–145.

242. Frymoyer JW, Newberg A, Pope MH, Wilder DG, Clements J, MacPherson B. Spine radiographs in patients with low-back pain. An epidemiological study in men. *J Bone Joint Surg Am* 1984; 66:1048–1055.

243. Valkenburg HA, Haanen HCM. The epidemiology of low back pain. In: White A, Gordon S, eds. *Symposium on idiopathic low back pain*. Miami: CV Mosby, 1980:9–22.

244. Salminen JJ, Erkintalo MO, Pentti J, Oksanen A, Kormano MJ. Recurrent low back pain and early disc degeneration in the young. *Spine* 1999; 24:1316–1321.

245. Videman T, Nummi P, Battie MC, Gill K. Digital assessment of MRI for lumbar disc desiccation. A digital versus subjective assessments and digital intensity profiles versus discogram and macroanatomic findings. *Spine* 1994; 19:192–198.

246. Sward L, Hellstrom M, Jacobsson B, Nyman R, Peterson L. Disc degeneration and associated abnormalities of the spine in elite gymnasts. A magnetic resonance imaging study. *Spine* 1991; 16:437–443.

247. Symmons DP, van Hemert AM, Vandenbroucke JP, Valkenburg HA. A longitudinal study of back pain and radiological changes in the lumbar spines of middle aged women. I. Clinical findings. *Ann Rheum Dis* 1991; 50:158–161.

248. Mundt DJ, Kelsey JL, Golden AL, et al, for the Northeast Collaborative Group on Low Back Pain. An epidemiologic study of sports and weight lifting as possible risk factors for herniated lumbar and cervical discs. *Am J Sports Med* 1993; 21:854–860.

249. Videman T, Sama S, Battie MC, et al. The long-term effects of physical loading and exercise lifestyles on back-related symptoms, disability, and spinal pathology among men. *Spine* 1995; 20:699–709.

250. Battie MC, Videman T, Gibbons LE, et al. 1995 Volvo award in clinical sciences. Determinants of lumbar disc degeneration: A study relating lifetime exposures and magnetic resonance imaging findings in identical twins. *Spine* 1995; 20:2601–2612.

251. Sambrook PN, MacGregor AJ, Spector TD. Genetic influences on cervical and lumbar disc degeneration: A magnetic resonance imaging study in twins. *Arthritis Rheum* 1999; 42:366–372.

252. Arnoldi CC, Brodsky AE, Cauchoix J, et al. Lumbar spinal stenosis and nerve root entrapment syndromes. Definition and classification. *Clin Orthop* 1976; 115: 4–5.

253. Arbit E, Pannullo S. Lumbar stenosis: A clinical review. *Clin Orthop* 2001; 384:137–143.

254. Porter RW. Spinal stenosis and neurogenic claudication. *Spine* 1996; 21:2046–2052.

255. Hall S, Bartleson JD, Onofrio BM, Baker HL Jr, Okazaki H, O'Duffy JD. Lumbar spinal stenosis. Clinical features, diagnostic procedures, and results of

surgical treatment in 68 patients. *Ann Intern Med* 1985; 103:271–275.
256. Johnsson R, Herrlin K, Hagglund G, Stromqvist B. Spinal canal remodeling after thoracolumbar fractures with intraspinal bone fragments. 17 cases followed 1–4 years. *Acta Orthop Scand* 1991; 62:125–127.
257. Porter RW, Hibbert C, Evans C. The natural history of root entrapment syndrome. *Spine* 1984; 9:418–421.
258. Matsunaga S, Sakou T, Morizono Y, Masuda A, Demirtas AM. Natural history of degenerative spondylolisthesis. Pathogenesis and natural course of the slippage. *Spine* 1990; 15:1204–1210.
259. Macfarlane GJ. Generalized pain, fibromyalgia and regional pain: An epidemiological view. *Baillieres Best Pract Res Clin Rheumatol* 1999; 13:403–414.
260. Buskila D. Fibromyalgia, chronic fatigue syndrome, and myofascial pain syndrome. Curr Opin Rheumatol 2001; 13:117–127.
261. Wolfe F, Aarflot T, Bruusgaard D, et al. Fibromyalgia and disability. Report of the Moss International Working Group on medico-legal aspects of chronic widespread musculoskeletal pain complaints and fibromyalgia. *Scand J Rheumatol* 1995; 24:112–118.
262. Makela M, Heliövaara M. Prevalence of primary fibromyalgia in the Finnish population. *BMJ* 1991; 303(6796):216–219.
263. Croft P, Rigby AS, Boswell R, et al. The prevalence of chronic widespread pain in the general population. *J Rheumatol* 1993; 20:710–713.
264. Croft P, Schollum J, Silman A. Population study of tender point counts and pain as evidence of fibromyalgia. *BMJ* 1994; 309:696–699.
265. Greenfield S, Fitzcharles MA, Esdaile JM. Reactive fibromyalgia syndrome. *Arthritis Rheum* 1992; 35:678–681.
266. Taylor VM, Deyo RA, Goldberg H, Ciol M, Kreuter W, Spunt B. Low back pain hospitalization in Washington State: Recent trends and geographic variations. *J Spinal Disord* 1995; 8:1–7.
267. Sperber AD, Atzmon Y, Neumann L, et al. Fibromyalgia in the irritable bowel syndrome: Studies of prevalence and clinical implications. *Am J Gastroenterol* 1999; 94:3541–3546.
268. Benjamin S, Morris S, McBeth J, Macfarlane GJ, Silman AJ. The association between chronic widespread pain and mental disorder: A population-based study. *Arthritis Rheum* 2000; 43:561–567.
269. Okifugi A, Turk DC, Sinclair JD, Starz TW, Marcus DA. A standardised manual tender point survey. I. Development and determination of a threshold point for the identification of positive tender points in fibromyalgia syndrome. *J Rheumatol* 1997; 24:377–383.
270. Ledingham J, Doherty S, Doherty M. Primary fibromyalgia syndrome—An outcome study. *Br J Rheumatol* 1993; 32:139–142.
271. Hawley DJ, Wolfe F, Cathey MA. Pain, functional disability, and psychological status: A 12-month study of severity in fibromyalgia. *J Rheumatol* 1988; 15:1551–1556.
272. Felson DT, Goldenberg DL. The natural history of fibromyalgia. *Arthritis Rheum* 1986; 29:1522–1526.
273. Macfarlane GJ, Thomas E, Papageorgiou AC, et al. Natural history of chronic pain in the community: A better prognosis than in the clinic? *J Rheumatol* 1996; 23:1617–1620.
274. Hashemi L, Webster BS, Clancy EA. Trends in disability duration and cost of workers compensation low back pain claims (1988–1996). *J Occup Environ Med* 1998; 40:1110–1119.
275. Watson PJ, Main CJ, Waddell G, Gales TF, Purcell-Jones G. Medically certified work loss, recurrence and costs of wage compensation for back pain: A follow-up study of the working population of Jersey. *Br J Rheumatol* 1998; 37:82–86.
276. Thomae MK, Porteous JE, Brock JR, Allen GD, Heller RF. Back pain in Australian military helicopter pilots: A preliminary study. *Aviat Space Environ Med* 1998; 69:468–473.
277. Brown JJ, Wells GA, Trottier AJ, Bonneau J, Ferris B. Back pain in a large Canadian police force. *Spine* 1998; 23:821–827.
278. Smedley J, Egger P, Cooper C, et al. Manual handling activities and risk of low back pain in nurses. *Occup Environ Med* 1995; 52:160–163.
279. Bigos SJ, Battie MC, Spengler DM, et al. A longitudinal, prospective study of industrial back injury reporting. *Clin Orthop* 1992; 279:21–34.
280. Silverstein B, Kalat J. *Work-related disorders of the back and upper extremity in Washington State, 1990–1987.* Technical Report # 40-2-1999. Olympia, WA. Safety and Health Assessment and Research for Prevention Program, March 1999.
281. Guo HR, Tanaka S, Cameron LL, et al. Back pain among workers in the United States: National estimates and workers at high risk. *Am J Ind Med* 1995; 28:591–602.
282. Chaffin DB, Park KS. A longitudinal study of low-back pain as associated with occupational weight lifting factors. *Am Ind Hyg Assoc J* 1973;34:513–525.
283. Latza U, Kohlmann T, Deck R, Raspe H. Influence of occupational factors on the relation between socioeconomic status and self-reported back pain in a population-based sample of German adults with back pain. *Spine* 2000; 25:1390–1397.
284. Lee P, Helewa A, Goldsmith CH, Smythe HA, Stitt LW. Low back pain: Prevalence and risk factors in an industrial setting. *J Rheumatol* 2001; 28:346–351.
285. National Research Council and the Institute of Medicine. *Musculoskeletal Disorders and the Workplace: Low Back and Upper Extremities*. Panel on Musculoskeletal Disorders and the Workplace. Commission on Behavioral and Social Sciences and Education. Washington, DC: National Academy Press, 2001.
286. Fransen M, Woodward M, Norton R, Coggan C, Dawe M, Sheridan N. Risk factors associated with the transition from acute to chronic occupational back pain. *Spine* 2002; 27:92–98.
287. Cady LD, Bischoff DP, O'Connell ER, Thomas PC, Allan JH. Strength and fitness and subsequent back injuries in firefighters. *J Occup Med* 1979; 21:269–272.

288. Dueker JA, Ritchie SM, Knox TJ, Rose SJ. Isokinetic trunk testing and employment. *J Occup Med* 1994; 36:42–48.
289. Mostardi RA, Noe DA, Kovacik MW, Porterfield JA. Isokinetic lifting strength and occupational injury. A prospective study. *Spine* 1992; 17:189–193.
290. Magora A. Investigation of the relation between low back pain and occupation. 3. Physical requirements: Sitting, standing and weight lifting. *IMS Ind Med Surg* 1972; 41:5–9.
291. Svensson HO, Andersson GBJ. Low-back pain in 40- to 47-year-old men: Work history and work environment factors. *Spine* 1983; 8:272–276.
292. Wells J, Zipp JF, Schuette PT, McEleney J. Musculoskeletal disorders among letter carriers: A comparison of weight carrying, walking, and sedentary occupations. *J Occup Med* 1983; 25:814–820.
293. Arad D, Ryan MD. Back disorders and health problems among subway train operators exposed to whole-body vibration. *Aust Nurses J* 1986; 16:44–48.
294. Gilad I, Kirschenbaum A. About the risks of back pain and work environment. *Int J Ind Ergon* 1986; 1: 65–74.
295. Mandel JH, Lohman W. Low back pain in nurses: The relative importance of medical history, work factors, exercise, and demographics. *Res Nurs Health* 1987; 10:165–170.
296. Stobbe TJ, Plummer RW, Jensen RC, Attfield MD. Incidence of low back injuries among nursing personnel as a function of patient lifting frequency. *J Saf Sci* 1988; 19:21–28.
297. Estryn-Behar MM, Kaminski M, Peigne E, et al. Strenuous working conditions and musculoskeletal disorders among female hospital workers. *Int Arch Occup Environ Health* 1990; 62:47–57.
298. Alcouffe J, Manillier P, Brehier M, Fabin C, Faupin F. Analysis by sex of low back pain among workers from small companies in the Paris area: Severity and occupational consequences. *Occup Environ Med* 1999; 56:696–701.
299. Ory FG, Rahman FU, Katagade V, Shukla A, Burdorf A. Respiratory disorders, skin complaints, and low-back trouble among tannery workers in Kanpur, India. *Am Ind Hyg Assoc J* 1997; 58:740–746.
300. Waters TR, Baron SL, Piacitelli LA, et al. Evaluation of the revised NIOSH lifting equation. A cross-sectional epidemiologic study. *Spine* 1999; 24:386–394, discussion 395.
301. Suadicani P, Hansen K, Fenger AM, Gyntelberg F. Low back pain in steel plant workers. *Occup Med (Lond)* 1994; 44:217–221.
302. Gardner LI, Landsittel DP, Nelson NA. Risk factors for back injury in 31,076 retail merchandise store workers. *Am J Epidemiol* 1999; 150:825–833.
303. Kraus JF, Schaffer KB, McArthur DL, Peek-Asa C. Epidemiology of acute low back injury in employees of a large home improvement retail company. *Am J Epidemiol* 1997; 146:637–645.
304. Smedley J, Egger P, Cooper C, Coggon D. Prospective cohort study of predictors of incident low back pain in nurses. *BMJ* 1997; 314:1225–1228.
305. Punnett L, Fine LJ, Keyserling WM, Herrin GD, Chaffin DB. Back disorders and nonneutral trunk postures of automobile assembly workers. *Scand J Work Environ Health* 1991; 17:337–346.
306. Burdorf A, Govaert G, Elders L. Postural load and back pain of workers in the manufacturing of prefabricated concrete elements. *Ergonomics* 1991; 34:909–918.
307. Burdorf A, Naaktgeboren A, de Groot HCWM. Occupational risk factors for low back pain among sedentary workers. *J Occup Med* 1993; 35:1213–1220.
308. Bovenzi M, Betta A. Low-back disorders in agricultural tractor drivers exposed to whole-body vibration and postural stress. *Appl Ergon* 1994; 25:231–241.
309. Linton S. Risk factors for neck and back pain in a working population in Sweden. *Work Stress* 1990; 4:41–49.
310. Josephson M, Vingard E, for the MUSIC-Norrtalje Study Group. Workplace factors and care seeking for low-back pain among female nursing personnel. *Scand J Work Environ Health* 1998; 24:465–472.
311. Houtman ILD, Bongers PM, Smulders PGW, Kompier MAJ. Psychosocial stressors at work and musculoskeletal problems. *Scand J Work Environ Health* 1994; 20:139–145.
312. Leigh JP, Sheetz RM. Prevalence of back pain among fulltime United States workers. *Br J Ind Med* 1989; 46:651–657.
313. Snook SH, Campanelli RA, Hart JW. A study of three preventive approaches to low back injury. *J Occup Med* 1978; 20:478–481.
314. Lloyd MH, Gauld S, Soutar CA. Epidemiologic study of back pain in miners and office workers. *Spine* 1986; 11:136–140.
315. Clemmer DI, Mohr DL. Low-back injuries in a heavy industry. II. Labor market forces. *Spine* 1991; 16:831–834.
316. Damkot DK, Pope MH, Lord J, Frymoyer JW. The relationship between work history, work environment and low-back pain in men. *Spine* 1984; 9:395–399.
317. Wells JA, Zipp JF, Schuette PT, McEleney J. Musculoskeletal disorders among letter carriers. A comparison of weight carrying, walking and sedentary occupations. *J Occup Med* 1983; 25:814–820.
318. Marras WS, Lavender SA, Leurgans SE, et al. The role of dynamic three-dimensional trunk motion in occupationally-related back disorders: The effects of workplace factors, trunk position, and trunk motion characteristics on risk of injury. *Spine* 1993; 18: 617–628.
319. Marras WS, Lavender SA, Leurgans SE, et al. Biomechanical risk factors for occupationally related low back disorders. *Ergonomics* 1995; 38:377–410.
320. Magora A. Investigation of the relation between low back pain and occupation. V. Psychological aspects. *Scand J Rehabil Med* 1973; 5:191–196.
321. Andersson GB. Epidemiologic aspects on low-back pain in industry. *Spine* 1981; 6:53–60.
322. Andersson GB, Murphy RW, Ortengren R, Nachemson AL. The influence of backrest inclination and lumbar support on lumbar lordosis. *Spine* 1979; 4:52–58.

323. Nahit ES, Pritchard CM, Cherry NM, Silman AJ, Macfarlane GJ. The influence of work related psychosocial factors and psychological distress on regional musculoskeletal pain: A study of newly employed workers. *J Rheumatol* 2001; 28:1378–1384.
324. Andersson GB, Svensson HO, Oden A. The intensity of work recovery in low back pain. *Spine* 1983; 8:880–884.
325. Spengler DM, Bigos SJ, Martin NA, Zeh J, Fisher L, Nachemson A. Back injuries in industry: A retrospective study. I. Overview and cost analysis. *Spine* 1986; 11:241–245.
326. Bernard BP, ed. *Musculoskeletal disorders and workplace factors: A critical review of epidemiologic evidence for work-related musculoskeletal disorders of the neck, upper extremity, and low back*. Cincinnati, OH: National Institute for Occupational Safety and Health, US *Department of Health and Human Services*, 1997. Publication No. 97–141.
327. Bongers PM, Hulshof CT, Dijkstra L, Boshuizen HC, Groenhout HJ, Valken E. Back pain and exposure to whole body vibration in helicopter pilots. *Ergonomics* 1990; 33:1007–1026.
328. Boshuizen HC, Bongers PM, Hulshof CT. Self-reported back pain in tractor drivers exposed to whole-body vibration. *Int Arch Occup Environ Health* 1990; 62:109–115.
329. Johanning E. Back disorders and health problems among subway train operators exposed to whole-body vibration. *Scand J Work Environ Health* 1991; 17:414–419.
330. Boshuizen HC, Bongers PM, Hulshof CT. Self-reported back pain in fork-lift truck and freight-container tractor drivers exposed to whole-body vibration. *Spine* 1992; 17:59–65.
331. Bovenzi M, Hulshof CT. An updated review of epidemiologic studies on the relationship between exposure to whole-body vibration and low back pain (1986–1997). *Int Arch Occup Environ Health* 1999; 72:351–365.
332. Liles DH, Deivanayagam S, Ayoub MM, Mahajan P. A job severity index for the evaluation and control of lifting injury. *Hum Factors* 1984; 26:683–693.
333. Herrin GD, Jaraiedi M, Anderson CK. Prediction of overexertion in juries using biomechanical and psychophysical models. *Am Ind Hyg Assoc J* 1986; 47:322–330.
334. Norman R, Wells R, Neumann P, Frank J, Shannon H, Kerr M. A comparison of peak vs cumulative physical work exposure risk factors for the reporting of low back pain in the automotive industry. *Clin Biomech (Bristol, Avon)* 1998; 13:561–573.
335. Fathallah FA, Marras WS, Parnianpour M. The role of complex, simultaneous trunk motions in the risk of occupation-related low back disorders. *Spine* 1998; 23:1035–1042.
336. Davis KG, Heaney CA. The relationship between psychosocial work characteristics and low back pain: Underlying methodological issues. *Clin Biomech (Bristol, Avon)* 2000; 15:389–406.
337. Dehlin O, Berg S. Back symptoms and psychosocial perception of work among nursing aides in a geriatric hospital. *Scand J Rehabil Med* 1977; 9:61–65.
338. Ahlberg-Hulthen GK, Theorell T, Sigala F. Social support, job strain and musculoskeletal pain among female health care personnel. *Scand J Work Environ Health* 1995; 21:435–439.
339. Hultman G, Nordin M, Saraste H. Physical and psychological workload in men with and without low back pain. *Scand J Rehabil Med* 1995; 27:11–17.
340. Lagerstrom M, Wenemark M, Hagberg M, Hjelm EW. Occupational and individual factors related to musculoskeletal symptoms in five body regions among Swedish nursing personnel. *Int Arch Occup Environ Health* 1995; 68:27–35.
341. Hemingway H, Shipley MJ, Stansfeld S, Marmot M. Sickness absence from back pain, psychosocial work characteristics and employment grade among office workers. *Scand J Work Environ Health* 1997; 23:121–129.
342. Barnekow-Bergkvist M, Hedberg G, Janlert U, et al. Determinants of self-reported neck–shoulder and low back symptoms in a general population. *Spine* 1998; 23:235–243.
343. Skov T, Borg V, Orhede E. Psychosocial and physical risk factors for musculoskeletal disorders of the neck, shoulders, and lower back in salespeople. *Occup Environ Med* 1996; 53:351–356.
344. Hughes RE, Silverstein BA, Evanoff BA. Risk factors for work-related musculoskeletal disorders in an aluminum smelter. *Am J Ind Med* 1997; 32:66–75.
345. Toomingas A, Theorell T, Michelsen H, et al. Associations between self-rated psychosocial work conditions and musculoskeletal symptoms and signs. *Scand J Work Environ Health* 1997; 23:130–139.
346. Krause N, Ragland DR, Greiner BA, et al. Psychosocial factors associated with back and neck pain in public transit operators. *Scand J Work Environ Health* 1997; 23:178–186.
347. Papageorgiou AC, Macfarlane GJ, Thomas E, et al. Psychosocial factors in the workplace: Do they predict new episodes of low back pain? *Spine* 1997; 22:1137–1142.
348. Van Poppel MNM, Koes BW, Deville W, Smid T, Bouter LM. Risk factors for back pain incidence in industry: A prospective study. *Pain* 1998; 77:81–86.
349. Feyer AM, Williamson A, Mandryk J, et al. Role of psychosocial factors in work-related low-back pain. *Scand J Work Environ Health* 1992; 18:368–375.
350. Van der Wiede WE, Verbeek JHAM, Salle HJA, van Dijk FJH. Prognostic factors for chronic disability from acute low-back pain in occupational health care. *Scand J Work Environ Health* 1999; 25:50–56.
351. Hurri H. The Swedish back school in chronic low back pain. II. Factors predicting the outcome. *Scand J Rehabil Med* 1989; 21:41–44.
352. Bergenudd H, Johnell O. Somatic versus nonsomatic shoulder and back pain experience in middle age in relation to body build, physical fitness, bone mineral content, gamma-glutamyltransferase, occupational workload, and psychosocial factors. *Spine* 1991; 16:1051–1055.

353. Karasek RA, Theorell T. *Healthy work. stress, productivity and the reconstruction of working life*. New York, NY: Basic Books, 1990.
354. Burton AK, Tillotson KM, Symonds TL, Burke C, Mathewson T. Occupational risk factors for the first-onset and subsequent course of low back trouble. A study of serving police officers. *Spine* 1996; 21:2612–2620.
355. Bongers PM, de Winter CR, Kompier MA, Hildebrandt VH. Psychosocial factors at work and musculoskeletal disease. *Scand J Work Environ Health* 1993; 19:297–312.
356. Hoogendoorn WE, Bongers PM, de Vet HC, et al. Flexion and rotation of the trunk and lifting at work are risk factors for low back pain: Results of a prospective cohort study. *Spine* 2000; 25:3087–3092.
357. Loeser JD, Henderlite SE, Conrad DA. Incentive effects of workers' compensation benefits: A literature synthesis. *Med Care Res Rev* 1995; 52:34–59.
358. Leavitt F. The physical exertion factor in compensable work injuries. A hidden flaw in previous research. *Spine* 1992; 17:307–310.
359. Sander RA, Meyers JE. The relationship of disability to compensation status in railroad workers. *Spine* 1986; 11:141–143.
360. Hadler NM, Carey TS, Garrett J. The influence of indemnification by workers' compensation insurance on recovery from acute backache. North Carolina Back Pain Project. *Spine* 1995; 20:2710–2715.
361. Jamison RN, Matt DA, Parris WC. Treatment outcome in low back pain patients: Do compensation benefits make a difference? *Orthop Rev* 1988; 17:1210–1215.
362. Greenough CG, Fraser RD. The effects of compensation on recovery from low-back injury. *Spine* 1989; 14:947–955.
363. Dworkin RH, Handlin DS, Richlin DM, Brand L, Vannucci C. Unraveling the effects of compensation, litigation, and employment on treatment response in chronic pain. *Pain* 1985;23:49–59.
364. Sanderson PL, Todd BD, Holt GR, et al. Compensation, work status, and disability in low back pain patients. *Spine* 1995; 20:554–556.
365. Leavitt F. Comparison of three measures for detecting psychological disturbance in patients with low back pain. *Pain* 1982; 13:299–305.
366. Burns JW, Sherman ML, Devine J, et al. Association between workers' compensation and outcome following multidisciplinary treatment for chronic pain: Roles of mediators and moderators. *Clin J Pain* 1995; 11:94–102.
367. Simmonds MJ, Kumar S, Lechelt E. Psychological factors in disabling low back pain: Causes or consequences? *Disabil Rehabil* 1996; 18:161–168.
368. Taylor VM, Deyo RA, Ciol M, et al. Surgical treatment of patients with back problems covered by workers compensation versus those with other sources of payment. *Spine* 1996; 21:2255–2259.
369. Trief P, Stein N. Pending litigation and rehabilitation outcome of chronic low back pain. *Arch Phys Med Rehabil* 1985; 66:95–99.
370. Talo S, Hendler N, Brodie J. Effects of active and completed litigation on treatment results: Workers compensation patients compared with other litigation patients. *J Occup Med* 1989; 31:265–269.
371. Solomon P, Tunks E. The role of litigation in predicting disability outcomes in chronic pain patients. *Clin J Pain* 1991; 7:300–304.
372. Gallagher RM, Moore P, Chernoff I. The reliability of depression diagnosis in chronic low back pain. A pilot study. *Gen Hosp Psychiatry* 1995; 17:399–413.
373. Hunt HA, Habeck RV. *The Michigan Disability Prevention Study: Research highlights*. Kalamazoo, MI: Uphohn Institute for Employment Research, 1993.
374. Shannon HS, Walters V, Lewchuck W, et al. Workplace organizational correlates of lost-time accident rates in manufacturing. *Am J Ind Med* 1996; 29:258–268.
375. Krause N, Dasinger LK, Neuhauser F. Modified work and return to work: A review of the literature. *J Occup Rehabil* 1998; 8:113–139.
376. Strunin L, Boden LI. Paths of reentry: Employment experiences of injured workers. *Am J Ind Med* 2000; 38:373–384.
377. Wassell JT, Gardner LI, Landsittel DP, Johnston JJ, Johnston JM. A prospective study of back belts for prevention of back pain and injury. *JAMA* 2000; 284:2727–2732.
378. Hazard RG, Reid S, Haugh LD, McFarlane G. A controlled trial of an educational pamphlet to prevent disability after occupational low back injury. *Spine* 2000; 25:1419–1423.
379. Mierau D, Cassidy JD, Yong-Hing K. Low-back pain and straight leg raising in children and adolescents. *Spine* 1989; 14:526–528.
380. Burton AK, Clarke RD, McClune TD, Tillotson KM. The natural history of low back pain in adolescents. *Spine* 1996b; 21:2323–2328.
381. Harreby M, Nygaard B, Jessen T, et al. Risk factors for low back pain in a cohort of 1389 Danish school children: An epidemiologic study. *Eur Spine J* 1999; 8:444–450.
382. Salminen J, Pentti J, Terho P. Low back pain and disability in 14-year-old schoolchildren. *Acta Paediatr* 1992; 81:1035–1039.
383. Ebrall PS. The epidemiology of male adolescent low back pain in a north suburban population of Melbourne, Australia. *J Manipulative Physiol Ther* 1994; 17:447–453.
384. Gunzburg R, Balague F, Nordin M, et al. Low back pain in a population of school children. *Eur Spine* 1999; 8:439–443.
385. Taimela S, Kujala UM, Salminen JJ, Viljanen T. The prevalence of low back pain among children and adolescents. A nationwide, cohort-based questionnaire survey in Finland. *Spine* 1997; 22:1132–1136.
386. Brattberg G. The incidence of back pain and headache among Swedish school children. *Qual Life Res* 1994;3(Suppl 1):S27–S31.
387. Nissinen M, Heliövaara M, Seitsamo J, Alaranta H, Poussa M. Anthropometric measurements and the incidence of low back pain in a cohort of pubertal children. *Spine* 1994; 19:1367–1370.

388. Olsen TL, Anderson RL, Dearwater SR, et al. The epidemiology of low back pain in an adolescent population. *Am J Public Health* 1992; 82:606–608.
389. Troussier B, Davoine P, de Gaudemaris R, Fauconnier J, Phelip X. Back pain in school children. A study among 1178 pupils. *Scand J Rehabil Med* 1994; 26:143–146.
390. Balague F, Nordin M, Skovron ML, Dutoit G, Yee A, Waldburger M. Non-specific low-back pain among schoolchildren: A field survey with analysis of some associated factors. *J Spinal Disorders* 1994; 7:374–379.
391. Kristjansdottir G. Prevalence of self-reported back pain in school children: A study of sociodemographic differences. *Eur J Pediatr* 1996; 155:984–986.
392. Newcomer K, Sinaki M. Low back pain and its relationship to back strength and physical activity in children. *Acta Paediatr* 1996; 85:1433–1439.
393. Salminen JJ. The adolescent back. A field survey of 370 Finnish schoolchildren. *Acta Paediatr Scand Suppl* 1984; 315:1–122.
394. Salminen JJ, Erkintalo MO, Pentti J. Low back pain in adolescents. *Duodecim* 1994; 110:52–58.
395. Balague F, Dutoit G, Waldburger M. Low back pain in schoolchildren. An epidemiological study. *Scand J Rehabil Med* 1988; 20:175–179.
396. Jarvinen P, Aho K. Twin studies in rheumatic diseases. *Semin Arthritis Rheum* 1994; 24:19–28.
397. Gunzburg R, Fraser R, Fraser G. Lumbar intervertebral disc prolapse in teenage twins. *J Bone Joint Surg Br* 1990; 72:914–916.
398. Matsui H, Terahata N, Tsuji H, Hirano N, Naruse Y. Familial predisposition and clustering for juvenile lumbar disc herniation. *Spine* 1992; 17:1323–1328.
399. Varlotta GP, Brown MD, Kelsey JL, Golden AL. Familial predisposition for herniation of a lumbar disc in patients who are less than twenty-one years old. *J Bone Joint Surg Am* 1991; 73:124–128.
400. Videman T, Leppavuori J, Kaprio J, et al. Intragenic polymorphisms of the vitamin D receptor gene associated with intervertebral disc degeneration. *Spine* 1998; 23:2477–2485.
401. Balague F, Damidot P, Nordin M, et al. Cross-sectional study of the isokinetic muscle strength among schoolchildren. *Spine* 1993; 18:1199–1205.
402. Kujala UM, Salminen JJ, Taimela S, Oksanen A, Jaakkola L. Subject characteristics and low back pain in young athletes and nonathletes. *Med Sci Sports Exerc* 1992; 24:627–632.
403. Schofferman J, Anderson D, Hines R, Smith G, Keane G. Childhood psychological trauma and chronic refractory low-back pain. *Clin J Pain* 1993; 9:260–265.
404. Salminen JJ, Oksanen A, Maki P, Pentti J, Kujala UM. Leisure time physical activity in the young. Correlation with low-back pain, spinal mobility and trunk muscle strength in 15-year-old school children. *Int J Sports Med* 1993; 14:406–410.
405. Kujala UM, Taimela S, Oksanen A, Salminen JJ. Lumbar mobility and low back pain during adolescence. A longitudinal three-year follow-up study in athletes and controls. *Am J Sports Med* 1997; 25:363–368.
406. Sward L, Hellstrom M, Jacobsson B, Peterson L. Back pain and radiologic changes in the thoraco-lumbar spine of athletes. *Spine* 1990; 15:124–129.
407. Hellstrom M, Jacobsson B, Sward L, Peterson L. Radiologic abnormalities of the thoraco-lumbar spine in athletes. *Acta Radiol* 1990; 31:127–132.
408. Goldstein JD, Berger PE, Windler GE, Jackson DW. Spine injuries in gymnasts and swimmers. An epidemiologic investigation. *Am J Sports Med* 1991; 19:463–468.

CHAPTER

5

FUNCTIONAL CONTROL OF THE LOW BACK

Paul Hodges and Vladimir Janda

OUTLINE

OBJECTIVES

1. To discuss the requirements for functional control of the spine and pelvis.
2. To describe the role of the nervous system in low back control.
3. To outline the key strategies of feedforward and feedback control of the spine.
4. To consider the integration between muscle architecture and motor control strategies to maintain optimal control of the lumbar spine and pelvis
5. To overview the neuromuscular changes that have been identified in people with acute and chronic low back pain.
6. To consider the progression of clinical philosophies that has been developed for the exercise management of low back and pelvic pain.

INTRODUCTION

Exercise for low back pain has been used for many years with the assumption that improved control and support of the spine and pelvis will result in reduced pain and disability. This philosophy is based on a biomechanical model that argues that low back pain results from stimulation of nociceptors due to poor control of the spinal structures. Although early exercise interventions focused on changing the strength and endurance of the trunk muscles in order to improve "control," more recently the focus has shifted to consideration of control and coordination of the trunk muscles. Many and varied philosophies have evolved that incorporate factors such as reeducation of the dissociation between hip and lumbar movement,[1] correction of muscle length,[2,3] and reeducation of control of intrinsic and superficial muscles of the trunk.[4] These contemporary approaches to the management of the low back pain that address the motor control of the trunk muscles are gaining support from randomized clinical trials. To further complicate the issue of appropriate interventions for low back pain, recent emphasis has been placed on the neurobiology of pain, which questions the validity of a model that presumes a biomechanical etiology for pain. It is important to incorporate the complex interaction between biomechanical models and the other biological, psychological, and social elements of pain. The purpose of this chapter is to consider the requirements for control of the spine, the strategies used by the central nervous system to meet these requirements, changes in the system when people have low back pain, and finally, how these changes relate to clinical strategies for exercise management of low back pain.

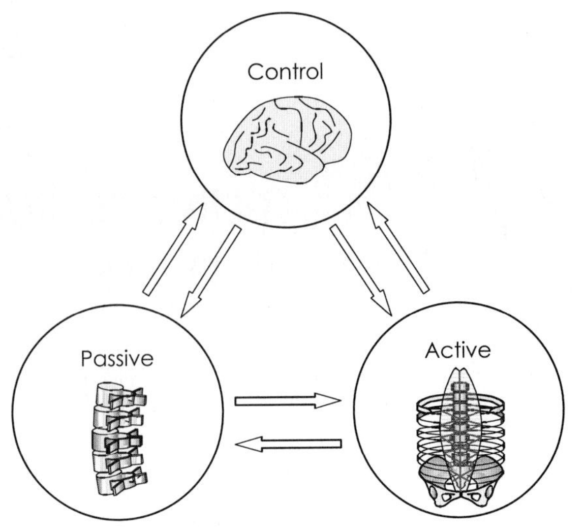

FIGURE 5–1. The three systems that contribute to lumbopelvic stability. (*Adapted from Panjabi.*[6])

REQUIREMENTS FOR CONTROL OF THE SPINE

The spine is inherently unstable and dependent on the contribution of muscle. When the spine is tested in vitro with passive elements intact, but with muscle removed, collapse occurs with compressive loading of as little as 90 N.[5] Thus, although passive elements of the spine provide a contribution to control of the spine, this is not sufficient to maintain stability. This led Panjabi[6] to propose a system that integrates the contribution of passive elements, muscle, and the control system that determines the requirements for stability and plans strategies to meet these demands (Fig. 5–1). The passive system involves all of the noncontractile elements of the spine including the ligaments, fascia, joint capsules, intervertebral discs, and noncontractile components of muscle. While passive elements provide their greatest contribution toward the end of range of motion, the contribution of this system is essential. The active system includes the contractile elements that surround the spine. All muscles that surround the spine contribute to its control. However, there has been considerable debate regarding which muscles provide the "greatest" contribution to the control of spinal motion, and the specific contribution of muscles to discrete elements of spinal control. This will be addressed in greater detail in subsequent sections. The neural or control system is responsible for control of muscle activity to meet the demands of spinal stability. In order to meet these demands the neural system must evaluate the status of stability and evaluate the demands for spinal control. If a disturbance or challenge to the spine is predictable, the neural system can control for this in advance of movement. If the disturbance is unpredictable, the control system initiates responses with varying levels of complexity, from simple inflexible reflex responses to complex malleable responses. In planning responses the neural system must consider the architectural properties of the trunk muscles and match the strategy with the biomechanical demands. In order to understand the strategies used by the neural system to meet the demands for control, it is essential to consider the biomechanical demands for control of the lumbar spine and pelvis.

Clinical Pearl: Changes in neural control have been identified in patients with low back pain which are similar to the changes seen in people with neurological disorders such as Parkinson disease and frontal lobe trauma.

Biomechanical Models of Spinal Control

Most models of spinal control consider Euler mechanics, which considers the control of the buckling forces. In this model the muscle system is required to act like guy ropes to maintain the spine upright in stable equilibrium.[7–9] Equilibrium refers to the situation in which the net force acting on the spine is zero. Stable equilibrium infers that if a perturbation is applied, equilibrium can be maintained.[10] This model is relatively static and is focused on the control of

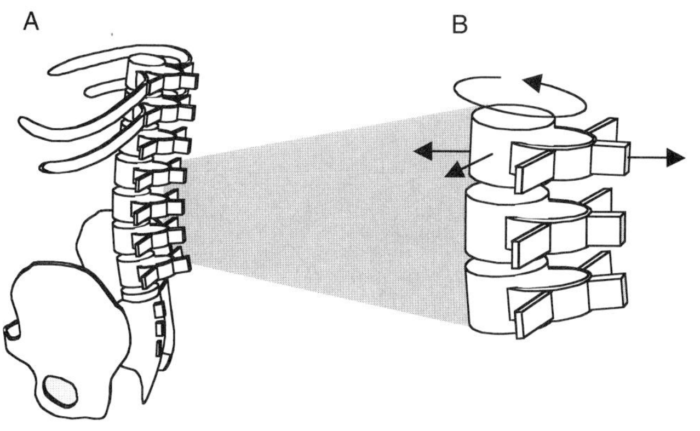

FIGURE 5–2. Components of trunk control. *A*. Control of lumbopelvic orientation. *B*. Control of intervertebral motion.

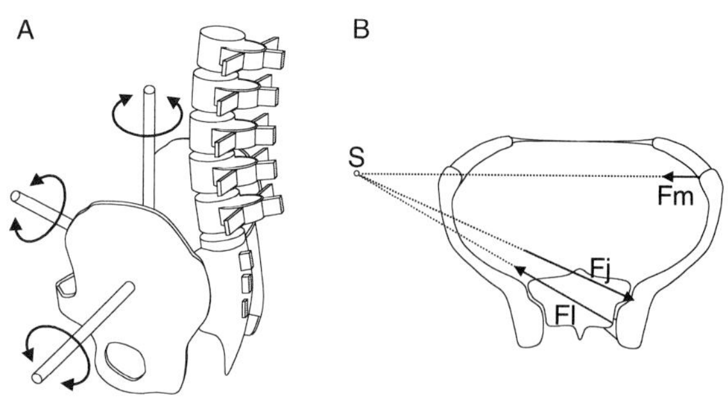

FIGURE 5–3. Components of pelvic control. *A*. Control of the orientation of the pelvis around three orthogonal axes (*Adapted from Snijders et al.*[17]). *B*. Control of the sacroiliac joints. The medial-directed force of transversus abdominis (Fm) is amplified by the lever formed by the ilium, resulting in a compressive force (Fj) at the anterior sacroiliac joint. Distraction force at the posterior aspect of the force is counteracted by the posterior sacroiliac ligament.

the orientation of the spine or its stability. In addition to the control of upright orientation, control of the spine is also dependent on the regulation of translation and rotation at the intervertebral level both in static positions and during movement (Fig. 5–2). It is this latter component that is implicated in many studies of instability. For instance during lifting, motion at a single intervertebral segment has been observed fluroscopically in association with pain,[11] and people with clinical signs of instability have been shown to have an abnormal relationship between translation and rotation at a specific intervertebral segment.[12] It has been argued variously that different muscles and strategies may be responsible for control of each of these elements of stability.[13–15]

An additional consideration is that the requirement for muscular control of the spine varies within the range of motion. Around the neutral position the spine exhibits least stiffness.[16] As such, it is in this region, called the *neutral zone*,[16] that the contribution of the muscle system is most critical. However, muscle activity is available and required throughout the range of motion, except in specific situations, such as at the end of lumbar flexion range of motion when paraspinal muscles are inactive, the so-called *flexion relaxation phenomenon*. In the neutral zone the spine is dependent on muscle, and it has been proposed that this postural region, or position, may increase in low back pain owing to injury or microtrauma.[16] The increase in this range may be responsible for irritation of pain-sensitive structures and requires a greater than normal control of spinal muscles to ensure optimal function.

Clinical Pearl: Although there is no clinical method to measure the neutral zone, it has been implicated as the key factor to be affected by injury to the passive elements of the spine.

Control of the Pelvis

The same principles of control of orientation and intersegmental motion also apply to the pelvis. At one level there is the need to control orientation of the pelvis around the three orthogonal axes; however, there is also the requirement to control the relationship between segments of the pelvis (Fig. 5–3). In upright positions the sacroiliac joint is subjected to considerable shear force as the mass of the upper body must be transferred to the lower limbs via the ilia.[17,18] The body has two mechanisms to overcome this shear force: one dependent on the shape and structure of the joint surfaces of the sacroiliac joints (form closure), which is wedge shaped with a high coefficient of friction, and the other mechanism involves generation of compressive forces across the sacroiliac joint via muscle contraction (force closure).[17] Similar to the spine, different muscles and recruitment strategies are likely to be involved in control of each aspect of stability of the pelvis.

Clinical Pearl: Similar muscles are involved in the control of the intersegmental control of the spine and pelvis.

NEURAL STRATEGIES FOR SPINAL CONTROL

If spinal control is to be optimal, strategies must be in place to control both spinal orientation and intervertebral translation and rotation. To some degree the control of these elements may be independent of each other, but must be interrelated. In order to meet these demands it is necessary for the nervous system to accurately detect the status of stability. Over a lifetime of movement experience the central nervous system builds up an abstract model that includes information of the body and how it is affected by internal and external forces. This is commonly referred to as the *internal model of body dynamics* or *virtual body*.[19,20] Using this model the central nervous system is able to predict the effect that movements and forces will have on the body to plan strategies *in advance of* (i.e., prior to) movement to prepare the trunk for predictable perturbations, and also to plan appropriate strategies of muscle activity to respond (i.e., afterward) quickly and appropriately to unexpected demands. The former type of control is commonly referred to as *feedforward* and the latter is *feedback* control.

Feedforward Control of Spinal Stability

In a feedforward system the central nervous system predicts the effect of a perturbation and initiates a sequence of muscle activity that is matched to the demands of the movement.[21] It has been established that these feedforward strategies involve muscle activity that counteracts

- the challenge to postural equilibrium of the entire body,
- the challenge to spinal orientation and alignment, and
- the challenge to intervertebral motion.

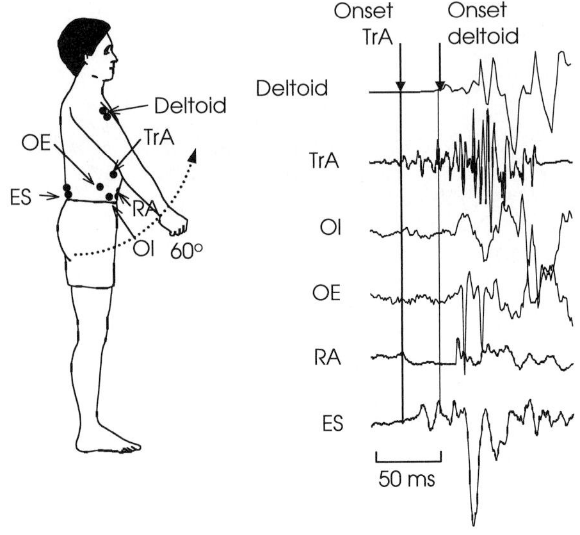

FIGURE 5–4. Feedforward control of trunk stability. Rapid arm movement is associated with a sequence of trunk muscle activity that varies between directions of limb movement. Onsets of activity of deltoid and the trunk muscles are shown. The deep muscle transversus abdominis is controlled separately and does not vary with movement direction *(Adapted from Hodges and Richardson.*[25]) Key: TrA - Transversus Abdominis; OI - Obliquus Internus Abdominis; OE - Obliquus Externus Abdominis; RA - Rectus Abdominis; ES - Erector Spinae.

It is the latter two that are of greatest importance for the spine. Numerous studies have investigated feedforward control of the spine.[15,22,23] A common model to investigate these responses is the investigation of the postural adjustment associated with rapid movement of a limb. In this task, reactive moments that are equal in magnitude but opposite in direction to the moments to move the arm.[24] In general, a sequence of muscle activity is initiated in advance of the muscle responsible for movement of the limb (such as deltoid). The activity of large superficial muscles (see below) is generally initiated in a manner that is predictable based on the direction of the limb movement. For instance, activity of the trunk extensor muscles is initiated in advance of flexion of the upper limb to prepare the spine for the flexion moment that is induced by the arm movement[15,22] (Fig. 5–4). There are two issues to consider. First, it is important to recognize that these responses do not aim to simply *stiffen* the spine and make it rigid. Instead, they are *movements*[24,26] (Fig. 5–5). It is well accepted that movement assists in the absorption and dissipation of forces, and minimizes energy expenditure.[27] As such by moving the spine in the direction opposite to the direction of reactive moments, the spine is able to dampen the reactive forces and reduce the impact on the spine. Thus, early activity of the paraspinal muscles with shoulder flexion is associated with a small trunk extension that is initiated prior to the onset of upper limb movement and the reactive flexion moment. The second issue to consider is that the finely tuned and direction-specific response of the trunk muscles is influenced by the predictability of the task. Notably, in situations in which the predictability is reduced, the superficial trunk muscles co-contract.[28] Studies of other tasks indicate that co-contraction is also associated with situations of high load.[29]

Clinical Pearl: Reduced movement and reduced movement variability are signs of poor control of the spine.

While the direction-specific activity of the superficial muscles is appropriate for control of the orientation of the spine, biomechanically these muscles have a limited ability to control intervertebral shear/translation and rotation. Studies of rapid voluntary limb movements provided an initial insight into the mechanisms used by the nervous system to control this element of stability. In these tasks, in association with the early activity of the superficial muscles to control the orientation of the spine, early activity of the deep intrinsic spinal muscles (such as transverus abdominis and the lumbar multifidus) has

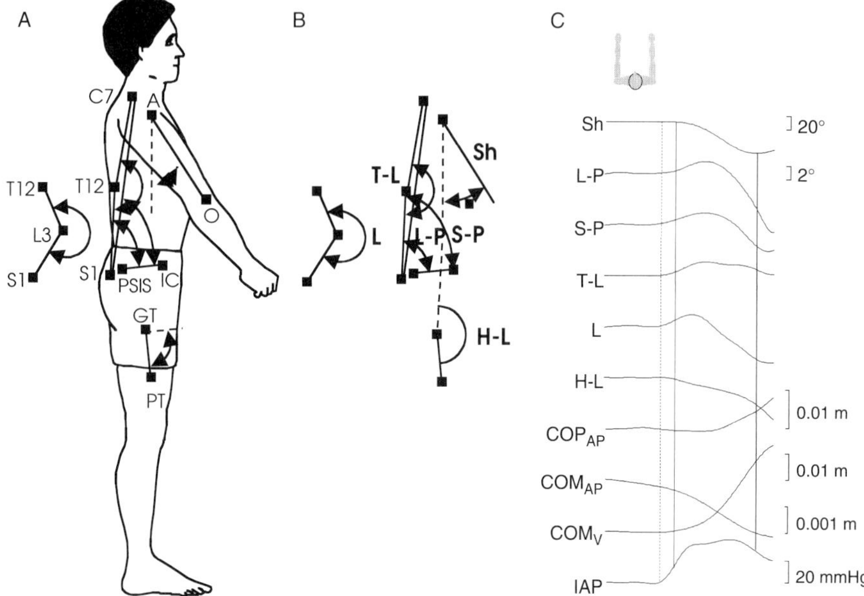

FIGURE 5–5. Postural responses use movement rather than simply making the spine rigid. The placement of markers to measure trunk motion and the angles that are measured are shown in Figure 5–5*A* and 5–5*B*, respectively. In Figure 5–5*C* the onset of arm movement is shown with a solid vertical line. The data indicate that when the arm is flexed rapidly at the shoulder (downward motion in *C*), the spine moves in the opposite direction initially and this spinal motion starts before the onset of movement. (*Adapted from Hodges et al.*[26])

been observed[15,30,31] (Fig. 5–4). However, unlike the direction-specific activity of the superficial muscles, the deep intrinsic spinal muscles were active in a manner that did not vary between the directions of limb movement, and therefore the direction of forces acting on the spine. Although the biomechanical and architectural properties of the trunk muscles are detailed later in the chapter, this observation is consistent with a strategy used by the central nervous system to initiate activity of the sleeve of muscles that surrounds the spine to stabilize the intervertebral segments.[14,15] These data suggest that the central nervous system uses separate muscles (deep versus superficial) and separate strategies (direction-specific and non-direction-specific) to control the different elements of stability and control of the spine and pelvis.

Clinical Pearl: Because the central nervous system uses separate strategies to control deep and superficial muscles, different strategies need to be used to retrain each system and it may be necessary to train them separately.

Recent studies have investigated the organization of the strategies for control of intervertebral motion and spinal orientation in more detail. These studies have confirmed that the strategies are controlled somewhat independently. That is, they are not two parts of the same command but are controlled by separate systems in the nervous system. For instance, when the preparation for rapid arm movement is reduced the reaction time for movement of the limb is increased (i.e., delayed) because of the increased time to plan the movement response. The activity of the superficial muscles is delayed along with the movement as the nervous system requires information of movement direction in order to plan the response of the superficial muscles.[32] However, the response of the deep intrinsic spinal muscles is not delayed. That is, the nervous system requires information that a movement will be performed but not its direction to plan the response of the deep intrinsic spinal muscles, and a response can be initiated with short latency, without delay for increased information processing. This finding supports the hypothesis that the different elements of spinal stability are controlled separately by the nervous system and led to the hypothesis that the deep muscle response may not be controlled by corticospinal systems.[14] However, recent studies have confirmed that there is corticospinal input to ongoing postural activity of the deep spinal muscles.[33] This is a critical consideration for clinical training of the trunk muscles as it suggests that the muscle control systems may require some degree of specificity in training.

Feedback Control of Spinal Stability

When a perturbation cannot be predicted by the nervous system, it must respond quickly and accurately to afferent input. The nervous system has several options for control of unexpected perturbations that range from simple inflexible reflex responses to more complex multisegmental responses that involve transcortical mechanisms. At the basic level of reflex responses there is evidence of rapid reflex activity in paraspinal[34] and abdominal muscles[35,36] in response to a mechanical tap to the muscle, akin to the stretch reflex to a tap to the quadriceps tendon. These simple

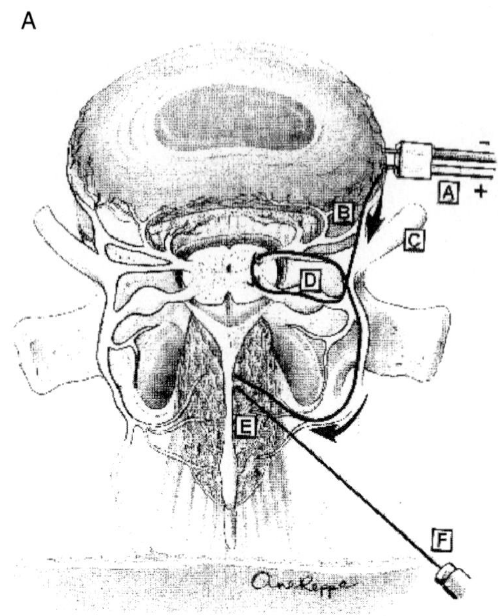

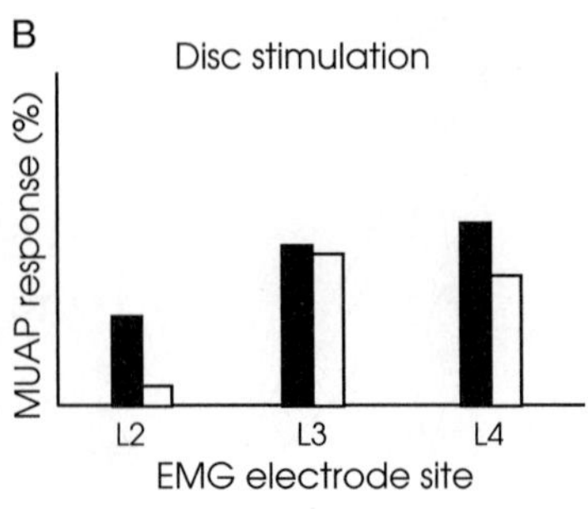

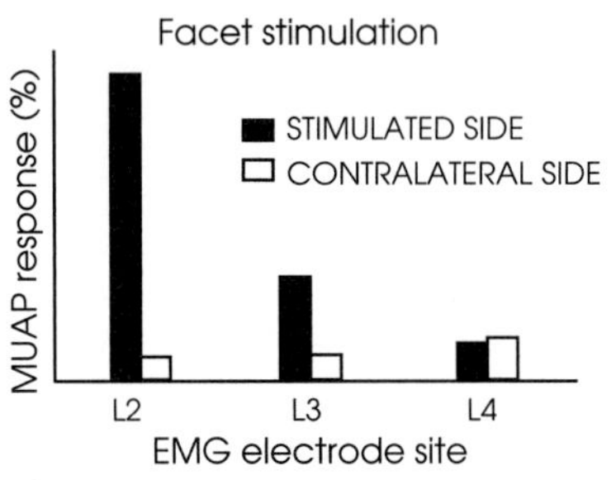

FIGURE 5–6. Muscle response to electrical stimulation of the intervertebral disc and facet joint. Electrical stimulation (*A*) of mechanoreceptors is associated with a short-latency response of the multifidus muscles (*B*). (*Adapted from Indahl et al.*[38])

responses are inflexible and represent a basic mechanism for the motor system to correct an error, for example, to resist an imposed stretch. However there appears to be some integration. For instance, reflex changes may occur in other related muscles, including those on the contralateral side of the body.[37] Other basic responses have been identified in response to electrical and/or mechanical stimulation of afferents in the ligaments, annulus, facet joint capsule, and sacroiliac joint in pigs, cats, and humans[38–42] (Fig. 5–6). In general, activity of multifidus was initiated with short latency, on both sides and over multiple spinal segments in response to the stimulus. The nature of the response was affected by the site of stimulation on the annulus[43] and sacroiliac joint,[39] and could be modified by injection of analgesic or saline into the facet joint capsule.

In a more functional context short-latency responses to muscle stretch have been identified in the abdominal[44] and paraspinal[45–47] muscles when subjects either catch an unexpected mass in hands or have a mass added to a harness over the shoulders (Fig. 5–7). These responses are generally specific to the direction of perturbation and represent a rapid response to prevent perturbation to the trunk. Notably, the refinement of the reflex response is dependent on the predictability of the task. When a load is added rapidly to the trunk the amplitude of paraspinal muscle activity is several times greater than the activity actually required to overcome the perturbation to the trunk.[48] At the other extreme, when the demands for spinal control are more predictable, for instance if a subject has visual input of the mass prior to acceptance of the loading, the characteristics of the response (i.e., amplitude and timing) can be more refined. For instance, when the predictability of adding a load to the upper limbs is increased the response of the multifidus muscle occurs earlier[45] and the deep and superficial components of the multifidus are controlled differentially,[46] with earlier activity of the deep portion which has been linked with the control of intervertebral motion.

Clinical Pearl: Although trunk muscle responses are initiated in response to afferent input, it is questionable whether these responses return spontaneously after an episode of pain.

It has also been suggested that short-latency postural responses may be initiated by sensory input in other regions of the body. Notably, activity of the deep abdominal muscle transversus abdominis occurs following addition of a mass to the arms, but with a latency that is too fast for the response to be initiated as a direct response to perturbation to the trunk (Fig. 5–8). This was interpreted to indicate that the response occurs as a result of excitation of afferents in the upper limb.[49] This is consistent with earlier data of postural responses in the leg muscles to upper limb perturbation that occur even after anaesthetization of the leg.[50]

Thus, the central nervous system involves complex strategies to integrate afferent input to initiate trunk muscle activity to optimize spinal control. It is also apparent that these postural responses frequently involve activity of the deep intrinsic spinal muscles, often in a manner that is not affected by the direction of forces acting on the spine. Conversely, activity of the superficial muscles is generally controlled in a manner that is specific to the direction of movement.

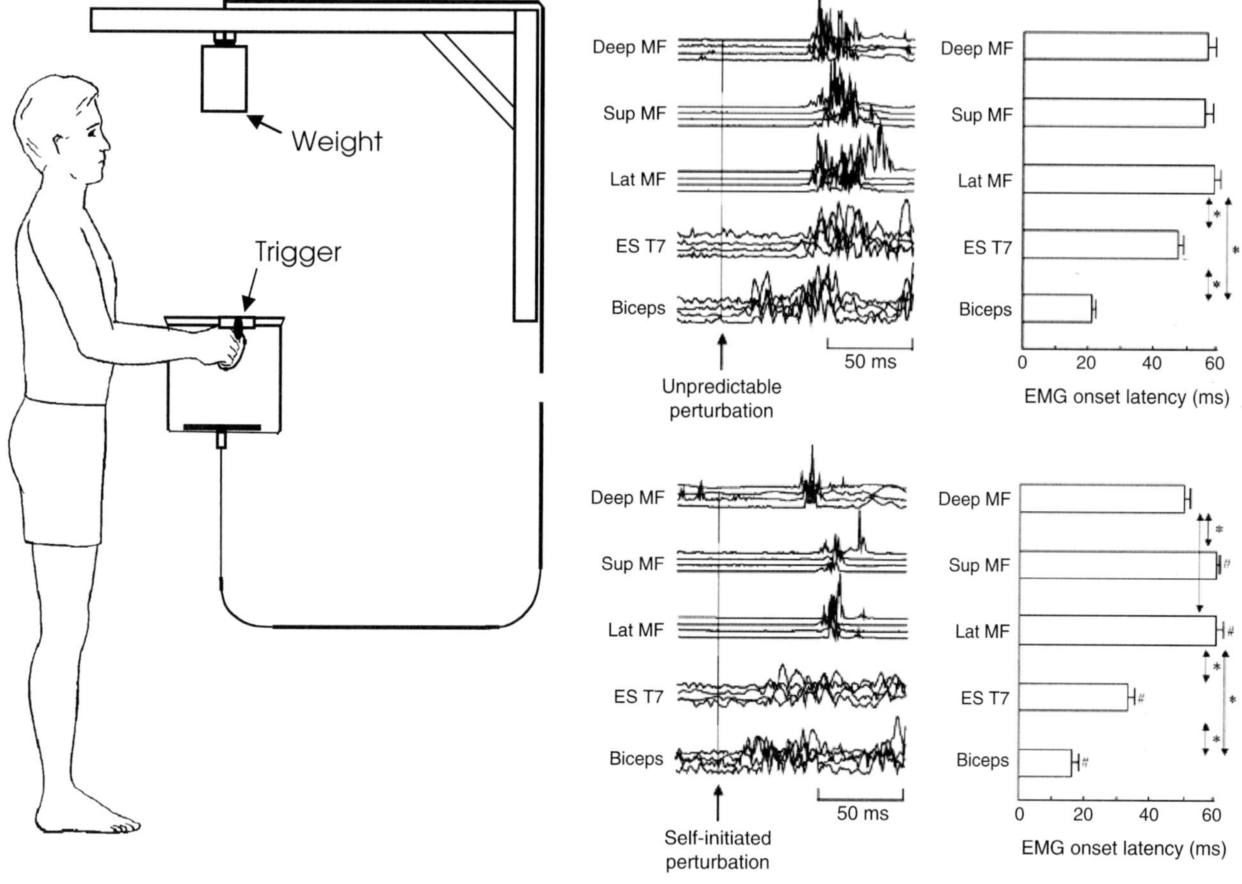

FIGURE 5–7. Response of the multifidus muscles to unexpected and self-initiated trunk loading. Data are shown up to four repetitions of catching a load in a bucket held in front of the body. The onset of the perturbation is shown by the vertical line. The mean data for the group are shown in the right panel. Note that the activity of deep, superficial, and lateral fibers of multifidus are active with the same latency when the loading is unexpected, but are active at different latencies when they initiate the loading themselves. (*Adapted from Moseley et al.*[46])

For instance, as described above, flexion loading of the trunk is associated with short-latency activity of the paraspinal muscles,[46] whereas extension loading induces flexor activity.[44] Other examples include the response of the trunk to unloading. When a load that tends to flex the trunk is removed from the trunk, activity of the extensor muscles must be reduced in order to maintain the trunk upright. Correspondingly, short-latency reduction in activity of the paraspinal muscles has been observed.[51,52] This unloading response is commonly argued to be due to removal of the contribution of spindle afferent input to muscle contraction[53] and thus is the opposite to a stretch reflex, but mediated by the same spinal networks. Similar to the loading responses these responses are also refined by increased predictability.[51]

At a more complex level the central nervous system also initiates complex patterns of activity of the trunk muscles that are highly integrated. A commonly investigated example is the response to movement of the support surface. In this task the overall equilibrium of the body is disturbed and a complex multisegmental response is required to move the center of mass of the body over the new base of support.[54] In this task, simple reflex responses are not sufficient to meet the demands for stability. For instance when the support is moved backwards, the trunk leans forwards and the paraspinal muscles are stretched (Fig. 5–9). However, if the trunk extended in response to this stretch the person would fall over (i.e., backwards). Instead the abdominal and hip flexor muscles must contract to flex the body and generate a hip torque sufficient to move the center of mass over the new base.[54] Thus, these responses require considerable integration and input from higher centers to plan the most appropriate strategy. An issue to consider in this task is that the goal of the body is more complex than just to maintain the orientation of the spine and intervertebral control. An additional level is added to the spectrum of control issues: control of body equilibrium. Thus the response of the trunk muscles to support surface translations moves the spine to restore

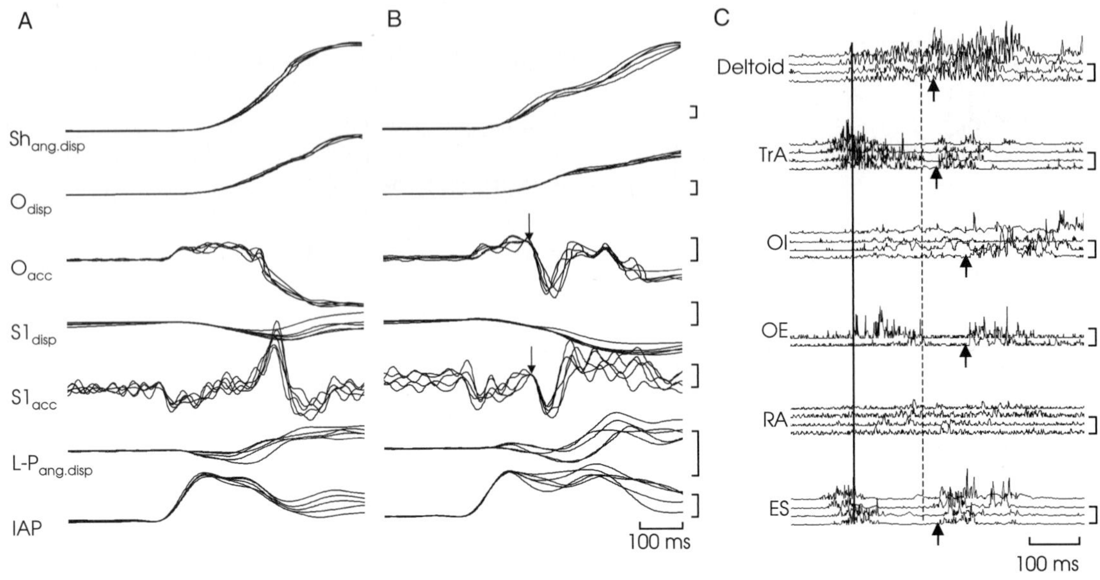

FIGURE 5–8. Raw movement data from a representative subject of limb movement without (*A*) and with (*B*) unexpected addition of load to the limb, and rectified electromyographic data with loading (*C*). Arrows indicate the onset of decreased acceleration of the olecranon and S1 markers (i.e., onset of the perturbation). In part *B* the solid line indicates the onset of limb movement and the dashed line indicates the deceleration of the limb. Arrows indicate the mean onsets of electromyogram for each muscle following the perturbation. Angular flexion and forward displacement is upwards. Note the short-latency increase in transversus abdominis electromyogram after the addition of the load to the arm. $Sh_{ang.disp}$: Shoulder angular displacement, O_{disp}: elbow linear displacement, O_{acc}: elbow acceleration, $L\text{-}P_{ang.disp}$: lumbopelvic angular displacement, $S1_{disp}$: S1 linear displacement, $S1_{acc}$: S1 acceleration. Calibrations—displacement: 15 cm, acceleration: 2.5 cm s^{-2}, angular displacement: 10 degree, IAP: 10 mmHg, EMG: 100 μV. IAP; Intra-Abdominal Pressure.

balance rather than just maintain spinal orientation and is specifically matched to the direction of perturbation. This provides another example of the strategy of the nervous system to use movement rather than simple stiffening. While the activity of the superficial muscles is closely linked to the direction of perturbation and the requirement to control equilibrium, the activity of the deep muscles is largely independent of the direction of perturbation.[33] Whether these responses are controlled by afferent input from proprioceptors or from vestibular or visual inputs is not completely understood. However, it is generally agreed that all systems contribute to the initiation and organization of the response.

Control of Muscle Stiffness

A third type of control strategy is related to both feedback and feedforward control and involves modulation of the "tone" in specific muscles, to provide an underlying degree of stability to the joints. This activity increases the stiffness of muscles that surround the joints.[9,13] Muscle stiffness is the property of muscles to act as springs (i.e., the ratio of length change to force change) and has viscoelastic and activity-related components. Muscle stiffness provides control of forces applied to a joint and contributes to control before even the shortest reflex response could be initiated.[56] It has been argued that postural stability may be controlled by modulation of stiffness of the ankle muscles.[57] Similarly, stability of the trunk may be controlled by stiffness of the spinal muscles. Importantly, the activity-related component of muscle stiffness is modulated by feedback from spindle and ligament afferents[56] (Fig. 5–10). It is the stretch reflex and the control of the gamma-motoneurons that control the sensitivity of the sensory component of the muscle spindles that control this system. In addition, the reflex activity of the multifidus muscle in response to stimulation of mechanoreceptors in the lumbar disc and ligaments[38–40] and supraspinous ligament in humans[42] may contribute to stiffness control. In terms of a feedforward contribution, repetitive movements are associated with tonic activity of the deep trunk muscles, which is consistent with the control of stiffness. Although the control of these movements is not completely understood,[58] it is likely that they involve a feedforward component owing to their predictability.[14]

Clinical Pearl: Tonic activity of the deep intrinsic spinal muscles contributes to muscle stiffness and is likely to provide a "first line of defense" for the spine against perturbation.

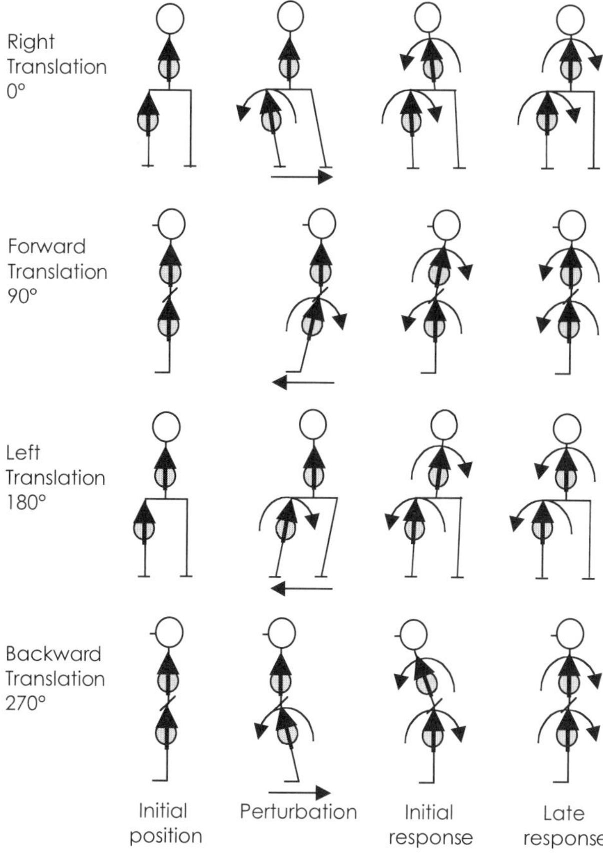

FIGURE 5–9. Postural perturbations from translation of the support surface. When the support moves, the base of support shifts from under the center of mass. When the support is moved quickly torque must be generated at the hip to move the mass over the new base of support. This involves contraction of muscles of the hip and trunk to extend the spine with forward translation and flex the spine with backward translation. (*Adapted from Huang et al.*[55])

Summary

The nervous system has a variety of strategies to modulate the stability of the spine that include feedforward and feedback mechanisms, as well as the modulation of muscles stiffness. In reality all movements involve a combination of mechanisms with some elements of functional movement that are predictable and some not. A key factor is that there is some differentiation in the control of orientation of the spine and intervertebral motion and the central nervous system draws on the architectural properties of muscle when planning strategies to control each element of stability.

MUSCULAR CONTRIBUTION TO SPINAL CONTROL

There has been considerable debate regarding the specific contribution of individual muscles to stability. Recent emphasis has been placed on identification of the muscles that provide the greatest contribution to stability and different authors have nominated muscles that they consider provide the greatest contribution to stability.[59,60] However, no biomechanical models encompass all of the elements of stability. Notably no model truly encompasses the control of spinal orientation and the fine-tuning of control of intervertebral shear/translation and rotation during movement. Thus, although a model may identify one specific muscle as being most critical for control, it is more likely that different systems may be responsible for control of individual elements of spinal stability, and a muscle that is optimal for control of one element may not be optimal for control of another. This was initially proposed by Bergmark[13] who argued that muscles could be divided into "local" and "global" systems, with the former system of muscle responsible for control of intervertebral stability, whereas the latter is

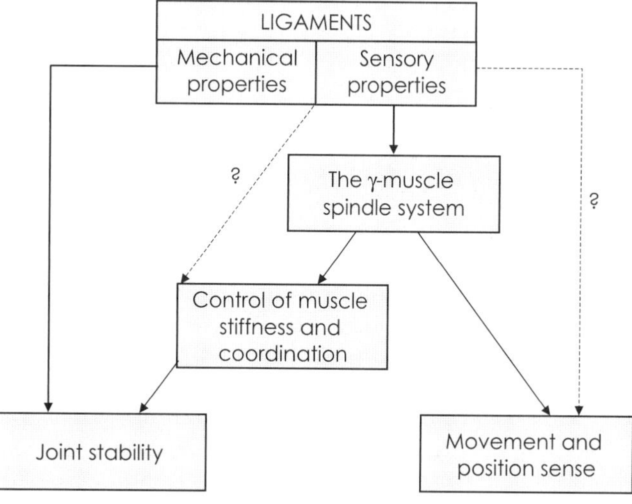

FIGURE 5–10. Contribution of ligaments to joint stability. In addition to the mechanical role of the ligaments in passive control of joint stability, they may also contribute to stability via sensory contributions to perception of joint position to assist in the planning of control strategies and by a contribution to the modulation of muscle stiffness via inputs to the gamma-motoneuron system. (Adapted from: Johansson H, Sjolander P, Sojka P. A sensory role for the cruciate ligaments. Clin Orth Rel Res 1991;268:161–178.)

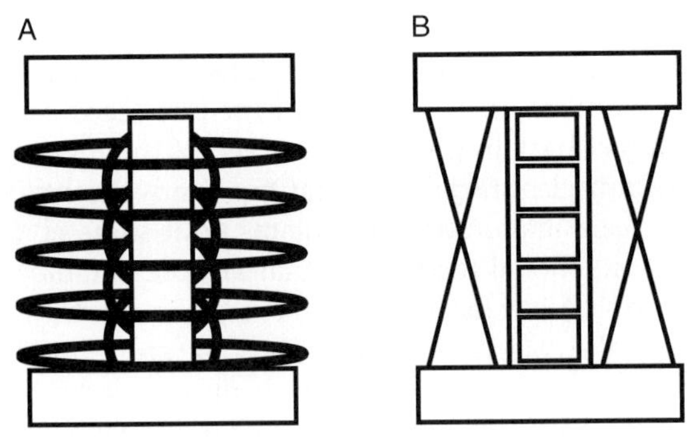

FIGURE 5–11. Local (*A*) and global (*B*) muscles of the lumbopelvic region.

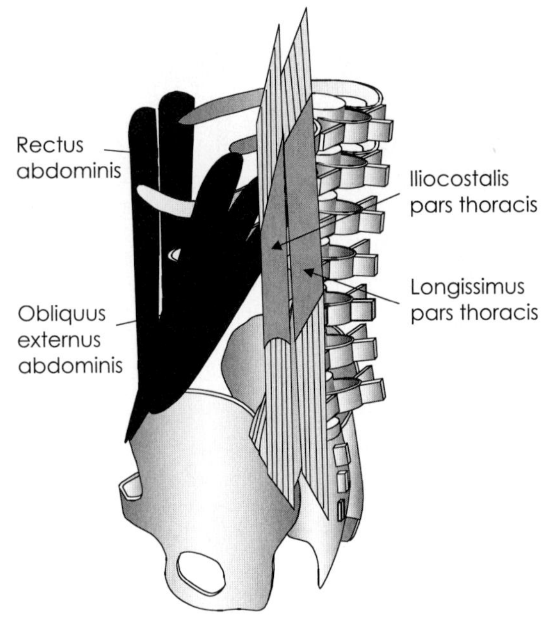

FIGURE 5–12. Anatomy of a major global muscles: rectus abdominis, obliquus externus abdominis, longissimus pars thoracis, iliocostalis pars thoracis.

responsible for control of orientation and load transfer across the spine (Fig. 5–11). Although any model that introduces a dichotomous classification system is likely to be too simplistic, the model provides a framework within which to understand how architectural properties of muscle can influence the contribution to stability. Notably, this will also influence how the muscles may be used by the nervous system to control stability and movement of the spine.

In Bergmark's model the local muscles are those that attach directly to the lumbar vertebrae and have the potential to specifically influence intervertebral motion. Panjabi considered that this segmental arrangement was an advantage to the nervous system in the sense that it is able to control the motion of a specific segment, as required.[6] Examples of local muscles are the lumbar multifidus and transversus abdominis (via the thoracolumbar fascia), although Bergmark did not include this latter muscle in his model. The global muscles are those that transcend the spine from the rib cage to the pelvis. These muscles generate torque at the spine but have a limited ability to control intervertebral shear and rotation. These muscles are ideal for control orientation of the spine and act like guy ropes to keep the spine upright. Examples of global muscles are the oblique abdominal muscles, rectus abdominis, and the long thoracolumbar erector spinae muscles.

Global Muscle Contribution to Spinal Control

There is considerable evidence in the literature to support the contribution of the global muscles to the control of the orientation of the spine. It is generally predictable based on the moment arm and direction of force provided by the muscles.[13,29] That is, flexors generate flexion torque and oppose extension (Fig. 5–12). Many studies provide data consistent with this proposal. For instance, as described above, activity of the "global" back extensors occurs in response to unexpected loading of the trunk that produces trunk flexion moment[45,61] and activity of the "global" abdominal muscles occurs with short latency after a support surface translation in sitting which causes the spine to extend.[62] In addition, it has been generally considered that antagonist trunk muscles are coactivated to stiffen the spine and prevent buckling.[63] This strategy has been most commonly identified in tasks associated with high load or with increased unpredictability. For example, greater activity of the superficial abdominal muscles has been demonstrated during isometric trunk tasks, than predicted by a biomechanical model[29]; antagonistic activity of obliquus exterus abdominis (OE) and obliquus internus abdominis (OI) has been recorded during lifting and isometric trunk efforts[29]; and coactivation is increased when a lifted load is unpredictable.[28] Activity of the global muscles, such as the lateral portion of the quadratus lumborum, has been linked to the control of spinal buckling, which is intrinsic to the Euler model of spinal stability. This has been indicated by increased quadratus lumborum activity with increased compressive load from holding a mass bilaterally in the hands.[64] It is important to note that although coactivation of the abdominal and extensor muscles increases the stability of the spine, this higher stability is traded off with the increased load on the passive structures of the spine.[65] Thus there is considerable evidence that the global muscles provide an important and critical role for the control of spinal stability, and contribute to both its feedforward and feedback control.

Clinical Pearl: Increased activity of global muscles may occur in association with high-level physical activity and respiratory disease, in addition to pain.

Limitations of the Global System

As indicated above, there are several limitations to the contribution of the global muscles to spinal stability. First, as the global muscles have no attachment to the vertebrae they can only influence intervertebral motion as a result of compressive forces from coactivation of antagonist muscles. While compression can assist in the control of shear and rotation forces, as mentioned above, this is associated with the cost of increased loading of the passive tissues.[63] The global trunk muscles generate torque at the trunk. This torque must be overcome by antagonist activation in order to keep the spine upright, and this coactivation results in a compressive load on the spine.[63,66–68] Excessive compression, which increases intradiscal pressure and loading through the posterior elements of the spine, has long been considered to be a risk factor for spinal degeneration and pain.[69] Excessive global muscle co-contraction during light functional tasks may even be indicative of inappropriate trunk muscle control in patients with back pain.[52] Others have argued that dysfunction in the passive stabilizing system may be indicated by increased levels of trunk muscle coactivation.[7]

Clinical Pearl: Overactivity of the global muscles is commonly observed in low back pain. While it presents an effective short-term strategy to limit spinal motion it may lead to long-term consequences for the health of the spine.

The second limitation of the global system is that the muscles of this system can only provide a nonspecific contribution to spinal control. That is, the global muscles cannot augment control selectively to a specific segment. Third, global muscles have a limited ability to control shear forces. This has been argued biomechanically,[70] and from in vivo studies. For example, when shear forces were imposed on the spine, there was no change in activity of the global muscles. Therefore, the authors reasoned that deeper local muscles must control this element.[71] A similar situation may exist in the sacroiliac joints. As mentioned previously, stability of the sacroiliac joints is dependent on compression,[17] although it is argued that this compression force is, to a large extent, provided by the large global muscles working in discrete synergies (e.g., the contraction of gluteus maximus with the diagonally opposed latissimus dorsi).[72] This is likely to be ineffective in light tasks in which these muscles are relatively inactive. Instead, horizontal forces produced by the local abdominal muscles (e.g., transversus abdominis) will compress and stabilize the sacroiliac joints.[17]

Fourth, antagonist global muscle coactivation results in a restriction of spinal motion or "rigidity" of the spine. It is known that in healthy subjects the central nervous system uses movement rather than simple stiffening of the spine to overcome challenges to stability [26,73] and reduce energy expenditure in many tasks.[27] A strategy of trunk stiffening, although requiring less complex neural control, would compromise optimal spinal function.

Clinical Pearl: It is critical to consider not only the motion of the spine, but also the adjacent segments. If the mobility of the hips and thoracic spine is compromised, this may lead to increased spinal motion to compensate.

Finally, trunk muscles are involved in functions other than spinal control and movement.[74] As the superficial abdominal muscles depress the rib cage and are involved in forced expiration,[75] increased activity of these muscles in people with pain may lead to compromised respiratory function, for example restricted movement of the chest wall. In contrast, local muscles have limited effect on rib cage motion.[75] Thus, reliance on global muscles for control may be problematic from a systemic point of view. In contrast, local muscles allow controlled spinal motion and have the ability to control individual segments rather that providing a general compressive force across the spine.

Clinical Pearl: Patients with low back pain may require specific education of coordination of the postural and respiratory functions of the trunk muscles.

Local Muscle Contribution to Spinal Control

Two local or deep intrinsic lumbopelvic muscles have specifically received attention in the literature: transversus abdominis and the lumbar multifidus. Transversus abdominis is a broad sheet-like muscle with extensive attachments to the lumbar vertebrae via the thoracolumbar fascia, and to the pelvis and rib cage (Fig. 5–13). The muscle fibers have a relatively horizontal orientation and, therefore, it has minimal ability to move the spine, although it may contribute to rotation.[76,77] Its contribution to spinal control is likely to involve modulation of intra-abdominal pressure and tensioning the thoracolumbar fascia. Transversus abdominis has been shown to be closely associated with control of intra-abdominal pressure,[44,76] and recent studies that have involved electrical stimulation of the diaphragm in humans[78,79] and transversus

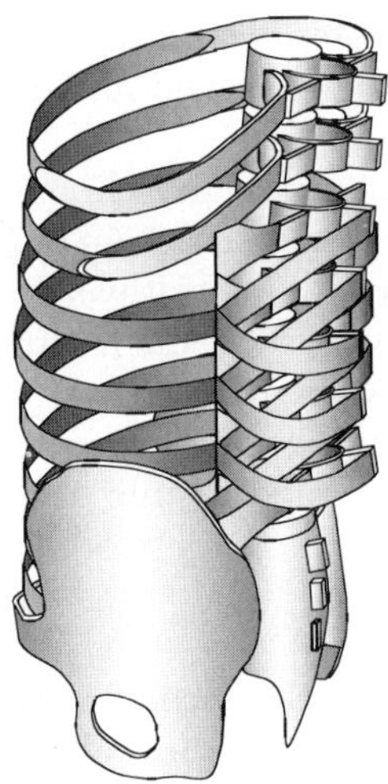

FIGURE 5–13. Transversus abdominis anatomy: Transversus abdominis has extensive attachment to the thoracolumbar fascia, rib cage, and iliac crest. Anteriorly the muscle attaches to the anterior abdominal fascias.

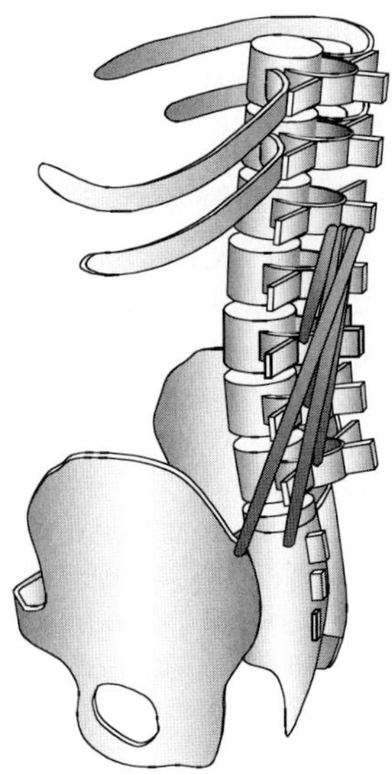

FIGURE 5–14. Multifidus anatomy: All fibers of multifidus arising from L1 are shown to demonstrate the change in fascicle length from the deep to superficial fibers of the muscle.

abdominis and the diaphragm in pigs[80] confirm that spinal stiffness is increased by intra-abdominal pressure. Fascial tension may directly restrict intervertebral motion or provide gentle segmental compression via the posterior layer of the thoracolumbar fascia.[81] Recent porcine studies confirm that the combined effect of intra-abdominal pressure and fascial tension is required for transversus abdominis to increase intervertebral stiffness, and the mechanical effect of its contraction is reduced if the fascial attachments are cut.[80] For sacroiliac support, transversus abdominis acts via the ilia to compress the sacroiliac joint anteriorly,[17] and this has been confirmed in vivo.[82]

Clinical Pearl: The effect of transversus abdominis on the spine is dependent /on bilateral contraction[80]; thus, asymmetrical function of this muscle in low back pain is likely to compromise the mechanical effect.

Multifidus has five fascicles that arise from the spinous process and lamina of each lumbar vertebra and descend in a caudo-lateral direction[83] (Fig. 5–14). The most superficial fibers cross up to five segments and attach caudally to the ilia and sacrum, while the deep fibers attach from the inferior border of a lamina and cross a minimum of two segments to attach on the mamillary process and facet joint capsule.[84] The superficial fibers are distant from the centers of rotation of the lumbar vertebrae, have an extension moment arm, and can control the lumbar lordosis.[83] In contrast, the deep fibers have a limited moment arm and a minor ability to extend the spine.[85] Multifidus can control intervertebral motion by generation of intervertebral compression[86] and control of shear forces.[83] The proximity of deep multifidus to the center of rotation results in compression with minimal extension moment. In addition, multifidus may contribute to the control of intervertebral motion by control of anterior rotation and translation of the vertebrae,[83] or via tensioning the thoracolumbar fascia as it expands on contraction.[87] Several studies have provided in vitro and in vivo evidence of the ability of multifidus to control intervertebral motion.[88,90]

Clinical Pearl: The deep fibers of multifidus are controlled independently of the superificial fibers[31] and are thought to be the most important to train in low back pain.

Other muscles that satisfy the criteria for local muscles are the interspinales, intertransversarii, posterior fibers of psoas, medial fibers of quadratus lumborum, and the lumbar portions of longissimus and iliocostalis. The interspinales and intertransversarii are small muscles that have a high density of muscle spindles and have been argued to have an important sensory rather than motor function.[89] The posterior fibers of psoas that attach to the transverse processes of the lumbar vertebrae have a minimal moment arm for spinal movement and have been argued to provide primarily an intersegmental compressive force,[90] and may have a primary function in intersegmental control.[91] The medial fibers of quadratus lumborum along with the lumbar erector spinae have one attachment to the transverse processes of the lumbar spine and thus have a segmental attachment such that these muscles may contribute to both elements of spinal control and have been implicated in spinal stability.[64]

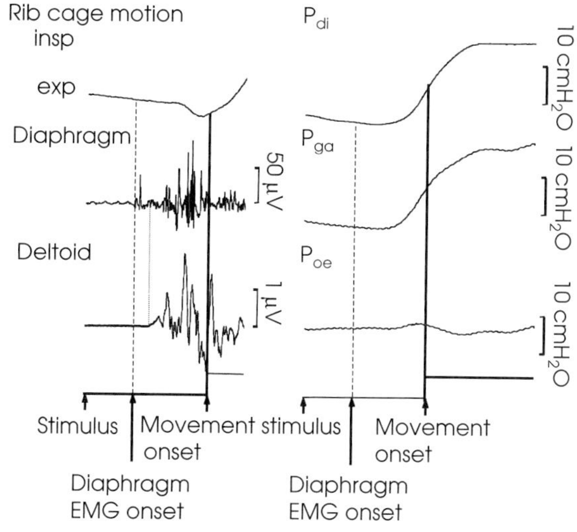

FIGURE 5–15. When a limb is moved, activity of the diaphragm muscle occurs in advance of the muscle responsible for limb movement (deltoid). In addition, there is an increase in gastric pressure (P_{ga}) that precedes the onset of arm movement. These data are consistent with a role of the diaphragm in postural control of the trunk. (*Adapted from Hodges et al.*[94])

Of the other abdominal muscles, obliquus internus has an attachment to the thoracolumbar fascia in a small proportion of people, thus providing a segmental attachment to the spine.[70] Anteriorly this muscle has fibers that are parallel to those of transversus abdominis and may contribute to the force closure of the sacroiliac joint.[17] However, despite the similarities to transversus abdominis there are distinct differences in control of these two muscles.

An important consideration is that for transversus abdominis to influence the stability of the spine via modulation of intra-abdominal pressure or increased tension in the thoracolumbar fascia, it is necessary for the roof and the floor of the abdominal cavity to contract. That is, the diaphragm and pelvic floor muscles must contribute to the postural response. Studies have confirmed that activity of these muscles occurs in conjunction with transversus abdominis during arm movements[74,92–94] (Fig. 5–15). However, their involvement in spinal control presents a challenge to the central nervous system to coordinate the respiratory and continence functions. Normal quiet respiration involves cyclical activity of the diaphragm, parasternal intercostal, and scalene muscles during inspiration, with expiration generated passively by the elastic recoil of the lung and chest wall.[75] However, when the demand for respiration is increased and the rate and depth of expiration is increased, abdominal muscles are phasically activated during the expiratory phase.[95] If respiration is increased involuntarily (e.g., hypercapnoea), transversus abdominis is recruited at lower minute ventilation than the other abdominal muscles.[96,97] Recent data indicate that this may vary between regions of the abdominal wall, with activity of the mid region of transversus abdominis recruited with lower respiratory demand (Urquhart D and Hodges, 2001). Studies of repetitive limb movements confirm that when the arm is moved repetitively to challenge the stability of the spine, tonic activity of the diaphragm and transversus abdominis is sustained, but is modulated with respiration to meet respiratory demands.[74,92] In a mechanical sense, the diaphragm and transversus abdominis co-contract tonically, yet during inspiration diaphragm increases its activity and shortens (concentric), and transversus abdominis decreases its activity and lengthens (eccentric). The converse pattern occurs during expiration. Recent data confirm that this coordination also occurs during natural repetitive movements such as locomotion.[98] This coordination occurs as if there is summation of the respiratory and postural drives to these muscles, which may occur at the motoneuron, providing a mechanism for the central nervous system to coordinate these functions (Fig. 5–16). However, when respiratory drive is increased by respiratory disease[99] or by breathing with an increased dead space to induce hypercapnoea[100] this coordination is compromised and tonic activity of the diaphragm and transversus abdominis is reduced.

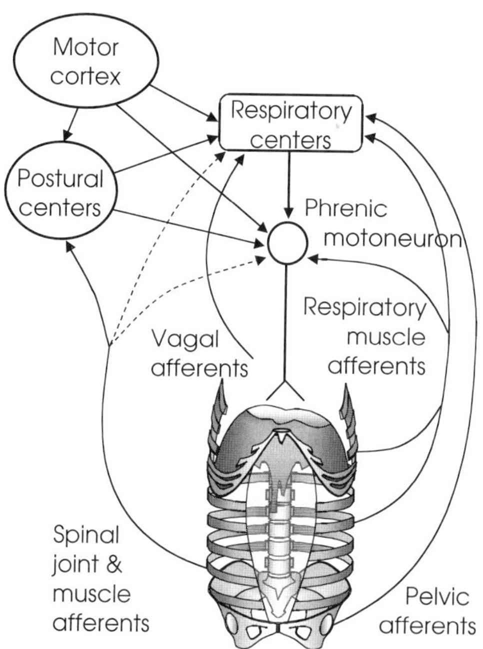

FIGURE 5–16. Organizational alternatives for the coordination of the postural and respiratory functions of the diaphragm. Postural inputs from the periphery and higher centers are summated with the respiratory drive from the pontine and medullary respiratory centers to coordinate the two drives. (*Adapted from Hodges et al.*[94])

Clinical Pearl: Patients who have respiratory disease in addition to low back pain may be more difficult to rehabilitate and may require consideration of timing of medication and training.

Similar to the coordination of postural control and respiration, the continence and stability function of the pelvic floor muscles must be coordinated. However, in most tasks the requirement for both of these functions is likely to be similar. For instance, activity of the pelvic floor muscles increases in tasks in which intra-abdominal pressure is increased, such as coughing,[101] which is consistent with the demand to control intra-abdominal pressure for spinal control.

Clinical Pearl: Rehabilitation of low back pain may require specific attention to the control of the pelvic floor muscles. If the patient suffers from incontinence, this may require specific attention.

Summary

Although any system of classification of muscles is likely to oversimplify the complex anatomical characteristics of the muscles of the spine and their differentiation in function for control of the spine, it provides a useful framework to consider the contribution of muscles to spinal stability and the organization of the postural responses by the central nervous system. It is likely that many muscles will not be so clearly categorized and may share features of both groups. Regardless of these criticisms, there is strong evidence that the local and global muscles are used relatively independently to control intervertebral motion and spinal orientation, respectively. It is important to consider that all muscles contribute to stability and control of the spine. However, each element of stability is best controlled by one group and the muscles of each group are unable to compensate for reduced activity in the other. However, when people have low back pain, changes in the coordination of the muscles systems have been observed. This is reviewed in the next section.

NEUROMUSCULAR CHANGES IN LOW BACK PAIN

When pain and injury are present, the strategies used by the central nervous system to control movement and/or posture and stability may be compromised. Early studies focused on the strength and endurance of the trunk muscles and many studies report decreased strength and endurance of the flexors and/or extensors of the trunk (e.g., ref. 102). However, other studies report no change, and it has been suggested that changes in these parameters are more related to physical activity level than they are to pain.[104] More recently, attention has focused on the potential for changes in the control of the trunk muscles. Numerous deficits in trunk muscle control have been identified. The mechanisms for these changes are poorly understood and could be due to changes at any level of the motor system. This section reviews the changes that occur in the motor control of the trunk in people with low back pain.

Changes in Feedforward Control of Movement and Stability of the Spine

As mentioned above, feedforward strategies are preplanned by the central nervous system and provide an opportunity to investigate changes in the organization of the planning of motor responses. Changes in feedforward strategies for postural control have been frequently identified in neurological disorders such as frontal lobe trauma and Parkinson disease.[104,105] Changes have also been identified in people with chronic low back pain. A common model for investigation of these changes has been the investigation of the activity of the trunk muscles in association with limb movement. As mentioned in an earlier section, limb movement is associated with activity of the global and local muscles of the trunk in advance of the movement of the limb in a manner that is matched to the demands of the limb movement.[15,30] Notably, in pain-free individuals the activity of the global muscles (such as the oblique abdominal muscles, rectus abdominis, and erector spinae) is dependent on the direction of movement,[15,22] but the activity of transverus abdominis is not specific to the direction of movement.[15,26] When people with low back pain perform the same task the onset of activity of transverus abdominis is delayed with movement of the arm[25] or leg[106] (Fig. 5–17).

Clinical Pearl: Irrespective of the specific pathology, delayed activity of transversus abdominis appears to be a consistent finding in low back pain.

There are several key findings to consider. First, the activity of the transversus abdominis fails to prepare the spine for the reactive forces from limb movements. On the basis of the in vivo and in vitro biomechanical studies described above[80,78,79,107] this would imply that it is the fine-tuning of control of intervertebral motion that is affected by this change. Second, the subjects selected for this study had a history of recurrent episodes of low back pain, but were pain-free at the time of testing. Thus, it is unlikely that the findings were simply due to avoidance of painful movements. Thirdly, although the

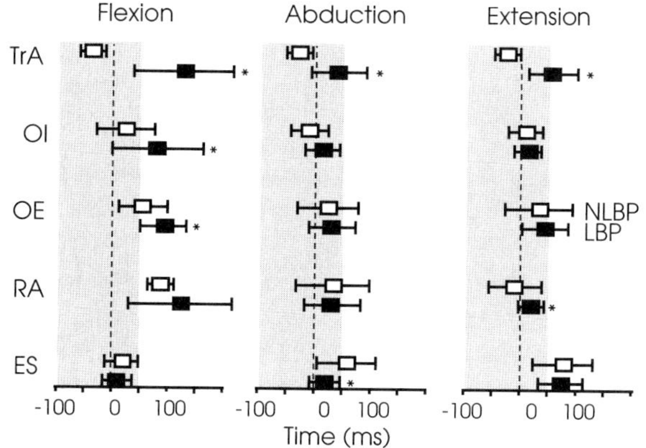

FIGURE 5–17. Onset of activity of the trunk muscles with movement of the arm in each direction for people with and without low back pain. The vertical dashed line indicates the onset of deltoid activity. With movement in each direction the onset of transversus abdominis (TrA) precedes the onset of deltoid in pain-free individuals, but is significantly delayed with each direction of movement. (*Adapted from Hodges and Richardson.*[25]) Key: TrA - Transversus Abdominis; OI - Obliquus Internus Abdominis; OE: Obliquus Externus Abdominis, Rectus Abdominis; Es-Erector Spinae; NLBP - Non Low Back Pain; LBP - Low Back Pain.

response of transversus abdominis was independent of the direction of movement in the control subjects, in the subjects with low back pain the response of these muscles was specific to the direction of movement with earlier activity during extension of the arm, along with the global abdominal muscles.[25] This finding suggests that the change in activity is not simply due to changes in excitability of the motoneuron (or other region of the central nervous system) or decreased conduction velocity somewhere in the motor pathway. The findings would suggest that there is a change in the planning of the motor response by the central nervous system. Fourthly, there was variable change in the superficial global muscles. Although there were specific changes in global muscle activity with specific movements in specific directions, this was not consistent.[25] Finally, further studies indicated that the threshold for activation of transverus abdominis was increased.[108] That is, no activity was recorded in this muscle until arm movement was performed at a faster speed than was required to initiate activity in pain-free controls.

Changes in Feedback Control of Movement and Stability of the Spine

Many studies have investigated feedback control strategies in low back pain and these studies have investigated a number of aspects from the sensory components and reflex control to more complicated control of voluntary movements. In many cases it is impossible to determine the exact component or components of the system that are responsible for the change in motor control. For instance, if the amplitude of activity of a muscle is modified during a movement task, it is difficult to determine whether the change results from inaccurate feedback from the periphery, inaccurate interpretation of normal feedback, or inability to initiate an appropriate command. However, behavioral studies provide insight into the nature of changes in motor control.

By definition, feedback mediated control strategies are dependent on accurate afferent input. One of the most commonly identified motor control deficits that have been identified in association with musculoskeletal pain and injury are sensory deficits. Numerous studies have investigated proprioception of the spine, and although there is variation in results, most agree that there is decreased acuity to spinal motion in low back pain,[109] and impaired ability to accurately reposition.[110,111]

Changes in a variety of reflex responses have been identified in musculoskeletal pain syndromes. Delayed activity of the erector spinae to trunk loading has been identified.[61,112] However, other studies suggest that the response of the erector spinae muscles is not increased in people with sciatica. When subjects are given some ability to predict the timing of the perturbation, pain-free subjects are able to shorten the reaction time, but people with low back pain cannot.[45] This may vary between components of the erector spinae group.[46] When subjects in a supported standing position have a mass attached to their back or front and are asked to maintain the upright posture, activity of the trunk muscles must reduce if the mass is suddenly removed. When this response has been investigated in people with low back pain they have a delayed offset of activity of global muscles such as the oblique abdominal and thoracolumbar erector spinae muscles and there is increased coactivation of these muscles[52] (Fig. 5–18). Notably, the delayed offset of activity was weakly correlated with performance of a balance task in sitting.

Clinical Pearl: Increased activity of superficial trunk muscles occurs consistently in low back pain, but there is variability between individuals in terms of the muscles that are overactive.

Changes in control of trunk muscle activity occur during ongoing functional movements. For instance, reduced amplitude of activity of multifidus has been identified during functional tasks in people with low back pain.[113,114] In contrast, there has been considerable debate in the literature regarding the presence of augmented activity of the paraspinal muscles.

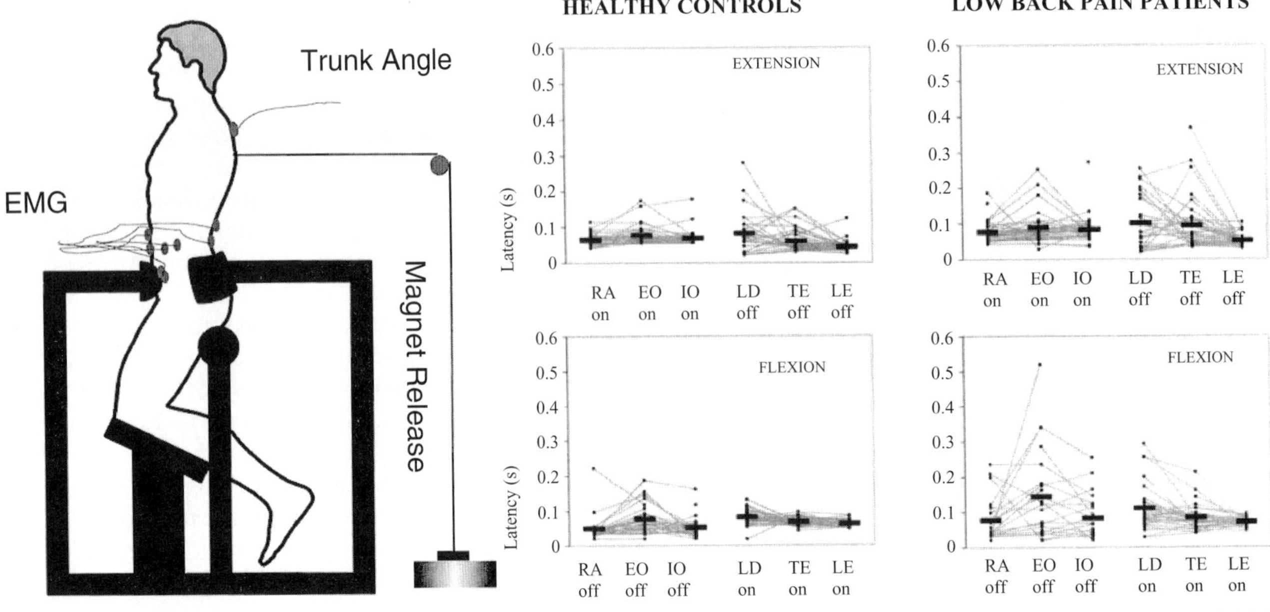

FIGURE 5–18. When a load is rapidly removed from the trunk, activity of the trunk muscles must reduce for the trunk to maintain an upright posture. When a load is removed from the back (bottom panels) activity of obliquus externus abdominis (EO) must reduce. This reduction in activity is delayed in a subset of people with chronic back pain (right bottom panel). (*Adapted from Radebold et al.*[52]) Key: RA - Rectus Abdominis; IO - Obliquus Internus Abdominis; LD - Latissimus Dorsi; TE - Thoracic Erector Spinae; LE - Lumbar Erector Spinae.

In general, these studies have had variable results with studies reporting increased,[115,116] decreased,[114] asymmetrical,[117] and no change in activity.[118] A consistent finding has been sustained activity of the erector spinae muscles at the end of range of spinal flexion, a point at which the erector spinae muscles are normally inactive (the "flexion relaxation" phenomenon), in people with low back pain.[119] This has been replicated by experimental pain[120] and has been shown to limit intervertebral motion.[121] During gait, the normal periods of silence in the erector spinae that normally occur in the period between heel strikes either have reduced duration or are absent.[122]

Numerous studies have investigated parameters of postural control in people with low back pain. These studies have identified impairments of balance when standing on one[123] or two legs[124] or sitting.[125] Furthermore, an increased risk of low back pain or recurrence of pain has been identified for people with poor performance in a test of standing balance.[126] These changes indicate a general reduction of the accuracy of the postural control system in these patients. Other more complex elements of control have also been found to be altered in low back pain. For instance, people with low back pain have a slower reaction time,[127] and slow reaction time has been associated with musculoskeletal injuries (including low back pain) in a variety of sports.[128]

Clinical Pearl: . . . an increased risk of low back pain or recurrence of pain has been identified for people with poor performance in a test of standing balance.

Interpretation of the Changes in Feedforward and Feedback Mechanisms

The changes in feedforward and feedback control of the spine suggest that the deep local muscles and the superficial global muscles are commonly affected in an opposite manner by the presence of pain. That is, activity of the global muscles is generally increased whereas activity of the local muscles is reduced. An important consideration is that while the response of the local muscles appears to be consistent across subjects, there is considerable variability in the response of the global muscles, but in the majority of cases activity of one or more global muscles is increased. This is consistent with the hypothesis of Cholewicki et al.[7] who suggested that excessive activity in the superficial muscles might be a measurable compensation for poor passive or active segmental support. This response is increasingly recognized in the literature.[129] Hypothetically, this reorganization may modify the efficacy of spinal control mechanisms. On the basis of the role of the local muscle system and the limitations of the global muscle system to control all elements of spinal stability this may lead to reduced efficiency of intervertebral control, increased spinal loading, and reduced spinal motion. Recent data is confirming these hypotheses.[129] It is important to consider the possible mechanisms for these changes and the timing of onset of the dysfunction relative to pain; that is, whether the motor control changes precede or follow the onset of pain.

Muscle Factors in Low Back Pain

While recent attention has been focused on the control of the trunk muscles in people with low back pain, it is still important to consider changes in other muscle factors. In addition to the changes in control of the paraspinal muscles, several studies have identified changes in morphology of the multifidus muscles that may be associated with changes in control. For example, studies report changes in muscle fiber composition,[130] and reduced cross-sectional area of multifidus has been identified as early as 24 hours after the onset of acute, unilateral low back pain.[131]

Other studies indicate that fatigability of the paraspinal muscles is increased during trunk extension efforts.[132,133] People with and without low back pain can be discriminated on the basis of electromyographic measures of such fatigability.[134] Consistent with the motor control data that suggest augmentation of activity of the trunk muscles in low back pain, recent data have suggested that the strength and endurance of the obliquus externus abdominis during rotation efforts is increased in low back pain.[135,136] Numerous other changes have also been identified. For instance decreased endurance of the back extensor muscles has been identified as a predictor of low back pain.[137] However, evaluation of fatigue and strength measures is complicated by motivation[138] and factors such as fear-avoidance behaviors.[132] In view of these findings clinical strategies must consider muscle factors in order to ensure optimal spinal control.

Clinical Pearl: People with and without low back pain can be discriminated on the basis of electromyographic measures of such fatigability.

Mechanism of Interaction of Pain and Motor Control

It is important to consider whether changes in motor control occur as a result of pain and injury or whether poor motor control strategies lead to inefficient spinal control, leading to microtrauma, nociceptor stimulation, and pain as suggested by Janda[3] and Farfan.[139] Although not a perfect model of clinical pain, numerous studies have investigated the effect of experimentally induced pain on motor control in many regions of the body. This stimulus is not capable of replicating all elements of pain. However, it provides an opportunity to investigate the response of the body to nociceptor stimulation and pain to determine whether those components of the pain experience may be responsible for the changes identified in clinical populations.

Clinical Pearl: People who are clumsy as children are more likely to have back pain as adults.

In terms of the trunk, back pain is commonly elicited experimentally by injection of hypertonic saline into the paraspinal muscles. When pain is induced in this manner and subjects perform rapid arm movements, the feedforward response of transverus abdominis is delayed in a manner similar to that identified in people with clinical pain[140] (Fig. 5–19). Changes in global muscle activity differed between individuals. However, in all subjects, activity of at least one superficial trunk muscle was increased. This variability of the superficial muscle response to pain is consistent with clinical observations.[4] In separate studies, loss of relaxation of the erector spinae muscles has been replicated during trunk flexion[120] and gait[122] by experimentally induced pain. Thus, it appears that pain can cause the changes in motor control. However, it is possible that this may not always be the case and motor control changes could also precede low back pain. Several authors have argued that poor control may lead to microtrauma and eventual injury.[6,7,139] Several studies have provided preliminary support for this hypothesis. For example, Janda[3] identified that many people with chronic back pain also had minor neurological signs associated with childhood clumsiness, and people with slow reaction times have been shown to have an increased risk of injury.[128]

The mechanism for pain and nociceptor stimulation to affect motor control is poorly understood. Pain could affect motor output at any level of the motor system including the cortex, the motoneurons, reflex pathways, and areas "upstream" of the motor cortex that are involved in motor planning. Studies have identified changes in motoneuron excitability,[141] decreased cortical excitability,[142] and changes in sensitivity of muscle spindles[143] in association with pain. However, the data from studies with variable preparation for movement suggest that the change in motor control identified in low back pain may be due to a change in motor planning, and not simple inhibition or transmission delays.[144] In a healthy population, when the preparation for movement is reduced, the reaction time of the arm movement is delayed. This is associated with a slowing of the response of the global abdominal muscles together with the limb movement, but there is no slowing of the response of transversus abdominis.[32] Instead, the response of transversus abdominis maintained a constant reaction time. This finding provides further evidence for differential control of the local and global muscles. However, when people with back pain perform that same task with

A

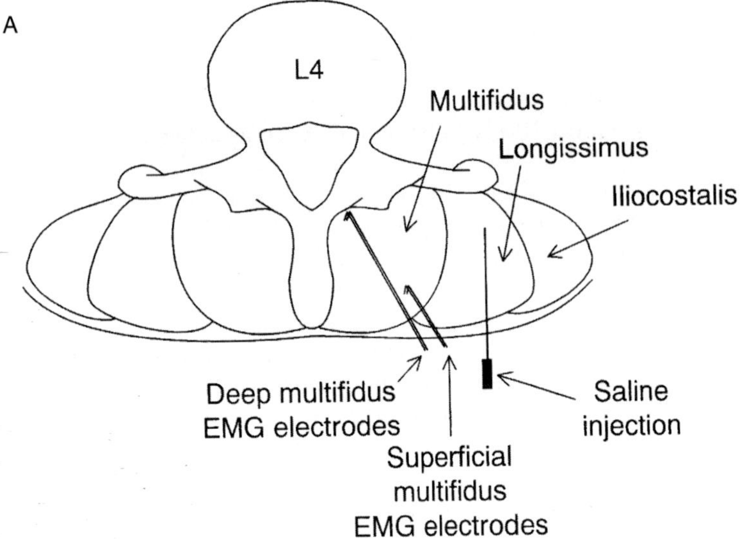

B

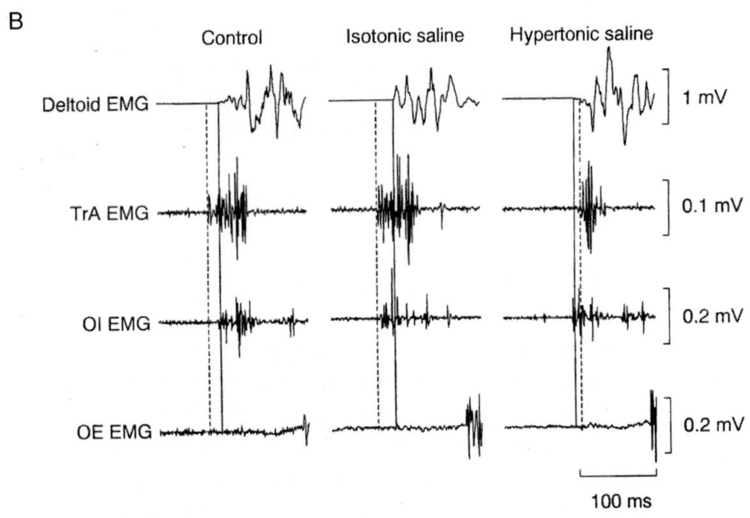

FIGURE 5–19. Effect of experimentally induced pain on motor control of transversus abdominis. Pain was induced by injection of hypertonic saline into the paraspinal muscles at the L4 level (*A*). When subjects rapidly moved an arm in response to a light the response of transversus abdominis (TrA) was initiated before deltoid in trials without pain and in trials with injection of non-painful isotonic saline (*B*). When the arm was moved during pain after injection of hypertonic saline, the onset of TrA activity was delayed. There was no change in activity of obliquus internus (OI) or externus (OE) abdominis for this subject. (*Adapted from Hodges et al.*[141])

variable preparation for movement, the activity of transversus abdominis is delayed along with the other abdominal muscles.[145] Taken together, these findings are likely to represent a change in motor planning. Consistent with this hypothesis, pain changes activity of areas of the brain involved in motor planning.[146]

Clinical Pearl: As the changes in control of the deep trunk muscles involve changes in the strategy used by the central nervous system to control these muscles, motor relearning strategies are likely to be required to rehabilitate this control.

Pain-Adaptation Model

These changes in motor control may be at least partially explained by the "pain-adaptation" model of Lund et al.[147] This model hypothesizes that movement velocity and amplitude are reduced in the presence of pain. In terms of limb and jaw movements this is associated with reduced agonist activity and increased antagonist activity.[148] In terms of the control of trunk stability, this model may suggest increased coactivation of the trunk muscles to increase trunk stiffness. This would be consistent with the prediction of Panjabi[6] and Cholewicki and McGill.[65] As outlined above, one response of the nervous system to pain is augmented activity of the superficial global muscles. In a pain-adaptation model this would be interpreted as an attempt by the central nervous system to splint and restrict motion of a region of the spine to protect it from injury or reinjury. As a result the deep muscle activity may be redundant and reduced, but at the expense of fine-tuning of segmental control. This hypothesis requires further investigation.

Contribution of Attention, Stress, and Fear

While the exact mechanism is unknown, pain may have a direct affect on motor planning or may affect planning as a result of the attention demanding nature of pain or stress associated with pain. In terms of attention, it has been argued that changes may arise owing to an inability to ignore unnecessary information and the affect that this would have on limited attention resources.[149] However, recent data indicate that the changes in control with rapid arm movements cannot be replicated by attention demanding or stressful tasks,[150] such as that induced by having subjects perform a Stroop color-word test under stressful and nonstressful conditions. Alternatively, fear of (re)injury or pain or avoidance of movement may be responsible for the changes in control.[151] Consistent with this proposal, when subjects perform rapid arm movements that are interspersed with painful electric shocks of unpredictable intensity and timing, some features of the activity of the trunk muscles associated with the movement, namely delayed transverus abdominis, are changed in a similar manner as that described for clinical and experimental pain.[150] Although this does not indicate that fear is responsible for the changes, the finding suggests that fear may at least replicate the changes identified in motor control in the presence of pain. This may be a mechanism for some individuals to have altered motor control of the trunk muscles after recovery of pain and may explain why some individuals go on to have recurrent episodes of pain.

Clinical Pearl: Fear of pain, in the absence of pain, may have similar effects on the motor system as actual pain and may be responsible for perpetuation of motor control deficits after recovery from an episode of pain.

Effect on Proprioception

Alternatively, pain may not directly affect motor control, but indirectly via the influence of pain on proprioception. In chronic pain, non-nociceptor mechanoreceptors may contribute to excitation of second-order nociceptor neurons[152] and pain may alter proprioceptive feedback.[153] Thus, pain may affect motor planning indirectly via inaccurate feedback and may influence feedforward responses as a result of development of an "internal model of body dynamics" that is built on faulty input.

Clinical Pearl: As deep intrinsic spinal muscles have a high density of muscle spindles, training of deep muscle control may lead to improvements of spinal proprioception.

Changes in Motoneuron Excitability

A final factor to consider is that motoneuron excitability may be altered in the presence of pain and injury. One factor that may change motoneuron excitability is reflex inhibition. The mechanism for reflex inhibition is generally considered to involve inhibition of the alpha motoneuron as a result of afferent input from effusion[154] or injury to joint structures.[155] For instance, when effusion is present in the knee the motoneuron excitability of quadriceps muscles is reduced.[156] Furthermore, this affects muscles to different degrees. For instance, the oblique fibers of vastus medialis are inhibited with lower volumes of effusion than other vasti muscles.[156] Reflex inhibition has also been argued to explain the rapid atrophy of multifidus in people with acute low back pain,[131] although this requires clarification. However this is unlikely to explain the changes in control as these changes represent a change in planning and not a simple delay in activation.

Clinical Pearl: Because reduced motoneuron excitability cannot explain the changes in deep muscle activity, simple strategies to increase activity of the muscles are unlikely to be sufficient to restore normal control and muscle be complemented in motor learning.

Summary

From this overview it appears that changes in motor control are a frequent finding in musculoskeletal disorders. Thus, it would seem logical that strategies aimed at restoring or augmenting (when the inherent structure of a joint may be impaired by injury or disease) normal motor control are likely to be an important part of management. The specific strategy that may be appropriate is likely to depend on the exact nature of the change in control. For instance, whether the change is one of motor planning or reflex inhibition the strategy is likely to vary.

CLINICAL CONSIDERATIONS FOR MOTOR CONTROL IN LOW BACK PAIN

In parallel with the advances in understanding of the physiology and pathophysiology of trunk control mechanisms there has been a progression of change in the strategies implemented for the management of low back pain. Early strategies commonly focused on the strength and endurance properties of the trunk muscles.[157] However, a range of options has been presented clinically to effect change in the motor system to improve clinical signs and symptoms. The aim of this section is not to provide an exhaustive summary, but to provide a broad overview of the variety of rationales that have been presented in the clinical literature and to consider the evolution of clinical techniques to contemporary approaches. Readers are encouraged to access the cited sources to obtain more detailed description of the various approaches.

In a very broad sense exercise interventions may be divided into two main groups. The first group revolves around the idea of the "muscle-tension" model of low back pain. The other group of strategies may be considered to have as their foundation a goal to improve movement. It must be remembered that these two groups are not mutually exclusive.

Muscle-Tension Models

The muscle-tension model asserts that pain occurs as a result of factors associated with increased muscle activity (e.g., increased metabolite concentration) and the clinical goal is to reduce the overactivity.[115] On this basis rationales have been developed using techniques such as electromyography as biofeedback to train patients to reduce muscle activity.[158] Although this technique received considerable popularity, more recent data suggest that the effect of biofeedback training is dependent on how well the patients *perceived* themselves to be able to control muscle tension rather than their actual ability to do so.[159] Another clinical rationale that may be included in this genre is trigger point therapies. Although the perceived mechanism and rationale differ from the relaxation techniques, the goal to reduce activity in localized areas of increased muscle activity is similar. The physiology of trigger points is not completely understood. However, they are argued to be regions of increased activity associated with gamma-motoneuron activity[160] (See Chapter 9 of this text.) A variety of techniques ranging from connective tissue techniques to needling procedures have been used. (See Chapter 23 of this text.)

Reeducation of Movement Patterns

There has been a historical progression of exercise aimed at the restoration of normal movement and control of the spine. Broadly these techniques have aimed to restore factors as broad as mobility and muscle length, proprioception, control of trunk muscle activity, and normal dissociation of hip, lumbar, and thoracic movement, or a combination of these techniques. Janda,[2,3] a key figure in the development of this clinical model of movement control, provided early insight into strategies to evaluate and retrain movement control. These strategies ranged from efforts to restore muscle length and restore normal proprioceptive input to the system. Janda described a range of "syndromes" such as the "distal (also "lower" or "pelvic") crossed syndrome" or "layered syndrome" which were argued to be associated with combinations of "shortened overactive" muscles and "lengthened underactive" muscles. It was argued clinically that the distal (or lower) crossed syndrome is associated with increased activity of the hip flexors and long erector spinae muscles and decreased activity of the abdominal and gluteal muscles. In the layer syndrome there is alternating layers of overactivity and underactivity. For example, in distal to proximal order, overactive hamstrings, underactive gluteals and low lumbar paraspinal muscles, overactive thoracolumbar erector spinae, underactive lower trapezius and overactive upper trapezius. In this model it was proposed that these combinations of muscle changes lead to suboptimal movement control. The assessment of patients also included identification of "soft" neurological signs such as low "tone." In terms of intervention attempts were made to restore the normal parameters of muscle length and activity. The latter element drew heavily on the hypothesis that increased proprioceptive input such as placing subjects on unstable surfaces (e.g., walking on balance sandals with a hard rubber hemisphere placed on the mid-sole) could be used to change the automatic control of the trunk muscles (see Chapter 30). Some evidence for this approach has come from a study that suggests that in healthy individuals the temporal activity of the gluteal muscles can be changed as a result of walking on balance shoes.[161]

In parallel with the approach of Janda, Kendall and McCreary developed an approach based on identification of postural types as well as length and strength of limb and trunk muscles.[162] Similar to the approach of Janda, the rehabilitation strategies involved exercises to lengthen and strengthen appropriate muscle groups.

In the past few decades a range of techniques or philosophies have developed that have either grown from these early ideas or developed in parallel. For example, Sahrman described a range of physiological effects on movement control such as poor ability to control muscles in their inner range and poor dissociation of movement of hip and lumbar movement.[1] On this basis a range of movement tasks are trained to restore dissociation of movement and techniques such as leg loading tasks are used to retrain the ability to hold the position of the pelvis and spine with added load. In parallel with these ideas Richardson and Jull[163,164] suggested strategies to more specifically investigate and control the motion of the pelvis and spine with feedback provided from an air-filled cuff placed under the spine. This device provided accurate feedback of position and could ensure that the *neutral* position was maintained. In general terms the *neutral spinal* position is a position of lumbar lordosis, thoracic kyphosis, and cervical lordosis (i.e., no flexion or extension, but rather maintaining the primary or secondary spinal curves). These authors also began to consider that the role of the intervention was to improve the stability of the spine and focused on control of the neutral position of the spine and control of this position with applied load. On the basis of research from the knee, these authors argued for tonic activation of specific trunk muscle and the benefits of weight bearing exercise.

Many other authors and clinicians considered the reeducation of neutral spinal position and control of this position during function. For example, Saal and Saal[165] undertook a clinical trial to investigate the effect of training neutral spinal position during a range of exercises that challenged the control of the lumbopelvic region and provided early evidence that this approach may lead to clinical improvement. Other approaches from Germany such as by Klein-Vogelbach[166] also has common elements of neutral spine, movement dissociation, and spinal control with external forces. Similarly, propioceptive neuromuscular facilitation techniques such as "rhythmic stabilizations" also satisfy these objectives. In this task external forces are provided with low load in alternating diagonal patterns as a patient aims to maintain a stable position[167] This model shares many feature with a popular ball exercises in which labile surface training is introduced by having a ball as part of the base of support (e.g., sitting on a ball). In this approach subjects learn to maintain the static neural posture with added proprioceptive cues from the support surface and other challenges are added such as movement of the limbs and trunk.[168]

More recently the beneficial effects of the neutral spinal position have been described for the minimization of spinal loading.[60] However, as movement of the spine is important for normal muscle function, it is important to consider that some of these approaches may be too static.

In view of the requirement for muscular control of the lumbar spine and pelvis it was proposed by Snijders, Vleeming, and coworkers[18,72] that posterior and anterior muscle systems are organized to provide a "sling" mechanism to support the spine and pelvis, particularly under high load. Posteriorly muscles such as latissimus dorsi and the contralateral gluteus maximus were considered important. Anteriorly the system involves the external oblique on one side and the contralateral internal oblique. A key feature of this system is the continuity of the fascial system and its ability to provide *force closure* to the pelvis and transfer load from the upper body to the ground via the spine.[18] As a result, interventions were developed that involved training into flexion or extension and rotation. One consideration has been that while these muscles slings may operate during high-load tasks, they may not be important in light activities. An extension of this model is the consideration that the paraspinal muscles contribute to the load transfer system because of the increase in fascial tension as a result of muscle expansion on contraction.[169] In this model it is considered that hypertrophy of the paraspinal muscles is an important outcome of treatment.

Other strategies have been based on the training muscle properties such as trunk extensor endurance. These strategies have been based on findings that endurance is reduced and subjects are trained in tasks such as prone trunk extension. There are preliminary indications of some clinical improvement from this strategy.[170] However, the mechanism is not completely clear as the performance of this task has been linked to parameters such as fear-avoidance beliefs.[171]

Recent Trends in Rehabilitation

On the basis of considerable evidence of motor control dysfunction in people with low back pain and the models of stability and instability proposed by Panjabi[6] the strategies for activation of the abdominal and paraspinal muscles have been refined. Rather than general education of control of lumbopelvic position, strategies now include attempts to retrain the specific control of different components of the muscle system.[4] A key issue is to commence rehabilitation by restoration of the control of the deep local muscles to optimize the control of intervertebral shear forces. These strategies are based on a motor relearning model and involve concepts of segmentation of movement so that the specific components of the system that are dysfunctional can be retrained and then integrated into the functional movement. These strategies also consider issues of simplification (such as performance of the task in supported positions) prior to functional integration, and accurate feedback of contraction that may be provided by palpation or ultrasound imaging (Fig. 5–20). A critical element of this approach is the progression through a range of exercises aimed at increasing load and complexity. As a general goal it is aimed to train patients to tonically activate the deep local muscles during a range of functions, to train coactivation of the local muscles, and to train early activity of these muscles. In many cases a major issue for training this control is to reduce the overactivity of the superficial muscles and train coordinated control of deep and superficial muscles to work appropriately to meet the demands of spinal control. Similar techniques are described by other authors.[172] Commonly, progression of exercise includes a range of strategies including leg loading, ball exercises, weight bearing exercise, etc.,[4] which are discussed in detail in later chapters of this text.

This approach has received support from randomized controlled clinical trials. For instance, back pain intensity and disability have been shown to improve following this intervention in people with chronic low back pain associated with a radiological diagnosis and spondylosis and spondylolysthesis.[172] Furthermore, following a first episode of acute low back pain,

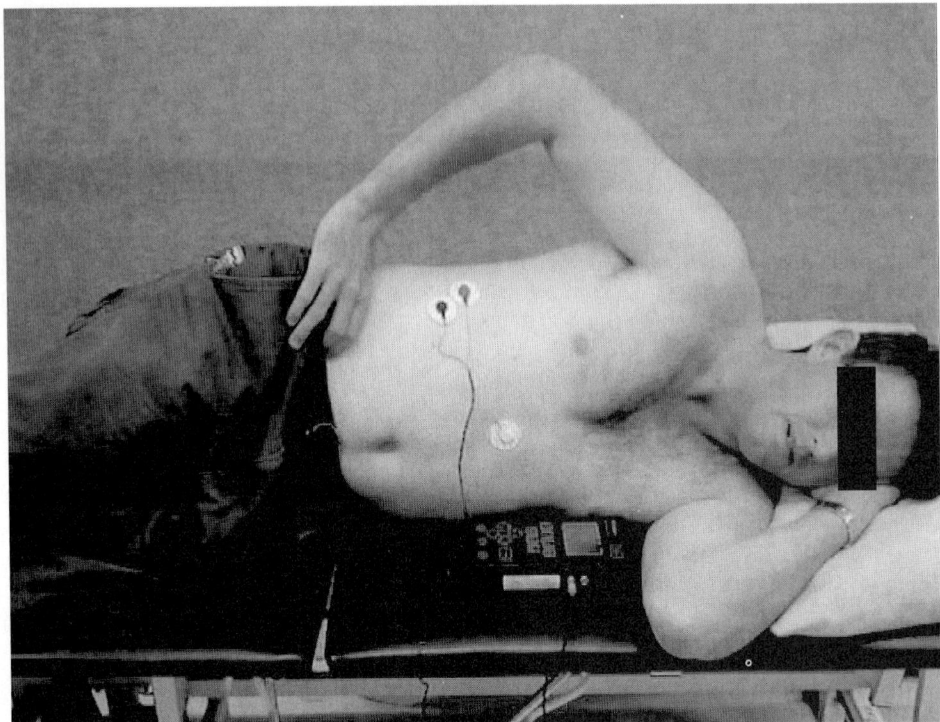

FIGURE 5–20. Clinical technique for training the independent activity of transversus abdominis. The performance of this skilled muscle contraction is simplified adopting a supported position. The patient is receiving feedback of contraction of transversus abdominis with palpation of the inferior abdominal wall and feedback of activity of obliquus externus abdominis with an electromyographic biofeedback unit.

people who have training of multifidus have been shown to have a reduced incidence of low back pain recurrence in the subsequent 3 years.[173,174] Further preliminary evidence is coming from additional trials of low back and pelvic pain.[175]

Another model has been proposed by McGill.[60] In this intervention attempts are made to minimize the load on the spine through techniques such as postural correction, while exercise interventions based on the Euler model of spinal stability are implemented. These strategies include activation of the quadratus lumborum and other global trunk muscles to control buckling forces at the spine. These strategies require investigation in randomized controlled clinical trials.

Trends for the Future

There are several major factors to consider for the future. These include issues such as the neurobiology of pain, psychological interventions, accurate patient selection and subgrouping. In the past few decades there has been increasing discussion of the neurobiology of pain. There is increasing realization that pain is associated with complex central and peripheral changes such as peripheral sensitization (e.g., due to release of inflammatory mediators and substances such as substance P) and central sensitization (e.g., due to neuroplastic changes in the dorsal horn and other regions of the nervous system and spinal windup). Although there is support for the biomechanical model of back pain in which poor control of passive elements leads to microtrauma, irritation of nociceptors, and pain, there is also realization that this is unlikely to explain the complexities of pain. With this understanding it is essential to consider that improvement of symptoms requires multimodal assessment and interventions including nonphysical ones (See Chapters 19 and 35). It is likely that with peripheral sensitization the margin for error in lumbopelvic control may be reduced and the accuracy of muscular control must be even better than for healthy individuals. In addition, there is increasing evidence that cognitive interventions can assist in changing central components. The link between manipulation of psychological parameters such as fear and the control of the trunk muscles[151] strengthens this idea. The optimal approach should include elements of both. The reader is referred to Butler[176] and Waddell[177] for review.

The second issue is that of patient selection. It is well accepted that the population with low back problem is heterogeneous and optimal efficacy of training is likely to be achieved when the treatment strategy is matched to the patient.[178] It is important to consider that although the changes in local muscle function are relatively consistent across individuals and not dependent on the specific nature of the pathology, there is considerable variation in the response of the superficial global muscles. For instance, optimal management is likely to include a combination of exercise, manual therapy techniques, education, and pain-relieving modalities. The ideal combination of these strategies will vary between individuals. The following chapters provide an overview of assessment and rehabilitation strategies that provide guidance for patient-specific management.

SUMMARY

1. Biomechanical and neurophysiological studies suggest that stability of the spine and pelvis is dependent on the control of intersegmental motion and orientation.
2. Different muscle systems and different strategies are used to control each of these elements.
3. When people have low back pain there is a general trend for activity of the deep local muscles to be impaired, while activity of the superficial muscles is augmented, although with variation between individuals.
4. Although the mechanism for this dysfunction is not completely understood, it is considered to be due to changes in motor planning.
5. Many strategies have been developed to deal with changes in control of the trunk muscles and these techniques are continuing to evolve.
6. There is increasing evidence that motor control interventions for the trunk muscles lead to positive clinical outcomes.
7. Future studies and clinical techniques must address the neurobiology of pain and the issue of accurate patient selection and subgrouping.

REFERENCES

1. Sahrmann S. *Diagnosis and treatment of movement impairment syndromes*. St Louis: Mosby, Inc., 2002.
2. Janda V. *Muscle function testing*. London: Butterworths, 1983.
3. Janda V. Muscles, central nervous motor regulation and back problems. In: Korr IM, ed. *The neurobiologic mechanisms in manipulative therapy*, 1st ed. New York: Plenum Press, 1978:27–41.
4. Richardson CA, Jull GA, Hodges PW, et al. *Therapeutic exercise for spinal segmental stabilisation in low back pain: Scientific basis and clinical approach*. Edinburgh: Churchill Livingstone, 1999.
5. Lucas DB, Bresler B. *Stability of the ligamentou spine*. Technical Report ESR. 11 No. 40. Berkeley: Biomechanics Laboratory, University of California, 1960.
6. Panjabi MM. The stabilizing system of the spine. Part I. Function, dysfunction, adaptation, and enhancement. *J Spinal Disord* 1992;5:383–389.
7. Cholewicki J, Panjabi MM, Khachatryan A. Stabilizing function of trunk flexor–extensor muscles around a neutral spine posture. *Spine* 1997;22:2207–2212.
8. Crisco JJ, Panjabi MM. The intersegmental and multisegmental muscles of the lumbar spine: A biomechanical model comparing lateral stabilising potential. *Spine* 1991;7:793–799.
9. Gardner-Morse M, Stokes IAF, Laible JP. Role of muscles in lumbar spine stability in maximum extension efforts. *J Orthop Res* 1995;13:802–808.
10. McGill SM. Low back exercises: Evidence for improving exercise regimens. *Phys Ther* 1998;78:754–765.
11. Cholewicki J, McGill SM, Norman RW. Lumbar spine loading during the lifting of extremely heavy weights. *Med Sci Sports Exerc* 1991;23:1179–1186.
12. Bogduk N, Amevo B, Pearcy M. A biological basis for instantaneous centres of rotation of the vertebral column. *Proc Inst Mech Eng [H]* 1995;209:177–183.
13. Bergmark A. Stability of the lumbar spine. A study in mechanical engineering. *Acta Orthop Scand* 1989;60:1–54.
14. Hodges PW. Is there a role for transversus abdominis in lumbo-pelvic stability? *Man Ther* 1999;4:74–86.
15. Hodges PW, Richardson CA. Feedforward contraction of transversus abdominis in not influenced by the direction of arm movement. *Exp Brain Res* 1997;114:362–370.
16. Panjabi MM. The stabilising system of the spine. Part II. Neutral zone and instability hypothesis. *J Spinal Disord* 1992;5:390–397.
17. Snijders CJ, Vleeming A, Stoeckart R, et al. Biomechanical modelling of sacroiliac joint stability in different postures. *Spine State Art Rev* 1995;9:419–432.
18. Snijders CJ, Vleeming A, Stoeckart R. Transfer of lumbosacral load to iliac bones and legs. Part 1. Biomechanics of self bracing of the sacroiliac joints and its significance for treatment and exercise. *Clin Biomech* 1993;8:285–294.
19. Gahery Y, Massion J. Co-ordination between posture and movement. *Trends Neurosci* 1981;4:199–202.
20. Gurfinkel VS. The mechanisms of postural regulation in man. *Sov Sci Rev F Physiol Gen Biol* 1994;7:59–89.
21. Belenkii V, Gurfinkel VS, Paltsev Y. Elements of control of voluntary movements. *Biofizika* 1967;12:135–141.
22. Aruin AS, Latash ML. Directional specificity of postural muscles in feed-forward postural reactions during fast voluntary arm movements. *Exp Brain Res* 1995;103:323–332.
23. Zattara M, Bouisset S. Posturo-kinetic organisation during the early phase of voluntary upper limb movement. I. Normal subjects. *J Neurol Neurosurg Psychiatry* 1988;51:956–965.
24. Bouisset S, Zattara M. A sequence of postural adjustments precedes voluntary movement. *Neurosci Lett* 1981;22:263–270.
25. Hodges PW, Richardson CA. Inefficient muscular stabilisation of the lumbar spine associated with low

back pain: A motor control evaluation of transversus abdominis. *Spine* 1996;21:2640–2650.

26. Hodges PW, Cresswell AG, Thorstensson A. Preparatory trunk motion accompanies rapid upper limb movement. *Exp Brain Res* 1999;124:69–79.
27. Perry J. *Gait Analysis: Normal and pathological function.* Thorofare, NJ: SLACK Inc., 1992.
28. van Dieen JH, de Looze MP. Directionality of anticipatory activation of trunk muscles in a lifting task depends on load knowledge. *Exp Brain Res* 1999;128:397–404.
29. Zetterberg C, Andersson GB, Schultz AB. The activity of individual trunk muscles during heavy physical loading. *Spine* 1987;12:1035–1040.
30. Hodges PW, Richardson CA. Contraction of the abdominal muscles associated with movement of the lower limb. *Phys Ther* 1997;77:132–144.
31. Moseley GL, Hodges PW, Gandevia SC. Deep and superficial fibers of lumbar multifidus are differentially active during voluntary arm movements. *Spine* 2002;27:E29–E36.
32. Hodges PW, Richardson CA. Transversus abdominis and the superficial abdominal muscles are controlled independently in a postural task. *Neurosci Lett* 1999;265:91–94.
33. Hodges PW, Smith M, Grigorenko A, et al. Trunk muscle response to support surface translation in sitting: Normal control and effects of respiration. Proceedings of the International Society for Posture and Gait Research, 2005.
34. Dimitrijevic MR, Gregoric MR, Sherwood AM, et al. Reflex responses of paraspinal muscles to tapping. *J Neurol Neurosurg Psychiatry* 1980;43:1112–1118.
35. Kondo T, Bishop B, Shaw CF. Phasic stretch reflex of the abdominal muscles. *Exp Neurol* 1986;94:120–140.
36. Myriknas SE, Beith ID, Harrison PJ. Stretch reflexes in the rectus abdominis muscle in man. *Exp Physiol* 2000;85:445–450.
37. Beith ID, Harrison PJ. Stretch reflexes in human abdominal muscles. Exp Brain Res 2004;159:206–213.
38. Indahl A, Kaigle A, Reikeras O, et al. Electromyographic response of the porcine multifidus musculature after nerve stimulation. *Spine* 1995;20:2652–2658.
39. Indahl A, Kaigle A, Reikeras O, et al. Sacroiliac joint involvement in activation of the porcine spinal and gluteal musculature. *J Spinal Disord* 1999;12:325–330.
40. Indahl A, Kaigle AM, Reikeras O, et al. Interaction between the porcine lumbar intervertebral disc, zygapophysial joints, and paraspinal muscles. *Spine* 1997;22:2834–2840.
41. Solomonow M, Zhou BH, Baratta RV, et al. Biomechanics of increased exposure to lumbar injury caused by cyclic loading. Part 1. Loss of reflexive muscular stabilization. *Spine* 1999;24:2426–2434.
42. Solomonow M, Zhou BH, Harris M, et al. The ligamento-muscular stabilizing system of the spine. *Spine* 1998;23:2552–2562.
43. Holm S, Indahl A, Kaigle A, et al. The neuromuscular role of mechanoreceptors in the porcione lumbar intervertebral disc. In: *Proceedings of the International Society for the Study of the Lumbar Spine*, Adelaide, Australia, 2000:263.
44. Cresswell AG, Oddsson L, Thorstensson A. The influence of sudden perturbations on trunk muscle activity and intra-abdominal pressure while standing. *Exp Brain Res* 1994;98:336–341.
45. Leinonen V, Kankaanpaa M, Luukkonen M, et al. Disc herniation-related back pain impairs feed-forward control of paraspinal muscles. *Spine* 2001;26:E367–E372.
46. Moseley GL, Hodges PW, Gandevia SC. External perturbation of the trunk in standing humans differentially activates components of the medial back muscles. *J Physiol* 2003;547:581–587.
47. Wilder DG, Pope MH, Seroussi R, et al. Sudden, unstable rotation responses to an overload in the lumbar spine. In: *Proceedings of International Society for Study of the Lumbar Spine*, 1987:76.
48. Marras WS, Rangarajulu SL, Lavender SA. Trunk loading and expectation. *Ergonomics* 1987;30:551–562.
49. Hodges PW, Cresswell AG, Thorstensson A. Perturbed upper limb movements cause short-latency postural responses in trunk muscles. *Exp Brain Res*, 2001;138:243–250.
50. Marsden CD, Merton PA, Morton HB. Anticipatory postural responses in the human subject. *J Physiol (Lond)* 1977;275:47P–8P.
51. Hodges P, Moseley G, Gandevia S. Differential control of the deep and superficial compartments of multifidus is dependent on input from higher centres.In: *VIIth International Physiotherapy Congress*, Sydney, 2002.
52. Radebold A, Cholewicki J, Panjabi MM, et al. Muscle response pattern to sudden trunk loading in healthy individuals and in patients with chronic low back pain. *Spine* 2000;25:947–954.
53. Angel RW, Eppler W, Iannone A. Silent period produced by unloading of muscle during voluntary contraction. *J Physiol* 1965;180:864–870.
54. Horak F, Nashner LM. Central programming of postural movements: Adaptation to altered support-surface configurations. *J Neurophysiol* 1986;55:1369–1381.
55. Huang QM, Hodges PW, Thorstensson A. Postural control of the trunk in response to lateral support surface translations during trunk movement and loading. *Exp Brain Res* 2001;141:552–559.
56. Johansson H, Sjolander P, Sojka P. A sensory role for the cruciate ligaments. *Clin Orthop Relat Res* 1991;268:161–178.
57. Winter DA, Patla AE, Prince F, et al. Stiffness control of balance in quiet standing. *J Neurophysiol* 1998;80:1211–1221.
58. Zedka M, Prochazka A. Phasic activity in the human erector spinae during repetitive hand movements. *J Physiol* 1997;504:727–734.
59. Cholewicki J, VanVliet IJ. Relative contribution of trunk muscles to the stability of the lumbar spine during isometric exertions. *Clin Biomech (Bristol, Avon)* 2002;17:99–105.
60. McGill S. *Low back disorders: Evidence based prevention and rehabilitation*. Champaign, IL: Human Kinetics Publishers, Inc., 2002.

61. Wilder DG, Aleksiev AR, Magnusson ML, et al. Muscular response to sudden load. A tool to evaluate fatigue and rehabilitation. *Spine* 1996;21:2628–2639.
62. Lucas DB. Mechanics of the spine. *Bull Hosp Jt Dis Orthop Inst* 1970;31:115–131.
63. Gardner-Morse MG, Stokes IA. The effects of abdominal muscle coactivation on lumbar spine stability. *Spine* 1998;23:86–91.
64. McGill S, Juker D, Kropf P. Quantitative intramuscular myoelectric activity of quadratus lumborum during a wide variety of tasks. *Clin Biomech (Bristol, Avon)* 1996;11:170–172.
65. Cholewicki J, McGill SM. Mechanical stability of the *in vivo* lumbar spine: Implications for injury and chronic low back pain. *Clin Biomech* 1996;11:1–15.
66. Lavender SA, Tsuang YH, Andersson GBJ, et al. Trunk muscle cocontraction: The effects of moment direction and moment magnitude. *J Orthop Res* 1992;10:691–700.
67. Mirka GA, Marras WS. A stochastic model of trunk muscle coactivation during trunk bending. *Spine* 1993;18:1396–1409.
68. Thelan DG, Schultz AB, Ashton-Miller JA. Co-contraction of lumbar muscles during the development of time-varying triaxial movements. *J Orthop Res* 1995;13:390–398.
69. Nachemson A, Morris JM. In vivo measurement of intradiscal pressure: Discometry, a method for the determination of presure in the lower lumbar discs. *J Bone Joint Surg* 1964;46-A:1077–1092.
70. Bogduk N. *Clinical anatomy of the lumbar spine and sacrum*, 3rd ed. London: Churchill Livingstone, 1997.
71. Raschke U, Chaffn DB. Trunk and hip muscle recruitment in response to external anterior lumbosacral shear and moment loads. *Clin Biomech* 1996;3:145–152.
72. Vleeming A, Pool-Goudzwaard AL, Stoeckart R, et al. The posterior layer of the thoracolumbar fascia: Its function in load transfer from spine to legs. *Spine* 1995;20:753–758.
73. Hodges PW, Cresswell AG, Daggfeldt K, et al. Three dimensional preparatory trunk motion precedes asymmetrical upper limb movement. *Gait Posture* 2000;11:92–101.
74. Hodges P, Gandevia S. Changes in intra-abdominal pressure during postural and respiratory activation of the human diaphragm. *J Appl Physiol* 2000;89:967–976.
75. DeTroyer A, Estenne M. Functional anatomy of the respiratory muscles. In: Belman MJ, ed. *Respiratory muscles: Function in health and disease*. Philadelphia: WB Saunders Co., 1988:175–195.
76. Cresswell AG, Grundstrom H, Thorstensson A. Observations on intra-abdominal pressure and patterns of abdominal intra-muscular activity in man. *Acta Physiol Scand* 1992;144:409–418.
77. Urquhart DM, Hodges PW. Differential activity of regions of transversus abdominis during trunk rotation. Eur Spine J. 2005;14:393–400.
78. Hodges PW, Cresswell AG, Daggfeldt K, et al. In vivo measurement of the effect of intra-abdominal pressure on the human spine. *J Biomech* 2001;34:347–353.
79. Hodges PW, Eriksson AEM, Shirley D, Gandevia SC. Intra-abdominal pressure can directly increase stiffness of the lumbar spine. J Biomed 2005;38(9):1873–1880.
80. Hodges P, Kaigle-Holm A, Holm S, et al. Intervertebal stiffness of the spine is increased by evoked contraction of transversus abdominis and the diaphragm: In vivo porcine studies. *Spine* 2003;28:2594–2601.
81. Gracovetsky S, Farfan H, Helleur C. The abdominal mechanism. *Spine* 1985;10:317–324.
82. Richardson CA, Snijders CJ, Hides JA, et al. The relation between the transversus abdominis muscles, sacroiliac joint mechanics, and low back pain. *Spine* 2002;27:399–405.
83. Macintosh JE, Bogduk N. The detailed biomechanics of the lumbar multifidus. *Clin Biomech* 1986;1:205–231.
84. Lewin T, Moffett B, Viidik A. The morphology of the lumbar synovial joints. *Acta Morphol Neerlanco Scandinav* 1962;4:299–319.
85. Panjabi MM, Abumi K, Duranceau J, et al. Spinal stability and intersegmental muscle forces. A biomechanical model. *Spine* 1989;14:194–200.
86. Wilke HJ, Wolf S, Claes LE, et al. Stability increase of the lumbar spine with different muscle groups: A biomechanical in vitro study. *Spine* 1995;20:192–198.
87. Gracovetsky S, Farfan HF, Lamy C. A mathematical model of the lumbar spine uing an optimised system to control muscles and ligaments. *Orthop Clin North Am* 1977;8:135–153.
88. Kaigle AM, Holm SH, Hansson TH. Experimental instability in the lumbar spine. *Spine* 1995;20:421–430.
89. Nitz AJ, Peck D. Comparison of muscle spindle concentrations in large and small human epaxial muslces acting in parallel combinations. *Am Surg* 1986;52:273–277.
90. Bogduk N, Pearcy M, Hadfeild G. Anatomy and biomechanics of psoas major. *Clin Biomech* 1992;7:109–119.
91. Gibbons S. Biomechanics and stability mechanisms of psoas major. In: Vleeming A, Mooney V, Gracovetsky SA, et al, eds. *4th Interdisciplinary World Congress on low back pain pelvic pain*. Montreal, Canada: European Conference Organisers, 2001.
92. Hodges P, Gandevia S. Activation of the human diaphragm during a repetitive postural task. *J Physiol* 2000;522:165–175.
93. Hodges PW, Butler JE, McKenzie D, et al. Contraction of the human diaphragm during postural adjustments. *J Physiol* 1997;505:239–248.
94. Hodges PW, Sapsford RR, Pengel HM. Feedforward activity of the pelvic floor muscles precedes rapid upper limb movements. In: *VIIth International Physiotherapy Congress*, Sydney, Australia, 2002.
95. Campbell EJM. An electromyographic study of the role of the abdominal muscles in breathing. *J Physiol (Lond)* 1952;117:222–233.
96. DeTroyer A, Estenne M, Ninane V, et al. Transversus abdominis muscle function in humans. *J Appl Physiol* 1990;68:1010–1016.
97. Hodges PW, Gandevia SC, Richardson CA. Contractions of specific abdominal muscles in postural tasks

are affected by respiratory maneuvers. *J Appl Physiol* 1997;83:753–760.

98. Saunders S, Rath D, Hodges PW. Respiratory and postural activation of the trunk muscles changes with mode and speed of locomotion. Gait and Posture 2004;20:280–290.
99. Hodges PW, McKenzie DK, Heijnen I, et al. Reduced contribution of the diaphragm to postural control in patients with severe chronic airflow limitation. In: *Proceedings of the Annual Sceintific Meeting of the Thoracic Society of Australia and New Zealand*, Melbourne, Australia, 2000.
100. Hodges PW, Heijnen I, Gandevia SC. Reduced postural activity of the diaphragm in humans when respiratory demand is increased. *J Physiol* 2001;537:999–1008.
101. Deindl F, Vodusek D, Hesse U, et al. Activity patterns of pubococcygeal muscles in nulliparous continent women. *Br J Urol* 1993;72:46–51.
102. Shirado O, Kaneda K, Ito T. Trunk-muscle strength during concentric and eccentric contraction: A comparison between healthy subjects and patients with chronic low back pain. *J Spinal Disord* 1992;5:175–182.
103. Thorstensson A, Arvidson Å. Trunk muscle strength and low back pain. *Scand J Rehabil Med* 1982;14:69–75.
104. Paltsev YI, El'ner AN. Preparatory and compensatory period during voluntary movement in patients with involvement of the brain of different localisation. *Biofizika* 1967;12:142–147.
105. Rogers MW, Kukulka CG, Soderberg GL. Postural adjustments preceding rapid arm movements in parkinsonian subjects. *Neurosci Lett* 1987;75:246–251.
106. Hodges PW, Richardson CA. Delayed postural contraction of of transversus abdominis associated with movement of the lower limb in people with low back pain. *J Spinal Disord* 1998;11:46–56.
107. Tesh KM, ShawDunn J, Evans JH. The abdominal muscles and vertebral stability. *Spine* 1987;12:501–508.
108. Hodges PW, Richardson CA. Altered trunk muscle recruitment in people with low back pain with upper limb movement at different speeds. *Arch Phys Med Rehabil* 1999;80:1005–1012.
109. Taimela S, Kankaanpaa M, Luoto S. The effect of lumbar fatigue on the ability to sense a change in lumbar position. A controlled study. *Spine* 1999;24:1322–1327.
110. Brumagne S, Cordo P, Lysens R, et al. The role of paraspinal muscle spindles in lumbosacral position sense in individuals with and without low back pain. *Spine* 2000;25:989–994.
111. Gill KP, Callaghan MJ. The measurement of lumbar proprioception in individuals with and without low back pain. *Spine* 1998;23:371–377.
112. Magnusson M, Aleksiev A, Wilder D, et al. Unexpected load and asymmetric posture as etiologic factors in low back pain. *Eur Spine J* 1996;5:23–35.
113. Lindgren K-A, Sihvonen T, Leino E, et al. Exercise therapy effects on fuctional radiographic findings and segmental electromyographic activity in lumbar spine instability. *Arch Phys Med Rehabil* 1993;74:933–939.
114. Sihvonen T, Lindgren KA, Airaksinen O, et al. Movement disturbances of the lumbar spine and abnormal back muscle electromyographic findings in recurrent low back pain. *Spine* 1997;22:289–295.
115. Arena JG, Sherman RA, Bruno GM, et al. Electromyographic recordings of 5 types of low back pain subjects and non-pain controls in different positions. *Pain* 1989;37:57–65.
116. Wolf SL, Basmajian JV. Assessment of paraspinal electromyographic activity in normal subjects and chronic low back pain patients using a muscle biofeedback device. In: Asmussen E, Jorgensen K, eds. *Biomechanics IV B*. Baltimore: University Park Press, 1977:319–324.
117. Cram JR, Steger JC. EMG scanning in the diagnosis of chronic pain. *Biofeedback Self Regul* 1983;8:229–241.
118. Collins GA, Cohen MJ, Naliboff BD, et al. Comparative analysis of paraspinal and frontalis EMG, heart rate and skin conductance in chronic low back pain patients and normals to various postures and stresses. *Scand J Rehabil Med* 1982;14:39–46.
119. Shirado O, Ito T, Kaneda K, et al. Flexion-relaxation phenomenon in the back muscles. A comparative study between healthy subjects and patients with chronic low back pain. *Am J Phys Med Rehabil* 1995;74:139–144.
120. Zedka M, Prochazka A, Knight B, et al. Voluntary and reflex control of human back muscles during induced pain. *J Physiol (Lond)* 1999;520:591–604.
121. Kaigle AM, Wessberg P, Hansson TH. Muscular and kinematic behavior of the lumbar spine during flexion–extension. *J Spinal Disord* 1998;11:163–174.
122. Arendt-Nielsen L, Graven-Nielsen T, Svarrer H, et al. The influence of low back pain on muscle activity and coordination during gait: A clinical and experimental study. *Pain* 1996;64:231–240.
123. Luoto S, Aalto H, Taimela S, et al. One-footed and externally disturbed two-footed postural control in patients with chronic low back pain and healthy control subjects. A controlled study with follow-up. *Spine* 1998;23:2081–2089.
124. Byl NN, Sinnott PL. Variations in balance and body sway in middle-aged adults: Subjects with healthy backs compared with subjects with low back dyfunction. *Spine* 1991;16:325–330.
125. Radebold A, Cholewicki J, Polzhofer GK, et al. Impaired postural control of the lumbar spine is associated with delayed muscle response times in patients with chronic idiopathic low back pain. *Spine* 2001;26:724–730.
126. Takala E, Viikari-Juntura E. Do functional tests predict low back pain? *Spine* 2000;25:2126 –2132.
127. Luoto S, Heliövaara M, Hurri H, et al. Static back endurance and the risk of low-back pain. *Clin Biomech* 1995;10:323–324.
128. Taimela S, Kujala UM. Reaction times with reference to musculoskeletal complaints in adolescence. *Percept Mot Skills* 1992;75:1075–1082.
129. Marras WS, Davis KG, Ferguson SA, et al. Spine loading characteristics of patients with low back pain compared with asymptomatic individuals. *Spine* 2001;26:2566–2574.
130. Rantanen J, Hurme M, Falck B, et al. The lumbar multifidus muscle five years after surgery for a

lumbar intervertebral disc herniation. *Spine* 1993;18:568–574.

131. Hides JA, Stokes MJ, Saide M, et al. Evidence of lumbar multifidus muscle wasting ipsilateral to symptoms in patients with acute/subacute low back pain. *Spine* 1994;19:165–177.
132. Biederman HJ, Shanks GL, Forrest WJ, et al. Power spectrum analysis of electromyographic activity: Discriminators in the differential assessment of patients with chronic low back pain. *Spine* 1991;16:1179–1184.
133. Roy SH, DeLuca CJ, Casavant DA. Lumbar muscle fatigue and chronic low back pain. *Spine* 1989;14:992–1001.
134. Roy SH, DeLuca CJ, Snyder-Mackler L, et al. Fatigue, recovery, and low back pain in varsity rowers. *Med Sci Sports Exerc* 1990;22:463–469.
135. Ng JK, Richardson CA, Parnianpour M, et al. EMG activity of trunk muscles and torque output during isometric axial rotation exertion: A comparison between back pain patients and matched controls. *J Orthop Res* 2002;20:112–121.
136. Ng JK, Richardson CA, Parnianpour M, et al. Fatigue-related changes in torque output and electromyographic parameters of trunk muscles during isometric axial rotation exertion: An investigation in patients with back pain and in healthy subjects. *Spine* 2002;27:637–646.
137. Biering-Sørensen F. Physical measurements as risk indicators for low-back trouble over a one year period. *Spine* 1984;9:106–119.
138. McNeill T, Warwick D, Andersson G, et al. Trunk strengths in attempted flexion, extension, and lateral bending in healthy subjects and patients with low-back disorder. *Spine* 1980;5:529–538.
139. Farfan HF. *Mechanical disorders of the low back.* Philadelphia: Lea & Febiger, 1973.
140. Hodges P, Moseley G, Gabrielsson A, Gandevia SC. Acute experimental pain changes postural recruitment of the trunk muscles in pain-free humans. *Exp Brain Res* 2003;151:262–271.
141. Matre DA, Sinkjaer T, Svensson P, et al. Experimental muscle pain increases the human stretch reflex. *Pain* 1998;75:331–339.
142. Valeriani M, Restuccia D, Di Lazzaro V, et al. Inhibition of the human primary motor area by painful heat stimulation of the skin. *Clin Neurophysiol* 1999;110:1475–1480.
143. Pedersen J, Sjolander P, Wenngren BI, et al. Increased intramuscular concentration of bradykinin increases the static fusimotor drive to muscle spindles in neck muscles of the cat. *Pain* 1997;70:83–91.
144. Hodges PW. Changes in motor planning of feedforward postural responses of the trunk muscles in low back pain. *Exp Brain Res* 2001;141:261–266.
145. Hodges P. Changes in motor planning of feedforward postural responses of the trunk muscles in low back pain. *Exp Brain Res* 2001;141:261–266.
146. Derbyshire SW, Jones AK, Gyulai F, et al. Pain processing during three levels of noxious stimulation produces differential patterns of central activity. *Pain* 1997;73:431–445.
147. Lund JP, Donga R, Widmer CG, et al. The pain-adaptation model: A discussion of the relationship between chronic musculoskeletal pain and motor activity. *Can J Physiol Pharmacol* 1991;69:683–694.
148. Svensson P, Arendt-Nielsen L, Houe L. Sensory-motor interactions of human experimental unilateral jaw muscle pain: A quantitative analysis. *Pain* 1995;64:241–249.
149. Luoto S, Taimela S, Hurri H, et al. Mechanisms explaining the association between low back trouble and deficits in information processing. A controlled study with follow-up. *Spine* 1999;24:255–261.
150. Mosely GL, Nicholas MK, Hodges PW. Pain differs from nonpainful attention-demanding or stressful tasks in its effect on postural control patterns of trunk muscles. *Exp Brain Res* 2004;156:64–71.
151. Vlaeyen JW, Linton SJ. Fear-avoidance and its consequences in chronic musculoskeletal pain: A state of the art. *Pain* 2000;85:317–332.
152. Siddall PJ, Cousins MJ. Pain mechanisms and management: An update. *Clin Exp Pharmacol Physiol* 1995;22:679–688.
153. Capra NF, Ro JY. Experimental muscle pain produces central modulation of proprioceptive signals arising from jaw muscle spindles. *Pain* 2000;86:151–162.
154. Stokes M, Young A. The contribution of reflex inhibition to arthrogenous muscle weakness. *Clin Sci* 1984;67:7–14.
155. Ekholm J, Eklund G, Skoglund S. On reflex effects from knee joint of cats. *Acta Physiol Scand* 1960;50:167–174.
156. Spencer JD, Hayes KC, Alexander IJ. Knee joint effusion and quadriceps reflex inhibition in man. *Arch Phys Med Rehabil* 1984;65:171–177.
157. Kendall PH, Jenkins JM. Exercises for backache: A double blind controlled trial. *Physiotherapy* 1968;54:154–157.
158. Flor H, Haag G, Turk DC, et al. Efficacy of EMG biofeedback, pseudotherapy, and conventional medical treatment for chronic rheumatic back pain. *Pain* 1983;17:21–31.
159. Holroyd KA, Penzien DB, Hursey KG, et al. Change mechanisms in EMG biofeedback training: Cognitive changes underlying improvements in tension headache. *J Consult Clin Psychol* 1984;52:1039–1053.
160. Travell JG, Simons DG. *Myofascial pain and dysfunction. The trigger point manual.* Baltimore: Williams & Wilkins, 1983.
161. Bullock-Saxton JE, Janda V, Bullock MI. Reflex activation of gluteal muscles in walking with balance shoes: An approach to restoration of function for chronic low back pain patients. *Spine* 1993;18:704–708.
162. Kendall FP, McCreary EK. *Muscles: Testing and function*, 3rd ed. Baltimore: Williams & Wilkins, 1983.
163. Richardson CA, Jull GA, eds. *An historical perspective on the development of clinical techniques to evaluate and treat the active stabilising system of the lumbar spine.* Melbourne, Australia: Australian Journal of Physiotherapy, 1995.

164. Richardson CA, Jull GA, Hodges PW, Hides JA. Therapeutic exercise for spinal segmental stabilisation in low back pain: Scientific basis and clinical approach. Edinburgh: Churchill Livingstone, 1999.
165. Saal JA, Saal JS. Nonoperative treatment of herniated lumbar intervertebral disc with radiculopathy: An outcome study. *Spine* 1989;14:431–437.
166. Klein-Vogelbach S. *Therapeutic exercises in functional kinetics: Analysis and instruction of individually adaptable exercises*. Berlin: Springer-Verlag, 1991.
167. Voss DE, Ionta MK, Myers BJ. *Proprioceptive neuromuscular facilitation: Patterns and techniques*. New York: Lippincott Williams & Wilkins, 1985.
168. Creager CC. *Therapeutic exercises using the Swiss ball: Executive physical therapy*, 1994.
169. Porterfield JA, DeRosa C. *Mechanical low back pain—Perspectives in functional anatomy*, 2nd ed. Amsterdam: Elsevier, 1998.
170. Chok B, Lee R, Latimer J, et al. Endurance training of the trunk extensor muscles in people with subacute low back pain. *Phys Ther* 1999;79:1032–1042.
171. Mannion AF, Dolan P, Adams MA. Psychological questionnaires: Do "abnormal" scores precede or follow first-time low back pain? *Spine* 1996;21:2603–2611.
172. O'Sullivan PB, Twomey LT, Allison GT. Evaluation of specific stabilizing exercise in the treatment of chronic low back pain with radiologic diagnosis of spondylolysis or spondylolisthesis. *Spine* 1997;22:2959–2967.
173. Hides JA, Jull GA, Richardson CA. Long term effects of specific stabilizing exercises for first episode low back pain. *Spine* 2001;26:243–248.
174. Hides JA, Richardson CA, Jull GA. Multifidus muscle recovery is not automatic after resolution of acute, first-episode low back pain. *Spine* 1996;21:2763–2769.
175. Stuge B. Veierod MB, Laerum E. Vollestad. The efficacy of a treatment program focusing on specific stabilizing exercises for pelvic girdlpain after pregnancy: a two year follow-up of a randomized clinical trial. SPINE 2004 May 29(10):E197–203.
176. Butler DS. *The sensitive nervous system*. The Adelaide: NOI Group Publications, 2000.
177. Waddell G. *The back pain revolution*. Edinburgh: Churchill Livingstone, 1998.
178. O'Sullivan PB. Lumbar segmental "instability": Clinical presentation and specific stabilizing exercise management. *Man Ther* 2000;5:2–12.

PART

II

LOW BACK SYNDROMES

CHAPTER

6

THE INTERVERTEBRAL DISC AND ITS SYNDROMES

Dennis R. Skogsbergh and Matthew H. Kowalski

OUTLINE

OBJECTIVES

1. To understand the normal development and dynamics of the lumbar intervertebral disc.
2. To detail the pathophysiology of internal disc disruption syndromes and their clinical presentation.
3. To present the utilization of advanced diagnostic imaging techniques and the nomenclature used to describe visualized intervertebral disc abnormalities.
4. To investigate the most useful clinical examination procedures.
5. To characterize the treatment and management options for the stage and classification of disc disruption.

INTRODUCTION

The intervertebral discs (IVDs) and vertebral end plates, together with their associated restraining ligaments, create part of a unique joint found only between adjacent vertebrae. This symphyseal joint provides intrinsic static stabilization of the spine by anchoring adjacent segments together. The skeletal musculature has been shown repeatedly to be the major structure that generates forces capable of maintaining dynamic spine stability under various conditions.[1–4] The physical properties of the IVD (resiliency and elasticity) also allow for limited movement and the absorption of shock and distribution of loads, which occurs even during normal weight bearing. Vertical stresses are exerted on the cartilaginous end plates, loads are transferred to the nucleus pulposus and anulus fibrosus, and the forces are dissipated in an isotropic manner.

During aging, the discs may undergo striking alterations in volume, shape, structure, and composition that may alter their mechanical properties and influence intervertebral motion. Probably no other spinal component undergoes such a striking transformation, as does the IVD.

As the IVD ages it becomes more susceptible to a variety of pathological conditions and clinical scenarios. Some of these conditions are directly linked to the disc, but others are indirectly related. Some have clinical symptoms while others may be silent. Root compression is only one possible pain source. Bogduk suggested that less than 30% of lower back problems are related to nerve root compression.[5] Others believe that true nerve compressive involvement is as low as 1%.[6] Furthermore, there are a number of pain-sensitive structures in very close proximity to the IVD that may produce confusing symptoms and confounding clinical findings. In some cases, the identification of a specific pain generator is impossible. This chapter is designed to help sort through these issues and provide the foundation for better understanding of disorders of the lumbar IVD and clearer clinical pathways of management.

Specific issues related to the posterior facet joints, sacroiliac joints, and lumbar spinal stenosis are covered elsewhere in the ensuing chapters.

THE STRUCTURE OF THE IVD

The IVD is a very specialized connective tissue complex. The nucleus contains a sparse cellular population, but an abundant extracellular matrix composed of an elaborate framework of macromolecules filled with water. These various cellular components are responsible for synthesizing macromolecules and repairing the framework.[7–9] Indeed, the structural integrity of the disc depends greatly upon its macromolecular chemistry.

Since the mature disc lacks a significant blood supply, cellular metabolism must rely on the ability of nutrients and wastes to move through the disc and its matrix. Both the composition and the organization of the macromolecular framework and matrix water content are important variables for adequate transport. The most important of these is the concentration of proteoglycans.

Collagen and proteoglycans are the primary structural components of the macromolecular framework. Collagen gives tensile strength to the tissue, and the proteoglycans through their water bonding afford stiffness and resilience. The various matrices of the disc differ significantly in their relative amounts of these two components. For instance, collagen makes up approximately 70% of the dry weight of the outer anulus, but less than 20% of the dry weight of the central nucleus. On the other hand, proteoglycans represent only 3% of the outer anulus, but up to 50% of the nucleus (in a child).

Grossly the disc consists of three distinct parts: an outer part or *anulus fibrosus*, and an inner *nucleus pulposus* "sandwiched" by two *cartilage end plates*. The normal outer anulus is arranged with densely packed, highly oriented, and concentrically arranged collagen fibril lamellae. The outer fibers are mostly Type I collagen consisting of up to 20 lamellae.[10] Outer lamellae are attached to the anterior longitudinal ligament. Posteriorly and laterally the anulus is thinner than the anterior portion. Inner anular fibers are attached to the cartilage end plate. These fibers are composed of Type II collagen.[11] They also have lamellae with a rich ground substance of proteoglycans that increases their capacity to resist compression.[12] The inner anulus is less well organized and more fibrocartilaginous, and forms a transitional zone between the anulus and the central nucleus. There is no distinct separation of

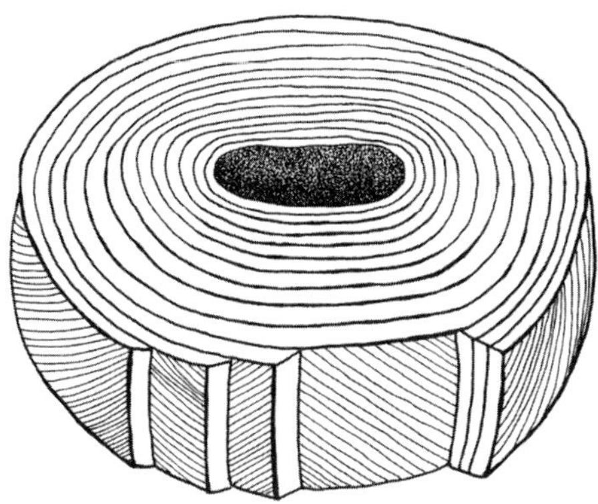

FIGURE 6–1. Schematic representation of the concentrically arranged lamellar rings of the normal lumbar anulus fibrosus. Note that the fiber arrangement of each consecutive ring alternates in the opposite direction. This layout provides greater stiffness and less deformation under compressive and torsional loading.

anulus from the nucleus or cartilage end plates.[13] Collectively, the taut anular fiber arrangement does not allow large proteoglycan molecules from the nucleus to pass through even under heavy loading.

The anular lamellar rings are parallel to one another, with the orientation of the fibers forming an angle of 25–30 degrees with the bony vertebral rim (Fig. 6–1). Each consecutive concentric layer angularly alternates in the opposite direction. Such a configuration enables the anulus to sustain forces of compression, torsion, flexion, and extension. This also affords greater stiffness and lower deformation and energy dissipation.[14]

Relationship of the Anulus Fibrosus to the Posterior Longitudinal Ligament

Grossly the posterior longitudinal ligament (PLL) is denticulate in appearance. It is narrow over the posterior aspect of lumbar vertebral bodies, but flares laterally at each disc space onto the anulus. It has a layered arrangement of superficial and deep components (superficial fibers are most posterior). At the mid-vertebral level the superficial layer of the PLL is much wider than the deep layer. It also becomes wider as the PLL progresses cranially. The long central fibers of the PLL are 8–10 mm wide. They attach to the anulus at the vertebral margins but not to the mid-anulus.

The *peridural membrane* is a fibrovascular sheath external to the dura that lines the vertebral canal. This membrane passes under the superficial layer of the PLL as it attaches to the undersurface of the deep layer. Collectively the deep PLL layer and the peridural membrane attach loosely to a midline bony septum.[15]

The proteoglycan content of the IVD declines with age. This probably reflects a reduced synthesis of these macromolecules. Hydrostatic pressure experiments by Hutton et al. show that pressure inversely affects the synthesis of collagen and proteoglycans (increasing pressure reduces synthesis).[16] Any reduction in proteoglycan content may have significant detrimental consequences for the disc's ability to resist mechanical loads and thus predisposes it to anular delamination and abnormal collagen fiber strain.

The biological intricacies of IVD aging and degeneration are undergoing extensive study. Traditionally, biomechanical factors were considered the key generators of degeneration. The degree to which biological and biomechanical mechanisms interplay remains to be determined. Kang and others have demonstrated increasing evidence that biochemical events may play an integral role in the process of degeneration.[17,18]

Cartilaginous vertebral end plates form the superior and inferior boundaries of the disc proper. Initially the end plates are composed of hyaline-like cartilage about 3 mm thick. Perinatally the end plates are vascularized but their blood supply declines rapidly and dramatically, with little remaining by age 4.[19] The avascular nucleus pulposus receives some of its nutrition by diffusion from the adjacent vertebral subchondral bony sinusoids through the end plates. Vascular contact points perforate the central aspect of the end plate. With aging these may calcify and alter the permeability of the end plates.[20] The relationship between degeneration of the end plates and the initiation of degenerative alteration of the nucleus pulposus has been established. From a structural standpoint, the end plates are the weakest of the three components of the healthy IVD.

The nucleus pulposus is about 88% water at birth. By age 77 it normally decreases to 69%. By comparison, the newborn anulus is about 78% water versus 70% water at age 30, after which it tends to remain constant.[21] There is a lower concentration of collagen in the nucleus (Type II) that is smaller and more loosely arranged. It has an abundant ground substance consisting of 65% hydrophilic nonaggregated proteoglycans. In the lumbar spine, the nucleus resides slightly posterior to the geometric center.

Innervation of the IVD

Cavanaugh et al. also reported that the superficial anulus of the disc is richly innervated with small nerve fibers that correspond to A-delta and C fiber size range, that are associated with transmitting pain signals.[22] The recurrent meningeal nerve (sinuvertebral nerve) innervates the posterior anulus and PLL while the sympathetic chain innervates the lateral and anterior aspect of the anulus.[23] General somatic afferent nerves and general visceral afferent nerves, running with sympathetic efferent fibers, innervate the outer third of the anulus fibrosus.[24] In degenerated discs the identification of nerve elements reaches the inner third and sometimes into the nucleus pulposus.

The dorsal root ganglion may be a mediator of sensory environment at the motion segment. An IVD with anular disruption may be sensitized to further irritation. Fibers whose cell bodies reside in the dorsal root ganglion may release the neurotransmitters into the region of the anulus. This could lead to increased nociceptive stimulation and heightened sensitivity of the patient.

DEVELOPMENT AND MATURATION OF THE LUMBAR IVD

Both the volume and shape of the disc exhibit changes during development and growth, and then again after skeletal maturity is achieved. After birth the disc rapidly increases in height and diameter, keeping pace with vertebral body enlargement. After maturation varying degrees of altered disc volume, thinning, and protrusion occur. As might be expected, changes in disc structure and composition both precede and accompany the gross alterations of morphology. Indeed, changes in disc size, vascular supply, and chemical composition begin during growth, well before there is any gross evidence of disc degeneration on imaging studies.

Every component of IVD tissue (including the cartilage end plates) changes from birth through old age, but the most extensive alteration occurs in the nucleus pulposus. The number of viable cells, concentrations of proteoglycans, and water content all progressively decline. This is accompanied by fragmentation of the aggregating proteoglycans. All discs eventually develop similar age-related changes. However, the rate and extent of such changes vary considerably between individuals, and even within the same spine. Some discs transform more rapidly or more slowly relative to expected time sequences.

The Newborn

In the newborn disc distinct hyaline cartilage end plates separate the nucleus pulposus from the vertebral bodies. The outer rim of the anulus consists of dense circumferential layers of collage fibrils that penetrate the periphery of the cartilage plates. Small blood vessels may be found between the lamellae of the outer anulus (especially posterolaterally) and adjacent to the cartilage end plates. An occasional blood vessel may penetrate into the inner anulus.

The nucleus fills almost half the disc and consists primarily of notochordal tissue. A soft gelatinous, clear matrix surrounds clusters of notochordal cells. The matrix of the nucleus contains few collagen fibrils and even more rare sheets of elastin embedded in an abundant network of highly hydrated proteoglycans.

Childhood and Adolescence

The sources and pathways for nutrition change very early in life. During skeletal growth the volume of the disc increases many times over, thereby increasing the distance between the nucleus and any peripheral vasculature. At the same time, the blood vessels of the anulus and vertebral cartilage end plate become progressively smaller and less numerous.

During this phase of development the notochordal cell population also diminishes. More collagen fibrils appear in the nucleus and the collagen fibrils of all disc components increase in diameter. By adolescence, proteoglycan populations consist of short clusters and non-aggregated proteoglycans. While the fibrocartilaginous components of the anulus increase in size, the nucleus still comprises about half of the disc and is easily distinguished from the inner anulus. At this time on magnetic resonance imaging (MRI) there is a low signal intensity zone transversely across the equator of the nucleus of the IVD reflecting a fibrous tissue plate (Fig. 6–2*A* and 6–2*B*).

Adulthood

By skeletal maturity, many of the disc's peripheral blood vessels have disappeared. The outer anulus remains about the same relative size, but the fibrocartilaginous inner layer expands centrally, mostly at the expense of the nucleus. Myxomatous degeneration develops in portions of the anulus with a loss of the normal collagen fibrilar organization. At this time, minute fissures and cracks begin to appear. The nucleus becomes firmer with an increase in the diameter of the collagen fibrils, and the fibrous plate becomes more obvious. By this time very few notochordal cells (perhaps none) remain. Proteoglycan and water concentrations continue to decrease slowly.

Between 23 and 40 years of age, there also is gradual mineralization of the end plate cartilage and porosity for nutrient transfer begins to decrease. By age 60 only a thin layer of bone separates the disc from the vascular channels that were previously in direct contact with the cartilage. As a result of this course of progressive end plate densification, nutrient channels are slowly obliterated. This process may significantly compromise IVD nutrition.

Collectively, these age-related modifications of the IVD after skeletal maturity contribute to the changes in disc volume, shape, and resilience. This multiplex results in diminished resistance to axial, shearing, and torquing loads and represents the very factors that increase the probability of disc herniation and other disc disruption syndromes. There are numerous factors that are thought to contribute to or accentuate age-related change in the IVD (Table 6–1), as well as issues that may be responsible for a decline in cellular nutrition (Table 6–2).

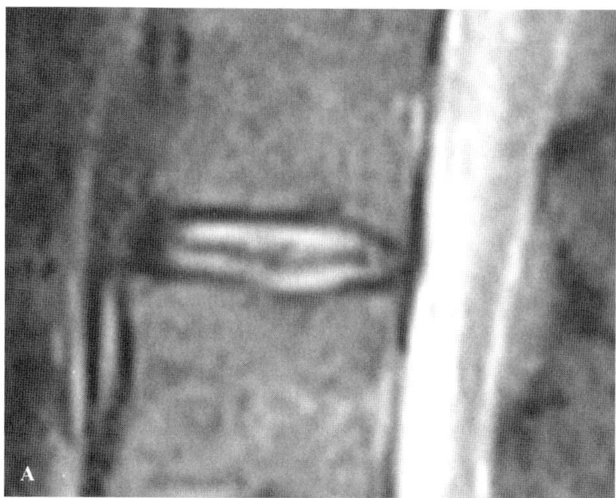

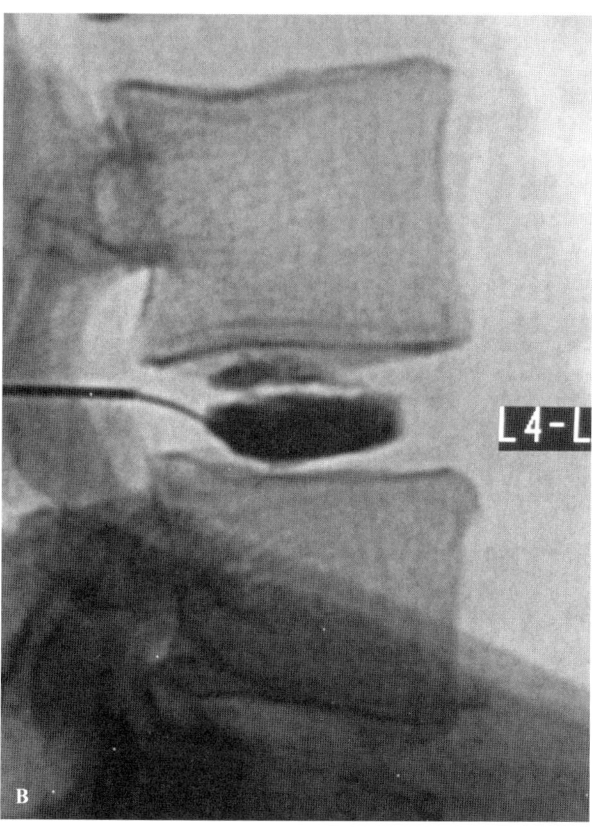

FIGURE 6–2. *A.* Sagittal T2-weighted MRI of the lumbar spine in a normal 14-year-old male. There is high signal intensity of the IVD proper with a horizontal low signal band across the mid-portion of the disc, which represents the normal fibrous equatorial plate. *B.* Normal lateral discogram scout of a different patient. There is normal morphology of the L4–L5 lumbar IVD with typical containment of the injectate. The horizontal zone through the disc's mid-sector represents the fibrous equatorial plate of a mature nucleus.

The Elderly

In the aged individual the entire disc inside the outer anular lamellae gradually becomes a stiffer plate of fibrocartilage. Disc height continues its slow decline and more prominent fissures and clefts form in its center. Marginal proliferative changes may develop at the discovertebral and ligamentous attachments (see Chapter 7 for a discussion of degenerative disease and stenosis).

TABLE 6–1. Factors Contributing to Age-related Changes

- Declining nutrition
- Decreasing concentration of viable cells
- Cellular senescence
- Accumulation of degraded matrix macromolecules
- Fatigue failure of the matrix (the most critical event responsible for change in the central disc and its matrix)
- Decline in the number and size of arteries
- Calcification of the end plate cartilages
- Accumulating degraded matrix macromolecules
- Rising lactate concentration
- Decreased pH levels that compromise cell metabolism and biosynthetic functions that may cause cell death

Clarification on Terminology

The understanding and use of terms often varies within and across disciplines. In this chapter the term '**disc disruption**' refers to intrinsic disruption within the disc consisting of radial tears and varying degrees of morphological change in the anular contour. It is used in distinction from the use of the term '**disc derangement**' by those familiar with the McKenzie school wherein a shifting of the nucleus pulposus with or without an alteration of the anular architecture is implied (see Chapter 15). Elsewhere the terms '**internal disc derangement**' and '**internal disc disruption**' are usually used synonymously.

TABLE 6–2. Factors Contributing to Decline in Cellular Nutrition

Indirect factors
- Increased loading due to demanding physical activities
- Immobilization
- Vibration
- Spinal deformity

Direct vascular compromise
- Smoking
- Vascular disease
- Diabetes

THE MECHANISM OF INTERNAL DISC DISRUPTION

Normal spinal movement requires loading and deformation of discs followed by recovery of disc shape. As an osmotic system, the disc is sensitive to load, pressure, and the concentration of proteoglycans and normal physiological loading provides for fluid transfer. Maintaining the upright posture decreases disc height by hydrostatically driving water (and waste) out of the disc matrix. Prolonged recumbency then restores the original disc shape and volume as water (and nutrients) returns to the hydrophilic nuclear matrix, a process known as *imbibition*. In this manner there is a significant variation in disc hydration, morning through evening. The ebb and flow of water to and from the nucleus continuously changes the mechanical response of the disc to loading.

The IVD has been shown to undergo changes in its height and viscoelastic properties as a result of several mechanisms. The fluid contents of the disc change over a routine 24-hour period.[25–29] This occurs as a result of compressive forces from prolonged standing or sitting,[27,30–32] and because of cyclic, vibratory, or prolonged loading.[33–36]

When deformation and reduced thickness of the disc are substantial, there may be an increased laxity of the posterior joints, and resultant increase in range of intervertebral motion. Such a situation may increase the likelihood of injury.

Frequent changes in posture improve fluid exchange, but maintaining high-pressure postures like sitting and standing may actually inhibit disc nutrition. A sedentary, inactive lifestyle correlates well with the natural course of early and progressive disc degeneration. At the opposite extreme, an overly aggressive lifestyle may result in disc damage that may hasten the degenerative cascade. Moderation in physical demand appears to be the most practical action to aid disc nutrition within a reasonable and safe range.

Repeatedly the spinal musculature had been shown to be the major factor that generates forces capable of dynamically stabilizing the spine under various loading conditions.[1–4] In addition, a recent model has come to light that reveals how the musculature of the abdominals, multifidi, diaphragm, and pelvic floor can co-contract and pressurize the abdomen and increase spinal stability. This "pressurized canister" concept has gained acceptance over the past decade. This is addressed in detail in Chapter 4 and in later chapters. However, all the intricacies of such dynamic stability of the spine during occupational activities and normal activities of daily living are not fully understood, and remove injury at times occurs during simple unloaded movements.

Coactivation of agonist and antagonist muscles seems to stiffen spinal segments and maintain stability in the presence of both external and internal loads. If the laxity developed by creep in the viscoelastic tissues is relatively small, then muscular co-contraction may adequately compensate. [The phenomenon of deformation of viscoelastic materials when a constant load is applied over time is known as "creep" deformity. For instance, the time-dependent change in disc height in the evening after day-long loading compared to a morning measurement is due to such behavior.]

The creep induced in the viscoelastic tissues of the spine as a result of repetitive loading (such as lumbar flexion) desensitizes, or fatigues, the mechanoreceptors within. This is manifested by dramatically diminished muscular activity, allowing increased exposure to instability and injury, even before there is fatigue of the musculature.[37] For example, in this animal study, within the first 5 minutes of continuous brisk cyclic loading of the lumbar spine in moderate anterior flexion there was a reduction of the stabilizing muscular reflexes by up to 85%. If this occurs similarly in humans, the spine may easily be exposed to destabilizing injury. In the same study, the reflex stabilizing effect was not restored even after a 10-minute rest period. This process appears to diminish or eliminate the ability of the nervous system to monitor relative intersegmental motion and recruit the necessary forces to compensate for any destabilizing motion. Actual muscle fatigue could be a compounding factor.

There is one period in *midlife* where clinical disc symptoms and syndromes arise at a higher frequency and intensity than any other. This is not surprising considering that any existing age-related changes make the tissues less able to recover from deformation and more vulnerable to progressive fatigue failure. Fatigue failure of the matrix consists of fissures, cracks, myxoid degeneration, and fragmentation of proteoglycans and disruption of collagen fibrils.

Since the disc often exhibits some internal disruption as early as the teenage years, there may be varying degrees of displacement and bulging of the anulus. But during midlife the risk of herniation is highest. At this time the disc still has the ability to hydrostatically transmit loads, the anulus already has some tears and fissures, and relatively high levels of activity remain. In the young the ability of the disc to dissipate load is very high but the anulus is more likely to be strong enough to provide adequate containment. At the opposite end of the spectrum, the anulus in the elderly has more fissures, but houses a dehydrated nucleus that is less capable of expansion. Even in cases where degeneration approaches 100%, the spine is stiffer, but it is often less painful. Unfortunately, at this stage there may be additional pain generators from facet disease and spinal stenosis (see Chapter 7).

One popular theoretical model describes the progressive degenerative changes of the anulonuclear complex as comprised of three transitional phases:[38] (1) *dysfunction* (with circumferential and radial tears of the IVD), (2) *instability* (internal disruption and disc resorption), and (3) *restabilization* (marginal osteophytes and traction spurs).

Yu et al. correlated the internal architecture of lumbar IVDs with MRI findings and cryomicrotomy using fresh frozen cadaveric spines.[39,40] They were the first to correlate the findings and conclude that MRI was an accurate means for investigating anular tears of the lumbar disc. They classified tear patterns into concentric, transverse, and radial (see Fig. 6–3*A* and 6–3*B*). A concentric (*circumferential*) tear is a crescent-like or oval cavity associated with rupture of the short transverse fibers connecting the concentric lamellar layers in the anulus fibrosus (interlaminar delamination), and they are most commonly seen peripherally in the anterior and posterior sectors of the disc.[41] A *radial tear* is a fissure extending from the nucleus toward the outermost surface of the anulus. *Transverse tears* (peripheral) rupture Sharpey's fibers near their attachment to the ring apophysis. Transverse tears occur early in life and lead to secondary degenerative changes. Kim concluded that these peripheral tears are most likely to occur during extension under preload.[42]

There are two basic types of IVD prolapse: *anular protrusion* (displaced nuclear material causes the outer anulus to bulge, but it remains "contained" within the anular perimeter), and *nuclear extrusion* (nuclear material escapes from the disc proper and is considered "noncontained").

Adams and Hutton describe two basic mechanisms for disc prolapse.[49] The first and more typical mechanism is gradual and progressive, resulting from a compressive force of lesser magnitude applied repetitiously to a spine in flexion (e.g., frequent bending and lifting). The second is less common and occurs suddenly, usually associated with a traumatic event when a high compressive force is abruptly applied to the spine while in an unfavorable position (commonly a forward bend combined with a twisting movement). For a disc to prolapse, a fissure or channel (radial tear) is required for the passage of nuclear material to the periphery.

In nondegenerated discs the nucleus pulposus has been shown to migrate slightly posteriorly during flexion and anteriorly in extension.[43] Tensile stress in the anulus fibers of an intact disc changes, varying from a maximum at the inner layer to a minimum at the outer layer. Pressure on the inner anulus may be greater in the morning after the disc has been in a relatively unloaded state when the nucleus is saturated with fluid, and at its maximum volume and height.

Ito summarizes the pathology of internal disc disruption as being characterized by inner anulus disruption in the form of a radial fissure.[44] Work by Aspden and Porter suggests that isolated fragments of coalesced nuclear material may increase focal inner anular stresses, or facilitate the disruption process.[45] When there is fiber failure at the innermost layer, stresses concentrated at the zone of failure are displaced to the immediately adjacent fibers.[46] Fatigue loading of a disc wedged in flexion can chronically distort the lamellae and propagate tears producing or increasing posterolateral radial fissures.[47] Hyperflexion

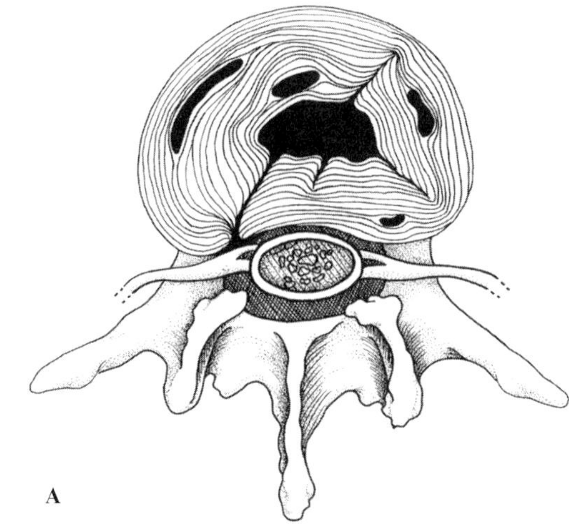

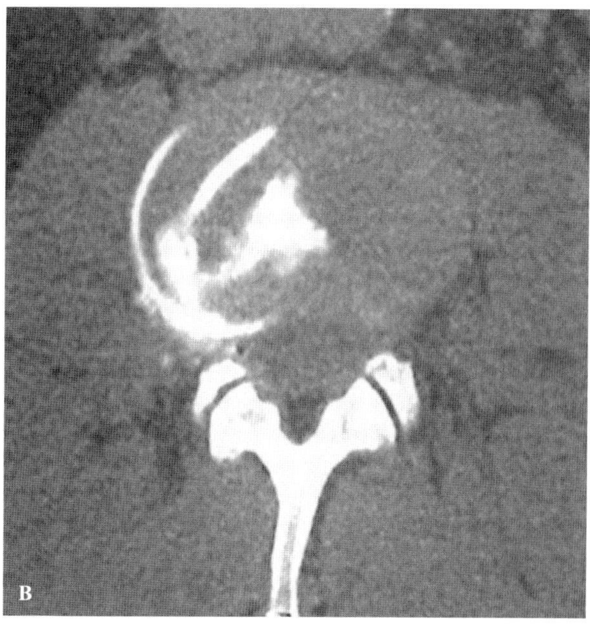

FIGURE 6–3. *A.* Schematic illustration of a lumbar disc showing several types of disruptions and abnormalities of the anular integrity. *Concentric tears* represent delamination of concentric lamella. They are crescent shaped. In contrast, *radial tears* pass transversely from the nucleus to the periphery. For a disc to prolapse, a radial tear is necessary. In this illustration there is a complete radial tear on the right side with collection of extruded nuclear material adjacent to the exiting nerve root. *B.* Postdiscography CT examination, L4–L5. On the right side there are both circumferential (concentric) and radial tears.

with substantial axial load may produce disc prolapse.[48] Cyclical compression and flexion has been shown to produce peripheral migration of nuclear material in younger discs, but this should not be expected in more degenerated discs.[49]

After significant anular fiber failure or herniation, there is stress redistribution so that the compressive load must increase in order to rupture more fibers. This may actually work as a protective mechanism to offset catastrophic collapse of the collagen fiber fences.[50] Clearly, any fiber failure insufficient to produce immediate prolapse may be the beginning of a gradual prolapse when the cellular mechanisms of repair are inadequate.

When the anulus tears sufficiently to extend to the periphery of the disc and allows the escape of its contents, a radial fissure is completed and the disc is technically ruptured. It is not, however, necessarily prolapsed and intruding spatially into the confines of the spinal canal.

Pain and/or paresthesia may occur with nerve root compression or chemical nerve irritation. However, the disc itself may become a pain generator as a result of inflammatory biochemical degradation of the disc matrix, as the result of chemical irritation of the nerve endings in the outer fibers of the anulus.[41,51] More than 70% of the fissures that reach the outer third of the anulus have been reported to be associated with pain.[52]

Stages of Disc Prolapse: A Model

Adams and Hutton further describe several stages of gradual prolapse of a disc[49]:

Stage I The first stage (self-selection of the disc) really means a disc that is predilected for tear. For instance, discs that have a softer and more "pulpy" nucleus along with a posterior anulus that is much thinner than the anterior are at increased risk. This equates best with younger discs at L5–S1 and L4–L5 that would show a relative posterior position of the nucleus pulposus on discography. No discogenic pain is present at this level and other diagnostic tests such as MRI would be normal.

Stage II In the second stage repeated activities of bending and lifting gradually distort the posterior inner anular lamellae. The inner lamellae become tightly curved and packed together posterolaterally. The nucleus follows this line of distortion and migrates peripherally as has been seen in specimens, and on MRI and discography. However, in Stage II the lamellar layers have not been breached. Upper lumbar discs infrequently pass this stage.

Stage III In the third stage the lamellae are breached. The nuclear pulp migrates through a narrow, and sometimes tortuous, channel through the lamellae. The final barrier consists of the outermost lamellae and theadhering PLL. The nuclear pulp must penetrate these tightly packed lamellae of the posterior anulus in order to escape. Any remaining collagen can present a formidable barrier to penetration. This distance may be only 2 or 3 mm in the posterolateral corners (typically somewhat thicker centrally). The disc may stretch and bulge outwards in response to the pressure of the migrating pulp producing an anular protrusion. In mature discs with a mostly fibrotic nucleus, this may be the final stage. The Stage III disc is most frequently responsible for symptom reproduction when injected (discography). The leaking disc may occur in Stage III or IV.

Most radial fissures are not visible on MRI as such. Some may appear bright on T2-weighted, fat saturation, and STIR (short tau inversion recovery) sagittal and axial MRI images (see Fig. 6–4*A* and 6–4*B*). These areas have been termed high-intensity zones (HIZs). Localized anular disruption and generalized loss of central disc signal intensity on MRI suggests that a radial tear can induce generalized physical and chemical changes involving the proteoglycans of the nucleus pulposus and inner portion of the anulus. The abnormal signal of the HIZ actually represents fluid or mucoid material of nuclear origin associated with granulation tissue and neovascularization that is entrapped between the torn fibers of the outer anulus and the PLL complex.

Several studies looking at the correlation between LBP (low back pain) and IVD architecture and morphology have been attempted by using MRI and post-discography CT (computerized tomography-see Chapters 16 and 17). The lessons of discography and cryomicrotomy have greatly improved our understanding of common disc lesions that we see on MRI.

It is believed that many radial tears are responsible for symptoms.[58] It is speculated that with progression of a tear to the periphery, inflammatory substances can reach the outer anulus and the free nerve endings.[51] "Awake discography" may identify discogenic pain segments in the lumbar spine by having the patient compare any provoked pain response with their typical pain patterns, and also by observing the morphological changes subsequently visualized on post-discography-CT.

The validity of discography in demonstrating certain morphological abnormalities of the IVD, and more specifically anular radial tears, has been well established by previous post-mortem studies[39,59] and surgical correlations.[60] Its validity as a clinical test, confirming its ability to isolate the pain generator, has been more controversial. More recently Walsh

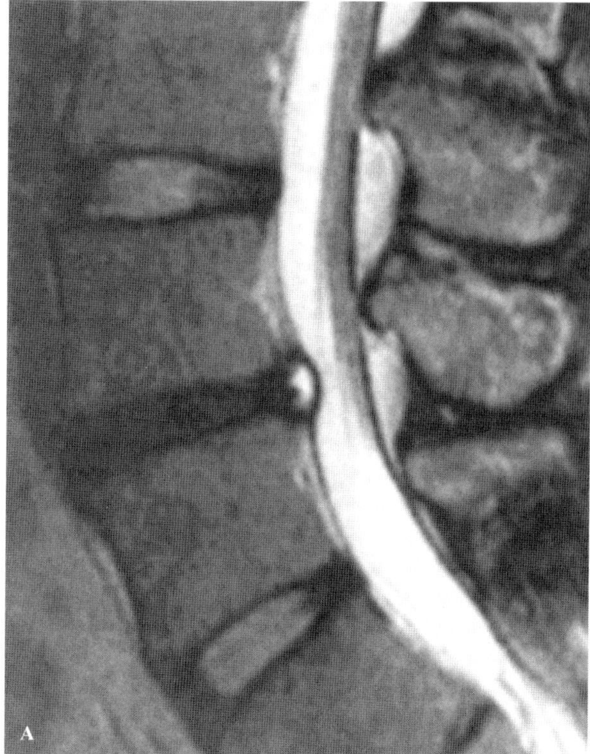

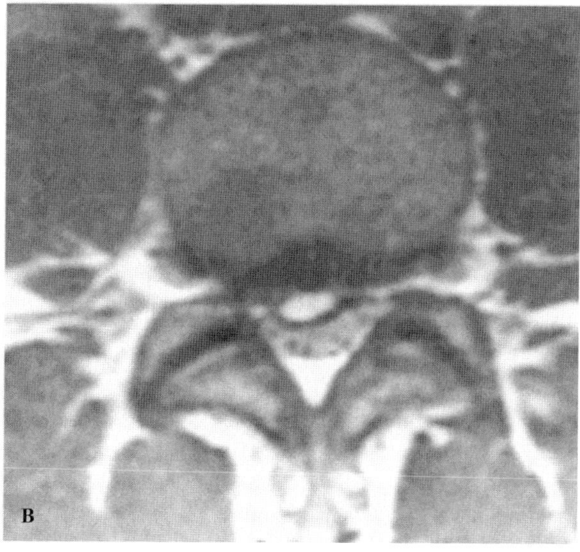

FIGURE 6–4. High-intensity zone (HIZ). *A.* Mid-sagittal T2-weighted lumbar image. *B.* Axial T2-weighted image through the mid portion of the L4–L5 disc. This L4–L5 disc exhibits overall low signal intensity with slight decrease in its vertical dimension. There is some modest focal posterior protrusion centrally. In this sector of the disc at its anular interface, note the high signal zone. This represents the localized internal disruption associated with a radial tear. Focal fluid, mucoid material, or granulation tissue produces the high signal appearance.

et al., after confirming adequate intranuclear positioning with anteroposterior and lateral fluoroscopy, found no false positives.[61] Notwithstanding its invasiveness, MRI cannot replace the "gold standard" of discography, which remains the only direct means of evaluating pain character and the precise level of pain production.

It also may be confusing to consider that bulges and protrusions of the disc are fundamentally distinct anatomical and clinical entities. Nomenclature based purely on the morphology of posterior disc contours may create artificial anatomicopathological entities that discount the possibility of symptomatic internal disc disruption. Crock reported internal disc disruption as a prominent source of somatic LBP. He characterized this situation as disruption of the internal disc architecture, discogenic lumbar pain in the absence of peripheral disc shape abnormality, and the absence of nerve root compression on CT-myelography.[20] In fact, back and leg pain may derive from multiple potential sources irrespective of the imaged pathoanatomy.

As it turns out, there is strong correlation between an HIZ and concordant pain produced by discography. More than 70% of fissures that reach the outer third of the anulus were associated with pain provocation.[52,62] An HIZ is believed to be a marker of internal disc disruption and back pain, and back and leg pain without true radiculopathy.[63] Noxious stimulation of the disc results in lower back and referred extremity radiation.[64] These findings were corroborated by Schellhas et al.[65] The HIZ usually enhances on MRI with contrast (Gd-DPTA), indicating granulation tissue or neovascularization. By definition, Stage III abnormalities are never seen in a normal disc, but they may be present in asymptomatic patients.[53,66]

Stage IV Stage IV represents extrusion (noncontainment) of nuclear pulp. The pulp may appear at the mouth of the fissure, but quite commonly extends beyond the final barrier, migrating and collecting elsewhere.

In some cases, the body's reaction to these changes is neovascularization and infiltration by macrophages.[67,68] Blood vessels form in extruded tissue and also enter the degenerated disc. This action tends to reduce the size of some masses and may explain reduction of symptoms. Larger disc protrusions have a greater tendency to regress in size.[69,70] This occurs in up to 56% of complete prolapses,[71] but is seen less frequently in incomplete prolapses (37.5%) and in only 11.3% of protrusions.[72]

Stage V The disc does not continue to leak pulp indefinitely. In Stage V the ruptured disc achieves some degree of stability. For instance in mature discs with fibrotic nuclear lumps, herniation is most unlikely because there can be no passage of the nucleus except under extreme loading circumstances. Even in less fibrotic discs a 10% loss of disc fluid makes it difficult to propagate an anular tear. Therefore, nuclear extrusion and anular protrusion are expected to occur in normal and slightly degenerated discs, but not in severely degenerated discs. This stage is not necessarily painless as such; rather it implies that leaking ceases and there is no further significant or progressive posterior migration/bulging.

While one would expect a direct progression through these sequences, the actual rates and extents of alteration vary considerably between spines and even within different levels of the same spine. This makes the clinical correlation of an individual pathoanatomical change difficult or impossible.

Previous mention of the importance of the cartilaginous end plate relationships was made, which now need some amplification as to its place in the disc-maturation model.

Schmorl's Nodes

Symptomatic extrusion of disc material is most common posteriorly and posterolaterally. However, anterior, lateral, and intraspongiosal herniation also occurs. Any one of these scenarios may be painful. The latter of these herniations (intraspongiosal) with central prolapse of nuclear material into the spongiosa of the adjacent vertebral body is commonly known as a *Schmorl's node*. Anterior disruption of the rim apophysis (limbus) by prolapsing disc material may also occur. A similar situation may develop posteriorly, with associated disc herniation with or without posterior rim fracture.

The Schmorl's node has been reported to be the most common lesion of the IVD, indeed of the whole spine. Males are predilected. The most common location is thoracolumbar. Theories regarding the development of Schmorl's nodes include developmental (embryonic defects, ossification gaps, vascular channels, and notochordal extrusion defects form points of weakness), degenerative (sites of weakness because of aging in the cartilaginous end plate), pathological (diseases causing vertebral body or end plate weakness), and trauma. In an acute scenario, Schmorl's nodes are often associated with pain.

Clinical Pearl: In an acute setting, a Schmorl's node is commonly associated with pain.

Only a few studies suggest a direct causal relationship to acute traumatic episodes. The highest percentage of recorded cases occurs in motorcyclists and in association with jumping sports. Such loading may precipitate an acute focal and symptomatic end plate fracture/herniation by the well-hydrated and delineated nucleus pulposus. On MRI, nuclear material may be seen bending into and through the defect in the subchondral plate. Such cases may exhibit sudden-onset, localized, nonradiating back pain. It is assumed that inflammatory changes may be induced by intraosseous fracture and biological reactions to intraspongiosal disc material might cause pain.[73] Symptomatic cases have demonstrated the presence of vertebral body marrow edema on MRI. Any relationship to trauma may be important in the medicolegal setting.

Small Schmorl's nodes are difficult to detect with conventional radiography and only 30%–50% are visible.[74] In time, Schmorl's nodes are usually associated with moderate degenerative change at the motion segment.[75,76]

Posterior vertebral body rim fractures may be associated with posterior herniations at the same level. This may cause significant LBP and radiculopathy in adolescents and young adults, similar to an acute disc prolapse alone. Rarely they present with neurogenic claudication due to spinal stenosis in older patients. Occasionally these lesions may appear to be incidental findings. The rim fracture may be central (often larger with broad-based disc herniation) or posterolateral (fragments small with focal herniation). Plain radiographs are diagnostic in about 40% of cases. CT is more reliable, showing the fracture fragment and vertebral defect in most cases (Fig. 6–5). However, the fracture fragment may be overlooked on MRI. An accurate diagnosis is important, as the surgical

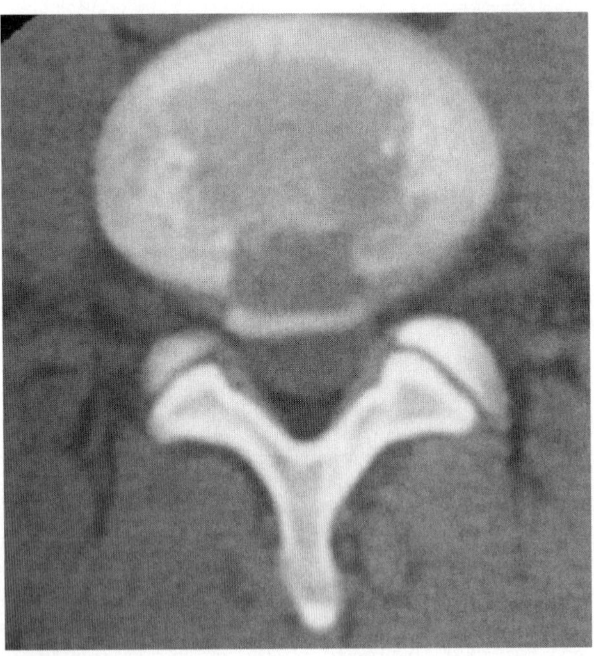

FIGURE 6–5. Seventeen-year-old male with a posterior vertebral body rim fracture. An axial lumbar CT image shows the disrupted posterior vertebral rim margin. Sagittal reconstructed views showed the bony fragments attached to the IVD. Central involvement is often larger and seen with broad-based herniation. Conventional radiographs are diagnostic in only 40% of cases. Bony fragments are often not visualized on MRI.

technique for disc herniation may be inappropriate for end plate fractures.[77]

Clinical Pearl: Posterior vertebral body rim fractures are a significant cause of LBP and radiculopathy in adolescents and young adults. Occasionally these lesions may appear to be incidental findings. Conventional radiography is diagnostic in only 40% of cases, and CT is most reliable.

IMAGING OF THE IVD

High-quality conventional radiography is helpful for the initial assessment of gross osseous morphology, vertebral alignment, intervertebral spacing, and intersegmental stability. However, intrinsic changes in the IVD largely go undetected on the conventional radiograph until gross thinning and marginal stress-related reactions occur. Routine radiography is therefore limited, with many disc conditions escaping early detection, leading to a possible delay in their diagnosis. The uncertainties and ambiguities of disc pathology largely may be clarified by various advanced imaging studies, possibly allowing for earlier appropriate treatment options.

The clinical strength of MRI lies in its excellent soft tissue contrast resolution, direct multiplanar imaging, lack of ionizing radiation, and the potential to characterize pathological tissue.

Clinical Pearl: The potential of MRI to characterize pathological tissue helps clarify the uncertainties and ambiguities of IVD pathology.

Aging and degeneration produce classical MRI appearances in signal intensity and morphological character. The hallmark finding of degeneration is decrease in signal of the intrinsic aspect of the disc on T2-weighted images (remember that this sequence portrays water as bright or high signal). This produces a "dark disc" appearance. Depending upon the extent of degeneration, there may also be measurable thinning of the disc and marginal hypertrophic changes and end plate reactions.

Reaction to degenerative disc disease may occur at the adjacent discovertebral interface, and may take on several forms.[78] *Type I* change consists of vascular-reactive marrow and edema (intermediate to low signal intensity on T1-weighted and high or bright signal intensity on T2-weighted). *Type II* end plate change, representing progressive fatty marrow replacement, demonstrates a zone of high signal intensity on both T1-weighted and T2-weighted images. *Type III* change, representing bony accretion and sclerosis, appears low signal on both T1-weighted and T2-weighted images. Type III pattern may appear on conventional radiographs when sufficiently advanced.

Discs that exhibit intrinsic disruption and correlate with discogenic pain syndromes are best predicted by Type II end plate changes and the presence of an HIZ. Type I changes may relate to discogenic pain and perhaps instability.[79,80]

Most lumbar IVD herniations are seen in discs that exhibit degenerative changes. T1-weighted axial images show the midline herniations well because of epidural fat displacement. There is good contrast between the disc posteriorly and the bright cerebrospinal fluid on T2-weighted images. Focal abnormal anular contours measuring 3 mm assuredly have nuclear material that has reached the margin.

Mass appearance of a disc herniation should always be correlated with the cross-sectional mensuration of the canal and relationship to descending and exiting nerve roots. In some instances pre- or post-compressive edema of the involved nerve root may be apparent.

The space occupying mass effect of a disc protrusion into the spinal or foraminal canal is virtually always greater in appearance on MRI and CT imaging than the actual dimension. A cap of inflammatory reaction or granulation tissue contributes to the appearance of mass effect. This tissue enhances with the administration of intravenous gadolinium. There may be some prognostic significance in such cases as these types of discs are more likely to exhibit resorption, and decrease in size.[81]

Nomenclature Used to Describe Lesions of the IVD

The terminology used for the reporting of visualized abnormalities on imaging studies is varied and often confusing.[82] Diagnostic categories of disc abnormalities are best based on understood pathological categories, e.g. normal, developmental variation, degeneration, infection, etc. Normal discs are so defined without knowledge of the clinical situation. This includes the fibrous plate that develops at the equator of the disc as the result of age-related changes, producing a bilocular appearance on discography (Fig. 6–2*B*).

The general term *herniation* has been used to describe some degree of disc extension beyond the vertebral margin. This extension may include nuclear material, anulus, and even bony tissue. Convention implies a *focal herniation* to be less than 25% of the disc's circumference, whereas *broad-based herniation* means 25%–50% of the disc's circumference (Fig. 6–6).

Herniations may take the form of *protrusion* or *extrusion*.[82] In a *protrusion* the greatest dimension in any direction between the edges of disc material that

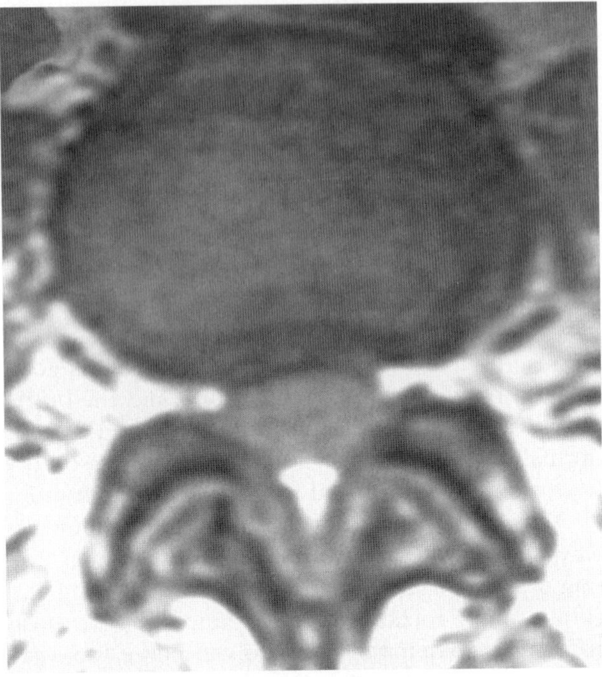

FIGURE 6–6. Axial MRI showing a broad-based (about 50% of the circumference) herniation, with about 4 mm of intrusion into the confines of the spinal canal.

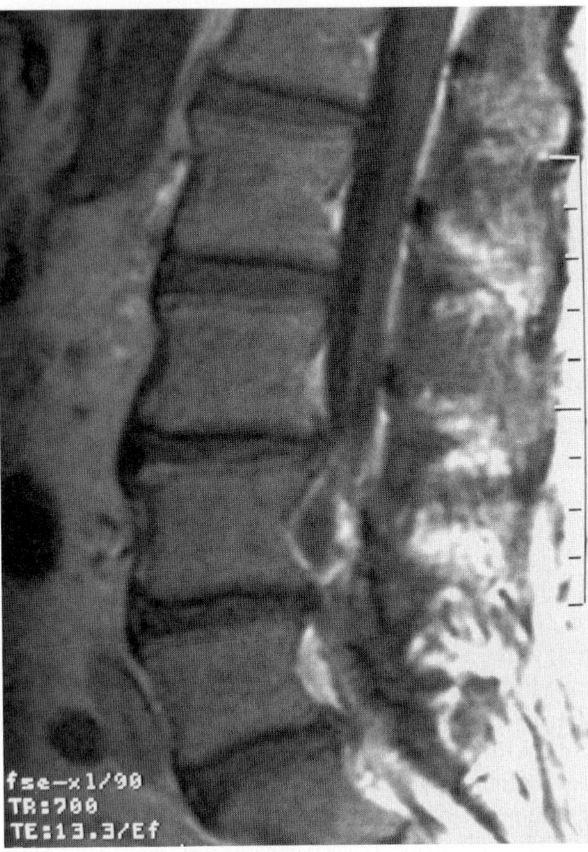

FIGURE 6 7. Sagittal, contrast-enhanced, T1-weighted image. There is a large sequestered disc fragment completely isolated from the patent disc, seen lying posterior to the L4 vertebra. The fragment is surrounded by halo of higher signal probably representing granulation tissue.

extends beyond the vertebral margin is less than the distance between the edges of the base (in the same plane). *Extruded* discs exhibit the distance between the edges of the disc material beyond the vertebral margin to be greater than the distance between the base, in the same plane. In a given disc there may be characteristics of both protrusion and extrusion depending on the plane of imaging. In such instances the designation *extrusion* should be used. In cases of extrusion, when there is a loss of continuity with the parent disc, the term *sequestration* is usually applied (Fig. 6–7). Examples of various imaging appearances are shown in Figures 6–6, 6–7, 6–9, 6–10, 6–11, and 6–12. Despite the quest for reliable descriptive terms for the pathoanatomical appearances, Modic et al. found no correlation between pain and disability on the one hand and disc size, behavior, or type of disc herniation on the other.[83]

Any degree of caudal or cephalad migration of the fragment is measured. In Figure 6–8 there is a huge extruded L4–L5 central and left paracentral mass in a normal-sized spinal canal with caudal displacement about 11 mm, but it retains connection with the parent disc. The remaining neural elements at this level have been displaced posteriorly and to the right. This young female patient had mild LBP and moderate left leg radiation without hard neurological findings. Lumbar stabilization, physiotherapeutic modalities, and changes in her activities of daily living reduced pain and peripheral manifestations. In some cases, irrespective of the size of herniation, symptoms may recur and surgery may be necessitated for a future episode that is nonresponsive to similar measures including epidural steroid injections.

In addition to the morphological description of these disc changes there should also be a comparison with the relative size of the intruded space and not just measurement of the protrusion itself. Spinal canal size varies significantly (see Fig. 7–1*A* to 7–1*E* and Fig. 7–2*A* to 7–2*B*). Small protrusions into tight canals have greater mass effect than those into normal, or large canals. Reported findings like "... a large 12 mm extrusion, left paracentral in location, that fills two thirds of the canal and extends to the intervertebral foramen" has more descriptive power than "... a 12 mm left paracentral disc herniation."

Whether or not the IVD wall contains the protrusion is not always clear on the imaging study and the MRI criteria for the differentiation of supraligamentous and subligamentous herniations are not reliable.[84] Remember that the PLL is largely a

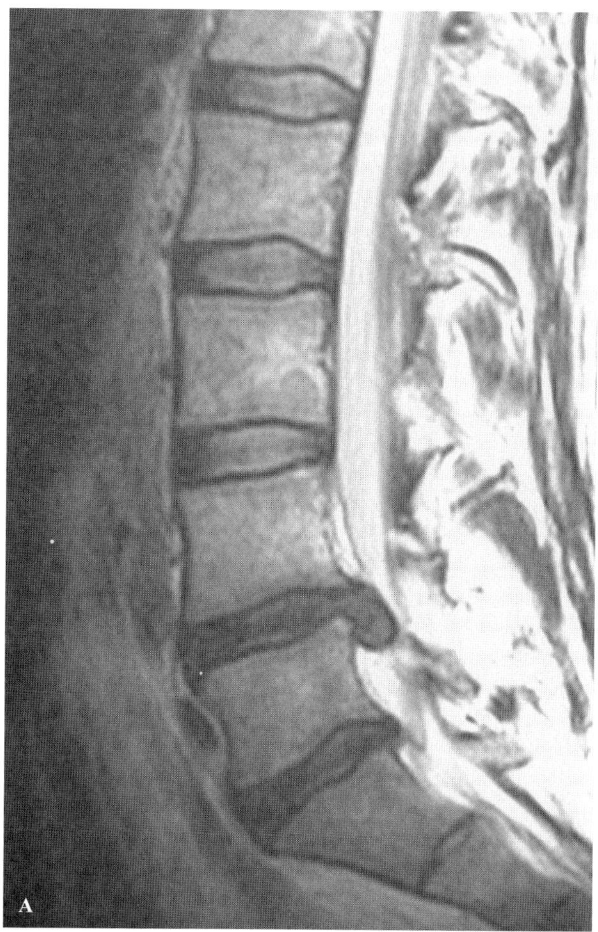

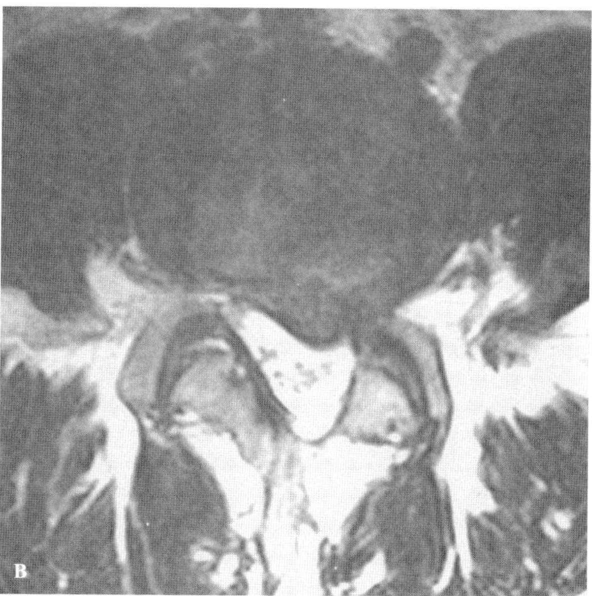

FIGURE 6–8. There is a huge extruded L4–L5 central and left paracentral mass. The spinal canal is normal sized. There is caudal displacement about 11 mm, but it retains a connection with the parent disc. The neural elements at this level have been displaced posteriorly and to the right. The L5–S1 disc also is abnormal in this patient but any mass effect is small.

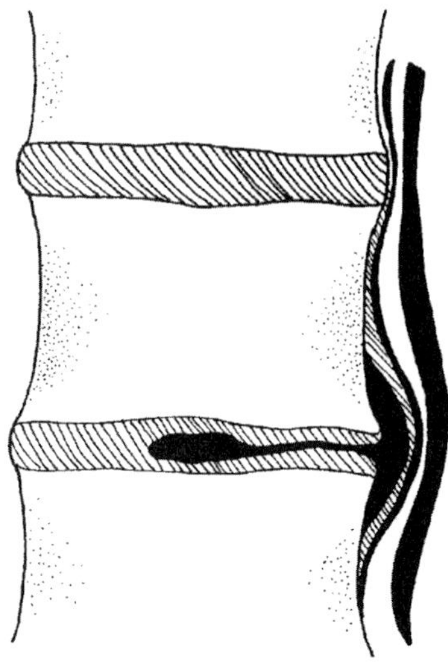

FIGURE 6–9. Schema suggesting an extrusion through anular fibers with collection behind the cephalad and caudal vertebrae and under the PLL/peridural membrane. This midline structure may also limit shift of the mass from side to side. This attachment is variable in location, extent, and strength, which allows for significant individual variation. *(After Wiltse.*[15]*)*

midline structure, with or without solid connection in the midline, and weak attachment to the anulus. Also, the fibrovascular peridural membrane attaches to the deep layer of the PLL. Nuclear material that breaks through the anulus may readily collect beneath these collective restraints. Indeed, this is the likely explanation for relative containment of fragments and hematoma formation to one side or the other (Fig. 6–9). This however does not always occur, as there are several anatomical variations of these connections.

Other observations are also important. The signal character of the protruded material suggests the degree of disc hydration, a factor that may be of predictive value relative to resorption and shrinking of the herniation. That is, the greater the hydration, the more likely the mass effect of the herniation will be reduced (Fig. 6–10). It is important to observe any impact of the mass on vital structures within the neural canals. These include the distortion and shifting of the thecal sac, the relationship of the descending and exiting nerve roots, and any degree of swelling of the nerve roots proper.

Several different signal intensities are present posterior to the L4 segment in Figure 6–11. In part there is extruded disc material, but also a significant hematoma formation. This often occurs following stripping of the epidural veins. Blood and inflammatory exudates are walled-off in the adjacent area. It should be recalled that the veins of Batson's plexus lie on the posterior surface of the peridural membrane and penetrate it in many places, forming the basivertebral veins. These easily may be disrupted as

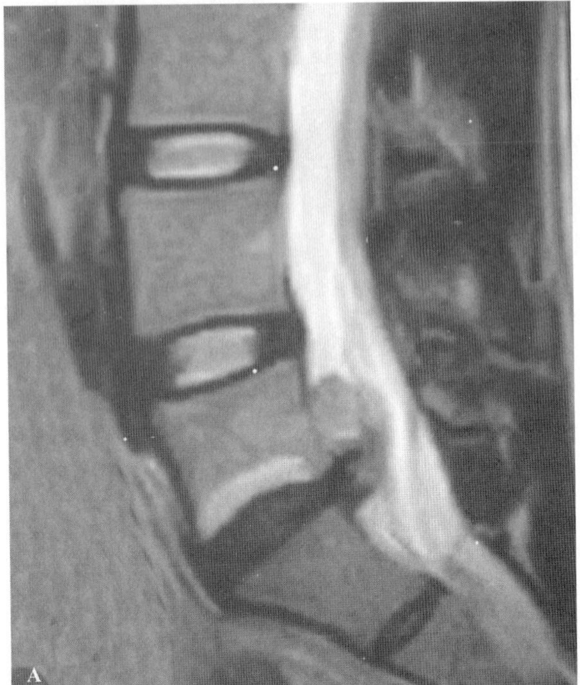

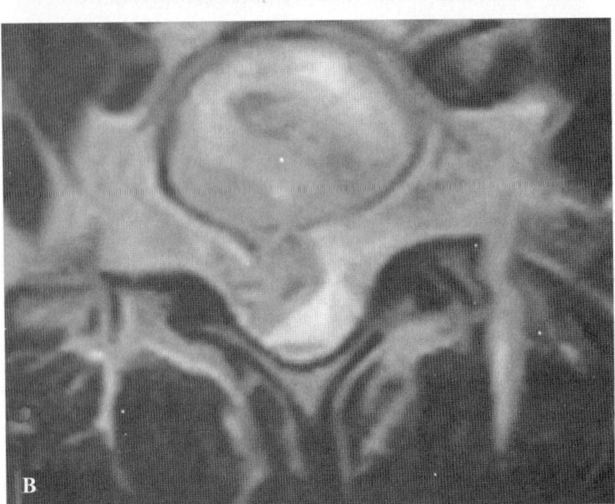

FIGURE 6–10. *A.* Mid-sagittal T2-weighted image. *B.* Axial T2-weighted image through the L5–S1 disc. The L5–S1 disc exhibits uniform low signal and there is high signal paralleling the L5 inferior end plate (fatty marrow replacement). Posteriorly there is anular low signal prominence opening into an area of intermediate signal and a huge mass effect occupying more than 50% of the spinal canal and extending proximally to lie behind the L5 vertebra. Note the signal continuity with the parent disc. The higher signal of this huge herniation (higher degree of hydration) correlates well with the tendency toward resorption and shrinkage over time.

the peridural membrane/PLL confluence is displaced by protruding disc tissue. Subsequently, the combined mass may significantly regress as the hematoma resolves and the discal tissue is resorbed. If the nucleus portion of a herniated mass actually perforates the PLL it may be subject to a stronger neovascularization

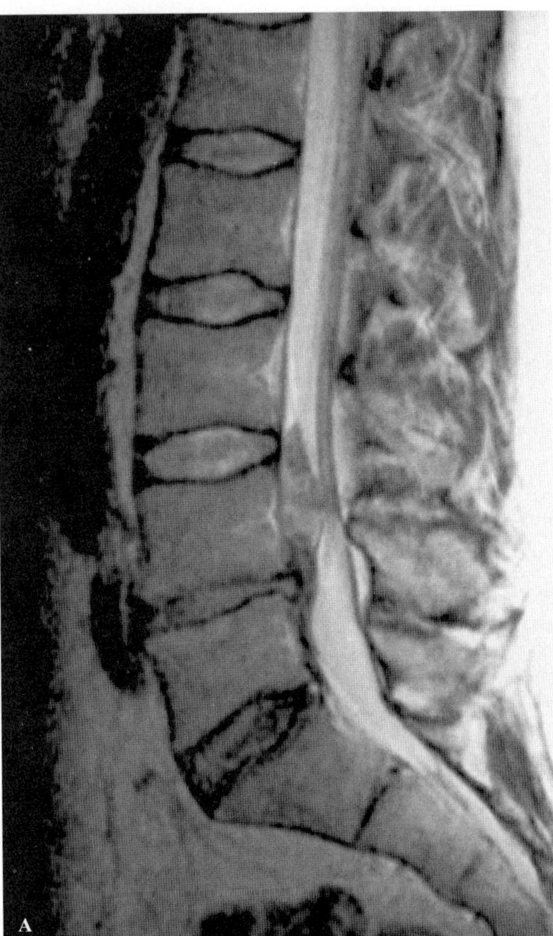

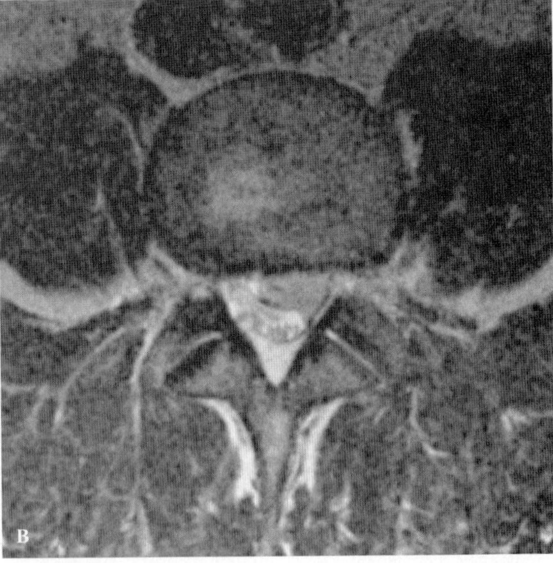

FIGURE 6–11. *A.* Mid-sagittal T2-weighted lumbar MRI. *B.* Axial T2-weighted image through the lower L4 body. The L4–L5 disc exhibits decreased signal and decrease in height. Posteriorly there is a lower signal mass adjacent to the disc. There also is a tenting of the dura over an intermediate signal area that extends as high as the lower border of L3. These mixed signals represent extruded disc material and hematoma. As the hematoma regresses, the overall mass effect will reduce significantly.

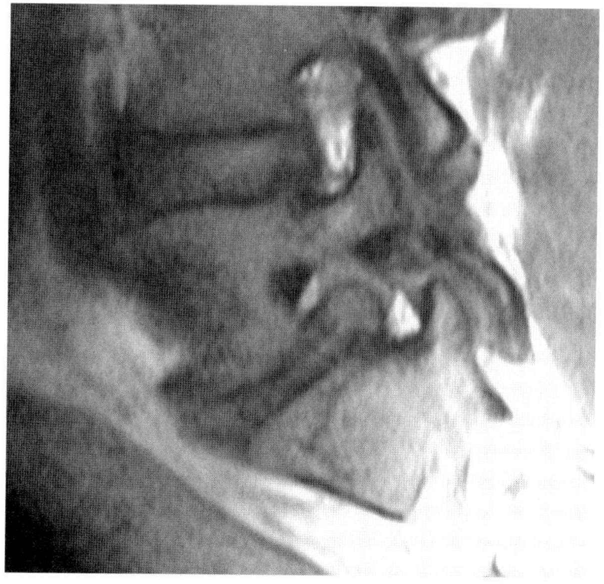

FIGURE 6–12. Parasagittal MRI through the intervertebral foramen. There is a large IVD extrusion impaling the exiting nerve root high in the foramen. The disc exhibits decreased vertical dimension.

reaction than it would otherwise, thus increasing the potential for resorption.[85]

It now appears that most cases of radiculopathy are more the result of inflammation (chemical and edematous factors), and not by compressive events alone. Either is possible. Figure 6–12 shows an intraforaminal protrusion that has significant mass effect on the exiting nerve root. On the sagittal image the exiting nerve root appeared enlarged, possibly reflecting an inflammatory reaction.

About 3% of patients have conjoined nerve roots or perineural cysts.[86] Either may confuse the clinical picture or place the root(s) at greater risk for entrapment. Nerve root anomalies should be suspected in cases of failed disc surgery.[87]

THE CLINICAL ASSESSMENT OF LUMBAR IVD DISRUPTION

The effort to categorize patients with LBP, with or without limb pain, has frustrated clinicians for almost a century. One needs only to witness the abundance of orthopedic and neurological examination procedures (often with eponymic references) to attest to this difficulty. Furthermore, the recent advent of advanced diagnostic imaging and physiological evaluative studies has shifted focus away from the art and science of the physical examination.

The fact that many asymptomatic subjects demonstrate clinically insignificant findings with advanced imaging modalities raises the question of whether these studies can discriminate between asymptomatic and symptomatic lesions.[88,89] This observation led Morris et al. to conclude: "Increasingly sophisticated radiology must be matched by improved clinical diagnosis if we wish to remain doctors caring for patients, rather than become technicians operating on radiologic abnormalities."[90]

Performing an effective examination in a meaningful sequence and timely fashion is the foundation of responsible patient management. Selection of relevant examination components is accomplished by knowledge of the sensitivity, specificity, and predictive value of the various interview interrogatives and examination procedures. When coupled with the appropriate imaging, a more accurate diagnosis may be formulated.

Practical clinical assessment of patients with suspected symptomatic disc disruption is designed to accomplish the following: (1) rule out those disorders that mimic disc disruption, (2) identify pain generators, (3) grade any neurological impairment, (4) define comorbid conditions or complicating factors that may influence patient management or clinical course, and (5) triage the patient for the appropriate treatment.

Anatomical Considerations (Nerve Root and Intervertebral Foramen)

Various combinations of pain, paresthesia, and weakness in the lumbopelvic region and lower limbs may result from IVD disruption. In order to better understand the clinical expression of a lumbar disc disruption, a brief review of the relevant anatomy is helpful.

The spinal cord ends at the conus medullaris (L1–L2 disc space) below which the lumbar and sacral nerve roots and rootlets descend inferiorly within the subarachnoid space of the lumbar cistern. Before exiting the neural foramen, the dorsal and ventral roots (rootlets) are accompanied by the radicular arteries and radicular veins within a dural root sleeve. This union occurs approximately at the level of the IVD of the cephalad vertebra. For example, the union of the L4 nerve occurs at L3–L4, then courses inferiorly and exit at the L4–L5 intervertebral foramen (IVF). A mixed spinal nerve is formed within the distal aspect of the funnel-shaped dural root sleeve at the level of the intervertebral foramen. At the lateral edge of the IVF, the dural sleeve becomes continuous with the epineurium of the mixed spinal nerve.[23]

Lumbar nerve roots are numbered by the vertebra below which they leave the spinal canal. That is, the L4 root exits between L4 and L5. The roots typically exit high in the intervertebral foramen, close against the pedicle. The IVD is located caudal to the exiting spinal nerve. Therefore, herniation of the disc at the level of a departing nerve may spare the exiting nerve root, but create a mass effect on the descending nerve root of the caudal level before it enters the IVF. On the other

TABLE 6–3. The Intervertebral Foramen, Their Occupying Nerve Roots, and the Spinal Nerve That May Be Affected by Disc Abnormality at That Level

Intervertebral Foramen/ Disc	Exiting Nerve Root	Nerve Root Affected by Paracentral HNP	Nerve Root Affected by Intraforaminal HNP
L2–L3	L2	L3	L2
L3–L4	L3	L4	L3
L4–L5	L4	L5	L4
L5–S1	L5	S1	L5

hand, when an intraforaminal herniation occurs, both the exiting and descending roots may be compressed (Table 6–3).

Clinical Pearl: The IVD is located caudal to the exiting spinal nerve. Herniation at the level of an exiting nerve root may spare that root, but create a mass effect on the descending nerve root of the caudal level before it enters the IVF.

History and Pain Distribution

The underlying pathological changes of lumbar disc disruption usually develop progressively and build without patient awareness. Symptoms may surface either insidiously or suddenly. The distribution of pain and other symptoms often provides insight into the severity and location of the disc lesion, and may be the most important factor in defining the anatomical diagnosis and prognosis.

Distribution of Pain in Internal Disc Disruption Internal disruption of a disc may present with pain across the lumbosacral junction that radiates to the upper buttock and groin. Extension into the posterior thigh is less common and rarely occurs below the knee.

Distribution of Pain in Disc Protrusion When a disrupted IVD protrudes, any resulting pattern of pain and/or paresthesia bears a relationship to its horizontal location. Central protrusions tend to cause LBP only; lateral protrusion may produce leg pain only; and intermediately located lesions may result in both back and lower limb involvement.[91] Leg pain may either be of referred or radicular origin. Referred pain does not necessarily follow the sciatic distribution. Radicular pain implies a specific nerve root source. The sensitivity (.98) and specificity (.88) of leg pain as the first indication of nerve root irritation is good.[92]

Clinical Pearl: Central disc protrusions tend to cause back pain only; lateral protrusions may produce leg pain only; intermediately located lesions may result in back and leg pain.

When nerve root involvement occurs, the distribution of limb pain appears to be of value in determining the pattern of the underlying disc pathology. For instance, patients who present with leg pain only, or with leg pain greater than back pain, have an extruded disc fragment at surgery (96% and 85% respectively). Also, patients with an extruded fragment usually experience improvement or resolution of the LBP as the leg pain develops.[93]

Pain distribution is valuable as it often suggests the level of a disc lesion. With monoradiculopathy, the involved vertebral level may be correctly predicted in up to 93% of cases.[94] When more than one nerve root becomes involved, the diagnostic value of pain distribution decreases.

Radicular pain does not always follow a clear dermatomal distribution. Pain projection to the first sacral nerve root distribution is the most common of all lumbar disc herniations and has been found to be an unreliable indicator of the level of disc herniation. On the other hand, pain projection along the L5 nerve root distribution has a predictive value equivalent to myelography for an L4–L5 disc lesion.[95]

Upper lumbar radiculopathy (L1–L3) radiates into the groin or anterior thigh. In these cases there is a gamut of differential diagnostic considerations that include primary hip and pelvis pathology, lumbar radiculopathy, femoral neuropathy, diabetic neuropathy, joint dysfunction from the sacroiliac and zygapophyseal joints, and myofascial pain syndromes.[96]

Pain diagrams are useful in documenting the location of back and lower limb pain. With L4–L5 lesions, 68% of patients mark the anterior leg (but 23% of those with an L5–S1 lesion mark this region). Posterior foot pain is marked in 85% of cases with L5–S1 lesions.[97]

The Physical Examination

Physical assessment attempts to identify the pain-generating tissue(s) and grade any degree of neurological impairment. This should include inspection, palpation, observed range of motion, posture and gait, neurological function screening and selective tissue stress tests.

Posture, Motion, and Palpation

Trunk listing or pelvic shift is commonly seen in disc syndromes, and is named by the direction of shift of the cephalad region. For instance, when the patient is bent to the right and unable to stand erect, a right lateral antalgia or list exists. Unfortunately, there is poor correlation between trunk list and the topographical location of a disc lesion (i.e., central, intermediate, lateral). However, it has been suggested that those patients with a gravity-induced trunk list (i.e., no list is present while recumbent) may have a worse prognosis for conservative management.[98,99] Takahashi et al. measured a twofold greater nerve root pressure at surgery in those patients with a trunk list.[100]

Patients with symptomatic disruption tend to avoid isolated lumbar flexion. Instead, forward bending may be accomplished through flexion of the hips and knees. The so-called Minor's sign is a nonspecific protective movement pattern that is observed while patients rise from seated positions. The patient self-supports on the healthy side, placing one hand on his or her back (the other on the thigh) and then simultaneously flexes the knee and extends the thigh of the affected limb while continuing to weight bear on the healthy side and "crawls" up the thigh.[101]

Palpation findings tend to be nonspecific, but patients with radiculopathy may have tenderness along the course of the sciatic nerve. Sitting is often uncomfortable and may elicit pain in the buttock and posterior thigh from pressure onto the sciatic nerve. Compression over the sciatic notch (the midpoint on a line drawn from the posterior superior iliac spine and ischial tuberosity) is frequently tender. Discrimination should be made from piriformis tenderness.

The common peroneal nerve, as it passes behind the proximal fibula, may also be tender to palpation. Patients frequently complain of burning, stinging, or aching pain in this region when lower lumbar or sacral nerve root irritation is present.

Neurological Assessment

Spinal nerve root irritation/inflammation may elicit pain into the corresponding dermatome. Compression of a spinal nerve causes varying combinations of sensory alterations (numbness, tingling, and hypesthesia), deep tendon reflex abnormality, and true or perceived muscular weakness.

The most significant expression of neural compromise is loss of bowel and/or bladder control (*cauda equina syndrome*), a situation that should prompt immediate surgical attention (see Table 6–4). In these cases symptoms occur acutely in about one third of patients. Symptoms become established in less than 24 hours in almost all cases. Most patients have bilateral leg pain, often one side worse than the other. Weakness in the foot and inability to stand is also common. Urological problems including retention or incontinence and saddle hypalgesia/anesthesia are typical. Bowel and sexual function abnormalities may not be recognized in the short development time frame. Prompt recognition of the clinical presentation and decompression is critical. About 60% of patients with

TABLE 6–4. Possible Bowel, Bladder, and Sexual Dysfunction Symptoms in Cauda Equina Syndrome

- Bowel
  - Unable to discriminate between feces and flatus
  - Soiling
  - Loss of desire to evacuate
- Bladder (urodynamic)
  - Retention (incomplete bladder emptying, straining to empty)
  - Irritation (nocturia, daytime frequency, urgency, urge incontinence)
  - Obstructive (weak stream, hesitancy, postmicturation dribbling)
- Sexual dysfunction
  - Difficult ejaculation
  - Incomplete erection
  - Vaginal anesthesia

bladder paralysis from cauda equina syndrome obtain incomplete recovery.[102]

Clinical Pearl: *Cauda equina syndrome* symptoms occur acutely without a history of back complaint in about one third of patients. In about 90% the symptoms are established in less than 24 hours. Most have bilateral leg pain, often worse on one side. Lower extremity weakness and inability to stand is common. Urological, bowel, and sexual function abnormalities may not be recognized in the short development time frame. Prompt recognition of the clinical presentation and decompression is critical.

Neurological assessment includes reflex, motor, and sensory testing (see Table 6–5 for a summary of neurological findings). Throughout this examination, consideration must be given to the patient's age, general health, and comorbidities that may alter the findings. The examiner also should bear in mind that some neural deficits may not be clinically definable, even in the presence of confirmed true nerve root compression/inflammation, and severe dermatomal pain.

Sensation Testing

Loss of sharp/dull discrimination or hypesthesia occurs in 38%–65% of patients with confirmed disc disruption (Table 6–6). However, pinprick sensibility testing of a dermatome is highly subjective and frequently misleading, and the accuracy of sensory findings in identifying the level of nerve compression may be as low as 50%.[106] When sensory deficits are present, they are usually accompanied by dermatomal pain projection and motor or reflex disturbance.[95]

TABLE 6–5. **Summary of Neurological Findings**

Herniation Level	Reflex	Sensation	Myotome	Pain Distribution
L3–L4	Patellar	Anterior thigh and medial foot (L4)	Quadriceps	
L4–L5	Medial Hamstring	Dorsum of the foot and web between the first and second digit (L5)	Extensor Hallucis	Anterior leg
L5–S1	Achilles	Lateral foot/small toe	Peroneal	Posterior foot

There is disagreement on the peripheral sensory distribution of the spinal nerve roots on published dermatomal maps, and studies of limb sensibility deficits from herniated lumbar discs often prove unrewarding. Because there is less dermatomal overlap along the distal distribution of a nerve root, these areas are targeted in the examination to help localize the level of a lesion: the lateral foot and small toe (S1), dorsum of the foot and web between the first and second digit (L5), and the anterior thigh and medial foot (L4).

Clinical Pearl: The far distal distributions of the peripheral sensory nerve roots are more reliable for localization because there is less dermatomal overlap.

Overall the positive predictive value for determination of disc herniation level based on sensory deficit findings is of limited value, but it is better for sensory deficits along the L5 dermatome than at S1 (.69 versus .50 positive predictive value, respectively).[107] Despite the relatively low sensitivity of traditional sharp/dull sensibility testing, it should not be eliminated from the clinical examination. It may be useful when ruling out other disorders such as peripheral neuropathy or compartment syndromes.

Motor Assessment

One should always inspect for objective signs of denervation such as atrophy or fasciculations in the corresponding myotome. Fasciculations may be elicited by lightly tapping the affected muscle (percussive myotonia). The impact of nerve root compression on the motor system is assessed through manual isometric strength testing of target muscles that are innervated in greater concentration from a single nerve root (Table 6–7). Manual strength assessment is highly variable and subjective, and as much as 25% of strength must be lost in order to be detected manually. Therefore subtle strength loss may easily be missed.[108] The patient may be asked to perform a short squat, heel walk, or toe walk. Subtle strength loss may be revealed by the fatigue characteristics by repeating these same maneuvers.[109] Pain-induced weakness (nociceptive inhibition) during muscle testing limits the usefulness of manual strength testing.

Clinical Pearl: Manual strength assessment is subjective and highly variable. As much as 25% strength loss is necessary to be detected. Repeated heel and toe walk maneuvers may help to detect subtle strength loss.

Considering the relative frequency of disc herniations at L4 and L5, strength of the extensor hallucis longus (EHL) must always be assessed. EHL loss is the primary objective indicator of possible L5 nerve root compression.

Patients with upper lumbar disc disruption with root involvement are more likely to have motor loss versus those with lower lumbar herniations. The quadriceps group is more frequently involved than any other muscle group.[110]

TABLE 6–6. **Summary of Examination Findings in Patients with Confirmed Lumbar Disc Herniation**[103]

Study	+SLR (%)	+XSLR (%)	Decreased Sensibility (%)	Paresis (%)	Achilles Areflexia (%)	Patellar Areflexia (%)	No Neurological Signs (%)
Spengler et al.[104]	96	60	—	37	41	—	22
Jonsson and Stromqvist[105]	88	23	65	50	49	11	—
Kortelainen et al.[95]	94	—	38	45	52	7	20
Vucetic and Svensson[103]	85	30	44	28	29	11	30

TABLE 6–7. Innervation of the Lower Extremity Musculature

Muscle	Motion	Nerve Levels	Key Level(s)
Iliopsoas	Hip flexion	L2–L3	L2–L3
Quadriceps*	Knee extension	L2–L4	L3–L4
Hamstrings*	Knee flexion	L5–LS1	S1
Tibialis anterior*	Ankle dorsiflexion	L4–L5	L4–L5
Gastrocnemius/soleus	Ankle plantarflexion	S1–S2	S1–S2
Peroneus longus	Foot eversion	L4–S1	L5–S1
Extensor hallucis longus*	Great toe extension	L5–S1	L5
Flexor hallucis longus	Great toe flexion	L5–S2	

*Recommended as part of routine motor assessment.

Muscle Stretch Reflexes (Deep Tendon Reflexes) An asymmetrically attenuated or absent muscle stretch reflex may be indicative of nerve root compression/inflammation. At the very minimum, the Achilles and quadriceps responses should be graded. The Achilles response correlates to the S1 nerve root and quadriceps response to L4 nerve root level. The absence of reflex deficit, however, does not rule out nerve root involvement (Table 6–8).

The patellar response is rarely affected by herniations at L5–S1 and infrequently at L4–L5.[95] If the descending S1 nerve is compressed by a herniation on its way to the L5–S1 intervertebral foramen, the patellar reflex may be lost. The Achilles reflex may be affected by L4–L5 herniations as well. High lumbar herniations rarely affect the Achilles response.[111,112]

Inclusion of the medial hamstring reflex in the neurological examination has been recommended on the basis of its high positive predictive value of L4 herniations (85%–89%), which tests the L5 nerve root.[113] In comparison, the positive predictive value of the Achilles reflex (S1) was 67%–84% (see Table 6–7 for a summary of the neurological findings).

Orthopedic Examination

Physical examination procedures used to evaluate individuals with suspected discogenic or nerve root pain rely on provocative compression, irritation, or stretching of sensitive tissues in an attempt to reproduce the patient's complaints. The two major structures that are assessed for reactivity are the disc and the nerve roots. For instance, local, central lumbosacral junction pain produced by overpressure at L5 relates more closely to disc disruption than to sacroiliac joint dysfunction.

Discogenic Pain Provocation One of the greatest challenges in clinical assessment of the patient with LBP is encountered when attempting to determine the tissue origin of nonradicular pain. Diagnostic consideration must be given to the nonmusculoskeletal structures, dura, osseous structures, sacroiliac joints, facet articulations, myofascial tissues, and the IVD itself.

A provocative discogram is considered the "gold standard" for determining pain of discogenic origin. Its use is often reserved as a presurgical study for patients failing a well-designed and executed conservative management program (see Chapter 17 for an in-depth consideration of the issues of discography). Physical examination procedures have been correlated with discography that may satisfy diagnostic curiosities in patients who are not clear surgical candidates. Correlations between discography, MRI and, physical examination findings have identified noninvasive procedures that offer promise in identifying pain of discogenic origin and predicting the degree of disc disruption.[114–117]

TABLE 6–8. The Prevalence of Reflex Deficit in Cases of Confirmed HNP

	L2–L3	L3–L4	L4–L5	L5–S1
Patellar, absent or weak; Hakelius and Hindmarsh[111]		14%	36%	3%
Achilles, absent or weak; Hakelius and Hindmarsh[111]		0%	14%	60%
Patellar, absent or weak; Kortelainen et al.[95]	37%	43%		6%

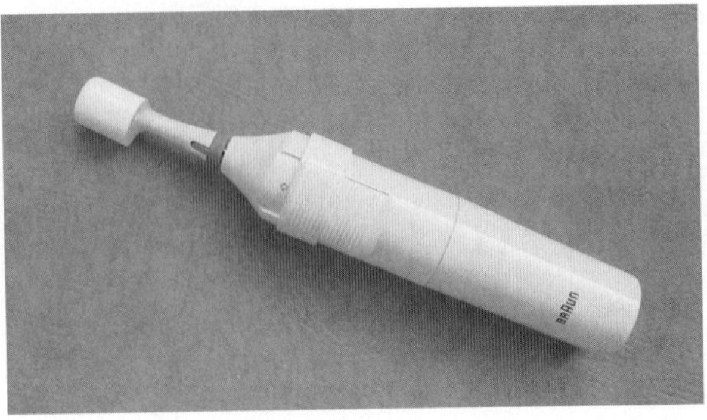

FIGURE 6–13. Braun™ electric toothbrush modified and fabricated with a blunted end used to deliver vibratory stimulation at the spinous process. This may elicit the pain associated with internal disc disruption. Such vibratory pain provocation agrees with discographic provocation in 70.9% of discs. This figure rises to 81.3% when relying on the vibratory pain provocation of discs with mild to moderate disruption on MRI.

Using a modified Braun™ electric toothbrush fabricated with a blunted end (Fig. 6–13) to deliver vibratory stimulation at the spinous process (in a lateral recumbent patient, symptomatic side down) may elicit the pain associated with internal disc disruption. Such vibratory pain provocation agrees with discographic provocation in 70.9% of discs. In contrast, the specificity of MRI compared with discographic findings was only 55.7%. This figure rises to 81.3% when relying on the vibratory pain provocation of discs with mild to moderate disruption. Sensitivity of the combined evaluation (MRI and vibratory test) was 85.9% and accuracy was 83.0%.[114]

When applied to patients without previously operated backs and prolapsed discs, a sensitivity of .96 and specificity of .72 may be expected. Prolapsed, but discographically painful discs are expected to be painless during the vibration test.[115] On the other hand, in cases of total anular rupture, a negative pain response does not exclude symptomatic anular damage.[117]

Clinical Pearl: In the presence of a partial IVD tear demonstrated on MRI, the bony vibration test helps determine the clinical significance of the lesion. The result of this test provides nearly the same information as provocative discography, *in the absence of prior back surgery*.

Pain responses during positional loading testing have also been correlated to provocative discography findings and provide some insight into the integrity of the anulus. The McKenzie assessment process has demonstrated the ability to reliably differentiate discogenic from nondiscogenic pain, and a competent from incompetent anulus.[116] Ninety-one percent of patients who experienced pain upon discography and centralization of pain on positional testing were found to have an intact anular wall. In contrast, only 54% of patients who had a positive discogram and peripheralized were found to have an intact anulus.

Neural Provocation Tests

Provocative neural tests attempt to produce neural tension, increase nerve root compression, increase intrathecal pressure, or cause dynamic changes in cerebrospinal fluid and epidural venous plexus pressure. These procedures may enhance radiating pain, paresthesia or sensory loss along the corresponding dermatome, in the lower back pain, or a combination of both.

Neural Tension Tests The most studied nerve tension sign is the straight-leg raising (SLR) test, referred to as the Lasegue's test by Forst (one of Lasegue's pupils) in 1864.[118] During this maneuver the examiner elevates the relaxed, straight leg of a supine patient and notes the location and pattern of any symptoms induced. The neck and contralateral lower limb should be in a neutral position. Reproduction or aggravation of lower limb pain or paresthesias along the distribution of an affected nerve root is considered a positive test. Maximal tension is placed on the S1 and L5 nerve roots. Traction upon the L4 nerve root is dependent on the concentration of sciatic nerve contribution. The lumbar nerve roots move about 4–8 mm within the IVF. Normally, the nerve roots remain stationary during the initial 30–40 degrees of straight leg elevation from horizontal. Rapid nerve root movement then occurs until 70 degrees of elevation, after which there is minimal, if any, further translation.[119]

Passive SLR also stresses the lumbopelvic and lower limb structures, including the hamstrings, hip, sacroiliac joint, lumbar paraspinal muscles and facet joints, for example. These should be considered in a differential diagnosis.

The degree of neural traction during limb elevation decreases with advancing age as a result of shortening of the spinal canal.[120]

SLR has been found to be positive in up to 96% of cases with confirmed herniated nucleus pulposis (HNP),[121] but *the absence of a positive SLR does not rule out the presence of an HNP*[91,122] and has been reportedly negative in up to 33% of confirmed cases.[123,124] Tables 6–9 and 6–10 summarize the specificity, sensitivity, positive and negative predictive values of the SLR and XSLR tests (see below).

Clinical Pearl: The absence of a positive SLR maneuver does not rule out disc herniation.

SLR is also performed on the asymptomatic limb, usually prior to the symptomatic side. If symptom

TABLE 6–9. Summary of Pooled Sensitivity and Specificity Assessments for SLR and XSLR

	SLR		XSLR	
Resource	**Sensitivity**	**Specificity**	**Sensitivity**	**Specificity**
Deville et al.[125]	.91	.26	.29	.88
van den Hoogen et al.[126]	1.0–.88	.11–.44	.23–.44	.86–.95
Andersson and Deyo[127]	.97–.72	.66–.11	.42–.23	1.0–.85

reproduction/exacerbation occurs in the affected limb during elevation of the symptom-free side, the result is documented as a positive "well leg raise," or "positive crossed leg raise" sign (XSLR). This sign is more often seen with very large disc extrusions and sequestration that often present in the "axilla" of the nerve root. Correlation with a poorer outcome to conservative management has been made.[99,128]

The XSLR is present in up to 40% of patients with a confirmed lumbar disc herniation[123] and one study identified a tendency toward centrally located protrusions.[91] Tables 6–8 and 6–9 summarize the specificity, sensitivity, positive and negative predictive values of the SLR and XSLR tests.

Severe limitation in SLR (under 30 degrees) appears more common with extruded/sequestered disc fragments.[129] A positive SLR has a nearly linear correlation with parameters that signify the level of pain, e.g., pain at rest, pain at night, pain upon coughing, and reduction of walking capacity.

A positive postoperative SLR has correlation with the degree of surgical success.[130] On 2-year assessment, those patients with a positive postoperative SLR had a reoperation rate of 18% compared to a 4.5% rate among those without a positive postoperative SLR.[131]

Restriction of limb elevation by hamstring tightness limits the validity of the SLR. In instances of overly tight hamstrings, neural slack may be removed through passive neck flexion or ankle dorsiflexion.

Patients under age 30 have an increased tendency for a positive SLR.[121] A negative test, however, excludes the presence of a disc herniation to a higher degree of probability. After age 30, the diagnostic value of a positive SLR increases, but a negative test does not exclude the diagnosis.[121]

Patients with upper lumbar involvement may experience no pain provocation or even relief upon SLR testing. In order to stretch the upper lumbar nerve roots, tension is transmitted through the femoral nerve. Tension may be applied to the L4 and L5 root through the femoral nerve traction test. During this maneuver, the patient lies on the affected side with the neck fully flexed (placing tension on the cauda equina). The painful extremity is gently hyperextended to approximately 15 degrees at the hip, followed by passive knee flexion of about 90 degrees. Pain along the anteromedial thigh, groin, or hip may be indicative of an upper lumbar nerve root involvement. A crossed femoral nerve stretch test may also be present, with the patient remaining on the symptom side, which is the equivalent of the XSLR.[132,133] The same maneuver may be accomplished with the patient laying prone, while applying counterpressure on the buttock ("bent-knee pulling" test).[134]

Confirmatory Maneuvers Several helpful confirmatory maneuvers also may be performed in conjunction with the SLR in order to rule out pain sources other than the lumbar nerve roots. For instance, after the SLR is performed, the straightened limb is lowered several degrees, until the pain abates and

TABLE 6–10. Positive and Negative Predictive Values of SLR and XSLR

	SLR		XSLR	
	+ Predictive Value	**− Predictive Value**	**+ Predictive Value**	**− Predictive Value**
Deville et al.[125]	.89 (.86)*	.33 (.86)	.92 (.82)	.22 (.82)
Andersson and Deyo[127]	.67†	.57	.79	.44

*Value in parentheses represents the prevalence.
†Considering a 60

passive ankle dorsiflexion is performed (Braggard's or Fajersztajn's test).[135,136] Neck flexion or medial hip rotation (Bonnet's test)[137] may be used in conjunction with the SLR.

The bowstring (Cram) maneuver is an excellent confirmatory test performed after a positive SLR. The knee and hip are flexed and pain abates. Manual thumb pressure is then applied to the popliteal region (posterior tibial nerve). Reproduction of back and/or leg pain is reportedly more specific for nerve root compression from a herniated lumbar disc.[138] A variation of the bowstring test may be performed in the sitting position. While the patient sits in an erect position, the examiner slowly extends the affected lower limb to the point of pain reproduction. Sciatic nerve tension is then relieved by slightly bending the knee, and posterior tibial nerve compression is applied in the popliteal fossa. Jugular compression may also be substituted for popliteal compression, which increases intrathecal pressure.[139] These seated tests are reported to be more specific for nerve root compression, as the myofascial structures of the lumbar spine and hip are not stressed while sitting.

Clinical Pearl: The bowstring sign is an excellent confirmatory maneuver, and is performed after a positive SLR. It is more specific for nerve root involvement as the myofascial structures are stressed differently with this test.

Neural provocation and confirmatory movements may be combined or "stacked" in order to elicit more subtle nerve root irritation. An example is the "slump test" during which the patient sits on the examination table while the affected limb is passively straightened, internally rotated, and the ankle dorsiflexed while at the same time the neck is actively flexed and the patient performs a Valsalva maneuver.[140]

Clinical Pearl: Combining the leg signs into a single maneuver increases sensitivity. For instance, SLR performed with ankle dorsiflexion, hip adduction, and internal rotation is more sensitive than each maneuver performed individually.

Alteration in Jugular Venous Pressure Application of jugular vein compression is another means to elicit or relieve the extremity symptoms resultant from disc herniation and nerve root compression. Originally, this test was performed using a blood pressure cuff around the neck inflating to 40 mmHg.[141] Today, light paratracheal pressure on the external jugular veins is used to dampen the venous return. Operative studies have demonstrated that jugular venous pressure produces engorgement of the upper attachment of the extradural nerve, carrying it laterally.[112] The patient should be told to expect a typical feeling of intracranial pressure. Any change in limb symptoms should be reported.

Neural Compression Testing For identifying cases of subtle neural compression, Herron and Pheasant use a "prone knee flexion provocation test." The patient lies prone on the examination table and the knees are bilaterally hyperflexed by the examiner so that the heels approximate the buttock. After maintaining this position for 45–60 seconds, the knees are extended and the reflexes (Achilles and patellar) and strength (EHL, tibialis anterior, gastrocnemius/soleus) are reassessed. Increase in distal weakness or reflex attenuation/obliteration is considered a positive test. This maneuver may be more applicable to cases of suspected stenosis.[142]

Intrathecal Pressure Changes Discogenic radicular pain that is aggravated by coughing, sneezing, and bearing down (each being a Valsalva maneuver) has been referred to as Dejerine's triad. Coughing and sneezing raise the intra-abdominal pressure that distends the epidural venous plexus, which is in continuity with the veins on the posterior abdominal wall. Coughing displaces the thecal sac cranially for up to one to two disc spaces, tractioning the nerve roots. Simultaneously, the activated musculature of the "pressurized canister" (abdominals, multifidii, pelvic floor, and thoracoabdominal diaphragm) cause increased intradiscal pressure.[143] Patients with leg pain and/or paresthesia upon coughing have been found to be more likely to have extruded/sequestered herniations.[129]

In many instances treatment can be initiated with a high degree of diagnostic certainty upon completion of the examination. Clinical suspicions may arise that warrant diagnostic investigations beyond the core orthopedic and neurological examination (e.g., patients who do not respond to a reasonable trial of therapy, have undergone prior surgery, present with coexisting health concerns, or react uncharacteristically to the clinical evaluation). Diagnostic imaging and laboratory studies, while important in their own right, do not replace a thorough history and physical examination.

MANAGEMENT OF DISC DISRUPTION SYNDROMES

The current body of knowledge regarding IVD pathology and management has advanced substantially during the past decade. Understanding of the natural history of disc disruption has narrowed the selection criteria for those needing surgical intervention. Patients once categorized as candidates for surgery may now be effectively managed conservatively with equal, or better outcomes. In the absence of bladder or bowel incontinence (cauda equina syndrome) or progressive neurological deficit, most patients are suitable for a 2- to 3-month trial of conservative management before proceeding with surgery.[144]

The Natural History of Herniated Lumbar Discs

Disc disruptions exhibit a positive natural history for clinical improvement.[145] Nevertheless there may be questions that confront the clinician when managing patients with symptomatic disc disruptions. Will strength and sensory loss return? How long should conservative care extend before opting for surgery? What are the risks of permanent nerve damage or adhesions? What if surgery is delayed? Until recently, these questions have remained unanswered. There is also the question of when surgery may be premature? Findings on advanced imaging studies, acute symptoms, and patient insistence often prompt unnecessary surgery. In Weber's epic 10-year prospective study, "60 percent of the operated patients may have been submitted to an unnecessary procedure."[146]

Change in the Mass Effect of Herniated Discs Regression in the size of an extruded nucleus with abatement of radiculopathy is common.[147] In one series of herniated and sequestered discs demonstrated on CT imaging, 76% regressed or completely resolved. Large extrusions are expected to decrease to a greater degree than bulging discs.[148] Maximum shrinkage of extrusions is observed in the cephalocaudad dimension and to a lesser degree in the anteroposterior dimension. Clinical improvement and morphological change, however, do not necessarily follow a parallel time course. While the precise mechanism by which resorption of herniated nuclear material is not totally understood, neovascularization and macrophage infiltration have been observed.

Patterns of Symptom Resolution Saal et al. described three clinical improvement patterns with time frames of clinical and symptom resolution that may assist in patient education and treatment selection.[149]

Pattern I has mild neurological deficits such as sensory loss with or without a single grade of motor loss and will improve in 6–12 weeks. Abolished muscle stretch reflexes rarely return to normal.

Pattern IA begins with acute, severe pain, often with a combination of low back and lower limb pain. The acute phase persists for 1–2 weeks with or without the assistance of treatment. A relatively painless mild neurological deficit may remain that resolves over the following 6–12 weeks.

Pattern IB begins with acute, severe pain and is often associated with neurological deficit that does not abate despite the passage of time and nonoperative management. This pattern is frequently associated with a sequestered fragment.

Pattern 2 begins insidiously and is moderate in pain intensity. It remains constant until treated. Effective treatment may require several months and has the highest recurrence rate of these improvement patterns. Pattern 2 corresponds to contained disc herniations or small extrusions (moderate neurological loss, such as absent muscle stretch reflex with more than one grade of motor loss; complete resolution in 3–6 months with a gradual improvement of motor strength).

Pattern 3 begins insidiously with mild to moderate pain. The duration is 6–12 weeks and the symptoms spontaneously resolve. This represents small, contained herniations, but may be associated with all types (severe neurological loss to Grade 3 or below and may require as much as 1 year to full, or occasionally partial recovery).[149]

Residuals and Response to Treatment Appropriately selected patients with uncontained herniations may be treated without surgery, if the patient can tolerate the symptoms for the first 2 months. It is rare for patients with uncontained herniation to require surgery in the first 4 months or more after the onset of symptoms.[44]

Other interesting related statistical information is found in the literature. For instance, the prognosis is better if the anulus is ruptured versus bulged, if there is no preoperative comorbidity (uncontrolled hypertension, unstable angina, etc.), and when the patient is male.[150] Women and patients with severely limited SLR tend to have a higher operation rate, and males and younger patients have a better outcome to nonoperative management.[148] Also, physically fit patients have a better outcome at 4 years, regardless of the treatment chosen.[146] The conservative management of far lateral disc herniations is successful in about 70% of cases.[151]

In general, patients with symptomatic disc disruptions may be advised that, with or without surgery, existing muscle weakness will progressively improve over the first 4 years, but some degree of weakness remains in less than 10% of patients. Thirty-five percent of patients may continue to have sensory deficit at 10-year follow-up. Furthermore, there is no pain or spinal mobility difference at 10-year follow-up between surgically and nonsurgically managed patients.[146] Also, nonsurgical management does not appear to lead to perithecal or perineural fibrosis.[69]

Conservative Management Strategies

Considering the favorable outcome of disc herniations, clinicians must give consideration to the goals of treatment, and work to expedite the natural history,

TABLE 6–11. Conservative Treatment Options for Patients with Symptomatic Disc Disruption

Pharmacological	Physical Treatment	Minimally Invasive
NSAIDs	Positional release	Epidural steroids
Oral steroids	McKenzie exercises	Selective nerve root block
Non-narcotic analgesics	Williams exercises	Laser ablation
Narcotic medications	Manipulation/mobilization	Nucleoplasty
Anticonvulsants	Manual	
	Mechanical assisted	
	Exercise programs	
	Therapeutic modalities	
	Traction	
	Braces	
	Bed rest	

provide pain relief, reduce the potential for surgery, improve quality of life, and limit the loss of productivity.

There are many conservative treatment options, many of which are discussed in greater detail elsewhere in this text. Little uniformity, however, is observed among professionals providing spine care. The care modality selected is most likely to reflect the discipline of the patient's entry contact into the health-care system. Conservative strategies may be subdivided into pharmacological, physical medicine, and minimally invasive approaches (see Table 6–11). A number of alternative and eclectic treatments also are available.

Two broad diagnostic categories are encountered when treating patients with disc pathologies: (1) primary discogenic pain and (2) radiculopathy with or without discogenic pain. Each may prompt different therapy selections. Regardless of how the treatment is balanced with complimentary procedures, the most important underlying principle is to "centralize," "stabilize," and "mobilize." Whether the pain is of radicular or referred origin, symptom relief should be pursued using the concept of *centralization*. Then, as soon as possible, core exercises, lumbopelvic stabilization exercises, and later cardiovascular fitness aid in restoring functional capacity. Patients should be motivated to actively participate in the recovery process and to remain *mobile* to avoid reliance on passive care efforts. Finally, passive mobilization techniques are administered to restore optimal articular function and myofascial flexibility (Table 6–12).

The Centralization Phenomenon The phenomenon known as *centralization* was described by McKenzie[152] as a recession of radiating symptoms (pain or paresthesia) from the periphery to the midline during mechanical load assessment or treatment. The reference point of "peripheral" is dynamic and may begin as far distally as the leg or foot, or as proximal as the buttock. As the symptoms centralize and regress proximally, they may become intensified, improve, or remain the same. On the other hand, *peripheralization* means increasing distal symptomatology. Centralization is the desired result of treatment. Activities that cause peripheralization are to be avoided and those that result in centralization are performed more frequently.

Centralization has proved to be a useful tool in assessment and treatment of patients with acute and chronic central, radicular, and referred pain syndromes. It has value in predicting patient's prognosis and in correlation with advanced imaging findings. Despite clinical experience level and training, when operational definitions are used (i.e., "centralization,"

TABLE 6–12. Conservative Strategies Based upon Phase of Treatment

Centralize	Stabilize	Mobilize
Positional release (flexion and extension protocols)	Core exercises	Mobilization
Epidural steroid injections	Lumbopelvic stabilization exercises	Manipulation
Oral anti-inflammatory agents	Bracing/taping	Mechanized tables
Selective nerve root blocks		
Activity modulation		Cardiovascular conditioning

"peripheralization," or "status quo"), the reliability of judgment of centralization during movement testing is excellent (87.8%).[153]

Clinical Pearl: The concept of centralization is fundamental in the assessment and treatment phase. Its value in predicting outcome is significant.

Even at the initial assessment, the concept of centralization has proved to be a valuable tool in predicting the outcome and prognosis of both patients with acute LBP and patients with chronic LBP. In general, centralizers have a better rating improvement in pain intensity and return to work rate following an interdisciplinary work-hardening program compared to noncentralizers.[154] In the acute state, noncentralizers have a tendency toward chronicity. Those classified as noncentralizers continued to report pain symptoms, have extended activity interference or downtime at home, and continued to use health-care resources. Having leg pain at intake was also a predictor of those who had high sick leave and downtime at work (four times greater than those without it)[155] (see Chapter 15 for details of McKenzie assessment protocols, and Chapter 22 for McKenzie treatment protocols).

Exercise-Based Programs Injury and reflex pain inhibition may result in loss of dynamic and anatomical stability of the lumbar spine. Recent investigations have identified key dynamic stabilizer muscles that may be trained and rehabilitated to volitionally override this loss. Through a skillfully designed and administered rehabilitation program, patients may attain greater functional stability, relieve LBP, and reduce risk of recurrence.

Clinical Pearl: A well-designed and administered spine stabilization rehabilitation program is a vital component of the early treatment plan.

Low impact aerobic exercises such as walking or swimming are recommended early on. Core stabilizer muscle activation should also be initiated on the first point of contact in order to minimize loss of dynamic stabilization control (see Chapters 28 and 29). As core stability is gained, progressive functional perturbations are added to challenge and progress core stabilization. Finally, endurance, strength, and task-specific training is completed to restore functional capacity. Ergonomic advice is provided throughout the course of care.

A cohort retrospective study of patients with lumbar disc herniation and radiculopathy treated by back school and stabilization training demonstrated a 90% good to excellent outcome and 92% return to work rate among patients. Of those patients with neurological loss, extruded fragments and seeking second opinion, there were good to excellent outcomes in 87% and 83% of patients with a 100% return to work rating.[156]

Physiotherapeutic Modalities Physical medicine therapeutic modalities such as cold/thermal agents and transcutaneous electrical nerve stimulation are often administered to patients experiencing painful disc disruption. Although these agents may provide temporary palliation and assist the short-term therapeutic process, none have proved to independently contribute to cumulative therapeutic progress.

One study suggested that therapeutic ultrasound aids in decreasing the LBP associated with a disc herniation.[157] Patient tolerance to manual procedures may be improved after administration of cryo, thermal, or electrical modalities.

The duration of passive therapeutic modality usage should be limited in order to avoid fostering clinician dependence. When beneficial, patients may use ice or heat at home.

Spinal Orthoses and Bracing The use of spinal orthoses remains a topic of debate among spine care practitioners. Although it is generally accepted that elastic corsets are of little value in preventing low back injury, some back pain sufferers report a reduction in pain and a sense of greater stability while wearing a lumbar corset.

Patients with chronic discogenic LBP may benefit from a rigid custom lumbar jackets, such as the "chair-back" type brace. Factors to consider when selecting a brace include ease of application, patient fit/comfort, compliance, and cost. There tends to be an inverse relationship between comfort and degree of motion restriction.[158] Off-the-shelf products are also available that closely match the support of custom products. Unloading braces are also available that are designed to apply continuous low-grade traction to the lumbar spine.

Kinesiotaping™ may be used in conjunction with other therapies. Using a highly adhesive tape with strong tensile properties, two parallel paraspinal strips are applied along each side of the spine, on top of a previously taped "X" that crosses at L3. When the patient attempts to flex the lumbar spine, pulling of the tape provides mechanoreceptive feedback and an enhanced sense of positional awareness.

Traction Traction has been shown to separate vertebrae, decrease intradiscal pressure,[159] reduce electromyographic paraspinal activity,[160] and retract herniated disc material.[161] Presumably, traction reduces the size of a disc herniation and decompresses nerve roots. Clinicians must be aware that if traction is applied so that the back muscles contract, disc pressures may increase rather than decrease.[162]

Only two decades ago, patients with disc disruption pain were hospitalized for several weeks in order to administer continuous lumbar traction, a practice that has never proven effective. A controlled trial of continuous lumbar traction in the treatment of back pain and sciatica showed similar improvements in both the treated and control groups.[163]

Various forms of traction may be used in the management of disc disruption. Simple inexpensive home units are available, while sophisticated devices are quite costly. A number of different patient positions may be assumed while applying traction forces. Included are inverted, standing, prone, or supine. Forces may be applied by the patient (auto-traction), clinician, mechanically, or in combination.

Home inversion devices have shown to distract the lower lumbar intervertebral spaces between 0.3 and 4.0 mm. Although these devices make home lumbar traction practical, patients should be under medical supervision because of the possible side effects including hypertension and headache.[164] In one study, periorbital and pharyngeal petechiae, persistent headaches, persistent blurred vision, and contact lens discomfort were also reported.[165]

Traction may also be accomplished through an unloading device that is used while the patient is ambulatory on a treadmill. The degree of unloading can be adjusted to a percentage of the body weight.

Spinal Manipulation Manipulation includes various manual procedures including those with unloaded spinal motion, manually assisted passive motion, and manipulation. The latter includes both standard static high-velocity, low-amplitude (HVLA) thrusting and dynamic motion-assisted HVLA. Some techniques require the use of specially equipped tables that assist in delivering the treatment force.

Debate continues regarding the appropriateness of delivering an HVLA thrust and would consider it to be a relative or absolute contraindication, or of questionable value.[149] Practitioners of spinal manipulation need to be cognizant of a number of reported professional liability cases claiming injury to the lumbar discs during spinal manipulation. Rather than regarding manipulation to be unconditionally safe and effective in the treatment of all cases of lumbar disc herniation, consideration must be given to the biomechanics of manipulation as they apply in an individual patient's condition.[166]

Triano contends that skilled manipulative procedures can be performed safely and successfully in these types of cases using clinical judgment following provocative testing procedures of patient tolerance.[167] The authors' own similar experience with complex cases has demonstrated great success in carefully selected patients using clinically appropriate techniques.

A variety of manipulative procedures have been described in the literature and are taught in institutions of manual therapy. The examiner must first identify a clinically significant functional spinal lesion. This lesion may be at the level of the disc herniation, at an adjacent motor segment, or in a remote location. Patient position for receiving treatment include prone, side posture, or supine.

In preparation for a side-posture manipulation, the patient is positioned in a lateral recumbent position lying on the scapula and posterolateral buttock. The functional lesion is positioned away from the plinth. Slight gapping of the facet articulations may be achieved through passive hip flexion. Before administering any manipulative force, graded premanipulative stressing is performed. Low-grade oscillatory stresses within the functional boundaries of the joint determine anticipated patient tolerance to the procedure. If the patient is intolerant to the premanipulative stressing, or if peripheralization of pain occurs, position modification is made and premanipulative tolerance reassessed. With proper positioning in the absence of peripheralization or marked increased local pain, a short-amplitude, high-velocity manipulative force focused on a specific spinal segment is often possible.

Side posture lumbar techniques may produce significant rotational components. On the other hand, sacroiliac joint techniques may be applied with little rotatory force. Axial rotation and compressive disc loading has been implicated as a risk for anular tear. The orientation of the posterior facets may prevent rotation necessary for anular injury.[168] The work of Adams and Hutton maintains that rotation is limited to 2–3 degrees, barring facet fracture.[169] While only 2–3 degrees of rotation occurs because of facet contact, in some cases of severe disc degeneration, up to 7.7 degrees may be possible.[170]

Cassidy questioned how the small amounts of rotation induced by side posture manipulation could damage or irritate a healthy disc. Observations of 14 HNP patients receiving a 2- to 3-week regimen of daily side posture manipulation revealed 13 of them to obtain significant clinical improvement and relief of pain. The appearance of the disc herniation on CT did not change following manipulation.[171]

Manipulation is not without remotely possible complication, the most serious of which has been cauda equina syndrome. Lumbar radiculopathy with disc extrusion is not a categorical contraindication to HVLA manipulation, but the suspicion of cauda equina syndrome or progressive neurological deficit warrants surgical consultation. If a patient responds adversely to a manual procedure, reassessment and treatment modification is necessary.

The mechanism by which manipulation might reduce a disc herniation remains unclear. For those patients with active pain generators at articular components, improvement following manipulation likely relates to the restoration of optimal arthrokinematics of mechanically dysfunctional joints.

There is a paucity of studies investigating the administration of spinal manipulation to patients with symptomatic disc disruption. Careful examination of the literature on this topic makes it clear that it is difficult to compare the results of the studies because of the various techniques used. No controlled trial of HVLA treatment has been reported.

There are a number of case reports that detail successful relief of radicular pain following spinal manipulative procedures, or treatment including spinal manipulation.[172,173] Manipulation may be performed under general anesthesia or combined with other treatment modalities such as epidural steroid injections.

In a priori analysis of patients treated at a chiropractic care clinic, 44 of 3531 patients satisfied the clinical diagnostic criteria of lumbar disc herniation with radiculopathy and had sufficient documentation to estimate outcome. Manipulation was administered to 93%. Thirty-three of the 44 patients reported improvement in their condition and demonstrated an increase in straight-leg raising and lumbar spine motion.[174]

Mensor administered rotary lumbar mobilizations under anesthesia as one component in the management of patients clinically diagnosed with disc herniations. Of 205 patients, 52% achieved satisfactory results (27% excellent and 24% good).[175] Using a variety of mobilization and gentle manipulation procedures, Kuo and Luo reported a 76.8% "acceptable result" following treatment. Unfortunately, the details of this study were not clearly reported.[176]

Manipulation under Anesthesia Manipulation under general anesthesia has been administered for lumbar HNP as early as 1964. Immediate pre- and postmanipulation under anesthesia myelograms were performed in one investigation. More than 50% of patients experienced immediate sciatic pain reduction. Significant improvements were observed in deep tendon reflexes, sensory changes, and SLR testing. Of those patients with positive myelograms prior to manipulation, about 30% improved. During surgery, patients were also placed in a side posture manipulation position. Neither the nerve root nor the disc protrusion moved perceptibly, but the laminae separated by as much as 5 mm, markedly stretching the lower fibers of the ligamentum flavum and the superior lateral joint capsule. The best results were observed in the patient group without myelographic evidence of disc protrusion.[177]

Using SLR and lumbar range of motion as objective outcomes, Nwuga compared the results of manipulation versus conventional therapy (diathermy, pelvic tilt exercises, postural education, and lifting instructions) for patients with myelographic and electrodiagnostically confirmed lumbar disc herniations. The manipulation treatment group (MTG) received side posture oscillatory mobilization and the conventional treatment group (CTG) received diathermy, isometric exercises, and lifting/postural education. In all outcomes parameters, the MTG patient's outcomes exceeded those of the other group. The mean improvement in SLR increased 39 degree in the MTG, compared to 4 degree in the CTG. Total flexion and extension improvements were 34 degree versus 13degree respectively.[178]

Outcome comparison between spinal manipulation and chemonucleolysis for lumbar HNP favored the cost-saving benefits of manipulation. Equal 12-month outcomes were achieved, although manipulation/flexion-distraction provided a better short-term relief and disability benefit.[179]

Case studies have been published on the positive outcomes of flexion-distraction therapy, a therapeutic concept introduced by McManus and later promoted and expanded by Cox, in treating patients with lumbar disc herniations.[172,173,180–182] For this procedure, the patient is positioned prone on a table that is designed to allow the practitioner to administer controlled flexion, extension, side bending, rotation, flexion, and axial distraction forces through a mobile pelvic section. Straps may be used to secure the ankles in order to amplify the mobilization. By placing the heel of the hand on interspinous space the mobilization force may be concentrated on a spinal region or level. Also, the thoracic section of the table may be adjusted to modify the treatment force. Some tables are motorized and are used to accomplish continuous passive end range spinal motion.

Epidural Steroid Injections Epidural steroid injections (ESIs) are commonly used in an attempt to relieve back and lower limb pain associated with disc disruption with or without nerve root involvement. This topic is addressed in detail in Chapter 24. The therapeutic mechanism appears to be reduction in inflammation of the affected neural tissues and neighboring structures. Once limited to patients with radicular pain, ESI may also be administered to those with primary low back and buttock pain.

Two injection routes may be used: a direct spinal approach at the level of the disc disruption, or at the sacrococcygeal hiatus (caudal approach). The procedure is performed under local anesthesia and mild general sedation is optional. It is recommended that the procedure be performed under fluroscopic guidance. When performed without fluroscopic guidance, up to 35% are administered to the incorrect location compared to only 3% with fluoroscopic visualization.

The ESI procedure tends to be well tolerated. Only about 12% of patients rate them to be significantly uncomfortable. Early satisfaction is reported, but satisfaction tends to decrease 3 months after the procedure, with 17% unsatisfied and 48%–50% reporting good to excellent satisfaction. Immediate improvement is greater than that measured at 3 months.[183] The complication rate is rather low with adverse responses including dural tap (2.5%), transient headache (2.3%), and transient increase in pain (1.9%). There are no long-term adverse events recorded.[184] Improvement may not be noted for 6 days following the injection.[185] In general, the number of injections provided annually is limited to three. Some practitioners order three simultaneously, spaced 2 weeks apart. Others prefer to proceed with individual injections and await clinical response. Many patients prosper with a single injection.

Viton et al. also reported a statistically significant decrease in mean VAS score following periradicular corticosteroid injections for lumbar radiculopathy in 90% of patients. At 90-day follow-up, 85% continued to report a significant improvement.[186]

Few studies demonstrate long-term benefits of lumbar epidural steroid injections for radicular pain. Papagelopoulos et al. reported that early pain relief may be anticipated after injections in 80% of patients and that 68% were asymptomatic at long-term follow-up.[187] The odds ratio for short-term near or total relief was 2.79 (95% CI) and for long-term relief was 1.87.[184]

From these various data, it appears that ESIs may provide some short benefit to some patients with acute radiculopathy.

Clinical Pearl: Any short-term benefit that is gained may significantly aid the patient in tolerating symptoms during management and the natural history evolution.

Conservative Management of Discogenic Pain/Disc Disruption Syndrome There is another clinical pattern of internal disc disruption in addition to the more classical disc protrusion/extrusion syndromes. This pattern includes those patients who have an extended history of recurrent episodic, or even chronic, pain. For some time symptoms may have been successfully managed with manipulation. As recurrences occur, however, the results and pattern of symptomatic improvement changes, and manipulation becomes progressively less effective, and possibly aggravating. Benefits attained from a procedure may be only transient. These types of cases tend to exhibit back pain greater pain, and acute radicular symptoms are uncommon. Response to ESI is often minimal. It is likely that this pattern compare with the "instability" phase of disc degeneration in the Kirkaldy-Willis scheme. In a study of 10 such cases, Triano found some temporary relief in 80%.[188]

There is no data on the long-term treatment of these cases with nonoperative means. The natural history, of course, would predict eventual stabilization. The ineffectiveness of manipulation and persistent and often disabling pain often impels the frustrated patient to have a spinal fusion procedure. For conservative management to succeed, the primary treatment strategy must shift strongly to stabilization efforts. While continuous passive motion, manual, and physiotherapeutic modalities may be beneficial early on, they become less important except to control symptoms following exacerbation. Bracing may be helpful at times of stressful activity. In actual practice, patients improve following implementation of two major strategies: first, extended and advanced stabilization rehabilitation; second, and often most important, the patient must be willing to make substantial changes in their occupational or avocational activities.

Intradiscal Electrothermal Therapy (Anuloplasty) Intradiscal electrothermal therapy (IDET) or anuloplasty is a recently developed technique which is an alternative to interbody fusion for patients with chronic discogenic LBP. It is discussed in depth in Chapter 24, with further commentary in Chapter 34. The objective of the procedure is denervation of painful tissue and improvement of motion segment stability. Through the administration of a controlled dosage of thermal energy to the region of an anular tear, IDET may shrink collagen, cauterize granulation tissue, and coagulate nerve tissue to provide relief.

Patient selection for IDET is strict. It may be recommended for patients with chronic LBP (>6 months) who have exhausted conservative management options including ESI/oral steroids, who do not have neural tension signs, and have a positive provocative discogram.

Saal and Saal describe the protocol for IDET.[189] While under local anesthesia and using fluoroscopic guidance, a 17-guage thin-wall needle is placed into the center of the disc to be treated. A navigable intradiscal catheter with a temperature-controlled thermal resistive coil is then deployed through the needle and maneuvered intradiscally under two-plane fluoroscopic control. The catheter is placed adjacent to the inner posterior anulus.

The catheter temperature is then gradually raised to 90°C over a course of 13 minutes and maintained for 4 minutes to heat the adjacent tissues to 60–65°C.

A prophylactic dosage of cefazolin is administered to prevent infection.

Patients undergoing IDET typically begin to experience varying levels of improvement within 2–3 months that continues until about 6 months. Improvements have been measured in pain severity, sitting tolerance, analgesic consumption, and return to work in 75%–80% of patients in controlled trials.

There have been two published randomized controlled trials of IDET.[189,190] Both demonstrated statistically significant improvements in pain level. In the study by Saal and Saal, 80% improved.[189] Karasek and Bogduk demonstrated that a decrease in VAS of at least 50% correctly predicted return to work in all cases. Sixty percent of patients appreciated at least 50% reduction in pain, and 23% reported total relief.[190] A 2-year minimum follow-up study demonstrated a statistically significant improvement in pain, physical function, and quality of life.[191]

IDET is not without potential complications. One case of cauda equina syndrome was reported in the literature following the procedure when the thermal catheter was accidentally placed into the spinal canal. Although it was successfully relocated prior to the heating protocol, the complication was permanent.[192] The number of reported cases of complication from IDET is expected to rise as it gains popularity and clinicians of varying skill begin to perform the procedure.

Precisely how IDET works remains unclear. Human cadaver studies of the acute effects of IDET on motor unit biomechanics and anular architecture have produced conflicting results. In one study, spinal stiffness was found to *decrease* by 6%–12% after the heating protocol, and in no case did it increase spinal stiffness.[193] In another study, there was no significant change in the stability of the spine before and after IDET, and that the spinal segments were not destabilized.[194]

Does IDET alter the anulus? One study found that the anular architecture was not grossly affected in the vicinity of the catheter by the heating protocol. The temperatures sufficient to denature collagen (60–65°C) were not achieved at any site other than the catheter itself during the described protocol. The author concluded that the acute effects of IDET are limited to a small area around the catheter (1–2 mm).[193] Yet, in another study, there was denaturation shrinkage and coalescence of anular collagen. Extensive collagen disorganization, decreased quantity of collagen, collagen fibrils shrinkage, and chondrocyte damage were all seen when compared to the controls. IDET was found to raise temperatures sufficiently to induce collagen denaturation and coalescence.[195]

Further investigation into the outcomes, indications, and physiologic response to IDET must be made. Currently, it appears to be a useful procedure for a select group of patients with LBP. The histology and loading studies performed to date have been on cadaver samples and may not accurately reflect in vivo changes. Although stabilization could not be demonstrated in the current study, stiffening may occur after biological remodeling.[193]

Surgical Management of Painful Lumbar Disc Disruption

As previously stated, the natural history of disc disruption favors long-term recovery. However, patients who undergo laminectomy/discectomy report higher short-term (1 year) satisfaction and improved quality of life and physical function than those who opt to avoid surgery.[196] For a complete discussion of surgical issues, see Chapters 32 and 33. Few nonsurgically treated patients experience worsened pain or require subsequent surgery and 20% of the surgically treated patients report no improvement.[145]

Based on work capacity, neurological deficits, pain, and spinal mobility, surgery appears to provide patients with a greater early improvement over nonsurgically managed patients. This improvement favors the surgically treated patient over 4 years, but, by 10 years, there is little difference between the two groups.[146]

Patients treated surgically for discogenic pain undergo a variety of fusion procedures or prosthetic disc replacement.

Postoperative Imaging

For several weeks after surgery, the MRI appearance of immature scar and hematoma may be very similar to that of the original HNP and interpretation must be made with great care. Features seen at this time in asymptomatic patients may be similar to those in failed back surgery syndrome.[197] This extradural soft tissue mass effect usually decreases 2–6 months postoperatively, but occasionally may be seen for as long as 1 year. Afterwards there is progressive loss of enhancement and resorption or contraction of the soft tissue mass on sequential MR studies.

Epidural fibrosis may be in continuity with the parent disc, producing a mass effect. The epidural scar, however, is usually irregularly marginated compared with the smoother configuration of a recurrent herniation. A hypointense rim adjacent to the increased signal intensity of the new herniation may demarcate a recurrent disc herniation. Peripheral enhancement at the site of the original disc herniation usually decreases by 3 months postoperatively.

Both symptomatic and asymptomatic patients may demonstrate nerve root enhancement perioperatively and postoperatively. The use of contrast in postoperative differentiation of reherniation is somewhat controversial. Mullin et al. claim that its routine use adds little diagnostic value and may be confusing.[198]

Postoperative discitis, which occurs in 1.3%–10% of cases, is indicated by decreased signal intensity within the vertebral body marrow on T1-weighted images, hyperintensity on T2-weighted images, and enhancement of vertebral marrow after intravenous injection of gadolinium. However, similar findings may be present after extensive discectomies, especially if cortical end plate curettage was done. Grand et al. found that 18.5% postoperative hypointense end plates enhanced with gadolinium in absence of infection.[199]

High-resolution CT is the premier imaging modality for the evaluation of subtle areas of end plate destruction. Only later are changes of indistinctness or destruction of the cortical end plate detectable with conventional radiography. Epidural abscesses may also occur.

Differentiating normal postoperative changes from discitis often requires correlation with the erythrocyte sedimentation rate (ESR) to exclude discitis. Normally, the ESR returns to baseline within 4 months. In many instances, percutaneous aspiration or core biopsy is required to make the diagnosis of discitis.

SUMMARY

1. The lessons learned from biomechanics research and histopathological and cryomicrotome studies compliment our understanding of the nature of the IVD pathology that present clinically and on advanced imaging studies. This understanding is integral for the proper selection of management strategies and outcome goal determination.
2. IVD disruptions may produce different clinical patterns including both radiculopathic and discogenic. The presentation and treatment of these basic syndromes are distinctive. Skilled sorting of the clinical findings and selection of appropriate treatment yields excellent outcomes with both conservative and surgical approaches.
3. When the clinical examination, performed in a meaningful sequence with relevant tests and confirmatory procedures, is combined with historical and imaging essentials, the patient with LBP (with or without leg pain) can be properly categorized.
4. Discography permits striking demonstration of internal morphological abnormalities of the IVD. MRI also allows great insight into the uncertainties and ambiguities of discal pathology. However, the varied terminology used to describe the visualized abnormalities often adds to clinical confusion. As it turns out, IVD protrusions, bulges, and internal disruption are not fundamentally different pathological entities. Imaging nomenclature that discriminates purely on the basis of the morphology of the disc's contour may promote ignorance regarding the possibility of symptomatic internal disc disruption. Furthermore, many asymptomatic patients have significant imaging abnormalities and clinical correlation is always necessary.
5. The selection criteria for those patients requiring surgical intervention has narrowed based on our knowledge of the natural history of disc disruption. In the absence of bowel and bladder symptoms, or progressive neurological loss, most patients are suitable for a 2- to 3-month trial of conservative treatment. The determinations for individual treatment options are usually straightforward.

REFERENCES

1. Bogduk N, Macintosh JE. The applied anatomy of the thoracolumbar fascia. *Spine* 1984;9(2):164–170.
2. Gardner-Morse MG, Stokes IA. The effects of abdominal muscle coactivation on lumbar spine stability. *Spine* 1998;23(1):86–91.
3. Granata KP, Marras WS. The influence of trunk muscle coactivity on dynamic spinal loads. *Spine* 1995;20(8):913–919.
4. Zetterberg C, Andersson GB, Schultz AB. The activity of individual trunk muscles during heavy physical loading. *Spine* 1987;12(10):1035–1040.
5. Bogduk N. The lumbar disc and low back pain. *Neurosurg Clin North Am* 1991;2(4):791–806.
6. Mooney V. Presidential address. International Society for the Study of the Lumbar Spine. Dallas, 1986. Where is the pain coming from? *Spine* 1987;12(8):754–759.
7. Humzah MD, Soames RW. Human intervertebral disc: Structure and function. *Anat Rec* 1988;220(4):337–356.
8. Nitobe T, Harata S, Okamoto Y, et al. Degradation and biosynthesis of proteoglycans in the nucleus pulposus of canine intervertebral disc after chymopapain treatment. *Spine* 1988;13(11):1332–1339.
9. Mendel T, Wink CS, Zimny ML. Neural elements in human cervical intervertebral discs. *Spine* 1992;17(2):132–135.
10. Ghosh P. Basic biochemistry of the intervertebral disc and its variation with ageing and degeneration. *J Man Med* 1990;5:48–51.
11. Bibby SR, Jones DA, Lee RB, et al. The pathophysiology of the intervertebral disc. *Jt Bone Spine* 2001;68(6):537–542.
12. Jahnke MR, McDevitt CA. Proteoglycans of the human intervertebral disc. Electrophoretic heterogeneity of the aggregating proteoglycans of the nucleus pulposus. *Biochem J* 1988;251(2):347–356.
13. Inerot S, Axelsson I. Structure and composition of proteoglycans from human annulus fibrosus. *Connect Tissue Res* 1991;26(1–2):47–63.

14. Galante JO. Tensile properties of the human lumbar annulus fibrosus. *Acta Orthop Scand* 1967; (Suppl 100:1–91).
15. Wiltse LL, Fonseca AS, Amster J, et al. Relationship of the dura, Hofmann's ligaments, Batson's plexus, and a fibrovascular membrane lying on the posterior surface of the vertebral bodies and attaching to the deep layer of the posterior longitudinal ligament. An anatomical, radiologic, and clinical study. *Spine* 1993;18(8):1030–1043.
16. Hutton WC, Elmer WA, Boden SD, et al. The effect of hydrostatic pressure on intervertebral disc metabolism. *Spine* 1999;24(15):1507–1515.
17. Kang JD, Stefanovic-Racic M, McIntyre LA, et al. Toward a biochemical understanding of human intervertebral disc degeneration and herniation. Contributions of nitric oxide, interleukins, prostaglandin E2, and matrix metalloproteinases. *Spine* 1997;22(10):1065–1073.
18. Gruber HE, Hanley EN Jr. Observations on morphologic changes in the aging and degenerating human disc: Secondary collagen alterations. *BMC Musculoskeletal Disord* 2002;3(1):9.
19. Ahsan R, Tajima N, Chosa E, et al. Biochemical and morphological changes in herniated human intervertebral disc. *J Orthop Sci* 2001;6(6):510–518.
20. Crock HV. Internal disc disruption. A challenge to disc prolapse fifty years on. *Spine* 1986;11(6):650–653.
21. Gower WE, Pedrini V. Age-related variations in protein polysaccharides from human nucleus pulposus, annulus fibrosus, and costal cartilage. *J Bone Joint Surg Am* 1969;51(6):1154–1162.
22. Cavanaugh JM, Kallakuri S, Ozaktay AC. Innervation of the rabbit lumbar intervertebral disc and posterior longitudinal ligament. *Spine* 1995;20(19):2080–2085.
23. Cramer GD, Darby SA. *Basic and clinical anatomy of the spine, spinal cord, and ans*. St Louis, Mosby, 1995:193–194.
24. Freemont AJ, Peacock TE, Goupille P, et al. Nerve ingrowth into diseased intervertebral disc in chronic back pain. *Lancet* 1997;350(9072):178–181.
25. Adams MA, Dolan P, Hutton WC. Diurnal variations in the stresses on the lumbar spine. *Spine* 1987;12(2): 130–137.
26. Botsford DJ, Esses SI, Ogilvie-Harris DJ. In vivo diurnal variation in intervertebral disc volume and morphology. *Spine* 1994;19(8):935–940.
27. Dolan P, Benjamin E, Adams M. Diurnal changes in bending and compressive stresses acting on the lumbar spine. *J Bone Jt Surg Br* 1993;75(Suppl):22.
28. Dunlop RB, Adams MA, Hutton WC. Disc space narrowing and the lumbar facet joints. *J Bone Joint Surg Br* 1984;66(5):706–710.
29. Eklund JA, Corlett EN. Shrinkage as a measure of the effect of load on the spine. *Spine* 1984;9(2):189–194.
30. Hedman TP, Fernie GR. In vivo measurement of lumbar spinal creep in two seated postures using magnetic resonance imaging. *Spine* 1995;20(2):178–183.
31. Leivseth G, Drerup B. Spinal shrinkage during work in a sitting posture compared to work in a standing posture. *Clin Biomech (Bristol, Avon)* 1997;12(7–8):409–418.
32. Twomey L, Taylor J. Flexion creep deformation and hysteresis in the lumbar vertebral column. *Spine* 1982;7(2):116–122.
33. Adams MA, Dolan P, Hutton WC, et al. Diurnal changes in spinal mechanics and their clinical significance. *J Bone Joint Surg Br* 1990;72(2):266–270.
34. Ekstrom L, Kaigle A, Hult E, et al. Intervertebral disc response to cyclic loading—An animal model. *Proc Inst Mech Eng [H]* 1996;210(4):249–258.
35. Goel VK, Voo LM, Weinstein JN, et al. Response of the ligamentous lumbar spine to cyclic bending loads. *Spine* 1988;13(3):294–300.
36. Keller TS, Hansson TH, Holm SH, et al. In vivo creep behavior of the normal and degenerated porcine intervertebral disk: A preliminary report. *J Spinal Disord* 1988;1(4):267–278.
37. Solomonow M, Zhou BH, Baratta RV, et al. Biomechanics of increased exposure to lumbar injury caused by cyclic loading. Part 1. Loss of reflexive muscular stabilization. *Spine* 1999;24(23):2426–2434.
38. Yong-Hing K, Kirkaldy-Willis WH. The pathophysiology of degenerative disease of the lumbar spine. *Orthop Clin North Am* 1983;14(3):491–504.
39. Yu SW, Haughton VM, Sether LA, et al. Comparison of MR and discography in detecting radial tears of the anulus: A postmortem study. *AJNR Am J Neuroradiol* 1989;10(5):1077–1081.
40. Yu SW, Sether LA, Ho PS, et al. Tears of the anulus fibrosus: Correlation between MR and pathologic findings in cadavers. *AJNR Am J Neuroradiol* 1988;9(2):367–370.
41. Osti OL, Vernon-Roberts B, Moore R, et al. Annular tears and disc degeneration in the lumbar spine. A post-mortem study of 135 discs. *J Bone Joint Surg Br* 1992;74(5):678–682.
42. Kim Y. Prediction of peripheral tears in the anulus of the intervertebral disc. *Spine* 2000;25(14):1771–1774.
43. Fennell AJ, Jones AP, Hukins DW. Migration of the nucleus pulposus within the intervertebral disc during flexion and extension of the spine. *Spine* 1996;21(23):2753–2757.
44. Ito T, Takano Y, Yuasa N. Types of lumbar herniated disc and clinical course. *Spine* 2001;26(6):648–651.
45. Aspden RM, Porter RW. Localized stresses in the intervertebral disc resulting from a loose fragment. A theory for fissure and fragment. *Spine* 1999;24(21):2214–2218.
46. Brinckmann P. Injury of the annulus fibrosus and disc protrusions. An in vitro investigation on human lumbar discs. *Spine* 1986;11(2):149–153.
47. Adams MA, Hutton WC. The effect of fatigue on the lumbar intervertebral disc. *J Bone Joint Surg Br* 1983;65(2):199–203.
48. Adams MA, Hutton WC. Prolapsed intervertebral disc. A hyperflexion injury 1981 Volvo Award in Basic Science. *Spine* 1982;7(3):184–191.
49. Adams MA, Hutton WC. Gradual disc prolapse. *Spine* 1985;10(6):524–531.

50. Lu YM, Hutton WC, Gharpuray VM. Do bending, twisting, and diurnal fluid changes in the disc affect the propensity to prolapse? A viscoelastic finite element model. *Spine*1996;21(22):2570–2579.
51. Saal JS, Franson RC, Dobrow R, et al. High levels of inflammatory phospholipase A2 activity in lumbar disc herniations. *Spine* 1990;15(7):674–678.
52. Sachs BL, Vanharanta H, Spivey MA, et al. Dallas discogram description. A new classification of CT/discography in low-back disorders. *Spine* 1987;12(3):287–294.
53. Buirski G. Magnetic resonance signal patterns of lumbar discs in patients with low back pain. A prospective study with discographic correlation. *Spine* 1992;17(10):1199–1204.
54. Gibson MJ, Buckley J, Mawhinney R, et al. Magnetic resonance imaging and discography in the diagnosis of disc degeneration. A comparative study of 50 discs. *J Bone Joint Surg Br* 1986;68(3):369–373.
55. Horton WC, Daftari TK. Which disc as visualized by magnetic resonance imaging is actually a source of pain? A correlation between magnetic resonance imaging and discography. *Spine* 1992;17(6 Suppl):S164–S171.
56. Schneiderman G, Flannigan B, Kingston S, et al. Magnetic resonance imaging in the diagnosis of disc degeneration: Correlation with discography. *Spine* 1987;12(3):276–281.
57. Simmons JW, Emery SF, McMillin JN, et al. Awake discography. A comparison study with magnetic resonance imaging. *Spine* 1991;16(6 Suppl):S216 S221.
58. Moneta GB, Videman T, Kaivanto K, et al. Reported pain during lumbar discography as a function of anular ruptures and disc degeneration. A re-analysis of 833 discograms. *Spine* 1994;19(17):1968–1974.
59. Adams MA, Dolan P, Hutton WC. The stages of disc degeneration as revealed by discograms. *J Bone Joint Surg Br* 1986;68(1):36–41.
60. Milette PC, Melanson D. A reappraisal of lumbar discography. *J Can Assoc Radiol* 1982;33(3):176–182.
61. Walsh TR, Weinstein JN, Spratt KF, et al. Lumbar discography in normal subjects. A controlled, prospective study. *J Bone Joint Surg Am* 1990;72(7):1081–1088.
62. Vanharanta H, Sachs BL, Ohnmeiss DD, et al. Pain provocation and disc deterioration by age. A CT/discography study in a low-back pain population. *Spine* 1989;14(4):420–423.
63. Aprill C, Bogduk N. High-intensity zone: A diagnostic sign of painful lumbar disc on magnetic resonance imaging. *Br J Radiol* 1992;65(773):361–369.
64. O'Neill CW, Kurgansky ME, Derby R, et al. Disc stimulation and patterns of referred pain. *Spine* 2002;27(24):2776–2781.
65. Schellhas KP, Pollei SR, Gundry CR, et al. Lumbar disc high-intensity zone. Correlation of magnetic resonance imaging and discography. *Spine* 1996;21(1):79–86.
66. Ricketson R, Simmons JW, Hauser BO. The prolapsed intervertebral disc. The high-intensity zone with discography correlation. *Spine* 1996;21(23):2758–2762.
67. Carreon LY, Ito T, Yamada M, et al. Neovascularization induced by anulus and its inhibition by cartilage endplate. Its role in disc absorption. *Spine* 1997;22(13):1429–1434.
68. Ito T, Yamada M, Ikuta F, et al. Histologic evidence of absorption of sequestration-type herniated disc. *Spine* 1996;21(2):230–234.
69. Saal JA, Saal JS, Herzog RJ. The natural history of lumbar intervertebral disc extrusions treated nonoperatively. *Spine* 1990;15(7):683–686.
70. Maigne JY, Rime B, Deligne B. Computed tomographic follow-up study of forty-eight cases of nonoperatively treated lumbar intervertebral disc herniation. *Spine* 1992;17(9):1071–1074.
71. Yasuma T, Arai K, Yamauchi Y. The histology of lumbar intervertebral disc herniation. The significance of small blood vessels in the extruded tissue. *Spine* 1993;18(13):1761–1765.
72. Pai RR, D'sa B, Raghuveer CV, et al. Neovascularization of nucleus pulposus. A diagnostic feature of intervertebral disc prolapse. *Spine* 1999;24(8):739–741.
73. Hamanishi C, Kawabata T, Yosii T, et al. Schmorl's nodes on magnetic resonance imaging. Their incidence and clinical relevance. *Spine* 1994;19(4):450–453.
74. Fahey V, Opeskin K, Silberstein M, et al. The pathogenesis of Schmorl's nodes in relation to acute trauma. An autopsy study. *Spine* 1998;23(21):2272–2275.
75. Pfirrmann CW, Resnick D. Schmorl nodes of the thoracic and lumbar spine: Radiographic-pathologic study of prevalence, characterization, and correlation with degenerative changes of 1,650 spinal levels in 100 cadavers. *Radiology* 2001;219(2):368–374.
76. Wagner AL, Murtagh FR, Arrington JA, et al. Relationship of Schmorl's nodes to vertebral body endplate fractures and acute endplate disk extrusions. *AJNR Am J Neuroradiol* 2000;21(2):276–281.
77. Beggs I, Addison J. Posterior vertebral rim fractures. *Br J Radiol* 1998;71(845):567–572.
78. Modic MT. Degenerative disorders of the spine. In: Masaryk TJ, Ross JS, eds. *Magnetic resonance imaging of the spine*. St. Louis: Mosby, 1994:80–150.
79. Braithwaite I, White J, Saifuddin A, et al. Vertebral end-plate (Modic) changes on lumbar spine MRI: Correlation with pain reproduction at lumbar discography. *Eur Spine J* 1998;7(5):363–368.
80. Weishaupt D, Zanetti M, Hodler J, et al. Painful lumbar disk derangement: Relevance of endplate abnormalities at MR imaging. *Radiology* 2001;218(2):420–427.
81. Komori H, Okawa A, Haro H, et al. Contrast-enhanced magnetic resonance imaging in conservative management of lumbar disc herniation. *Spine* 1998;23(1):67–73.
82. Fardon DF, Milette PC. Nomenclature and classification of lumbar disc pathology: Recommendations of the combined task forces of the North American Sspine Society, American Society of Spine Radiology,

and American Society of Neuroradiology. *Spine* 2001;26(5):E93–E113.

83. Modic MT, Ross JS, Obuchowski NA, et al. Contrast-enhanced MR imaging in acute lumbar radiculopathy: A pilot study of the natural history. *Radiology* 1995;195(2):429–435.
84. Silverman CS, Lenchik L, Shimkin PM, et al. The value of MR in differentiating subligamentous from supraligamentous lumbar disk herniations. *AJNR Am J Neuroradiol* 1995;16(3):571–579.
85. Ozaki S, Muro T, Ito S, et al. Neovascularization of the outermost area of herniated lumbar intervertebral discs. *J Orthop Sci* 1999;4(4):286–292.
86. Prestar FJ. Anomalies and malformations of lumbar spinal nerve roots. *Minim Invasive Neurosurg* 1996; 39(4):133–137.
87. Neidre A, MacNab I. Anomalies of the lumbosacral nerve roots. Review of 16 cases and classification. *Spine* 1983;8(3):294–299.
88. Wiesel SW, Tsourmas N, Feffer HL, et al. A study of computer-assisted tomography. I. The incidence of positive CAT scans in an asymptomatic group of patients. *Spine* 1984;9(6):549–551.
89. Jensen MC, Brant-Zawadzki MN, Obuchowski N, et al. Magnetic resonance imaging of the lumbar spine in people without back pain. *N Engl J Med* 1994;331(2):69–73.
90. Morris EW, Di Paola M, Vallance R, et al. Diagnosis and decision making in lumbar disc prolapse and nerve entrapment. *Spine* 1986;11(5):436–439.
91. Xin SQ, Zhang QZ, Fan DH. Significance of the straight-leg-raising test in the diagnosis and clinical evaluation of lower lumbar intervertebral-disc protrusion. *J Bone Joint Surg Am* 1987;69(4):517–522.
92. Deyo RA, Rainville J, Kent DL. What can the history and physical examination tell us about low back pain? *JAMA* 1992;268(6):760–765.
93. Pople IK, Griffith HB. Prediction of an extruded fragment in lumbar disc patients from clinical presentations. *Spine* 1994;19(2):156–158.
94. Albeck MJ. A critical assessment of clinical diagnosis of disc herniation in patients with monoradicular sciatica. *Acta Neurochir (Wien)* 1996;138(1):40–44.
95. Kortelainen P, Puranen J, Koivisto E, et al. Symptoms and signs of sciatica and their relation to the localization of the lumbar disc herniation. *Spine* 1985;10(1):88–92.
96. Nadler SF, Campagnolo DI, Tomaio AC, et al. High lumbar disc: Diagnostic and treatment dilemma. *Am J Phys Med Rehabil* 1998;77(6):538–544.
97. Vucetic N, Maattanen H, Svensson O. Pain and pathology in lumbar disc hernia. *Clin Orthop* 1995;(320):65–72.
98. Porter RW, Miller CG. Back pain and trunk list. *Spine* 1986;11(6):596–600.
99. Khuffash B, Porter RW. Cross leg pain and trunk list. *Spine* 1989;14(6):602–603.
100. Takahashi K, Shima I, Porter RW. Nerve root pressure in lumbar disc herniation. *Spine* 1999;24(19):2003–2006.
101. Minor LS. Uber eine bewegungsprobe und bewegungstorung bei lumbalshemerz und bei ischias. *Deutche Med Wochenschr* 1898;24:363–382.
102. Postacchini F. Management of herniation of the lumbar disc. *J Bone Joint Surg Br* 1999;81(4):567–576.
103. Vucetic N, Svensson O. Physical signs in lumbar disc hernia. *Clin Orthop* 1996;(333):192–201.
104. Spengler DM, Ouellette EA, Battie M, et al. Elective discectomy for herniation of a lumbar disc. Additional experience with an objective method. *J Bone Joint Surg Am* 1990;72(2):230–237.
105. Jonsson B, Stromqvist B. Symptoms and signs in degeneration of the lumbar spine. A prospective, consecutive study of 300 operated patients. *J Bone Joint Surg Br* 1993;75(3):381–385.
106. Weise MD, Garfin SR, Gelberman RH, et al. Lower-extremity sensibility testing in patients with herniated lumbar intervertebral discs. *J Bone Joint Surg Am* 1985;67(8):1219–1224.
107. Jensen OH. The level-diagnosis of a lower lumbar disc herniation: The value of sensibility and motor testing. *Clin Rheumatol* 1987;6(4):564–569.
108. Mayer TG, Gatchel RJ. *Functional restoration for spinal disorders: The sports medicine approach.* Philadelphia: Lea & Febiger, 1988.
109. Yeomans SG. Spinal and orthopedic and neurological testing. In: Yeomans SG, ed. *The clinicl application of outcomes assessment.* Stamford: Appleton & Lange, 2000:171.
110. Aronson H. Herniated upper lumbar discs. *J Bone Joint Surg Am* 1963;45:311–317.
111. O'Connell J. Protrusions of the lumbar intervertebral discs. A clinical review based on five hundred cases treated by excision of the protrusion. *J Bone Joint Surg Br* 1951;33:8–30.
112. Hakelius A, Hindmarsh J. The significance of neurological signs and myelographic findings in the diagnosis of lumbar root compression. *Acta Orthop Scand* 1972;43(4):239–246.
113. Jensen OH. The medial hamstring reflex in the level-diagnosis of a lumbar disc herniation. *Clin Rheumatol* 1987;6(4):570–574.
114. Vanharanta H, Ohnmeiss DD, Aprill CN. Vibration pain provocation can improve the specificity of MRI in the diagnosis of symptomatic lumbar disc rupture. *Clin J Pain* 1998;14(3):239–247.
115. Yrjama M, Vanharanta H. Bony vibration stimulation: A new, non-invasive method for examining intradiscal pain. *Eur Spine J* 1994;3(4):233–235.
116. Donelson R, Aprill C, Medcalf R, et al. A prospective study of centralization of lumbar and referred pain. A predictor of symptomatic discs and anular competence. *Spine* 1997;22(10):1115–1122.
117. Yrjama M, Tervonen O, Kurunlahti M, et al. Bony vibration stimulation test combined with magnetic resonance imaging. Can discography be replaced? *Spine* 1997;22(7):808–813.
118. Dimitrijevic D. Laseque sign. *Neurology* 1952;2:453–454.
119. Charlney J. Orthopedic signs in the diagnosis of disc

protrusion: With special reference to the straight-leg-raising test. *Lancet* 1951;260:186–192.

120. Goodard M, Reid J. Movements induced by straight leg raising in the lumbosacral roots, nerves and plexus, and in the intrapelvic section of the sciatic nerve. *J Neurol Neurosurg Psychiatry* 1965;28: 12–18.
121. Spangfort EV. The lumbar disc herniation. A computer-aided analysis of 2504 operations, *Acta Orthop Scand* 1972;142(Suppl.)5–79.
122. Ramamurthi B. Absence of limitation of straight leg raising in proved lumbar disc lesion: Case report. *J Neurosurg* 1980;52(6):852–853.
123. Kosteljanetz M, Bang F, Schmidt-Olsen S. The clinical significance of straight-leg raising (Lasegue's sign) in the diagnosis of prolapsed lumbar disc. Interobserver variation and correlation with surgical finding. *Spine* 1988;13(4):393–395.
124. Kosteljanetz M, Espersen JO, Halaburt H, et al. Predictive value of clinical and surgical findings in patients with lumbago-sciatica. A prospective study (Part I). *Acta Neurochir (Wien)* 1984;73(1–2):67–76.
125. Deville WL, van der Windt DA, Dzaferagic A, et al. The test of Lasegue: Systematic review of the accuracy in diagnosing herniated discs. *Spine* 2000;25(9):1140–1147.
126. van den Hoogen HM, Koes BW, van Eijk Joint, et al. On the accuracy of history, physical examination, and erythrocyte sedimentation rate in diagnosing low back pain in general practice. A criteria-based review of the literature. *Spine* 1995;20(3):318–327.
127. Andersson GB, Deyo RA. History and physical examination in patients with herniated lumbar discs. *Spine* 1996;21(24, Suppl):10S–18S.
128. Hudgins WR. The crossed straight leg raising test: A diagnostic sign of herniated disc. *J Occup Med* 1979;21(6):407–408.
129. Jonsson B, Stromqvist B. Clinical appearance of contained and noncontained lumbar disc herniation. *J Spinal Disord* 1996;9(1):32–38.
130. Jonsson B, Stromqvist B. The straight leg raising test and the severity of symptoms in lumbar disc herniation. A preoperative evaluation. *Spine* 1995;20(1):27–30.
131. Jonsson B, Stromqvist B. Significance of a persistent positive straight leg raising test after lumbar disc surgery. *J Neurosurg* 1999;91(1, Suppl):50–53.
132. Dyck P. The femoral nerve traction test with lumbar disc protrusions. *Surg Neurol* 1976;(3):163–166.
133. Nadler SF, Malanga GA, Stitik TP, et al. The crossed femoral nerve stretch test to improve diagnostic sensitivity for the high lumbar radiculopathy: 2 case reports. *Arch Phys Med Rehabil* 2001;82(4):522–523.
134. Jabre JF, Bryan RW. Bent-knee pulling in the diagnosis of upper lumbar root lesions. *Arch Neurol* 1982;39(10):669–670.
135. Braggard K. Umber das laseguesche phaenomen. *Muenched Med Wehnsehr* 1928;75:387–389.
136. Fajersztajn J. Ueber das gekreuzte isciasphanomen wiener. *Wein Klin Wochenschr* 1901;14:41–47.
137. Breig A, Troup JD. Biomechanical considerations in the straight-leg-raising test. Cadaveric and clinical studies of the effects of medial hip rotation. *Spine* 1979;4(3):242–250.
138. Cram R. A sign of sciatic nerve root pressure. *J Bone Joint Surg Br* 1953;35:192–195.
139. Deyerle WM, May VR. Sciatic tension test. *So Med J* 1956;49:999–1005.
140. Johnson EK, Chiarello CM. The slump test: The effects of head and lower extremity position on knee extension. *J Orthop Sports Phys Ther* 1997;26(6):310–317.
141. Arid RB, Naffziger HC. Prolonged jugular compression, a new diagnostic test of neurologic value. *Trans Am Neurol Assoc* 1940;66:45–48.
142. Herron LD, Pheasant HC. Prone knee-flexion provocative testing for lumbar disc protrusion. *Spine* 1980;5(1):65–67.
143. Epstein B Epstein J. Efffect of anatomic variations in lumbar vertebra and spinal canal on cauda equina and nerve root syndromes. *AJR Am J Roentgenol* 1964;91:1055–1063.
144. Postacchini F. Results of surgery compared with conservative management for lumbar disc herniations. *Spine* 1996;21(11):1383–1387.
145. Atlas SJ, Deyo RA, Keller, RB et al. The Maine Lumbar Spine Study, Part III. 1-year outcomes of surgical and nonsurgical management of lumbar spinal stenosis. *Spine* 1996;21(15):1787–1794.
146. Weber H. Lumbar disc herniation. A controlled, prospective study with ten years of observation. *Spine* 1983;8(2):131–140.
147. Ellenberg M, Reina N, Ross M, et al. Regression of herniated nucleus pulposus: Two patients with lumbar radiculopathy. *Arch Phys Med Rehabil* 1989;70(12):842–844.
148. Bush K, Cowan N, Katz DE, et al. The natural history of sciatica associated with disc pathology. A prospective study with clinical and independent radiologic follow-up. *Spine* 1992;17(10):1205–1212.
149. Saal JA. Natural history and nonoperative treatment of lumbar disc herniation. *Spine* 1996;21(24, Suppl):2S–9S.
150. Vucetic N, Astrand P, Guntner P, et al. Diagnosis and prognosis in lumbar disc herniation. *Clin Orthop* 1999;(361):116–122.
151. Rust MS, Olivero WC. Far-lateral disc herniations: The results of conservative management. *J Spinal Disord* 1999;12(2):138–140.
152. McKenzie RA. *The lumbar spine: Mechanical diagnosis and therapy.* Waikanea, New Zealand: Spinal Publications, 1981.
153. Fritz JM, Delitto A, Vignovic M, et al. Interrater reliability of judgments of the centralization phenomenon and status change during movement testing in patients with low back pain. *Arch Phys Med Rehabil* 2000;81(1):57–61.
154. Long AL. The centralization phenomenon. Its usefulness as a predictor or outcome in conservative treatment of chronic law back pain (a pilot study). *Spine* 1995;20(23):2513–2520.

155. Werneke M, Hart DL. Centralization phenomenon as a prognostic factor for chronic low back pain and disability. *Spine* 2001;26(7):758–764.
156. Saal JA, Saal JS. Nonoperative treatment of herniated lumbar intervertebral disc with radiculopathy. An outcome study. *Spine* 1989;14(4):431–437.
157. Nwuga VC. Ultrasound in treatment of back pain resulting from prolapsed intervertebral disc. *Arch Phys Med Rehabil* 1983;64(2):88–89.
158. Buchalter D, Kahanovitz N, Viola K, et al. Three-dimensional spinal motion measurements. Part 2. A noninvasive assessment of lumbar brace immobilization of the spine. *J Spinal Disord* 1988;1(4):284–286.
159. Ramos G, Martin W. Effects of vertebral axial decompression on intradiscal pressure. *J Neurosurg* 1994,81(3):350–353.
160. Nosse LJ. Inverted spinal traction. *Arch Phys Med Rehabil* 1978;59(8):367–370.
161. Onel D, Tuzlaci M, Sari H, et al. Computed tomographic investigation of the effect of traction on lumbar disc herniations. *Spine* 1989;14(1):82–90.
162. Andersson GB, Schultz AB, Nachemson AL. Intervertebral disc pressures during traction. *Scand J Rehabil Med Suppl* 1983;9:88–91.
163. Pal B, Mangion P, Hossain MA, et al. A controlled trial of continuous lumbar traction in the treatment of back pain and sciatica. *Br J Rheumatol* 1986;25(2):181–183.
164. Haskvitz EM, Hanten WP. Blood pressure response to inversion traction. *Phys Ther* 1986;66(9):1361–1364.
165. Gianakopoulos G, Waylonis GW, Grant PA, et al. Inversion devices: Their role in producing lumbar distraction. *Arch Phys Med Rehabil* 1985;66(2):100–102.
166. Slosberg M. Side posture manipulation for lumbar intervertebral disk herniation reconsidered. *J Manipulative Physiol Ther* 1994;17(4):258–262.
167. Triano J. The mechanics of spinal manipulation. In: Herzog W, edr. *Clinical biomechanics of spinal manipulation*. New York: Churchill Livingston, 2000:92–190.
168. Ahmed AM, Duncan NA, Burke DL. The effect of facet geometry on the axial torque-rotation response of lumbar motion segments. *Spine* 1990;15(5):391–401.
169. Adams MA, Hutton WC. The relevance of torsion to the mechanical derangement of the lumbar spine. *Spine* 1981;6(3):241–248.
170. Gudavalli MR, Triano JJ. Effects of combined motions on the posterior ligaments of the spine. *JNMS* 1997;5(4):150–156.
171. Cassidy JD, Thiel HW, Kirkaldy-Willis WH. Side posture manipulation for lumbar intervertebral disk herniation. *J Manipulative Physiol Ther* 1993;16(2):96–103.
172. Morris CE. Chiropractic rehabilitation of a patient with S1 radiculopathy associated with a large lumbar disk herniation. *J Manipulative Physiol Ther* 1999;22(1):38–44.
173. Bergmann TF, Jongeward BV. Manipulative therapy in lower back pain with leg pain and neurological deficit. *J Manipulative Physiol Ther* 1998;21(4):288–294.
174. Stern PJ, Cote P, Cassidy JD. A series of consecutive cases of low back pain with radiating leg pain treated by chiropractors. *J Manipulative Physiol Ther* 1995;18(6):335–342.
175. Mensor M. Non-operative treatment, including manipulation, for lumbar intervertebral disc syndrome. *J Bone Joint Surg* 1955;37(A):925–936.
176. Kuo PP, Loh ZC. Treatment of lumbar intervertebral disc protrusions by manipulation. *Clin Orthop* 1987;(215):47–55.
177. Chrisman D, Mittnacut A, Snook G A study of the results following rotatory manipulation in the lumbar intervertebral disc syndrome. *J Bone Joint Surg* 1964;46A(3):517–524.
178. Nwuga VC. Relative therapeutic efficacy of vertebral manipulation and conventional treatment in back pain management. *Am J Phys Med* 1982;61(6):273–278.
179. Burton AK, Tillotson KM, Cleary J. Single-blind randomised controlled trial of chemonucleolysis and manipulation in the treatment of symptomatic lumbar disc herniation. *Eur Spine J* 2000;9(3):202–207.
180. Cox JM, Hazen LJ, Mungovan M. Distraction manipulation reduction of an L5–S1 disk herniation. *J Manipulative Physiol Ther* 1993;16(5):342–346.
181. Hession EF, Donald GD. Treatment of multiple lumbar disk herniations in an adolescent athlete utilizing flexion distraction and rotational manipulation. *J Manipulative Physiol Ther* 1993;16(3):185–192.
182. Neault CC. Conservative management of an L4–L5 left nuclear disk prolapse with a sequestrated segment. *J Manipulative Physiol Ther* 1992;15(5):318–322.
183. Bowman SJ, Wedderburn L, Whaley A, et al. Outcome assessment after epidural corticosteroid injection for low back pain and sciatica. *Spine* 1993;18(10):1345–1350.
184. Watts RW, Silagy CA. A meta-analysis on the efficacy of epidural corticosteroids in the treatment of sciatica. *Anaesth Intensive Care* 1995;23(5):564–569.
185. Benzon HT. Epidural steroid injections for low back pain and lumbosacral radiculopathy. *Pain* 1986;24(3):277–295.
186. Viton JM, Peretti-Viton P, Rubino T, et al. Short-term assessment of periradicular corticosteroid injections in lumbar radiculopathy associated with disc pathology. *Neuroradiology* 1998;40(1):59–62.
187. Papagelopoulos PJ, Petrou HG, Triantafyllidis PG, et al. Treatment of lumbosacral radicular pain with epidural steroid injections. *Orthopedics* 2001;24(2):145–149.
188. Triano J. *SMT in painful disc syndrome*. Washington, DC: North American Spine Society, 1995.
189. Saal JS, Saal JA. Management of chronic discogenic low back pain with a thermal intradiscal catheter. A preliminary report. *Spine* 2000;25(3):382–388.
190. Karasek M, Bogduk N. Twelve-month follow-up of a controlled trial of intradiscal thermal anuloplasty for back pain due to internal disc disruption. *Spine* 2000;25(20):2601–2607.
191. Saal JA, Saal JS. Intradiscal electrothermal treatment for chronic discogenic low back pain: Prospective outcome study with a minimum 2-year follow-up. *Spine* 2002;27(9):966–973.

192. Hsia AW, Isaac K, Katz JS. Cauda equina syndrome from intradiscal electrothermal therapy. *Neurology* 2000;55(2):320.

193. Kleinstueck FS, Diederich CJ, Nau WH, et al. Acute biomechanical and histological effects of intradiscal electrothermal therapy on human lumbar discs. *Spine* 2001;26(20):2198–2207.

194. Lee J, Lutz GE, Campbell D, et al. Stability of the lumbar spine after intradiscal electrothermal therapy. *Arch Phys Med Rehabil* 2001;82(1):120–122.

195. Shah RV, Lutz GE, Lee J, et al. Intradiskal electrothermal therapy: A preliminary histologic study. *Arch Phys Med Rehabil* 2001;82(9):1230–1237.

196. Atlas SJ, Deyo RA, Keller RB, et al. The Main Lumbar Spine Study, Part II. 1-year outcomes of surgical and nonsurgical management of sciatica. *Spine* 1996;21(15):1777–1786.

197. Van Goethem JW, Van de KE, Biltjes IG, et al. MRI after successful lumbar discectomy. *Neuroradiology* 1996;38(Suppl 1):S90–S96.

198. Mullin WJ, Heithoff KB, Gilbert TJ, et al. Magnetic resonance evaluation of recurrent disc herniation: Is gadolinium necessary? *Spine* 2000;25(12):1493–1499.

199. Grand CM, Bank WO, Baleriaux D, et al. Gadolinium enhancement of vertebral endplates following lumbar disc surgery. *Neuroradiology* 1993;35(7):503–505.

CHAPTER

7

THE STENOTIC SYNDROMES

Dennis R. Skogsbergh and Matthew H. Kowalski

OUTLINE

OBJECTIVES

The objectives of this chapter are to

1. appreciate the factors contributing to lumbar spinal stenosis;
2. improve clinical recognition and differentiation of the problem;
3. understand the importance of diagnostic imaging;
4. learn how to monitor disease progression; and
5. identify and select treatment options for optimal outcomes.

INTRODUCTION

Lumbar spinal stenosis is one of the most frequently encountered and clinically important degenerative disorders in the aging population.[1] In the United States, the fastest growing segment of the population is over 80, and this trend is expected to continue over the next 50 years.[2] This trend is global. The world's population over 60 constitutes about 20%, and by 2050 it is estimated to be 33%. The majority of the world's elderly population reside in Asia while only 25% live in Europe.[3] Today the fact that humans are living longer has created an increased focus on improved identification and management of age-related disorders such as spinal stenosis.

Better diagnostic imaging techniques and emergent surgical procedures have contributed to an increase in the number of patients diagnosed with lumbar stenosis and those receiving surgical intervention. A 1994 study revealed that the greatest increase in spinal surgery rates was for spinal stenosis, which quadrupled during the study years.[4] Furthermore, hospitalization rates more than tripled for spinal stenosis, whereas most other spine-related diagnostic categories dropped.

Lumbar spinal stenosis is a complex clinical disorder. The anatomical, diagnostic imaging, functional, symptomatic, and clinical attributes do not always agree. Surgery for spinal stenosis was performed as early as the late 1800s, but an understanding of the underlying pathophysiology did not truly begin to emerge until the late twentieth century. Verbiest is credited for first differentiating stenosis from "developmental narrowing" of the spinal canal.[5] Meta-analysis of the literature from that time until 1992 concluded: "The most definitive finding of this literature synthesis was the poor scientific quality of the literature."[6] Fortunately, more recent investigations have provided a better understanding of the pathophysiology and diagnosis of this disorder.

CLASSIFICATION OF SPINAL STENOSIS

Lumbar spinal stenosis includes any type of narrowing of the spinal canal, nerve root canals (or tunnels), or intervertebral foramina. It may be local, segmental, or generalized and may be caused by bone, soft tissue, or both, in any combination.[7] The two broad subdivisions of congenital/developmental and acquired[7] was further extensively expanded to include etiology, level of entrapment, anatomic location, and the compressive anatomy (Table 7–1).[8]

The neurogenic symptoms in each subcategory are indistinguishable, as the underlying pathophysiology appears identical regardless of the pathoanatomy. The most widely occurring type of spinal stenosis is acquired and degenerative.

An understanding of normal spinal growth, anatomy, and mechanics provides insight into the development and progression of stenosis.

ANATOMY OF THE SPINAL CANAL

The lumbar spinal canal consists of a central spinal canal and two lateral (root) canals, also called *recesses*. Stenosis may present in any location, and in any combination.

TABLE 7–1. Classification of Stenosis According to Pathology

Congenital–developmental stenosis

- Idiopathic
- Achondroplastic
- Hypochondroplastic
- Marquio's mucopolysaccharisosis
- Dysplasias associated with lax atlantoaxial joints (metratropic dwarfism, spondyloepiphyseal dysplasia, Kniest's disease, multiple epiphyseal dysplasia, chondrodysplasia punctata
- Down's syndrome (C1–C2 instability)
- Hypophosphatemic vitamin D-resistant rickets

Acquired stenosis

- Degenerative
  - Central portion of spinal canal
    - Disc herniation
    - Ligamentum flavum hypertrophy
    - Facet hypertrophy, posterior epidural fat compression
    - Facet/ligamentum flavum cysts
  - Peripheral portion of canal, lateral recess, and nerve canals (tunnels)
  - Degenerative spondylolisthesis
- Combined—any possible combination of congenital–developmental stenosis, degenerative stenosis, and herniations of the nucleus pulposus
- Spondylolisthetic/spondylolytic
- Iatrogenic
  - Post laminectomy
  - Post fusion (anterior and posterior)
  - Post chemonucleolysis
- Posttraumatic, late changes, compression fractures
- Miscellaneous
  - Ankylosing spondylitis
  - Calcification of ossification of the ligamentum flavum
  - Diffuse idiopathic skeletal hyperostosis
  - Conjoined origin of lumbosacral nerve roots
- Metabolic
  - Paget's disease
  - Epidural lipomatosis (Cushing's syndrome or long-term steroid therapy)
  - Acromegaly
  - Flourosis
  - Calcium pyrophosphate deposition disease

The Central Spinal Canal

The anterior wall of the central spinal canal is formed by the posterior border of the vertebral body–intervertebral disc interface and the posterior longitudinal ligament. Laterally, the central canal opens to the lateral recess. The superomedial portion of the superior articulating facet and capsule next border the central canal. The inferior articular process of the cephalad vertebra of the motion segment is located posteriorly and medially and contributes to the lateral osseous wall of the central canal.[1] Posteromedially projecting laminae, with an attached ligamentum flavum, complete the posterior arch. The normal thickness of the ligamentum flavum is about 4 mm centrally, but it thins laterally as it joins the facet capsule.[8,9] It is normally under a slight pretension while the spine is in a neutral position.

Size and Shape of the Central Canal The *midsagittal diameter* is the shortest distance between the dorsal aspect of the vertebral body and the ventral spinolaminar junction. Normally, the midsagittal diameter at the cephalad border of the laminar junction is narrower than that at the caudad border. The *interpedicular diameter* (*transverse diameter*) is the widest distance between the medial aspects of the pedicles.

The sagittal diameter is determined early in life, but interpedicular dimension growth continues to increase until skeletal maturity. The L1–L4 midsagittal canal diameter achieves adult size by 1 year of age. The L5 segment increases in size until age 4, at which time it actually is somewhat larger than the adult dimension. The spinal canal shape continues to evolve, reducing the L5 sagittal diameter until age 6, when it attains and maintains the same dimension into adulthood. The interpedicular diameter at L1 significantly increases until 10 years of age, while the others continue to grow until adulthood.[10]

Progressing caudally from L1 to L5, the pedicle lengths are shorter and the interpedicular distance is wider. At L1, the pedicles project directly posterior, and become more laterally oriented caudally, making the mature spinal canal wider and flatter in the lower lumbar and lumbosacral levels.[11]. The shape and size of the L5 and S1 canals are quite variable (Figs. 7–1A to 7–1F).[12,11]

Throughout most of the lumbar spine, the spinal canal is dome or bell shaped. Because of the orientation of the pedicles, the upper lumbar canals are more rounded, while the lower are more triangular. The trefoil (clover) shape is a variant that causes a narrower sagittal diameter (Fig. 7–2*A*). This occurs in 7% of cases at L4 and 15% at L5.[13] This variation may play a role in compression of the caudal nerve roots in the lateral recesses.[12,14]

The mean osseous dimensions of the lumbar spinal canal, lateral recess, and vertebral body vary among ethnic groups. As a general rule, sagittal measurements under 12 mm are considered abnormal. Transverse diameters appear more variable with the low end of normal being about 16 mm (Fig. 7–2*B*).[12,14]

The significant variations in spinal canal dimension among and between different races suggest that measurements of osseous spinal canal dimension per se may be of limited value in evaluating spinal stenosis.[12,14] Therefore, there are no mean values for lower limits of normal that appear valid for all populations. Furthermore, the osseous boundaries of the spinal canal do not accurately reflect the space available for the spinal canal contents. A spinal canal that measures under the recommended limit of normal may have sufficient room for the nerve roots in a patient with a stable lumbar spine and without degenerative disc pathology or thickening of the ligamentum flavum. However, if there is instability due to disc degeneration or spondylolisthesis, nerve roots may be affected even if the actual canal measurements are normal.[15]

Clinical Pearl: The osseous boundaries of the spinal canal do not accurately reflect the space available for the spinal canal.

Advanced diagnostic imaging and surgical findings have increased the awareness that osseous canal dimensions and encroachment are only one aspect of spinal stenosis. The concept of "spinal reserve capacity" helps clarify this issue. The spinal canal may be viewed as a container in which the contents (soft tissues and neural structures) occupy a given percentage. A reserve space (volume) is available to accommodate dynamic or structural change, and is necessary for tension-free movement of the neural contents. If the volume of the contents increases, or the container volume decreases, the reserve capacity is diminished. Obliteration of this reserve capacity is necessary for symptom expression.[16] Quantitative measurement of the canal is possible using digitized CT (computed tomography) or MRI (magnetic resonance imaging) images and ImageTool™, a public software (freeware) program.

The Lateral Spinal Canal

The lateral spinal canal connects the intraspinal space to the extraspinal space. Several terms are used interchangeably when referring to the lateral spinal canal. Included are "lateral recess," "subarticular gutter," and "nerve root canal." Lee et al. classified the lateral spinal canal into three zones: entrance zone, mid zone, and exit zone and described the content of each (Fig. 7–3).[17]

The *entrance zone* is located medial to, or underneath, the superior articular process. Its anterior wall is formed by the posterior surface of the disc, while the posterior wall is the superior articulating process and facet joint (covered by the ligamentum flavum). There is no true medial wall; rather the lateral dura forms its boundary. Contained within this zone is the lumbar nerve root, which is covered by the dura mater and

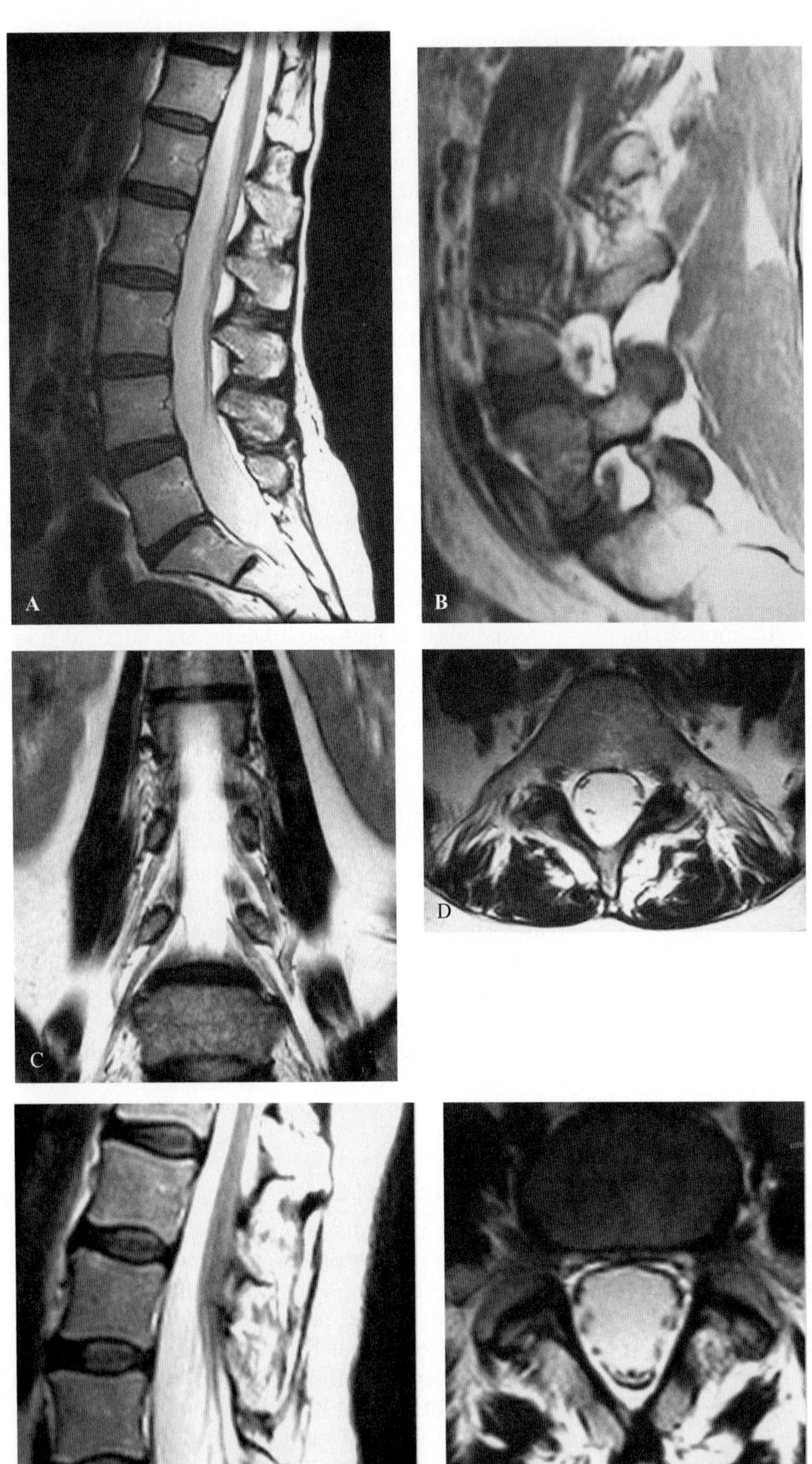

FIGURE 7–1. MRI characterization of the normal lumbar spine canal morphology. *A.* Midline sagittal T2-weighted image. *B.* Same spine, sagittal T2-weighted image through the intervertebral foramina. *C.* Same spine, coronal image through the plane of the pedicles. Note the nerve roots exiting beneath the pedicles. *D.* Same spine, axial T2-weighted image. For comparison the anteroposterior vertebral body/canal ratio is 1:0.8. *E.* A sagittal T2-weighed image showing a huge spinal canal in another case. *F.* Same spine, axial T2-weighted image. The vertebral body/canal ratio is 1:1.1.

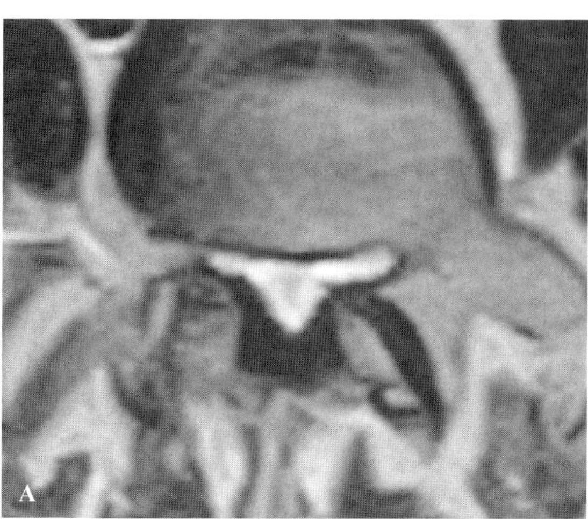

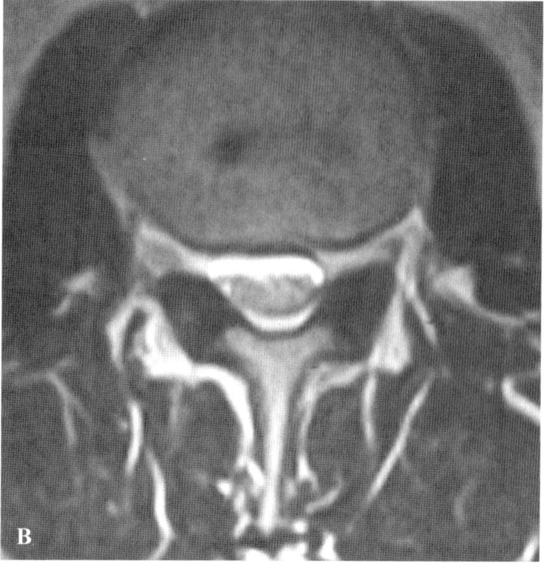

FIGURE 7–2. Lumbar spine MRI canal morphology. *A.* Axial T2-weighted image exhibiting a trefoil-shaped lumbar spinal canal variation. *B.* Axial imaging showing a developmentally small lumbar spinal canal. Note that the vertebral/body ratio is 1:0.3.

bathed in cerebrospinal fluid (CSF). Variations in the disc–body interface, pedicle length and size, length and slope of the superior articular process, and facet size determine the depth and length of the entrance zone. The entrance zone is the narrowest aspect of the lateral spinal canal.[18]

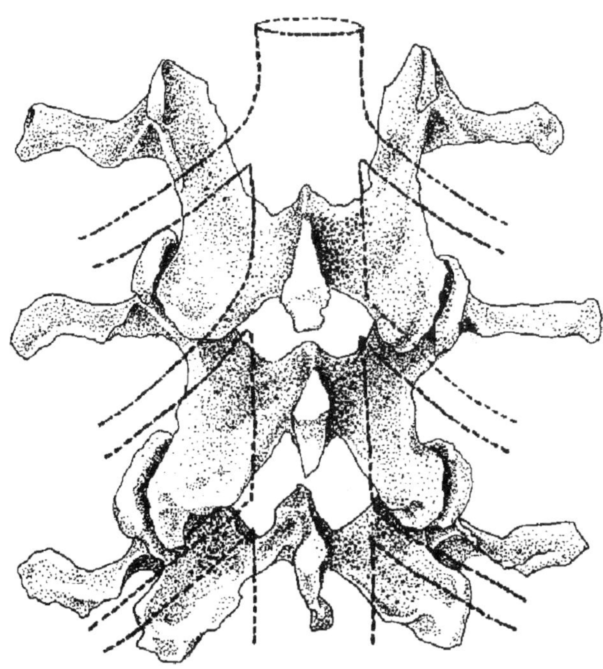

FIGURE 7–3. Zones of the lateral lumbar spinal canals. *(Redrawn from Lee et al.*[17]*)* The *entrance zone* is located medial to and underneath the superior articular process. The *mid zone* contains the dorsal root ganglion and is the region beneath the pars interarticularis part of the lamina and below the pedicle. The *exit zone* is essentially the intervertebral foramina proper.

The *mid zone* contains the dorsal root ganglion and is the region beneath the pars interarticularis sector of the lamina and below the pedicle. It is bordered anteriorly by the posterior aspect of the vertebral body and posteriorly by the pars interarticularis. Medially, the mid-zone is open to the central canal and is bordered by the dural sac. The free intrathecal roots are ensheathed by the meninges. The arachnoid membrane terminates at the medial border of the ganglion, but the dura is contiguous with the capsule of the ganglion and the perineurium of the segmental nerve.[19] The dorsal root ganglion is covered by a fibrous connective tissue extension of the dura mater and bathed in CSF.

The *exit zone* is essentially the intervertebral foramina. The intervertebral disc, posteroinferior vertebral body of the cephalad vertebra, and posterosuperior aspect of the caudal vertebra form the anterior border of the intervertebral foramen. The facet joint, formed by the adjoining superior and inferior articular processes, creates the posterior wall. The roof and floor are formed by the respective pedicles.

Nerve roots of the lower lumbar spine are larger and exit relatively smaller foramina, making the lower nerve roots more susceptible to compression.[20] One factor that determines the height of the intervertebral foramen is the posterior disc height. Compression of the exiting nerve root may occur when the posterior disc height is 4 mm or less and the foraminal height is 15 mm or less. Intraforaminal ligaments may be present in the foramen further cramping the neural contents.[21]

Postacchini reported that the width of the lateral recess depends on the length of the pedicles and shape of the vertebral canal. Vertebrae with short pedicles and a trefoil shape tend to have shallower lateral recesses.[12] A lateral recess height of 5 mm is considered normal.[18]

Spinal Mechanics Influencing Anatomy

Spinal movements and loading influence the volume and dimensions of the spinal canal. In general, flexion opens the spinal and neural foraminae, and extension has the opposite effect.[19] Flexion separates the laminae and causes thinning of the loaded ligamentum flavum. Extension of the spine results in posterior annular bulging, thickening of the unloaded ligamentum flavum, inferior sliding of the inferior articular process, and associated bulging of the facet joint.

Analysis of apathological cadaveric spines reveals that the capacity of the lumbar spinal canal increases 3.5–6.0 mL in flexion from maximal extension.[22] When compared to the neutral spine, extension has been shown to decrease the canal size by 11% and foraminal size by up to 15%, while flexion increases the foraminal cross-sectional area by 12%.[23] Using CT, Schonstrom demonstrated that the spinal dimensions increase when moving from extension to flexion and axial compression to distraction.[24] Cross-sectional area increased on average 40 and 50 mm^2 respectively, which corresponded to 16% and 19% of the canal dimension. The mid sagittal diameter decreased 2 mm from full flexion to extension.

Torsion of a vertebra with respect to the vertebra next below results in some posterior displacement of the lateral portion of the proximal vertebra with posterior bulging of the disc on the side toward the torsion. Rotation mainly affects the root canals, which narrow because of changes both in the soft tissues and vertebral displacement.[19] For example, posterior and right rotation of the L4 spinous process (e.g., left trunk rotation) may cause *bilateral* nerve root canal narrowing due to posterior vertebral displacement on the left and nerve root narrowing on the right (due to posterior disc displacement).

OVERVIEW OF SELECT STENOSIS CATEGORIES

Our present knowledge of the nature and etiology of spinal stenosis allows a classification according to associated pathology (Table 7–1). This may provide further insight into the disorder and aid the clinician in management.

Congenital/Developmental Lumbar Stenosis

Achondroplasia Achondroplasia is an autosomal dominant genetic disorder, although the majority of cases are new mutations. It is a disease of endochondral bone formation and a cause of dwarfism, with a prevalence rate between 0.5 and 1.5 per 10,000 births.[25] Abnormalities of ossification also cause significant appendicular deformity.

A decrease in height of the vertebral bodies accounts for the relative shortness of the whole spine.[26] Premature synostosis of the neurocentral synchondrosis leads to a very shallow spinal canal. The pedicles and laminae are short and thick and the transverse diameter is narrow. The achondroplastic spine tapers caudally.[26] The pedicles may be 30%–40% thicker in the achrondroplast and contribute to narrowing of the nerve root canal size. Thickening of the inferior facet may also occur and contributes to central narrowing.[27] The intervertebral discs tend to bulge posteriorly and laterally.[28] However, the spinal cord, conus medularis, and cauda equina are of normal size and may completely fill the spinal canal space, thereby obliterating the reserve capacity.

The bone changes responsible for achondroplastic spinal stenosis are present throughout the entire spine. A gibbus angulation may develop at the thoracolumbar junction, the most common site of myeloradiculopathy. Lumbosacral hyperlordosis is also common, which may functionally narrow the spinal canal. The majority of spinal stenosis-related symptoms occur in the fourth or fifth decades. The effects of trauma, degeneration, and posture are more consequential in this population because there is little to no spinal reserve capacity.[28]

Idiopathic Congenital Stenosis Congenital spinal stenosis is manifest primarily as narrowing of the anteroposterior diameter of the canal with normal development of the remaining skeleton (Figs. 7–2*B*, 7–5*A*, and 7–5*B*, and 7–13*A* to 7–13*E*). The reserve capacity of the spinal canal is compromised and there is little ability to accommodate for any degenerative changes that occur later. Indeed, its presence may remain anonymous until other temporal factors occur.

Environmental perturbations or prenatal/perinatal illnesses may override genetic regulation of spinal growth.[29,30] Prenatal stresses, such as parental malnutrition, protein deficiency, illness, or smoking, are believed to be primarily responsible.[29] Intrauterine factors are also associated with a small adult lumbar spinal canal. The most significant intrauterine factor is the length of gestation, which, if short (<37 weeks), adversely affects growth. Older maternal age and low placental weight have similar effects. Children of lower socioeconomic class parents also tend to have smaller canals. This may be because of low birth weight. The L3 level is the most affected by antenatal factors.[30] Familial stenosis has also been documented.[31]

Factors that influence spinal canal growth render it permanently stunted and, because the sagittal diameter is predominantly determined by 1 year of

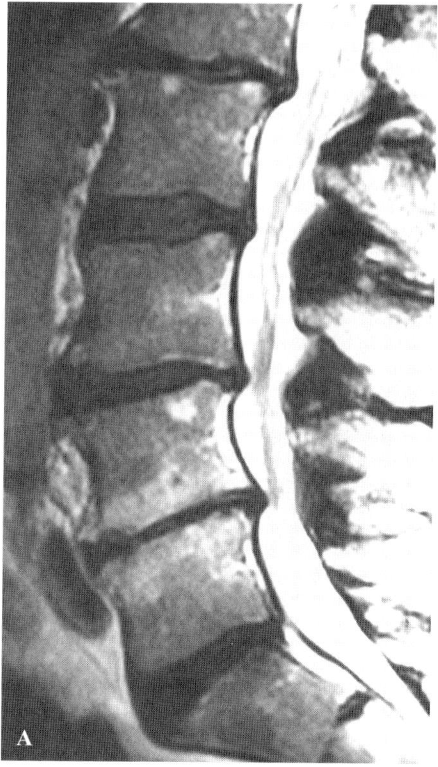

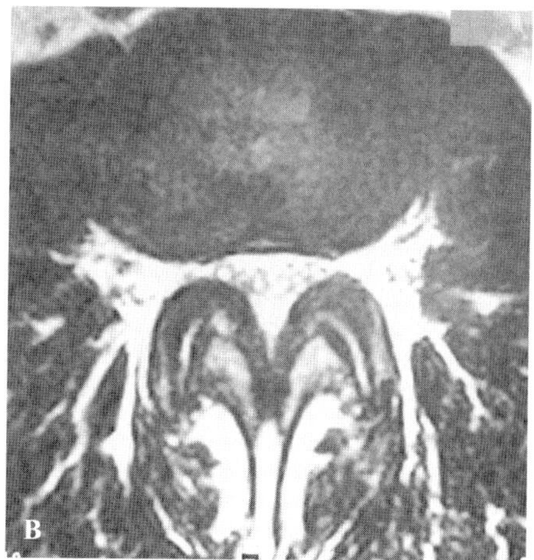

FIGURE 7–4. Multilevel degenerative disc disease and facet hypertrophy with narrowing of the central canal and lateral recesses in an elderly male patient. In this patient back pain was significantly greater than his occasional claudication. *A.* Sagittal T2-weighted image. There is moderate to advanced intervertebral disc degeneration with marginal osteophytic spurring and reactive end plate changes. No degenerative listhesis is evident. *B.* Axial T2-weighted image at the level of L4–L5. Hypertrophic posterior facets and decreased anteroposterior dimension cause the central canal and lateral recesses to be encroached symmetrically.

age, there is no time for "catch up" growth.[30] Most of these individuals become symptomatic between the third to fifth decades when early degenerative changes develop.[32]

Acquired Stenosis

Degenerative changes of the spine are responsible for the most common subcategory of spinal stenosis. These changes do not occur uniformly throughout the spine. Anterior and posterior sectors of the spinal canal may be affected individually or together, in any pattern. The greatest involvement is often at L4.

Degenerative Central Canal Stenosis Internal disc disruption may cause varying degrees of posterior annular bulging/protrusion. Intervertebral disc thinning and segmental hypermobility may increase stress loading on the posterior facet articulations. Periosteal reaction of the vertebral end plates and microinstability of the facet articulations trigger osteophyte formation along the posterior/posterolateral vertebral bodies, and hypertrophic changes of the facets (Figs. 7–4*A* and 7–4*B*, 7–5*A* and 7–5*B*, and 7–6*A* and 7–6*B*).[33]

Reactive remodeling of the articular processes is common. Anteromedial and posterolateral elongation

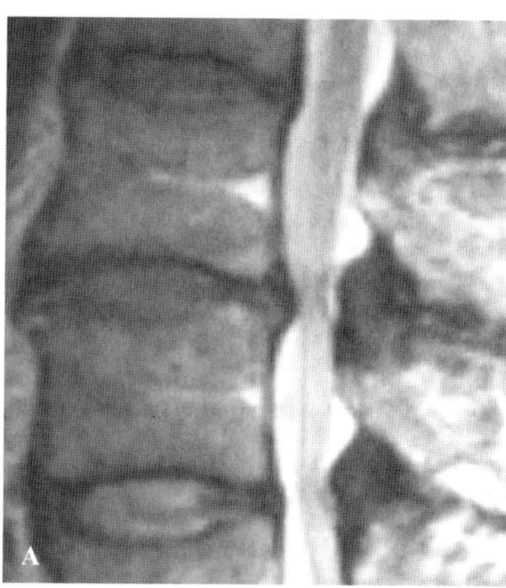

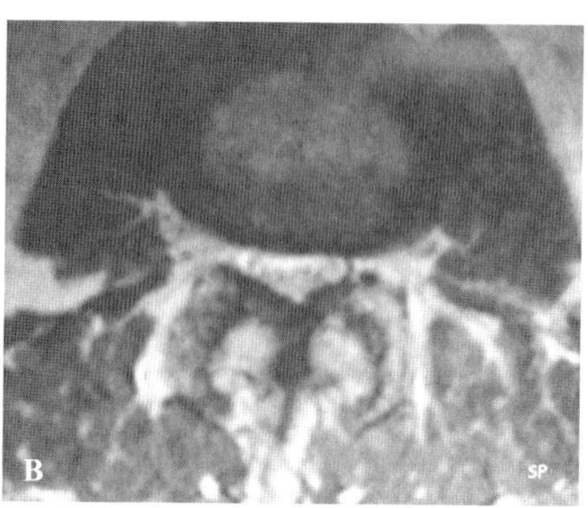

FIGURE 7–5. Multiple lumbar stenotic factors in a 59-year-old woman. There is a developmentally small canal associated with posterior disc protrusion, advanced facet disease, and flaval ligament thickening. *A.* Sagittal T2-weighted MRI. *B.* Axial T2-weighted MRI.

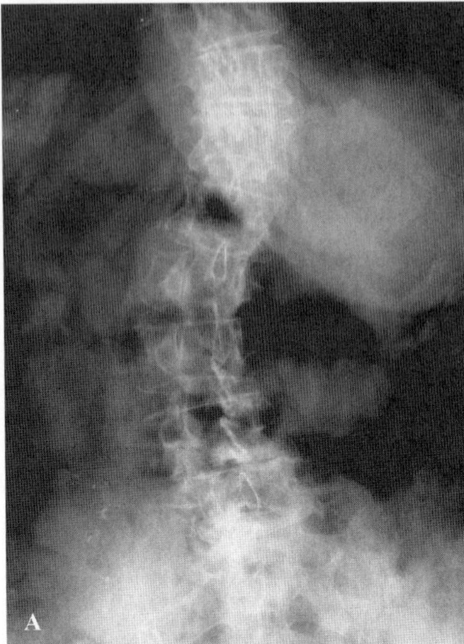

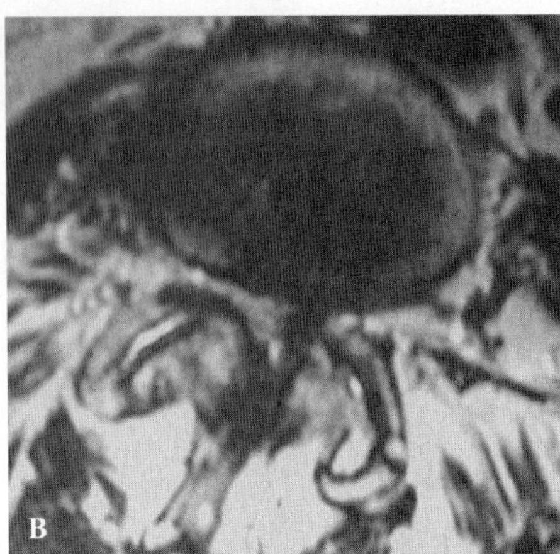

FIGURE 7–6. An elderly female patient with degenerative scoliosis and exaggerated degenerative changes, notably asymmetrical in development due to the lateral curve. *A*. Conventional radiograph showing dextrorotatory lumbar deviation and thoracolumbar compensation. There is marked intervertebral disc space loss in the lower levels. *B*. Axial MRI exhibits broad-based disc protrusion and advanced facet disease, greater on the left side. Note the fluid in the posterior joints. These types of changes may arise de novo in the elderly patient with degenerative disc disease and arthrosis, or sometimes in the patient with preexisting idiopathic scoliosis. These patients may complain of low back pain, but may also exhibit stenosis type complaints. The greatest degenerative changes tend to occur at L3–L4 and L4–L5. Two patterns of degenerative scoliosis emerge. One exhibits lumbar scoliosis having little rotational component. The other presents as progressive degenerative of a shorter segmental curve with greater degrees of rotation and also loss of the lordotic attitude.

promotes a transverse orientation.[19] Generally, superior articular process hypertrophy contributes to lateral canal stenosis and inferior articular process hypertrophy to central stenosis, although variations of both are quite common.

Clinical Pearl: Hypertrophy of the superior articular process is generally responsible for lateral canal stenosis while excrescences about the inferior articular process contribute to central stenosis.

Facet joint and disc space narrowing also shortens the lumbar spinal canal and decreases the overall volume of space available for the cauda equina.[1] Approximation of the adjacent laminae may reduce the resting pretension on the ligamentum flavum, causing it to thicken and bulge into the canal (Fig. 7–7*A* to 7–7*C*). Histological changes in the central ligamentum flavum include large fibrotic areas with decreased elastic and increased collagenous tissue. Small areas of chondroid metaplasia and regressive changes of the elastin fibers are seen. The fibrocartilaginous zone near the bone insertion often undergoes slight enlargement. Combined with ligamentum flavum calcifications, these changes reduce the elasticity of the ligament.[34] Calcium pyrophosphate dihydrate (CPPD) crystal deposition also has been identified in the ligamentum flava of 24.5% of specimens.[35] Patients with symptoms of spinal stenosis who were found to be CPPD positive may present with more acute symptoms than the CPPD negative cases. The diminished elastic properties of the ligamentum flavum also contribute to bulging into the canal with standing or lumbar extension. Insertional osteophytes may develop along the subpedicular aspect of the ligamentum flavum and hypertrophic thickening of the laminae develops.[19] Lamina thickness greater than 5 mm is considered abnormal.[9]

The dorsal fat pad appears to play an integral role in the development of anatomic stenosis. Narrowing of the interfacetal distance by facet hypertrophy, and thickening of the ligamentum flavum, forces the fat pad to move anteriorly, narrowing the sagittal diameter of the canal.[36] It remains unclear whether hypertrophic facets are responsible for pushing the ligamentum flavum into the canal or if canal narrowing is due to morphological changes within the ligament itself. In contrast, patients with developmentally large facets and posterior canal narrowing appear to have decreased epidural fat on a developmental basis and are not subject to the same thecal sac compression by the posterior fat pad.[37]

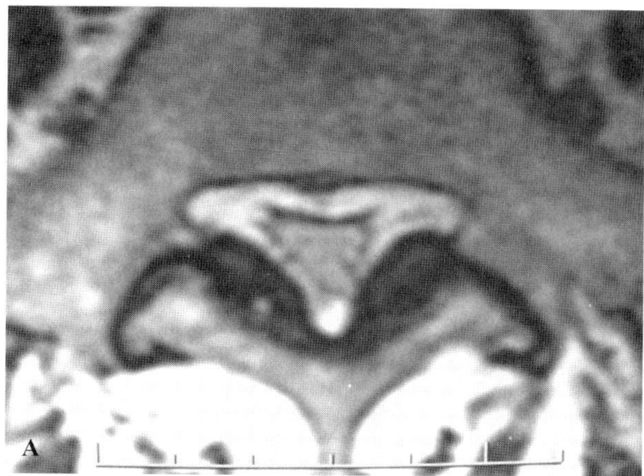

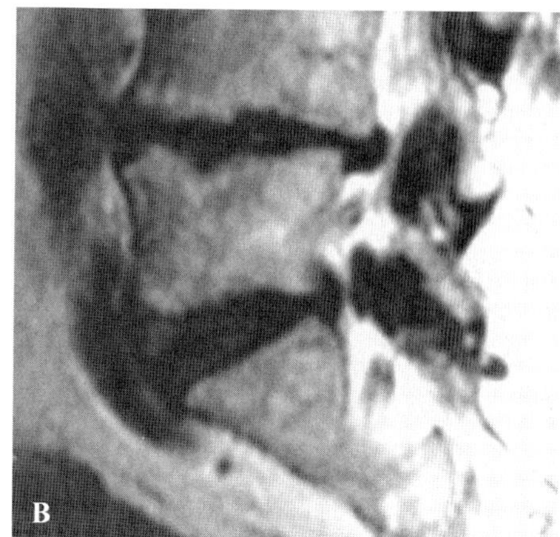

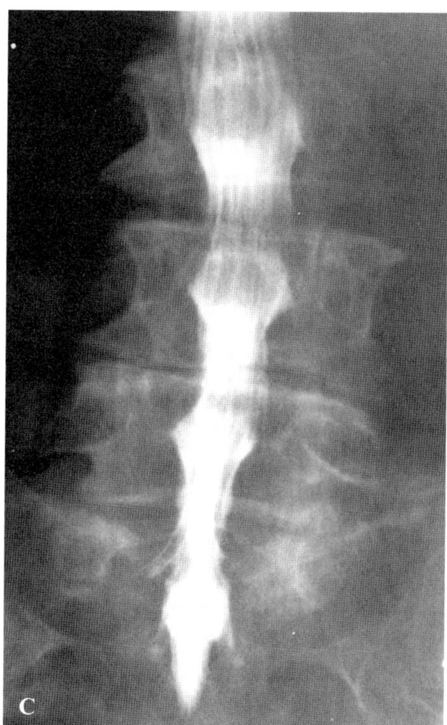

FIGURE 7–7. Lower lumbar spinal canal stenosis with ligamentum flavum hypertrophy. *A*. Axial T2-weighted MRI image showing flaval thickening, greater on the left side. *B*. Sagittal image through the lateral recess showing significant intrusion of the thickened ligament and some associated disc protrusion. There is multilevel involvement. *C*. Same case. Lumbar myelogram showing narrowing and distortion of the caudal sac and root sleeve cutoff.

Degenerative cysts in the region of a synovial facet joint or ligamentum flavum often produce a significant mass lesion and canal narrowing. These cysts may compress nerve roots, producing radiculopathy similar to that caused by focal intervertebral disc herniation (Fig. 7–8*A* and 7–8*B*). They may also produce intermittent activity-related pain that is more typical of lumbar stenosis.[1]

Degenerative Lateral Canal Stenosis Congenital and degenerative abnormalities in the posterolateral vertebral body, intervertebral disc, and pedicle and superior articular process influence the shape and size of the lateral spinal canal. Any of the three zones of the lateral canal may be affected. Entrance zone stenosis may be caused by marginal hypertrophy, as well as developmental variations in facet joint shape, size, and orientation.[17] Hypertrophy of the facets, posterolateral disc protrusion, fibrotic and calcified ("hard") discs, and vertebral body ridging represent acquired factors. Most commonly, the L4–L5 level is involved.[18,38] Congenitally large or anteriorly sloping facet joints and short pedicles may increase the consequence of acquired changes.

Mid-zone stenosis may result from fibrocartilaginous or bursal tissue hypertrophy at a spondylolytic defect.[17]

Exit zone intervertebral foraminal stenosis may occur from facet hypertrophy, intervertebral disc protrusion, or a combination of each. A correlation exists between the posterior disc height and the foraminal heights. Disc space narrowing parallels decreased foraminal height with associated subsidence and subluxation of the articular processes. The superior

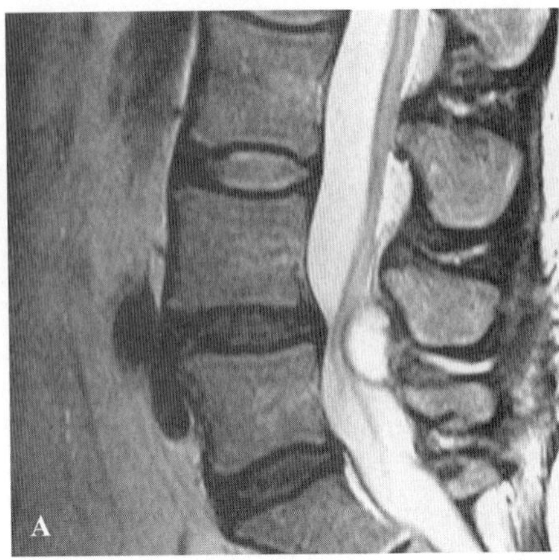

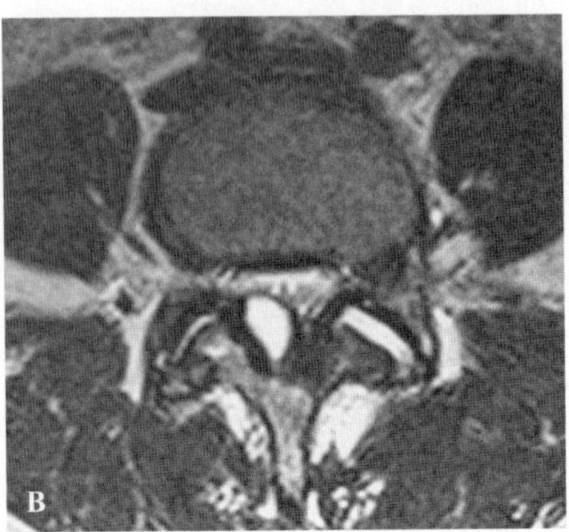

FIGURE 7–8. A large synovial facet cyst intrudes with significant mass effect into the spinal canal at L4–L5 on the right side. Note the slight anterior listhesis of L4 on L5, and loss of signal intensity of the L4–L5 and L5–S1 intervertebral discs. *A.* Sagittal T2-weighted MRI. *B.* Axial T2-weighted MRI showing bilateral facet disease and joint effusion in addition to the large cyst.

articular process of the caudad vertebra slides superior and anterior, causing the ligamentum flavum to bulge anteriorly and to encroach the nerve root.[20]

These types of degenerative changes at one vertebral level may produce symptoms along two nerve roots and confuse the clinical picture. For example, hypertrophic changes of the L5 superior articulating process may affect compression of both the L5 and the S1 nerve root.

Ciric et al. studied the vertical dimension of the lateral recess on polytomography and CT imaging.[18] Heights of 2 mm or less are considered diagnostic, and a height of 3 mm or less is highly indicative of a lateral recess stenosis. On the other hand, a lateral recess measuring 5 mm probably rules out lateral recess stenosis.

Bulging of the facet articulation during lumbar extension, combined with posterior bulging of the disc, narrows the region of the lateral recess and closes the anterolateral angles of the spinal canal. The opposite occurs during lumbar flexion.[36]

Spondylolisthesis Degenerative spondylolisthesis with anterior vertebral slippage, without pars interarticularis defect, is most common at L4–L5. When the L4–L5 facets are more sagittal in disposition there may be decreased resistance to shear stresses.[39] Anterior shift is resisted at L5–S1 by coronal facets joints and the iliolumbar ligament. Facet disease and remodeling are common in degenerative spondylolisthesis. Cartilage loss and facet remodeling allows for anterior translation in the absence of sagittal facet disposition.

As L4 slides anteriorly, the inferior aspect of the posterior arch approximates the posterosuperior end plate of L5, and may result in a guillotine-like compression of the thecal sac (Fig. 7–9*A* and 7–9*B*).

In these cases, any increased mobility tends to subside following natural spinal stabilization (i.e., spur formation, end plates sclerosis, and ligamentous ossification), which provides for an improved prognosis and amenability to conservative management.[40]

THE CLINICAL PROFILE: HISTORY AND PHYSICAL EXAMINATION

There is no gold standard examination procedure for lumbar spinal stenosis. Diagnostic imaging alone is not sufficiently discriminating. This is illustrated by the high incidence of false-positive findings of stenosis in an asymptomatic population: 21% of MRI studies[41] and 5% on CT examinations.[42] Furthermore, the severity of stenosis found on imaging studies does not correlate well with the clinical profile, either with regard to intensity of pain or clinical signs.[43–45] *Most often, lumbar spinal stenosis defies clear clinical identification and the patient history becomes the most powerful diagnostic tool.*

Clinical Pearl: Diagnostic imaging alone is not sufficiently discriminating to appraise clinical spinal stenosis.

Katz et al. presented a logical progression for diagnostic assessment.[32] First, other conditions that may be confused with spinal stenosis should be excluded. Second, if the clinical–anatomic diagnosis of spinal stenosis is made, then etiological factors should be identified. Finally, spinal stenosis may be associated with other pain syndromes besides neurogenic claudication and chronic nerve compression. These should be identified and their impact on the patient's disability assessed (see Table 7–1 and *Differential Diagnosis*).

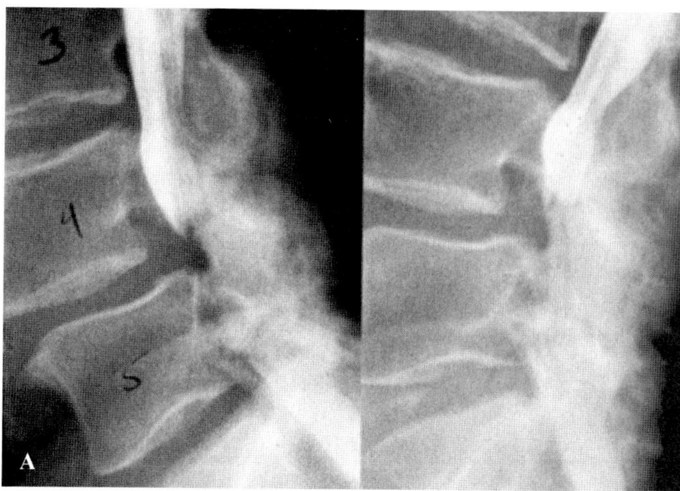

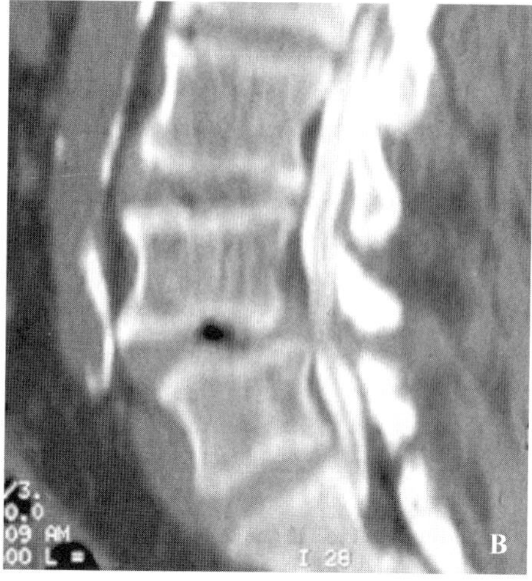

FIGURE 7–9. A 67-year-old male with degenerative spondylolisthesis, diffuse idiopathic skeletal hyperostosis, and mild stenotic symptoms relieved by successful sacroiliac joint manipulation and an exercise program. *A*. Myelogram with flexion and extension views. Note the myelographic cutoff at L4–L5 without evidence for intersegmental instability. *B*. Sagittal reformatted CT image showing small amount of contrast trailing through the L4–L5 sector only in the midline. Compression occurs by the disc anteriorly, ligamentum flavum posteriorly, and facet hypertrophy laterally.

Clinical Pearl: The patient history often becomes the most powerful diagnostic tool in clearer clinical identification of lumbar spinal stenosis.

The patient interview should be directed at defining the duration of symptoms (back and leg), activities that provoke and relieve the symptoms, impact on function and quality of life, presence of any advancing neurological deficits, and a self-assessment of health status.

Symptoms of Lumbar Spine Stenosis

The most common subjective complaints associated with symptomatic lumbar spinal stenosis are low back pain and leg symptoms. Those with congenital spinal stenosis generally become symptomatic earlier (third through fifth decades), whereas patients with degenerative stenosis become symptomatic later (sixth through eighth decades).[32] The mean age is about 67 years.[46] Some studies show a female preponderance of up to 65 %.[32,46] A possible explanation for a female predominance is the higher incidence of degenerative spondylolisthesis in the female population.

Symptoms of degenerative joint disease such as backache or stiffness characterize the back complaints. Vague lower limb symptoms develop insidiously and may persist for years before a definitive diagnosis is made. Patients may complain of lower limb pain, fatigue, weakness, paresthesias, cramping, or ataxia that progressively increase with prolonged ambulation or static standing. Bilateral symptoms may occur with central stenosis and unilateral radicular-like symptoms result from lateral nerve tunnel compression, the latter mimicking the symptoms of a neurocompressive disc herniation.

Patients typically endure years of back pain before the onset of claudication symptoms.[32] The word *claudication* is derived from the Latin verb *claudicare*, which means "to limp" or "to be lame."[47] The terminology associated with claudication is confusing. With claudication related to vascular abnormalities one would expect no change in leg pain with back movements, decreased pulses, bruits, stocking deficits, relief with standing and lying flat, and exacerbation with exercise. *Intermittent claudication* is discomfort in the lower extremity musculature that is prompted by exercise and relieved by rest. *Neurogenic (pseudo) claudication* is defined as calf pain with walking (as in patients with vascular claudication), but increased with lumbar spine extension and relieved with lumbar flexion.

Neurogenic claudication is reported in 62%–100% of cases.[43,48–50] An important characteristic of neurogenic claudication symptoms is relief upon forward bending or sitting. Maximal walking distances of less than 0.5 km are seen in 66 % of patients with central spinal stenosis.[51] Patients with more severe stenosis tend to have greater walking limitation, and may also complain of greater symptom aggravation with downhill walking. A strategy that provides relief for many is walking stooped behind a shopping cart. Bicycling distance is commonly unaffected and walking uphill is less provocative.

Clinical Pearl: Patients with more severe stenosis tend to have greater walking limitations and may also complain of greater symptom aggravation with

down-hill walking. A strategy that provides relief for many is walking stooped behind a shopping cart.

Differences in symptom profile exist between those with symptomatic central and lateral spinal stenosis. The symptoms of "pure" lateral stenosis are usually either radiculopathy or atypical leg pain (presents with sciatica and neurological symptoms or as a diffuse, bizarre pain in a nondermatomal distribution). Neurogenic intermittent claudication can also occur, but is more common with concomitant central canal stenosis.[52]

Subjective lower limb sensory abnormalities/paresthesias occur in 50%–75% of cases. Feelings of limb weakness are highly variable and occur in 33%–87%.[6,32,43,48]

Bladder dysfunction is reported in fewer than 12 percent,[6,43] and male sexual dysfunction such as impotence is possible. Walking-induced erections without sexual stimulation (priapism) are a rare and poorly understood symptom of lumbar spine stenosis that may be caused by parasympathetic dysfunction from compression in the lower lumbar spine. Patients may report associated urinary incontinence or an increased urge to void. These symptoms are usually relieved by surgical spinal decompression.[53–56]

Differential Diagnosis

The symptoms of spinal stenosis are shared with a number of other, potentially more consequential conditions. The primary differential diagnosis to consider is a comorbid claudication of vascular origin. In such cases it confuses and complicates both clinical identification and management. Vascular claudication is most notable in the gastrocnemius muscle, which, because of its high muscle fiber density per tissue unit and its large number of motor units per innervating neuron, consumes more oxygen per tissue unit than any other muscle in the body.[57]

Clinical Pearl: Vascular claudication is most notable in the gastrocnemius.

Neurological disorders such as diabetic or compressive neuropathy, primary demyelinating diseases such as multiple sclerosis, or chronic inflammatory demyelinating polyneuropathy should also be ruled out.[58] Functional, degenerative, or inflammatory musculoskeletal conditions affecting the intervertebral disc, facet articulations, sacroiliac joints, hips, and knees should all be considered. Visceral referred pain to the lower part of the back, such as retroperitoneal tumors, aortic aneurysms, peptic ulcers that penetrate posteriorly, and renal lesions all require differential consideration.[59]

Physical Examination

The physical examination for the suspected patient with lumbar stenosis should include peripheral vascular status; abdominal examination; spine, hip, knee, and ankle ranges of motion; motor and reflex grading; neural tension testing; and a sustained standing extension test. Functional assessment such as bicycle riding or walking capacity may serve as a baseline evaluation of entry-level endurance (see *Outcome Assessment*).

One should inspect for trophic changes consistent with peripheral vascular disease. These include shiny, thin distal extremity skin; diffuse loss of hair; poorly healing scars; and thin weak nails. The strength and quality of the dorsalis pedis and posterior tibial pulses and capillary refill should be assessed. Auscultation and palpation of the abdomen is performed to rule out bruits or a bounding abdominal aortic pulse.

Adaptive posturing is frequently observed in the advanced lumbar spinal stenosis population and a wide-based gait is common. Combined hip, knee, and lumbar flexion ("Simian stance" or ape-like) may be present while standing, and increases with ambulation distance.[60] Such posturing, when chronic, may contribute to shortening of the iliopsoas muscle, which limits hip extension. This compensatory posture is assumed to provide claudication relief by opening the sagittal spinal canal diameter and decompressing the affected nerve roots. Neurogenic claudication symptoms may be relieved, and ambulation distance increased, by stooping forward while walking or by riding on a bicycle. However, the absence of this finding is insensitive and does not differentiate whether the patient has either neurogenic or intermittent claudication.[61]

Lumbar spine ranges of motion are usually restricted, especially extension. When examining lumbar motion, observe for the quality as well as the quantity of motion. Trunk flexibility may be estimated with finger-to-floor or Schober's test. The latter measurement of a marked 10-cm spine segment, neutral compared to flexion, is reliable.[62]

Provocation of lower extremity symptoms during lumbar extension can be viewed as the physical examination equivalent of neurogenic claudication. Often, patients must maintain lumbar extension for 30–60 seconds in order to reproduce leg pain.[32] Attention should be paid to the patient's posture when performing this maneuver. Because of pain provoked during standing lumbar extension, there is a tendency to flex the knees while maintaining a straight or flexed lumbar spine. For this procedure the hands are placed on the buttocks to maintain stability, the knees are extended as fully as possible, and the patient is observed for lordotic extension.

The neurological examination is of limited value and is not specific in defining patients with lumbar stenosis. It is not possible to determine the side or extent of the spinal canal constriction from the neurological findings.[45] Indeed a normal neurological examination is present in approximately 18 percent of stenotic cases.[6] It is primarily performed to rule out other neural entrapment syndromes and define a baseline of neurological status. Deficits in Achilles muscle stretch reflexes are found in 43%–66% of cases and quadriceps (patellar) responses are affected in 18%–42%, but reflexes in general are commonly decreased in the elderly.[6,45,48] Inconsistencies between any loss of motor strength and compression level is seen in 23%–50% of cases. Motor deficits are more common in lateral recess stenosis (68%).[51]

Straight-leg raising (SLR) is positive in fewer than 50% of confirmed cases. A positive SLR is more likely indicative of a concomitant disc extrusion with nerve root involvement. Balance and vibratory sensation disturbances are common but were reported in only one study (66% and 80% of cases respectively).[49] Valsalva maneuvers generally do not influence the symptoms of either lateral recess stenosis[18] or central stenosis.[51] Fortunately, cauda equina syndrome is a rare complication.

The true value of the historical interview and physical examination is its ability to positively predict whether a patient has the condition in question. Considering the limited value of the clinical examination, how should one apply the history and physical examination findings effectively? Several statistical analyses can be used to determine the value of the history and physical examination. These include the sensitivity, specificity, and positive/negative likelihood ratios (LRs) (see Table 7–2)

The absence of pain while sitting is highly specific (.93). The most specific physical findings are a

TABLE 7–2. Value of the History and Physical Examination

	Sensitivity	Specificity	+LR	−LR
Factors from patient's history				
Age >65	.77	.69	2.5	0.33
Pain below buttocks	.88	.34	1.3	0.35
No pain when seated	.46	.93	6.6	0.58
Symptoms improved when seated	.52	.83	3.1	0.58
Symptoms worse when walking	.71	.30	1.0	0.96
Able to walk better when holding onto a shopping cart	.63	.67	1.9	0.55
Pain in legs worsened by walking and relieved by sitting	.81	.16	0.8	1.2
Best posture with regards to symptoms is sitting	.89	.39	1.5	0.28
Worst posture with regards to symptoms is standing/walking	.89	.33	1.3	0.33
Factors from the physical examination				
No pain with lumbar flexion	.79	.44	1.4	0.48
Thigh pain with 30 seconds of lumbar extension	.51	.69	1.6	0.71
Lower extremity weakness	.47	.78	2.1	0.68
Absent Achilles reflex	.46	.78	2.1	0.69
Factors from clinical diagnostic testing				
Improved walking tolerance with spinal flexion	.58	.91	6.4	0.46
Improved walking tolerance on inclined versus level treadmill	.50	.92	0.65	0.54
Earlier onset of symptoms on level versus inclined treadmill walking	.68	.83	4.1	0.39
Longer recovery time after level versus inclined treadmill walking	.82	.68	2.6	0.26

Note: Likelihood ratios (LRs) close to 1 indicate that a test does little to alter the diagnostic probability. A high LR (>5.0) indicates a test in which a positive result is helpful for ruling in the diagnosis, whereas a small negative LR (e.g., <0.30) is associated with tests in which a negative result is helpful in ruling out the diagnosis.[63]

wide-based gait and an abnormal result on the modified Romberg test (both >.90).[49]

Of all the extracted variables from the patient history, the most valuable are those concerning the postural nature of the patient's pain. The absence of pain when seated (6.6) or decrease of symptoms when seated (3.1) each have a high positive LR, and are therefore helpful in ruling in a diagnosis of lumbar spinal stenosis.

A small negative LR is found for patient reports of sitting being the best posture with regards to symptoms (0.28), and standing/walking being the worst postures (0.33). This means that the absence of these factors would be helpful in ruling out a diagnosis of lumbar spinal stenosis.

The sensitivity of improved walking tolerance with spinal flexion is low (.58), but the high specificity of this finding gives the test a high positive LR, making it a valuable piece of diagnostic data for ruling in lumbar spinal stenosis. The results of the two-stage treadmill test comparing neutral versus spine flexed also has a high positive LR for improved total walking time with the spine flexed (6.5). Table 7–2 is Fritz's statistical analysis of the history, physical examination, and objective testing results of patients with suspected lumbar stenosis.[63]

As an example, considering these data, a 75-year-old patient with no pain when seated, and a wide-based gait, but no thigh pain with lumbar extension, would have a 90% likelihood of having lumbar spinal stenosis.[49]

Functional Assessment

Although the physical examination frequently falls short when working toward a clinical diagnosis, functional assessment is both descriptive and prescriptive. Factors that may contribute to increased lordotic or torsional stresses to the lumbar spine need to be assessed and can be used to tailor treatment strategies.

Clinical Pearl: Functional assessment of the patient is not just descriptive. They are often prescriptive as well, and findings at examination can become valid treatment strategies.

Lateral or anteroposterior postural deviations may result from disturbances in any link of the lower functional kinetic chain. Assessment of standing postural symmetry may identify factors such as static pelvic unleveling. Gait analysis may reveal compensatory patterns or other abnormalities. Anterior pelvic tilting and an increased lumbar lordosis may be caused by tightness of the iliopsoas and erector spinae, and weakness in the rectus abdominis, gluteus maximus, and hamstring muscles. Imbalances in muscles of normal gross strength and flexibility may also be responsible. Poor reflexive control or weakness of the multifidi and transverse abdominis muscles results in functional stability compromise (see Chapter 4).

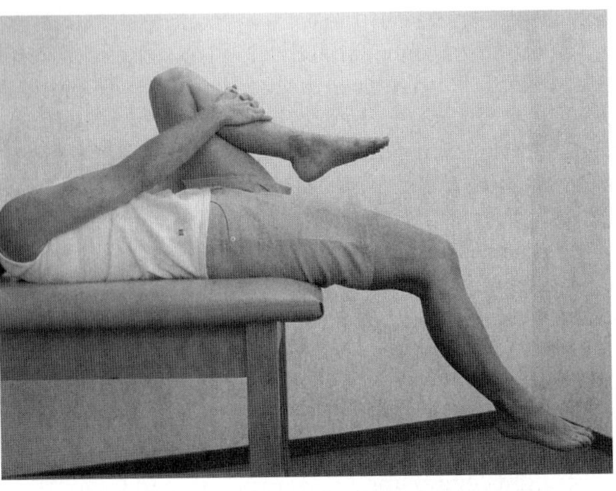

FIGURE 7–10. Thomas test. The patient lies supine with one thigh flexed and held against the chest. The low back and sacrum should be flat against the examining table, which places the pelvis in approximately 10 degree of posterior tilt. Care should be taken not to induce excessive posterior pelvic tilting, as a false reading will be obtained. In the absence of hip flexor shortness, the posterior aspect of the free thigh will fall to horizontal and the knee will flex to 80 degree.[64]

Soft tissue flexibility tests such as the modified Thomas test (Fig. 7–10), LSR, and piriformis stretch test are used to identify areas of soft tissue tightness. In the resting supine position, any degree of hyperlordosis may suggest erector spinae or psoas major shortening.

Gross hip mobility may be assessed with Patrick's maneuver (FABERE test). Capsular limitation or acetabular-femoral pathology may restrict motion with or without inguinal, gluteal, or medial thigh pain. Passive hip abduction with the knee straight and flexed to 90 degrees assesses the two and one joint adductor muscle respectively. Tightness may be associated with abductor weakness that causes gait abnormality.

The coordination quality of the hip extensor complex is evaluated as the prone patient lifts each thigh individually from the examination table. The normal activation sequence is (1) hamstrings/gluteus maximus, (2) contralateral lumbar erector spinae, and (3) ipsilateral lumbar erector spinae (see Chapter 4). Hyperextension of the lumbar spine indicates excessive erector spinae activity and/or weakness of the gluteus maximus muscles. Hip extension restriction points to tightness of the psoas major or hip capsule tightness. Abnormal muscle activation sequences may contribute to excessive lumbosacral extension during ambulation ("false hip extension") and warrant reeducation. Gross motor strength assessment of the hip extensors is also assessed.

Abdominal muscle strength assessment is performed with the patient lying supine with the legs extended. The ability of the spine to flex segmentally without substitution of the hip flexors is observed. Patients who raise their torso with an extended lumbar spine may have overactive iliopsoas muscles, tight erector spinae, and/or abdominal weakness.[64]

Diagnostic Imaging

The essential anatomicopathological concept of stenosis is space limitation and imaging has been used to portray those changes. Investigation of the spine patient with degenerative disease and suspected stenosis typically begins with properly positioned, high-quality conventional radiographs.

The usefulness of plain films is established but so are the limitations. They allow for general quantification of the significant bony abnormalities, disc interspace thinning, marginal spurring and facet disease, and clinical findings add suspicion of stenosis. However, central and lateral recess changes are often missed or underestimated (see Fig. 7–13*A* to 7–13*E*). Furthermore, critical landmark determination for the calculation of mid-sagittal bony diameters is often inaccurate and the cut-off guidelines should not be strictly applied. Nevertheless, the plain film examination provides for a preliminary staging as well as direction to other imaging procedures.

Clinical Pearl: Landmark determinations used for the calculation of mid-sagittal bony diameters are often inaccurate. The cut-off guidelines should not be strictly applied.

Since soft tissue abnormalities are poorly demonstrated on plain films, more accurate techniques are often needed for their assessment. For instance, the ligamentum flavum and degenerative facet joint cysts are not apparent on conventional imaging unless they contain some calcification. CT is well suited to exhibit the bony changes of stenosis at any site, flaval thickening, hypertrophy of bone grafts, facet cysts, and soft tissue calcifications.

CT is used commonly to assess the presence and severity of spinal stenosis. It is relatively inexpensive, readily available, and has few adverse effects. The internal structure of bone is exquisitely revealed and the contrast resolution is greater than plain film. Contrast of the soft tissue is also superior with CT.

Narrowing of the various canal dimensions must be associated with appropriate clinical manifestations as they vary significantly according to location, severity, and cause.[65] Cross-sectional mensuration of the thecal sac is possible, which correlates better with clinical stenosis.[66]

As might be expected, there may be disagreements between readers of CT scans. There is better agreement regarding mid-sagittal canal measurements than foraminal dimensions.[67] One study shows poor interexaminer agreement among surgeons regarding the presence and severity of lumbar spinal stenosis, even when individual features of stenosis, such as facet arthrosis, nerve root impingement, ligamentum flavum hypertrophy and disc protrusion, were addressed.[68]

There is continuing controversy as to the utilization of CT alone or in conjunction with myelography (CT-myelography) for the diagnosis of degenerative disease including stenosis. In many spine specialty centers today CT-myelography and CT-discography are extensively used to sort through and understand the various pain generators, especially when surgical procedures are being contemplated.

MRI adds additional information about intrinsic changes within the spinal cord, nerve rootlets, and related soft tissues, including epidural fibrosis, infection, and tumors. The goal of lumbar MRI evaluation in patients with radiculopathy or myeloradiculopathy is to identify the presence of, and provide relative contributions of, each stenotic component: canal dimensions and intrusion into the intervertebral canals at entrance, mid, or exit zones.

Alone, or in combination, today's advanced imaging is capable of providing detailed information regarding the site and extent of spatial intrusion into the spinal and foraminal canals, along with accurate mensuration of their diameters, areas and contents, as well as additional information regarding the status of the intervertebral discs, articular facets, thickness of epidural fat, etc.

Although CT and MRI are presently the most frequently used noninvasive imaging methods, imaging of a supine patient may not demonstrate the maximal spinal stenosis that has been shown by upright flexion–extension myelography. This procedure is not new. It has shown marked variation in the severity of lumbar dural sac stenosis during flexion and extension in some patients.

Underestimation of the diameter of the dural sac (by up to 30%) is found when CT-myelograms are compared with extension myelography. Myelography with extension positioning may be considered for patients whose symptoms are not explained by routine cross-sectional imaging studies to exclude positionally dependent spinal stenosis,[69] as long as no other upright technology is available.[70]

Currently there is much interest in dynamic loading, as well as weight-bearing and dynamic flexion–extension imaging. Axial loaded CT-myelography and MRI have been accomplished with the patient recumbent and loaded in a portable device.[71] In 66 of 84 patients investigated in another study, there was a statistically significant reduction of the dural sac cross-sectional area in at least one site during axial compression in slight extension.[72] With change from flexion to extension and distraction to compression, up to 16% area reduction can be expected, along with a reduction in the mid-sagittal canal diameter of 2 mm.[24]

In the past, positional MRI had to be variously obtained without weight-bearing or significant motion range. Using a mid-field strength scanner with the patient seated, Weishaupt et al. recently documented positionally related changes in the intervertebral canal measurements and nerve root compression not visible at conventional recumbent MRI.[73]

For the first time there is now an MRI system available with capabilities to image in the upright, recumbent, and other nontraditional positions (Fonar, 0.6 T). This opens investigation for patient scanning in clinically relevant positions that may unmask dynamically dependent pathoanatomical conditions.

Criteria for Diagnosing Symptomatic Lumbar Spinal Stenosis

Considering all of the ambiguities and potentially conflicting data, the clinician is faced with a formidable diagnostic challenge. Katz et al. proposed the following diagnostic criteria: (1) imaging evidence of impingement of the cauda equina and/or exiting nerve roots; and (2) one or both of the clinical syndromes of neurogenic claudication and chronic nerve root compression (radicular or polyradicular abnormalities in lower extremity reflexes, muscle strength, or sensation not explained by the presence of a generalized peripheral neuropathy).[32]

Pathophysiology of Claudication

The precise pathophysiology of neurogenic claudication remains unclear. Proposed mechanisms include compression of the cauda equina and/or nerve roots, increased epidural pressure, ischemia, venous stasis, and neural tension. Since there is some evidence to support each mechanism, a combined etiology is likely.

Spinal stenosis, central and lateral, may cause direct compression of the thecal sac, nerve roots, or both. Compression alone, however, is not sufficient to cause claudication symptoms. This is supported by the imaging findings of advanced stenosis in asymptomatic individuals, and the absence of symptoms at rest in those patients with intermittent claudication. Interestingly, patients with even severe stenosis caused by one level disc extrusion do not typically experience claudication symptoms. This observation has led some investigators to conclude that more than one level of stenosis must be present for symptom expression to occur.

Most of the research into the pathophysiology of intermittent claudication has been completed during the past decade.

Histological and morphological characteristics of the human cauda equina with stenosis-induced intermittent claudication: Post-mortem sections demonstrate a loss in the number of neurons, particularly the large-caliber fibers. Empty axons are numerous and various degrees of demyelination are seen. Some small fiber regeneration may be present. Nonneural changes include interstitial fibrosis, thick-walled congested veins, and pia-arachnoid adhesions. As the descending nerve roots become adherent to each other, the cauda equina acquires an *hourglass* appearance. Distal to the compression site, myelin bubble formation (Schwann cell and endoneural fibroblast proliferation) indicates chronic demyelination.[74] The longitudinal radicular arteries appear to maintain their continuity during slowly developing compression, and pronounced compensatory arterial coils are more exaggerated adjacent to the lesioned area. These coils are believed to compensate for the immobilization of the roots at the point of the lesion, which could produce extra tension during flexion/extension of the lumbar vertebrae.[47] It is important to remember that the electrophysiological changes do not occur while large myelinated nerve fibers remain relatively intact.[74]

What are the events that lead to these morphological and histological changes and how do they affect the function of the cauda equina and nerve roots? Chronic nerve root compression causes large myelinated fiber degeneration and intrafascicular fibrosis. Wallarian degeneration becomes evident. The thin-walled venules of the intrinsic nerve root vasculature are particularly vulnerable to compression. When blood flow within a venule is impaired, there may be a reduced flow in the connected capillaries. Short-term compression results in reversible ischemic/nutritional deficit, whereas longer compression times result in a more permanent edema formation, even at very low pressures. If the pressure on a nerve root reaches a critical level, and the intrinsic vessels can no longer compensate, local ischemia of the nerve roots result. During increased demand, such as walking, "functional ischemia" develops.[75]

Edema formation around the nerve root can result from either rapid and slow onset compression. Generally, this is more pronounced in severity with rapid onset. Intraneural edema is formed by increased microvascular permeability and leakage of macromolecule-containing fluid into the endoneurial space. A "miniature compartment syndrome" may occur. Nutrient transfer and ionic balance in the endoneurial space is likely altered.[76]

Nerve impulse propagation impairment has been identified during experimental compression of the cauda equina. Rapid onset compression induces more pronounced impulse propagation deficits than does slow rate compression. There is, however, no significant change in propagation during the early stages of compression, either rapid or slow-rate. Theoretically, this indicates that there are no severe mechanical effects, such as disruption of axons, induced during the compression onset. Rather, nutritional deficits may be responsible for the impulse propagation deficit.[77]

Porter and Ward postulated that two levels of stenosis are necessary to produce claudication symptoms: either a two-level or multilevel central canal stenosis, or a one-level central stenosis and associated root canal stenosis.[78] Under this model, venous pooling and congestion, rather than arteriole compression, between the two levels causes ischemia of one or several nerve roots. One level central stenosis, with combined distal lateral canal stenosis causes congestion in only one nerve root (Fig. 7–11*B*). Two-level central stenosis may result in venous congestion between the two levels and more diffuse, bilateral symptoms (Fig. 7–11*A*). The incidence of neurogenic claudication in two-level stenosis versus one-level compression is statistically greater.[79] Electrophysiology laboratory investigations support the two-level compression model of intermittent claudication development.[80] The ischemia model was supported early on by Evans who tested intermittent claudication symptom onset in patients under varying oxygen tension. Claudication symptoms were provoked earlier under lower oxygen tension concentrations.[81]

If the anatomic changes associated with stenosis are constantly present, why do the symptoms occur only during ambulation and standing with extension? Changes in the size and shape of the spinal canal occur during upright weight bearing. Functional narrowing of the spinal canal decreases the reserve capacity available for the spinal contents and alters the epidural pressure. Epidural pressure is sensitive to changes in lumbar spine position and more marked in individuals with lumbar spinal stenosis. Epidural pressures have been measured in a series of positions. Lowest pressures occurred during recumbency. Sitting doubled and standing quadrupled the pressure. Prone extension caused a fivefold increase, but standing extension caused sixfold increase. Flexion, on the other hand, produced only 25% of the sitting value. In this study, all patients became symptomatic during sustained extension.[82]

The epidural pressure in patients with stenosis during simple walking was approximately 2.5 times

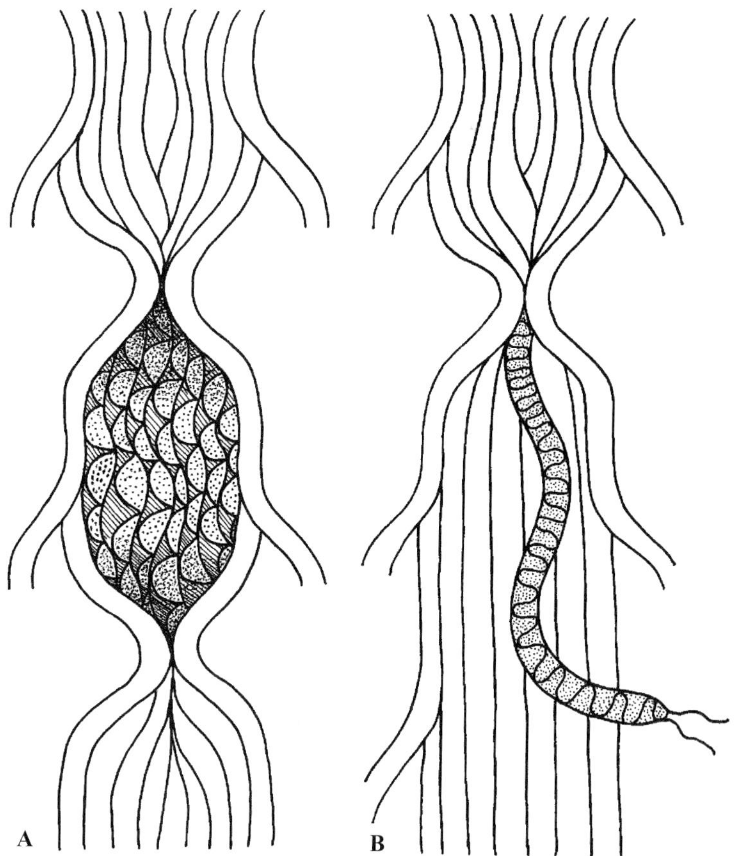

FIGURE 7–11. Schema of the significance of two-level stenosis pathology. *(Redrawn from Porter and Ward.*[78]*) A.* A two-level central canal stenosis is depicted with venous congestion and pooling in multiple nerve roots of the cauda equina between the two levels of stenosis. *B.* A one-level central stenosis with an associated single-level root canal stenosis producing venous congestion in a single nerve root.

that of the asymptomatic subject. Walking with slight forward bending reduced the epidural pressure measurements to a level very similar to that of asymptomatic individuals walking upright.[83] Myeloscopy of subjects walking compared to resting demonstrates relatively greater dilatation of the cauda equina blood vessels in patients with intermittent claudication when compared to a control group.[84]

The Theoretical Mechanism Summarized Chronic constriction of the cauda equina causes pia-arachnoiditis and leads to constrictive adhesions. These adhesions may lead to fixation, compromising the cauda equina biomechanical excursion that normally occurs during spinal movements. "Pigtailing" of the radicular arteries develop above and below the lesion to compensate for the fixation. Hypertrophic thickening of the pia-arachnoid membranes impair the permeability of the membranes. CSF flow becomes blocked from free percolation through the constricted segment and impairs nutrient/metabolite transfer. Under increased physiologic demand, the compressed segment is subject to relative ischemia, rendering it more mechanosensitive and responsive to chemical alterations. When blood flow is reestablished to the hypoxoic nerves there may be ectopic discharge and paresthesias or other symptoms.[47]

PROGNOSIS AND MANAGEMENT OF LUMBAR SPINAL STENOSIS

Introduction

Many of the conclusions regarding the efficacy of conservative management of lumbar spinal stenosis have been based on observation of the "natural history" of the disorder. For example, a 4-year observation of patients with symptomatic lumbar stenosis who either declined surgery or were rejected by the anesthesiologist revealed that the pain intensity of 70% was unchanged, 15% improved, and 15% worsened.[85] Walking capacity was unchanged in 33%, improved in 37% and worsened in 30%. Electrophysiological parameters were significantly worse in 38%. Analgesic usage dropped from 100% to 41% at follow-up.

Treatment for symptomatic lumbar stenosis includes a wide spectrum of conservative and surgical options. Generally, surgery is reserved for those patients with severe, intolerable symptoms (leg and/or back pain) or who demonstrate functionally significant or progressive neurological impairment.[86]

Clinical Pearl: Surgery is usually reserved for those patients with severe intolerble symptoms despite aggressive conservative management, or those who demonstrate functionally significant or progressive neurological impairment.

There is a paucity of controlled studies that assess the efficacy of conservative treatment, and those that compare surgical outcome to conservative management are observational in design. It is generally accepted that patients with mild to moderate symptomatic lumbar stenosis can be managed conservatively, and there is no evidence that a trial of conservative care negatively affects those patients who later require surgical intervention.[86]

Surgery appears to provide better short-term relief of spinal stenosis symptoms,[87] but long-term studies do not support a substantial difference from conservatively managed patients. Additionally, neurophysiological studies indicate that surgery does not halt slowly progressive deficits.[86,88] Patients with scoliosis did worse with treatment when compared with patients without scoliosis.[89]

Conservative Management

Patients with the diagnosis of stenosis often have had their pain chronically. The initial patient's questions of What do I have? Can it be fixed? What is the cost? How long will it take? are confronted. Attempts are then made to finalize a diagnosis.[90] Claudication symptoms and signs usually receive the greatest attention in this effort, but it is likely that the character and intensity of their complaints are more complex. In fact, they may be related to the cervical spine (e.g., tandem stenosis/myelopathy), adjoining (nonstenotic) lumbar areas, the sacroiliac joints, and the myofascial systems. Most often a constellation of physical, behavioral, socioeconomic, and psychological factors exist. Any successful management strategy must incorporate plans to bridge both physical and any emotional factors.[91]

The most robust goal should be to restore to full function with pain relief, or significant decrease in pain, with the abolition of pain medication, elimination of assistive devices, low or zero disability rating, job satisfaction with return to work and leisure activities without limitations, independence from the health-care system, prevention of reinjury, and optimum wellness.[92] This may require a multidisciplinary approach and an aggressive treatment program.

Simotas et al. conducted such a nonsurgical treatment program on a group of 49 nonrandomized patients who were tracked for a mean of 33 months using a validated lumbar spinal stenosis outcome assessment tool.[89] Treatments included therapeutic exercises, analgesics, and epidural steroid injections. Severity of central stenosis was radiographically rated as mild (12%), moderate (43%), and severe (45%). Pain severity was rated very severe in 65% while 35%

could walk for less than two blocks. During the course of treatment 19% of the patients were transferred to surgery because of pain intensity. At follow-up, 66% of surgical and 30% of nonsurgical patients reported no, or mild, pain. Thirty percent of nonsurgical and 56% of surgically treated patients reported sustained relief. Satisfaction ratings in the nonsurgical group were slightly higher (80% versus 66%).[89]

In a larger study by Onel et al., 145 patients received inpatient treatment for 1 month with combinations of ultrasound, diathermy, exercises, and synthetic calcitonin.[50] Before treatment, 100% of patients experienced pain on motion and neurogenic claudication. At follow-up, 91% were pain-free with motion, with an 89% improvement rating in walking capacity. With the exception of reflex deficit, all other neurological examination parameters were improved. Based on pain, spinal functional capacity, neurogenic findings, and neurogenic claudication, global improvement was excellent (52%), good (18%), mild (23%). Seven percent were not improved.

Rosomoff and Rosomoff reported improvement in 47 of 50 patients with lumbar stenosis, noting 32 experienced excellent pain relief with a nonsurgical multidisciplinary treatment. They observed that extensive spinal canal intrusion often had minimal impact on the condition, especially when the encroachment occurred gradually. This finding drove them to search for other potential pain generators. The ultimate success of their program was their focus on the nonstenotic issues, particularly those related to soft tissues. As such, this approach led them to encourage it as the treatment of choice for most patients with stenosis.[93] They also encouraged rapid referral of patients for such treatment when initial management in a primary care setting fails so that chronicity is avoided.[93]

While older patients are distinctly different from younger patients with chronic pain, they have been shown to evidence significant improvement with conservative management, usually as great as their counterparts in other age groups.[94]

Conservative care falls into several categories including patient education; stretching, strengthening, and cardiovascular-based programs; myofascial techniques; mobilization and manipulation; bracing; and medication including therapeutic injections.

While there is no single standardized treatment plan for conservative management of lumbar spinal stenosis, strategies can be individualized based on the severity and duration of symptoms, impact on function and quality of life, and functional physical examination parameters. A stepwise approach has been conceptually divided into three independent and overlapping phases: pain control, stabilization, and conditioning.[57] Any program may need to be modified so that it remains effective but avoids exacerbation of coexisting orthopedic conditions, such as osteoarthritis of the hips or knees.[95]

Clinical Pearl: There is no single standardized treatment plan for conservative management of lumbar spinal stenosis. Strategies are individualized based on the severity and duration of symptoms, impact on function and quality of life, and functional physical examination parameters.

Patient Education Patients should be counseled on the prognosis and pathophysiology of their problem. They should understand the signs indicating the need for surgery on an emergent basis. Other important recommendations include ergonomic issues applicable to activities of daily living. Workplace environmental strategies should focus on stress reduction and the promotion of postural health. Positive actions that reduce the lumbar lordosis, such as weight reduction or maintaining a slight posterior pelvic tilt while erect, should be beneficial. Prone sleeping positions should be avoided, unless a pillow is placed under the abdomen to promote neutral or slight lumbar flexion. When standing for prolonged periods, alternately placing one foot on a raised surface causes slight lumbar flexion that can reduce static stress during activities such as cooking or washing dishes. Sustained overhead reaching and the resulting lumbar extension should be avoided, and items frequently used prophylactically placed on lower surfaces. The patient needs to implement avoidance strategies for all pain-provoking positions and movements. Furthermore, the patient with stenosis needs to become increasingly aware of positions and movements that provoke their symptoms in order to avoid exacerbating the condition.

Stretches Diligence with frequent stretching has been shown effective in the patients with chronic pain, including geriatric patients. Stretches are performed in an aggressive manner, and not perfunctorily or with indifference. Results of stretching have included a significant improvement in functional abilities as measured by an increase in the static strength of the back extensors and in lumbar myoelectric signals, and a decrease in their pain levels by 2 weeks.[96]

Areas of soft tissue tightness need to be stretched patiently and frequently. At least three repetitions with hold times of 15–30 seconds or longer are performed a minimum of twice daily, with higher frequency if possible. Significant muscle shortening may require more sustained soft tissue elongation techniques. Selection of exercises is based on clinical examination findings, coupled with the patient's functional limitations. Comorbidities of knee and hip osteoarthritis require clinician creativity and customization of stretches and exercises.

Also helpful are facilitative muscle energy techniques such as contract-relax or hold-relax stretches, and manual/instrumented soft tissue release techniques. These along with physiotherapeutic modalities and heat can promote relaxation and increased tissue suppleness (see Chapter 24).

Exercise Exercises that improve core functional stability and slight flexion-bias are performed initially on a daily basis.[89] Transverus abdominis/lumbar multifidus co-contraction exercises in supine, seated, and standing are low strain, promote volitional control and body awareness, and are an excellent entry point into a spinal stabilization program. Extensive coaching and education is often necessary in order to improve co-contraction control. A clinician, therapist, or perhaps a personal trainer with appropriate training may be needed. Care should be taken to avoid any exercise or stretch that promote provocative lumbar extension (see Chapter 28).

Cardiovascular Conditioning Because of the prevalence of claudication symptoms during ambulation that limit walking capacity, other forms of cardiovascular exercise are substituted. A stationary bicycle is an excellent option. A "Peddlar" is a less expensive substitute. Swimming is a viable option for some but excessive lumbar extension should be avoided. Organized aquatherapy and aquatic-based programs also allow for practicing core spinal stabilization exercises while the water buoyancy reduces loading and dampens perturbations.

While walking on a treadmill, slight inclination (5–10 degrees) or a deloading harness can be used. The deloading harness, pneumatic belt, and mild lumbar traction have clinically enabled patients to exercise with reduced back and lower limb symptoms. As an alternative to the treadmill, patients may wear an aquatic belt and tread water in the pool.[57]

Manual Techniques No randomized trials currently exist for treatment of lumbar radicular syndromes by means of manipulation. Favorable observational data show that over 50% of symptoms in patients with symptom duration lasting months were improved at 2 weeks with spine manipulation.[97] Cassidy et al. also reported that 36% of patients with confirmed central canal stenosis were able to return to unrestricted, normal activities of daily living. The average duration of symptoms was 17 years and all patients had failed other operative and nonoperative forms of management.

Treatment of the complicated case is becoming commonplace in clinical settings where spine care is integrated and multidisciplinary. For instance, at the Texas Back Institute, Plano, TX, up to 45% of patients receive spine manipulation during the early postsurgical rehabilitation phase, or later during recurrent episodes of pain recurrence.[98] The challenge for the patient with stenosis is similar to those cases of lumbar fusion where the predominant pain generator and manipulable lesion is at the sacroiliac joints. Sacroiliac joint involvement is common following low back and hip surgery, as well as in patients with stenosis. Greenman estimated that 62.3% patients post-back surgery have sacroiliac joint complications requiring manipulation for resolution.[99] Empirically, manipulative treatment is successfully used in postsurgical settings and for radiculopathy, and application can be extrapolated with case-specific modifications for patients with stenosis. As experience continues to increase with these types of cases a better understanding of the frequency, threshold effect, dosage, and additive effects from combinations of treatments will be better understood.[100]

Manipulative treatment is designed to achieve local effects, including connective tissue lengthening, disruption of adhesions and restoration of motion and tissue stresses.[101] In cases of advanced degenerative joint disease there may be a permanent restriction of joint motion that is unaffected by manipulation efforts. Manual and mechanical-assisted spinal and sacroiliac joint mobilization techniques are useful in optimizing articular mobility at functionally restricted areas, particularly above and below the area of stenotic effect. Stress demands for motion may thereby be distributed more uniformly across the lumbar spine. Theoretically, continuous passive spinal motion not only improves the efficiency of nutrient transfer to the cauda equina and adjacent tissues but also improves joint ranges and muscle flexibility. Those patients with intersegmental instability, noted on flexion/extension stress radiographs, need special attention and treatment considerations that are similar to the care and caution necessary in postsurgical fusion cases.

Clinical Pearl: Manual and mechanical-assisted spinal and sacroiliac joint manipulation and mobilization techniques are useful in optimizating articular mobility at functionally restricted areas, particularly above and below the area of stenotic effect. Stress demands for motion may thereby be distributed more uniformly across the lumbar spine.

Appropriately administered manipulation enhances range of motion and reduces pain. Irrespective of the underlying mechanism, the clinical benefits from successful manipulation may be an asset during the overall rehabilitation process. Symptom relief and enhanced mobility often encourages hope and confidence so that the patient may continue and complete their rehabilitation without symptomatic recurrence or abandonment of treatment.[91]

Different manipulative procedures are available to treat the lumbar spine. The selection of the appropriate method is guided by considerations of the severity of the coexisting pathology, response to provocative joint preloading, history of previous treatment, provider skill, and preference. This process is called *procedure–patient matching*.[102]

The technical nature of matching control strategies and any complicating features requires professional diagnostic training, skill, and experience. Together, patient- and provider-centered control strategies provide a wide set of options for addressing a patient's specific problem. When used properly an appropriate set of conditions can be found to provide manipulation without risk. Indeed, there is no evidence of risk in performing these procedures as long as provocative maneuvers demonstrate tolerance prior to their delivery. Skill is not inconsequential and has been studied and reported by Triano et al.[103,104]

Other Motorized and Manual Techniques In addition to standard static high-velocity, low-amplitude manipulation (HVLA), other types of manual procedures are available including unloaded continuous passive spinal motion (CPM) in a variety of positions, and dynamic motion assisted passive motion (Fig. 7–12).

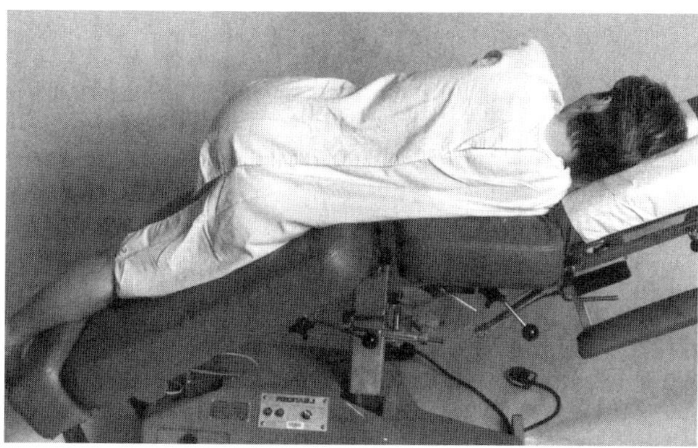

FIGURE 7–12. Right decubitus lumbar flexion CPM on a Leader™ motorized treatment table. The patient is positioned with the shoulder girdle perpendicular to the table surface. Pelvic orientation is somewhat forward and coupled with lumbosacral flexion CPM. Patient position may be varied to invoke the effects of motion coupling to achieve different local effects. These types of procedures may precede direct manipulative effort or be combined with HVLA procedures. A wide variety of manipulation control strategies are thereby available.[98]

Pharmacological Management Pharmacological inflammation control strategies may include prescription or over-the-counter anti-inflammatory agents such as ibuprofen, ketoprofen, naproxen sodium, or Cox-2 inhibitors. There are no controlled trials that evaluate the use of oral anti-inflammatory agents in the management of lumbar spinal stenosis. Pain-altering medications include tricyclic antidepressants and anticonvulsants.[89] Some reports suggest that patients with central stenosis are more responsive to nonsteroidal anti-inflammatory drugs than patients with lateral recess stenosis.[57]

Salmon calcitonin has been marginally beneficial in alleviating the symptoms of neurogenic intermittent claudication. The mechanism of this response is unclear and may not be completely due to the direct effects of calcitonin.

In severe cases, or those who are nonresponsive to conservative physical medicine approaches, a trial of epidural steroid injections may be attempted. The proposed pharmacological basis for epidural steroids includes suppression of chemical inflammatory mediators, capillary dilation, ectopic nerve discharge, and blocking of nociceptive nerve fibers.[89]

Surgical Management

A decision to proceed with surgical intervention is directed by several key determinants: patient–physician goal, relative risk versus benefit, patient age, and the ability to identify the appropriate region upon which to operate. In the absence of severe or advancing neurological compromise, surgery is not usually performed without an aggressive and comprehensive trial of conservative management.

Clinical Pearl: In the absence of severe or advancing neurological deficit, surgery is not usually performed without an aggressive and comprehensive trial of conservative management.

Surgery for symptomatic stenosis yields varied results. Turner's meta-analysis defined a 64% good to excellent outcome, which was reported in other studies.[88,105,106] Higher success rates were reported by Postacchini et al.[107] and Hansraj et al.[108]: 80% and 94% respectively.

Clinically, pain relief outweighs neurological deficit as the reason for surgery.[89] More than 80% of patients who underwent surgery reported pain relief as their primary goal.[87] Patients should be advised that claudication symptoms are more likely to improve over back pain because facet arthropathy and abnormal mechanics are not changed by the surgical procedure.[109]

Absolute indications include fecal or urinary control loss (cauda equina syndrome), acute foot drop, and sudden severe walking restriction. Relative indications for surgery are pain or heaviness in the legs, such that the patient's quality of life is poor despite an adequate nonoperative trial.[39] Decompressive procedures do not necessarily prevent neurophysiological deterioration.[88]

Clinical Pearl: Absolute indications for decompressive surgery include fecal or urinary control loss (cauda equina syndrome), acute foot drop, and sudden severe walking restriction.

Surgery is aimed at removing enough relevant compressive anatomy without compromising spinal stability. Unfortunately, deciding the relevancy of the various compressive factors is not easy. The most significant radiographically constricted level or region may not be the most clinically important.[33] Ultimately the degree of decompression performed will likely reflect the surgeon's operative findings, rather than be based solely on imaging.

Potential candidates for excision include varying degrees of marginal osteophytes, laminae, ligamentum flavum, articular facets, synovial cysts, hypertrophied pedicles, pars interarticularii, and herniated discs. Stenosis may be central, lateral, or combined, prompting combined procedures.

Laminectomy is the most common decompressive procedure (Fig. 7–13). It also may serve as a portal for other procedures such as facetectomy, pediculectomy, and discectomy.[52] Postacchini advised against discectomy as it may contribute to postsurgical instability.[110] Laminotomy, with resection of half of the superior and inferior laminae at the level of compression, is less invasive and is gaining popularity. It is reportedly most useful in treating unilateral stenotic compression. Foraminotomy is used to relieve symptoms of exit zone compression.

Partial undercutting facetectomy is used for lateral recess stenosis.[52] However, excision of more than 50% of the facet may increase the risk of postoperative instability.

Whether or not to also perform a fusion remains controversial. Arthrodesis options include anterior or posterior interbody fusion. For patients with stenotic symptoms less than 8 years, decompression without fusion may offer better results.[111] On the other hand, those having had symptoms present for more than 15 years, decompression with posterior instrumented fusion may be a better alternative.

Fusion may be necessary when more than 60% of one facet is removed or more than 50% of successive facets.[52] Of the patients with a degenerative spondylolisthesis, those who underwent athrodesis showed a higher proportion (80%) of satisfactory results than those without arthrodesis (40%).[107] Wiltse et al. recommended fusion in the patient past 60 years of age with degenerative spondylolisthesis.[112] Grob et al. compared the results of decompression with and without arthrodesis in patients presenting with symptomatic spinal stenosis without preoperative instability.[113] There was no difference in outcome, leading to the conclusion that fusion was not indicated in stenosis without preoperative instability.

Reoperation rates following decompressive surgery range from 9% to 23%.[105,106,114,115] The most common reason for a second surgery was persistent pain due to inadequate initial decompression.[38,107,116] Jenis and An identified overlooked foraminal stenosis as a common cause of persistent pain.[38] Also regrowth of the lamina may follow surgery.[107]

Spine surgery is not without risk. Complications may arise as a direct result of the procedure, or comorbities related to the age and health of the population. Iatrogenic stenosis, postoperative instability, postoperative infection, increased pain, dural tears, pars interarticularis fracture, disturbances in micturition, and retrograde ejaculation all have been reported. Operations for stenosis have the highest complication rate and duration of hospitalization among lumbar spine surgeries, primarily because of comorbid health issues.[117] Operated levels with spondylolisthesis are more likely to develop progressive spondylolisthesis after laminectomy.

Residual postsurgical lower back and limb pain is common. When surgical outcome fails to meet patient expectation or when comorbid functional pain remains, a trial of conservative management should be instituted. In appropriately selected cases, manipulation may be performed after fusions have been judged solid, usually between 3 and 6 months. Prior to that time mechanical treatment is limited to areas and methods that do not significantly load the healing fusion.[98,118] Cardiovascular and spinal stabilization decompensation also must be addressed for a safe return to function.

Clinical Pearl: When appropriately selected, manipulation may be performed after spine fusions have been judged solid, usually between 3 and 6 months. Prior to that time mechanical treatment is limited to areas and methods that do not significantly load the healing fusion.

Very few factors assist in predicting outcomes. Patient age, gender, duration of preoperative symptoms, presence of workers' compensation claim,[106] neurogenic claudication, prior back surgery, isthmic spondylolisthesis, number of levels of laminectomy, whether a fusion was performed,[6] and clinical and radiographic findings[86] all appear to have no predictive value.

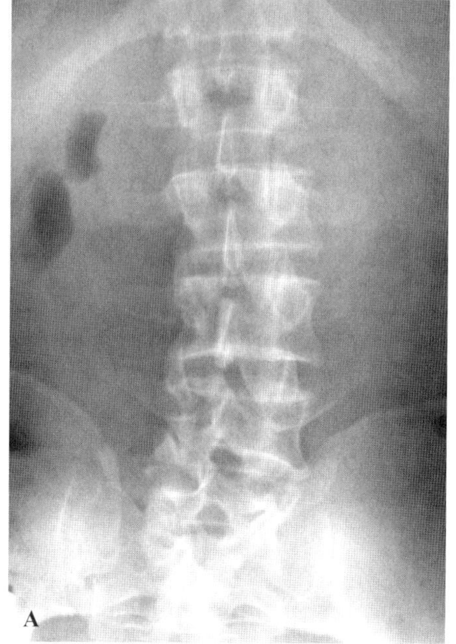

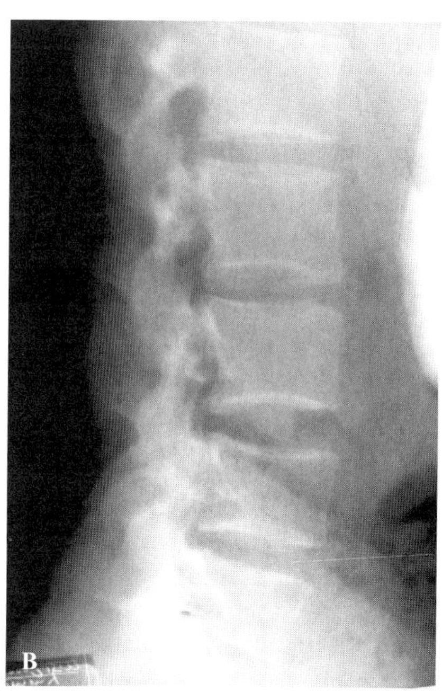

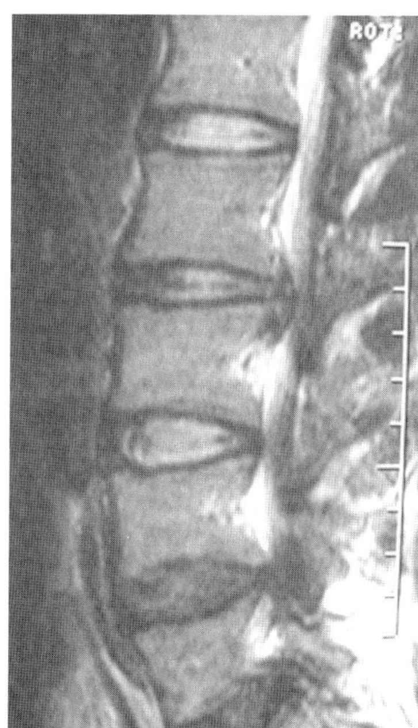

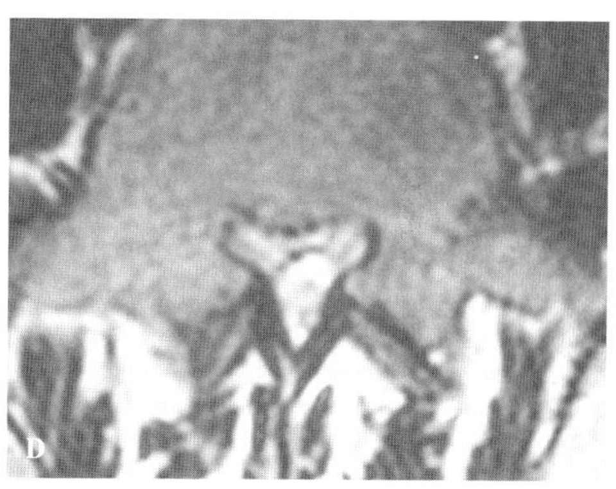

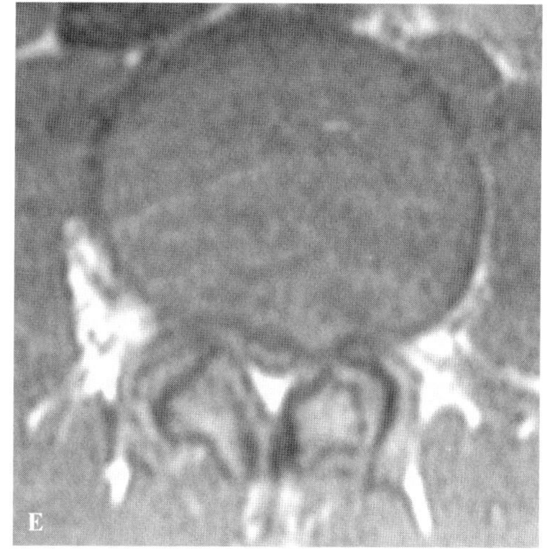

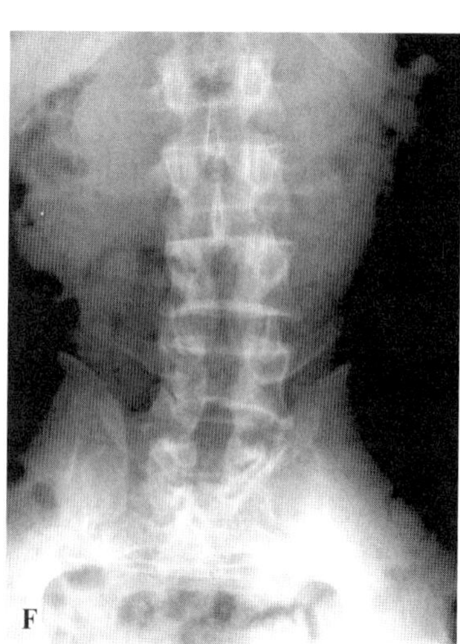

FIGURE 7–13. A 39-year-old man with stenotic leg complaints and some low back pain. His clinical course was unrelenting and he failed conservative management strategies. *A.* Anteroposterior conventional radiograph with developmentally abnormal lower lumbar appearance. *B.* Lateral conventional image showing general preservation of the intervertebral disc heights, but decreased anteroposterior canal dimension. *C.* Sagittal T2-weighted MRI showing small canal dimension and an L2–L3 disc protrusion. *D.* Axial MRI at the lumbosacral level. Here the lumbar canal is small and trefoil in configuration. *E.* Axial MRI image at the level of L2–L3. The canal at this level is also very small and there is left paracentral disc protrusion. *F.* Conventional anteroposterior postsurgical radiograph. A wide multilevel laminectomy and partial facetectomy was performed with good early clinical result.

The best candidate for surgery appears to be the patient with severe osteoligamentous compression (≤6 mm) of the neural structures, [115] severe leg symptoms, moderate or no neurological deficit, and, except for patients with degenerative spondylolisthesis, little or no back pain.[110] The most powerful preoperative predictors of greater satisfaction from surgery are greater walking capacity, milder symptoms, and the patient's report of good to excellent health before surgery.[119] Low cardiovascular comorbidity also favors a good outcome.

Outcome Assessment

Pain relief is the primary goal of patients receiving treatment for symptomatic spinal stenosis. Equally important objectives include improvement of function, life quality, and measures of patient/provider treatment satisfaction. Self-administered questionnaires and direct measurement of physical function appear most useful in the assessment of treatment outcome (see Chapter 14).

The visual analog scale (VAS) is the most simple and cost-effective tool to represent a patient's perception of pain intensity. It has several variations. One popular format is a 100-mm horizontal line with opposing descriptors at each end (e.g., "No Pain" and "Worse Pain Imaginable"). The patient is asked to place a vertical mark on the line at the point of pain intensity. Pain intensity is expressed as the measured value/100. Time requirements for administration are less than 1–2 minutes.

The Oswestry Low Back Pain Disability Index (ODI) and Roland–Morris-18 questionnaires are valid and reliable self-administered questionnaires that are commonly used to assess the impact of low back pain on an individual's function.[120,121] Each may require up to 5 minutes to administer and can be scored against the normal population; higher scores represent greater disability. Both questionnaires are of limited value in assessing disability resultant from stenosis. Neither takes into account the primary complaint associated with spinal stenosis, neurogenic claudication.

Stucki et al. created an instrument that is stenosis specific and addresses the outcome of surgery based on symptom severity, physical function, and satisfaction scales (Swiss Spinal Stenosis Score).[122] This instrument recently has been shown to be precise and condition specific when compared to ODI, Shuttle Walking Test (SWT), and the Oxford Claudication Score (OCS).[123] This questionnaire requires approximately 5 minutes to complete and can be used in longitudinal assessment of patients. We have modified it for use with conservative management (see Appendix).

Walking endurance may be used to assess a patient's baseline functional capacity and as a treatment outcome measurement tool. Care must be taken to insure that the patient's posture remains upright, as there is a tendency to flex forward and use the treadmill handrails. A walking speed of 1.2 mph and 0 degree of inclination are recommended. The time to symptom onset and total ambulation time are recorded. This tool has been used to assess the efficacy of decompressive surgery and is valuable in determining conservative treatment outcomes.[124] It has demonstrated good test–retest reproducibility.[125]

SUMMARY

1. Patients with lumbar spinal stenosis are *not* necessarily faced with progressive deterioration.
2. Conservative management *is* a viable option for patients with mild to moderate symptoms.
3. Delaying surgery, even in instances of severe pain, does *not* negatively impact the prognosis.
4. The 10-year outcome for those patients managed surgically and conservatively are *nearly identical.*
5. Surgery provides a much better *short-term* result than conservative management.
6. The level, degree, classification, and severity of lumbar spinal stenosis does *not* assist in evaluating the outcome of management.

REFERENCES

1. Spivak J. Degenerative lumbar spinal stenosis. *J Bone Joint Surg* 1998;80A(7):1053–1066.
2. US Census Bureau, 2000.
3. *World population prospects: the 2000 revision.* United Nations, 2001:1–34.
4. Taylor V, Deyo R, Cherkin D, et al. Low back pain hospitalizations: Recent United States trends and regional variations. *Spine* 1994;19(11):1207–1213.
5. Verbiest H. A radicular syndrome from developmental narrowing of the lumbar vertebral canal. *J Bone Joint Surg* 1954;36B(2):230–237.
6. Turner H, Ersek M, Herron L, et al. Surgery for lumbar stenosis. Attempted meta-analysis of the literature. *Spine* 1992;17(1):1–8.
7. Arnoldi C, Brodsky A, Cauchoix J et al. Lumbar spinal stenosis and nerve root entrapment syndromes: Definition and classification. *Clin Orthop* 1976;115: 4–5.
8. Dowart R, Vogler L, Helms C. Spinal stenosis. *Radiol Clin North Am* 1983;21:301–325.
9. Kirkaldy-Willis W, Paine K, Cauchoix J. Lumbar spinal stenosis. *Clin Orthop* 1974;99:30–50.
10. Papp T, Porter RW, Aspden RM. Trefoil configuration and developmental stenosis of the lumbar vertebral canal. *J Bone Joint Surg Br* 1995;77(3):469–472.
11. Dominisse G. Morphological aspects of the lumbar spine and lumbosacral region. *Ortho Clin North Am* 1975;6(1):163–175.

12. Postacchini F, Ripani M, Carpano S. Morphometry of the lumbar vertebrae: An anatomic study in two Caucasoid ethnic groups. *Clin Orthop* 1983;172:296–303.
13. Porter RW. Central spinal stenosis. Classification and pathogenesis. *Acta Orthop Scand* 1993;64(Suppl 251):64–66.
14. Eisenstein S. The trefoil configuration of the lumbar vertebral canal. A study of South African skeletal material. *J Bone Joint Surg* 1980;62B(1):73–77.
15. Uden A, Johnsson KE, Jonsson K et al. Myelography in the elderly and the diagnosis of spinal stenosis. *Spine* 1985;10(2):171–174.
16. Weisz GM, Lee P. Spinal canal stenosis. Concept of spinal reserve capacity: Radiologic measurements and clinical applications. *Clin Orthop* 1983;(179):134–140.
17. Lee CK, Rauschning W, Glenn W. Lateral lumbar spinal canal stenosis: Classification, pathologic anatomy and surgical decompression. *Spine* 1988; 13(3):313–320.
18. Ciric I, Mikhael MA, Tarkington JA et al. The lateral recess syndrome. A variant of spinal stenosis. *J Neurosurg* 1980;53(4):433–443.
19. Rauschning W. Pathoanatomy of lumbar disc degeneration and stenosis. *Acta Orthop Scand* 1993;64(Suppl 251):3–12.
20. Hasegawa T, An HS, Haughton VM et al. Lumbar foraminal stenosis: Critical heights of the intervertebral discs and foramina. A cryomicrotome study in cadavera. *J Bone Joint Surg Am* 1995;77(1): 32–38.
21. Cramer G, Skogsbergh D, Winterstein J et al. Accuracy and reliability of the identification of transforaminal ligaments of the lumbar intervertebral foramina by means of magnetic resonance imaging. *J Manipulative Physiol Ther* 2002;25(4):199–208.
22. Dai LY, Xu Y, Zhang W et al. The effect of flexion–extension motion of the lumbar spine on the capacity of the spinal canal. An experimental study. *Spine* 1989;14(5):523–525.
23. Inufusa A, An HS, Lim TH et al. Anatomic changes of the spinal canal and intervertebral foramen associated with flexion–extension movement. *Spine* 1996;21(21):2412–2420.
24. Schonstrom N, Lindahl S, Willen J et al. Dynamic changes in the dimensions of the lumbar spinal canal: An experimental study in vitro. *J Orthop Res* 1989;7(1):115–121.
25. Orioli IM, Castilla EE, Barbosa-Neto JG. The birth prevalence rates for the skeletal dysplasias. *J Med Genet* 1986;23(4):328–332.
26. Alexander E Jr. Significance of the small lumbar spinal canal: Cauda equina compression syndromes due to spondylosis. 5. Achondroplasia. *J Neurosurg* 1969;31(5):513–519.
27. Lutter LD, Longstein JE, Winter RB et al. Anatomy of the achondroplastic lumbar canal. *Clin Orthop* 1977;(126):139–142.
28. Morgan DF, Young RF. Spinal neurological complications of achondroplasia. Results of surgical treatment. *J Neurosurg* 1980;52(4):463–472.
29. Clark GA, Panjabi MM, Wetzel FT. Can infant malnutrition cause adult vertebral stenosis? *Spine* 1985;10(2):165–170.
30. Papp T, Porter RW, Craig CE et al. Significant antenatal factors in the development of lumbar spinal stenosis. *Spine* 1997;22(16):1805–1810.
31. Postacchini F, Massobrio M, Ferro L. Familial lumbar stenosis. Case report of three siblings. *J Bone Joint Surg Am* 1985;67(2):321–323.
32. Katz JN, Dalgas M, Stucki G et al. Diagnosis of lumbar spinal stenosis. *Rheum Dis Clin North Am* 1994;20(2):471–483.
33. Sheehan JM, Shaffrey CI, Jane JA. Degenerative lumbar stenosis: The neurosurgical perspective. *Clin Orthop* 2001;(384):61–74.
34. Postacchini F, Gumina S, Cinotti G et al. Ligamenta flava in lumbar disc herniation and spinal stenosis. Light and electron microscopic morphology. *Spine* 1994;19(8):917–922.
35. Markiewitz AD, Boumphrey FR, Bauer TW et al. Calcium pyrophosphate dihydrate crystal deposition disease as a cause of lumbar canal stenosis. *Spine* 1996;21(4):506–511.
36. Penning L, Wilmink JT. Posture-dependent bilateral compression of L4 or L5 nerve roots in facet hypertrophy. A dynamic CT-myelographic study. *Spine* 1987;12(5):488–500.
37. Herzog RJ, Kaiser JA, Saal JA et al. The importance of posterior epidural fat pad in lumbar central canal stenosis. *Spine* 1991;16(6, Suppl):S227–S233.
38. Jenis LG, An HS. Spine update. Lumbar foraminal stenosis. *Spine* 2000;25(3):389–394.
39. Bassewitz H, Herkowitz H. Lumbar stenosis with spondylolisthesis: Current concepts of surgical treatment. *Clin Orthop* 2001;(384):54–60.
40. Matsunaga S, Sakou T, Morizono Y et al. Natural history of degenerative spondylolisthesis. Pathogenesis and natural course of the slippage. *Spine* 1990;15(11):1204–1210.
41. Boden SD, Davis DO, Dina TS et al. Abnormal magnetic-resonance scans of the lumbar spine in asymptomatic subjects. A prospective investigation. *J Bone Joint Surg Am* 1990;72(3):403–408.
42. Wiesel SW, Tsourmas N, Feffer HL et al. A study of computer-assisted tomography. I. The incidence of positive CAT scans in an asymptomatic group of patients. *Spine* 1984;9(6):549–551.
43. Amundsen T, Weber H, Lilleas F et al. Lumbar spinal stenosis. Clinical and radiologic features. *Spine* 1995;20(10):1178–1186.
44. Herno A, Airaksinen O, Saari T. Computed tomography after laminectomy for lumbar spinal stenosis. Patients' pain patterns, walking capacity, and subjective disability had no correlation with computed tomography findings. *Spine* 1994;19(17):1975–1978.
45. Jonsson B, Annertz M, Sjoberg C et al. A prospective and consecutive study of surgically treated lumbar spinal stenosis. Part I. Clinical features related to radiographic findings. *Spine* 1997;22(24):2932–2937.
46. Atlas SJ, Deyo RA, Patrick DL et al. The Quebec Task Force classification for spinal disorders and the

severity, treatment, and outcomes of sciatica and lumbar spinal stenosis. *Spine* 1996;21(24):2885–2892.
47. Watanabe R, Parke WW. Vascular and neural pathology of lumbosacral spinal stenosis. *J Neurosurg* 1986;64(1):64–70.
48. Hall S, Bartleson JD, Onofrio BM et al. Lumbar spinal stenosis. Clinical features, diagnostic procedures, and results of surgical treatment in 68 patients. *Ann Intern Med* 1985;103(2):271–275.
49. Katz JN, Dalgas M, Stucki G et al. Degenerative lumbar spinal stenosis. Diagnostic value of the history and physical examination. *Arthritis Rheum* 1995;38(9):1236–1241.
50. Onel D, Sari H, Donmez C. Lumbar spinal stenosis: Clinical/radiologic therapeutic evaluation in 145 patients. Conservative treatment or surgical intervention? *Spine* 1993;18(2):291–298.
51. Jonsson B, Stromqvist B. Symptoms and signs in degeneration of the lumbar spine. A prospective, consecutive study of 300 operated patients. *J Bone Joint Surg Br* 1993;75(3):381–385.
52. Andersson GB. Surgical aspects on lateral spinal stenosis. Indications and principles. *Acta Orthop Scand Suppl* 1993;251:74–75.
53. Laha RK, Dujovny M, Huang PS. Intermittent erection in spinal canal stenosis. *J Urol* 1979;121(1):123–124.
54. Ram Z, Findler G, Spiegelman R et al. Intermittent priapism in spinal canal stenosis. *Spine* 1987;12(4):377–378.
55. Ravindran M. Cauda equina compression presenting as spontaneous priapism. *J Neurol Neurosurg Psychiatry* 1979;42(3):280–282.
56. Hopkins A, Clarke C, Brindley G. Erections on walking as a symptom of spinal canal stenosis. *J Neurol Neurosurg Psychiatry* 1987;50(10):1371–1374.
57. Nagler W, Hausen HS. Conservative management of lumbar spinal stenosis. Identifying patients likely to do well without surgery. *Postgrad Med* 1998;103(4):69–71.
58. Ginsberg L, Platts AD, Thomas PK. Chronic inflammatory demyelinating polyneuropathy mimicking a lumbar spinal stenosis syndrome. *J Neurol Neurosurg Psychiatry* 1995;59(2):189–191.
59. Spengler DM. Degenerative stenosis of the lumbar spine. *J Bone Joint Surg Am* 1987;69(2):305–308.
60. Simkin PA. Simian stance: A sign of spinal stenosis. *Lancet* 1982;2(8299):652–653.
61. Dong G, Porter RW. Walking and cycling tests in neurogenic and intermittent claudication. *Spine* 1989;14(9):965–969.
62. Williams R, Binkley J, Bloch R et al. Reliability of the modified-modified Schober and double inclinometer methods for measuring lumbar flexion and extension. *Phys Ther* 1993;73(1):33–44.
63. Fritz JM, Delitto A, Welch WC et al. Lumbar spinal stenosis: A review of current concepts in evaluation, management, and outcome measurements. *Arch Phys Med Rehabil* 1998;79(6):700–708.
64. Kendall F, McCreary E, Provance P. *Muscles: Testing and function*, 4th ed. Baltimore: Williams & Wilkins, 1993:162.
65. Mikhael MA, Ciric I, Tarkington JA et al. Neuroradiological evaluation of lateral recess syndrome. *Radiology* 1981;140(1):97–107.
66. Schonstrom N, Bolender N, Spengler D. The pathomorphology of spinal stenosis as seen on CT scans of the lumbar spine. *Spine* 1985;10(9):806–811.
67. Beers G, Carter A, Leiter B et al. Interobserver discrepancies in distance measurements from lumbar spine CT scans. *AJR Am J Roentgenol* 1985;144(2):395–398.
68. Drew R, Bhandari M, Kulkarni AV et al. Reliability in grading the severity of lumbar spinal stenosis. *J Spinal Disord* 2000;13(3):253–258.
69. Zander DR, Lander PH. Positionally dependent spinal stenosis: Correlation of upright flexion–extension myelography and computed tomographic myelography. *Can Assoc Radiol J* 1998;49(4):256–261.
70. Coulier B. Evaluation of lumbar canal stenosis: Decubitus imaging methods versus flexion–extension myelography and surface measurements versus the diameter of the dural sac. JBR-BRT 2000;83(2):61–67.
71. Danielson BI, Willen J, Gaulitz A et al. Axial loading of the spine during CT and MR in patients with suspected lumbar spinal stenosis. *Acta Radiol* 1998; 39(6):604–611.
72. Willen J, Danielson B, Gaulitz A et al. Dynamic effects on the lumbar spinal canal: Axially loaded CT-myelography and MRI in patients with sciatica and/or neurogenic claudication. *Spine* 1997;22(24): 2968–2976.
73. Weishaupt D, Schmid MR, Zanetti M. Positional MR imaging of the lumbar spine: Does it demonstrate nerve root compromise not visible at conventional MR imaging. *Radiology* 2000;215:247–253.
74. Yoshizawa H, Kobayashi S, Morita T. Chronic nerve root compression. Pathophysiologic mechanism of nerve root dysfunction. *Spine* 1995;20(4):397–407.
75. Olmarker K, Rydevik B, Holm S et al. Effects of experimental graded compression on blood flow in spinal nerve roots. A vital microscopic study on the porcine cauda equina. *J Orthop Res* 1989;7(6):817–823.
76. Olmarker K, Rydevik B, Holm S. Edema formation in spinal nerve roots induced by experimental, graded compression. An experimental study on the pig cauda equina with special reference to differences in effects between rapid and slow onset of compression. *Spine* 1989;14(6):569–573.
77. Olmarker K, Holm S, Rydevik B. Importance of compression onset rate for the degree of impairment of impulse propagation in experimental compression injury of the porcine cauda equina. *Spine* 1990;15(5):416–419.
78. Porter RW, Ward D. Cauda equina dysfunction. The significance of two-level pathology. *Spine* 1992;17(1): 9–15.
79. Sato K, Kikuchi S. Clinical analysis of two-level compression of the cauda equina and the nerve roots in lumbar spinal canal stenosis. *Spine* 1997;22(16):1898–1903.
80. Olmarker K, Rydevik B. Single- versus double-level nerve root compression. An experimental study on the porcine cauda equina with analyses of nerve

impulse conduction properties. *Clin Orthop* 1992;(279):35–39.

81. Evans JG. Neurogenic intermittent claudication. *Br Med J* 1964;2:985–7.
82. Takahashi K, Miyazaki T, Takino T et al. Epidural pressure measurements. Relationship between epidural pressure and posture in patients with lumbar spinal stenosis. *Spine* 1995;20(6):650–653.
83. Takahashi K, Kagechika K, Takino T et al. Changes in epidural pressure during walking in patients with lumbar spinal stenosis. *Spine* 1995;20(24):2746–2749.
84. Ooi Y, Mita F, Satoh Y. Myeloscopic study on lumbar spinal canal stenosis with special reference to intermittent claudication. *Spine* 1990;15(6):544–549.
85. Johnsson KE, Rosen I, Uden A. The natural course of lumbar spinal stenosis. *Clin Orthop* 1992;(279):82–86.
86. Amundsen T, Weber H, Nordal HJ et al. Lumbar spinal stenosis: Conservative or surgical management? A prospective 10-year study. *Spine* 2000;25(11):1424–1435.
87. Atlas SJ, Deyo RA, Keller RB et al. The Maine Lumbar Spine Study. Part III. 1-year outcomes of surgical and nonsurgical management of lumbar spinal stenosis. *Spine* 1996;21(15):1787–1794.
88. Johnsson KE, Uden A, Rosen I. The effect of decompression on the natural course of spinal stenosis. A comparison of surgically treated and untreated patients. *Spine* 1991;16(6):615–619.
89. Simotas AC, Dorey FJ, Hansraj KK et al. Nonoperative treatment for lumbar spinal stenosis. Clinical and outcome results and a 3-year survivorship analysis. *Spine* 2000;25(2):197–203.
90. Skogsbergh D, Chapman S. Dealing with chronic pain. *Top Clin Chiro* 1994;1(4):9–19.
91. Triano J, McGregor M, Skogsbergh D. Use of chiropractic manipulation in lumbar rehabilitation. *J Rehabil Res Dev* 1997;34(4):25–36.
92. Rosomoff H, Rosomoff R. Comprehensive multidisciplinary pain center approach to the treatment of low back pain. *Neurosurg Clin North Am* 1991;2(4):877–890.
93. Rosomoff HL, Rosomoff RS. Low back pain. Evaluation and management in the primary care setting. *Med Clin North Amer* 1999;83(3):643–662.
94. Cutler R, Fishbain D, Rosomoff R et al. Outcomes in treatment of pain in geriatric and younger age groups. *Arch Phys Med Rehabil* 1994;75(4):457–464.
95. Bodack MP, Monteiro M. Therapeutic exercise in the treatment of patients with lumbar spinal stenosis. *Clin Orthop* 2001;(384):144–152.
96. Khalil T, Asfour S, Martinez L et al. Stretching in the rehabilitation of low-back pain patients. *Spine* 1992;17(3):311–317.
97. Cassidy J, Kirkaldy-Willis W, McGregor M. Spinal manipulation in the treatment of low-back pain. In: Buerger A, Greenman R, eds. *Empirical approaches to the validation of spinal manipulation.* Springfield: Charles C. Thomas, 1985:119–148.
98. Triano J. The mechanics of spinal manipulation. In: Herzog W, ed. *Clinical biomechanics of spinal manipulation.* New York: Churchill Livingston, 2000:92–190.
99. Greenman PE. *Principles of manual medicine.* Baltimore: Williams & Wilkins, 1989.
100. Triano J. Studies on the biomechanical effect of a spinal adjustment. *J Manipulative Phys Ther* 1992;72(12): 885–92.
101. Twomey A. A rationale for the treatment of back pain and joint pain by manipulation. *Phys Ther* 1992;72(12):885–92.
102. Triano J, Skogsbergh D, McGregor M. Validity and basis of manipulation. In: White A, ed. *Spine care: Diagnosis and conservative management.* St Louis: Mosby, 1995:437–450.
103. Triand J. Rating skill in SMT. In: *International Conference on Spinal Manipulation*, Palm Springs, CA, 1994.
104. Biomechanical parameters of skill in lumbar SMT. In: *International Conference on Spinal Manipulation*, Palm Springs, CA, 1994.
105. Herno A, Airaksinen O, Saari T. Long-term results of surgical treatment of lumbar spinal stenosis. *Spine* 1993;18(11):1471–1474.
106. Tuite GF, Stern JD, Doran SE et al. Outcome after laminectomy for lumbar spinal stenosis. Part I. Clinical correlations. *J Neurosurg* 1994;81(5):699–706.
107. Postacchini F, Cinotti G, Gumina S et al. Long-term results of surgery in lumbar stenosis. 8-year review of 64 patients. *Acta Orthop Scand Suppl* 1993;251:78–80.
108. Hansraj KK, Cammisa FP, O'Leary PF et al. Decompressive surgery for typical lumbar spinal stenosis. *Clin Orthop* 2001;(384):10–17.
109. Grabias S. Current concepts review. The treatment of spinal stenosis. *J Bone Joint Surg Am* 1980;62(2):308–313.
110. Postacchini F. Management of lumbar spinal stenosis. *J Bone Joint Surg Br* 1996;78(1):154–164.
111. Niggemeyer O, Strauss JM, Schulitz KP. Comparison of surgical procedures for degenerative lumbar spinal stenosis: A meta-analysis of the literature from 1975 to 1995. *Eur Spine J* 1997;6(6):423–429.
112. Wiltse LL, Kirkaldy-Willis WH, McIvor GW. The treatment of spinal stenosis. *Clin Orthop* 1976;(115):83–91.
113. Grob D, Humke T, Dvorak J. Degenerative lumbar spinal stenosis. Decompression with and without arthrodesis. *J Bone Joint Surg Am* 1995;77(7):1036–1041.
114. Katz JN, Lipson SJ, Chang LC et al. Seven- to 10-year outcome of decompressive surgery for degenerative lumbar spinal stenosis. *Spine* 1996;21(1):92–98.
115. Jonsson B, Annertz M, Sjoberg C et al. A prospective and consecutive study of surgically treated lumbar spinal stenosis. Part II. Five-year follow-up by an independent observer. *Spine* 1997;22(24):2938–2944.
116. Getty CJ. Lumbar spinal stenosis: The clinical spectrum and the results of operation. *J Bone Joint Surg Br* 1980;62B(4):481–485.
117. Deyo RA, Cherkin DC, Loeser JD et al. Morbidity and mortality in association with operations on the lumbar spine. The influence of age, diagnosis, and procedure. *J Bone Joint Surg Am* 1992;74(4):536–543.
118. McGregor M, Cassidy JD. Post-surgical sacroiliac joint syndrome. *J Manipulative Physiol Ther* 1983;6(1): 1–11.

119. Katz JN, Stucki G, Lipson SJ et al. Predictors of surgical outcome in degenerative lumbar spinal stenosis. *Spine* 1999;24(21):2229–2233.
120. Fairbank JC. The use of revised Oswestry Disability Questionnaire. *Spine* 2000;25(21):2846–2847.
121. Stratford PW, Binkley JM. Measurement properties of the RM-18. A modified version of the Roland–Morris Disability Scale. *Spine* 1997;22(20):2416–2421.
122. Stucki G, Daltroy L, Liang MH et al. Measurement properties of a self-administered outcome measure in lumbar spinal stenosis. *Spine* 1996;21(7):796–803.
123. Pratt RK, Fairbank JC, Virr A. The reliability of the Shuttle Walking Test, the Swiss Spinal Stenosis Questionnaire, the Oxford Spinal Stenosis Score, and the Oswestry Disability Index in the assessment of patients with lumbar spinal stenosis. *Spine* 2002;27(1):84–91.
124. Deen HG, Zimmerman RS, Lyons MK et al. Use of the exercise treadmill to measure baseline functional status and surgical outcome in patients with severe lumbar spinal stenosis. *Spine* 1998;23(2):244–248.
125. Deen HG, Zimmerman RS, Lyons MK et al. Test–retest reproducibility of the exercise treadmill examination in lumbar spinal stenosis. *Mayo Clin Proc* 2000;75(10):1002–1007.

APPENDIX: SWISS SPINAL STENOSIS SCORE[122]

In the last month, how would you describe:

The pain you have had on average including pain in your back, buttocks, and pain that goes down the legs?
1. None
2. Mild
3. Moderate
4. Severe
5. Very Severe

How often have you had back, buttock, or leg pain?
1. Less than once a week
2. At least once a week
3. Everyday, for at least a few minutes
4. Everyday, for most of the day
5. Every minute of the day

The pain in your back or buttocks?
1. None
2. Mild
3. Moderate
4. Severe
5. Very Severe

The pain in your legs or feet?
1. None
2. Mild
3. Moderate
4. Severe
5. Very Severe

Numbness or tingling in your legs or feet?
1. None
2. Mild
3. Moderate
4. Severe
5. Very Severe

Weakness in your legs or feet?
1. None
2. Mild
3. Moderate
4. Severe
5. Very Severe

Problems with your balance?
1. No, I've had no problems with balance
2. Yes, sometimes I feel my balance is off, or that I am not sure footed
3. Yes, often I feel my balance is off, or that I am not sure footed

In the last month, on a typical day:
How far have you been able to walk?
1. Over 2 miles
2. Over 2 blocks, but less than 2 miles
3. Over 50 feet, but less than 2 blocks
4. Less then 50 feet

Have you taken walks outdoors or in malls for pleasure?
1. Yes, comfortably
2. Yes, but sometimes with pain
3. Yes, but always with pain
4. No

Have you been shopping for groceries or other items?
1. Yes, comfortably
2. Yes, but sometimes with pain
3. Yes, but always with pain
4. No

Have you walked around the different rooms in your house or apartment?
1. Yes, comfortably
2. Yes, but sometimes with pain
3. Yes, but always with pain
4. No

Have you walked from your bedroom to the bathroom?
1. Yes, comfortably
2. Yes, but sometimes with pain
3. Yes, but always with pain
4. No

How are you satisfied with:

The overall result of your back treatment?
1. Very satisfied
2. Somewhat satisfied
3. Somewhat dissatisfied
4. Very dissatisfied

Relief of pain following treatment?
1. Very satisfied
2. Somewhat satisfied
3. Somewhat dissatisfied
4. Very dissatisfied

Your ability to walk following treatment?
1. Very satisfied
2. Somewhat satisfied
3. Somewhat dissatisfied
4. Very dissatisfied

Your ability to do housework, yard work, or job following treatment?
1. Very satisfied
2. Somewhat satisfied
3. Somewhat dissatisfied
4. Very dissatisfied

Your strength in the thighs, legs, and feet?
1. Very satisfied
2. Somewhat satisfied
3. Somewhat dissatisfied
4. Very dissatisfied

Your balance, or steadiness on your feet?
1. Very satisfied
2. Somewhat satisfied
3. Somewhat dissatisfied
4. Very dissatisfied

CHAPTER

8

THE POSTERIOR JOINT SYNDROMES: ZYGAPOPHYSEAL AND SACROILIAC JOINTS

David Byfield, Peter McCarthy, Vincenzo Cascioli, Mark Webster, and Drew Heusch

OUTLINE

OBJECTIVES

1. To discuss the clinical importance of the posterior joint complexes with regard to low back disorders.
2. To define the functional anatomy of the zygapophyseal and sacroiliac joint complexes.
3. To describe the stabilizing aspects of the posterior joints.
4. To discuss the reliability and validity of various methods to assess the posterior joints.
5. To provide literature-based updates regarding objective confirmation of the posterior joints.

INTRODUCTION

The social impact of low back pain has been described as enormous and extremely costly in terms of treatment and lost productivity.[1,2] There is little doubt that low back pain affects the quality of life for a substantial number of people in contemporary Western society.[2,3] It has also been suggested that modern societies are currently facing an epidemic of lower back disability that until recently was rising exponentially.[1] The magnitude of this problem is clearly indicated when 60%–80% of the general population will suffer low back pain at some time during their lives and a large number of international studies show a point prevalence of back pain in the order of 17%–31%.[2] Consequently, owing to a cumulative lifetime incidence as high as 65%, it should not be unexpected that more than one half of the working population will suffer low back pain during their working life.[4]

Clinical Pearl: There is little doubt that low back pain affects the quality of life for a substantial number of people in contemporary Western society. It has also been suggested that modern societies are currently facing an epidemic of lower back disability that until recently was rising exponentially.

Chronic low back (CLB) pain represents the most rapidly growing cause of disability.[1,2,5] CLB pain has been identified as the leading cause of disability and consequently the most expensive health-care problem in the 30- to 50-year-old age group.[6] More alarming is the fact that there appears to be no evidence of any change in the nature, severity, or biological basis of back pain.[5] However, there is preliminary evidence that this trend may have stopped in the last few years, particularly in the United Kingdom, which are not the result of any biological changes but more likely due to social, cultural, and social security changes.[7] This state of affairs has been attributed, in part, to a lack of understanding of the pathophysiological and pathoanatomical principles associated with low back pain.[8] It is reasonable to assume that therapeutic intervention is going to have limited measurable value when the etiological factors are unknown. Musculoskeletal pain is multidimensional and multifactorial in nature, which represents a much wider view of the potential etiological parameters associated with low back pain.[9] Recent attempts by the back pain community have attempted to redirect and focus the attitude of the health-care providers into viewing the problem as more of a social dilemma rather than a single identifiable lesion.[2,7]

Clinical Pearl: Chronic back pain represents the most rapidly growing cause of any other form of disability.

Notwithstanding, the etiology of most spinal pain remains obscure and in most cases unknown,[8]which, as a result of the complexity of its pathogenesis, remains a poorly understood chain of events.[10] Even though there is little agreement upon the nature of the etiology of low back pain, clinical models, management strategies, and clinical guidelines have recently been developed in a number of countries on the basis of available best evidence regarding natural history, biomechanical characteristics, and therapeutic effectiveness.[11–16] There is no doubt that a sedentary lifestyle and escalating socioeconomic tensions have contributed to the problem in the industrialized world. In an attempt to address this issue, medical treatment and management of back pain has failed because of a seemingly passive role and a sustained focus on structural disorders. This seemingly limited approach has been supplanted by more clinically relevant functional, psychosocial, and environmental factors (biopsychosocial model) which define a more contemporary and comprehensive management strategy based upon best research evidence, clinical experience, and patient needs.[8,17–19] In addition to the low back pain problem, other conditions arising from the lumbopelvic region that extend to the lower extremities can magnify the problem in terms of clinical management and disability. Conditions that extend into the buttock, groin, and/or lower extremities can arise from a neurocompressive lesion, as was discussed in Chapters 6 and 7. Other etiological possibilities include vascular compromise, visceral disease, and myofascial issues, which will be discussed in detail in Chapters 9, 10, and 11. Another key region that can cause, in part or entirely, back, buttock, groin, and/or leg pain is commonly known as the posterior joints.

Clinical Pearl: The etiology of most spinal pain remains obscure and in most cases unknown, which, as a result of the complexity of its pathogenesis, remains a poorly understood chain of events.

It has been stated that the posterior spinal joints and the sacroiliac joints are a source of uncomplicated and referred mechanical low back pain.[20–23] The actual proportion of low back pain that can be attributed to a mechanical cause has been quoted as being anywhere between 20% and 70% of all low back pain sufferers.[20,24,25] This remarkable variation highlights the problem of precise diagnosis of the pain-producing structures within this region. Notwithstanding, the intervertebral disc, posterior joints, and the sacroiliac joints have been reported to be responsible for approximately 70% of all low back pain episodes.[20] It therefore stands to reason that the role of the posterior joints (intervertebral facet or zygapophyseal joints) and sacroiliac joints are integral in understanding the complex issues surrounding low back pain syndromes and effective management.[26–28]

Clinical Pearl: It has been stated that the posterior spinal joints and the sacroiliac joints are a source of uncomplicated and referred mechanical low back pain.

The understanding of both the concept and the frequency of occurrence of pain associated with the joint structures of the lower spine and pelvis has undergone a gradual evolution since the days of Mooney and Robertson[29]and before them Ghormley.[30] The concept of the "facet syndrome" initially coined by Ghormley in 1933 and revisited by Mooney and Robertson[29]indicated that the intervertebral disc did not explain all low back pain and referred leg complaints. Their contention at the time was that clinical evidence was emerging that suggested alternative posterior structures (i.e., posterior facet joint or zygapophyseal joints) were in fact a source of low back and leg pain. In *anatomical terms* posterior joint structures are commonly known as *zygapophyseal* ("*z*") *joints*[31]and clinically these structures are also referred to as *facet joints*.[29,32] There have been many authors since who have attempted to precisely identify the *facet syndrome*, a constellation of symptoms arising from the zygapophyseal joints, as clinical reality or mere professional myth.[24,32–38] Schwarzer et al.[37]found that facet joint infiltration is a good method for both diagnosis and treatment of lumbar facet syndrome of particularly those patients in the study group with spondyloarthrosis. Nonetheless, pinpointing the actual source of the pain has many associated problems. It is only by developing a greater understanding of the pathophysiology that a more accurate diagnosis and therefore appropriate management is possible. As mentioned previously, both the sacroiliac and zygapophyseal joints have been identified as a potential primary source of pain, thought to be a significant source of mechanical pain in patients suffering from CLB pain.[21,26,39] Resolving the actual cause of the problem from within such a multiplicity of pain-producing structures requires highly developed clinical and diagnostic skills as well as valid clinical instrumentation.

Clinical Pearl: Resolving the actual cause of the problem from within such a multiplicity of pain-producing structures requires highly developed clinical and diagnostic skills as well as valid clinical instrumentation.

As a consequence of the problems facing clinicians in this area, many different diagnostic procedures have been developed for use in patients with low back pain. Many of these diagnostic approaches are addressed in detail in this text. The array of procedures include medical history, clinical examination, plain film radiography, computed tomography (CT) scan, magnetic resonance imaging (MRI), bone scintigraphy ("bone scan"), diagnostic nerve root blocks, facet injections, functional tests in manual medicine, strength tests of trunk muscles, work-related performance, psychological and social evaluation including psychometric tests are examples of a few.

Despite such a vast number of available procedures, the scientific literature has not significantly changed its conclusion that in up to 85% of all low back pain episodes the cause remains unclear.[28] An additional confounding factor is that during the course of a low back pain episode the relevant factors could change. The patient's perception of the condition will depend on many nonmechanical factors that come under the umbrella of the psychosocial element of the biopsychosocial model of low back pain.[1] Thus, physical presentation of the cause is different from that of prognostic factors. Although there appear to be recognizable factors and even subgroups, there seems to be no consistently identifiable distribution of etiology in the population(s) of patients with low back pain. While individual social factors may be the one important factor in some patients, functional and structural factors may be significant in others. Clinical examination is important, but several problems occur in the evaluation of patients with low back pain. Because of their anatomical location and functional interrelationships, important pain-generating structures of the lumbopelvic spine, e.g., soft tissues, discs, or facet joints, are difficult to unequivocally discern with respect to their being the primary nociceptive source. Additionally, there are a few diagnostic tests available during clinical examination that do not rely on the patient's cooperation or communication and which specifically stress key pain-generating structures in isolation.

The terms "nonspecific or simple mechanical low back pain" or "syndrome" are clinically sound for the majority of patients, because they reflect the fact that the nociceptive etiology and precise pathophysiology are primarily unclear. It must be taken into consideration that these terms enjoy only limited acceptance by both patients and physicians. In reality, clinicians have an obligation to their patients to make a serious attempt to resolve this dilemma. In order to accomplish this, the clinician must employ all aspects of their knowledge, clinical experience, and the proper utilization of established and emerging diagnostic procedures. Is a precise diagnosis really necessary when a number of modalities have shown general success? These and more issues will be discussed in more detail throughout this chapter.

Clinical Pearl: Despite such a vast number of available procedures, the scientific literature has not significantly changed its conclusion that in up to 85% of all low back pain episodes the cause remains unclear.

NEUROLOGY AND NEUROANATOMY OF THE ZYGAPOPHYSEAL JOINTS OF THE LUMBAR SPINE

It is estimated that 15%–40% of CLB pain is due to the zygapophyseal joints.[40]

In order to delve deeper into the factors leading to such a significant percentage of such an international problem, a review of the anatomy is warranted.

Anatomy of the Dorsal Rami

The anatomy of the L1–L4 dorsal rami is different from that of the L5.[41]

L1–L4 Dorsal Rami At the L1–L4 levels, each dorsal ramus arises from the spinal nerve at about the level of the intervertebral disc. The L1–L4 dorsal rami project at almost a right angle to the spinal nerve. They are about 5 mm long and run dorsocaudally through the intertransverse space, deep to the intertransversarii mediales.

In the intertransverse space, each ramus usually divides into medial, lateral, and intermediate branches.[41]

Medial Branch The medial branch is largely sensory. Each lumbar medial branch innervates two adjacent zygapophyseal joints and supplies the fascicles of the multifidus and interspinous muscle and ligament (as per Bogduk) that arise from the spinous process with the same segmental number as the nerve.

These nerves run in a posterior direction on the posterior aspect of the base of the transverse process. The medial branch then passes through a tunnel formed by the mammilloaccessory ligament, a fibrous band connecting the mammillary process (on the dorsolateral surface of the superior articular process), and the accessory process (on the dorsal surface of the transverse process near its junction with the superior articular process). Beyond the mammilloaccessory ligament, the medial branch runs medially and caudally across the vertebral lamina to lie deep to multifidus and become embedded in loose areolar and adipose tissue. In this region further branches to the zygapophyseal joints arise (proximal, distal, and interspinous branches).[41]

Intermediate Branch The intermediate branch is mainly motor and runs dorsally and caudally from the intertransverse spaces. Distribution is to the longissimus muscle.[41]

Lateral Branch The lateral branch is mainly motor, providing efferent innervation to the iliocostalis muscle.

The lateral branch crosses the subjacent transverse process approximately opposite the level of the accessory process. It travels caudally, laterally, and dorsally through the iliocostalis lumborum to innervate this muscle. L1–L3 branches pierce the thoracolumbar fascia to become cutaneous, providing sensory input to the region of the upper buttocks. The L4 branch remains intramuscular.[41]

L5 Dorsal Ramus The L5 dorsal ramus is longer than those at higher levels. It arches over the rostral and dorsal aspect of the ala of the sacrum to lie in the groove formed by the junction of the ala with the root of the superior articular process of the sacrum. Along this course it divides into medial and intermediate branches. It lacks a lateral branch.[41]

Medial Branch The medial branch curves medially around the caudal aspect of the lumbosacral zygapophyseal joint, which it innervates, and ends in the multifidus.[41]

Intermediate Branch The intermediate branch innervates those fibers of longissimus thoracis that arise from the medial aspect of the dorsal segment of the iliac crest, and communicates with the S1 dorsal ramus.[41]

Zygapophyseal Joint

The facet joint itself is a true synovial joint with hyaline cartilage surfaces and a joint space enclosed in a fibrous capsule, lined with synovial membrane.

Two different levels of medial branches supply each zygapophyseal joint. Each medial branch supplies articular branches to the caudal aspect of the joint above it and to the rostral aspect of the joint below. For example, the medial branch of L3 innervates L2/3 and L3/4 zygapophyseal joints. There is no evidence of contralateral innervation.[42,43]

Synovial joints possess a dual pattern of innervation. Primary articular nerves are independent branches from larger peripheral nerves that specifically supply the joint capsule and ligaments; accessory articular nerves reach the joint after passing through muscular or cutaneous tissues to which they provide primary innervation. This results in the joint capsules containing the endings of nerves that arise from the same spinal segment and one level above, at least. These primary and accessory articular nerves terminate in a variety of encapsulated and unencapsulated nerve endings that are sensitive to mechanical, chemical, and thermal stimuli.[44]

Articular Capsule

The zygapophyseal joint capsule consists of an outer layer of dense connective tissue (fibrous capsule) and an inner discontinuous single or multilayered sheath of synovial cells (synovial layer intima). Both layers are separated by a vascular fatty connective tissue (subliminal layer).[45]

The fibrous capsule of the lumbar zygapophyseal joint is 1 mm thick, attaching 2 mm from the articular margins, and is quite strong. The capsule of the facet joint blends with the ligamentum flavum on its medial and superior aspects. At the superior and inferior ends of the lumbar zygapophyseal joint capsules are two subcapsular recesses containing fibroadipose meniscoids that project into the joint. Anatomically, the facet syndrome has been *connected* to this meniscus-like or plical structure of the zygapophyseal joint. It has been suggested that they protect exposed cartilaginous articular surfaces during movement.[46]

Capsular tissue is well supplied with capillaries and neural elements, at all spinal levels. Small myelinated nerve fibers and bundles of unmyelinated nerve fibers have been consistently found in the posterior joint capsule, in the adjacent part of the subintimal layer and in the adipose synovial plica. The capsule has substantial innervation by sensory (nociceptive and mechanoreceptive) and autonomic nerve fibers and has a structural basis for pain perception.[44,45,47–49]

Clinical Pearl: Capsular tissue is well supplied with capillaries and neural elements, at all spinal levels.

Until recently, it was believed that neural structures were not present in the ligamentum flavum, which forms the medial part of the capsule.[45,49] However, this was possibly the result of too few available studies on this tissue, in addition to this is the complexity of the structure especially in respect to its high proportion of elastin. Such tissue components make it difficult to resolve nerve tissue. On the macroscopic level, the ligamentum flavum has two layers, superficial and deep, in which the fibers are opposite. The direction of the fibers in the dorsal layer (superficial) is oriented craniomedially to caudolaterally at an angle between 15 and 30 degrees to the median line, the deeper fibers (the ventral layer) appear to be "strictly" aligned craniocaudally.[50]

In addition, the ligamentum flavum has close relations with a number of potentially important "pain sources." The fibers of the ligament have been described as merging into the capsular structures of the facets,[50] with its accepted innervation. In addition, the tendons of some erector spinae muscles attach close to the attachment point of the ligamentum flavum.[51] Microscopically, the predominance of flavum elastin fibers is unique among ligamentous tissue. The elastin confers active properties to this ligament in that it can deform in stretching (i.e., during forward flexion), but not kink on extension of the spine. Injury to this structure will obviously affect these properties and thus may have neurological sequelae. More recently there have been two reports that have suggested that the ligamentum flavum has an intrinsic innervation.[47,51] It was reported that protein gene product 9.5 immunoreactive nerve fibers (a general nerve marker that stains a large proportion of nerve fiber populations, often described rather loosely as a pan-neuronal marker; see Box 1) were detected in 72% of human lumbar spine ligamentum flavum specimens. Interestingly, these authors found more of the ligamentum flavum specimens to contain nerve fibers than either facet joint capsule (70%) or intervertebral disc (20%) samples.[47] The presence of such an innervation can be seen as a double-edged sword. As one grows older, the nerves in a tissue may atrophy and otherwise decrease in number; this can result in compromised tissue maintenance and subsequent degradation of tissue properties. Such change may be an additive factor in the production of back pain.

Box 1. Interpretation of the Presence of "Neuropeptide-Immunoreactive" Nerve Fibers

Almost every report of lumbar-sacral innervation in the past 15 years has tended to use antibodies to study the presence of nerves in the tissue. However, there are many peptides whose immunoreactivity has been found inside nerve fibres. How does one interpret the findings? Many of the peptides have been characterized so that the sequence and structure are known. Consequently, these compounds have been tested for biological activity. Currently, however, we know only a small part of the story. Many of these compounds appear to have some degree of specific receptor-mediated activity, not always purely related to nerve transmission, with many of the experiments being performed in animals. Therefore, we cannot directly extrapolate with respect to function in the lumbosacral spine of humans. It used to be thought that these compounds could be used to specifically "find and describe" particular types of nerve within a tissue. This is where the idea of relating substance P [SP] and calcitonin gene-related peptide [CGRP] with nociceptors originated. Again the experiments to describe this relationship were performed in rodents. However, this time there are differences in the expression of these compounds even within what appear closely similar species (rats and guinea pigs). It is therefore less realistic to assume that any tight relationship between the SP and CGRP immunoreactivity and nociceptors will hold up in humans. Indeed, there may not even be a tight relationship between sensory innervation and CGRP immunoreactivity, as it has been located in motoneurones. The crux of this is to warn the reader that although certain immunoreactivity to peptides has become synonymous with the presence of nociceptors, this may be subject to criticism and debate as there is little evidence available to support such a direct extrapolation to function in humans.

WHAT IS THE SIGNIFICANCE OF SP/CGRP RELEASE?

Taking the above into consideration, what do we know about the two main neuropeptides and what can we conclude about their potential significance to the tissues in which they are found? In deciding this, one must consider that there is evidence for the release of such substances into the periphery from the nerves that contain them (see McCarthy, 1998, for review). CGRP has been shown to be a vasodilator in a variety of tissues.[52,53] SP "compliments" the CGRP-induced vasodilation by causing extravasation of fluid and mast cell degranulation,[55] In addition, CGRP appears capable of causing neutrophil accumulation[55] which completes the basic requirements for an initial ***acute inflammatory reaction.***

Possible Role in Lumbar Spinal Tissues

In addition, the role of SP and CGRP may not be one that solely evolves around the issue of creating pain. Although this is a major issue from the point of view of "the patient" with back pain, SP and CGRP also can be seen to have a protective effect. Both of these peptides have an effect on the cartilage producing cells in order to cause an increase in synthesis of matrix proteins. These could be seen as crucial adjuncts to tendinous, ligamentous, and synovial tissue's capacity for adaptation and repair. A study of tissue from intervertebral discs adjacent to damaged (ruptured and surgically fused) discs showed an increase in the number of SP and CGRP immunoreactivity containing nerve fibres as well as an increased vascularization.[56] As these discs are under greater loading due to the relative immobility of the adjacent ones, it is only reasonable to assume they need to upregulate their matrix synthesis. Apart from physical stimulation, it would make sense for the system to also stimulate the growth of appropriate other tissues (nerves and vascular) to facilitate the process.

In addition to protein gene product 9.5 (PGP), other neuropeptide-immunoreactive fibers have been reported in facet joint capsule and related tissues in humans. These include substance P (SP), calcitonin gene-related peptide (CGRP), vasoactive intestinal polypeptide (VIP), and neuropeptide Y (NPY). Immunoreactivity to enzymes associated with the autonomic nerve supply to a tissue includes dopamine β-hydroxylase (DBH), which is involved in the creation of noradrenaline (norepinephrine, sympathetic) and choline acetyl transferase (ChAT), which is capable of creating acetylcholine (parasympathetic and limited sympathetic). There are problems in interpreting the origin and role of any nerve fibers revealed by these methods; this is explored further in Box 1.

Synovial Membrane

There seems to be a discrepancy of opinion regarding the innervation of the synovial membrane. Giles and Harvey[57] reported finding substance P immunoreactivity, possibly sensory nerve structures in the lumbosacral zygapophyseal joint synovial folds. A nociceptive function was suggested for these nerves, with a possible involvement in back pain originating in the facet joint.

Gronblad et al.[58] suggested that it is more likely that plical fold nerves mainly participate in local vasoregulation and the very few "sensory" neuropeptide nerves, which were only occasionally seen in this tissue, and never freely in the stroma, are of only minor importance. However, more recently,

Vandenabeele et al.[45] was not able to demonstrate any neural structures in the synovial membrane. Part of this discrepancy might arise from the understanding of what is meant by synovial membrane. Superficial regions might have an associated innervation whereas deeper layers (including the inner surface) might be less likely to have one. Therefore, the manner of selection might be expected to determine the outcome. This is only the view of the author based on experience (P.M.), however, without knowledge of the selection criteria used.

Articular Cartilage and Subchondral Bone

Histological examination of facets obtained from patients with degenerative spinal conditions demonstrated erosion channels extending through the subchondral bone and calcified cartilage into the articular cartilage. Immunostaining showed the presence of substance P-positive nerve fibers within these erosion channels, and also within marrow spaces.[59]

The presence of substance P-immunoreactive nerve fibers in these erosion channels may have several implications. Increased or abnormal loads may cause pain by activation of the nerve endings. Substance P causes the release of inflammatory mediators, which may effect the local environment of facet joint. This release may sensitize nociceptors to these peptides and other mediators, facilitating the formation of chronic pain states. Substance P may also affect the degenerative process through bone remodeling.[59]

Pain Maps for the Lumbar Facet Joints

Mooney and Robertson,[29] in a landmark study, injected the lumbar zygapophyseal joints with hypertonic saline to map their pain distribution. Indeed, the interest in this study was piqued because the lead author was the volunteer subject for the study. Initially upon injection, the volunteer reported a local pain around the injection site. Within approximately 20 seconds, the hypesthesia radiated down the lower back, greater trochanter, and to the posterolateral thigh. No radiation proximally up the back occurred.

The L3–L4 zygapophyseal joint seems to produce pain more laterally down the lower back, buttock, and lower limb. Pain patterns of L4–L5 and L5–S1 were difficult to distinguish from each other, and were more posteriorly distributed. Interestingly, the pain distribution maps differed in asymptomatic and symptomatic subjects (see Fig. 8–1).[29]

Neurology and Neuroanatomy of the Sacroiliac Joint

Hilton's law states that a joint may receive innervation from any nerve that crosses it. Thus, the sacroiliac joint

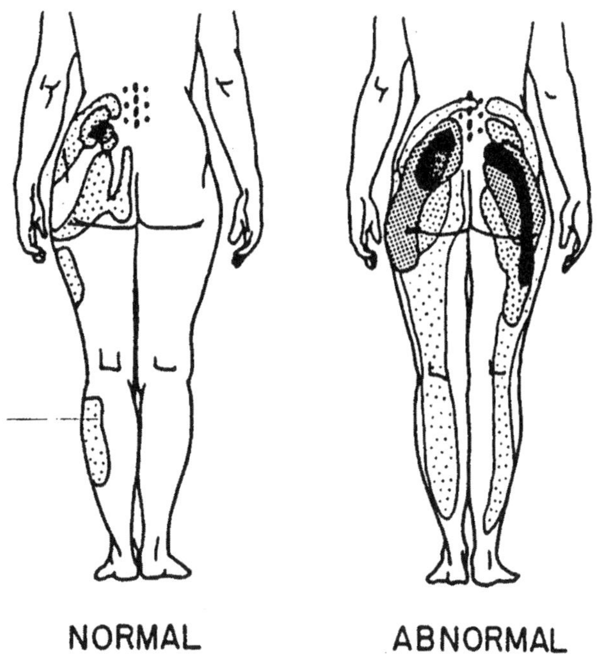

FIGURE 8–1. Pain referral patterns produced by intra-articular injections of hypertonic saline in asymptomatic (normal) and symptomatic (abnormal) patients. (*Adapted from Mooney & Robertson,*[29] *with permission)*

may be innervated from as cephalad as L2 and as caudad as S3 or S4 and from both anterior and primary rami. This extensive source of innervation explains their associations with low back, buttock, proximal thigh, and groin pain.[60]

Solonen[61] suggests that the sacroiliac joint receives innervation from the neighboring nerve trunks, including the lumbosacral plexus, superior gluteal nerve, dorsal rami of S1 and S2, and sometimes the obturator nerve.

Similar to the above, other studies have concluded that the nerve filaments in the sacroiliac joint are derived from the ventral rami of L4 and L5, from the superior gluteal nerve, and from the dorsal rami of L5, S1, and S2.[62,63]

Horwitz[64] found that the sacroiliac ligaments contained branches from the dorsal rami of S1 and S2.

A study on fetuses has shown a significant number of neurofilaments that could only be found in the dorsal mesenchyme.[65]

A recent study found no nerve branches from the sacral plexus or obturator nerve supplying the ventral part of the sacroiliac joint. It was noted that many small blood vessels (which stain in a similar manner to peripheral nerves), which appeared to be derived from the sacral plexus, entered the ventral ligaments of the sacroiliac joint. Dissection of the dorsal aspect of the joint revealed nerve branches derived from the loops connecting S1–S4 dorsal rami.[66]

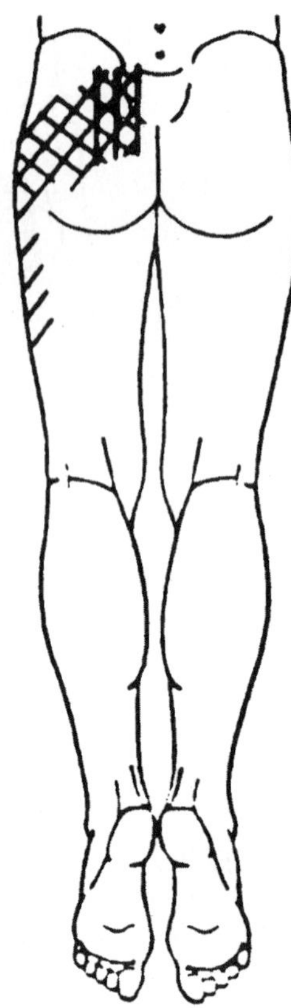

FIGURE 8–2. Composite sacroiliac joint referral map illustrating the area of intersectional overlap (common to all 10 volunteers).

Clinical Pearl: It would appear that the nerve supply to the sacroiliac joint is both complex and extensive including dorsal and ventral rami from L3 to S4 levels.

Pain Maps for the Sacroiliac Joints

Pain referral maps generated from asymptomatic volunteers following sacroiliac injections demonstrated hypesthesia locally over the posterior superior iliac spine, extending approximately 10 cm caudally and 3 cm laterally from the posterior superior iliac spine (see Fig. 8–2).[67] The sensory changes in the figure are more consistent with the distribution of dorsal rami than with that of ventral rami.[66]

POSTERIOR JOINT COMPLEX—STABILITY AND FUNCTIONAL CONSIDERATIONS

Introduction

The posterior joint complex of the lumbopelvic spine has been the subject of great debate and contention over the past decades particularly with respect to the largely enigmatic neurobiomechanical function and pain-generating properties. It is the least understood region of the spine and the most controversial with respect to overall function, complexity, and role in low back pain.[68] There is some speculation at present regarding the true function of these structures, and the exact role in the pathogenesis of low back pain is unclear at this stage.[18] The role of the sacroiliac joint, for instance, as a source of low back pain is still the subject of great debate and controversy among health-care professionals.[69–73] There is still a poor understanding of the actual pathogenesis of mechanical pain syndromes and a lack of objective diagnostic evidence to support this view. Nonetheless, many clinicians have always contested the fundamental role of the sacroiliac joint and posterior facet joints in the production of low back and leg pain. This supposition is strengthened by the functional anatomy, histology, and understanding of the pathomechanics of the sacroiliac and posterior facet joints, which has provided a rational basis for manipulative intervention.[71,74,75] This view has been reinforced recently by research that indicates that sacroiliac joint mechanoreceptors may play more of a nociceptive rather than a proprioceptive role at specific thresholds than was previously thought.[39] Further research in this area may shed some light on this matter that has considerable clinical interest. Considerable research efforts have recently been made investigating the role of both the lumbar zygapophyseal (z) and sacroiliac joints in the genesis of low back pain.[21,26,37,60,76] The results of this work have considerable clinical implications particularly for those engaging in spinal manipulative therapy, providing additional rationale for effective clinical intervention and management of low back pain.

Sacroiliac Joint—Biomechanical and Functional Considerations

Even though attempts have been made to describe and measure sacroiliac motion, discussions regarding joint biomechanics are still largely speculative and its biomechanical function is still regarded as variable and uncertain.[72,77,78] A recent model describing lumbopelvic stability has been proposed that incorporates a comprehensive interplay between the various structures of this region.[68] This model is based primarily upon the anatomical and biomechanical properties of several structures within the lumbopelvic (sacroiliac and lumbosacral facet joints) region that provide both form and force stability via anatomical characteristics and compressive friction properties. These concepts will be discussed in more detail later in this chapter.

In order to appreciate the functionally comprehensive nature of the above-noted model, a review of a prior model by Illi[79] may be helpful. Illi's model provided the rationale for a number of examination procedures, such as Gillet's tests,[23] and manipulative techniques for the pelvic/sacroiliac region[80,81] Illi's reciprocal motion model proposed that compensatory and equivalent movement of the innominates creates predictable sacral motion. Illi suggested that as one innominate flexes (i.e., the PSIS moves posterior and inferior), the ipsilateral sacral base moves anterior and inferior (*"nutates"*) and as the other innominate extends (i.e., PSIS moves anterior and superior), the sacral base on that side moves posterior and superior ("counter-nutates") predominantly via the *x*-axis of motion. During gait this would be described as a continuous motion or a figure-of-eight rocking motion with simultaneous nutation and counter-nutation taking place within the same movement cycle in response to the flexion and extension of the individual innominate structures as per a gait cycle predominantly via the *x*-axis of movement.[81] This reciprocal movement model underpinned several standing motion palpation tests used by clinicians for decades[82] and provided a clinically feasible structure to determine specific manipulative interventions based upon the observed lack of motion detected via these clinical testing procedures. This model depicts a predominantly structural osseous interplay, which ignores the important stabilizing characteristics of local myofascial tissues and the inherent interlocking features of the region that contribute to its stiffness, known respectively as *"force closure"* and *"form closure."* The more contemporary functional model of the sacroiliac/lumbosacral joint incorporates a host of functional components ranging from anatomical characteristics to soft tissue nature, which will be discussed in greater detail throughout this chapter.

Clinical Pearl: The anatomical and biomechanical properties of several structures within the lumbopelvic (sacroiliac and lumbosacral facet joints) region that provide both form and force stability via both inherent anatomical characteristics and compressive friction properties.

The sacroiliac joints, owing to their mobility and somewhat vertical orientation, contribute to the static and dynamic challenges necessary during standing gait and other posturally demanding tasks. They also paradoxically provide support for the trunk and guide overall movements. The sacroiliac joints also function to provide elasticity to the pelvic ring, serve as a buffer between the lower limbs and spine, contribute to the proprioceptive and nociceptive output of the joint capsule, and transfer large loads during weight bearing and locomotion. Recent studies have demonstrated that contrary to previous thought, the sacroiliac joint has less proprioceptive function, suggesting that the mechanosensitive receptors in the capsule are in effect nociceptive in nature.[39] One could argue that in all tissues there is probably a greater potential for nociception than proprioception based upon the proportions of each neuron type present. This once again reinforces the fact that the sacroiliac joint may be a source of mechanical pain in humans. The results of a study investigating double block techniques and the value of sacroiliac pain provocation tests concluded that the sacroiliac is an uncommon but real source of low back pain and that the accuracy of common provocation tests is highly questionable.[22] They did however go on to say that the sacroiliac joint should be included in a differential diagnosis when managing mechanical nonspecific low back pain, despite the fact that to isolate a distinct "sacroiliac syndrome," based upon the evidence, was currently untenable.

Clinical Pearl: The sacroiliac joint should be included as a potential source of pain in a differential diagnosis when managing mechanical nonspecific low back pain.

The sacroiliac joints are mobile, diarthrodial, transferring loads from the spine to the pelvis and providing support for the trunk.[68] This joint complex provides elasticity to the pelvic ring, serves as a buffer between the lower limb and the spine, and functions both as an organ of proprioception and nociception. In terms of mechanics, recent evidence suggests that sacroiliac joint mobility is minimal and variable, particularly influenced by increasing age and gender. Movement has been found to be greatest around the transverse axis (*x*-axis) in the order of 2.5 degrees with a mean translation of 0.7 mm (Fig. 8–3).[83] A more recent investigation found that the sacroiliac joints in the elderly were mobile, allowing up to 4 degrees of rotation,[84] whereas other researchers have established that rotation of the sacrum was much less in the sacroiliac joints of males (0.6–1.2 degrees) than of females (1.9–2.8 degrees).[85]

In terms of biomechanical characteristics, the sacroiliac joint in comparison to a lumbar motion segment can withstand 6× more medially directed and 7× more lateral bending force, whereas the lumbar motion segment is capable of withstanding 20× more axial compression and 2× more axial torsion.[71] Therefore, it can be surmised that the sacroiliac joints, from an anatomical and biomechanical perspective, seem to be more prone to axial compression and torsional loading, which are integral components during the execution of normal daily activities. These activities typically involve forward bending, lifting, and twisting the trunk.[68,71,72,78] This evidence holds considerable clinical implications particularly when attempting to identify the primary pain generator and apply the appropriate therapeutic modalities.

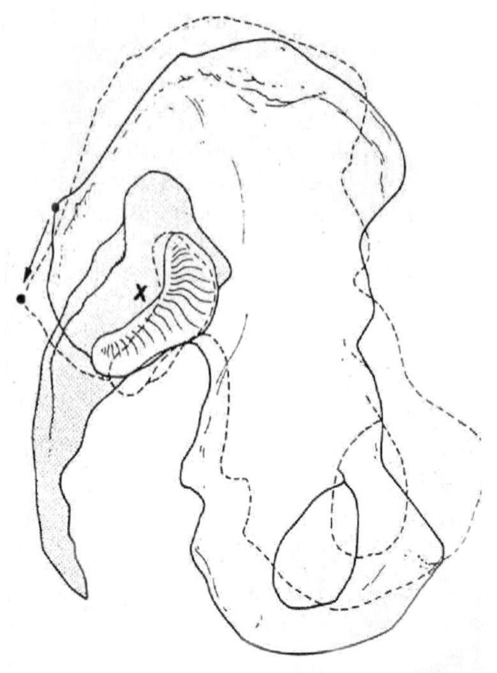

FIGURE 8–3. Illustration of the primary axis of motion of the sacroiliac joint.

Functional stability appears to be a paramount necessity for efficient movement and less mechanical stress on pain-sensitive structures.[68,86,87] A shear prevention system defined by anatomical form and force closure structures to create self-locking mechanism has been proposed for sacroiliac joint stability.[68] The wedge-shaped sacrum, rough articular cartilage, and the multiple articular grooves and ridges are all designed to reduce shear forces in the range of 1750 N while the lumbosacral ligaments, thoracolumbar fascia, and related musculature (multifidus, piriformis, gluteus maximus, and iliopsoas) via ligamentous attachments increase joint compressive forces and overall stability.[68,88–90] These authors have suggested that insufficient self-locking may result because of joint capsule and ligamentous laxity (i.e., faulty form closure mechanism), muscle weakness, and inadequate coordination between various key muscle structures (i.e., faulty force closure mechanism). It would appear that active rehabilitation aimed at restoring functional capacity to these structures would be an appropriate methodology particularly in light of the underlying rationale for the instability and the outcomes of a specific and graded exercise program.[91] Furthermore, there is promising evidence regarding the importance of both strength and endurance characteristics of soft tissues required for spinal stability and optimal function.[92] This concept fits well with Panjabi's[86] spinal stability model and its various components. This model supports the fact that most back injuries are not due to frank trauma but more likely to be the result of trivial events, unstable movements, and associated motor control errors causing inappropriate muscle activation and aberrant joint motion.[87,93] Therefore, the cornerstone of lumbopelvic rehabilitation is trunk muscular endurance (extensor/flexor/lateral flexor) and sensorimotor training.[87,93] Such an approach provides patients with the skills necessary to sustain a variety of trunk postures over a period of time and improve reaction times appropriately to sudden shifts in movement as a result of changes in terrain and environment.[87,93] Furthermore, these programs are considered safe and effective for all age groups as a prevention strategy for mechanical back pain.[81] Lumbopelvic rehabilitation strategies and methods are discussed in detail in later chapters of this textbook.

Clinical Pearl: Functional stability appears to be a paramount necessity for efficient movement and less mechanical stress on pain-sensitive structures.

The mechanical influence of musculoligamentous interplay has been closely associated with various kinematic chains influencing sacroiliac joint mobility.[68,94] It is their contention that contraction of the gluteus maximus, for example, could strongly affect the nature of sacroiliac joint motion via its attachment to the sacrotuberous ligament. This could shed some light on the etiology of mechanical irritation of the sacroiliac joint by way of asymmetrical contraction of these large stabilizing muscles. More recently, researchers are reporting that contraction of the transversus abdominis significantly decreases the laxity of the sacroiliac joint improving overall stability of this structure as has been shown within the lumbar spine for the treatment of low back pain.[95] Other groups are demonstrating the functional integration and role of various structures related to the lumbosacral region and the links between the legs, spine, and arms during the performance of various activities of daily living.[96] It has come to light that the function of the long dorsal sacroiliac ligament has anatomical relations with the erector spinae muscles, the posterior layer of the thoracolumbar fascia, and the sacrotuberous ligament providing a mechanical and neurophysiological (via the mechanoreceptors) connection transferring loads between the upper and lower body.[96,97] This may have significant clinical implications with respect to patients with nonspecific mechanical low back pain as a result of dysfunction of the facet and sacroiliac joints. In fact, there has been some suggestion that posterior pelvic pain in pregnant women may occur as a result of disturbed muscle function in a response to nociceptive stimulation during gait,[98] which could imply an impairment of the stability cycle at the lumbopelvic level.[82] The concept of functional stability and biomechanical integration is extremely important clinically in understanding the complexity of low back posterior joint pain syndrome presentation and its influence on other related joint complex dysfunction.[99] Furthermore, the functional stability scenario especially for the lumbar spine has clinical implications, particularly when specific segmental muscle stabilizer atrophy (i.e., multifidus) persists without recovery after the acute pain resolves, leaving the individual susceptible to recurrent episodes.[100] In addition, a recent clinical trial found a significant decrease in recurrent low back pain episodes in the specific exercise group targeting the multifidus via transversus abdominis compared with the control group employing advice and medication.[101] This particular situation underpins the need to instigate a rehabilitation program immediately in order to restore segmental functional stability to control recurrent pain episodes.[91]

Clinical Pearl: The cornerstone of lumbopelvic rehabilitation is trunk muscular endurance (extensor/flexor/lateral flexor) and sensorimotor training.

The fact that the multifidus extends throughout the lumbar spine and caudally as far down to cross the sacroiliac joints indicates its role in posterior joint

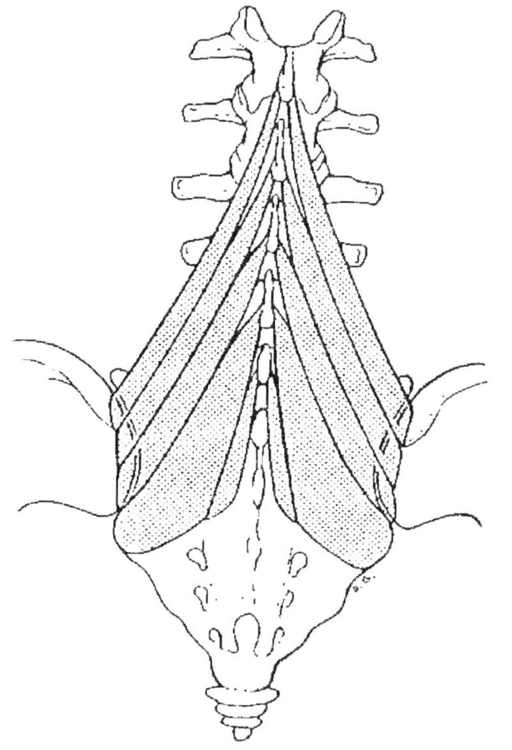

FIGURE 8–4. Demonstration of the expanse of the multifidus muscle as a primary stabilizer of the lumbopelvic region.

stability (Fig. 8–4). In addition, it has recently been demonstrated that asymmetric laxity of the sacroiliac joints in pregnancy related pelvic pain has been identified as a possible predictive indicator for those who may suffer moderate to severe postpartum back pain.[102] These investigators have developed a reliable Doppler imaging technique capable of detecting asymmetric laxity in the sacroiliac joint.[103] This same team of researchers have also determined that a pelvic belt placed high in the pelvis at the level just below the anterior superior iliac spine seems to influence sacroiliac joint laxity in normal females.[104] Laxity in the joint was influenced more by the position of the belt rather than the tension in the belt, which may contribute to a better understanding of the management of low back pain in pregnant and postpartum patients.[104] The effect of the belt is thought to enhance the "self-bracing" forces around the joints and the line of action of the belt is compared to that of the piriformis muscle. The role of these stabilizing structures and the responsibility of clinicians to introduce appropriate management strategies become more apparent as more evidence comes to light. Moreover, it has been stated that very little attention has been given to the role of these influential soft tissue structures during spinal manipulation therapy[105] and it is only recently becoming more apparent that their role is pivotal in stabilizing spinal structures during various activities to resist deformation. Nevertheless, McGill[93] has postulated that the extremely high mechanical loads characteristic of this region (lumbosacral and sacroiliac joints) could potentially lead to microfailure of the tendon-periosteum attachment of these soft tissues and corresponding extensor aponeurosis, resulting in a local pain response. This may explain the local tenderness associated with the tissues of this region during examination, which may be totally unrelated to joint dysfunction.[92]

Since the sacroiliac joint displays extremely small movements, it is unlikely that the response to manual therapy is simply a reduction of a misalignment.[71,106] Rather, it was implied that the role of a high-velocity, low-amplitude manipulation lies in restoring the balance between joint kinematics and associated muscle function, which subsequently normalizes the arthrokinetic reflex and breaks the pain cycle. It could well be that active stimulation and stretch of these large pelvic muscle structures create a reflex myofascial relaxation and pain inhibition. These concepts would certainly support the notion that skilled manipulation is mandatory to discriminate the complex interaction of so many influential and pain-sensitive structures.

Clinical Pearl: The concept of functional stability and biomechanical integration is extremely

important clinically in understanding the complexity of low back posterior joint pain syndrome presentation and in recognizing the influence of other related joint complex dysfunction.

Biomechanical models of lifting seem to ignore the influence of the pelvic mechanism and lower limbs as part of an integrated regional system that functions in harmony transferring and distributing loads safely. The controversy surrounding the merits and utility of various lifting techniques rages on and there is still doubt as to which particular skill provides an advantage for workers. There are others who suggest that biomechanically there is very little difference between the two most common lifting techniques (stoop vs. squat) in terms of axial compression and anterior shear forces.[107] It has also been suggested that the enormous ergonomic effort to promote the squat lift technique throughout industry has demonstrated very little in terms of a decrease in the incidence of occupational back pain.[1,16,87] McGill[87] has presented biomechanically sound principles with respect to lifting safely, such as avoiding full end-range lumbar flexion, flexing from the hips, and keeping the object close to the body during the lifting action to protect sensitive structures and maintain neutral spine stability. It appears that it may not matter how one lifts (stoop, squat, or variation), rather that the individual maintains a *stable neutral spine via trunk muscle bracing* and flexes forward and backward via the hip joints. This evidence-based approach to lifting could very well revolutionize occupational health and safety programs with respect to education and workplace prevention.

Clinical Pearl: It may not matter how one lifts (stoop, squat, or variation), but more importantly that the individual maintains a stable neutral spine via trunk muscle bracing. This approach could revolutionize occupational health and safety programs with respect to education and workplace prevention.

Moreover, lifting is a complex mechanical effort that cannot be viewed upon as a function of the lumbar spinal elements in isolation. Conservative care practitioners of low back syndromes are, of course, deeply interested in the mechanics of the pelvic ring and in particular the sacroiliac joints especially during common functional activities. Snijders et al.[108] goes some way toward redressing the balance and deals, almost exclusively, with the role of the sacroiliac joints and the pelvic ring in the transfer of upper body loads to the legs.

As mentioned previously, Pool-Goudzwaard et al.[68] have thoroughly described how the sacroiliac joints resist very large shear loads imposed upon them and how the joints' form and force management systems are well designed for these tasks. The flat nature of these joints makes them well suited for the transfer of large bending moments but susceptible to shear forces, which would tend to displace the sacrum inferiorly with respect to the iliac bones. It is important to remember that up to 60% of the body weight is supported by the sacrum. These authors view the pelvis as an arched structure. They describe a mechanism whereby displacements of the sacrum are reduced to a minimum by a constant compressive force across the sacroiliac joints—the "self-bracing" effect.[68] This mechanism is dependent not only on joint compression but on friction forces within the joint (ridges and groves; joint cartilage characteristics), sacral wedge angle, and the influence of muscles and ligaments. The architecture and mechanical properties of the passive structures, such as the ligaments, arch structure, joint cartilage, and ridges and grooves, provide the stabilizing component of form closure. The dynamic tissues provide further stability via force closure. The authors also show that if the pelvis is treated as an arch, the intrinsic stability and mechanical function of the sacroiliac joints do not depend on an intact "pelvic ring." They go on to suggest that by far the greatest factor in sacroiliac joint stability is the compressive forces acting across the joint surfaces. These forces, together with the propeller-like orientation of the sacral surfaces, will resist sacral slipping. Of greatest interest perhaps to clinicians is the suggestion that forces generated within certain pelvic muscles, particularly the gluteus maximus and piriformis, can markedly increase the compressive forces across the joint and thus improve overall stability. This reinforces the contribution of these structures from a clinical perspective and even more importantly strengthens the need for additional strategies in the case management plan.[92] According to more recent evidence asymmetrical loading via large pelvic muscles may contribute to mechanical incongruity, which in turn may predispose the pain-sensitive structures to additional mechanical stress, which in turn could cause mechanical/nociceptive pain.[102,103] By the same token it would seem logical that in order to manipulate or adjust these joints, one should exploit the influence these muscles have on their related articulation. It is the authors' opinion that the passive tension within these myofascial structures may therefore be of greater importance to manipulative skills than the final "thrust" itself and therefore a working knowledge of the mechanical properties and effects of muscular tissues is essential to all manipulative clinicians. Snijders et al.[108] also hypothesize that, through connections with the lumbodorsal fascia, other muscles such as the latissimus dorsi may work in synergy with the gluteus maximus, under certain loading conditions, to support the sacroiliac joints. McGill[109] has more recently described the functional anatomy of the lumbar spine. Through his detailed experimental efforts he highly rates the role of the latissimus dorsi in contributing to the stabilization (stiffening) and extension of the lumbar spine owing to its attachment to each lumbar spinous process via the lumbodorsal fascia and insertion into the humerus. This certainly highlights the need for clinicians to revise rehabilitation strategies to include training these vital structures and include them in a more comprehensive and practical program so as to improve back stability and efficiency.[91] Work over the last decade has emphasized the importance of various stabilizers of the low back region. McGill[109] regards training the "big four" stabilizers of the lumbopelvic region, including (1) rectus abdominis, (2) obliques, (3) transversus abdominis, and (4) quadratus lumborum as core elements of any rehabilitation and prevention program. In addition, the sacrotuberous ligament is also thought to play a central role in sacroiliac joint stability. Vleeming et al.[94] suggested that, through connections with the long head of biceps femoris, the straight-leg raising (SLR) test can directly affect the sacroiliac joint. Thus pain elicited by the SLR test may reflect sacroiliac dysfunction rather than nerve root irritation. This may be supported by the fact that 99% of those under the age of 65 who experience pain are most likely to report nociceptive (mechanical) pain only as opposed to approximately 1% who report neuropathic pain characteristics.[110] Furthermore, the stabilizing effect of gluteus maximus may be partly mediated through tension in the sacrotuberous ligament.[94] This is hardly a surprising function of the ligament; however, the concept that through attachments with the lumbodorsal fascia, gluteus maximus, and biceps femoris muscles this stabilizing function may be modified certainly provokes clinical and research interest. The limited view that muscles and ligaments subserve entirely separate functions may well be outdated particularly in light of Panjabi's stability model, which clearly illustrates the close and interdependent interaction of the various active and passive structures under the control of the nervous system to ensure overall joint and functional stability (see Chapter 5, Fig. 5–1).[86] Moreover, the sacroiliac joints have been compared to a multidirectional force transducer, presuming the existence of mechanoreceptors in the surrounding ligaments, which means that there are two "sensors" in the path of considerable force streams being transferred by the pelvis from the upper body to the legs. It has been suggested that the spinal ligaments will act more like strain gauges than force transducers and that the large deformations that occur in these tissues around the neutral position will better stimulate receptor cells than the forces (stress) generated as a consequence of load.[86] The information generated by these sensors can then be used via the neural subsystem to modify muscular responses to imposed loading or postural/positional shifts (the active subsystem) and restore mechanical stability instantly if it has been compromised.

Clinical Pearl: Panjabi's stability model clearly illustrates the close and interdependent interaction of the various active and passive structures under the control of the nervous system to ensure overall joint and functional stability.

It is very apparent that these researchers view articular stability (lumbar and sacroiliac joints) as an active process rather than a passive or static resistance to imposed demands.[111] Furthermore, it seems likely that one can influence this mechanism externally through alterations to muscular tone and rehabilitation or by indirect stimulation of mechanoreceptors, a possible effect of manipulation. This does provide a strong case for a multidimensional approach to back pain management and prevention.

Spinal, and many other, ligaments possess the ability to vary their stiffness throughout a range of movement.[86] This viscoelastic behavior allows greater movement within and around the neutral position but progressively limits motion toward the end of the range. The region of relative ligamentous laxity around the neutral position has been termed the *neutral zone* (NZ) and that part of the range of motion associated with increasing ligament stiffness the *elastic zone* (EZ) (Fig. 8–5).[86] This is particularly relevant when referring to a lumbar motion segment with its multiplanar motion characteristics (Fig. 8–6). Spinal motion segment stability is necessary during the performance of common movements such as those

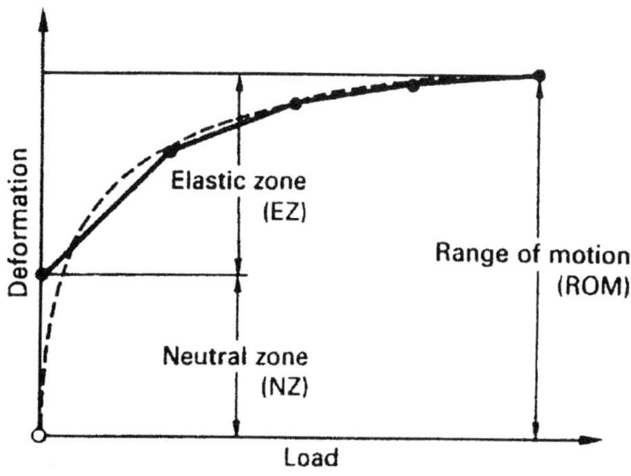

FIGURE 8–5. Illustration of the nonlinear load deformation curve of soft tissues and joints. High flexibility is described by the neutral zone (NZ) and the region of relative stiffness is defined by the elastic zone (EZ) throughout the physiological range of motion. *(Adapted from Byfield et al.,[82] with permission.)*

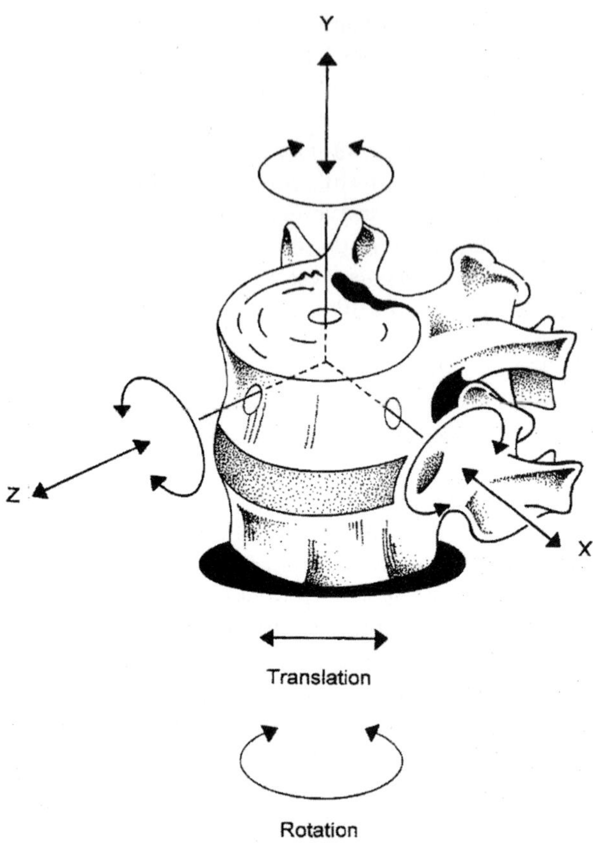

FIGURE 8–6. Illustration of a typical lumbar motion segment with multiple axes of motion. *(Adapted from Byfield et al.,[82] with permission.)*

required during a lifting action which requires sagittal plane rotation around the x-axis (Fig. 8–7).

This biphasic nature of spinal motion allows minimum energy expenditure for movements around the neutral position, but provides opposition to potentially damaging movements at the end of range and is vital in understanding the concept of spinal and pelvic stability during normal activities of daily living.[111] Utilizing data from a previous study,[112] Panjabi[86] suggests that although an individual's overall range of spinal motion may be within normal limits, an increase in the NZ would indicate instability. This "region of low bending moment" is a fairly constant proportion of the range and therefore should not be expected to change under normal circumstances.[113] For clinicians that utilize manual techniques such as mobilization and manipulation, segmental instability is one entity that will be encountered clinically, particularly with today's understanding of spinal function and stability concepts. Consequently, if an increase in the NZ characterizes instability, then perhaps a reduction of this "region of low bending moment" at a segmental level can characterize the spinal dysfunction or manipulable lesion.[111]

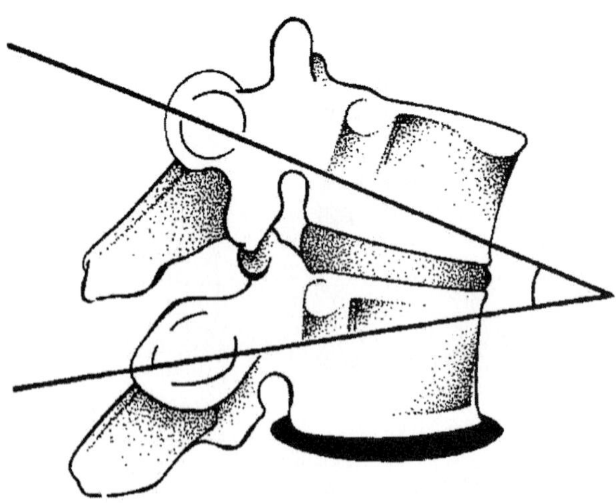

FIGURE 8–7. Illustration of a typical lumbar motion segment during rotation around the x-axis during trunk flexion and extension. *(Adapted from Byfield et al.,[82] with permission.)*

Clinical Pearl: Although an individual's overall range of spinal motion may be within normal limits, an increase in the NZ would indicate instability.

This certainly has clinical implications in terms of joint stability and the role of the various functional components in this particular scheme. This particular model does however highlight the basis for understanding lumbopelvic stability, case management, and rehabilitation and injury prevention. It also emphasizes a more global mechanical view of these pain syndromes.

Sacroiliac Joint—Clinical Considerations

Despite the lack of objective evidence to define the role of the sacroiliac joint in mechanical low back pain, its pathogenesis, some diagnostic criteria, and the treatment of the sacroiliac syndrome have been described in detail.[69,77,114]

Sacroiliac joint dysfunction is prevalent in the population. Sacroiliac disorders have been implicated in 50%–70% of adults presenting with low back pain,[70] whereas 26% and 33.5% of a sample of school-aged children had low back pain and some form of sacroiliac joint dysfunction, respectively.[115] The older age group of students (12–17 years) had a 41.5% prevalence of sacroiliac dysfunction, which is lower than that reported for adults but represents a very high incidence for a young age group population. The role of the sacroiliac joint as a mechanical source of pain during pregnancy has also been established.[102–104,116] Even though the true pathophysiology of the sacroiliac joint and the etiology of the pain remain unclear, there is a growing body of evidence that suggests a positive response to manipulative intervention. Even though there is no compelling data supporting any specific treatment approach as of yet, there still appears to be more support for manipulative management.[73]

Biomechanical Considerations (Disc and Facet)

Several chapters in this textbook address lumbopelvic biomechanical issues, especially Chapter 3. However, this is a very broad and complex topic. As such, there are a number of excellent textbooks currently published highlighting in detail the biomechanics of the lumbopelvic region.[92,117,118] These publications provide essential supplemental reading in the region of back pain and functional rationale concerning the intervertebral disc and facet joints that extend well beyond the scope of this particular chapter.

Clinical Pearl: It has been reported that the origin of the most severe and chronic pain is most likely the posterior aspect of the intervertebral disc and the associated posterior longitudinal ligament, structures that can be damaged by repetitive and heavy lifting.

Nevertheless, it has been reported that the origin of the most severe and chronic pain is most likely the posterior aspect of the intervertebral disc and the associated posterior longitudinal ligament, structures that can be damaged by repetitive and heavy lifting.[119] The zygapophyseal (z) or facet joints have also been identified as common sites of pain (as mentioned previously) and are easily damaged by twisting[20,119] or as a result of functional instability due to inability to react appropriately to postural or other daily activity demands.[87] McGill[87] suggests that most back injury occurs as a result of trivial movements due to functional instability rather than frank trauma. This view coincides with Panjabi's multidimensional spinal stability model, which has active, passive, and neural control elements.[86]

Clinical Pearl: Most back injury occurs as a result of trivial movements due to functional instability rather than frank trauma.

Early studies have demonstrated that forced rotation of the intervertebral joints in vitro will produce a torsional injury.[120,121] Cassidy et al.[122] indicate that the direct relationship between torsion and disc failure is an erroneous notion. They contend that the intervertebral disc is well suited to withstand rotation based upon, among other factors, the orientation of the annular fibers. However, evidence is now emerging which states that about 25% of the population have asymptomatic lumbar disc herniations, which would be considered for surgical intervention if they were symptomatic.[123] More recently Boos et al.[124] established that an age, sex, and risk factor matched group of asymptomatic individuals had a substantially higher prevalence of disc herniation (76%) than previously reported in an unmatched group. Disc herniations have been reported to occur in 20%–36% of asymptomatic volunteers.[124] From a clinical perspective Dickson and Butt[123] indicate that inducing a disc herniation during lumbar rotary spinal manipulation is simply not tenable, which coincides with more recent conclusions following a systematic review of the literature that the risk of a disc herniation as a result of spinal manipulation is extremely rare.[125] This could very well reflect and illustrate that the structures of the lumbar spine are biologically and biomechanically well designed and very capable of withstanding and transferring significant mechanical loads while performing normal tasks of daily living. In addition, investigators have cautioned clinicians attributing a particular anatomical finding found on imaging and designating this as the patient's source of pain.[126] Boos and Lander[127] reinforce this opinion particularly from the point of view of imaging modalities in the diagnosis of low back pain disorders. Their review concluded that methodological flaws exist in various imaging studies (e.g., patient selection, design) and they caution spine specialists to be very critical in their interpretation of these studies paying particular attention to patient selection, sample size, and the reasoning behind clinical recommendations.

Clinical Pearl: Investigators have cautioned clinicians attributing a particular anatomical finding found on imaging and designating this as the patient's source of pain.

Torsional loads that normally damage the facet joints have been shown to have no effect on the integrity of the disc.[128] Under normal conditions within the physiological range of movement, there is minimal strain on the disc. Excessive torsional strain will be resisted by the intact facet joint,[129] which if applied repetitively may disrupt the axis of motion, increasing the lateral shear across the plane of the disc, causing torsional failure and peripheral tears in the annulus.[130]

Nonetheless, the intervertebral disc is not totally exempt from injury. It has been reported that the disc will prolapse (i.e., defined as herniation of the nucleus beyond the periphery of the annulus, extending into the neural canal) as a result of a sudden hyperflexion action, sometimes associated with industrial lifting accidents.[131] The disc has also been demonstrated to prolapse gradually over a period of time owing to cumulative microtrauma under repetitive compression and flexion loads often being the focus of occupational disability.[132] These two mechanisms, sudden or insidious, are common etiological processes seen clinically

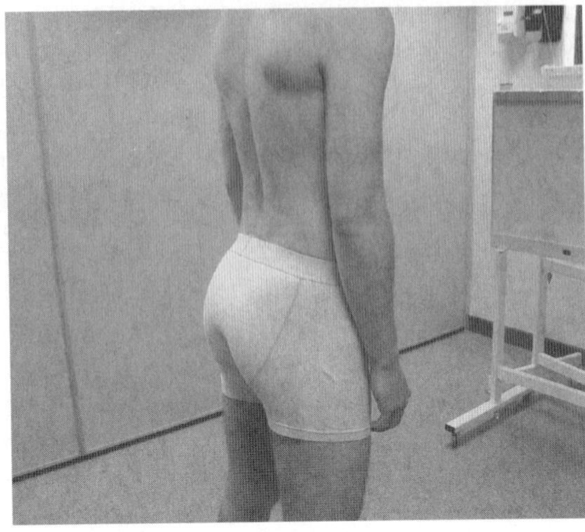

FIGURE 8–8. Illustration of the neutral lordosis recommended during various activities to ensure stability and reduce spinal injuries.

with patients presenting with both acute and chronic back pain.

The lumbar spine in a neutral lordotic posture can sustain very large forces as a result of the tension developed in the posterior ligamentous system, which includes the joint capsules and interspinous and supraspinous ligaments.[133] On the other hand and more recently, McGill[92] has emphasized the need to maintain a *"neutral spine"* or *lordosis* (that mid-range position between extreme flexion and extreme extension as determined by pelvic forward and backward tilt) during the performance of a number of common tasks, which provides more inherent stability (Fig. 8–8). The neutral spine or lordosis concept is defined as a lordotic lumbar spine which typically avoids extreme end-range motion in either flexion or extension, thereby avoiding excessive compressive and shear loads at the discal and facet levels.[87]

Clinical Pearl: The neutral spine or lordosis concept is defined as a lordotic lumbar spine which typically avoids extreme end-range motion in either flexion or extension, thereby avoiding excessive compressive and shear loads at the discal and facet levels when performing essential tasks of daily living.

It is however becoming increasingly clear that the complexity of these joint structures is interdependent and forms a multi-joint complex including two sacroiliac joints, the lumbosacral articulation, symphysis pubis, and hip joints bilaterally. The posteroligamentous and myofascial stabilizing systems are an intricate system of poorly understood tissues whose overall function and role until more recently had eluded researchers for some time. The complicated interaction of these various posterior joint complexes makes this an intriguing clinical dilemma and challenge from both a diagnostic as well as a functional management perspective.

Summary

This section has presented a view that the posterior joint system that includes the facet (z) joints and the sacroiliac joints are part of a functional kinematic chain. This section also emphasized that this system is stabilized by functional properties of the region based upon Panjabi's stability model concept.

ORTHOPEDIC ASSESSMENT—RELIABILITY AND VALIDITY

It is becoming increasingly important in clinical practice to diagnose a health problem appropriate and to treat effectively following best practice and evidence-based guidelines. Low back pain is no different from other health-care problems in this respect. There is an ever-increasing body of evidence concerning treatment strategies for back problems. However, there is a growing realization of the very real difficulties faced by clinicians dealing with low back pain in making an accurate anatomical diagnosis,[1,28,134] together with the growing awareness of the importance of other nonorganic factors in the development of CLB pain and disability which come under the banner of the biopsychosocial model of pain management.[1] This is discussed in detail in other chapters of this textbook.

Only some subgroups of low back pain have a clearly identifiable anatomical or pathological cause, such as fracture or intervertebral disc herniation. In the majority of cases, a specific pathological or anatomical cause of low back pain cannot be accurately identified.[28,135] This has resulted in difficulties in subdividing and classifying "mechanical" or "nonspecific" low back pain, leading to confusion and communication problems among health professionals.[136]

Clinical Pearl: Only some subgroups of low back pain have a clearly identifiable anatomical or pathological cause, such as fracture or intervertebral disc herniation.

The patient's clinical presentation forms the basis of the diagnostic process and subsequent management strategy. The clinical presentation refers to a group of signs and symptoms, or objective data and subjective complaints. In low back pain there is a large overlap and similarity in the clinical presentation between the different subclassifications. The interrelationship of spinal and pelvic kinematics also results in a high proportion of low back pain suffers who have more than one coexisting clinical low back syndrome. The occurrence of multiple clinical syndromes and the similarity of clinical presentation confuse the clinical picture, making the diagnostic process prone to misinterpretation and error.[23,67,137]

Clinical Pearl: The patient's clinical presentation forms the basis of the diagnostic process and subsequent management strategy.

Diagnostic studies, such as plain film radiographs and MRI scans, have been shown to be of limited value in the diagnosis and management of the majority of low back sufferers in the absence of specific clinical indications. They may in fact result in more confusion than assistance because of the high incidence of false-positive findings.[138,139]

The Clinical Examination: Reliability Issues

Clinicians tend to emphasize the importance of the art of clinical examination. However, one should be cautious not to overestimate the reliability of information gained from this important but relatively subjective clinical skill. There are numerous areas for potential error and misinterpretation with most forms of clinical examination procedures.

Numerous authors caution clinicians about overrating the reliability of clinical examinational procedures.[140–142] It is important to remember that general acceptance and usage of an examinational procedure or clinical test does not confer reliability, sensitivity, or specificity.[140] The limitations of clinical examination were analyzed in the Agency for Health Care Policy and Research (AHCPR) guidelines and the values for sensitivity and specificity were reported for various medical history and examinational procedures.

Clinical Pearl: It is important to remember that general acceptance and usage of an examinational procedure or clinical test does not confer reliability, sensitivity, or specificity.

The majority of orthopedic tests are not specific, although they have been designed with specific conditions in mind. Most are prevocational tests relying on the reproduction of the patients' complaint of pain to be classed as positive. Performing them requires stress being placed on a number of anatomical structures rather than just one specific area. For example, orthopedic tests for the sacroiliac joints (Yeoman's and Gaenslen's tests) place stress on the hip joints and lumbar spine as well as the surrounding myofascial tissues, therefore making interpretation potentially prone to misinterpretation, as pain could be elicited from a number of sources.

There is also sometimes confusion and variations in the literature as to how to actually perform certain orthopedic tests. Together with the interpretation and the value of the procedures, even with classical and commonly used clinical tests such as the passive straight-leg raise should raise doubts regarding clinical utility.[141,143]

The difficulty in the interpretation of clinical symptoms, the in-built errors in physical examination procedures and findings, and the lack of a accepted standardized classification system may explain some of the difficulties faced by clinicians in dealing with low back pain and other neuromusculoskeletal problems. These type of problems have led Pedersen[144] to describe the concept of a *functional diagnosis and clinical impression* when dealing with neuromusculoskeletal problems.

Orthopedic Assessment for Posterior Facet Syndrome

Irritation of the lumbar facet joints by electrostimulation and hypertonic saline injections has been shown to produce both spinal and referred lower extremity pain in low back pain suffers and normal volunteers.[24,29,32,76,145] The pain patterns provoked by such stimulation of structures in or around the facet joints at different spinal levels appear to vary greatly between individuals and are not characteristic enough to be of diagnostic value by themselves. However, certain guidelines can be suggested based on the available research. First, the absence of refereed pain should not be regarded as excluding the facet joint as a source of pain. Second, it is reasonable to infer a low lumbar (L3/L4 to L5/S1) origin for pain radiating into the lower extremity. Third, spinal pain felt locally in the midline and paraspinal region is unlikely to be referred from a different spinal level other than that closest to the site of pain, and finally, coccygeal pain is unlikely to be of facet joint origin.

The *symptoms* of a classic facet syndrome are

- Hip and buttock ache pain
- Cramping leg pain primarily above the knee
- Low back stiffness especially in the morning or with inactivity
- Absence of paresthesia
- Transient sharp pains with sudden movement

The *signs* of a classic facet syndrome are

- Local paralumbar tenderness
- Pain on spinal hyperextension
- Absence of neurological deficit
- Absence of nerve root tension signs
- Hip, buttock, or back pain on passive SLR[33,146]

Presently, there are no documented pathognomonic, noninvasive radiological or physical examination findings that allow one to definitively diagnose a posterior facet syndrome.[27] The gold-standard diagnostic procedure for posterior facet syndrome has been the use of facet blocks with varying volumes of local anaesthetic and in some cases cortisone injections (see Chapter 17). Most facet block techniques reported in the literature have involved either periarticular or intra-articular injection of the joints.[35] Results of this form of injection have generally been favorable within the literature, but to date there are very few randomized controlled prospective studies, and false-positive test results have been reported to be as high as 38% with this type of procedure.[76]

Although there are no noninvasive, pathognomonic findings in facet joint-mediated pain, clinicians must approach the formation of a working diagnosis in a rational and systematic fashion. Each clinician relies upon a constellation of findings from patient information and physical examination to form their clinical impression and diagnosis of a patient.

Clinical Pearl: Although there are no noninvasive, pathognomonic findings in facet joint-mediated pain, clinicians must approach the formation of a working diagnosis in a rational and systematic fashion.

In an attempt to establish an objective and more accurate set of diagnostic criteria for the facet syndrome, Helbig and Lee[32] formulated a scorecard system in which clinical features are given points.

Scoring is as follows:

Back pain associated with groin or thigh pain	+30 points
Localized paraspinal tenderness	+20 points
Reproduction of pain with extension–rotation	+30 points
Significant corresponding radiographic changes (i.e., facet asymmetry or DJD)	+20 points
Pain below knee	−10 points

All patients scoring 60 points or more (100 possible points) showed a positive and prolonged response to facet block injections. It was concluded that this scoring system improves diagnostic accuracy and predictability of successful response to facet joint injection. It is possible that such a system of diagnostic parameters may help clinicians in the identification and management of facet syndrome patients.[147] However, further research is needed on the reliability of the facet syndrome diagnostic scorecard as the research has questioned its usefulness.[76]

Neurological Findings Objective physical findings usually implicate no neurological abnormalities; deep tendon reflexes however have been reported in a number of cases to be diminished following isotonic saline inject into the lower lumbar facet joints, which have returned following facet block injections.[29] This reduction in the reflex excitability has been attributed to possible inhibition of the anterior horn cells by noxious stimuli arising from irritated posterior facet joints.[33]

Sensory testing is generally within normal limits, though there may be reports of hypoalgesia or hyperalgesia (or both) in the skin overlying the pain distribution.[35] These sensory changes are subjective rather than objective and may be a reflex phenomenon that is not a true loss of sensation. Muscle weakness may also be present on examination due to pain inhibition rather than true neurological motor deficit. Objective lower extremity neurological findings on examination should exclude the posterior joints as the primary diagnosis in the majority of cases. Any associated bladder and bowel dysfunction requires prompt referral for neurological or surgical evaluation.

Physical Findings

Range of Motion Forward flexion is generally described as being pain-free in patients suffering from facet syndrome, though in some cases patients may show mild restriction with postural deviation toward the side of pain as a result of paraspinal muscle spasm. Hypertonicity of the hamstring muscle may also limit the normal range of forward flexion as might pain due to associated concomitant conditions.[35]

Extension and extension with rotation to the side of discomfort are usually reported to provoke pain due to the approximation of the irritated facet joint articular surfaces.

Biomechanical Intersegmental Assessments (Motion Palpation, Static Palpation) Spinal palpation is an important clinical tool in the assessment and diagnosis of spinal and pelvic pain syndromes.[142] The detection of spinal intersegmental dysfunction and tenderness at the involved spinal level or levels are major prerequisites for the diagnosis of a posterior facet syndrome. However, the clinical evaluation of spinal intersegmental mobility and the palpation of bony landmarks are controversial and have been shown to be of varied reliability. Furthermore, the detection of spinal tenderness has been shown to be more reliable and consistent than assessing segmental mobility.[141,142]

Clinical Pearl: The clinical evaluation of spinal intersegmental mobility and the palpation of bony

landmarks are controversial and have been shown to be of varied reliability.

Although the identification of segmental mobility has been shown to be subjective, because of poor inter-examiner reliability, it forms the most frequently used technique by practitioners of spinal manipulation in the detection of spinal dysfunction. Peterson and Bergmann[90] advocate the use of the "PARTS" acronym in the evaluation of spinal joint dysfunction but warn that physical joint examination procedures depend upon the skill of the examiner and are susceptible to errors in performance and/or interpretation.

Isolation of Motion Segment Dysfunction (PARTS) Goal: To identify and define the specific dysfunction and specific tissues involved

P *Pain* (location, quality, and intensity) or tenderness produced by palpation and pressure over specific structures and soft tissues.

A *Asymmetry* of segmental components identified by static palpation of specific anatomical structures.

R *Range of motion* decreases in or loss of specific movements (active, passive, and accessory) distinguished through motion palpation techniques.

T *Tone, texture, and temperature* changes in specific soft tissues identified through palpation.

S *Special tests* or procedures linked to a technique system.

Palpation of the facet joints should ideally be performed by motion palpation in a weight-bearing (i.e., sitting) position and by static palpation in a non-weight-bearing (i.e., recumbent) position. This allows the examiner to assess the influence of paraspinal muscle hypertonicity on spinal mobility, allowing a better assessment of facet joint dysfunction.[142]

Orthopedic Examinations As previously mentioned there are no documented pathognomonic orthopedic tests for the diagnosis of facet syndrome. There are however a number of physical examination procedures that are useful clinically in helping differentiate and confirm the presence or absence of facet joint irritation as part of a complete physical examination. The reader is directed to the history and physical examination (see Chapter 12) for a more complete summary of examination procedures. However, a brief review of the tests utilized for the topic of this chapter is presented to provide a more complete and contiguous overview.

Kemp's Test The Kemp's maneuver is probably the most commonly described and used test in the differentiation and diagnosis of a lumbar posterior facet syndrome, though it is nonspecific.[148–150] This provocational procedure can be performed with the patient either seated or standing. The seated maneuver is described in Chapter 12, and the standing test is explained below.

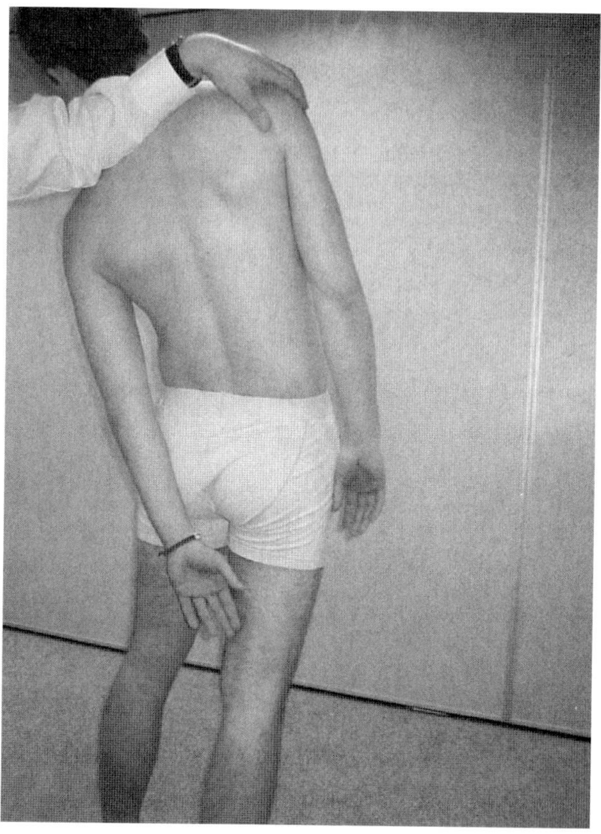

FIGURE 8–9. Standing Kemp's test is a classic orthopedic test, which is designed to compress the facet joints on the side of lateral flexion.

Standing Kemp's Test The examiner instructs the patient to place the back of one hand on the ipsilateral buttock region and then slide the hand down the posterior thigh toward the knee. This produces extension, rotation, and lateral flexion of the lumbar spine and thus compresses the lower lumbar facet joints on the side of lateral flexion. The examiner may place additional stress by pressing downwards on the patient's shoulders, adding axial compression (see Fig. 8–9).

Straight-Leg Raising Test Straight-leg raising (SLR) test, being primarily a nerve root tension test, is almost always normal and negative for nerve root tension signs in posterior facet syndrome. However, due to the fact that it not only stresses the lower lumbar nerve roots but also places a stress on the surrounding structures, it may be limited because of hypertonicity of the ipsilateral hamstrings muscles resulting in posterior thigh and/or buttock discomfort on being stretched.[33,35] The SLR may also be limited by the production of nonradiating low back pain resulting from stretching of the lower lumbar musculoligamentous or facet capsular structures. Finally, it must be stressed that the *SLR should be a passive procedure on the part of the patient*, and that activation of the lumbopelvic stabilizers, either intentionally or unintentionally, compromises the dynamics of the test, rendering it practically useless. To avoid confusion, the clinician may wish to call this test the *passive* SLR.

Sacroiliac Joint Disorders Similar to that of the posterior facet joints, studies using intra-articular injections of noxious stimuli have shown that the sacroiliac joint can be a source of pain. The referral patterns extend over the region of the joint and into the buttock and thigh.[67,151] Pain patterns of patients with sacroiliac joint pain are quite diverse and can even encompass the calf and foot.[21] Known causes of sacroiliac joint pain include spondyloarthropathy, crystal and pyogenic arthropathy, fracture of the sacrum, and diastasis resulting from, among other causes, pregnancy or childbirth. **More controversial is the entity of sacroiliac joint dysfunction syndrome. This term is used to explain pain from a sacroiliac joint that exhibits no demonstrable pathology, but which is presumed to have some form of biomechanical dysfunction that causes pain.[140] To date, no causal connection between an increased or decreased range of motion of the sacroiliac joint and low back pain has ever been identified.[152]**

The classic *symptoms* of a sacroiliac syndrome are

- Aching pain over the back of the sacroiliac joint
- Variable discomfort usually radiating into the buttock, as well as diffusely into the posterior proximal thigh, rarely extending below the knee
- Additional variable discomfort into the groin, anterior pelvis, or anterior proximal thigh
- Absence of paresthesia
- Transient sharp pains on certain movements

Orthopedic Assessment for Sacroiliac Joint Syndrome

As with posterior facet syndromes there are no documented pathognomonic, noninvasive radiological, histological, or physical examination findings that allow one to definitively diagnose a sacroiliac syndrome. There are many tests documented in the manual medicine literature for detecting sacroiliac dysfunction. Unfortunately a large proportion of these tests would appear to be nonspecific and difficult to interpret. The majority of the tests that have been investigated have shown questionable diagnostic reliability.[134,140,153–159]

The clinical *signs* of a classic sacroiliac joint syndrome are

- Local tenderness over the posterior aspect of the sacroiliac joint
- Pain on mechanically stressing the joint
- Pain on forward flexion
- Hamstring tightness
- Absence of neurological deficit
- Absence of nerve root tension signs
- Aberrant sacroiliac movement pattern
- Hyperesthesia over the ipsilateral buttock extending into the posterolateral thigh[66]

More controversial is the entity of sacroiliac joint dysfunction syndrome. This term is used to explain pain from a sacroiliac joint that exhibits no demonstrable pathology, but which is presumed to have some form of biomechanical dysfunction that causes pain.[140] To date though no causal connection between an increased or decreased range of motion of the sacroiliac joint and low back pain has ever been identified.[152]

Motion Palpation

As with posterior facet syndrome, motion palpation procedures are generally considered an important form of assessment of sacroiliac joint function. The use of palpation to detect small variations of movement however is subjective. It has poor inter-examiner reliability and low specificity.[152] A system of sacroiliac motion analysis that is commonly used in manual therapy to assess such function is known as the Gillet test.[153] Lewit and Alies[159] however pointed out a number of limitations with these procedures and a number of other studies have shown poor reliability in the assessment of sacroiliac motion using these procedures.[134,140,155]

The most reliable indicators for sacroiliac dysfunction would appear to be a history of pain over the sacroiliac joint combined with tenderness over and around the joint on palpation.[134] With regards to prevocational sacroiliac stress tests, Laslett and Williams[152] found the Sacroiliac Posterior Shear or "Thigh Thrust" test to have the highest level of interexaminer reliability when compared to six others. This type of test has also been shown to have a good level of sensitivity and specificity.[160]

Positive sacroiliac stress tests are significant only when the clinical history and other physical findings rule out other causes of low back pain and support the diagnosis of sacroiliac involvement. Localized pain over the sacroiliac joint combined with three or more sacroiliac stress tests giving positive findings will allow an examiner to make the diagnosis of sacroiliac joint syndrome with more confidence.[23]

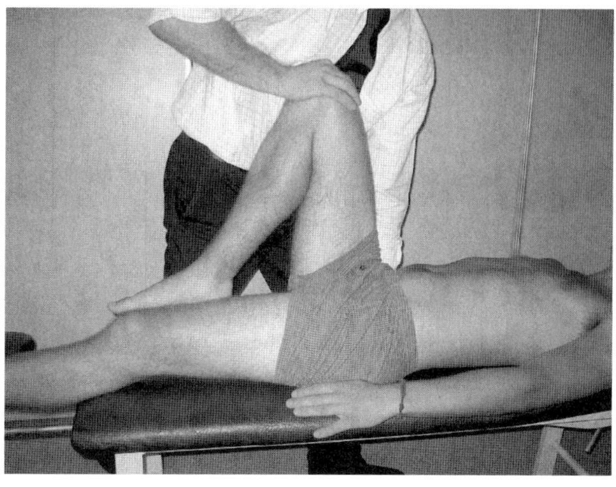

FIGURE 8–10. The Posterior Shear test applies a posterior shearing stress to the sacroiliac joint and ligaments by applying axial compression through the femur. This test is believed to stress not only the sacroiliac joint and associated ligaments, but also the hip joint.

Posterior Shear ("Thigh Thrust") Test The patient lies supine and the examiner stands at the painful side. The hip is flexed to 90 degrees and the knee is flexed. The examiner applies a posterior shearing stress to the sacroiliac joint and ligaments by applying axial compression through the femur. This test stresses not only the sacroiliac joint and associated ligaments, but also the hip joint. Excessive adduction of the hip should be avoided since flexion and adduction combined is normally uncomfortable. Some authors believe that this test in particular puts strain on the iliolumbar ligament and that if the thigh is maximally flexed and adducted toward the opposite shoulder, axial pressure falls on the posterior sacroiliac ligaments. If the thigh is pushed toward the same shoulder, axial pressure is believed to tense the sacrotuberous ligament (see Fig. 8–10).[161]

Straight-Leg Raise and Double Leg Raise Tests The examiner performs a passive single straight-leg raise and nonradiating localized low back pain is provoked. The examiner notes the angle at which pain is produced. The examiner then passively raises both legs simultaneously and again notes the angle at which pain is provoked.

If the angle at which the pain is felt is higher on the double straight-leg raise than on the single, the lesion is assumed to be more likely due to sacroiliac involvement.

The rationale behind this provocative test is that on performing a single passive straight-leg raise the order of joint movement is generally accepted to be hip movement first followed by the sacroiliac joint and then the lumbosacral junction. However, when both legs are raised simultaneously the sequence of joint movement is assumed to change to the hip joints followed by the lumbosacral junction and then the sacroiliac joints, since on performing the double straight-leg raise there is minimal torque produced between the innominate bones.

It must be emphasized that this is a passive test on the part of the patient, and that the examiner must lift the entire weight of the lower extremities. Otherwise, the patient would necessarily brace the lumbopelvic region to lift the legs, compromising the isolation of the various pain-generating tissues and rendering the test invalid.

Goldthwaite's Test With the patient supine the examiner places their cephalic hand under the patient at the lumbosacral junction while performing a passive straight-leg raise with the caudal hand. If low back pain is elicited before movement is felt by the cephalic at the lumbosacral junction, a sacroiliac or hip problem is suspected. If pain is produced as the lumbosacral junction starts to move then a lumbosacral lesion is suspected.

Adam's and Supported Adam's Tests Adam's test is active forward flexion of the lumbar spine by the patient in the standing position. If this action provokes nonradiating low back pain, the source may be either the lumbar spine or the sacroiliac joints. To differentiate these options, the examiner performs the Supported Adam's test where the patient stands with their back to the examiner who stabilizes the sacroiliac joints by firmly contacting the patient's sacrum with the examiner's lateral thigh while holding the patient firmly round the anterior aspect of the pelvis. The patient is instructed to flex forward again. Of course, overall flexion should be subsequently reduced as movement at the sacroiliac joints and hips is now restricted. If this reduction of movement at the sacroiliac joints reduces the level of pain on forward flexion, a sacroiliac joint lesion is suspected. If the pain is not reduced, or perhaps even increases with this maneuver, then the suspected pain generator would be the lumbar or lumbosacral spine.

Yeoman's Test The patient is prone. With one hand, the examiner stabilizes the effected sacroiliac joint. With the other hand the examiner flexes the ipsilateral knee to 90 degrees. The examiner then hyperextends (generally beyond 10 degree) the ipsilateral thigh, lifting it off the examination table. Pressure is maintained over the affected sacroiliac joint. The reproduction of local sacroiliac pain may indicate sacroiliac irritation. The examiner should be aware that this procedure would also produce some extension and therefore compression of the lumbosacral junction facet joints and also the ipsilateral hip, and so pain from these sources must be ruled out. The clinician can also contact the lateral ala of the sacrum, just medial to the sacroiliac joint in order to allow for sacroiliac shearing as the thigh is extended. Moreover, there is a wide variation in the way these tests are described in the literature, which describes no pressure placed over the target joint to pressure just placed over the sacroiliac joint or the method described above. This does create some confusion but reinforces the fact that orthopedic tests should not be used in isolation in formulating a diagnosis as a result of the variation in methodology and performance.

Nachlas' Test The patient is prone. The examiner exerts pressure with the cephalic hand over the pelvis to prevent hip flexion and then passively flexes the involved side knee to the point where pain is felt or resistance is met. This procedure stretches the quadriceps and may produce a stretching sensation in the front of the thigh. It also stresses the ipsilateral sacroiliac joint and may therefore provoke localized sacroiliac pain if the joint is irritated. The test is also used as a nerve tension test, as it stretches the femoral nerve and upper lumbar nerve roots (L1–L4); therefore these sources must be ruled out.

Hibbs' Test The patient is prone. The examiner stabilizes the unaffected side of the pelvis with one hand. With the other hand, the examiner grasps the ankle of the affected leg and flexes the knee to 90 degrees, without elevating the thigh from the examination table. The examiner then slowly pushes the flexed lower leg laterally, causing internal rotation of the affected femoral head. The reproduction of local sacroiliac pain may indicate irritation of the joint. Of course, this procedure also stresses the ipsilateral hip joint and surrounding musculature; therefore pain from these sources must also be ruled out.

Gaenslen's Test The patient is supine on the examination table, with the side of complaint close to the edge of the table. The examiner instructs the patient to flex the knee of the nontest side to the chest maximally and hold the knee against the chest. The other leg is extended at the hip by having the patient hanging the leg over the side of the examination table. The examiner then applies a downward pressure over both of the knees. This procedure stresses both sacroiliac joints, especially on the side of the hip extension, and may produce pain over the sacroiliac joint if irritated. This test also stresses the hip joints and the psoas muscle on the side of hip extension, which are possible pain sources.

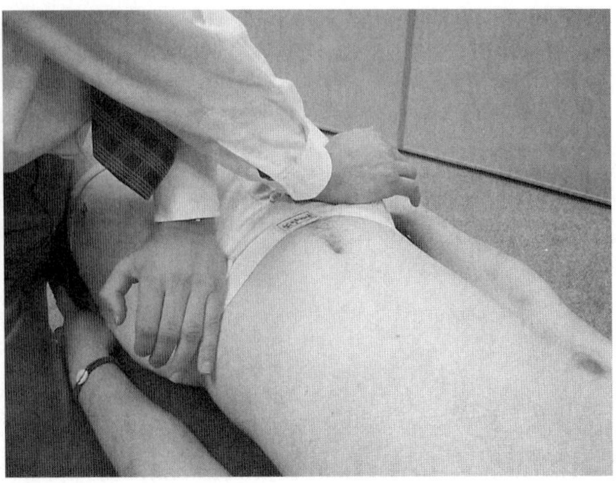

FIGURE 8–11. Sacroiliac Gapping test is designed to stress the anterior ligaments of the sacroiliac joints bilaterally.

Gapping (Sacroiliac Stretch) Test The patient lays supine on the examination table, with the legs together. The hips are neutral and knees are extended. With crossed arms in a scissor-like manner, the examiner place both hands on the opposite anterior superior iliac spines of each ileum. A downward and lateral pressure is applied to both ilia. This test stresses the anterior ligaments of the sacroiliac joints bilaterally and may reproduce sacroiliac pain in the case of strained anterior ligaments and/or sacroiliac joint inflammation (see Fig. 8–11).

Sacroiliac Squish Test The patient is supine on the examination table, with the legs together. The hips are neutral and knees are extended. The examiner takes a bilateral contact over the lateral aspect of both anterior superior iliac spines and applies a lateral to medial pressure in an anterior to posterior direction. This procedure stresses the posterior sacroiliac ligaments. Pain in the sacroiliac, buttock, or thigh region may indicate a sprain of these ligaments (see Fig. 8–12).

Patrick's FABERE Test This test is traditionally used as a hip stress test, but, as previously mentioned, due to the fact that most prevocational orthopedic tests stress more that one structure, can also be used to assess the sacroiliac joints. The patient is supine on the examination table, with the legs slightly apart. The hips are neutral and knees are extended. The examiner abducts and externally rotates the target leg, then flexes that knee, and places the ankle across the lower thigh of the opposite leg. The target knee is then lowered toward the examination table, effectively extending the target thigh. This procedure places stress on the ipsilateral hip and joint capsule together with the hip flexor musculature and sacroiliac joint. Pain in the anterolateral

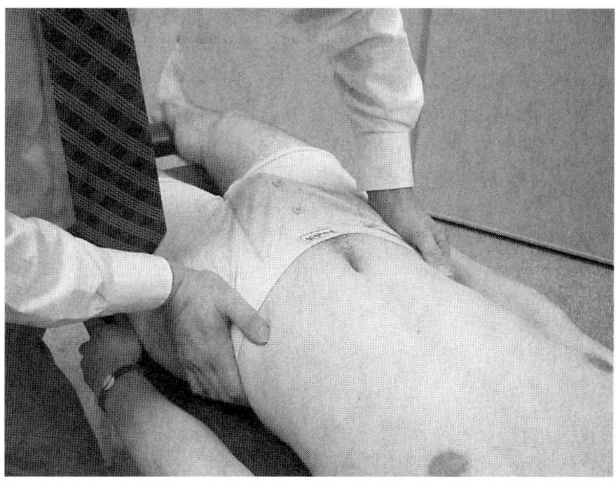

FIGURE 8–12. The Sacroiliac Squish test is designed to stress the posterior sacroiliac ligaments. Pain in the sacroiliac, buttock, or thigh region may indicate a sprain of these ligaments.

aspect of the hip may indicate a hip pathology. Pain around the sacroiliac and/or gluteal region may be the result of sacroiliac joint irritation or pathology (see Fig. 8–4).

Summary

This section has presented a detailed account of the clinical orthopedic evaluation of posterior joint syndromes. There are a number of views concerning the reliability and validity of various procedures utilized in the clinical appreciation of this region, which indeed require further investigation. Current methods though questionable still follow the basis of best practice and appropriate clinical interpretation.

RECENT DEVELOPMENTS IN OBJECTIVE CONFIRMATION

The present reliance on subjective clinical assessment for confirming a diagnosis as being either sacroiliac or posterior joint syndrome is unsatisfactory, as most clinicians would agree. A number of quantifiable modalities have been embraced in respect of clarifying this diagnostic dilemma; these include computerized tomography (CT) with or without myelography, selective sacroiliac or facet blocks (see Chapter 17), magnetic resonance imaging (MRI) (see Chapter 16), surface electromyography (sEMG) (see Chapter 17), and noncontact infrared telethermometry or thermography (IRT) (see Chapter 18). Only the last two modalities are noninvasive and free from potential adverse reactions.[162–165] Additionally, there is no guarantee that the specified muscle is the source of the signal when using sEMG in the lumbosacral region. Although CT combined with myelography and MRI are used for assessing lumbar disc herniations, they cannot regularly provide images when patients are standing or walking. New technologies are emerging, however, and multipositional (spinal extension, neutral, and flexion) standing MRI machines are rapidly becoming available in the United States (see Chapter 16). To date, reliable normative studies regarding multipositional standing MRI are not yet available. Ido et al.[166] used upright lateral myelography as a measure against upright CT with myelography and concluded that the upright position seemed to be the most reliable method for assessing patients with lumbar disc herniations, especially those at the L4–L5 level, whose neurological symptoms developed during standing or walking.

IRT is another diagnostic option with the enviable benefit of being noninvasive. Based on the scientific evidence to date, IRT is not recommended for clinical use, as it is still considered experimental owing to high sensitivity but poor specificity. Nevertheless, IRT continues to be a tempting topic. Recent and ongoing research by two of the authors provide hope that IRT will one day hold a greater degree of diagnostic reliability.

SUMMARY/CONCLUSIONS

1. This chapter has attempted to portray the posterior joint complex as an integrated and complicated neurobiomechanical unit that is functionally well designed, providing key aspects of dynamic lumbopelvic stability under physiological circumstances.
2. There is clear evidence that the zygapophyseal joints and the sacroiliac joints are capable of producing mechanical nociceptive pain that typically presents as a variety of clinical syndromes.
3. The posterior joint syndromes may be typically distinctive in their clinical presentation consisting of generalized nonspecific diffuse dull pain with various patterns of referred pain above the knee into the buttock, groin, and anterior and posterior thigh regions without any hard neurological signs or any other functional deficit.
4. It is the authors' opinion that pain can be generated from a number of anatomical locations, which may explain the varied patterns seen clinically.
5. Methods utilized in differentiating the various pain generators were discussed, allowing the clinician to be better able to localize the pain generator or generators. The increasing knowledge of these structures and their integrated function allows clinicians to establish a reasonably accurate diagnosis, generating a sensible and definite management plan. Often, multimodal treatment strategies become necessary in difficult cases, which are addressed in later chapters.

The concept of functional stability has provided clinicians with greater understanding of back pain from an evidence-based perspective. This approach also assists clinicians in developing meaningful prevention strategies for patient populations disabled by various low back syndromes, as will be also discussed in later chapters.

REFERENCES

1. Waddell G. The problem. In: Waddell G, ed. *The back pain revolution.* London: Churchill Livingstone, 1998:1–8.
2. Waddell G. Prevalence of low back pain. *Eur J Chiropractic* 2002;49:28–32.
3. Kelsey JL. Idiopathic low back pain: Magnitude of the problem. In: White AA, Gordon SL, eds. *American Academy of Orthopaedic Surgeons symposium on low back pain.* Toronto: CV Mosby, 1982:5–8.
4. Cassidy JD, Wedge JH. The epidemiology and natural history of low back pain and spinal degeneration. In: Kirkaldy-Willis WH, ed. *Managing low back pain*, 2nd ed. London: Churchill Livingstone, 1988:3–14.
5. Waddell G. Simple low-back pain: Rest or active exercise? *Ann Rheum Dis* 1993;52:317–319.
6. Spengler DM, Bigos SJ, Martin NA, et al. Back injuries in industry: A retrospective study. Part 1. Overview and cost analysis. *Spine* 1986;11:241–245.
7. Waddell G, Aylward M. Low back pain, disability and social security benefits: A literature review and analysis. Department of Social Security Research Report. London: Department of Social Security, 2001.
8. Waddell G. A new clinical model for the treatment of low-back pain. *Spine* 1987;12:632–644.
9. Troup J.D.G. and Videman T. Inactivity and the aetiopathogenesis of musculoskeletal disorders. *Clin Biomech* 1989;4:173–178.
10. Acker PD, Thiel HW, Kirkaldy-Willis WH. Low back pain: Pathogenesis, diagnosis and management. *Am J Chiropractic Med* 1990;3:19–24.
11. Kirkaldy-Willis WH, Wedge JH, Yong-Hing K, et al. Pathology and pathogenesis of lumbar spondylosis and stenosis. *Spine* 1978;3:319–328.
12. Rosen M, Breen A, et al. Management guidelines for back pain [Appendix B]. In: Report of a Clinical Standards Advisory Group Committee on Back Pain. London, England: Her Majesty's Stationary Office (HMSO), 1994.
13. Bigos S, Bowyer O, Braen G, et al. Acute low back pain problems in adults. Clinical Practice Guidelines No. 14. Rockville MD: Agency for Health Care Policy and Research, Public Health Service, US Department of Health and Human Services, 1994.
14. Royal College of General Practitioners [RCGP]. *Clinical guidelines for the management of acute low back pain.* London: RCGP, 1996.
15. Manniche C, Gam A. Low back pain: Frequency, management and prevention from an HAD perspective. *Danish Health Technol Assess* 1999;1(1).
16. Waddell G, Burton AK. *Occupational health guidelines for the management of low back pain at work—Evidence review.* London: Faculty of Occupational Medicine, 2000.
17. Vernon H. Chiropractic: A model of incorporating the illness behaviour model in the management of low back pain patients. *J Manipulative Physiol Ther* 1991;14:379–389.
18. Liebenson CS. Pathogenesis of chronic back pain. *J Manipulative Physiol Ther* 1992;15(5):299–308.
19. Waddell G. Modern management of spinal disorders. *J Manipulative Physiol Ther* 1995;18:590–596.
20. Bogduk N. The anatomical basis for spinal pain syndromes. *J Manipulative Physiol Ther November* 1995;18(9):603–605.
21. Schwarzer AC, Aprill CN, Bogduk N. The sacroiliac joint in chronic low back pain. *Spine* 1995;20: 31–37.
22. Maigne JY, Aivaliklis A, Pfefer F. Results of sacroiliac joint double block and value of sacroiliac pain provocation tests in 54 patients with low back pain. 9 *Spine* 1996;21:1889–1892.
23. Quon JA, Bernard TN Jr, Burton CV, Kirkaldy-Willis WH. The site and nature of the lesion. In: Kirkaldy-Willis WH, Bernard TN Jr, eds. *Managing low back pain*, 4th ed. London: Churchill Livingstone, 1999:122–152.
24. Hourigan CL, Bassett JM. Facet syndrome: Clinical signs, symptoms, diagnosis and treatment. *J Manipulative Physiol Ther* 1989;12(4):293–297.
25. Newton W, Curtis P, Witt P, Hobler K. Prevalence of subtypes of low back pain in a defined population. *J Fam Pract* 1997;45:331–335.
26. Schwarzer AC, Aprill CN, Bogbuk N. The sacroiliac joint in chronic low back pain. *Spine* 1994;20: 31–37.
27. Dreyfuss PH, Dreyer SJ, Herring SA. Contemporary concepts in spine care: Lumbar zygapophyseal (facet) joint injections. *Spine* 1995;20(18):2040–2047.
28. Dudler J, Balague F. What is the rational diagnostic approach to spinal disorders? *Best Pract Res Clin Rheumatol* 2002;16:43–57.
29. Mooney V, Robertson J. The facet syndrome. *Clin Orthop Relat Res* 1976;115:149–156.
30. Ghormley RK. Low back pain with special reference to the articular facets with presentation of an operative procedure. *J Am Med Assoc* 1933;C1:1773–1777.
31. Bogduk N. The zygapophysial joints. In: *Clinical anatomy of the lumbar spine and sacrum.* London: Churchill Livingstone, 1997:33–41.
32. Helbig T, Lee C. The lumbar facet syndrome. *1988; Spine* 13:61–64.
33. Lippitt AB. The facet joint and its role in spine pain. *Spine* 1984;9(7):746–750.
34. El-Khoury GY, Renfrew DL. Percutaneous procedures for the diagnosis and treatment of lower back pain: Diskography, facet-joint injection, and epidural injection. *Am J Roentgenol* 1991;157:685–691.
35. Jackson RP. The facet syndrome. Myth or reality? *Clin Orthop* 1992;279:110–121.
36. Revel ME, Listrat VM, Chevalier XJ, et al. Facet joint block for low back pain: Identifying predictors

of a good response. *Arch Phys Med Rehabil* 1992; 73:824–828.
37. Schwarzer AC, Aprill CN, Derby R, Fortin J, Kine G, Bogduk N. Clinical features of patients with pain stemming from the lumbar zygapophysial points. Is the lumbar facet syndrome a clinical entity? *Spine* 1994;19:1132–1137.
38. Revel M, Poiraudeau S, Auledley GR, et al. Capacity of the clinical picture to characterize low back pain relieved by facet joint anesthesia. Proposed criteria to identify patients with painful facet joints. *Spine* 1999;23:1972–1976.
39. Sakamoto N, Yamashita T, Takebayashi T, Sekine M, Ishii S. An electrophysiologic study of mechanreceptors in the sacroiliac joint and adjacent tissues. *Spine* 2001;26(20):E468–E471.
40. Dreyer JD, Dreyfuss PH. Low back pain and the zygapophysial (facet) joints. *Arch Phys Med Rehabil* 1996;77:290–300.
41. Bogduk N, Wilson AS, Tynan W. The human lumbar dorsal rami. *J Anat* 1982;134(2):383–397.
42. Bogduk N, Long DM. Percutaneous lumbar medial branch neurotomy: A modification of facet denervation. *Spine* 1980:5(2):193–200.
43. Bogduk N. Nerves of the lumbar spine. In: *Clinical anatomy of the lumbar spine and sacrum*. London: Churchill Livingstone, 1997:127–143.
44. McLain RF, Pickar JG. Mechanoreceptor endings in human thoracic and lumbar facets joints. *Spine* 1998;23(2):168–173.
45. Vandenabeele F, Creemers J, Lambrichts I, Robberechts W. Fine structure of vesiculated nerve profiles in the human lumbar facet joint. *J Anat* 1995;187:681–692.
46. Dreyfuss P, Tibiletti C, Dreyer SJ. Thoracic zygapophyseal joint pain patterns. A study in normal volunteers. *Spine* 1994;19:807–811.
47. Bucknill AT, Coward K, Plumpton C, et al. Nerve fibers in lumbar spine structures and injured spinal roots express the sensory neuron-specific sodium channels SNS/PN3 and NaN/SNS2 *Spine* January 15, 2002;27(2):135–140.
48. Vandenabeele F, Creemers J, Lambrichts I, Lippins P, Jans M. Encapsulated Ruffini-like endings in human lumbar facet joints. *J Anat* 1997;191:571–583.
49. Ashton IK, Ashton BA, Gibson SJ, Polak JM, Jaffray DC, Eisenstein SM. Morphological basis for back pain: The demonstration of nerve fibers and neuropeptides in the lumbar facet joint capsule but not in ligamentum flavum. *J Orthop Res* 1992;10:72–78.
50. Grifka J, Witte H, Schulze H, Heers G, Bohlen J, Recknagel S. The lumbar ligamentum flavum. Anatomic characteristics with reference to microdiscotomy [in German]. *Z Orthopedische Grenzgeb*. July–August 1997;135(4):328–334.
51. Viejo-Fuertes D, Liguoro D, Rivel J, Midy D, Guerin J. Morphologic and histologic study of the ligamentum flavum in the thoraco-lumbar region. *Surg Radiol Anat* 1998;20(3):171–176.
52. Holzer P, Guth PH. Neuropeptide control of rat gastric mucosal blood flow: Increase by calcitonin gene-related peptide and vasoactive intestinal polypeptide, but not substance P and neurokinin A. *Circ Res* 1991;68:100–105.
53. Buckley TL, Brain SD, Rampart M, Williams TJ: Time-dependent synergistic interactions between the vasodilator neuropeptide, calcitonin gene-related peptide (CGRP) and mediators of inflammation. *Br J Pharmacol* 1991;103:1515–1519.
54. Holzer P. Capsaicin: Cellular targets, mechanisms of action and selectivity for thin sensory neurons. *Pharmacol Rev* 1991;43:143–201.
55. Sung C-P, Arleth AJ, Aiyar N, Bhatnagar PG, Lysko PG, Feuerstein G. CGRP stimulates the adhesion of leukocytes to vascular endothelial cells. *Peptides* 1992;13:429–434.
56. Freemont AJ, Watkins A, Le Maitre C, et al. Nerve growth factor expression and innervation of the painful intervertebral disc. *J Pathol* July 2002;197(3): 286–292.
57. Giles LGF, Harvey AR. Immunohistochemical demonstration of nociceptors in the capsule and synovial folds of human zygapophysial joints. *Br J Rheumatol* 1987;26:362–364.
58. Gronblad M, Korkala O, Konttinen YT, et al. Silver impregnation and immunohistochemical study of nerves in lumbar facet joint plical tissue. *Spine* 1991; 16(1):34–38.
59. Beaman DN, Graziano GP, Glover RA, Wojtys EM, Chang V. Substance P innervation of lumbar spine facet joints. *Spine* 1993;18(8):1044–1049.
60. Daum WJ. The sacroiliac joint: An underappreciated pain generator. *Am J Orthop* 1995:24:475–478.
61. Solonen KA. The sacroiliac joint in the light of anatomical, roentgenological and clinical studies. *Acta Orthop Scand* 1957;27(Suppl):1–127.
62. Nakagawa T. A study on the distribution of nerve filaments over the iliosacral joint and its adjacent region. *J Jpn Orthop Assoc* 1966;40:419–430.
63. Ikeda R. Innervation of the sacroiliac joint. Macroscopical and histological studies. *Nippon Ika Daigaku Zasshi* 1991;58:587–596.
64. Horwitz MT. The anatomy of (a) the lumbosacral nerve plexus—its relation to variations of vertebral segmentation, and (b) the posterior sacral plexus. *Anat Rec* 1939;74:91–107.
65. Grob KR, Neuhuber WL, Kissling RO. Innervation of the sacroiliac joint of the human. *Z Rheumatolgische* 1995;54:117–122.
66. Fortin JD, Kissling RO, O'Connor BL, Vilensky JA. Sacroiliac joint innervation and pain. *Am J Orthop* 1999;28:687–690.
67. Fortin DF, Dwyer A, West S, Pier J. Sacroiliac joint: Pain referral maps upon applying a new injection/arthrography technique. Part 1. Asymptomatic volunteers. *Spine* 1994;19(13):1475–1482.
68. Pool-Goudzwaard AL, Vleeming A, Stoeckart R, Snijders CJ, Mens JMA. Insufficient lumbopelvic stability: A clinical, anatomical and biomechanical approach to "a-specific" low back pain. *Manual Ther* 1998;3:12–20.
69. Kirkaldy-Willis WH. The site and nature of the lesion. In: Kirkaldy-Willis WH, ed. *Managing low back pain*, 2nd ed. London: Churchill Livingstone, 1988:133–154.

70. Chapman-Smith D. Sacroiliac dysfunction. *Chiropractic Rep* 1990;5:1–6.
71. Bernard TN, Cassidy JD. The sacroiliac syndrome: Pathophysiology, diagnosis, and management. In: Frymoyer JW, ed. The adult spine: Principles and practice. New York: Raven Press, 1991:2107–2130.
72. Cassidy JD. The pathoanatomy and clinical significance of the sacroiliac joints. *J Manipulative Physiol Ther* 1992;15:41–42.
73. Chapman-Smith D. The sacroiliac joints revisited. *Chiropractic Rep* 1993;7:1–6.
74. Bowen V, Cassidy JD. Macroscopic and microscopic anatomy of the sacroiliac joint from embryonic life until the eighth decade. *Spine* 1981;6:620–628.
75. Vleeming A, Stoeckart R, Volkers ACW, et al. Relation between form and function in the sacroiliac joint. Part 1. Clinical anatomical aspects. *Spine* 1990; 15:130–132.
76. Schwarzer AC, Derby R, Aprill CN, Fortin J, Kine G, Boguk N. Pain from the lumbar zygapophysial joints: A test of two models. *J Spinal Disord* 1994;7:331–336.
77. McGregor M, Cassidy JD. Post-surgical sacroiliac syndrome. *J Manipulative Physiol Ther* 1983;6: 1–11.
78. Cassidy JD, Mierau DR. Pathophysiology of the sacroiliac joint. In: *Principles and practice of chiropractic*, 2nd ed. California: Appleton and Lange, 1992:211–224.
79. Illi F. The vertebral column: Lifetime of the body. Chicago: National College of Chiropractic, 1951.
80. Byfield D. Pelvic/sacroiliac manipulative skills. In: Byfield D, ed. *Chiropractic manipulative skills*, 1st ed. Oxford: Butterworth-Heinemann, 1996:129–146.
81. Peterson DH, Bergmann TF. Principles of adjustive technique. In: Peterson DH, Bergmann TF, eds. *Chiropractic technique*, 2nd ed. London: Mosby, 2002:97–174.
82. Byfield D. Basic lumbopelvic palpation and landmark identification skills. In: Byfield D, Kinsinger S, eds. *A manual therapist's guide to surface anatomy and palpation skills*. Oxford: Butterworth-Heineman, 2002:45–72.
83. Sturesson B, Selvik G, Uden A. Movements of the sacroiliac joints: A roentgen stereophotogrammetric analysis. *Spine* 1989;14:162–165.
84. leeming A, Van Wingerden JP, Dijkstra PF, et al. Mobility in the sacroiliac joints in the elderly: A kinematic and radiological study. *Clin Biomech* 1992;7:170–176.
85. Brunner C, Kissling R, Jacob HAC. The effects of morphology and histopathologic findings on the mobility of the sacroiliac joint. *Spine* 1991;16: 1111–1117.
86. Panjabi MM. The stabilizing system of the spine. Part 1. Function, dysfunction, adaptation and enhancement. Part 2. Neutral zone and instability hypothesis. *J Spinal Disord* 1992;5:383–397.
87. McGill SM. Low back exercises: Evidence for improving exercise regimens. *Phys Ther* 1998,78:754–765.
88. DonTigny RL. Function and pathomechanics of the sacroiliac joint. A review. *Phys Ther* 1985;65:35–44.
89. Harrison DE, Harrison DD, Troyanovich SJ. The sacroiliac joint: A review of the anatomy and biomechanics with clinical implications. *J Manipulative Physiol Ther* 1997;20:607–617.
90. Peterson DH, Bergmann TF. The spine: Anatomy, biomechanics, assessment, and adjustive techniques. In: Peterson DH, Bergmann TF, eds. *Chiropractic technique*, 2nd ed. London: Mosby, 2002:175–339.
91. Byfield D. Spinal rehabilitation and stabilization for the geriatric with back pain. In: Gleberzon BJ, ed. *Chiropractic care of the older patient*, Oxford: Butterworth-Heinemann, 2001:407–440.
92. McGill S. *Low back disorders: Evidence-based prevention and rehabilitation*. Canada: Human Kinetics, 2002:45–136.
93. Jull GA, Richardson CA. Motor control problems in patients with spinal pain: A new direction for therapeutic exercise. *J Manipulative Physiol Ther* 2000;23:115–117.
94. Vleeming A, Stoeckart R, Snijders CJ. The sacrotuberous ligament: A conceptual approach to its dynamic role in stabilizing the sacroiliac joint. *Clin Biomech* 1989;4:201–203.
95. Richardson CA, Snijders CJ, Hides JA, Damen L, Pas MS, Storm J. The relation between the transversus abdominis muscles, sacroiliac joint mechanics, and low back pain. *Spine* 2002;27:399–405.
96. Vleeming A, Pool-Goudzwaard AL, Hammudoghlu D, Stoeckart R, Snijders CJ, Mens JMA. The function of the long dorsal sacroiliac ligament. Its implication for understanding low back pain. *Spine* 1996;21:556–562.
97. Vleeming A, Pool-Goodzwaard AL, Stoeckart R, van Wingerden J-P, Snijders CJ. The posterior layer of the thoracolumbar fascia. Its function in load transfer from spine to legs. *Spine* 1995;20:753–758.
98. Sturesson B, Uden G, Uden A. Pain pattern in pregnancy and "catching" of the leg in pregnant women with posterior pelvic pain. *Spine* 1997;22:1880–1884.
99. Cibulka MT, Sinacore DR, Cromer GS, Delitto A. Unilateral hip rotation range of motion asymmetry in patients with sacroiliac joint regional pain. *Spine* 1998;23:1009–1101.
100. Hides JA, Richardson CA, Jull GA. Multifidus recovery is not automatic after resolution of acute, first-episode low back pain. *Spine* 1996;21:2763–2769.
101. Hides JA, Jull GA, Richardson CA. Long-term effects of specific stabilising exercises for first-episode low back pain. *Spine* 2001;26:E243–E248.
102. Damen L, Buyruk HM, Guler-Uysal F, Lotgering FK, Snijders CJ, Stam HJ. The prognostic value of asymmetric laxity of the sacroiliac joints in pregnancy-related pelvic pain. *Spine*, 2002;27:2820–2824.
103. Damen L, Stijnen T, Roebroeck ME, Snijders CJ, Stam HJ. Reliability of sacroiliac joint laxity measurement with Doppler imaging of vibrations. *Ultrasound Med Biol*, 2002;28:407–414.
104. Damen L, Spoor C, Snijders CJ, Stam HJ. Does a pelvic belt influence sacroiliac joint laxity? *Clin Biomech* 2002;17:495–498.

105. Schneider MJ. Soft tissue effects of sacroiliac and lumbosacral joint manipulation. *Chiropractic Tech* 1992;4:136–142.
106. Tullberg T, Blomberg S, Branth B, Johnsson R. Manipulation does not alter the position of the sacroiliac joint. A roentgen stereophotogrammetric analysis. *Spine* 1998;10:1124–1129.
107. Van Dieen JH, Hoosemans MJM, Toussaint HM. Stoop or squat: A review of biomechanical studies on lifting technique. *Clin Biomech* 1999;14:685–696.
108. Snijders CJ, Vleeming A, Stoeckart R. Transfer of lumbosacral load to iliac bones and legs. *Clin Biomech* 1993;8:285–301.
109. McGill S. Normal and injury mechanics of the lumbar spine. In: McGill S, ed. *Low back disorders: Evidence-based prevention and rehabilitation*. Canada: Human Kinetics, 2002:87–136.
110. Seaman DR, Cleveland C. Spinal pain syndromes: Nociceptive, neuropathic, and psychologic mechanisms. *J Manipulative Physiol Ther* 1999;22:458–472.
111. Kondracki M. Some biomechanical considerations in manipulative skills training. In: Byfield D, ed. Chiropractic manipulative skills. Oxford: Butterworth-Heinemann, 1996:22–31.
112. Yamamoto I, Panjabi MM, Crisco T, et al. Three-dimensional movements of the whole lumbar spine and lumbosacral joint. *Spine* 1989;14:1256–1260.
113. Dolan P, Adams M. Influence of lumbar and hip mobility on the bending stresses acting on the lumbar spine. *Clin Biomech* 1993,8:185–192.
114. Cassidy JD, Mierau DR. Pathophysiology of the sacroiliac joint. In: Haldeman S, ed. *Principles and practice of chiropractic*, 2nd ed. California: Appleton and Lange, 1992:211–224.
115. Mierau DR, Cassidy JD, Hamin T, et al. Sacroiliac joint dysfunction and low back pain in school aged children. *J Manipulative Physiol Ther* 1984,7:81–84.
116. Berg G, Hammer M, Moller-Nielsen J, et al. Low back pain during pregnancy. *Obstet Gynecol* 1988;71: 71–75.
117. Bogduk N. *Clinical anatomy of the lumbar spine and sacrum*, 3rd ed. London: Churchill Livingstone, 1997: 81–100.
118. Adams MA, Bogduk N, Burton K, Dolan P. Mechanical function of the lumbar spine. In: *The biomechanics of back pain*. London: Churchill Livingstone, 2002:131–158.
119. Adams MA. Biomechanics of low back pain. *Pain Rev* 1996;3:15–30.
120. Farfan HF, Cossette JW, Robertson GH, et al. The effects of torsion in the lumbar intervertebral joints: The role of torsion in the production of disc degeneration. *J Bone Joint Surg* 1970;52:468–497.
121. Farfan HF. Torsion and compression. In: *Mechanical disorders of the lumbar spine*. Philadelphia: Lea & Febiger, 1973:74–92.
122. Cassidy JD, Thiel HW, Kirkaldy-Willis WH. Side posture manipulation for lumbar intervertebral disc herniation. *J Manipulative Physiol Ther* 1993;16:96–103.
123. Dickson RA, Butt WP. Minisymposium: Surgery for back pain. (i) Clinical/radiological evaluation Part 1. *Curr Orthop* 1992;6:3–11.
124. Boos N, Rieder R, Schade V, Spratt KF, Semmer N, Aebi M. 1995 Volvo Award in clinical sciences. The diagnostic accuracy of magnetic resonance imaging, work perception, and psychosocial factors in identifying symptomatic disc herniations. *Spine* 1995; 20:2613–2625.
125. Haldeman S, Rubenstein SM. Cauda equina syndrome in patients undergoing manipulation of the lumbar spine. *Spine* 1992;17:1469–1473.
126. Jensen MC, Kelly AP, Brant-Zawaaski MN. MRI of degenerative disease of the lumbar spine. *Mag Imaging Q* 1994;10:173–190.
127. Boos N, Lander PH. Clinical efficacy of imaging modalities in the diagnosis of low back pain disorders. *Eur Spine J* 5:2–22.
128. Adams MA, Hutton WC. The relevance of torsion to the mechanical derangement of the lumbar spine. *Spine* 1981;6:241–248.
129. Stokes LA. Mechanical function of the facet joints in the lumbar spine. *Clin Biomech* 1988;3:101–105.
130. Bogduk N, Twomey LT. Nerves of the lumbar spine. In: *Clinical anatomy of the lumbar spine*, 2nd ed. London: Churchill Livingstone, 1991:107–120.
131. Adams MA, Hutton WC. Prolapsed intervertebral disc—A hyper-flexion injury. *Spine* 1982;7:184–191.
132. Adams MA, Hutton WC. Gradual disc prolapse. *Spine* 1985;10:524–531.
133. Adams MA, Hutton WC. Has the lumbar spine a margin of safety in forward bending? *Clin Biomech* 1986;1:3–6.
134. Herzog W, Read LJ, Conway PJW, Shaw LD, McEwen MC. Reliability of motion palpation procedures to detect sacroiliac joint fixation. *J Manipulative Physiol Ther* 1989;12:86–92.
135. Nachemson A. Our challenge for the next millennium. *J Orthop Sci* 1998;3:191–193.
136. Cedraschi C, Nordin M, Nachemson AL, Vischer TL. Health care providers should use a common language in relation to low back pain patients. *Clin Rheumatol* 1998;12(1):1–15.
137. Binkley J, Finch E, Hall J, Black T, Gowland C. Diagnostic classification of patients with low back pain: Report on survey of physical therapy experts. *Phys Ther* 1993;73(3):138–150.
138. Wiesel SW, Tsourmas N, Feffer HL, et al. A study of computer-assisted tomography. I. The incidence of positive CAT scans in an asymptomatic group of patients. *Spine* September 1984;9(6):549–551.
139. Boden SD, Davis DO, Dina TS, et al. Abnormal magnetic resonance scans of the lumbar spine in asymptomatic subjects. *J Bone Joint Surg* 1990;72:403–408.
140. Dreyfuss P, Michaelsen M, Pauza K, McLarity J, Bogduk N. The value of medical history and physical examination in diagnosing sacroiliac joint pain. 9 *Spine* 1996;21:2594–2602.
141. Strender L, Sjoblom A, Sundell K, Ludwig R, Taube A. Interexaminer reliability in physical

examination of patients with low back pain. *Spine* 1997;22:814–820.

142. Byfield D, Clancy M, Kelly L. Diagnostic palpation and anatomical landmark location—Clinical concepts and the evidence: In: Byfield D, Kinsinger S, eds. *A manual therapist's guide to surface anatomy and palpation skills*. Oxford: Butterworth-Heineman, 2002: 1–33.
143. Rebain R, Baxter D, McDonough S. A systematic review of the passive straight leg rasing test as a diagnostic aid for low back pain 1989 to 2000. *Spine* 2002;27:388–395.
144. Pedersen PE. The clinical history. In: Haldeman S, ed. *Principles and practice of chiropractic*, 3rd ed, 132–139 McGraw-Hill, London, 2004.
145. Marks R. Distribution of pain provoked from lumbar facet joints and related structures during diagnostic spinal infiltration. *Pain* 1989;39:37–40.
146. Souza TA. Lumbopelvic complaints. In: Souza TA, ed. *Differential diagnosis and management for the chiropractor*, 2nd ed. Maryland: Aspen, 2001:109–151.
147. Panzer DM. Facet subluxation syndrome. In: Gatterman MI. *Foundations of chiropractic: Subluxation*, 1st ed. London: Mosby, 1995:415–427.
148. Gatterman MI, Panzer DM. Disorders of the lumbar spine. In: Gatterman MI. *Chiropractic management of spine related disorders*. London: William & Wilkins, 1990:129–175.
149. Cipriano JJ. Lumbar orthopaedic tests. In: Cipriano JJ, ed. *Photographic manual of orthopaedic and neurological tests*, 4th ed. Philadelphia: Lippincott Williams & Wilkins, 2003:250–293.
150. Evans CR. The lumbar spine. In: Evan CR, ed. *Illustrated orthopedic physical assessment*, 2nd ed. London: Mosby, 2001:471–618.
151. Fortin JD, Dwyer AP, West S, Pier J. Sacroiliac joint pain referral maps upon applying a new injection/arthrography technique. Part 2. Clinical evaluation. 9 *Spine* 1994;20:31–37.
152. Laslett M, Williams W. The reliability of selected pain provocation tests for sacroiliac joint pathology. *Spine* 1994;19(11):1243–1249.
153. Gillet H, Leikens M. *Belgian chiropractic research notes*, 11th ed. Huntingdon Beach, CA: Motion Palpation Institute, 1981.
154. Potter NA, Rosthstein JM. Intertester reliability for selected clinical test of the sacro-iliac joint. *Phys Ther* 1985;65(11):1671–1675.
155. Carmichael JP. Inter and intra-examiner reliability of palpation or sacroiliac joint dysfunction. *J Manipulative Physiol Ther* 1987;10:164–171.
156. Ratannen P, Airaksinen O. Poor agreement between so called sacroiliac tests in ankylosing spondylitis. *J Manual Med* 1989;4:62–64.
157. Van Duersen JM, Partijn J, Ockhuysen AL, Vortman BJ. The value of some clinical tests of the sacro-iliac joint. *J Manual Med* 1990;5:96–99.
158. Mior SA, McGregor M, Schutt B. The role of experience in clinical accuracy. *J Manipulative Physiol Ther* 1990;13:68–71.
159. Lewit K, Rosina A. Why yet another diagnostic sign of sacroiliac movement restriction? *J Manipulative Physiol Ther* 1999;22(3):154–160.
160. Ostgaard HC, Zetherstrom G, Roos-Hansson E, Savansberg B. The posterior pelvic pain provocation test on pregnant women. In: Vleeming A, Mooney V, Snijders CJ, Dorman T, eds. Conference Proceedings. *First interdisiplinary world congress on low back pain and its relation to the sacroiliac joint*. San Diego, CA, 1992: 5–6.
161. Ombregt L, ter Veer HJ. Applied anatomy of the sacroiliac joint. In: Ombregt L, Bisschop P, ter Veer HJ, eds. *A system of orthopaedic medicine*, 2nd ed. London: Churchill Livingstone, 2003:941–954.
162. Haughton VM, Eldevik DP, Ho K, Larson SJ, Unger GF. Arachnoiditis from experimental myelography with aqueous contrast media. *Spine* 1978; 3(1):65–69.
163. Haughton VM, Eldevik DP, Magnaes B, Amundsen P. A prospective comparison of computed tomography and myelography in the diagnosis of herniated lumbar disks. *Radiology* 1982;142:103–107.
164. Gutterman P, Bezier HS. Prophylaxis of post-myelogram headaches. *J Neurosurg* 1978;49:869–872.
165. Lasser EC, Lamkin GE. Effects of intrathecal injection of diatrizoate on dopamine receptors. *Acad Radiol* 2002;9(7):826–829.
166. Ido K, Shiode H, Sakamoto A, et al. The validity of upright myelography for diagonsing lumbar disc herniation. *Clin Neurol Neurosurg* 2002;104(1):30–35.

CHAPTER

9

MYOFASCIAL PAIN IN LOW BACK SYNDROMES

Michael Schneider and Craig E. Morris

OUTLINE

OBJECTIVES

1. To understand the nature of myofascial pain and trigger points.
2. To understand the etiological aspects of myofascial pain.
3. To understand the secondary nature of myofascial pain with other pain syndromes.
4. To understand the referred nature of myofascial pain.
5. To understand how to detect myofascial trigger points.
6. To understand the stereotypical myofascial pain patterns of key low back syndrome muscles.
7. To understand strategies for the treatment of myofascial trigger points.
8. To understand the perpetuating factors of myofascial pain.

INTRODUCTION

Previous chapters have addressed the basic anatomical, biomechanical, epidemiological, and functional aspects of the lumbopelvic region. Others have reviewed various complications that can give rise to chronic disabling conditions that essentially stem from specific passive symptom generators.

Chapter 5 provided an overview of the mechanisms regarding motor control and coordination of the musculature of the lower back. It described how the nervous system evaluates the status of spinal stability, and the dynamic changes occurring in the active control of various muscles in order to maintain this stability. Also discussed was *global* muscle dysfunction, i.e., how various pairs or groups of muscles fail to adequately control spinal stability. It also touched upon the rehabilitative exercises helpful in reestablishing sensorimotor control of those muscles.

Panjabi's renowned model[1] of an inherent spinal stabilization system was previously referenced. It is composed of three components: the active (muscle), passive (osteoligamentous), and control (neural) elements. In this model, the passive elements of the spine become the pain generators when their nociceptors are excited owing to poor or inadequate muscular support. Muscles are not seen as primary pain generators themselves, but rather as indirectly causing pain by virtue of their failure to actively stabilize the passive tissues. Rehabilitative training,[2–5] in this model, is focused on improving the nervous system's control and coordination of muscles, thereby improving joint stability and lessening pain.

Other chapters of this textbook discuss various primary pain-generating tissues in the lower back that cause local or referred pain into the inguinal region, buttocks, hip, and lower extremities, such as intervertebral disc lesions, central canal and lateral recess stenosis, and lumbar zygapophyseal and sacroiliac joints. It is important to note that all of these pain-sensitive structures are considered *passive elements* of the intrinsic spinal stabilization system. What about the *active element* of this stabilization system, that is, muscle tissue itself? Aside from the consequences leveled on passive tissues by muscular dysfunction, can muscle tissue itself be a direct or an indirect pain generator? If so, what are the etiological and perpetuating factors associated with such phenomena?

This chapter will focus on a different type of muscle dysfunction—the *focal* type of muscle dysfunction known as *myofascial trigger points* (TrPs), in which only a portion or subsection of a muscle becomes taut and "nodular." While this might superficially seem to be a somewhat simple topic to cover, the ensuing text will disprove such a notion by discussing the etiological, perpetuating, diagnostic, therapeutic, and complicating factors associated with TrPs.

Myofascial Pain Syndrome Defined

Most people have experienced one or more common types of *acute* muscle pain, such as postexercise muscle soreness, muscle cramps, or mild muscular strain injuries. These simple types of muscle pain usually resolve simply, with self-monitored care such as rest and perhaps heat applications. However, more problematic is the major type of *chronic* muscle pain known as *myofascial pain syndrome (MPS)*, which is caused by localized areas of muscle dysfunction known as *myofascial trigger points (TrPs)*.

The term MPS can be confusing, because there are two different meanings in common usage within the health-care community. The *general* meaning relates to the usage of the term MPS to describe *any regional pain disorder that seems to emanate from any soft tissue*. Many clinicians who are well versed in myofascial treatment procedures would object to this nonspecific usage of the term MPS. The *specific* meaning, to which this author will refer throughout the remainder of this chapter, defines MPS to describe *a characteristic referred pain pattern from a specific skeletal* muscle.[6,7] A diagnosis of MPS in this specific sense requires the clinical identification of TrPs that reproduce the pain pattern described by the patient.

FOCAL VERSUS GLOBAL MUSCLE DYSFUNCTION

It is important to recognize that some type of muscle dysfunction is typically involved with all or almost all cases of low back pain. Muscle dysfunction can be simply defined as an abnormal change in muscle tone, either increased (hypertonic) or decreased (hypotonic). When one or several entire muscles undergo abnormal changes in overall tone, the term *global* muscle dysfunction is used to describe this clinical scenario. Janda,[8,9] for example, used the terms muscle tightness/weakness to describe one type of muscle dysfunction in which a muscle weakens as it becomes tight and relatively short. It is important to note that these globally dysfunctional muscles typically do not generate pain.

In distinction to global muscle dysfunction where an entire muscle becomes tight or weak, *the TrP phenomenon is a more focal type of muscle dysfunction*, in which only a small portion of fibers within a muscle become taut and hypertonic. The overall tone and length of a muscle harboring TrPs are not necessarily abnormal; only one (or possibly more) focal subsection(s) of muscle fibers is affected. This type of focal muscle dysfunction is typically associated with *myofascial pain*, which occurs in a specific pattern that is characteristic for each skeletal muscle. Later in this chapter there will be a comprehensive discussion of the proposed mechanisms underlying the development of TrPs and myofascial referred pain.

The Functional Neuromusculoskeletal System

The term *neuromusculoskeletal* (NMS) *system* aptly describes how muscles, joints, and bones are functionally interrelated via the central and peripheral nervous system. It is through muscles that the brain controls all movements of the body. Therefore it should follow that alterations in muscle tone occur as a *neurological* reflex response to irritation of spinal nerves, zygapophyseal joints, discs, or ligaments.[10] Muscles respond in reflex fashion to pain emanating from any of these passive elements of the spinal stabilization system. Such somato-somato reflex responses are typically seen in acute low back presentation by paraspinal muscle hypertonicity.

When muscle dysfunction occurs as a result of pain-induced somato-somato reflexes, there is typically neural excitation or inhibition of the entire muscle via increased or decreased alpha motor neuron activity. Examples include inhibition of quadriceps/excitation of hamstrings with an anterior cruciate ligament tear[11] and inhibition of multifidus/excitation of iliocostalis with acute disc herniation.[12] This type of global muscle dysfunction is typically verified by surface electromyographic (EMG) changes in the entire muscle's motor activity. Hodges et al.[13] recently performed an interesting experiment in which patients received noxious saline injections into the lumbar longissimus muscle to induce experimental muscular low back pain. The EMG activity of various trunk muscles was then assessed, with a consistent inhibition of the transversus abdominis noted.

Clinical Pearl: In distinction to global muscle dysfunction where an entire muscle becomes tight or weak, the TrP phenomenon is a more focal type of muscle dysfunction, in which only a small portion of fibers within a muscle become taut and hypertonic.

EMG Aspects of TrPs

Interestingly, focal muscle dysfunction presents a very different EMG picture compared to global muscle dysfunction. In the case of focal dysfunction, only fine wire EMG needle penetration directly into the nidus, or epicenter, of the TrP yields any abnormal EMG activity. The muscle fibers adjacent to the TrP "nodule" do not typically show any changes in EMG activity,[14] which casts doubt on reflex alpha motor neuron activity as the mechanism underlying the taut band or TrP. However, some authors[15,16] believe that dysfunctional gamma motor neurons may be implicated in the genesis of TrP and taut band formation, a theory that will be explored more fully later in this chapter.

In addition to the neurological reflexes that trigger changes in muscle function, there is also a *biomechanical* aspect of muscle tone that can be viewed from static and dynamic perspectives. Frequent positioning in prolonged postures may lead to muscle tightness and weakness from *static* shortening or lengthening, respectively. For example, frequent and prolonged sitting with the knees and hips maintained in a relaxed, flexed position might lead to tightness of the iliopsoas and hamstring muscles. Such inactivity also would tend to lengthen their antagonists, the gluteus maximus, and quadriceps. Kendall et al.[17] coined the terms *adaptive shortening* and *stretch weakness* to describe static changes in global muscle tone and compromised function.

Clinical Pearl: Kendall coined the terms *adaptive shortening* and *stretch weakness* to describe static changes in global muscle tone and compromised function.

Of course, muscle tightness and weakness may also develop in a *dynamic* manner, from overuse.[9] For example, a deconditioned office worker who spends numerous hours bending over picking up bricks to build a wall in his backyard would logically develop focal or global muscle dysfunction in the key low back muscles associated with this activity. Therefore, in the case of dynamic muscle overuse syndromes, discrete areas of focal TrP activity are more likely to be associated with the global muscle tightness.

In summary, it has been briefly stated that changes in muscle tone occur dynamically and passively, that such changes can occur globally or in a focal manner, and that such changes accompany low back pain. The focal nature of muscle dysfunction is that which is associated with MPS. In order to understand more about the etiology of MPS, a more in-depth review of muscle physiology is presented.

WHAT IS MUSCLE TONE?

As noted above, neurological and biomechanical causes of muscle dysfunction can lead to the development of localized TrP nodules and taut bands within certain muscles. Muscles prone to repetitive overuse or prolonged contraction are likely to develop TrPs and myofascial pain. Furthermore, dynamic changes in the overall tone of muscles (global dysfunction) often precede the specific and discrete focal changes detected as TrPs. In order to better understand the localized nature of the TrP phenomenon and myofascial pain, it may be helpful to first look at the issue of muscle tone, and the mechanisms by which functional changes in muscle tissue occur.

Any discussion of muscle dysfunction requires the conceptual model of *muscle tone*, which can be defined in simple terms as *resistance to stretch.*[18] Therefore, any increase or decrease in muscle tone will necessarily exhibit a proportional increase or decrease in resistance to stretch. In the clinical setting, muscles can be viewed as being normotonic (normal tone), hypertonic (increased tone), or hypotonic (decreased tone). What constitutes "normal tone" is debatable; different muscles develop different levels of tone based on the demands placed upon them by such factors as physical activity and posture. Muscles that are used frequently or regularly may adapt by developing increased tone (hypertonicity), whereas other muscles may develop decreased tone (hypotonicity) due to disuse.[19]

Muscle Tone: Dynamic and Nondynamic Aspects

There are two basic mechanisms by which muscles exhibit tone, or resistance to stretch. The first is *neurological* or *dynamic*, and relates to motor neuron activity that can increase or decrease the contractile components of muscle tissue. The term *dynamic* refers to the ability of the central nervous system (CNS) to rapidly alter the level of muscle tone based upon the needs of the NMS system.[18] The second mechanism underlying muscle tone is *biomechanical* or *nondynamic*, and relates to the mechanical properties of myofascial tissue itself such as the integrity of the ground substance, density of collagen fibers, and length of muscle fibers, fascia, and tendinous tissue. The term *nondynamic* refers to the fact that the body cannot inherently control or make immediate changes in the biomechanical component of myofascial tissue. In other words, nondynamic myofascial tissue is that which is incapable of contracting and decontracting directly via neurochemical stimulation. As such, the nondynamic tissue is also called the noncontractile myofascial tissue.

Despite the definition above, which on the surface would appear to be quite straightforward, *muscle tone* is a problematic term that connotes various interpretations depending upon the reference source. Most clinicians would concur that muscle "tone" is a combination of the *biomechanical* properties of the myofascial tissues (pliability, flexibility, ground substance, etc.) and the *neurological* degree of muscle contraction. Mense and Simons[18] describe these two properties of muscle tone as viscoelasticity and contractility, respectively.

Alpha and Gamma Motor Neurons

Contractility of skeletal muscle integrates two types of motor efferent innervation: the *alpha* motor neurons that stimulate muscle contraction, which is recordable by EMG studies, and the *gamma* motor neurons that cause contraction of the muscle spindles' intrafusal fibers, but do *not* cause any detectable EMG changes. Increased gamma, not alpha activity, may be the underlying cause of *hypertonic* or *facilitated* musculature,[20] which will be discussed later.

As previously noted, changes in muscle tone may occur on a "global" or "focal" level. *Global* changes in muscle tone involve the entire muscle and most of its associated fibers. *Focal* changes in muscle tone are typically found as the *taut bands* noted in association with myofascial TrP activity. These taut bands are thought to represent "islands" of hypertonic fascicles or bundles of muscle fibers found within a "sea" of otherwise relatively normotonic muscle fibers. It is also interesting to note that focal muscle dysfunction manifests only as focal *hypertonicity*, unlike globally dysfunctional muscles that can be either tight/hypertonic or weak/hypotonic. For some unknown reason, taut bands are always "tight strands," and never appear as "hypotonic strands."

TrPs: "Areas of Muscle Incoordination"

In the case of the focal hypertonicity seen with TrPs and taut bands, it almost appears as if a subsection of muscle fibers have become dissociated from the surrounding fibers within the same muscle, which lead Janda[9] to term TrPs "areas of muscle incoordination." One unresolved paradox is that TrPs and taut bands are frequently found in globally hypotonic muscles such as the gluteus medius. The muscle fibers within the taut band seem hypertonic and shortened, yet the vast majority of muscle fibers within the remainder of the gluteus medius seem hypotonic. This type of muscle incoordination is likely due to alterations in neural control of muscle tone mediated by gamma and alpha motor neurons through the muscle spindles. This "muscle spindle theory" of TrP formation will be covered later in this chapter.

Clinical Pearl: Muscle tone is defined as "resistance to stretch," and is controlled by neurological (dynamic) and biomechanical (nondynamic) mechanisms.

Thixotropic Nature of Muscle

Muscle tissue has a curious mechanical property of becoming more pliable and flexible with repeated movement. This physical property is known as *thixotropy*,[18] which is the ability of a substance to become less viscous when stimulated before reverting back to its viscous state following the stimuli. An example of a thixotropic substance would be gelatin, which becomes more liquid when warmed after being removed from the refrigerator and then again returns to a gel once it becomes chilled following a return to the refrigerator. Similarly, athletes have empirically capitalized on the thixotropic nature of muscle by warming up before exercise and competition, allowing their muscles to move more freely and with less resistance to stretch.

The specific mechanism underlying the thixotropic nature of muscle tissue is still undetermined. The most widely accepted model is a tendency for actin and myosin filaments to bind together when a muscle has been inactive for some period of time.[18,21] However, there may be other explanations involving biochemical changes in the connective tissues and ground substance of the muscles and their investing fascia.

Certain soft tissue treatment techniques that involve prolonged or repeated stretching of myofascial tissues are based upon the premise that they can make therapeutic changes by breaking adhesions, releasing contractures, scars, or other fascial "restrictions."[22–25] Practitioners of these techniques speak of feeling the tissues "melt apart" in their fingers, or sensing a "release of tension" while applying static stretching to the tissues. It is plausible that these empirical observations may be related to changes made in the thixotropic nature of myofascial tissues; however, there is a paucity of basic science data confirming the existence of these purported fascial restrictions, scars, or myofascial adhesions.

Neural Reflexes

A more likely explanation for the dramatic and almost instant pain relief experienced by some patients after manual myofascial therapy is that *neural reflexes* have been somehow altered, leading to dynamic changes in muscle tone. Nimmo[25] referred to this as the *neuromechanical* nature of manipulation, mobilization, soft tissue therapy, or any type of manual treatment in which a mechanical force was applied to the tissues of the human body, eliciting a neural response.

Neurological reflexes are very much involved with the maintenance of muscle tone and tension, more so than is generally appreciated in general practice. This statement is readily demonstrated by the following simple maneuver. A patient with bilateral hamstring tightness, 60 degrees or less on the straight-leg test, will be a sufficient subject. Perform some type of therapeutic stretch on the right hamstrings in order to increase the range of motion to about 80 or 90 degrees. Then recheck the left hamstring with the straight-leg test; most likely it has dramatically increased to about 70 or 80 degrees *without any specific stretching of that muscle.*

The results of this clinical observation cannot be explained by connective tissue shortening alone; there must be some type of neurological reflex underlying this "cross-over" change in muscle tone. Therefore, the resting *tone* of any given muscle is not merely due to the inert thixotropic properties of the muscle tissue itself, but is more likely to represent a combination of its biomechanical (thixotropic) properties and some degree of neural activation of motor neurons.[26] It is this neural aspect of manual soft tissue techniques that often is neglected in discussions about the possible mechanisms of action underlying manual therapy.

Manual Reflex Techniques

The above clinical experiment shows the relationship of neural reflexes to global muscle tightness, but what about the focal hypertonicity found with taut bands and TrPs? Janda[8,9,27–29] and Lewit[30] have empirically noted that manual reflex techniques such as postisometric relaxation (PIR) can eliminate TrPs, presumably from some type of reflex neural inhibition of motor neuron activity coupled with a slow and gentle muscle lengthening designed to avoid stretch reflex. The method of spray and stretch (S&S) was developed by Travell and Simons[6,7] to eliminate TrPs; the cold from fluorimethane spray was thought to inhibit pain and motor neuron activity, while the specific stretch was thought to biomechanically lengthen and disrupt the TrP nodule.

It is important to note that *both PIR and S&S techniques do not involve any specific manual pressure applied directly over or to the TrP nodule.* They are considered neural reflex techniques, presumably because they affect muscle tissue by alteration in the dynamic control of muscle tone. This leads to an intriguing question: Do the TrP nodule and associated taut band represent a focal area of neurologically mediated muscle hypertonicity? Or do they merely represent a focus of biomechanically shortened muscle fibers that are somehow contracted from adhesions or fascial restrictions? The apparent beneficial effect of PIR and S&S would seem to favor a neurological mechanism. This controversy over neurological vs. biomechanical mechanisms of action in the TrP phenomenon will be covered in greater detail later on.

Clinical Pearl: It is important to note that both PIR and S&S techniques *do not* involve any specific manual pressure applied directly over TrP nodule and therefore must be affecting muscle tone through neurological mechanisms of action.

Spasm versus Hypertonicity

Another important distinction is the palpably increased tone of taut bands, which should not be misrepresented as *spasm*, although it is tempting to think of them as areas of "mini-spasm." Spasm describes a type, or subset, of global hypertonicity and refers to the involuntary contraction of muscle tissue due to increased *alpha* motor nerve activity.[31] Muscle spasm represents a true state of neurologically mediated, global hypertonicity. Therefore, true muscle spasm involves the majority of fibers or an entire muscle belly, and such a muscle will exhibit increased EMG activity.[26]

Clinicians often use the term *spasm* inappropriately to describe *any type* of palpable increased muscle *tension* or *tone*, such as the taut bands found in association with myofascial TrP activity or the tense erector spinae muscles found in the absence of low back pain. Because of the multivariate etiology of increased muscle tone, it is often clinically presumptuous in the typical office setting to assume that all increased tone would be due to increased *alpha* motor nerve activity, or spasm. The correct term for this palpable tension is the generic term *hypertonicity*, not spasm.[9] Please make note of this important statement: *muscles in spasm are always tight, but not all tight muscles are in spasm*. For example, it is extremely common to find patients with tight hamstring muscles evidenced by pronounced restriction of supine straight-leg raising; yet there may be no detectable increased EMG activity over these tight hamstrings. A muscle may feel hard and ropey, with multiple TrPs embedded within taut bands, yet surface EMG over the muscle shows no significantly increased electrical activity. Therefore, it is important to recognize that there are several ways in which muscle tone or tension can be increased, short of true spasm.

Another common flaw in terminology is the erroneously synonymous use of the terms spasm and spastic. While spasm has already been defined, the term spastic refers to muscle dysfunction and movement patterns associated with upper motor neuron lesions. As such, a patient may have a spastic gait, but not a spasmodic gait.

Jacob[32] discusses one simple clinical observation that clearly demonstrates the flawed assumption of muscle spasm as a common clinical entity. Spasmodic muscles always limit the ability of their associated joints to move. Therefore, a spasmodic lumbar erector spinae would pull the spine into lordosis and prevent forward flexion. Yet in common cases of acute low back pain one does not typically see this presentation. The patient with acute central low back pain often has taut and tender muscle fibers palpable in the erector spinae muscles; however, the lumbar lordosis is *decreased*, inconsistent with the *increased* lordosis one would expect with *spasm* of these muscles.

Muscle spasm is *not* usually a primary musculoskeletal condition. Spasm is almost invariably a *secondary reflex phenomenon* caused by a primary pain generator in some other tissue that triggers the reactive spasm. Examples include the rectus abdominis and oblique abdominal muscle spasm seen with acute appendicitis (a viscerosomatic reflex), and the hamstring spasm observed with acute tears of the cruciate ligaments of the knee (a somatosomato reflex). Of course, the exception to this scenario occurs when the muscle itself is injured, in which case it would be both the primary musculoskeletal condition causing the secondary reflex phenomenon of spasm. Therefore, whenever a clinician observes frank muscle spasm, it is important that he or she avoids *clinical myopia* by looking both within and beyond that muscle for the primary pathological or inflamed tissue that is triggering the neurological reflexes that lead to this spasm. Direct treatment applied to a spasmodic muscle, without addressing the primary pain generator that is causing the reflex spasm, is subject to failure and recurrence of the spasm.

Clinical Pearl: Clinicians often use the term *spasm* inappropriately to describe any type of palpable increased muscle tension or tone, which is more appropriately termed *hypertonicity*.

PROPRIOCEPTORS AND MUSCLE DYSFUNCTION

As noted above, a muscle *at rest*, even one that may be hypertonic, does not necessarily exhibit any EMG activity.[18] This may seem contradictory to what is observed in clinical practice. After all, what practitioner has not palpated hypertonic musculature of patients who lie relaxed on the examination table? If their muscles are not showing increased EMG activity, from where does this palpable increased muscle tone come?

The answer, at least for the dynamic part of muscle tissue, seems to lie in the realm of muscle tissue receptors that mediate neurological control of muscle tone.

To appreciate the place of these receptors in the greater context of NMS function requires a brief review. Simply stated, in order for the CNS to control muscle function and thereby coordinate the NMS system, it must follow this sequence of events: it first must be capable of receiving sensory input, or *afferentation*, from the *peripheral receptors.* Then it must *process and integrate that* sensory input into a meaningful response. Finally, *coordinated motor output*, or *efferentation*, to the appropriate skeletal musculature is necessary to carry out the intended response.[33] Without quality incoming information, this cycle of the NMS system cannot function.

Focal muscle dysfunction, which involves the formation of discrete TrPs, involves a localized area of *muscle ischemia* that theoretically activates the chemical *nociceptors* and causes pain. In contrast, global muscle dysfunction, which involves changes in motor neuron activity to muscles and/or changes in the overall length of muscles, does not typically involve an ischemic process and therefore does not activate the chemical nociceptors. For this reason global muscle tightness or weakness is typically a painless phenomenon. However, despite the differences in focal and local dysfunction, both tend to alter muscular *tension and length*, mechanical forces that stimulate activity of the muscle *proprioceptors.*

Proprioception

The term *proprioceptor* was coined by Sherrington[34] in the early 1900s as an all-inclusive term for all of the peripheral receptors found in ligaments, muscles, tendons, and joints that relayed sensory information to the CNS for regulation of motor control and coordination. Specifically, these proprioceptors comprise various types of *mechanoreceptors.* Ruffini endings, Pacinian corpuscles, and Golgi tendon organ-like endings are the mechanoreceptors[33] found within ligaments and joints that sense the degree of joint capsule pressure and distension, thereby apprising the CNS of joint position, angulation, and movement. The mechanoreceptors found within musculotendinous tissue are the muscle spindles and Golgi tendon organs that sense the degree of muscle length and tension, respectively.[32]

Golgi Tendon Organs

The sensory input from Golgi tendon organs (GTO) and muscle spindles (MS) is neurologically wired via spinal cord reflexes to specific motor nerve outputs, which have different effects on muscle function. The GTOs are found in the tendons and myotendinous junctions of skeletal muscles, and chiefly "sense" the degree of *tension* that is imposed upon the tendons by muscle contraction. For this reason, GTOs are *stimulated* whenever muscles contract, since contraction causes increased tendon tension. Stimulation of GTOs causes reflex *inhibition* of alpha motor neuron output back to the muscle in which they reside.

This inhibitory nature of GTOs lead early researchers to theorize that only intense muscle contractions would stimulate GTOs; otherwise muscle contraction would always lead to counterproductive agonistic muscle inhibition. It was even purported that GTOs served only one purpose: the protective function of telling the CNS to inhibit muscle contraction that was close to exceeding the tensile limits of the tendon. However, it is now known that GTOs are stimulated very readily by even small degrees of muscle contraction,[26,35] but the excitatory effects from MS and other descending pathways from the brainstem and cerebellum usually overpower this inhibitory effect. Any motor output from the spinal cord is orchestrated by a complicated mixture of both inhibitory and excitatory signals from multiple parts of the CNS.

Muscle Spindles

MS are much more complicated than GTOs in several ways. Spindles are basically *length detectors,* and are stimulated during elongation or lengthening of muscle fibers. Therefore *inhibition* of spindle activity occurs during muscular contractions (which shortens the motor unit), whereas rapid elongation of muscle fibers will stimulate spindle activity. MS, unlike GTOs, are *excitatory* in nature, causing reflex *excitation* of the alpha motor neurons to the muscle in which they reside. MS function establishes the neurophysiological rationale for orthopedic muscle stretch reflex tests such as the knee jerk reflex. Quadriceps contraction occurs in response to the quick stretch on the quadriceps muscle caused by the reflex hammer. Incidentally, this is why the proper term for the group of tests that include the knee jerk response has evolved from deep tendon reflexes to *muscle stretch reflexes.*

The MS also represents a unique type of peripheral receptor in the human body. Although technically considered sensory receptors, spindles have both a *sensory and a motor function.* This unique dual function of spindles requires distinct sensory and motor neural pathways to and from the CNS, known as the *gamma afferent and efferent systems* respectively.[36] This seems contradictory: How could a sensory receptor have any type of motor or efferent function? The answer to this seeming paradox lies in the microanatomy of the spindle structure. Spindles contain small "mini-muscle fibers" known as *intrafusal* (IF) muscle fibers, and the tension of these IF fibers are controlled by *gamma* motor neurons. There are also sensory nerve endings that detect changes in length of the MS cells, which transmit impulses to the spinal cord via gamma *afferent* neurons.

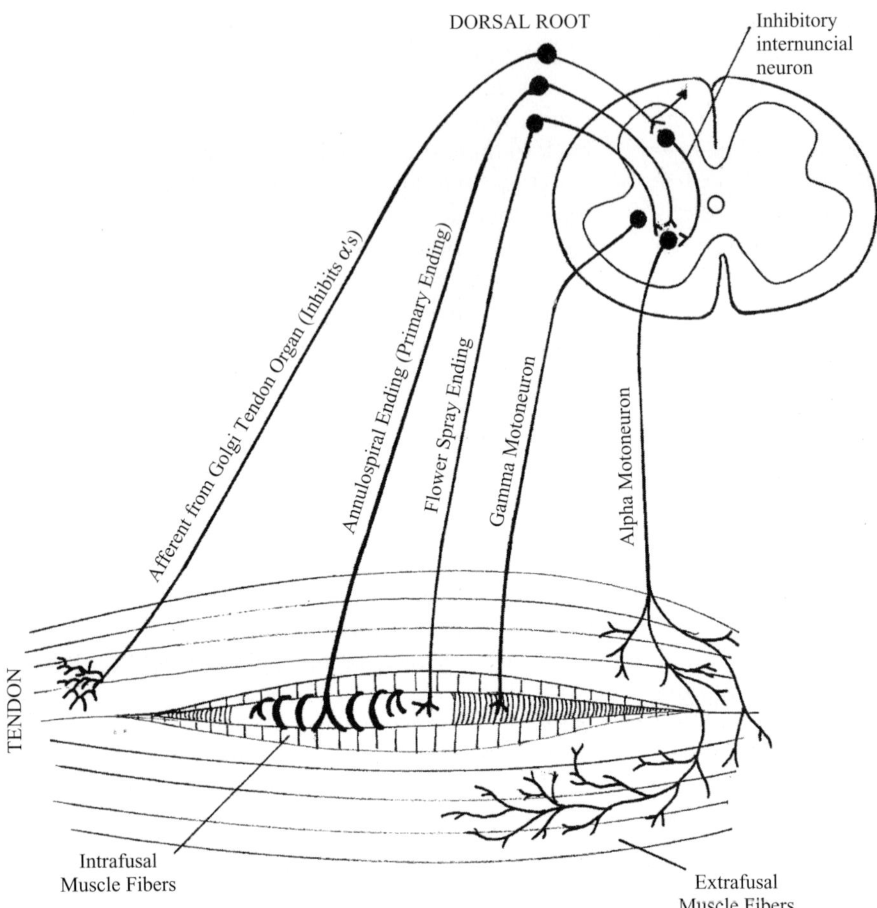

FIGURE 9–1. Muscle proprioceptors: the Golgi tendon organ (GTO) and muscle spindle (MS). The GTO *inhibits* and the MS *excites* the alpha motor neuron of the muscle in which these proprioceptors reside. The gamma motor neurons only create tension within the intrafusal fibers of the MS, whereas alpha motor neurons generate voluntary skeletal muscle fiber (extrafusal) contraction. (*From Jones.*[37])

The IF fibers found invested within the spindle need to be contrasted with the *extrafusal* (EF) muscle fibers, which represent the skeletal muscle cells themselves. Much confusion arises during discussions about the differences between IF and EF fibers. Simply put, the term *fusal* refers to the fusiform shape of the MS; hence, "intra"-fusal fibers are those found internally within the substance of the MS cells, whereas "extra"-fusal fibers lie external to the spindle cells. In reality, the term *extrafusal fiber* is synonymous with the term *skeletal muscle fiber*. The contractile elements of the EF fibers are actin–myosin microfilaments found within the skeletal muscle cells, whose degree of contractility is controlled by alpha motor neurons. *Alpha* motor neuron activity, a conscious mechanism, controls skeletal muscle contraction; *gamma* motor neurons, a subconsciously mechanism, control the tension of IF MS fibers. Figure 9–1 provides an overview of the GTO and MS afferents, and gamma–alpha efferents to muscle.

Clinical Pearl: The MS represents a unique type of peripheral receptor in the human body, because it has both a sensory and a motor function, controlled by afferent and efferent gamma neurons respectively.

The Gamma System

The gamma system provides the CNS with a mechanism by which to control the responsiveness of the muscular system.[20] The CNS is constantly matching the degree of length and tension it senses in the spindles with the amount of skeletal muscle contraction, integrating this proprioceptive information to make judgments about the readiness of the muscle for action. If the IF fibers of the spindles are stimulated (tensioned) by gamma motor neurons, but the skeletal muscle fibers are not proportionally activated by the alpha system, then the CNS is ready for action and the skeletal muscle will contract very rapidly. This state of increased responsiveness is known as *facilitation*, defined as a neurologically mediated increase in muscle contractibility.

The gamma system is intimately related to the alpha system, as increased tension in MS lead to early activation of muscle contraction. Therefore, signals from the motor cortex that control muscle function simultaneously activate *both* alpha and gamma motor neurons, co-contracting EF and IF fibers.[26] In addition, nociceptive input from the skin, joints, ligaments, discs, and other peripheral tissues often causes reflex muscle responses through the alpha–gamma systems.[38]

This seemingly ubiquitous nature of the alpha–gamma motor response has led to the *final common input hypothesis*.[20,39] This hypothesis suggests that information mediated by MS and the gamma system is shaped not only by changes in muscle length, but also to a larger extent by signals arising from the segmentally innervated joints, discs, and ligaments. In other words, all peripheral receptor input to the spinal cord is integrated into some type of gamma response, which results in altered muscle tone. In this manner, the gamma spindle system may be viewed as an integrative system that conveys polymodal feedback to the CNS about all types of NMS tissues, and through intricate spinal reflexes may coordinate muscular responses to peripheral NMS injury. The proprioceptive input from joint capsules and ligaments therefore leads to reflex changes in muscle tone, with the gamma system providing the appropriate muscular responses by which joint stability can be preserved when the passive tissues are injured.

The gamma system may also provide an explanation for the discrete nature of the taut band and TrP nodule. Hubbard and coworkers[14,15] proposed that TrPs and taut bands may be caused by dysfunctional MS, which are somehow maintaining a low-level activation of small numbers of muscle fibers. This *dysfunctional muscle spindle theory* helps to explain the lack of surface EMG activity over TrPs, because there is very little alpha motor neuron activation. Manual techniques such as deep pressure, stripping massage, and stretching may not merely act mechanically; they may also influence the MS and "reset" the degree of muscle tone through neurological mechanisms that are still poorly understood.

Proprioceptors are likely part of the explanation for the clinical effectiveness of the manual technique of PIR,[30,40,41] which appears to be capable of eliminating taut bands and TrPs. It is likely that this procedure utilizes the inherent spinal cord circuits of the gamma–alpha system to achieve its clinical effects. The muscle being treated is isometrically contracted for several seconds, during which time the MS activity is quieted (i.e., muscle contraction reduces tension on the IF fibers of the spindles) and GTOs are excited. This mechanism is known as *post-contraction inhibition*. Relaxation of the entire muscle with gentle elongation will ensue, after the decreased gamma activity of the quieted spindles and inhibition from GTOs allows for concurrent diminished alpha activity.

There is a continuous interplay involving neurological circuits between nociceptors, alpha and gamma motor neurons, as well as joint and muscle proprioceptors. According to the final common input theory, MS are responsive to input from all proprioceptors and nociceptors surrounding joints, and set the overall tone of muscle that move the respective joint(s). Therefore, it should not be surprising to find that lumbar zygapophyseal joint and lumbar disc nociceptive stimulation should invariably lead to some type of secondary reflex muscle dysfunction, which may manifest as the appearance of myofascial TrPs. These secondary TrPs may linger around as myofascial pain even after the primary zygapophyseal joint or disc problem has been corrected.

The above discussion helps to establish the conceptual model of *focal* muscle dysfunction, the taut bands and TrP "knots" in which only certain subsections of the muscle tissue undergo an apparent shortening or hypertonic change. The entire muscle is not in spasm, for reasons discussed earlier. This model then helps to set the base for various theories about how and why this occurs. As such, this is the topic of the next section, which will discuss the phenomena of focal muscle dysfunction, known more commonly as myofascial TrPs.

Clinical Pearl: The "final common input"theory proposes that all proprioceptive and nociceptive stimuli from joints, muscles, and ligaments synapse on gamma motor neurons provide the final control of muscle tone around joints through modification of MS excitability.

MECHANISMS OF MUSCLE PAIN

Nociception and the perception of pain occupy an a priori position in the hierarchy of sensory stimuli; it provokes the nervous system to respond by causing immediate muscular responses. The *nociceptors* are specialized peripheral receptors that provide sensory information about actual or potential tissue damage, and with sufficient stimulation will lead to the emotional state known as *pain*. Pain and nociception are not synonymous terms, as the same nociceptive stimulus applied to different people will lead to different perceptions.[35] Furthermore, nociceptive stimulation must reach a threshold before the sensation of pain is experienced, although subthreshold levels may indeed reflexively initiate local or systemic responses despite the absence of pain. Pain is an unpleasant *emotional experience* associated with the perception of actual or potential tissue damage; it serves an important protective function by warning us of injury that has occurred or should be avoided. Unlike other sensations, pain has a distinct urgency and primitive quality that is responsible for emotional, affective, and behavioral reflex responses, obviously survivalistic qualities that, on a broad scale, might promote the survival of a species.

There are three major types of nociceptors that respond to different types of stimuli: *thermal*, *mechanical*, and *chemical*. Thermal nociceptors respond to extremes of temperature such as intense heat or cold. Mechanical nociceptors are activated by intense pressure applied to the skin or muscle. Both thermal and mechanical nociceptors conduct their signals via *thinly myelinated A delta fibers*, and are responsible for the perception of very localized pain. Chemical nociceptors are stimulated by various biochemical exudates of tissue trauma or ischemia, and transmit their signals to the CNS via *nonmyelinated C fibers* that are responsible for vague, diffuse, and poorly localized pain. The "fast" or "first" pain that is felt immediately after an injury is transmitted by A delta fibers from the mechanical and thermal nociceptors, whereas the "slow" or "second" pain that develops later on after injury is transmitted by C fibers from the chemical nociceptors.[26]

Muscle Pain

Most muscle pain is caused by chemical irritation of nociceptors. These chemical irritants can come from several potential sources: external trauma to muscle cells (strains, contusions), intrinsic microtrauma to muscle cells from overuse, or localized TrPs. Therefore, the focal muscle dysfunction of TrPs causes pain, whereas the global muscle dysfunction seen with adaptive shortening and stretch weakness is relatively painless. Pain is caused by activation of the muscle *nociceptors* by the chemical by-products of the energy crisis found in the region of the TrP. Dysfunction, both focal and global forms, is due to abnormal stimuli arising from muscle *proprioceptors* when the shortened or lengthened state of these tissues activates MS and GTO in ways that disrupt normal control of muscle function by the CNS.

The *perception of pain* will lead to reflex and voluntary changes in motor neuron activity, and thereby causes reflexogenic spasm, hypertonicity, or hypotonicity in muscles far distant from site of actual nociception. For example, stepping on a sharp tack while walking in barefeet will trigger reflex hypertonic changes in the hip flexor muscles, which contract to flex the leg up away from the painful tack, as well as hypotonic changes in the antagonistic hip extensors.[35] These reflex motor responses are nothing more than a mechanism by which the body attempts to rid itself of pain, a response called pain avoidance behavior.

First and Second Pain

The sharp attribute of "first pain" is well localized; the patient knows precisely where the area of injury has occurred. In the example above, the individual who stepped on a tack clearly recognizes exactly where the tack is lodged in his or her foot. However, the dull attribute of "second pain" is very poorly localized, and one has difficulty discerning the specific location from where this deep aching sensation is emanating. Once the tack is removed, the sensation changes and the whole foot throbs and aches, replacing the perception of the specific, pointed pain where the tack entered the foot. The initial sharp localized pain was due to stimulation of *mechanical* nociceptors when the skin and subdermal tissues were injured: the transformation to diffuse widespread pain being caused by activation of *chemical* nociceptors once biochemical exudates sufficiently infiltrated the region of the injured tissue.

"Second pain" involves the perception of a deep, dull ache that is transmitted from chemical nociceptors via *nonmyelinated* axons (C fibers). This dull aching type of pain is characteristic of myofascial referred pain, and will lead to involuntary reflex responses as well as conscious pain avoidance behaviors. Eventually, chronic pain may lead to a more complex clinical scenario, where the mere *thought of pain* can produce motor neuron changes, *in anticipation* of any future movements that might provoke pain. Chronic, nagging pain ultimately activates the *limbic system*, which in turn generates powerful motor reflex responses that attempt to avoid pain at any price to the NMS system.[26]

It is important to note that different types of muscle responses result from different types and sources of pain. When a patient's superficial tissues (such as the skin) are irritated by mechanical or thermal stimuli (stepping on a tack or hot coal) the resulting nociceptive input to the spinal cord triggers chiefly the *flexor withdrawal reflex*, as noted in the above example. This reflex response occurs because of integrated circuits within the spinal cord that involve several muscles both in the painful and contralateral nonpainful limb.[42] These spinal cord mediated motor responses to painful stimuli represent the most simple and primitive example of pain avoidance behavior.

Reflex inhibition from myofascial TrPs is probably one of the most commonly seen types of muscle dysfunction. When a muscle that harbors a TrP becomes activated within a particular movement pattern, the additional contraction of the already contracted sarcomeres with the TrP nodule causes further irritation of the chemical nociceptors. This nociceptive stimulus causes spinal cord interneurons to *inhibit motor neuron* activity back to that muscle. In a sense, this is a form of autogenic pain avoidance; the muscle somehow has "learned" to avoid contracting at full intensity. Therefore, muscles that contain TrPs may not contract to their full maximal effort in order to avoid further damage or pain. Clinically, this may be seen upon manual muscle testing where this muscle "gives way" just short of full exertion, or upon observation of repeated movements where the muscle begins to reduce its activity after several repetitions.

"Chemical" Nature of Myofascial Pain

Myofascial referred pain from TrPs has the distinct quality of a deep, dull, aching type of pain and therefore is likely to be due chiefly to activation of chemical nociceptors. A common example of chemically mediated muscle pain is the *delayed onset muscle soreness (DOMS)*[4] that everyone has experienced the day after a vigorous exercise program. The frequent and/or intense muscle contractions do not stimulate nociceptors immediately, because it takes several hours for the biochemical by-products of muscle metabolism and microtrauma (bradykinins, histamines, lactic acid, prostaglandins, etc.) to accumulate and stimulate chemical nociceptors. When intense muscle contraction occurs in the absence of sufficient blood and oxygen supply, such as heavy weight lifting without associated aerobic exercise, the resulting ischemia leads to even faster accumulation of irritating muscle metabolites and a quicker onset of DOMS.

While DOMS can be thought of as "global muscle pain," since all or large portions of the muscle are painful, TrPs are areas of focal muscle dysfunction that are believed to be maintained by an ischemic "energy crisis" within a localized region of muscle. This localized area of metabolic overactivity and ischemia from the TrP nodule also generates the noxious by-products noted above. Most of these chemical by-products of ischemia are intense irritants of free sensory nerve endings, and thereby activate the chemical nociceptors to send a barrage of sensory stimuli to the spinal cord. TrPs are therefore focal sources of muscle ischemia that stimulate chemical nociception and cause muscle pain that is often perceived as widespread and diffuse. The nature of pain perceived from TrPs appears to manifest itself in specific *myofascial referred pain patterns*, which are amazingly consistent and reproducible to each individual skeletal muscle.

Clinical Pearl: ... TrPs are areas of focal muscle dysfunction that are believed to be maintained by an ischemic "energy crisis" within a localized region of muscle.

Coexisting Pain Generators

Bogduk and Simons[43] discussed in detail the concept that muscle and joint pain are often coexisting generators of pain, causing a composite muscle/joint referred pain pattern. This is because the nociceptors arising from muscles and joints (and viscera) at one spinal cord level share some common neural pathways to the brain. For example, a levator scapulae TrP typically refers pain along the posterior neck near the superior medial angle of the scapulae. The C4–C5 zygapophyseal joint has a referred pain pattern that also encompasses the posterior neck and upper trapezius/levator scapulae region. Spinal nerves at the C4–C5 spinal cord level innervate the levator scapulae. The logical conclusion is that referred pain is perceived not according to what tissue (muscle or joint) is causing the nociceptive input, but according to which *spinal nerves* are stimulated and the nature of their *segmental spinal cord interconnections.*

TrP Referral Zones

Knowledge of the key low back TrPs and their associated myofascial referred pain patterns (Table 9–1) can greatly aide the clinician in the differential diagnosis of low back pain syndromes. The deep, aching nature of muscle pain in many ways overlaps with a similar quality of joint pain, which is also poorly localized. It is again quite likely that many painful low back conditions represent a *composite referred pain pattern* consisting of both muscle and joint nociceptive input. TrPs in many low back muscles may cause the symptoms of low back pain and/or associated referred myofascial pain into the buttock, groin, or leg. TrPs in the upper lumbar erector spinae muscles, for example, may cause referred pain and tenderness in the tissues overlying the lower lumbar zygapophyseal and sacroiliac joints. The unwary clinician who merely palpates these tissues and observes localized tenderness can erroneously assume that this tenderness is caused by underlying zygapophyseal or sacroiliac joint dysfunction.

Referred Pain and Other Centrally Mediated Phenomena

The phenomenon of *referred pain*[26] may occur chiefly at the level of the spinal cord due to *sensory convergence.* Figure 9–2 shows an enlarged view of the spinal cord with sensory fibers arising from segmentally related

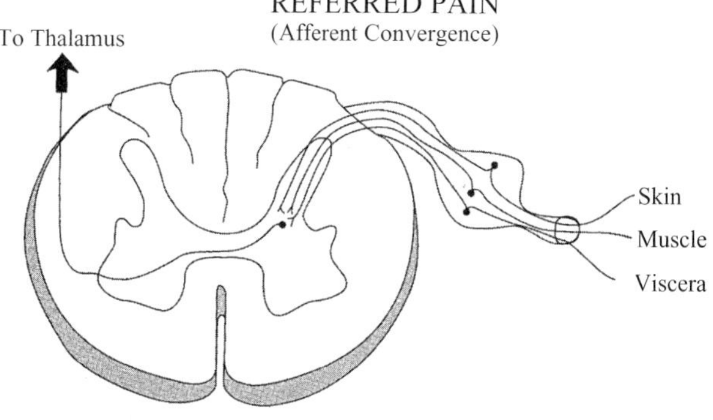

FIGURE 9–2. The sensory afferent convergence model of referred pain. Multiple sensory afferents synapse on a single spinothalamic projection neuron, which "confuses" the sensory cortex of the brain as to the actual source of the nociceptive input. The resulting sensation is referred pain to an area distal to the painful myofascial TrP.

muscles, joints, and viscera. Notice how the three incoming sensory axons synapse on one spinothalamic neuron, which travels up to the thalamus and cortex to trigger the perception of "pain." According to this simple *convergence projection theory*,[35] referred pain occurs as a result of this convergence of several (sensory afferent) neurons onto a single projection (spinothalamic) neuron. The brain cannot theoretically differentiate between the sensory input from the various receptors in the various peripheral tissues, leading to the phenomenon of referred pain. This would explain the previously discussed issue of muscle and joint pain causing similar or overlapping referred pain phenomena, based upon similar innervation from the same spinal cord level.

However, there are other neurological mechanisms at play that may cause even more interesting clinical phenomena, such as *hyperalgesic zones*, *referred tenderness*, and *autonomic reactions*. The sequelae of these scenarios include increased skin sensitivity and increased pain upon palpation and reactions that include altered pilomotor and sudomotor responses, respectively. In chronic situations such as long-standing TrPs in a muscle, the repeated activation of the chemical nociceptors (small C fibers) causes these axons to release *substance P* and other neuropeptides at their synapses in the dorsal horn of the spinal cord. Substance P is highly excitatory, and lowers the threshold for excitation of projection neurons and spinal interneurons in the cord. Once the dorsal horn interneurons become hyperexcitable, they may be activated by a lesser degree of sensory stimulation, a process called *spinal windup*, leading to a situation or phenomenon known as *central sensitization*.[44]

Clinical Pearl: The phenomenon of referred pain may occur chiefly at the level of the spinal cord because of sensory convergence. Other interesting clinical phenomena such as hyperalgesic zones, referred tenderness, and autonomic reactions may also be related to sensory spillover in the spinal cord.

With a state of central sensitization, increased excitability of dorsal horn neurons can lead to a number of clinically observed phenomena noted above. The incoming sensory input from mild to moderate palpatory pressure applied to the skin over the referred pain zone may trigger the perception of "pain," owing to lowered threshold for activation of spinal interneurons in the presence of central sensitization. These are seen clinically as *hyperalgesic zones*[30] or areas of *referred tenderness*,[45] both of which can be traced back to central sensitization of the segmental dorsal horn neurons. For example, quadratus lumborum TrPs typically cause referred pain into the buttock. After some time, the buttock may actually become tender to light palpation, exhibiting hyperalgesia and referred tenderness. The patient will be fooled into believing that the primary problem is in the buttock, because it is literally tender to the touch; yet this tenderness merely represents a "neurological illusion" of primary pain in that area of referred pain.

Various autonomic phenomena can also be associated with sensitization of spinal cord interneurons, some of which synapse in the lateral horn of the thoracic and upper lumbar spinal cord levels. The lateral horn is the location of all the *preganglionic sympathetic* neurons, and stimulation of these neurons will lead to segmentally related sympathetic responses such as pilomotor ("goosebumps") reactions, vasodilation (flushing) or vasoconstriction (blanching), sudomotor (sweat gland activation), etc. Many clinicians have empirically observed and discussed these autonomic phenomena associated with joint dysfunction and spinal manipulation/mobilization. Travell and Simons reported that these autonomic phenomena are often associated with myofascial TrP activity in certain muscles.

In summary, stimulation of chemical nociceptors causes most types of clinically observed muscle pain. The pain associated with myofascial TrPs is thought to be due to biochemical exudates secondary to the localized ischemic "energy crisis" in an area of focal muscle dysfunction. When nociceptive impulses become chronic, or of sufficient strength and intensity, they are likely to cause various neurological reflexes to occur, including referred pain patterns, referred tenderness, central sensitization, spinal windup, and possibly sympathetic responses. The next section will review the myofascial referred pain patterns of key low back and lower extremity muscles that are implicated in many cases of low back pain and pseudoradicular symptoms.

THE TrP PHENOMENON: THEORETICAL ASPECTS

Over the past 50 years, a plethora of hypotheses and theories have surfaced which claim to provide mechanisms by which muscles develop discrete TrPs. One of the oldest theories implicates a vicious *pain–spasm–pain cycle*.[25] Nociceptive stimuli from a TrP causes reflex activation of alpha motor neurons back to the same muscle, causing further irritation and spasm within the area of the TrP and completing the vicious cycle.

A corollary to the above theory was the idea that various biochemical exudates build up in the region of the TrP, causing sensitization of nociceptors, as well as reflex vasoconstriction that contributes to focal ischemia. Therefore, the *composite theory*[21,45] reasons that overactivity of spastic muscle fibers in an ischemic environment would lead to a focal stasis of muscle metabolites such as bradykinins, hyaluronic acid, and other chemical irritants known to stimulate nociceptors. Nociceptive input to the spinal cord leads to reflex motor changes, which leads to more nociception to complete the vicious cycle.

Many clinicians over the years empirically observed clinical success in eliminating TrPs and their associated referred pain patterns by various methods of manual pressure applied directly over the TrP nodules. In keeping with these theories about the pain–spasm–pain cycle and stasis of biochemicals within the TrP, it has been suggested that the clinical success of these manual techniques was due to two basic mechanisms of action. First, it is believed that deep manual pressure may cause hyperstimulation of nociceptors, which results in reflex inhibition of motor neuron activity, and eventual breakdown of the vicious pain–spasm–pain cycle.[25]

Secondly, it has been suggested that the reflex vasodilation observed over the skin following application of deep pressure methods is evidence of similar vasodilation in the deeper muscle fibers, which "flushes out" the accumulated noxious biochemical metabolites in the area of the TrP. Ridding the local TrP area of these chemical exudates would decrease the irritation of local nociceptors and thereby reduce pain.

Energy Crisis (Focal Ischemia) Hypothesis

Simons put forth a more current and comprehensive theory about the metabolic and biochemical dysfunction that accompanies the TrP phenomenon, to which he has applied the term *energy crisis hypothesis*.[21] This theory holds that the TrP nodule represents a focal area of muscular incoordination in which a circumscribed set of sarcomeres become "stuck," by virtue of persistent locking of a focal group of actin–myosin myofilaments. Muscle contraction occurs when calcium ions are released from the muscle membrane causing the initiation of actin–myosin cross-bridges. During muscle relaxation, these cross-bridges are broken when the calcium ions are pumped back into the muscle membrane, which requires energy supplied by ATP. Therefore, a lack of ATP due to decreased blood flow or ischemia in the region of the TrP could conceivably cause dysfunction of this "calcium pump" and lead to problems with release of actin–myosin cross-bridges. This could explain the focal nature of the TrP nodule as being an area of contracted sarcomeres.

The energy crisis hypothesis also suggests that in the presence of focal ischemia, blood oxygen levels will be reduced to the muscle tissue. This would lead to accumulation of various metabolites such as lactic acid, owing to a shift from aerobic to anaerobic metabolism as the body attempts to produce ATP molecules needed to release the contracted sarcomeres. As this anaerobic metabolic process continues, noxious metabolites continue to sensitize the local free nerve endings causing the pain and hyperalgesia that is clinically found over TrPs. Since the anaerobic metabolic pathway cannot produce as many ATP molecules as the aerobic Kreb's cycle, a vicious cycle of ischemic oxygen debt and anaerobic metabolism will perpetuate itself. Incidentally, these ischemic tissues lead to the realization over the past few years that the commonly used TrP treatment term *ischemic compression* is incorrect (see *"TrP Pressure Release" versus "Ischemic Compression"* below).

Sciotti et al. published some preliminary data that both supports and refutes various aspects of this energy crisis hypothesis. Using a microdialysis technique in the TrPs of upper trapezius muscles of human volunteers, they have found evidence of a disturbance in the local metabolic milieu and regionalized blood flow in TrP nodules. Interstitial lactate levels were found to be consistently elevated about 30% greater in the interstitium around TrPs when compared to control upper trapezius muscle tissue.[46] However, they have also reported a consistent finding of a paradoxical *increase* in local blood flow in the region of TrPs, compared to the contralateral normal muscle tissue.[47] One explanation for this seeming paradox is that these data may reflect an intrinsic self-protection mechanism, in which an attempt is being made to compensate for the perceived local ischemia by increasing local blood flow. Again, these data are quite preliminary and may not be considered definitive confirmation of an ischemic TrP model at this time.

The energy crisis theory fits in nicely with some clinically observed phenomena. First, most manual soft-tissue techniques involve some deep pressure or type of gliding/stripping massage, which typically causes reactive reflex vasodilation soon after the manual technique has been applied. Massage therapists are used to explaining to their clients that massage helps to increase blood flow through muscles, thereby "washing away" lactic acid and other noxious chemicals.[24] This is the explanation also used to explain the therapeutic benefit of heating pads, saunas, and hot showers for the treatment of sore and painful muscles. It is quite possible that manual massage and heat do indeed increase regional blood flow through the area of muscle tissue being treated, thereby bringing fresh oxygen to the area and restoring normal aerobic metabolism. Likewise, increased venous and lymphatic drainage from the region of the TrP may actually "wash out" noxious metabolic substances such as lactic acid.

The energy crisis hypothesis could also be used to explain how other and adjunctive modalities such as ultrasound, microcurrent stimulation, and needle injection are therapeutically beneficial in relieving TrPs. Ultrasound has both thermal and nonthermal effects; the thermal effects basically perform the same metabolic function as deep heat. The nonthermal effects include a micromassage effect on cells and interstitial fluids, as well as increased ATP synthesis by mitochondria in the cells stimulated by low-level ultrasound.[48] Microcurrent electrical stimulation is also noted to stimulate increased cellular ATP synthesis,[49] by mechanisms that are not completely understood.

"TrP Pressure Release" versus "Ischemic Compression"

Many types of manual pressure techniques have surfaced over the years that all involve the application of some type of static pressure directly over TrP nodules. As noted earlier in this chapter, the term *ischemic compression* is no longer considered an accurate description for these various types of manual pressure. The term ischemic compression was based on the conceptual model that deep pressure held statically for up to 2 minutes would create an ischemic "nerve block" by depriving the nociceptors around the TrP of oxygen and thereby disrupting the pain–spasm–pain cycle.

However, in light of Simons' more current energy crisis model[21,45] describing the TrP as an area of focal ischemia, it is now thought that deep manual pressure has an alternative mechanism of action. After all, what is the point of producing ischemia to an already ischemic TrP? Instead, compression causing hyperstimulation of nociceptors with reflex motor inhibition and reflex vasodilation are alternative theories for the benefits of manual pressure techniques. For this reason, the recommended use of a new term "TrP pressure release" is preferred over the outdated "ischemic compression" to describe the direct manual pressure techniques used to release TrPs and taut bands.[45]

Clinical Pearl: The term "ischemic compression" is being replaced from the soft tissue literature by the new term "TrP pressure release" to describe any manual technique that involves application of focal pressure over TrP nodules.

The MS Hypothesis and Other Neurological Mechanisms

Although the energy crisis hypothesis helps explain many of the clinical features of the TrP phenomenon, it does not address the CNS and its control over muscle tissue. Massage therapists have been taught over the years that an area of ischemic muscle tissue is a source of pain generation that evokes spinal cord reflexes, leading to increased motor nerve output to the muscle, which irritates the muscle further and leads to a vicious cycle of "pain–spasm–pain."[24,25] Essentially, this theory relies on an energy crisis model leading to a neurological dysfunction model of, and ultimately to, muscle dysfunction and pain; as one explores the neurological aspects of muscle dysfunction and the TrP phenomenon, some apparent discrepancies begin to surface.

It is known from basic science animal research that TrPs can be palpated in peripheral muscles in which the sensory and motor nerves have been surgically severed, effectively denervating the muscle from the CNS.[50] If the nerve supply to a muscle has been completely abolished, and TrP activity in that muscle continues, how can one evoke a pain–spasm–pain cycle as the underlying mechanism? Travell reports palpation of TrPs in some patients *after death*, until the time that rigor mortis made palpation for TrPs impossible[6] (J.G. Travell, personal communication, 1992). Therefore, in order to explain these seeming paradoxes about TrP phenomenon, it becomes necessary to extend beyond a simplistic pain–spasm–pain model.

Since motor nerves control muscles, it would seem logical to look at EMG data to provide us with clues about how the nervous system participates in muscle dysfunction and TrP formation. It may come as a surprise to learn that muscles that contain TrPs do not necessarily exhibit any increased *surface* EMG activity. However, *fine needle* EMG studies have clearly found specific and localized regions of increased electrical activity directly within TrP nodules, but not in the taut band outside of the discrete TrP region.[14] Although the TrP itself is a potent source of EMG spikes of spontaneous electrical activity (SEA), surface EMG shows no proportional increased electrical activity of the muscle in which the TrP resides. However, when fine needle electrodes are left inserted into upper trapezius TrPs and adjacent nonaffected muscle fibers in patients subjected to psychological stress, the TrPs exhibit increased SEA but the adjacent tissue remained electrically silent.[16]

Hubbard and Berkoff[14] were the first to demonstrate this spontaneous EMG activity within TrPs, while at the same time failing to show any increased EMG activity in the taut band or adjacent muscle tissue. They interpreted these findings as evidence that *MS dysfunction* was the culprit, and suggested that sympathetic and/or gamma motor pathways were responsible for causing this extremely localized contraction of muscle tissue known as the TrP. They further suggested that traumatic damage to a small number of MS might set in motion dysfunction of a specific set of muscle fibers around the area of the damaged spindles.[15] Why such a focal set of MS would become dysfunctional when the remaining tissues remain normal is still an open question.

Clinical Pearl: One extremely important consideration is whether or not TrPs represent some type of *primary* biomechanical shortening of muscle tissue, or rather some type of *secondary* neurological reflex phenomenon.

One very interesting finding is that TrPs are invariably found in the mid-belly portion of skeletal muscles, and often directly within the motor end-plate zone.[51] According to the current theory put forth by Simons,[45,52] TrPs form in the area of muscle tissue directly near neuromuscular junctions or motor end plates. It is in this area of the muscle where the terminal endings of alpha motor neurons interface with skeletal muscle, and initiate depolarization of the sarcolemmal membrane causing muscle contraction.[26] Simons proposes that repeated release of acetylcholine at the neuromuscular junction causes a focal area of ischemia[21,45] ("energy crisis") to develop in which localized actin–myosin cross-links cannot be released due to inadequate ATP stores. In this sense, Simons' model conceptualizes the TrP "knot" as a focal area of myofibrils that have been mechanically bound together as a type of functional *contracture*, not neural-mediated hypertonicity.

Spondylogenic Reflex Syndrome

The concept of the nervous system as a contributor of TrP formation is intriguing and may explain many empirical observations made by clinicians who have noted a relationship between the axial skeleton and peripheral soft tissues that cannot be explained by a simple radicular model. The term *spondylogenic reflex syndrome* was promulgated by Dvorak, Dvorak and coworkers,[53,54] to describe reflex relationships between specific joints of the axial skeleton and peripheral muscles and soft tissues. The concept is that faulty joint position or motion (segmental dysfunction) will cause reflexogenic changes in muscle tone and possible trophic changes in other soft tissues. This is the basis for the various reflex zones of referred tenderness or hyperalgesia known as "hyperalgesic zones,"[4,30] "paravertebral points" described by Maigne,[55] so-called periosteal points,[56] and the "tender points" discussed in the strain–counterstrain system.[37]

One extremely important consideration is whether or not TrPs represent some type of primary biomechanical shortening of muscle tissue, or rather some type of secondary neurological reflex phenomenon. If TrPs are indeed merely focal areas of muscle tightness or contracture, then they should not go away without a focal treatment such as injection, deep manual pressure, or stripping massage techniques. Yet many clinicians have empirically noticed that TrPs and taut bands do go away with various reflex techniques such as PIR, facet joint manipulation, and joint positioning techniques. In these cases where the TrP itself was never directly treated, one must consider that the muscle tone was changed via neurological reflexes. Even in the case of manual techniques applied directly over TrPs, the results of such focal pressure or stripping may do more than merely "pull apart" tight muscle tissue; they may have a neurological mechanism of action.

Clinical Pearl: . . . Janda's use of the term *muscle incoordination* to describe myofascial TrPs seems to be quite appropriate.

One possibility to consider is that TrPs may initially form due to neurological reflex overactivation of a focal set of myofilaments, which at some point become perpetually "locked" through the energy crisis model proposed by Simons. Once an intense ischemic condition has developed, and a shift to anaerobic metabolism has occurred, the TrP nodule may persist because of failure of the actin–myosin myofilaments to release from one another. At this point in the process, it would no longer require the nervous system's active participation in the process of maintaining the TrP nodule. This theory would explain the apparently paradoxical nature of EMG activity within the TrP and taut band, the animal studies in which the spinal nerves were severed, and even Travell's finding of TrP nodules in fresh cadavers. Tsai et al.[57] report an interesting case of a patient with infectious sacroiliitis who developed gluteal TrPs on the ipsilateral side of the sacroiliitis, presumably because of some type of somato-somato reflex activity. Once the infection was healed, the TrP activity did not go away until treated by focal needle injection.

In conclusion, Janda's use of the term *muscle incoordination*[9] to describe myofascial TrPs seems to be quite appropriate. It appears that a particular subset of muscle fibers within the taut band and TrP "knot" is somehow functionally incoordinated from the remainder of the fibers within the muscle belly. There are clear differences of EMG activity noted within the TrP nidus, the adjacent taut band, and surrounding normotonic muscle tissue. In addition, biochemical analysis of the interstitial fluids found within the TrP region is clearly different from surrounding muscle tissue. Unfortunately, many of the previously discussed theories about the formation of TrPs are just that: *theories*. The truth regarding the true underlying mechanisms of the TrP phenomenon remains unclear, and clearly this is an area ripe for further basic science research.

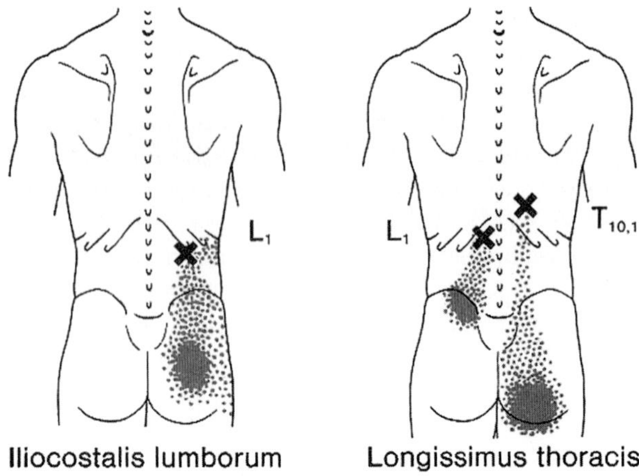

FIGURE 9–3. The thoracolumbar erector spinae mass consists of two muscles, the longissimus and the iliocostalis. Note how TrPs in the upper lumbar/lower thoracic region cause referred pain over the lower lumbar and sacroiliac joint regions. (Reproduced with permission from Travell and Simons, 1992)

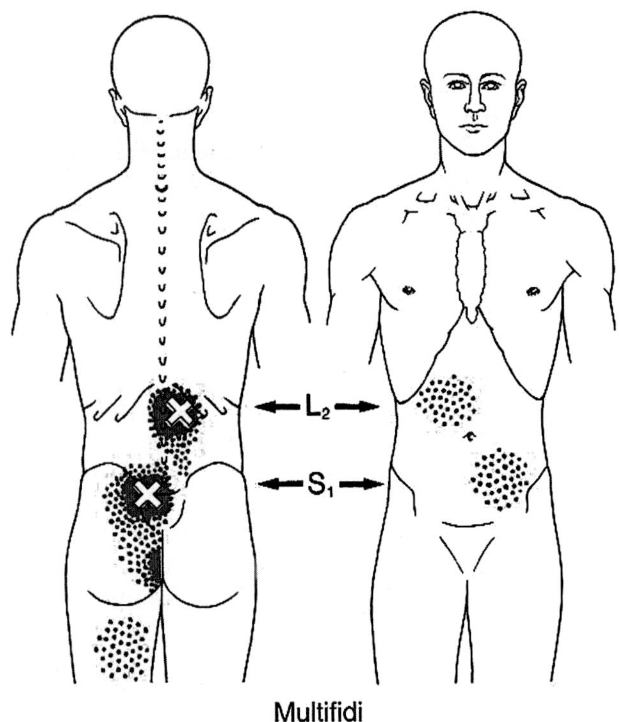

FIGURE 9–4. The thoracolumbar multifidi tend to refer pain to the spinous process at the same level as the TrP, although lumbar TrPs may also refer pain to the ipsilateral anterior abdominal region at the same level. Sacral region TrPs can refer pain to the coccygeal region. (Reproduced with permission from Travell and Simons, 1992)

MYOFASCIAL REFERRED PAIN PATTERNS OF KEY MUSCLES

It is impossible within one textbook chapter to provide an in-depth explanation of the various aspects of muscle dysfunction that may accompany each type of low back pain. However, for the purpose of brevity and clarity, it is possible to provide an overview of key muscles associated with low back syndromes and their respective referred myofascial pain patterns. Figures 9–3 to 9–20 present key lumbopelvic muscles associated with myofascial pain and their respective referral zones. The clinical importance and remembering each muscle's specific referred pain patterns cannot be overstated. Please be aware that chronic MPS frequently involves several muscles, and so an overlap of referral zones is not unusual and should be anticipated.

For a complete and comprehensive treatise on focal muscle dysfunction, TrPs, and the myofascial pain patterns implicated in low back and lower extremity pain, the reader is referred to the two-volume textbook series by Travell and Simons.[7,45] The first edition of Volume 2 addresses the lumbar spine and lower extremity muscles.[7] The second edition of Volume 1 provides updated information on the etiology and treatment for MPS and addresses the abdominothoracic diaphragm, a muscle that has gained recent notoriety in the understanding of the pressurized canister covered in Chapter 5.

Clinical Pearl: Figures 9–3 to 9–20 present key lumbopelvic muscles associated with myofascial pain and their respective referral zones. The clinical

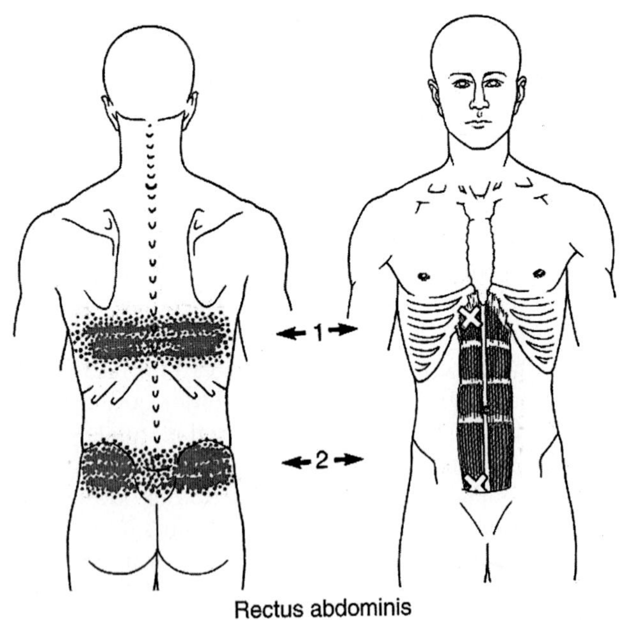

FIGURE 9–5. The rectus abdominis, although located on the anterior side of the body, has an unusual myofascial referred pain pattern horizontally across the lumbar region. Note that upper recti TrPs refer pain across the thoracolumbar region, and lower recti TrPs refer pain across the lower lumbar region. (Reproduced with permission from Travell and Simons, 1992)

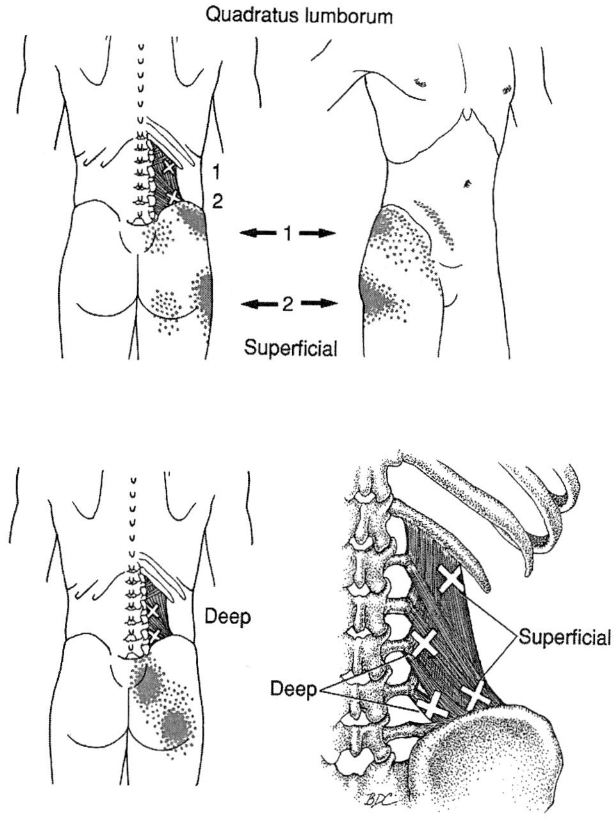

FIGURE 9–6. The quadratus lumborum (QL) consists of superficial and deep fibers. TrPs in the superficial fibers refer pain into the regions of the lateral iliac crest and trochanter, whereas TrPs in the deep QL fibers predominantly refer pain over the sacroiliac joint and into the lower buttock regions. (Reproduced with permission from Travell and Simons, 1992)

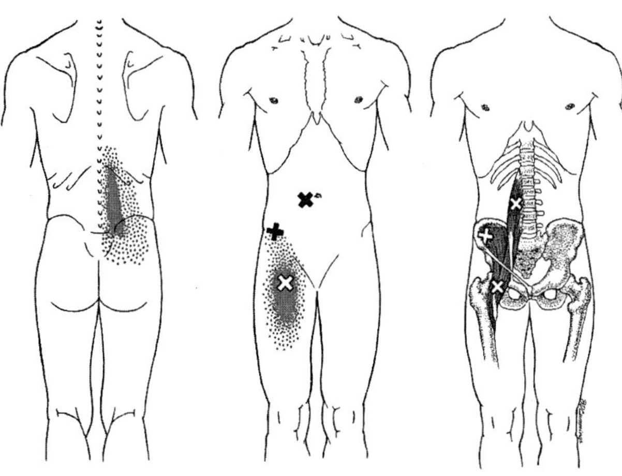

FIGURE 9–7. The iliopsoas is really three separate muscles, the psoas major, the psoas minor, and the iliacus. However, both psoas muscles can be functionally integrated regarding myofascial pain. TrPs in the psoas refer pain longitudinally along the ipsilateral lumbar spine and TrPs in the iliacus (and distal psoas) refer pain into the anterior thigh and groin, which may mimic L3 radiculopathy. (Reproduced with permission from Travell and Simons, 1992)

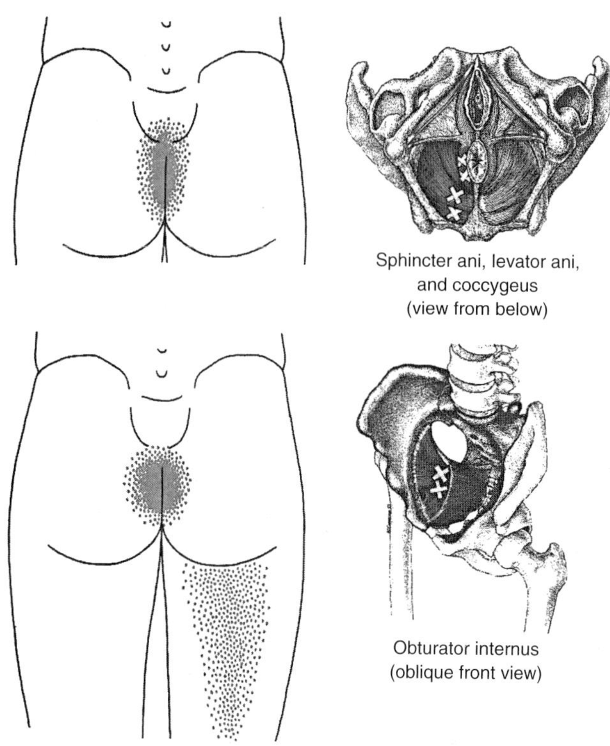

FIGURE 9–8. Muscles of the pelvic floor include the coccygeus, levator ani, and obturator internus. TrPs in these muscles refer pain over the sacrum and coccyx, and occasionally into the posterior thigh. (Reproduced with permission from Travell and Simons, 1992)

importance and remembering each muscle cannot be overstated. Please be aware that chronic MPS frequently involves several muscles, and so an overlap of referral zones is not unusual and should be anticipated.

Referred and Local TrP Pain

Various types of neurological reflex phenomena are associated with myofascial TrPs. Most important is the *characteristic pattern* of referred pain for each skeletal muscle in the human body.[7,45] These patterns of *myofascial referred pain* are amazingly consistent among

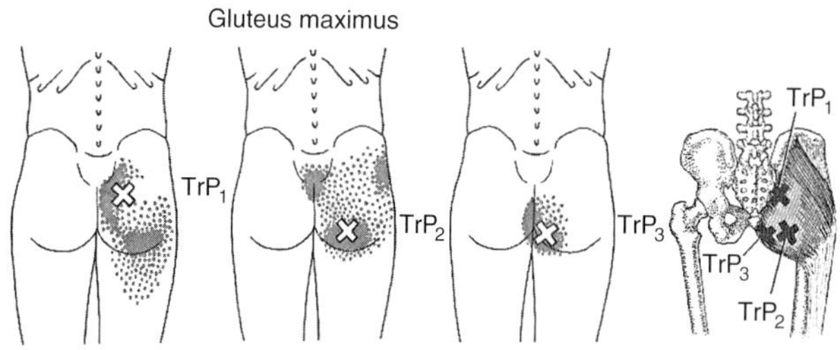

FIGURE 9–9. Gluteus maximus TrPs may refer pain anywhere in the ipsilateral buttock, over the sacrum, and sacroiliac joint. (Reproduced with permission from Travell and Simons, 1992)

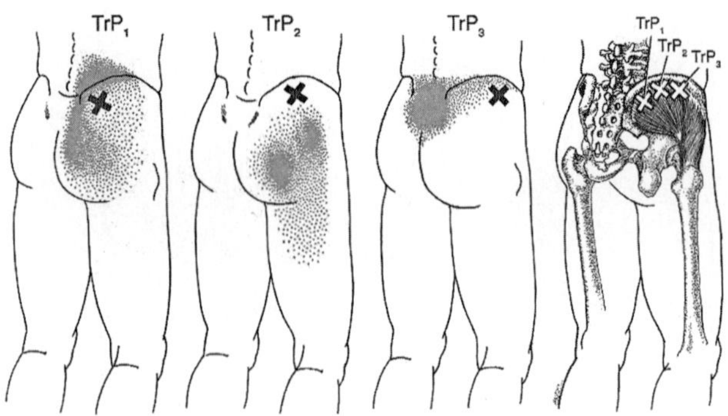

FIGURE 9–10. Gluteus medius TrPs cause intense referred pain over the ipsilateral sacroiliac joint, sacral base, and lower lumbar facet joints. (Reproduced with permission from Travell and Simons, 1992)

patient populations, and serve as important diagnostic criteria similar to the dermatomal patterns seen with inflamed nerve roots and the *scleratogenous* referred pain patterns seen with inflamed joints, discs, and ligaments. Various wall charts have been published which depict these myofascial referred pain patterns in vivid color for patient education.[58] It is not unusual in the clinical setting to walk into an examination room and have a patient exclaim, "That's it! That's my problem right here!" as they are found pointing to a particular TrP and its associated color-coded referred pain pattern on the wall chart.

Practically speaking, lumbopelvic myofascial pain can be separated into two categories: muscles that refer pain *locally* to the lumbar and buttock region, and those that refer pain *distally* into various parts of the

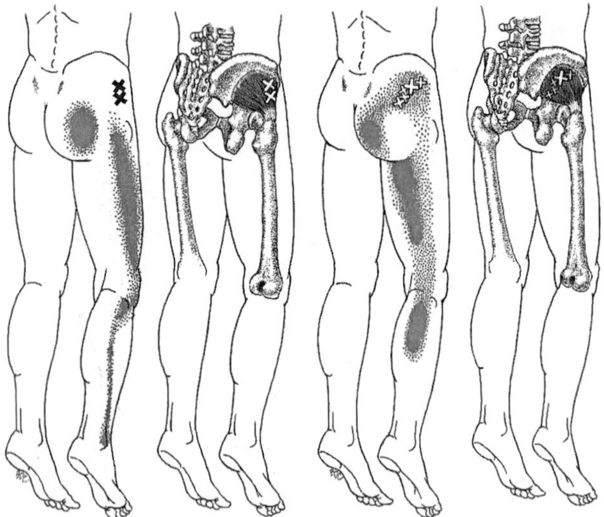

FIGURE 9–11. The gluteus minimus may contain TrPs in the *midbelly* that refer pain down the posterior thigh, or in the *anterior* belly that refer pain along the lateral thigh. These referred pain patterns may mimic S1 or L5 radiculopathy. (Reproduced with permission from Travell and Simons, 1992)

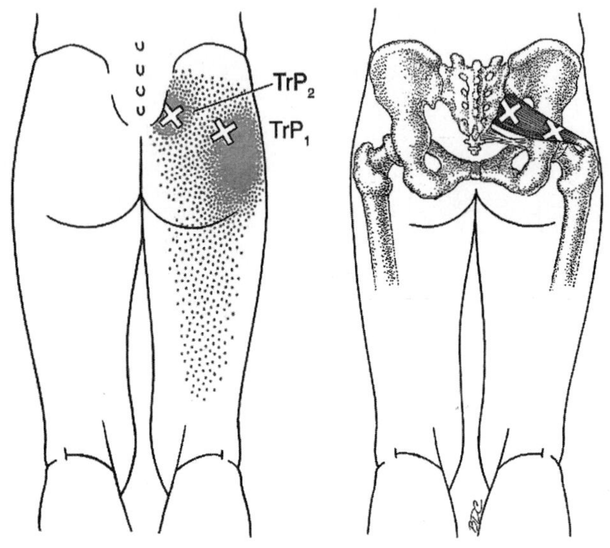

FIGURE 9–12. The piriformis may contain TrPs that cause referred pain deep into the ipsilateral buttock and along the posterior thigh. (Reproduced with permission from Travell and Simons, 1992)

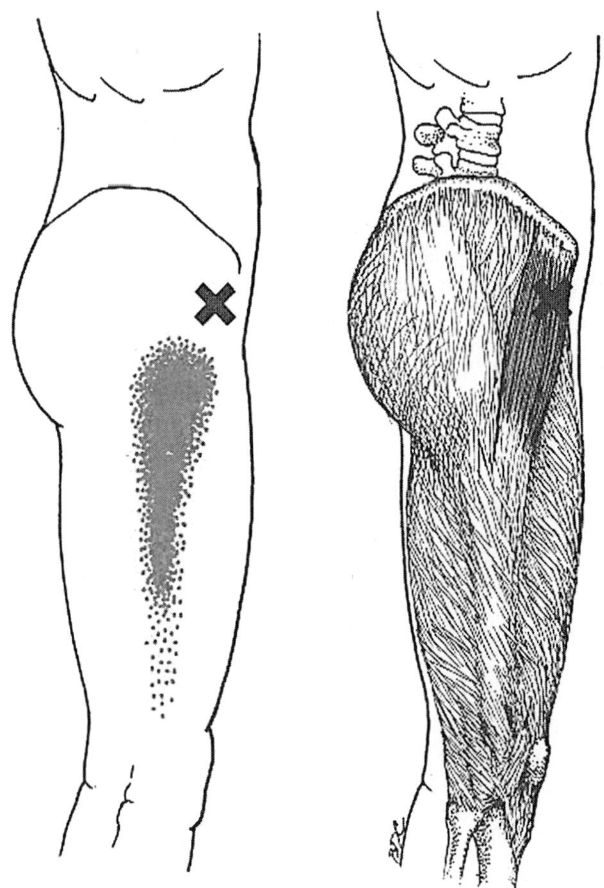

FIGURE 9–13. TrPs in the tensor fascia lata are found just lateral to the anterior superior iliac spine (not the lateral thigh), and refer pain along the lateral thigh within the proximal L5 dermatome. (Reproduced with permission from Travell and Simons, 1992)

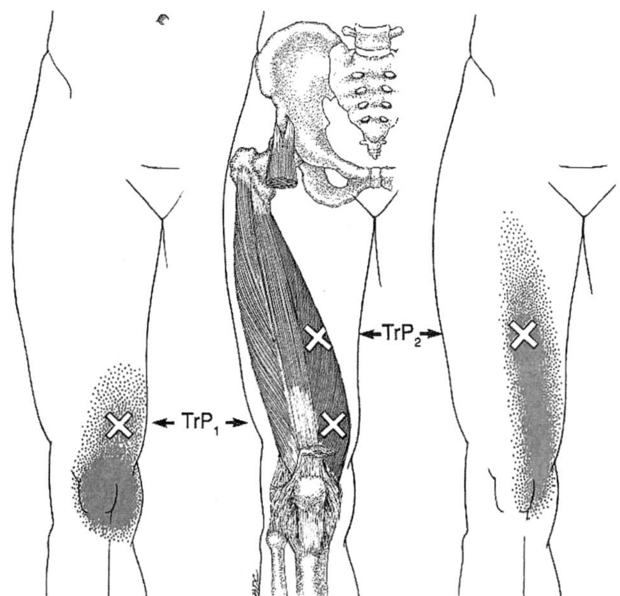

FIGURE 9–14. Vastus medialis TrPs may refer pain to the patella and medial knee, or cause a more diffuse referred pain pattern over the anteromedial thigh mimicking an L3 radiculopathy. (Reproduced with permission from Travell and Simons, 1992)

lower extremity. These latter referred pain patterns may mimic the symptoms of a lumbar radiculopathy; hence, the term for this clinical scenario is a *pseudoradicular* syndrome.[8,30]

Table 9–1 provides an overview of key myofascial pain patterns of the lumbopelvic musculature. This table includes the myofascial referred pain patterns and the associated muscles that cause local lumbar

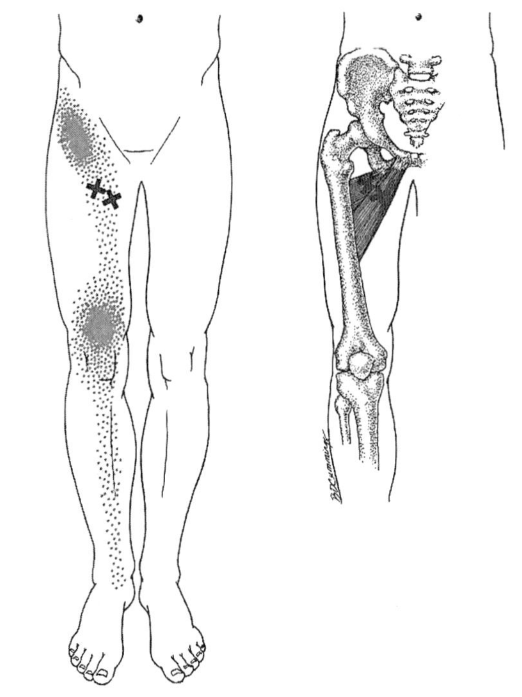

FIGURE 9–16. Adductor longus and brevis TrPs refer pain into the ipsilateral groin and along the anteromedial thigh mimicking an L3 dermatomal pattern. (Reproduced with permission from Travell and Simons, 1992)

and buttock pain and also those muscles whose TrPs refer pain into the lower extremity, causing so-called *pseudoradicular symptoms*. An in-depth understanding of these myofascial referred pain patterns is considered to be vital for the differential diagnosis of low back syndromes.

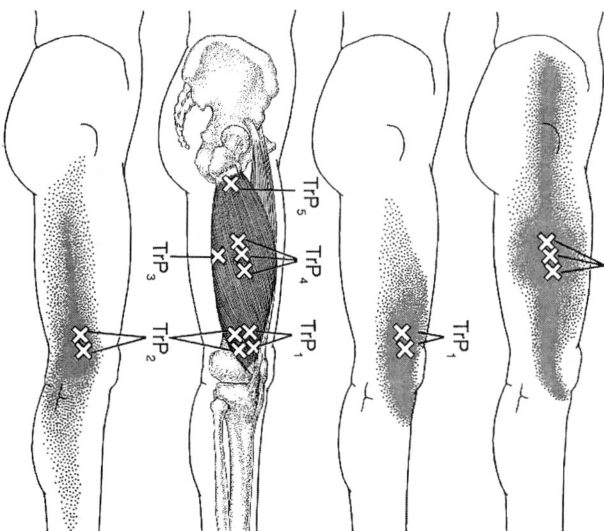

FIGURE 9–15. Vastus lateralis TrPs can be found anywhere along the lateral thigh muscle mass, and refer pain along the lateral thigh mimicking an L5 dermatomal pattern. (Reproduced with permission from Travell and Simons, 1992)

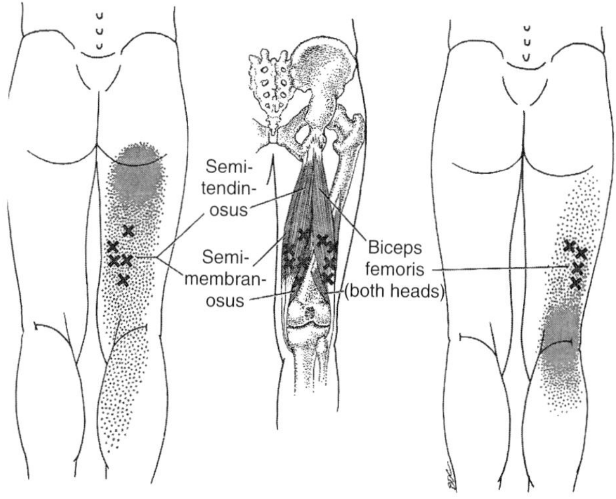

FIGURE 9–17. The hamstring group consists of the medial semimembranosus and semitendinous, and the lateral biceps femoris. TrPs in any of these muscles may refer pain up into the region of the ischial tuberosity and lower buttock, or along the posterior thigh mimicking an S1 radiculopathy. (Reproduced with permission from Travell and Simons, 1992)

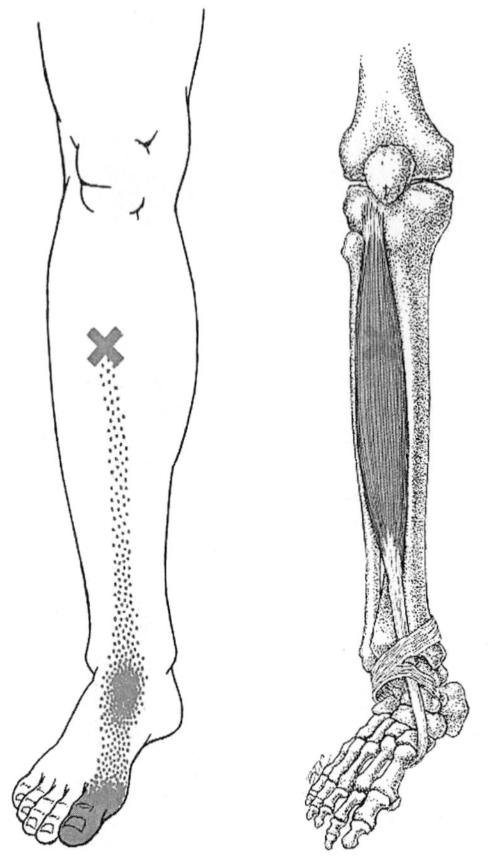

FIGURE 9–18. TrPs in the tibialis anterior cause referred pain along the distal anterior tibia, extending into the great toe, thus mimicking an L5 dermatomal pattern. (Reproduced with permission from Travell and Simons, 1992)

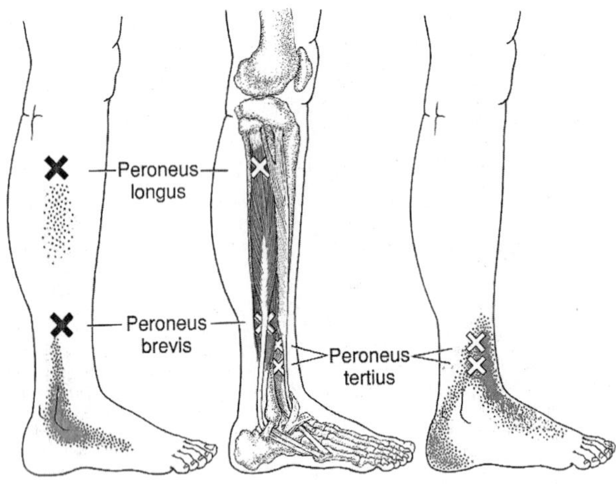

FIGURE 9–19. The peroneus longus, brevis, and tertius may contain TrPs that cause referred pain along the lateral lower leg into the lateral ankle, mimicking a distal L5 dermatomal pattern. (Reproduced with permission from Travell and Simons, 1992)

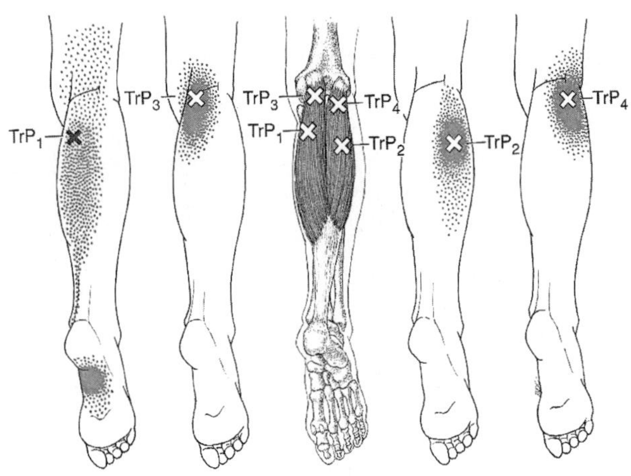

FIGURE 9–20. TrPs in the gastrocnemius cause referred pain in the region of the popliteal fossa and distally along the posterior lower leg into the sole of the foot, mimicking a distal S1 dermatomal pattern. (Reproduced with permission from Travell and Simons, 1992)

Various manual examination and treatment techniques for finding and eliminating myofascial TrPs and taut bands will be covered in subsequent chapters of this textbook, and therefore will not be included here. However, it is important to discuss the various clinical features of TrPs that distinguish these areas of focal muscle dysfunction from other types of global muscle tightness or weakness.

Clinical Pearl: Myofascial referred pain patterns are amazingly consistent and characteristic for each skeletal muscle. The key muscles involved with low back pain and their respective referred pain patterns are listed in Table 9–1.

CLINICAL FEATURES OF TrPs

As mentioned previously, myofascial TrPs usually develop in muscles that have been subjected to prolonged contraction, repetitive overuse, remained in a prolonged shortened position, or that have been injured by blunt trauma or overstretching (strain). TrPs may also develop in muscles whose tone has been altered secondary to somatosomatic and viscerosomatic reflex mechanisms (as previously discussed). In light of these factors, it is important to review some of the general clinical features of myofascial TrPs.

The first issue is the *character of pain* associated with myofascial pain disorders and TrPs. The type of pain perceived by patients with myofascial TrPs is typically poorly localized and of an aching nature. Rarely, if ever, does the patient with myofascial TrPs complain of sharp, localized pain. Nor do they complain of electrical shock-type sensations, shooting pains, numbness, or deep throbbing types of pain. Sharp localized

TABLE 9–1. **Common Myofascial Referred Pain Patterns**

Muscle	Myofascial Referred Pain Pattern
	Muscles That Cause Lumber and Buttock Pain
Thoracolumbar erector spinae	Local low back pain locally over TrP location. Referred pain over sacroiliac (SI) joint and superior buttock region.
Multifidi	Spinous processes at same level of TrP; ipsilateral abdominal lower quadrant; sacral TrPs refer pain to coccyx.
Quadratus lumborum	Superficial TrPs refer pain over iliac crest and greater trochanter; deep TrPs refer pain over SI joint and mid-lower buttock region.
Iliopsoas	Referred pain over ipsilateral erector spinae, ipsilateral groin, and anterior thigh.
Rectus abdominis	Referred pain horizonatally across lumbar region bilateraly.
Muscles of the pelvic floor (obturator internus, levator ani, coccygeus, etc.)	Referred pain over the sacrum, lower buttock, and proximal posterior thigh.
Gluteus maximus and medius	Gluteus maximus refers pain over SI joint and buttock; gluteus medius refers pain up into the lower lumbar region, over SI joint and sacrum, and mid-buttock.
	Muscles That Cause Pseudoradicular Symptoms (Hip, Thigh, and Leg Pain)
Gluteus minimus	Referred pain over lower buttocks, greater trochanter, posterolateral thigh and calf.
Piriformis (and other lateral hip rotators)	Referred pain over lower buttocks and posterior thigh; purported to entrap sciatic nerve and cause pseudo-sciatica.
Tensor fasciae latae	Referred pain over greater trochanter and lateral thigh.
Quadriceps femoris	Referred pain along anatomy of each muscle, i.e., vastus lateralis refers pain along lateral thigh.
Adductors longus, brevis, magnus	Referred pain along medial thigh and calf.
Hamstrings	Referred pain up toward ischium and down posterior thigh and calf.
Tibialis anterior	Referred pain along anterior lower leg to great toe.
Peroneii	Referred pain along lateral lower leg to lateral malleolus.
Gastrocnemius/soleus	Referred pain along posterior calf, heel, and plantar foot.

Source : From Travell and Simons.[6,7]

pain is more indicative of a specific zygapophyseal joint problem, intervertebral disc lesion, insertional tendonitis, or even bursitis. The exception to this comment is the localized pain that is felt over the TrP nodule *upon deep palpation*; however, the patient does not typically present to the clinic with this as a chief complaint.

Often the patient with myofascial pain will describe a *referred pain pattern*, which is quite characteristic to the experienced clinician, but quite confusing to the patient. He or she notices that the lower back and buttock region is sore and achy, but is unable to find the area of perceived pain while palpating the region. This is the hallmark of referred pain: the perception of pain in a body region that is anatomically distant from the pain generator. Of course, the patient may accidentally encounter some muscle "knots" that are very painful and tender, and reproduce some of the referred pain pattern.

MPS and Cold Sensitivity

Myofascial pain from TrPs is often provoked by cold temperature, such as air conditioning or cold drafts. Prolonged exposure to the cold during outdoor winter activities may likewise agitate underlying TrPs. The phenomenon of shivering while cold is the body's inherent mechanism for preserving heat; the frequent muscle contractions generate increased metabolic activity that generates heat. Any exposure to cold that causes a skeletal muscle to shiver or contract may provoke underlying TrPs to become painful and symptomatic. A patient living in an arctic region, for example, might report the acute onset of low back pain shortly after waiting outside in the wintertime for a bus, while wearing a winter jacket that did not cover his or her lower lumbar region. The office worker in an air-conditioned room with a vent directly over his or her right shoulder might develop an acute onset of upper trapezius TrP pain.

Conversely, patients with TrPs often report feeling better after being warmed by a hot shower, by use of a heating pad, or with an application of liniment. Athletes have found empirically that postexercise heat applications relieve muscle soreness. In addition, muscles feel more pliable and flexible after being heated and will stretch more easily, the underlying mechanism of which is likely due to changes in the thixotropic nature of myofascial tissues. The patient who reports pain relief with activities or warm environments may be describing myofascial pain from underlying TrPs.

Muscles that harbor TrPs are often painfully restricted from reaching their fully elongated position and/or may be inhibited from optimal contractile capacity or endurance. These symptoms are usually provoked as the patient attempts to use the muscle with TrPs, such as performance of lifting or bending when TrPs are present in the lumbar erector spinae, glutei, or multifidi.

Maintaining a muscle in a prolonged shortened state may also contribute to TrP formation, and also to the aggravation of existing TrPs. For example, the office worker who sits all day without using the backrest may overload the erector spinae, leading to muscular adaptive shortening. As the musculature adapts to this shortened position, it may develop discrete focal areas of shortening that lead to the birth of TrPs. This same office worker may also prefer to cross his or her legs routinely in one direction, and lean all of the body weight onto one buttock. In this position, one iliac crest is chronically elevated, allowing for shortening of the ipsilateral quadratus lumborum that may develop TrPs by a similar mechanism.

MPS: Five Defining Criteria

Simons and coworkers[45,52] have established five basic criteria for determining the presence of active or latent myofascial TrPs:

1. The presence of a painful muscle TrP "nodule"
2. Referred pain elicited upon digital examination of the TrP
3. A palpable taut band
4. A local twitch response elicited upon snapping the taut band
5. Verbal confirmation from the patient: "That's my pain"

The three minimum criteria necessary to make a diagnosis of myofascial pain are the presence of a palpable taut band in which a TrP nodule is found, accompanied by the patient's recognition of the pain pattern.

Clinical Pearl: The three minimum criteria necessary to make a diagnosis of myofascial pain are:

1. **presence of taut palpable band**
2. **TrP nodule within that band**
3. **patient recognition of pain pattern.**

FOCAL MUSCLE DYSFUNCTION: TAUT BANDS AND TrPs

As previously discussed, global muscle dysfunction and focal myofascial TrP activity are typically associated with any type of low back pain syndrome regardless of the primary pain generator. Therefore, clinicians must consider and examine the key muscles in Table 9–1 that are known to refer pain into the lumbar region, groin, buttocks, and lower extremity for the presence of myofascial TrPs that may be causing myofascial referred pain. This section will provide a more detailed discussion about how TrP nodules and taut bands are thought to develop as areas of focal muscle dysfunction.

Clinical expertise regarding assessment and treatment of myofascial pain requires clinical training that no textbook can teach. Nevertheless, an attempt to cover the key aspects of this topic is made in the hope of presenting a base of information from which one may grow. One should be forewarned that the palpatory aspects of myofascial assessment are less than pleasant for the patient, and distinctly challenging for the clinician in training.

One important clinical finding with myofascial pain is the presence of the tender TrP "nodule," or nidus, itself. In addition to a local pain response, a referred symptom such as pain may also be provoked. Clinicians experienced in assessment of TrPs routinely note that the palpable traits of the TrP nidus are unique.

Second, the nodules will be located within the stringy *taut bands* that encapsulate TrPs. The taut band represents a sort of intermediate zone of hypertonicity, demonstrating increased tone that is surrounding muscle tone, but less than the nidus. Of course, one tends to locate the nidus by first locating the larger taut band.

Third, vigorous cross-fiber palpation of the taut bands will elicit a *local twitch response*, which has been demonstrated to be a neurological reflex mediated at the spinal cord level. The importance of the twitch response, considered a pathognomonic finding for a TrP, cannot be overstated. The inexperienced clinician will roll over the muscle and erroneously believe that the target muscle rushed from underneath their finger during the end stage of the cross-fiber palpation. Only with repetition and slowing the technique will one learn that the muscle seems to rush at the same speed, regardless of how quickly or slowly the cross-fiber palpation occurs! Congratulations are in order, because the myofascial twitch response was just isolated and appreciated. Once this is understood, the clinician will have gained an invaluable diagnostic tool that will be utilized for the remainder of their clinical life. The manual examination chapter (Chapter 13) will address various techniques for assessing the twitch response based on regional morphological challenges.

Trigger Points versus Tender Points

Please note that the terms (and abbreviations) trigger point (TrP) and tender point (TeP) are not synonymous.[59] *Tender points (TeP)* are found in *fibromyalgia syndrome (FMS)*, a syndrome that will be discussed later in the chapter, and merely represent areas of cutaneous hyperalgesia. Biopsy studies of TePs have failed to show any specific abnormality of the myofascial tissues in the area of complaint.[60,61] This absence of any discernible tissue changes in TePs has led to the current theory that patients with FMS have a problem with CNS processing of pain, not a problem with their peripheral soft tissues.[44,62] *Trigger points (TrPs)* are found in *myofascial pain syndrome (MPS)*, and have shown specific biochemical and histological abnormalities upon needle aspiration and biopsy.[14,46] In addition, TrP nodules exhibit SEA upon needle EMG examination,[14] clearly defining them as areas of focal muscle dysfunction.

In contrast to TePs, TrPs have a very distinctive texture, like palpable small nodules or "muscle knots" found within a taut band of skeletal muscle tissue. As previously mentioned, the center of the TrP is known as the *nidus*. TePs do not exhibit any type of tissue texture change, and merely exhibit tenderness or hyperalgesia upon light palpation. For these and other reasons, it is important to recognize that the outdated abbreviation TP is no longer appropriate for usage in the scientific literature as it fails to differentiate between the TePs of FMS and the TrPs of MPS.[59] As such, it should also be removed from clinical charting and reporting and be replaced by the updated abbreviations TrP and TeP.

TrPs may be found in any skeletal muscle within the human body; however, muscles that are prone to repetitive overuse (microtrauma) or frank injury (macrotrauma) seem to be more likely to develop TrPs. Since the lumbar spine is one of the most commonly injured and painful musculoskeletal regions in the human body, TrP activity and muscular dysfunction are routinely found in the lumbopelvic musculature.

Active versus Latent TrPs

TrPs can have different properties and can therefore be subdivided and organized accordingly. One important scheme divides *active and latent TrPs*. Active TrPs are found in patients who have a current complaint of pain, which is reproduced by deep manual palpation over the offending TrP nodule. In short, *active* TrPs will cause *active symptoms* in a patient. *Latent* TrPs, on the other hand, may reside in muscles that are *not* actively causing any symptoms. Individuals do not typically perceive spontaneous pain or symptoms from latent TrPs at rest or during typical activities of daily living. However, while probing the muscles, the clinician finds a TrP nodule that is quite painful to the patient. The TrP is clearly present in the muscle tissue, but for some reason, it does not generate any pain or symptoms unless provoked by digital pressure.

Clinical Pearl: Please note that the terms (and abbreviations) trigger point (TrP) and tender point (TeP) are not synonymous.

Primary versus Secondary (Satellite) TrPs

TrPs are also classified as *primary* or *secondary*. A *primary* TrP is caused by direct trauma, repetitive overuse, or some other type of mechanical muscular strain, and is thought to act as a primary pain generator. *Secondary* TrPs, on the other hand, develop as a result of reflex neural phenomena and are often found in areas of referred pain from inflamed joints or other deep somatic tissues. They do *not* act as primary pain generators but *do* complicate musculoskeletal dysfunction. Secondary TrPs are also known as *satellite* TrPs because they often surround primary TrPs. Secondary or satellite TrPs may develop as a form of reflex motor dysfunction in the referred pain zones of primary TrPs, which further complicates the differential diagnosis of which muscle is the primary pain generator. While the subject of primary versus secondary TrPs may seem more academic than practical, such agreement on terminology allows for universal understanding of the today's concepts until further knowledge on the subject comes to light.

Clinical Pearl: Secondary or satellite TrPs may develop as a form of reflex motor dysfunction in the referred pain zones of primary TrPs.

Referred Tenderness and Autonomic Phenomena

Other curious reflex phenomena are *referred tenderness*, in which the area of referred pain is actually hyperalgesic or literally tender to palpation, and *autonomic phenomena* in which sympathetic reflex reactions previously addressed may occur in association with TrPs.[45] Referred tenderness can fool even the most astute clinician at times into erroneously believing this is an area of primary pain generation. For example, TrPs in the upper trapezius typically refer pain into the suboccipital region, which may cause tenderness and hyperalgesia over the suboccipital muscles. Inadvertently, a clinician may palpate this region and elicit a painful response from the patient. Solely on the basis of this pain response, the clinician may manipulate the upper cervical joints or perform soft tissue techniques on the suboccipital muscles, when in fact these tissues are not dysfunctional but merely regions of referred tenderness.

Some of these neurological reflex phenomena, especially referred tenderness and autonomic reflex reactions, may be the basis of many empirically derived "reflex point" approaches to treatment. In these systems, the clinicians understand that regions of referred tenderness are not areas of primary pain generation, but rather secondary mechanisms to a primary symptom generator, typically an irritated spinal or extremity joint, located elsewhere. This is likely the mechanism underlying the so-called "tender points" in strain–counterstrain technique,[37] the "paravertebral points" described by Maigne,[55] and the "zones of irritation" or "myotendinoses" described by Dvorak.[54] Various treatments for myofascial pain and TrPs will be addressed in later chapters, especially Chapter 23.

Reflex Motor Dysfunction

Another important clinical consequence of neurological reflexes involved with TrPs is the phenomenon of *reflex motor dysfunction*.[21,45] It appears that TrPs communicate with the CNS in such a way that muscle contraction is altered, thereby causing muscle dysfunction. This can be manifested as obvious inhibition of maximal muscular effort such as the buckling sensation of the knee with vastus medialis TrPs, or instability of one-legged standing with gluteus medius/minimus TrPs.

A TrP in one muscle may cause reflex facilitation of another muscle, typically within its referred pain zone. An interesting example is described by Mense and Simons,[18] in which they monitored EMG activity over the deltoid and upper trapezius muscles, while a painful TrP was palpated in the ipsilateral infraspinatus muscle. Irritation of the infraspinatus TrP by deep palpation caused *increased* EMG activity in the deltoid, but not the upper trapezius, indicating some type of selective *somato-somato* reflex activity between the infraspinatus and deltoid muscles.

TrP TREATMENT: INJECTIONS VERSUS "DRY NEEDLING"

Several chapters of this textbook will address various aspects of management of MPS. Notably, Chapter 23 will discuss several manual approaches for treatment of this fascinating and complex topic. Nevertheless, a brief discussion regarding manual reflex techniques was already presented in order to present relevant material pertaining to this chapter. In the same manner, minimally invasive therapeutic interventions for MPS will be covered here.

Needle injection of TrPs has been used for years with clinical success for the treatment of TrPs, and was popularized by Travell and Simons who espoused the use of procaine as the preferred injectate. Travell utilized procaine, not because of any specific therapeutic effect on the TrP, but rather because it was found to reduce postinjection soreness in her patients compared to other medications (J.G. Travell, personal communication, 1992). They did, however, warn of the use of long-lasting steroid injections into TrPs, considering these to be contraindicated medications.

Several studies have looked at the clinical effectiveness of various injected substances such as corticosteroids, anesthetics, saline solution, and even "dry needling" in which no substance was injected,[63] although longer postinjection soreness period has been reported with "dry needling." No significant differences in clinical effectiveness have been observed between injecting various medications, saline, or "dry needling" TrPs, which spawned the current opinion that it does not matter whether or not any substance is injected into TrPs, but rather the effect of the needle itself on the TrP. Lewit published an excellent review article[64] entitled "The needle effect in the relief of myofascial pain," which clearly discusses this issue in detail.

A recent trend in medicine is the injection of the clostridium botulinum toxin, called Botox, into TrPs. This toxin has its effect on the neuromuscular junction, where it competes for the acetylcholine receptor sites of the muscle membrane, thereby blocking the ability of the motor neuron to stimulate muscle contraction.[26] This topic is discussed in the pain management treatment chapter (Chapter 24). The big question, in light of the efficacy of "dry needling," is whether or not injections of this chemical are really necessary for the routine treatment of TrPs, especially when previous studies have shown that the "needle effect" is quite potent regardless of the presence or absence of injectate. Of course, "dry needling" is a skill that requires the clinician be capable both of isolating TrPs and also directing the needle tip to the nidus.

PERPETUATING FACTORS IN MYOFASCIAL PAIN

Multiple aspects of MPS and the TrP phenomenon have now been discussed, including the etiological aspects, clinical presentations, discerning criteria, and theoretical topics. If myofascial pain were only an acute condition that would typically self-resolve in the acute stage just like simple postexercise soreness, then it would engender little interest in the clinical forefront of chronic pain syndromes. It is the ubiquitous and chronic nature of MPS that justifies the depth of explanation provided in this chapter. As such, emphasis must be placed on the perpetuating factors of MPS, those issues that provide a fertile environment for persistent TrP activity and also the expansion of the condition via secondary TrPs.

The TrP is an area of focal muscle hypertonicity that is chronically maintained by a variety of perpetuating factors that either increase the neural activation of motor neurons or adversely affect the metabolism of muscle tissue. These perpetuating factors include long-term physical overload from poor posture or repetitive strain, somato-somato reflexes (nociception, articular dysfunction, etc.), viscerosomatic issues (renal colic, biliary colic, cardiac, "McBurney's point" in appendicitis, etc.), nutritional or metabolic issues (vitamin inadequacies, thyroid disorders, glucose handling disorders, etc.; see below), and neuroemotional issues (limbic system dysfunction, etc.). Some of these topics will be addressed in detail in later chapters, while others are discussed below.

Somato-Somato Reflexes

Nociception and its effect in the somato-somato reflex events of TrP formation were previously discussed. However, it is important to clarify that chronic nociception spawns chronic secondary myofascial pain owing to repeated facilitation of segmental motor neurons in the spinal cord.[7] Pain is well known to cause reflex stimulation of the flexors of the limbs, known as the flexion withdrawal response,[26] and TrPs may represent focal areas of such muscular reflexes responses. Another cause is articular dysfunction, which is also thought to cause spinal motor neuron facilitation via the previously discussed "common final input theory."[20,65] This theory purports that abnormal tension in the periarticular tissues (ligaments, joint capsule, etc.) stimulates mechanoreceptors that synapse on gamma motor neurons and thereby increases muscle tone. Articular dysfunction and the various assessment and therapeutic approaches to address this common problem are discussed in detail in Chapters 13, 20, 23, and 26.

It was stated earlier in the chapter that TrPs are often initiated owing to mechanical overload. One cause of recurrent and/or prolonged overload occurs with postural compromise. Simons and Travell stated, "...poor posture in various forms is a powerful activator and perpetuator of myofascial TrPs."[43] Chronic poor posture may cause irritation of the periarticular ligaments and joint capsules from prolonged stress and strain, thereby activating the same neural mechanisms at play with articular dysfunction ("common final input theory"). Also, chronic poor posture may involve inappropriate muscular effort or repeated muscular contractions, both of which cause direct biomechanical overload of certain muscle fibers.

Postural overload in the lumbopelvic region can occur while standing, walking, or sitting. Pelvic position, hyper- or hypolordotic lumbar spine, use of nonsupported seating, postures at work and sport, asymmetries in posture and gait, leg length discrepancies are only a few topics that can cause overload and lead to chronic myofascial pain by these mechanisms. Several of these topics will be discussed in Chapter 13.

Somatovisceral and Viscerosomatic Reflexes

The topic of somatovisceral and viscerosomatic reflexes is not without controversy. While few would contest that flank muscle hypertonicity can arise secondary to renal dysfunction, or "kidney colic," the topic of visceral dysfunction stemming from somatic causation and, conversely, restoring visceral dysfunction via treatment of somatic tissues remains beyond the reason of many schools of thought.

Simons and Travell devote an entire chapter of their textbook to a detailed discussion of the abdominal muscles and their associated somatovisceral and viscerosomatic reflexes.[45] They discuss numerous cases of abdominal TrP activation that have been noted in association with acute appendicitis, peptic ulcer, ulcerative colitis, and diverticulitis, which probably occur through a modified version of the previously mentioned nociceptive flexion withdrawal reflex. Pain triggers reflex changes in muscle tone; it does not matter whether the painful source is an inflamed visceral organ, joint, tendon, ligament, or muscle.

More controversial is the notion that pain emanating from somatic tissues, such as muscles and joints, may cause reflex changes in visceral function or tone. Nansel and Szlazak published a review article[66] about this subject, and concluded that visceral and somatic pains were often difficult to distinguish from one another due to spinal cord convergence of afferent neurons. They were highly critical of the conceptual model of somatovisceral reflexes, stating that the nervous system seems more designed toward muscles responding in reflex fashion to visceral pain, but not the other way around. Yet Simons et al.[45] provide a review of the somatovisceral literature that cites examples of TrPs in the oblique abdominals causing diarrhea, belching, dysmenorhea, or nausea. Travell claimed to have empirically found a specific TrP location in the pectoralis major that is associated with a type of ectopic cardiac arrhythmia (somatovisceral reflex), and that successful elimination of this TrP immediately restored normal cardiac rhythm.[67]

The debate about somatovisceral and viscerosomatic reflexes is apt to continue for some time. Certainly the concern for all clinicians should be TrPs that are perpetuated by underlying visceral disease, and the appropriate management of both the visceral problem and the myofascial problem. Nevertheless, the neurophysiological principles discussed in this chapter make no distinction of a unidirectional reflexive interaction between visceral, somatic, and emotional interactions that lead to, among other things, muscle dysfunction. As such, an understanding of these topics helps to better appreciate the perpetuating factors involved in myofascial pain. For the purposes of clarification, a couple of such perpetuating factors will be discussed to establish thought processes that form the basis for clinical and assessment strategies discussed later in this text.

PERPETUATING FACTORS: METABOLIC AND ENDOCRINE ASPECTS OF MYOFASCIAL PAIN

General Concepts about Biochemistry, Metabolism, and Muscle Function

It is important to recognize that muscle tissue is extremely active metabolically, and requires several essential vitamins and minerals to function properly. Also, adequate amounts of oxygen and blood flow are important to maintain normal muscle function.[68] This is why patients with arterial blockages in the lower extremities develop intermittent vascular claudication (as opposed to neurogenic claudication) during walking, the leg musculature becoming starved for oxygen, nutrients, and minerals. In the absence of these nutrients, the foot, calf, and/or thigh muscles may cramp, remaining in a shortened state as the sarcomeres are unable to separate owing to an inability to replenish ATP levels and return calcium to the sarcoplasmic reticulum (calcium pump failure).

In a sense, the TrP may represent a localized area of "intermittent claudication" when the local ischemia blocks the supply of adequate calcium and ATP to release the locked actin–myosin molecules. Therefore, if the Simons "energy crisis" theory[21,45] of TrPs is correct, any metabolic or endocrine problem that affects muscle metabolism is likely to perpetuate or aggravate TrP and muscle pain. Nearly 50% of chronic myofascial pain is perpetuated or confounded by vitamin inadequacies.[45] For this reason, it becomes necessary to review some of the more common nutritional and endocrine inadequacies seen in clinical practice.

Simons et al.[45] state that the most detrimental nutritional deficiencies found in patients with myofascial pain are inadequacies of the water-soluble vitamins B and C, as well as the key minerals calcium, iron, and potassium. Magnesium deficiencies are also considered to have an adverse effect on normal muscle function. All of these nutritional deficiencies are commonly seen in patients who smoke, drink moderate to excessive amounts of alcohol, have chronic diseases, and/or have poor dietary habits.

Vitamins and minerals play an essential role in normal muscle metabolism, because they act as coenzymes or cofactors in many metabolic pathways, especially the *aerobic* Kreb's cycle. The mitochondria in muscle cells generate the ATP, and their most efficient engine uses the Kreb's cycle to generate this power supply.[68] Any reduction in ATP output will result in muscular tendency toward early fatigue, and possibly pain or cramps from muscular ischemia.

B Vitamins

The water-soluble B vitamins are essential cofactors in many of the metabolic pathways involved with the oxidative metabolism of glucose (Kreb's cycle). Therefore, these vitamins are critical for normal energy production within all cells of the body, especially muscle and nerve cells. For this reason, B vitamin deficiencies will rapidly cause various types of metabolic dysfunction. A comprehensive discussion of each B vitamin is beyond the scope of this chapter; however, a brief description of key B vitamin deficiencies associated with myofascial pain and their associated symptoms are listed below[69]:

Vitamin B_1 (thiamine): Deficiency will cause peripheral neuropathy characterized by decreased pain and temperature perception in the lower extremities, as well as loss of vibration sense. Nocturnal calf cramps are also commonly seen in B_1 deficiency. Thiamine appears to potentiate the effectiveness of thyroid hormone, which is also essential for normal muscle metabolism.

Vitamin B_6 (pyridoxine): Deficiency may interfere with production of almost all neurotransmitters, especially serotonin and norepinephrine, involved with pain processing. B_6 is an essential cofactor in lipid and amino acid metabolism, which influences the formation of hemoglobin molecules. Some peripheral neuropathies such as carpal tunnel syndrome appear to be correlated with low B_6 tissue levels.

Vitamin B_9 (folic acid): Deficiency will impair the synthesis of DNA, causing megaloblastic anemia to occur as a result of dysfunction during the duplication of immature bone marrow cells. Folic acid is essential to the growth of all cells, and therefore during pregnancy its deficiency can lead to various birth defects, especially of the neural tube.

Vitamin B_{12} (cobalamin): Deficiency is linked with folic acid, as both vitamin B_{12} and B_9 are functionally related in the same enzymatic and metabolic pathways. They both are required for DNA synthesis in rapidly dividing cells, such as erythrocytes and gastrointestinal (GI) tract cells. B_{12} and B_9 are also cofactors in the fatty acid synthesis that is critical for nerve myelin formation. Both B_{12} and B_9 deficiencies will cause *pernicious anemia*, a megaloblastic anemia in which immature erythrocytes are formed due to impaired DNA synthesis. Neurological symptoms may also develop in B_{12} and B_9 deficient states that are similar to mild demyelination: loss of vibratory and position sense, peripheral neuropathy, and weakness/ataxic gait. It is conjectured that these neurological symptoms are related to impairment of myelin synthesis.

In general, multiple B vitamin deficiencies are seen together clinically and usually are related to poor dietary intake. Strict vegetarians are frequently vitamin B_{12} deficient, as B_{12} is only derived from animal products. In contrast, vitamin B_9 is found in both animal and vegetable foods. Excessive alcohol intake also is linked to rapid depletion of all B vitamins. B vitamin deficiencies can perpetuate muscle pain syndromes directly by interfering with normal mitochondrial energy production, causing anemias that decrease oxygenation to muscle tissue, or indirectly by interfering with normal nerve function.

Vitamin C

Vitamin C is an especially important cofactor in a number of metabolic pathways. First, it is essential to the production of *collagen* molecules, acting as a reducing agent in the conversion of the amino acids lysine and proline into the procollagen molecule. Without adequate vitamin C, the collagen necessary to maintain a firm blood vessel wall becomes inadequate and the patient experiences *capillary fragility* with easy bruising. This could have a detrimental effect on the highly vascular muscles, which would be more easily injured during minor trauma and lead to TrP formation. Simons et al.[45] reported that postexercise soreness can be markedly reduced by vitamin C supplementation prior to the strenuous physical event. Apparently, microtrauma to muscle fibers is part of the mechanism involved with postexercise soreness and stiffness.

Vitamin C is also part of the metabolic pathways involved with the synthesis of the neurotransmitters epinephrine and serotonin, both of which are important in pain processing. Ascorbic acid also is involved in the stress responses of the body; tissue levels of vitamin C in the adrenal gland are extremely high, as it participates in the formation of the adrenal corticosteroids. Deficiencies of vitamin C may therefore play a role in compromising normal pain processing and the immune responses of the body. Smoking appears to dramatically lower tissue ascorbic acid levels, and may represent one of the most common causes of vitamin C deficiency.

Clinical Pearl: Nearly 50% of chronic myofascial pain is perpetuated or confounded by vitamin inadequacies.

Minerals

As previously noted, several minerals and trace elements are also essential components to normal muscle function. *Iron* is an essential part of the hemoglobin and myoglobin molecules, which transport oxygen to the muscle fibers. The lack of normal oxygen levels being supplied to active muscle tissue may lead to anaerobic metabolism, ischemia, and postexercise muscle soreness. Iron deficiency is most common in females because of menstruation, but found in both males and females because of internal bleeding disorders such as GI ulcers. Iatrogenic causes such as prolonged use of nonsteroidal anti-inflammatory drugs are shockingly common causes of upper GI ulceration/bleeding and often initially manifest as an unexplained anemia.[69] Lack of adequate iron will lead to either *microcytic* anemia characterized by inadequately small erythrocytes or *normocytic* anemia in which the erythrocytes contain an inadequate amount of hemoglobin. Anemia will lead to decreased work capacity, fatigue, and impaired muscle energy production.

Calcium is another essential mineral involved directly with muscle contraction, as well as normal nerve transmission. Calcium is used as a cofactor in the process of binding and releasing the actin–myosin cross-links, and therefore inadequate calcium can disrupt the normal process of muscle contraction. As noted earlier, the TrP phenomenon is thought to be a localized dysfunction of certain actin–myosin links being bound together. Without sufficient calcium ions and ATP, these actin–myosin links cannot be released and will be maintained in a constantly locked state. Calcium ions are also involved with the nerve transmission, as they are involved in calcium-gated channels in the postsynaptic membranes. Lack of calcium can disrupt normal nerve transmission at the neuromuscular junction, leading to spontaneous discharge of nerves, known as *calcium-deficient tetany*.[69]

Magnesium also plays an important role as a catalyst of many steps of the Kreb's cycle, and therefore is a critical mineral for energy production by mitochondria. Lack of magnesium may slow down the oxidative metabolism of carbohydrates, leading to symptoms of fatigue and low energy. Anecdotal reports[42] have surfaced regarding magnesium deficiencies causing chronic fatigue and FMS, although hard data are lacking that prove a cause–effect relationship. Endurance athletes such as long distance runners or cyclists can exhibit pronounced magnesium deficiencies after intense exercise, probably because of loss through excessive perspiration. Studies of magnesium supplementation and exercise indicate that this mineral can improve the efficiency of aerobic metabolism and improve cardiovascular performance.

Although vitamin and mineral deficiencies are obvious detriments to normal muscle function, there are also *metabolic and endocrine disorders* that adversely affect muscle cell metabolism. Among the most important endocrine problems to be discussed is *hypothyroidism*, which can manifest itself in many ways. Inadequate thyroid hormone levels will lead to a state of general *hypometabolism*, and any disorder that reduces cellular metabolism will ultimately lead to reduction of energy production and muscle function.

Essentially, thyroid hormone influences cellular growth, energy production, and energy consumption throughout all tissues of the body, by several mechanisms, including increased protein and RNA production, increased activity of metabolic enzymes, and increased ATP production by enhancement of cellular membrane function in mitochondria. As noted earlier, active muscle tissue contains large amounts of mitochondria that must produce enough ATP molecules to drive muscle function. Therefore, muscle pain, weakness, and fatigue are some of the first clinical symptoms of hypothyroid states. Other symptoms of this globally hypometabolic disorder include cold intolerance, low body temperature, dry skin, loss or thinning of the hair, inability to lose weight, and myxedema.[68]

There are various manifestations of thyroid disorders, including *primary hypothryoidism* in which the thyroid gland basically produces less than adequate amounts of thyroid hormone, and *secondary hypothyroidism* in which the pituitary is not producing enough thyroid-stimulating hormone. These conditions are simply diagnosed with standard blood tests and treated with thyroid hormone supplementation. There are also more subtle, and commonly misdiagnosed, types of thyroid dysfunction that require some special attention.[70,71] Disorders of *peripheral conversion* exist, which involve presumably genetic defects that disrupt normal thyroid hormone metabolism. These disorders generally involve enzyme deficiencies that create hypothyroid-type symptoms. The depth and complexity of these disorders extend beyond the parameters of this chapter. Those readers who are interested in a detailed discussion of the effects of thyroid hormone on muscle metabolism are referred to Lowe,[72] who published a comprehensive textbook that looks at the connections between muscle pain, fatigue, and fibromyalgia, and their association with inadequate thyroid function.

Dietary alterations of carbohydrate and protein metabolism may also adversely affect muscle function. These subtle dietary abnormalities are often misdiagnosed or ignored by general practitioners, unless a very astute clinician takes the time to perform a comprehensive case history, which includes questions about diet and exercise. Patients who consume large amounts of refined carbohydrates and low amounts of protein may create some marked symptoms. After a rich intake of carbohydrates, the pancreas is stimulated to release large amounts of insulin. As insulin levels rise, blood glucose levels sharply drop, leading to a condition known as *reactive hypoglycemia*, which can cause profound symptoms such as sweating, shaking, trembling, and muscle twitching. This type of patient often falls into the vicious cycle of eating carbohydrate-rich foods (candy, donuts, soda) to get immediate relief of the symptoms of reactive hypoglycemia, which only perpetuates the increased insulin release and ensuing lowered blood glucose. Worse yet, some of these patients may develop a condition known as *insulin resistance*, in which insulin levels remain high but blood glucose levels also remain elevated, because the peripheral target cells are no longer responsive to insulin.[73] Insulin resistance may lead to adult onset diabetes and a whole host of other complicating factors.

Disorders of protein metabolism and diet can likewise have adverse affects on muscle physiology. Too little protein may lead to a weakened immune system and loss of muscle mass. Protein supplies the body with the essential amino acids; they are termed "essential" because they are vital to many enzymatic reactions in several organ systems. In patients who perform intense physical exercise, which causes microtrauma to their muscles, inadequate protein consumption may lead to a diminished ability for muscle cells to repair themselves. This is especially true in endurance athletes such as long distance runners, cyclists, and triathletes, as well as those persons performing intense weight training activities. Sears and Lawren[73] recommends that the appropriate amount of daily protein intake varies based upon physical activity and amount of lean muscle mass, with a minimum of 0.5 g of protein per pound of lean muscle for sedentary persons with a maximum of 1.0 g of protein per pound of lean muscle for intense athletes.

This section has only touched briefly on the subject of vitamin/mineral deficiencies, endocrine and metabolic disorders, and their respective effects on muscle metabolism and function. This brief overview will hopefully stimulate the reader to review the subjects of nutrition and endocrinology, as these biochemical factors are often key issues involved with the perpetuation of chronic MPS. Although this biochemical aspect of muscle metabolism and pain is very important, there is one last subject about muscle pain that needs to be covered, and that is the link between emotional states and muscle tension.

Clinical Pearl: This brief overview will hopefully stimulate the reader to review the subjects of nutrition and endocrinology, as these biochemical factors are often key issues involved with the perpetuation of chronic MPS.

PERPETUATING FACTORS: THE LIMBIC SYSTEM AND MYOFASCIAL PAIN

Health and wellness can be divided into three categories: physical, chemical, and mental. Previous sections of this chapter have covered the biomechanical (physical) and metabolic/endocrine (chemical) aspects of muscle pain and dysfunction. This section will now look at the connection between muscle tension and emotional states.

The limbic system is a ring of structures (limbus means *ring* in Latin) around the base of the cerebral cortex that consists of several brain centers, including the hypothalamus, amygdala, hippocampus, and cingulate cortex.[26] It is thought that these deep centers collectively represent the oldest and most primitive portion of the cerebral cortex, and the areas from which our emotional reactions and behavioral responses to sensory stimuli arise.[74] The limbic system appears to be the switchboard for the fight or flight motor responses to potentially dangerous sensory stimuli. In simpler animal species, any dangerous situation in the environment would activate the limbic system, leading to automatic motor responses such as running away or freezing to "play dead."

Although humans have much more voluntary control over their motor responses to sensory stimuli than lower animals, the human limbic system still exerts a subconscious yet powerful influence on muscle function. Most clinicians have observed anxious patients who often exhibit widespread muscle tension. This type of global muscle hypertonicity was considered by Janda[9] to be a form of limbic system-mediated muscle dysfunction. Such dysfunction targets specific regions where the limbic system affects muscle tone: the suboccipitals, the jaw muscles, the scapular elevators, the pelvic floor muscles, and the diaphragm. Smooth muscles may also be affected by the limbic system's effect on parasympathetic and sympathetic function; cardiac muscle tone and GI motility (functional irritable bowel syndrome) are often part of the anxiety–stress reaction.

Since this type of "emotional" muscle dysfunction occurs in multiple muscles, full body massage and stretching techniques are often the most beneficial types of manual treatment. Focal soft tissue techniques such as deep pressure points, acupressure, and transverse friction massage can eliminate focal areas of muscle dysfunction (TrPs), but are not as helpful as full body massage due to the widespread nature of the global muscle dysfunction. Psychotherapy and relaxation techniques are also beneficial to these patients. Some may require pharmaceutical treatment in the form of antidepressants, anxiolytics, or "muscle relaxants" (most of which are CNS depressants).

This anxious response occurs when the limbic system is activated, and in turn activates the excitatory portion of the brainstem that controls the gamma system (MS). When multiple muscles in the body have their spindle activity turned up, essentially the body is preparing the entire musculoskeletal system for a flight or fight response. As stated earlier, this increased gamma motor neuron activity may not be detectable by standard EMG studies, and hence an apparent contradiction; the patient is describing increased muscle "tone" and "tension" but the examiner using EMG cannot detect any overt muscle hypertonicity (from alpha motor neurons). Yet the manual therapy practitioner can readily palpate tissue and texture changes in the muscles of these patients, often manifesting as multiple areas of taut bands and TrPs. One might alternatively call this type of muscle dysfunction *global hypertonicity*, in which the clinical finding is numerous areas of taut bands and TrPs in multiple muscles, often bilaterally in the neck, jaw, and upper quarter.

It is plausible to speculate that maintenance of prolonged global muscle tension due to limbic system agitation could set the stage for TrP formation in certain muscles. As such, these factors would logically hold a key role in the recurrence and perpetuation of chronic MPS. Therefore, one should be certain to look for chronic emotional dysfunction in the patient with chronic muscle dysfunction. In such cases, treatment of the musculoskeletal dysfunction without addressing the psychological component would typically result in short-term TrP reduction, but long-term frustration as the TrPs return following the next emotional upset.

As discussed above, the fight or flight response seems to activate certain key muscles of the head, jaw, and upper extremity, as well as the diaphragm and pelvic floor muscles. Many clinicians have empirically noted that these muscles often develop TrPs in the absence of any direct trauma or repetitive overuse, and the limbic system dysfunction may be the culprit in these cases.

Fibromyalgia Syndrome

Extreme limbic system dysfunction may lead to another clinical problem known as FMS,[61] a condition often confused with MPS. Patients with FMS do not necessarily complain of being tight all over, but chiefly complain of *fatigue and widespread pain.* Upon physical examination, it becomes readily apparent that patients with FMS exhibit an abnormally low tolerance for any type of firm palpation or deep pressure applied to their muscles and soft tissues. They will typically vocalize their pain, and stop clinicians from performing any type of manual therapy that employs pressure.

This curious clinical finding of widespread hyperalgesia is in distinct contrast to the patient who is merely "tight all over" and often enjoys firm, deep palpation of their muscles stating it "hurts in a good way." There is no such thing as a "good hurt" to a patient with FMS, who complains of pain with even the lightest applied pressure. The patient with FMS therefore notes pervasive tenderness and exhibits a form of *global hyperalgesia.*

A diagnosis of FMS is defined[75] by the American College of Rheumatology (ACR) by two simple criteria: (1) widespread pain of greater than 3–6 months duration and (2) at least 11 of 18 points on the body that are tender to less than 4 kg of pressure. Widespread pain is defined as being bilateral, above and below the waist, and in the axial skeleton. The 18 TeP locations are merely predesignated locations on the body for examination purposes, and were chosen arbitrarily by a panel of ACR physicians at a consensus conference. As previously mentioned, the TePs of FMS should not be confused for the TrPs found in the focal type of muscle dysfunction discussed earlier.[59]

After 25 years of research, the etiology of FMS and its associated TePs remains elusive. However, some important findings have surfaced in the literature. First, attempts to find any histological evidence of muscle or soft tissue pathology have failed.[76] Second, studies that tried to correlate differences between pain thresholds over the 18 designated "tender points" and other "control points" have failed to show any statistically significant differences.[77,78] Lastly, patients with FMS show lowered thresholds to pain *all over their bodies*, not just the TeP locations, when compared to healthy controls.[79]

Hyperalgesia Versus Allodynia

This absence of any soft tissue pathology in FMS has led to the growing concept that the etiology of FMS may lie in the realm of *CNS dysfunction of pain processing pathways*, not muscle dysfunction. Two neurological terms are pertinent to any discussion of FMS. *Hyperalgesia* is a state in which the patient has a lowered threshold to *painful* stimuli, whereas *allodynia* is a state in which the patient perceives pain from normally *nonpainful* stimuli. Essentially, hyperalgesia is merely a variant form of a lowered pain threshold. Allodynia is far more pathological, because the patient complains of pain to mild stimuli that are not normally painful, such as soft brushing, light touch, etc. By definition, FMS can be alternatively labeled as some type of *widespread hyperalgesia or allodynia*. Both of these conditions are usually thought of as being mediated by abnormalities of the CNS. Therefore, it is logical to look at FMS as possibly being a *neurological* disorder, rather than a musculoskeletal disorder.

Russell[80] states that "a careful review of the histological and ultrastructural muscle biopsy studies has failed to reveal any primary abnormality in skeletal muscle characteristics of FMS." He suggests that since FMS does *not* appear to be caused by any peripheral muscle or soft tissue pathology, we should consider a *neurochemical* pathogenesis of FMS. Cerebrospinal fluid analysis of FMS has clearly shown a statistically significant increased substance P[81] and diminished serotonin[82] levels when compared with normal control patients, which help to explain some attributes of this condition.

Substance P is a neuroactive polypeptide that is released by nociceptive neurons and is known to lower the threshold for excitation at synapses. Serotonin is an important neurotransmitter in the neural pathways from the limbic system to the *descending antinociceptive system (DANS)*.[83] It is the DANS that dampen the background "noise" of low-level sensory stimuli (especially nociception) from being perceived by the brain as "pain." Failure of the DANS (due to serotonin deficiency) to inhibit incoming sensory stimuli and increased substance P levels exciting synapses would result in hyperalgesia, or in its extreme form, allodynia.[84] Russell has suggested that the term *fibromyalgia* is basically a misnomer, because the pain associated with this condition does not appear to be emanating from fibrous or muscular tissues. He has therefore proposed[61] that the term FMS be replaced with the term *widespread allodynia*, which more accurately describes the neurological sensitization underlying this pain processing disorder.

Clinical Pearl: The absence of any specific soft tissue pathology in FMS has led to the growing concept that the etiology of FMS may lie in the realm of *CNS dysfunction of pain processing pathways*, not muscle dysfunction.

This concept of FMS as a form of centrally mediated allodynia is apparently gaining momentum within the literature. Patients with FMS as a group have demonstrated significant sleep disorders due to various types of posttraumatic stress disorders, and often suffer from clinical depression and/or anxiety syndromes.[85,86] Their nervous systems have essentially malfunctioned to the point where the DANS no longer functions normally, with the ensuing symptom complex of widespread allodynia. If the TePs of FMS are indeed just peripheral locations that represent a more centrally mediated problem with pain processing pathways, one would not expect these patients to respond well to soft tissue therapy, since the primary problem is not in the soft tissues. Indeed, this is what typically is seen in clinical practice; FMS with true widespread allodynia rarely respond well to myofascial release, muscle stretching, therapeutic exercise, and the like.

Yet anecdotal reports abound about purported cures for FMS by utilizing various manual treatment methods. In cases where the patient has true CNS malfunction leading to widespread allodynia, it seems dubious that any manual treatments would have any substantial long-term therapeutic benefit. However, there may be an alternative explanation for these clinical results; they may simply be cases of misdiagnosis. If a patient presents to a physician with two or three areas of complaints (such as neck, low back, and shoulder pain) with some overlapping referred pain patterns, then that patient might be misdiagnosed with FMS. In reality, the patient has a musculoskeletal problem that is quite amenable to manual treatment. Unfortunately, a successful outcome may lead to the faulty conclusion that he or she was cured of FMS.

A similar sort of situation occurs in the natural health-care fields of nutrition, homeopathy, herbology, and naturopathy, wherein these practitioners also claim to have found the "cure" for FMS. There are many functional or metabolic problems that may lead to the symptoms of widespread pain and fatigue, which could easily be mistaken for FMS. A simple example is reactive hypoglycemia; this patient complains of a feeling of low energy, inability to concentrate, vague aches in the muscles—symptoms that occur when he or she has not eaten for a few hours. A clinician could easily misdiagnose this patient with FMS, especially when the clinician does not take the time to perform a comprehensive case history and fails to order any blood tests. Now this patient sees a nutritionist, starts eating properly, starts taking some vitamins, and is miraculously cured of "FMS."

A full and detailed discussion about FMS is beyond the scope of this chapter. The reader is referred to a comprehensive article cowritten by the author,[59] which proposes a new paradigm for the differential diagnosis of FMS from other disorders that mimic FMS. In summary, it is the author's opinion that FMS is really not a type of muscle dysfunction, but rather a type of CNS dysfunction in which the patient perceives pain from nonpainful stimuli (allodynia).

SUMMARY

1. This chapter has emphasized the multivariate etiological aspects and ubiquitous nature of myofascial pain and dysfunction.
2. Myofascial TrPs are a type of FOCAL muscle dysfunction.
3. The etiology of TrPs is thought to be a combination of neurological dysfunction and focal ischemia.
4. The focal ischemia is due to prolonged activation and fatigue of certain motor units, resulting in contracture of certain sarcomeres due to lack of ATP to drive the calcium pump and release the actin-myosin cross bridges.
5. Focal techniques such as deep pressure, stripping massage, transverse friction, and even modalities such as dry needling, laser, and ultrasound all have the common denominator of causing focal vasodilation which may relive the focal ischemia.
6. The neurological aspect of TrP formation has been documented by increased needle EMG activity from within the TrP nidus, but not in the adjacent taut band.
7. Reflex techniques such as PIR may release TrPs through a neurological mechanism of action, without directly treating the TrP nodule itself.
8. TrPs are palpable as a lumpy nodule, and always found within an associated taut band. Tender areas of muscle that do not have such a texture change may be "tender points" associated with fibromyalgia syndrome . . . which is NOT a type of muscle dysfunction.
9. The pain of active myofascial TrPs is likely coming from the focal ischemia, i.e. chemical exudates from the area of ischemia such as prostaglandins, bradykinins, etc. are exciting the nociceptors in the adjacent muscle tissue.
10. Latent TrPs are not painful at rest, because the concentration of these chemicals is not high enough to excite the nociceptors. However, when these muscles are used frequently it will "activate" the TrPs and when the concentration rises sufficiently, pain will ensue.
11. TrPs can only be diagnosed by palpation of muscles that are suspect due to characteristic referred pain patterns. Other than needle EMG, there is no other diagnostic test to find TrPs.
12. Perpetuating factors, including metabolic/nutritional disorders and physical/postural stresses/strains must be addressed for long-term relief of myofascial pain.
13. Referred pain patterns from myofascial TrPs can fool clinicians. Pseudo-radicular pain patterns in the lower extremities may be caused by TrPs in the lumbo-pelvic muscles.
14. It is important to include a palpatory examination of the lumbopelvic muscles for TrP activity in all cases of low back pain.

REFERENCES

1. Panjabi M. The stabilizing system of the spine. *J Spinal Disord* 1992;5:383–389.

2. Stude D. *Spinal rehabilitation.* New York: McGraw-Hill, 1999.
3. McGill SM. *Low back disorders: Evidence-based prevention and rehabilitation.* Champaign: Human Kinetics, 2002.
4. Murphy D. *Conservative management of cervical spine syndromes.* New York: McGraw-Hill, 2000.
5. Richardson C, Jull G, Hodges P, Hides J. *Therapeutic exercise for spinal segmental stabilization in low back pain.* London: Churchill Livingstone, 1999.
6. Travell JG, Simons DG. *Myofascial pain and dysfunction: The trigger point manual. Volume 1. Upper half of body.* Baltimore: Williams & Wilkins, 1983.
7. Travell JG, Simons DG. *Myofascial pain and dysfunction: The trigger point manual. Volume 2. The lower extremities.* Baltimore: Williams & Wilkins, 1992.
8. Janda V. Muscle weakness and inhibition (pseudoparesis) in back pain syndromes. In: Grieve GP, ed. *Modern manual therapy of the vertebral column.* London: Churchill Livingstone, 1986.
9. Janda V. Muscle spasm—A proposed procedure for differential diagnosis. *J Manual Med* 1991;6:136–139.
10. Indahl A, Kaigle AM, Reikeras O, Holm SH. Interaction between the porcine lumbar intervertebral disc, zygapophysial joints, and paraspinal muscles. *Spine* 1997;22(24):2834–2840.
11. Barrack RL, Munn BG. Effects of knee ligament injury and reconstruction on proprioception. In: Lephart S, Fu FH, eds. *Proprioception and neuromuscular control in joint stability.* Windsor: Human Kinetics, 2000;197–211.
12. Leinonen V, Kankaanpaa M, Luukkonen M, Hanninen O, Airaksinen O, Taimela S. Disc herniation-related back pain impairs feed-forward control of paraspinal muscles. *Spine* 2001;26(16):E367–E372.
13. Hodges PW, Moseley GL, Gabrielsson A, Gandevia SC. Experimental muscle pain changes feedforward postural responses of the trunk muscles. *Exp Brain Res* July 2003; 151(2):262–71.
14. Hubbard DR, Berkoff GM. Myofascial trigger points show spontaneous needle EMG activity. *Spine* 1993; 18(13):1803–1807.
15. Hubbard DR. Chronic and recurrent muscle pain: Pathophysiology and treatment, and review of pharmacologic studies. *J Musculoskeletal Pain* 1996;4(1/2): 123–143.
16. McNulty W, Gervitz R, Berkoff G, Hubbard D. Needle electromyographic evaluations of trigger point response to a psychological stressor. *Psychophysiology* 1994;31:313–316.
17. Kendall F, McCreary E, Provance P. *Muscles: Testing and function.* Baltimore: Williams & Wilkins, 1993.
18. Mense S, Simons DG. *Muscle pain.* Baltimore: Lippincott Williams & Wilkins, 2001.
19. Lewit K. Chain reactions in the locomotor system in light of co-activation patterns based on developmental neurology. *J Orthop Med* 1999;21(1):52–57.
20. Johansson H. Reflex integration in the gamma motor system. In: Boyd I, Gladden M, eds. *The muscle spindle.* London: Macmillan Press, 1985:297–301.
21. Simons D. Clinical and etiological update of myofascial pain from trigger points. *J Musculoskeletal Pain* 1996;4(1/2):93–121.
22. Leahy P. Improved treatments for carpal tunnel and related syndromes. *Chiro Sports Med* 1995;9(1):6–9.
23. Leahy PM. *Active Release Techniques: Soft tissue management system for the upper extremity* [Technique manual and videotape series]. Colorado Springs, CO: Self-published by the author, 1996.
24. Prudden B. *Pain erasure.* New York: Ballantine Books, 1980.
25. Schneider MJ, Cohen JH, Laws S, eds. *The collected writings of Nimmo and Vannerson: Pioneers of chiropractic trigger point therapy.* Pittsburgh, PA: Self-published by the editors, 2001.
26. Kandel ER, Schwartz JH, Jessell TM. *Principles of neural science.* New York: McGraw-Hill, 2000.
27. Janda V. Muscles, central nervous motor regulation, and back problems. In: Korr I, ed. *Neurobiological mechanisms in manipulative therapy.* New York: Plenum Press, 1978.
28. Jull GA, Janda V. Muscles and motor control in low back pain: Assessment and management. In: Twomey LT, Taylor JR, eds. *Physical therapy of the low back.* London: Churchill Livingstone, 1987;172–192.
29. Janda V. *Muscle function testing.* London: Butterworths, 1983.
30. Lewit K. *Manipulative therapy in rehabilitation of the motor system.* London: Butterworths, 1985.
31. *Stedman's medical dictionary.* Baltimore: Williams & Wilkins, 1976.
32. Jacob G. Course notes. In: *No nonsense rehab and mobilization.* Pittsburgh, PA: University of Pittsburgh, May 2003:100.
33. Lephart S, Fu F, eds. *Priopriocеption and neuromuscular control in joint stability.* Windsor: Human Kinetics, 2000.
34. Sherrington CS. *The integrative action of the nervous system.* New Haven: Yale University Press, 1947.
35. Leonard CT. *The neuroscience of human movement.* St Louis, MO: Mosby, 1998.
36. Knutson G. The role of the gamma motor system in increasing muscle tone and muscle pain syndromes: A review of the Johannson/Sojka hypothesis. *JMPT* 2000;23(8):564–572.
37. Jones LH. *Jones strain–counterstrain.* Boise: Jones Strain-Counterstrain, Inc., 1995.
38. Johansson H, Sjolander P, Sojka P. A sensory role for the cruciate ligaments. *Clin Orthop* 1991;268:161–178.
39. Johansson H, Pedersen J, Bergenheim M, Djupsjobacka M. Peripheral afferents of the knee: Their effects on central mechanisms regulating muscle stiffness, joint stability, and proprioception and coordination. In: Lephart SM, Fu FH, eds. *Proprioception and neuromuscular control in joint stability.* Champaign: Human Kinetics, 2000;5–22.
40. Lewit K. Postisometric relaxation in combination with other methods of muscular facilitation and inhibition. *Man Med* 1986;(2):101–104.
41. Greenman P. *Principles of manual medicine,* 2nd ed. Baltimore: Williams & Wilkins, 1996.

42. Benarroch EE, Westmoreland BF, Daube JR, Reagan TJ, Sandok BA. *Medical neurosciences*, 4th ed. Philadelphia: Lippincott Williams & Wilkins, 1999.
43. Bogduk N, Simons D. Neck pain: Joint pain or trigger points? In: Voeroy H, Merskey H, eds. *Progress in fibromyalgia and myofascial pain*. Amsterdam: Elsevier Science, 1993:267–273.
44. Salter M. The neurobiology of central sensitization. *J Musculoskeletal Pain* 2002;10(1/2):23–33.
45. Simons DG, Travell JG, Simons LS. *Myofascial pain and dysfunction: The trigger point manual. Volume 1. Upper half of body*, 2nd ed. Baltimore: Williams & Wilkins, 1999.
46. Sciotti V, Mittak V, Finn M, DiMarco L, Hickner R. The biochemical profile of myofascial trigger points: A clinical microdialysis study. *J Chiropractic Educ* 1999; 13(1):41–42.
47. Sciotti V, Mittak V, Finn M, DiMarco L, Hickner R. Interstitial fluid lactate and local blood flow in trapezius muscle trigger points. *J Chiropractic Educ* 2000; 14(1):19–20.
48. Frieder S, Weisberg J, Fleming B, Stanek A. A pilot study: The therapeutic effect of ultrasound following partial rupture of Achilles tendons in male rats. *JOSPT* 1988;10(2):39–45.
49. Cheng N, Van Hoof H, Bockx E, et al. The effects of electric currents on ATP generation, protein synthesis, and membrane transport in rat skin. *Clin Orthop Relat Res* 1982;171:264–272.
50. Hong CZ, Yu J. Spontaneous electrical activity of rabbit trigger spot after transection of spinal cord and peripheral nerve. *J Musculoskeletal Pain* 1998;6(4): 45–58.
51. Hong CZ. Current research on myofascial trigger points—Pathophysiological studies. *J Musculoskeletal Pain* 1999;7(1/2):121–129.
52. Simons DG. Diagnostic criteria of myofascial pain caused by trigger points. *J Musculoskeletal Pain* 1999; 7(1/2):111–120.
53. Schneider W, Dvorak J, Dvorak V, Tritschler T. *Manual medicine: Therapy*. Stuttgart, Germany: Georg Thieme Verlag, 1988.
54. Dvorak J, Dvorak V. *Manual medicine: Diagnostics*. Suttgart, Germany: Georg Theime Verlag, 1984.
55. Maigne R. Low back pain of lumbar origin. *Arch Phys Med Rehabil* 1980;61:389–395.
56. Chaitow L. *Soft tissue manipulation*. Wellingborough, UK: Thorsons Publishing Group, 1987.
57. Tsai WC, Wang TG, Hong CZ. Myofascial trigger points in the ipsilateral gluteal muscles associated with pyogenic sacroiliitis: A case report. *J Musculoskeletal Pain* 1999;7(3):73–82.
58. Smolders J. *The trigger point charts*. Huntington Beach, CA: MPA Provider Services.
59. Schneider MJ. Tender points/fibromyalgia vs. trigger points/myofascial pain syndrome: A need for clarity in terminology and differential diagnosis. *J Manipulative Physiol Ther* 1995;18(6):398–406.
60. Russell I. Neurochemical pathogenesis of fibromyalgia syndrome. *J Musculoskeletal Pain* 1996;4(1/2):61–92.
61. Russell I, ed. *Clinical overview and pathogenesis of the fibromyalgia syndrome, myofascial pain syndrome, and other pain syndromes*. Binghamton, NY: Haworth Press, 1996.
62. Hendriksson K. Is fibromyalgia a central pain state? *J Musculoskeletal Pain* 2002;10(1/2):45–57.
63. Garvey T. A prospective, randomized, double-blind evaluation of trigger point injection therapy for low back pain. *Spine* 1989;9:962–964.
64. Lewit K. The needle effect in the relief of myofascial pain. *Pain* 1979;6:83–90.
65. Johansson H. Role of knee ligaments in proprioception and regulation of muscle stiffness. *J Electromyogr Kinesiol* 1991;3:158–179.
66. Nansel D, Szlazak M. Somatic dysfunction and the phenomenon of visceral disease simulation: A probable explanation for the apparent effectiveness of somatic therapy in patients presumed to be suffering from true visceral disease [see comments]. *J Manipulative Physiol Ther* 1995;18(6):379–397.
67. Travell JG. *Office hours: Day and night*. New York: The World Publishing Co., 1968.
68. Guyton AC. *Medical physiology*, 5th ed. Philadelphia: W.B. Saunders, 1976.
69. Rakel RE. *Textbook of family practice*. Philadelphia: W.B. Saunders, 1990.
70. Brady D. Functional thyroid disorders. Part I. Dynamic chiropractic. March 20, 2000;2:11–12.
71. Brady D. Functional thyroid disorders. Part II. Dynamic chiropractic. April 17, 2000;25:40–41.
72. Lowe J. *The metabolic treatment of fibromyalgia*. Boulder, CO: McDowell Publishing Co., 2000.
73. Sears B, Lawren W. *The zone*. New York: HarperCollins Publishers, Inc., 1995.
74. Goldstein J. *Chronic fatigue syndromes: The limbic hypothesis*. Binghamton, NY: Haworth Medical Press, Inc., 1993.
75. Wolfe F, Smythe H, Yunus M, et al. The American College of Rheumatology 1990 criteria for the classification of fibromyalgia. *Arthritis Rheum* 1990;33(2):160–172.
76. Yunus MB, Kalyan-Raman UP, Masi AT, Aldg JC. Electromicroscopic studies of muscle biopsy in primary fibromyalgia syndrome: A controlled and blinded study. *J Rheumatol* 1989;16:97–101.
77. Pillemer S, ed. *The fibromyalgia syndrome: Current research and future directions in epidemiology, pathogenesis, and treatment*. Binghamton, NY: Haworth Press Inc., 1994.
78. Pillemer S, ed. *The neuroscience and endocrinology of fibromyalgia*. Binghamton, NY: Haworth Press, Inc., 1998.
79. Staud R, Vierck CJ, Cannon RL, Mauderli AP, Price DD. Abnormal sensitization and temporal summation of second pain (wind-up) in patients with fibromyalgia syndrome. *Pain* 2001;91(1/2):165–175.
80. Russell I, edr. *MYOPAIN '95: Abstracts from the 3rd World Congress on myofascial pain and fibromyalgia*. Binghamton, NY: Haworth Press Inc., 1995.
81. Russell IJ, Orr MD, Littman B, et al. Elevated

cerebrospinal levels of substance P in patients with fibromyalgia syndrome. *Arthritis Rheum* 1994;37:1593–1601.

82. Russell IJ, Vaeroy H, Javors M, Nyberg F. Cerebrospinal fluid biogenic amine metabolites in fibromyalgia/fibrositis syndrome and rheumatoid arthritis. *Arthritis Rheum* 1992;35:550–556.
83. Sandkuhler J. The organization and function of endogenous antinociceptive systems. *Prog Neurobiol* 1996;50(1):49–81.
84. Mense S. Neurobiological concepts of fibromyalgia—The possible role of descending spinal tracts. *Scand J Rheumatol Suppl* 2000;113:24–29.
85. Turk D. Suffering and dysfunction in fibromyalgia syndrome. *J Musculoskeletal Pain* 2002;20(1/2): 85–96.
86. Walen HR, Oliver K, Groessl E, Cronan TA, Rodriguez VM. Traumatic events, health outcomes, and health care use in patients with fibromyalgia. *J Musculoskeletal Pain* 2001;9(2):19–38.

CHAPTER

10

RED FLAGS FOR SERIOUS DISEASE IN LOW BACK SYNDROMES

Donald R. Murphy, Gideon Letz, and Craig E. Morris

OUTLINE

OBJECTIVES

1. To define clinical "Red Flags."
2. To emphasize the importance of clinical "Red Flags" in the management of low back syndromes.
3. To explain those low back patients with the greatest risk of serious underlying condition.
4. To clarify the clinical factors that lead one to practically suspect a serious underlying condition.
5. To explain key aspects of the history and examination that can help to determine the presence of a serious underlying condition.
6. To provide case studies to assist the reader how to practically assess for clinical "Red Flags."

INTRODUCTION

An important goal in the initial assessment of any patient complaining of low back pain (LBP), with or without leg symptoms (i.e., the so-called low back syndromes), is to determine whether the pain is due to a serious underlying spinal or nonspinal condition. Because of the potentially harmful nature of these serious disorders, they have become known as "red flags." Lumbopelvic and/or leg symptomatology may be the most prominent, or only, symptom, especially early in the process. Delay in the diagnosis and appropriate management will not only prolong the symptoms but may compromise the ultimate outcome of treatment.

Fortunately, the incidence of these conditions is quite low. For example, spinal malignant neoplasms occur in less than 1% of patients with LBP.[1] However, even an incidence this low would mean that a spine specialist is likely to see several cases per year. In fact, the rarity of these conditions is exactly why attention to the exclusion process for these "red flag" conditions must be incorporated into the routine evaluation of *every* LBP patient.

This chapter will present a systematic approach to the evaluation of patients with LBP, which will allow timely detection and initial management of these red flag conditions. They can be divided into five pathophysiological categories[2–5]:

1. *Fracture:* Fractures may be traumatic or "pathologic," i.e., related to osteopenia or bony infiltration by tumor.
2. *Tumor:* Primary spine tumors can be benign or malignant and are relatively rare compared to metastatic lesions.
3. *Infection:* Any infectious process involving spinal elements is potentially catastrophic. Infection of the bone (osteomyelitis) can occur with

disseminated tuberculosis, coccidiomycosis, or any bacterial septicemia. Other infections of the spine include epidural abscess, subdural empyema, and discitis, all typically occurring as surgical complications.

4. *Cauda equina syndrome:* Compression of the spinal cord can be caused by tumor or disc herniation.
5. *Abdominal disease:* Pathology in the abdomen, pelvis, or retroperitoneal space can present with lumbar pain as the primary symptom. Examples include aortic aneurysm, renal disease, endometriosis, and pelvic inflammatory disease.

HISTORY

There are certain factors in the patient's *history* that should raise the physician's level of suspicion that a serious or potentially life-threatening illness is present (see Table 10–1).

A patient with back pain following major trauma, such as a fall or a motor vehicle collision, should be immediately evaluated for spinal fracture. Most typically the history would involve a fall onto the buttocks or directly onto the lumbar spine, with the spine in a flexed position.[6] This may cause compression fracture of one or more vertebral bodies. Rarely, in the presence of violent trauma, a burst fracture of the vertebral body may occur which can cause neurological injury. Epidural hematoma may also occur after severe trauma.

In elderly patients or patients on long-term steroids who may have osteopenia or osteoporosis, less significant trauma may produce compression fracture. Another group at risk is adolescent and preadolescent athletes, such as gymnasts, who perform extreme loading activities at end-range and may develop *pars* fractures. (Sport-specific injuries are covered in greater detail in Chapter 30.)

Clinical Pearl: In elderly patients or patients on long-term steroids who may have osteopenia or osteoporosis, less significant trauma may produce compression fracture.

In general, those patients who are under 20 or over 50 years of age have the greatest likelihood of having a serious illness causing LBP. As with many of the factors discussed in this chapter, it is important to note that the majority of patients in these age groups who visit the spine physician will not have serious disease. Such risk factors should only be used to raise the level of suspicion for the clinician without creating undue anxiety for the patient.

TABLE 10–1. **Red Flags for Serious or Potentially Life-Threatening Illness: History**

Historical Feature	Suggestive of
Major trauma such as motor vehicle collision or fall from a height	Fracture
Minor trauma or strenuous lifting in an older or potentially osteoporotic patient	Fracture
Age over 50 or under 20	Tumor or infection
History of cancer	Metastasis
Constitutional symptoms such as recent fever chills or unexplained weight loss	Infection or tumor
Pain worse at night	Tumor
Recent bacterial infection, IV drug use, or immune suppression (e.g., from steroids or other immunosuppressive drugs, HIV infection)	Infection
No significant improvement after >1 month of conservative care	Tumor
Pain that has no mechanical exacerbating or remitting factors	Infection or tumor
Patient is on anticoagulant therapy	Epidural hematoma
Saddle anesthesia	Cauda equina syndrome
Sudden onset of bowel and/or bladder dysfunction	Cauda equina syndrome
Bilateral progressive neurological deficit covering several dermatomes	Cauda equina syndrome
Severe, disabling pain in child or adolescent	Tumor or infection
Male, age >60, abdominal pain, atherosclerotic disease risk factors (History of hypertension, smoker, obesity family history)	Abdominal aortic aneurysm

Clinical Pearl: In general, those patients who are under 20 or over 50 years of age have the greatest likelihood of having a serious illness causing LBP.

Those patients who have a previous history of cancer should be examined closely for the possibility of metastatic disease. In fact, there are some who feel that new onset of LBP in a patient with a history of cancer should be assumed secondary to metastatic disease until proven otherwise.[7] There are certain malignant tumors that tend to metastasize to bone, and so patients who have a history of these cancers are of particular concern (see Table 10–2).

TABLE 10–2. Carcinomata That Have a Predilection for Metastasis to Bone

Breast	Lung
Prostate	Thyroid
Kidney	Bladder
Endometrium	Cervix
Melanoma	Lymphoma

Source: Adapted from Ferri.[8]

The patient should be asked about constitutional symptoms such as recent fever, chills, or weight loss (defined at greater than 10 lb within 6 weeks), any of which would suggest infection or malignancy. Unexplained weight loss, when associated with malignancy, typically occurs with normal or decreased food intake and, in some cases, is coupled with increased caloric requirement.[8] The concern about infection in patients with recent fever or chills should be more acute in those who report a history of risk factors such as recent bacterial infection, intravenous (IV) drug use, or immune suppression secondary to drug treatment or HIV infection.

Clinical Pearl: The patient should be asked about constitutional symptoms such as recent fever, chills, or weight loss (defined at greater than 10 lb within 6 weeks), any of which would suggest infection or malignancy.

Pain that results from a tumor frequently is worse at night. While this is hardly specific for neoplasm, it should be noted, particularly if it is found in the presence of other red flags. It may be helpful to determine whether the pain awakens the patient as opposed to the patient waking and then being unable to return to sleep because of pain, with the second scenario *suggesting* a joint-related condition.

Some studies have found that tumor is more likely to be found in patients whose pain has been present for greater than 1 month, in spite of conservative treatment.[9,10] There certainly are many patients whose pain does not resolve within 1 month of treatment, and who do not have a tumor. But this factor should cause the physician to consider further investigation.

It is important to meticulously question the patient about what makes the pain better or worse. A patient with *mechanical* LBP will usually report that certain movements or positions increase the intensity of the pain, while other positions provide relief. The absence of remitting factors should raise concern for tumor or infection. It is important to note that in many acute patients with mechanical causes of pain, their distress is such that the pain seems unrelenting. But careful questioning often reveals that certain times of the day or postural positions provide relief.

Clinical Pearl: A patient with *mechanical* LBP will usually report that certain movements or positions increase the intensity of the pain, while other positions provide relief.

Severe, unrelenting pain in a child or adolescent is a red flag for tumor or infection (see Case #2).[11]

In patients who are on anticoagulant medications, there is an increased risk of epidural hematoma. This will often cause severe, unrelenting pain that is not relieved by rest. This can also occur after spine trauma or after surgery.[7]

A relatively uncommon (1%–15% of all cases of disc herniation[12,13]) but potentially devastating disorder that can occur in patients with LBP is *cauda equina syndrome*. It is important when taking the history to ask the patient about a saddle distribution (i.e., perineum and proximal, medial thighs) of anesthesia, loss of bowel or bladder function, or bilateral neurological deficit covering several dermatomes. In cauda equina syndrome, the bladder dysfunction can be in the form of urinary retention or incontinence. Typically, retention occurs first, followed by incontinence.[14]

In patients over 50, especially those with risk factors for atherosclerotic vascular disease (smoking, hypertension, obesity, positive family history), the physician should consider abdominal aortic aneurysm (AAA) in the differential diagnosis of LBP. Patients with AAA often have no symptoms, but once they develop symptoms, there is >80% mortality rate within 1 year. The "expanding" aneurysm may present with lumbar pain with radiation to the flank or groin. The pain may be intermittent and mild or may be continuous and increasing in intensity. The clinician should also enquire about such symptoms as a pulsating sensation in the abdomen, coldness, or discoloration in the legs and feet, and claudication.[15]

EXAMINATION

As with the history, meticulous examination can reveal clues that raise the index of suspicion that a serious or potentially life-threatening illness is present (see Table 10–3). In patients with fracture or infection, palpation of the spinous process may reveal exquisite tenderness. It is particularly important to use percussion to detect this. The reflex hammer is useful for this purpose.

Fever is a particularly important finding. In fact, fever in the presence of LBP should be considered to be spinal infection until proven otherwise.[16] This is because some infections, especially epidural abscess,

TABLE 10–3. Red Flags for Serious or Potentially Life-Threatening Illness: Examination

Finding	Suggestive of
Pinpoint tenderness of the spinous process	Fracture or infection
Fever	Infection
Multisegmental neurological deficit	Cauda equina syndrome
Hyperreflexia with upgoing toes	Myelopathy
Abdominal bruit, pulsating abdominal mass	Abdominal aortic aneurysm
Absent lower extremity pulses	Abdominal aortic aneurysm

can be rapidly progressive and fatal. Concern is further heightened if the patient is an IV drug user, has had recent surgery, or has had a recent infection.[17]

Clinical Pearl: Fever is a particularly important finding. In fact, fever in the presence of LBP should be considered to be spinal infection until proven otherwise.

Multisegmental neurological deficit demonstrated on neurological examination would suggest radiculopathy involving several nerve roots. This raises the possibility of cauda equina syndrome and may necessitate further investigation.

A thorough neurological examination, at least involving the level of the nervous system at or below the area of complaint, should be undertaken. Hyperreflexia with upgoing toes is a sign of upper motor neuron involvement and may signify a conus lesion or a tumor in the lower thoracic spinal cord. It is important to localize the lesion by examining higher in the central nervous system, specifically looking at Hoffmann's signs, scapulohumeral reflex,[18] jaw jerk, and sensory level in addition to looking for other signs of upper motor neuron involvement such as pronator drift and spasticity and clonus in the extremities.[19]

Auscultation and palpation of the abdominal aorta should be performed on all patients with LBP over the age of 50. The purpose of this is to identify a bruit or expansile pulse. In addition to palpating the abdominal aorta, the lower extremity pulses (i.e., dorsal pedis and posterior tibial) should be examined.

MANAGEMENT OF SUSPECTED "RED FLAG" PATIENTS

The specific history and examination findings highlighted here are indicators of risk for serious conditions. However, it is the totality of the clinical picture that must be considered when formulating the initial treatment plans.

When vertebral fracture is suspected, plain film radiography is the imaging modality of choice. It should be remembered, however, that in the acute stage, fracture is not always evident, especially if film quality is not optimal. In cases where plain films are negative, but there is still concern that a fracture may be present, computed tomography (CT) scan has greater sensitivity. There are those patients, especially older patients with osteoporosis, in whom compression fracture may be seen on routine plain films, but the age (i.e., recent versus pre-existing) of the fracture cannot be determined. Bone scan (scintigraphy) is most useful in this situation because it detects metabolic activity, which may be associated with active healing.

Clinical Pearl: In cases where plain films are negative, but there is still concern that a fracture may be present, CT scan has greater sensitivity.

In patients at risk for tumor, it is best to obtain plain films and blood tests, which should include erythrocyte sedimentation rate (ESR). If the ESR is greater than 20 mm, or if the x-ray is suggestive of malignancy, magnetic resonance imaging (MRI) should be obtained for clarification.[9] Plain films are fairly reliable in demonstrating bone tumors, but are not 100% sensitive. Bone scan may also improve the sensitivity of the investigation as well, owing to increased metabolic activity of the neoplasm. Urinalysis can be helpful, as proteinuria will often be seen in patients with multiple myeloma.

Clinical Pearl: If the ESR is greater than 20 mm, or if the x-ray is suggestive of malignancy, MRI should be obtained for clarification.

If infection is strongly suspected (e.g., fever and elevated white blood cells and ESR), MRI should be obtained immediately because of the possibility of epidural abscess. The patient should be admitted, or sent to a hospital Emergency Department. When these studies are inconclusive, lumbar puncture is often useful. Epidural abscess requires immediate surgical decompression and IV antibiotic therapy.

In suspected cauda equina syndrome, an MRI should be performed immediately with referral to a spine surgeon for possible surgical decompression. If the treating physician does not have admitting privileges, the patient should be sent to the emergency department of the closest hospital and a call should be made to the attending physician or the triage nurse apprising them of the diagnostic concern, so that MRI can be ordered and the spine surgeon on call can be contacted.

Clinical Pearl: In suspected cauda equina syndrome, an MRI should be performed immediately with referral to a spine surgeon for possible surgical decompression.

If AAA is suspected, abdominal ultrasound is the imaging modality of choice, although x-ray, CT, and MRI can also show pathology. The greatest incidence of aneurism occurs in the aorta, with the most common site being the abdomen, specifically between the levels of L2–L4. The most frequent age group is between 60 and 80, with a male/female ratio of 4:1. A measurement of 3.8-mm diameter on a lumbar plain film is diagnostic of AAA, while lesions greater than 5.0 mm are generally considered surgical. It is important to note that 50% of lesions measuring greater than 6.0 mm rupture. Case management recommendations vary, depending on the source. Some authorities recommend surgical consultation for cases AAA of 5 cm or greater, while some surgeons feel that this recommendation should be lower.[20–22] The authors recommend that the spine physician coordinate follow-up with the patient's primary care provider and/or a vascular surgeon for all patients with AAA as soon as the diagnosis is made.

In cases in which upper motor neuron signs are noted on examination, such as hyperreflexia, positive Babinski's test, and spasticity, an attempt should be made to localize the lesion. Once this is accomplished, MRI of the appropriate central nervous system region should be obtained. Further evaluation will depend on these initial imaging findings.

CASE STUDIES

The following case studies are provided to allow the reader to follow a clinical continuum of "red flag" protocol and management strategies. These are adapted from references 16, 19, and 23.

Case #1

This 71-year-old retired football coach was seen complaining of LBP and bilateral leg "numbness" of 2 weeks' duration. He reported a history of LBP nearly his entire life, although he stated that his current pain is the worst that he has had. He had been active in sports his whole life, to which he attributed his history of LBP; however, he was not able to attribute any particular event to his current level of pain. He had been building a stone lighthouse at his home for the 2 weeks prior to his initial visit, which involved lifting and carrying large boulders. He was still engaging in this project the day of his visit.

He had been treated by multiple spine physicians in the past for his previous episodes of LBP and always responded well to manipulative treatments, although the pain would always recur some time after. At the onset of the current episode, he saw his primary care practitioner (PCP) who ordered blood testing, which reportedly was negative. His PCP referred him to a neurologist. The neurologist performed an electromyography/nerve conduction velocity examination and diagnosed "neuropathy." He later saw an orthopedic surgeon, who took radiographs and sent him for physical therapy. The orthopedist also prescribed hydrocodone and methocarbamol. The patient did not fill the physical therapy prescription, and the medications did not make a difference in his pain.

The patient stated that he had vomited daily for the past week and had had very little appetite. He also had been awakening in a cold sweat each night for the past week. He had assumed these symptoms were side effects of the medications.

He described the pain as being "sharp," becoming "burning" at times, and located in his lumbosacral area without radiation or referral. He also described "numbness" in a stocking distribution extending to his mid calf. He denied the presence of muscle weakness in the lower extremities as well as difficulty with bowel or bladder function, painful urination, blood in the urine, and gastrointestinal complaints.

Past medical history was remarkable for recurrent LBP and a fracture to his left fibula while skiing several years ago. He was not taking any medication other than the muscle relaxants. Review of systems was remarkable for occasional neck pain. He did not smoke or drink alcohol and he walked and jogged for exercise. Family history was unremarkable.

During history taking, it was noticed that the patient would occasionally stop talking and appear to be confused, before continuing the conversation.

Examination revealed a well-nourished man who appeared to be agitated and "sick." He tremored frequently and breathed heavily. He moved gingerly and was antalgic in flexion. His tongue was almost completely coated in white and his skin was somewhat pale.

Temperature was 102.6°F. Straight leg raise was negative bilaterally. He had difficulty balancing on heel, toe, and tandem walking, although he was able to perform these maneuvers. Romberg's position revealed falling to the left. Examination of cranial nerves II–XII was within normal limits. Pupils were round, equal, and reactive to light and accommodation. Sensory examination to pinprick in the upper and lower extremities was unremarkable. Motor strength was 5/5 bilaterally throughout. Muscle stretch reflexes were 2+ and symmetric throughout, with the exception of the ankle jerks, which were absent bilaterally. Plantar responses were downgoing bilaterally. Rapid alternating movements, finger-to-nose movements, and heel-to-shin movements were carried out without evidence of dysmetria or tremor. Abdominal examination, including auscultation of the abdominal aorta, revealed no tenderness, masses, or bruits.

Because of the apparent mild mental status changes noted during history taking, the patient's son, who had driven him to the appointment, was asked privately if he had noticed any unusual behavior in his father. The patient's son related that both he and the patient's wife had become concerned that the patient seemed "out of it" at times and would frequently repeated himself and "talk nonsense."

Primarily based on the presence of fever and mental status changes, it was suspected that the patient had a central nervous system infection, with the most likely possibility being encephalitis. It was suspected that the LBP was simply a recurrence of his previous mechanical disorder. He was told that he should return immediately to his PCP and that a call would be placed to this doctor to apprise him of the suspected diagnosis and to recommend hospital admission. The patient and his son both stated that they did not wish to return to the PCP, and so it was recommended that they go immediately to the emergency department of the local teaching hospital.

At the hospital, a brain CT scan was ordered, which was negative. Abdominal ultrasound revealed mild hepatomegaly and thickening of the wall of the gall bladder, consistent with chronic cholecystitis. Radiographs of the cervical spine and chest were unremarkable. Echocardiogram was also negative. Blood work revealed normal white blood cell count but elevated polymorphonuclear cells and a few bands, as well as the presence of gram-positive cocci on culture, consistent with staphylococci. Lumbar MRI revealed some abnormal signal at L5–S1, but the patient was moving too much to confirm this finding. While in the hospital, the patient rapidly developed progressive motor loss in the lower extremities, along with incontinence. Repeat MRI of the lumbar spine demonstrated an epidural abscess at the level of L5–S1. There was no evidence of associated discitis or osteomyelitis.

Immediate surgery was performed to decompress the spinal canal. At surgery, frank pus was noted under pressure around L5–S1. The abscess was irrigated and a laminectomy was performed. Pathology analysis revealed the involved organism to be *Staphylococcus aureus*. The patient was placed on a 6-week course of IV nafcillin. The patient had complete recovery with no neurological sequelae.

Case #2

This patient was an 11-year-old girl who complained of LBP. The pain began 3 months prior to her initial visit after diving off her father's shoulders into shallow water. She struck her head and felt immediate pain in her lower back. She did not feel any neck pain at that time or any time after. Recurrent episodes of pain had developed since that time, which had become progressively worse. She described the pain as being a constant dull ache, which became sharp with all spinal movements. The pain had progressed to the point that she was not able to sleep in her bed and had to sleep in a reclining chair. Standing was the most comfortable position she could find. She also felt relief with the application of moist heat. The pain was located in the mid-lumbar spine bilaterally and she described referral of pain into her lower abdominal quadrants bilaterally. She denied the presence of numbness, parasthesia, motor weakness, difficulty with bowel or bladder function, and constitutional symptoms.

Past medical history was unremarkable. She denied previous injury or accident. She was not taking any medications. Review of systems and family history were unremarkable.

Examination revealed a well-nourished girl who appeared to be in acute pain. She was quite agitated and did not cooperate well in giving her history. Her mother had to assist in extracting information. She was alert and oriented times three and was antalgic in flexion and left lateral flexion and held a moist heating pack to her back, which she was reluctant to allow to be removed. Complete examination was not possible as the patient refused to lie down either prone or supine, stating that the pain did not allow her to do so. Neurological examination was performed in the seated position and revealed normal sensation to pinprick in the upper and lower extremities. Motor strength was 5/5 bilaterally throughout. Muscle stretch reflexes were 2+ and symmetric throughout. Plantar responses were downgoing bilaterally. Rapid alternating movements were carried out without evidence of dysmetria or tremor. Blood pressure was 130/80 in the left arm and oral temperature was 98.5°F.

As complete examination could not be carried out, the patient was told that she should rest in bed for 2 days and return to the office on the third day. She was instructed to apply ice packs for 30 minutes on, 1 hour off interval.

The following day the patient's treating chiropractor was away, and so he placed a telephone call to the patient's mother and she reported that the patient was still complaining of severe pain and now had a "slight fever." She also stated that the patient had vomited twice. The ice seemed to help her to feel more comfortable. She was told to continue with the ice and to monitor the patient's temperature and vomiting.

Another call was placed the following day and the patient's mother explained that the pain was much reduced and the patient was afebrile and had not vomited again. However, she stated that the patient reported that her left leg felt as if it was "giving way" when she bore weight on it. She stated that her sensation was intact. She was told to take the patient immediately to the emergency room. The clinical suspicion at this point was meningitis or Guillain-Barre syndrome.

The patient was admitted and examination findings at that time were normal with the exception of 4+/5 weakness in the left lower extremity. Plain film x-rays of the lumbosacral spine and left hip were negative. Lumbar puncture revealed 13 white cells with 77% polymorphonuclear cells and 5 red cells, glucose 53. Despite the slightly elevated cerebrospinal fluid white blood cell count, Gram stain did not reveal any infectious process. This elevation is likely to relate to some meningeal irritation. White count was 8500, hemoglobin 13.9, and platelets 302,000. The following day she was found to have upgoing toes (positive Babinski's test).

Somatosensory-evoked potentials revealed no cortical potentials on the left side upon stimulation in both the upper and lower extremities. The cervical potential from upper limb stimulation was normal and therefore there was some consideration to possible lesion of the brain stem or thalamocortical projections. However, normal CT scan of the head coupled with the absence of clinical findings in the head or cranial nerves lead to the conclusion that the lack of cortical potential from the upper limb stimulation was likely due to technical considerations.

MRI scans of the thoracic, lumbar, and sacral spines were ordered, which revealed a mass at approximately the T9–T10 region. She was worked up for pheochromocytoma, which was negative. Laminectomy and laminoplasty were performed and a large astrocytoma was found expanding the spinal cord. This was removed and the patient was maintained on steroids with a slow taper. Pathological analysis revealed the tumor to be of grade I. She was discharged to home 1 week later in stable condition.

Case #3

The patient was a 52-year-old crossing guard who was referred by her internist with a complaint of weakness of the right lower extremity, which had started 8 months previously. She first noticed it when walking. She found that her right foot would start to "drag" about 40 minutes into her walk. Over time the weakness became progressively more pronounced and occurred earlier in the walk, until it would start after approximately 20 minutes. She stated that she had some "soreness" in the right lumbosacral area but no significant lower back pain. She denied motor loss as well as bowel or bladder difficulties, abdominal pain or lower extremity swelling, coldness, or discoloration related to the weakness. She did not experience weakness during any other activities.

Past medical history was remarkable for asthma for which she took albuterol. Review of systems was remarkable for hot flashes, some increase in urinary frequency of recent onset, and occasional anxiety and depression. She was married with two children. She did not smoke, drank two glasses of wine per night, and walked for exercise. Family history was unremarkable.

Examination revealed a well-nourished, pleasant woman who appeared to be in no acute distress. Blood pressure was 125/80 on the left. Temperature was 98.7°F. Pulse was 72 per minute. Respirations were 16 per minute.

The straight leg raise and well leg raise were negative. Heel and toe walking were within normal limits, but she had difficulty with tandem walking. Romberg's position was held with eyes closed without difficulty. Examination of cranial nerves II–XII was within normal limits. Pupils were round, equal and reactive to light and accommodation. Funduscopic examination was unremarkable. Sensory examination to pinprick in the upper and lower extremities was unremarkable. Vibration sense was absent bilaterally in the feet and reduced bilaterally in the hands. Motor strength was 5/5 bilaterally throughout with the exception of the right tibialis anterior and extensor hallucis longus, which were both 4+/5. Muscle stretch reflexes were 3+ and symmetric throughout. Plantar responses were upgoing bilaterally. Tromner's signs were present bilaterally. Scapulohumeral reflexes were present bilaterally. Jaw jerk was normal. There were four or five beats of clonus in the ankles bilaterally. Spasticity was noted in the lower extremities with rapid knee flexion bilaterally. No clonus was noted in the upper extremities. There was no evidence of pronator drift.

Because of the upper motor neuron findings that were present on examination, which was localized to below the brain stem, a cervical MRI was ordered, with the suspicion of cervical spondylotic myelopathy, or some other cervical myelopathic process.

The MRI revealed a sharp kyphosis in the mid cervical spine with spondylosis at C4–C5 and disc bulge at C5–C6, both of which encroached on the spine cord. There was mild cord atrophy at the C4–C5 level, and hyperintensity could be seen on the T2 weighted images. These findings were suggestive of cervical spondylotic myelopathy except that the hyperintensity within the spinal cord was in the posterior aspect of the cord, rather than in the anterior, which was the site of compression on the cord. Because hyperintensity in the posterior cord is a characteristic finding in multiple sclerosis, a brain MRI was ordered. This demonstrated multiple small, circumscribed deep white matter subependymal T2 hyperintensities, characteristic of multiple sclerosis. The diagnosis was confirmed with lumbar puncture. She was started on interferon self-injection therapy.

Case #4

The patient was a returning 29-year-old female who presented with acute left-sided LBP with some radiation to the ipsilateral gluteal region. The pain began 2 days before and seemed to progressively worsen. Her symptoms were unrelenting and minimally affected by movement or changing positions. Her pain did not waiver throughout the day, and she did note that the pain awakened her at night. Over-the-counter nonsteroidal anti-inflammatory drugs (NSAIDs) provided minimal pain relief. Dejerine's triad (coughing, sneezing, or straining) was negative for increased symptoms to the buttock or leg.

Past history was remarkable for three, nondebilitating low back episodes over a 5-year period, all of which responded well with conservative management at the spine physician's clinic within 2–4 weeks. Prior conservative treatment consisted of NSAIDs, manipulation, patient education, and exercise. The patient was also remarkable for two prior episodes of bladder infections. She denied any recent trauma, any history of cancer, any prolonged steroid use, or any prior surgery. In addition to the above-mentioned NSAIDs, her only other medication was birth control pills. She stated that she underwent her annual pelvic examination and Pap smear less than 6 months before, both of which were normal. Review of systems and family history were otherwise unremarkable.

Examination revealed a well-nourished, pleasant woman who appeared to be in mild acute distress due to her pain and sleep deprivation. Blood pressure was 131/86 on the left. Temperature was 99.7°F. Pulse was 82 per minute. Respirations were 20 per minute.

Static postural evaluation revealed the patient to be slightly antalgic, leaning to the left from the waist. Thoracolumbar mobility was reduced by 20% in right lateral flexion, 50% in bilateral rotation, and 10% in forward flexion, although these motions provoked little additional pain. Instead, the patient felt as though her left low back region restricted her motion. Neurological examination, including reflex, sensory, and motor functions, of the lower extremities was within normal limits. Orthopedic testing failed to provoke a significant increase in pain. Palpation was remarkable for rigidity of the left paraspinal musculature, which extended the patient's flank. Percussion lateral to the L1–L3 region provoked increased left-sided pain, which the patient felt was "deep" (i.e., as apposed to being superficial tenderness). Abdominal palpation revealed mild tenderness and hypertonicity of the left lateral musculature, but was otherwise unremarkable. Palpation of the thoracic, lumbar, sacroiliac, and coccyx revealed mild dysfunction, with generalized diminished segmental motion in the lower thoracic, lumbar, and left sacroiliac. However, no tenderness was noted of these regions, nor did springing palpation of the joints (see Chapter 13) provoke pain.

The initial differential diagnosis was kidney colic secondary to kidney infection. The diagnosis was based upon the patient's unrelenting symptoms, the lack of recent trauma, the rather rapid onset, the low-grade fever, the minimal skeletal examination findings, the significant left-sided rigidity, and the prior history of bladder infections. A urinalysis was performed in the office, which revealed an elevated leukocyte count. This was considered sufficiently confirmatory of the differential diagnosis to warrant immediate referral, and so the patient's primary physician was called and the patient sent directly there for follow-up. The patient was instructed to contact the spine physician's office following the visit with her primary physician. She was instructed to return if her back pain persisted after her infection resolved.

CONCLUSION

Assessment for "red flags," potentially serious underlying conditions such as systemic disease, fracture, and neurological compromise, should be the first step in the diagnostic triage of patients with low back syndromes. Surprisingly, the majority of back care physicians polled in a recent study failed to properly screen for red flags.[24] Such a startling finding emphasizes the importance of maintaining a consistent clinical regimen.

Clinical Pearl: Surprisingly, the majority of back care physicians polled in a recent study failed to properly screen for red flags.

Red flag screening is typically presented as a part of an initial comprehensive evaluation. It is important to remember, however, that disease processes may first become clinically apparent at any time after the initial examination. Therefore, the clinician must always be alert for signs suggesting the presence of a red flag condition. Perhaps the most challenging case for the clinician is that of the returning patient, whose symptoms mimic prior episodes of mechanical LBP that responded well to conservative care. Although the patient may assume that his/her symptoms are simply a recurrence of a previous musculoskeletal condition, the clinician cannot make such an assumption. Case #4 (presented earlier in this chapter) illustrates the need for clinicians to remain vigilant for red flags conditions.

The red flag screening process need not be cumbersome. For example, Bogduk and McGuirk developed an effective history-based screening questionnaire that typically required less than 1 minute to complete.[25] The reader is also referred to the acute and chronic algorithms presented in Chapter 31 to better understand how the red flag screening process can be incorporated into the overall evaluation and management of patients with LBP.

Clinical Pearl: ...the time taken during the history and examination helps to build a strong doctor–patient bond, as patients appreciate the clinician who takes the time to carefully enquire, listen, examine, and then clearly explain their findings and recommendations.

Ruling out red flags provides the patient and clinician with multiple benefits. The patient is triaged in a manner that expedites appropriate treatment. The treating physician can be confident that conservative care can be expected to provide therapeutic benefit and if it does not, the index of suspicion for red flag conditions must be increased. Ruling out red flags also helps to reduce the inappropriate utilization of costly imaging studies. The clinician can utilize the results of the red flag screening to explain to the patient why a thorough evaluation does not necessarily involve advanced imaging or other diagnostic testing. The clinician can also use the red flag screening process to reassure the patient that there is no evidence of a serious underlying condition and that his/her symptoms are likely to respond well to conservative care. Finally, the time taken during the history and examination helps to build a strong doctor–patient bond, as patients appreciate the clinician who takes the time to carefully enquire, listen, examine, and then clearly explain their findings and recommendations.

Because only a small percentage of patients will have positive red flag findings, this creates a temptation for the busy clinician to inadvertently bypass the screening process. Nevertheless, it remains the professional responsibility of every clinician to be consistently vigilant and incorporate the red flag screening process into the routine evaluation of *every* low back syndrome patient.

SUMMARY

1. Assessment for clinical "Red Flags" those with serious underlying conditions, represents the first stage of the diagnostic triage.
2. The patient history represents a critical opportunity to assess for clinical "Red Flags."
3. The examination provides supporting documentation for suspected clinical "Red Flags."
4. The clinician must always be alert for clinical "Red Flags," among established patients.
5. The time taken to rule out clinical "Red Flags" helps to build a strong patient-doctor relationship, as patients appreciate thorough care.
6. It has been reported that a majority of clinicians in one study failed to assess for clinical "Red Flags," suggesting that this crucial part of diagnostic triage is being forsaken.

REFERENCES

1. Deyo RA, Diehl AK. Cancer as a cause of back pain: Frequency, clinical presentation and diagnostic strategies. *J Gen Int Med* 1988;3:230–238.
2. Bigos S, Bowyer O, Braen G, et al. *Acute low back problems in adults.* Clinical Practice Guidelines No. 14. Rockville, MD: Agency for Health Care Policy and Research, Public Health Service, US Department of Health and Human Services, December 1994. AHCPR Publication No. 95-0642.
3. Nachemson A, Vingard E. Assessment of patients with neck and back pain: A best-evidence synthesis. In: Nachemson A, Johnsson. E, eds. *Neck and back pain: The scientific evidence of causes, diagnosis, and treatment.* Philadelphia: Lippincott Williams & Wilkins, 2000:191–193.
4. Cessna RM. Dangerous back pain. *JACA* 1988;22:65–66.
5. Schofferman L, Schofferman J, Zucherman J, et al. Occult infections causing persistent low back pain. *Spine* 1989;14(4):417–419.
6. Yochum TR, Rowe LJ. *Essentials of skeletal radiology.* Baltimore, MD: Williams & Wilkins, 1987.
7. Swensen RS. A medical approach to the differential diagnosis of low back pain. *J Neuromusculoskeletal Syst* 1998;6(3):100–113.
8. Ferri FF, ed. *Ferri's clinical advisor.* St. Louis: Mosby, 2002.
9. Joines JD, McNutt RA, Carey TS, Deyo RA, Rouhani R. Finding cancer in primary care outpatients with low back pain. A comparison of diagnostic strategies. *J Gen Intern Med* 2001;16:14–23.
10. Slipman CW, Patel RK, Botwin K, et al. Epidemiology of spine tumors presenting to musculoskeletal physiatrists. *Arch Phys Med Rehabil* 2003;84:492–495.
11. Grattan-Smith PJ, Ryan MM, Procopis PG. Persistent or severe back pain and stiffness are ominous symptoms requiring prompt attention. *J Paediatr Child Health* 2000;36:208–212.
12. Ahn UM, Ahn NU, Buchowski JM, Garrett ES, Siebern AN, Kostuik JP. Cauda equina syndrome secondary to lumbar disc herniation: A meta-analysis of surgical outcomes. *Spine* 2000;25(12):1515–1522.
13. Busse JW, Hsu WS. Rapid progression of acute sciatica to cauda equina syndrome. *J Manipulative Physiol Ther* 2001;24(5):350–355.
14. Shapiro S. Medical realities of cauda equina syndrome secondary to lumbar disc herniation. *Spine* 2000;25(3):348–351.
15. Crawford CM, Hurtgen-Grace K, Talarico E, Marley J. Abdominal aortic aneurysm: An illustrated narrative

review. *J Manipulative Physiol Ther* 2003;26(3):184–195.

16. Murphy DR, Carr BM. Spinal epidural abscess in a patient with chronic, recurrent low back pain: A case report. *J Neuromusculoskeletal Syst* 1999;7(2):70–73.
17. Hlavin ML, Kaminski HJ, Ross JS, Ganz E. Spinal epidural abscess: A ten year perspective. *Neurosurgery* 1990;27:177–184.
18. Shimizu T, Shimada H, Shirakura K. Scapulohumeral reflex (Shimizu): Its clinical significance and testing maneuver. *Spine* 1993;18:2182–2190.
19. Murphy DR, Williams DS. Complaint of foot drop leads to diagnosis of multiple sclerosis: A case report. *JACA* 2004;41(5):32–35.
20. Estes JE Jr. Abdominal aorta aneurysm: A study of one hundred and two cases. *Circulation* 1950;2:258–265.
21. Steinberg I, Stein HL. Visualization of abdominal aortic aneurysms. *Am J Roentgenol Radium Ther Nucl Med* November 1965;95(3):684–695.
22. Harger BL, Hoffman LE, Arkless R. Miscellaneous abdomen diseases. In: Marchiori DM, ed. *Clinical imaging with skeletal, chest and abdomen pattern differentials.* St. Louis: Mosby, 1999:979–984.
23. Murphy DR, Murphy LB, Tyszkowski RJ. Spinal astrocytoma in an 11 year old girl: A case report. *J Neuromusculoskeletal Syst* 1997;5(1):35–38.
24. McGlynn EA, Asch SM, Adams J, et al. The quality of health care delivered to adults in the United States. *NEMJ* 2003;348:2635–2645.
25. Bogduk N, McGuirk B. *Medical management of acute and chronic ow back pain. An evidence-based approach.* London: Elsevier, 2002.

CHAPTER

11

NONSPECIFIC LOW BACK PAIN AND CHRONIC LOW BACK SYNDROMES

Paul D. Hooper, Craig E. Morris, J. David Cassidy, and Niels Grunnet-Nilsson

OUTLINE

OBJECTIVES

1. To understand the nature of nonspecific low back pain.
2. To understand the subset of common diagnoses that currently fall under the heading of nonspecific back pain.
3. To understand the natural history of low back syndromes.
4. To understand the complex nature of chronic low back syndromes.
5. To understand the differences between disability and impairment.
6. To review and integrate four clinical flags into the understanding of chronic pain syndromes.

INTRODUCTION

In spite of recent developments in the understanding of anatomy and biomechanics, significant improvements in diagnostic procedures, and new, innovative treatment methods, low back pain is as prevalent today as it has ever been.[1,2] In addition, disability resulting from back pain is on the rise. Fortunately, for most individuals who suffer from back pain, recovery is quick and incapacity is limited.[3] As will be discussed later in this chapter, a significant number of individuals continue to suffer from recurring episodes of back pain, while a small group develops incapacitating problems.

Clinical Pearl: It is generally agreed that, for the vast majority of back pain sufferers, the etiological factors are not known.

Over the years, back pain has been associated with various anatomic structures and assorted pathologic changes. This includes low back pain due to the presence of a herniation and/or degeneration of an intervertebral disc, arthrosis of zygapophyseal joints, changes in myofascial structures, muscle weakness, and even autoimmune disorders. However, it is generally agreed that the etiological factors are not known among the vast majority of back pain sufferers. This was emphasized by Nachemson when he stated that only 20% of back pain can be traced to any specific tissue.[4] While some individuals claim to understand the "real cause" of back pain, it is fair to state that a great deal of back pain is most easily identified by a lack of any obvious pathological findings. The purpose of this chapter is to look at this category of back pain that represents the most common, and probably the least understood form of this familiar condition, i.e. nonspecific low back pain. In addition to looking at the nature of nonspecific back pain, this chapter will also discuss why a small percentage of patients end up among the ranks of the disabled.

Patient Presentation

Clear Clinical Picture When patients see a doctor, they present in one of several ways.[5] First, they may present with something that is very obvious or a clear clinical picture. An example is seen in the patient with a relatively minor wrist sprain. Advanced clinical skills are not required to assess the situation. The diagnosis is easy and treatment is uncomplicated. Patients typically recover quickly and completely. In terms of the patient with back pain, a young, otherwise healthy individual with a minor back sprain may provide an example of the typical back pain that is the subject of this chapter. Although there may be some disagreement regarding which particular tissues are the actual pain generators, it is clear with this individual that there is no overt pathology and/or anomalies that account for his or her pain. As with the minor wrist sprain, recovery is usually quick and seemingly complete.

Obvious Signs and Symptoms Some patients present with back problems that are difficult to diagnose. For instance, the patient who presents with an acute episode of low back pain may be in such pain that a thorough examination may not be possible. Additionally, the limited number of examination procedures that can be performed may all be positive because of severe pain. Consequently, the exact nature of the injury may not be readily determined. In such a case, it may actually be more important to establish what the patient does not have. Whether the patient has a joint or a muscle injury may not be critical when deciding on the type of treatment to be provided. However, knowing that the patient does not have a fracture or some form of serious pathology or "red flag" is crucial. While a tissue-specific diagnosis may not be readily available in such patients, there are obvious signs and symptoms that are present. These may include pain, limited range of motion, and muscle hypertonicity. When the precise diagnosis may not be readily apparent, and after more serious conditions have been effectively ruled out, treatment is used primarily to address the symptoms. Perhaps, as treatment progresses and the patient's condition improves, a more tolerable and thorough examination may better reveal the specific nature of the condition.

Problem Behind the Problem Another group of patients presents with a primary complaint that masks the complexity or seriousness of other problem(s). In these patients, a number of other conditions and/or concerns coexist with the back pain and complicate the clinical picture. Some of these additional conditions may be potentially serious and, in some instances, may even be life-threatening. These must be identified early in order to provide appropriate treatment. The clinician must be alert for the "red flags" that are seen with these conditions (see Chapter 10). In addition to potentially serious medical conditions, other concerns may be hidden by the magnitude of the primary complaint. An example of this occurs with the patient who presents with acute low back pain that coincides with some organ pathology (e.g., ovarian cyst). While the underlying visceral disorder may be a greater concern, the magnitude of the low back symptoms diverts the attention of both the patient and the clinician. Still other factors, such as psychosocial considerations, may simply make recovery more difficult.[6,7] When faced with such conditions, the clinician must determine whether additional assistance may be required in order to successfully evaluate and/or treat the patient. Also, when faced with the nonresponsive patient, the clinician must determine whether or not other conditions (i.e., comorbidities) complicate the clinical picture, whether the patient is doing something detrimental, or whether some other form of treatment might be more beneficial.

LOW BACK PAIN AS A WELL-DEFINED DISEASE

In order to better understand low back pain, it may be helpful to look at the following four characteristics of any well-defined disease. A well-defined disease is said to have four characteristics:

1. A similar set of signs and symptoms
2. An understanding of the etiology
3. An appreciation of the natural history
4. Treatment methods that are derived from a combination of #2 and #3

Although some may argue whether low back pain qualifies as a "well-understood disease," for the purposes of this chapter, nonspecific low back pain will be looked at in this context, i.e., as a well-understood disease. First, however, it is necessary to define what is meant by "nonspecific low back pain." Other terms used for this condition include mechanical low back pain, lumbalgia, and simple backache.

Providing a useful definition of *nonspecific back pain* is not an easy task. In fact, it is more readily defined by what it is not. Lindena et al. report on German guidelines that attempt to differentiate between "disease-related specific back pain and non-specific back pain of a more functional or mechanical origin"[8]. Waddell[9] states that "simple backache is mechanical, in the sense it varies with physical activity." Burton et al. list several common features of simple backache[10]:

- Backache is very common.
- There is no sign of serious damage or disease.
- No permanent weakness is likely.
- Recurrence is possible but does not mean reinjury.
- Activity is helpful, too much rest is not.

Snook[11] refers to nonspecific low back pain as an age-related disorder that is affected by differences in occupation, genetics, and personal behavior. However, nonspecific back pain is evident in almost all age groups. In addition, it is worth noting that while nonspecific back pain may be best defined by the absence of disease-related pain, certain conditions (e.g., scoliosis) may be present concurrently. This statement perhaps best describes the problem: "Uncertainty is the rule rather than the exception."[12] The reader is referred to Table 11–1 for a list of conditions that may be used to distinguish between disease-related back pain and nonspecific back pain.

Clinical Pearl: ...while nonspecific back pain may be best defined by the absence of disease-related pain, certain conditions (e.g., scoliosis) may be present concurrently.

TABLE 11–1. Nonspecific vs. Disease-Specific Back Pain

Nonspecific Back Pain	Disease-Specific Back Pain
Simple backache	Multiple myeloma
Lumbalgia	Metastatic carcinoma
Lumbar sprain/strain	Infection
Facet syndrome	Ankylosing spondylitis
Sacroiliac syndrome	Rheumatoid arthritis
Intervertebral disc syndrome	Fracture
Myofascial pain syndrome (e.g., piriformis syndrome)	Viscerogenic pain (e.g., kidney stones, ovarian cyst, abdominal aneurysm)
Dysfunctional segmental motion	Cauda equina syndrome

A Similar Set of Signs and Symptoms

Patients who present with lower back pain have signs and symptoms that are relatively similar. One of the more practical methods of characterizing the various types of low back pain is that developed by the Quebec Task Force (QTF).[13] Although this classification system is somewhat dated, the QTF places patients in 11 categories based on their symptom picture (see Table 11–2). Because of this excellent design, the QTF remains a worthwhile format for a strategic understanding of nonspecific back pain.

The first two categories are used to describe pain and symptoms that are present in the absence of any specific pathologic process. Perhaps Lewit's term "functional pathology" is most appropriate here.[14] Categories 3 and 4 may occur in the absence of significant structural pathology, or they may be associated with degenerative changes in the disc, facet joints, or other spinal structures. Although it is generally agreed that there is no strong correlation between structural changes seen on X-rays and the presence or absence of back pain, Categories 5 through 9 are associated with specific and obvious pathologies, in other words, those pathologies that can be seen on plain film radiographs and with magnetic resonance imaging (MRI) and computed tomography (CT) studies. Category 10, low back pain associated with chronic pain, involves a complex interaction of factors, not

TABLE 11–2. The Quebec Task Force Classification

1	local low back pain with no radiation
2	Low back pain with some radiation into the proximal extremity
3	Low back pain with radiation into the distal extremity
4	Low back pain with radiation and positive neurological findings
5	Low back pain with presumptive compression of spinal nerve roots – possibly associated with spinal instability and/or fracture
6	Low back pain with confirmation of compression of spinal nerve root
7	Low back pain associated with spinal stenosis
8	Low back pain associated with a postsurgical status of less than 6 months after intervention
9	Low back pain associated with a postsurgical status of greater than 6 months after intervention
10	Low back pain associated with chronic pain syndrome
11	Low back pain associated with other medical causes

Source: From Spitzer et al.[13]

all of which are physical. Finally, patients in Category 11 have low back pain that is secondary to some other medical condition, such as metastasis or ankylosing spondylitis. It is those patients in Categories 1 and 2, with the addition of some in Categories 3 and 4, who are of particular interest in this chapter. The 11 QTF categories will be revisited again later in this chapter.

Clinical Pearl: One of the more practical methods of characterizing the various types of low back pain is that developed by the Quebec Task Force (QTF).

Serious Conditions While the focus of this chapter is on patients with low back pain of mechanical origin, it is important to initially identify any individuals who have underlying disease and who need referral to a medical specialist. Several studies have suggested that this is a relatively easy step to accomplish, providing an adequate evaluation of the patient is performed. A recent study by McGlynn et al.[15] looked at the clinical management and preventive care for 30 common conditions, including back pain. The authors stated the majority of health-care providers appeared to leave out vital steps in the assessment of back pain, including the search for systemic disease and neurological compromise. The study found that clinicians who evaluate acute back pain often do not screen for red flags, i.e., signs of serious disease (see Chapter 10). They also concluded that more than half of the providers do not conduct a neurological examination. They suggest that the assessment of patients with low back pain should include

- Focused questions about red flags
- Performing a neurological screening and
- Performing a passive straight-leg raise test.

Clinical Pearl: Bogduk stated that when serious conditions escape detection, it is often due to inattention during the history.

In a similar study, Bogduk[16] stated that when serious conditions escape detection, it is often due to inattention during the history. In a study of 437 patients, McGuirk et al.[17] noted that physicians were able to catch all red flag conditions (1.4%) at the initial consultation. Once again, the reader is referred to Chapter 10 for a more detailed look at "red flags."

While these systemic conditions are serious, it is worth emphasizing that they are relatively rare, with nonspecific low back and/or leg pain representing some 97% of cases. Spinal conditions such as neoplasm, infection, etc., account for only 1% of cases, and back pain that is associated with some form of visceral disorder is found only 2% of the time.[18] As stated earlier, one of the more important aspects of differential diagnosis is understanding what the patient "does not" have. In other words, *nonspecific back pain is really a diagnosis of exclusion*. Once the more serious and/or potentially life-threatening conditions have been ruled out, the clinician is safe to continue.

Clinical Pearl: Spinal conditions such as neoplasm, infection, etc., account for only 1% of cases, and back pain that is associated with some form of visceral disorder is found only 2% of the time.

Functional Diagnoses While the term *nonspecific back pain* has been used for the category of back pain discussed in this chapter, in some patients functional conditions may be diagnosed. It is worth noting, however, that these conditions are not usually associated with any specific pathological structural changes. These conditions include facet syndrome, sacroiliac syndrome, postural syndrome, posterior derangement, myofascial pain, and dysfunctional segmental motion. It should be pointed out that these are conceptual clinical constructs that help some clinicians address nonspecific low back pain, but their validity has not been established.

1. Facet syndrome: Also referred to as posterior joint syndrome, and also the redundant posterior facet syndrome, this condition represents functional changes in the zygapophyseal joints. While this disorder is accepted by many, others argue its relevance. In 1992, Jackson stated that while the lumbar facet joints are very important biomechanically, the facet is not a common or clear source of significant pain and the facet syndrome is not a reliable clinical diagnosis.[19] Dreyer and Dreyfuss stated that although the histological basis for this condition has been established, the precise clinical etiology remains undetermined.[20] They also note that there are no unique identifying features in the history, physical examination, and/or radiographic imaging. In spite of this apparent confusion, recent studies estimate that 15%–40% of chronic low back pain due to the zygapophyseal joints.[21] For more information on this condition, the reader is referred to Chapter 8.
2. Sacroiliac syndrome: This condition includes back pain that is produced by changes in the function of the sacroiliac joint(s). Riddle and Freburger use the term *sacroiliac joint region dysfunction* to describe pain in or around the region of the sacroiliac joint which is presumed to be due to malalignment

or abnormal movement of the joints.[22] Bogduk states that anesthetic joint blocks can identify the sacroiliac joint as a source of pain in 20% of patients with chronic low back pain. In a recent review of the literature on examination procedures for the low back, Saal stated that over the past few decades, the sacroiliac joint has received varying degrees of interest as an important pain generator of low back pain.[23] Unfortunately, despite testimonials to the contrary, no diagnostic or physical examination criterion has established the diagnostic validity of this condition. For more information on the posterior joint syndromes (i.e., facet and sacroiliac), the reader is directed to Chapter 8.

3. Postural syndrome: Several authors have attempted to connect poor posture with the development of low back pain. Fahrni and Trueman[24] noted a lower incidence of back pain in ground dwelling or agrarian populations. They attributed this to the flexed position of the spine seen in the squatting position so common in these cultures. Similarly, Williams blamed back pain on the development of a lumbar lordosis and the negative impact this purportedly had on the intervertebral disc. He developed a protocol designed to treat low back pain by reducing the lumbar lordosis.[25] Williams' flexion exercises became a staple in both the treatment and prevention of back pain for many years.

   Like Williams, McKenzie also attributed low back pain to postural stresses.[26] It must be clarified that this is quite different from the postural syndrome discussed in the previous paragraph. McKenzie's postural syndrome describes pain provoked by non-disc-supporting spinal structures caused by postural overload. It is classically found in individuals who maintain prolonged postures, such as those who sit at computers for hours at a time. And, like Williams' flexion exercises, McKenzie's protocol has been a popular method of treating back pain for many years. Chapters 15 and 22 discuss McKenzie's approach in detail.

   Janda described the common pattern of muscle imbalance that contributes to the development of back pain.[27] According to Janda, *postural muscles*, those that are used to combat the forces of gravity, become shortened and strong with overuse, while their antagonists, called *phasic muscles*, tend to become lengthened and weak (see Table 13-1, Chapter 13). This leads to the development of the lower crossed syndrome, a postural condition that is commonplace in modern society owing to prolonged, constrained postures such as sitting.

4. Posterior derangement: McKenzie described intervertebral disc posterior bulging as a result of sustained flexion stress.[28] According to McKenzie, flexion caused a posterior migration of the annulus with resulting pain, which he called a posterior derangement (see Chapter 15). He also stated that continued postural stresses would ultimately cause a permanent change in the internal structure of the disc. His therapeutic approach, initially known as McKenzie's extension protocol, focused attention on the use of extension exercises and movements to evaluate, treat, and prevent low back pain and is discussed in Chapter 22.
5. Lumbar segmental instability: This is a type of chronic instability related to changes in the intervertebral disc and/or the vertebral body due to degenerative changes, tumor, or infection. The associated instability has been termed *mechanical instability*. This condition is characterized by pain that is usually made worse by activity and improved both by rest and by positioning the body in a way that minimizes spinal stresses. The pain pattern is said to implicate an exaggeration of reflex muscle activity that accompanies attempts to maintain an acceptable amount of stability.[29]

Complicating Factors In addition to serious medical conditions that must be identified, many patients with back pain are found to have additional problems that complicate or confound the clinical scenario. These may or may not directly affect the presenting complaint, but must be taken into account. These problems include both physical and psychosocial concerns. Some of the physical factors that may be identified include scoliosis, short leg syndrome, spondylolisthesis, osteoporosis, obesity, etc.

1. Scoliosis: In a recent article looking at risk factors for low back pain in adolescents, Kovacs et al. found an almost threefold association with scoliosis (odds ratio, OR = 2.87).[30] They also found a hereditary association with scoliosis in the parents. However, there was no association between the presence of scoliosis in parents and the presence of low back pain in children. Weinstein et al. looked at long-term studies of idiopathic scoliosis.[31] They noted a higher incidence of chronic back pain in the scoliosis group (61%) when compared to age- and sex-matched controls (35%). (For an explanation of OR, the reader is referred to Chapter 4.)
2. Short leg syndrome: Some authors have claimed an association between leg length inequality and the presence of low back pain. In the above-noted study by Kovacs et al., a weak association was seen

(OR = 1.26). In a case series of patients with lumbar disc herniations, ten Brinke et al. showed an association between leg length discrepancy and the side of radiating pain.[32] Interestingly, the relation was only significant in women. Others have previously argued that any such association is questionable.[33,34]

3. Spondylolisthesis: It is well known that there is an association between certain activities and the development of spondylolisthesis.[35] For example, certain athletes such as cricket bowlers and gymnasts have a high incidence of spondylolisthesis. Beutler et al. report on a 45-year follow-up study of 500 first-grade children to determine the natural history of spondylolysis and spondylolisthesis.[36] They report no difference in any health outcome in those individuals with or without pars defects. Also, there was no association between slip progression and low back pain. However, a far different situation exists in the case of an unstable spondylolisthesis. Such instability may likely result in surgery, which is described in detail in Chapter 34.
4. Osteoporosis: With more individuals reaching advanced age, the incidence of osteoporosis is increasing. However, in the absence of spinal fracture, a review of published research failed to demonstrate any correlation between osteoporosis and the development of back.[37]
5. Obesity: This is associated with a variety of health disorders, including a number of musculoskeletal conditions. In a recent study on obesity and low back pain, the authors state that there is a moderate association.[38] Deyo and Bass examined back pain and lifestyle factors such as smoking and obesity.[39] They reported a greater prevalence with increasing body mass index, with a substantial rise in the most obese. Bernard[40] and Frank et al.[41] note that obesity (or high body mass index) has only a weak association for low back pain. Whether the relationship is one of cause and effect or whether it is more indicative of the results of a sedentary lifestyle is unclear. It may also be that changes in lifestyle and activity levels that often accompany back pain lead to a general deconditioning that may increase the mechanical stresses on the lower back.
6. Yellow flags: In addition to various physical factors, there are numerous psychosocial issues that may coexist with back pain. These include such issues as litigation and compensation, poor job satisfaction, low education level, depression, etc. These are collectively referred to as "yellow flags" and are addressed in Chapter 19. While the physical factors are important in back injury, the psychosocial factors can play an important and often unrecognized role in the development and potential recovery of the patient. This will be discussed in more detail in the section on *Chronic Disability Syndromes*.
7. Comorbid conditions: Patients often present with more than one condition at the same time. For example, a patient with discogenic back and leg pain will often move with an antalgic posture. With time and persistent symptoms, the altered mechanics of this postural imbalance can lead to immobility and withdrawal from normal activities. The constant pain and associated limitations can lead to deconditioning and depression, both of which can further aggravate the low back pain.[42]

An Understanding of the Etiology

Although the true etiology of nonspecific back pain is often unclear, it is sometimes attributed to a specific event such as a lift or fall. This is unfortunate as it may give individuals affected by low back pain a sense that since the problem appeared to develop suddenly, it may in turn resolve quickly. In contrast to low back pain, other musculoskeletal disorders, particularly cumulative trauma disorders (CTDs) such as carpal tunnel syndrome, are not usually attributed to any single event but rather to a series of repeated activities. In the majority of cases, nonspecific low back pain is not associated with any particular traumatic event and the etiology is not known.

How Injuries Occur Back injuries occur in one of several ways. First, when the failure tolerance of the tissue is exceeded by the application of an unacceptable load, overload occurs.[43] Specifically, what structure fails remains unclear, although recent investigations have provided some interesting clues.[44] In addition to tissue failure that results from the application of a single load, tissue also fails when it is subjected to a constant and repetitive application of loads that, individually, are well within the tissue tolerance. The continued loading results in a gradual deterioration of tissue integrity. This is the case with CTDs, and there is increasing interest in considering back pain in such a manner. In fact, it may be more appropriate to look at back pain in this way. Rather than being the result of a single event, it is likely that a significant number of back problems develop gradually over a period of time. Then, when the individual is unprepared, a seemingly trivial activity precipitates the onset of an episode of back pain. A typical example might occur when an individual reaches to retrieve a pencil and "sprains" his back.

Clinical Pearl: ...when the failure tolerance of the tissue is exceeded by the application of an unacceptable load, overload occurs.

It is worth pointing out that when living tissue is subjected to a repeated demand, an adaptive response is seen and the tolerance level of the tissue is increased. This is the basis of most exercise programs. However, this response is dependent upon a sufficient recovery period to allow for an adaptive response. Recent evidence suggests that this recovery period may be an important link in the development of CTDs.[45]

An Appreciation of the Natural History

One important aspect in the consideration of any well-understood disease is to be aware of what happens naturally, with or without intervention. In this regard, low back pain has long been considered to be a "self-limiting" condition.[46] In other words, much like the common cold, low back pain is believed to typically disappear on its own. Treatment therefore has not been considered to be important, at least during the acute episode. Consequently, the use of heroic, expensive, and/or invasive procedures, either diagnostic or therapeutic, has been considered to be unnecessary. Even the routine use of lumbar spine radiographs, previously considered a staple of the initial diagnostic process, is now often considered uncalled for due to cost and unnecessary patient exposure to radiation.

Clinical Pearl: While many consider nonspecific low back pain to be self-limiting, it would appear that, rather than recovering completely, many patients simply stop seeking care.

There is recent evidence, however, that forces a rethinking of the above perspective regarding the natural history of low back pain. While many consider nonspecific low back pain to be self-limiting, it would appear that rather than recovering completely, many patients simply stop seeking care.[46] In a study of 503 patients aged 18–60 with low back pain of less than 2 weeks duration, 50% of those on sick leave were back to work within 8 days. At 1-year follow-up, only 2% remained on sick leave. At first glance, this appears to support the view of back pain as self-limiting. However, although most went back to work, a full 45% continued to complain of pain 1 year later. Factors most significantly associated with a poor recovery were severity of initial symptoms, assessments by the general practitioner of susceptibility to develop chronic problems, and a history of previous low back pain causing work absence.[47]

Clinical Pearl: von Korff and Saunders (1996) found that one third of patients in primary care settings experienced intermittent or persistent pain of at least moderate severity at least 1 year after the initial episode.

Several other investigators have looked at the natural history of patients with low back pain. Coste et al. claimed that 90% of patients in a primary care setting recovered within 2 weeks.[3] McGuirk et al.[17] showed a high level of symptom resolution, while Croft et al.[48] stated that 40% of patients continued to complain of pain and disability 1 year after their initial episode. Similarly, von Korff and Saunders found that one third of patients in primary care settings experienced intermittent or persistent pain of at least moderate severity at least 1 year after the initial episode.[49]

Two systematic reviews have looked at the literature in this area. The first review by Hestbaek et al. states the following[50]:

- There is no evidence that 80%–90% of patients become pain-free within 1 month.
- 42%–75% of patients still had symptoms after 12 months.
- 44%–78% had relapses.
- 26%–37% of workers who underwent a back-related work absence experienced a relapse of work absence.
- Those with a previous history of back symptoms were twice as likely to experience further pain as those without a prior history.

The second review by Pengel et al. provided the following[51]:

- Most studies reported that acute back pain decreased rapidly, by between 12% and 48% of initial levels (average 58%) within 1 month.
- Pain continued to decrease, more slowly, until about 3 months.
- Two studies with longer follow-up found that pain levels remained nearly constant from 3 to 12 months.
- 68%–86% of subjects who were absent from work at baseline returned to work within 1 month. Among the studies that provided 12-month follow-up, the cumulative risk of recurrence at 1 year ranged from 66% to 84%.

It would appear, based on the above studies, that most patients are likely to recover from any given episode of back pain, with the median time to recovery being approximately 7 weeks. However, relapses are common and up to 80% of patients may remain disabled to some degree at 12 months. A small percentage (10%–15%) will be highly disabled (this group will be discussed later in this chapter). Of particular importance, the status of the patient at 2 months is a good indicator of their status at 12 months.[13] The clinician must consider that just because patients do not return for treatment or follow-up, it does not necessarily mean they have recovered. In fact, it is possible they have not recovered and simply do not return.

Clinical Pearl: The clinician must consider that just because patients do not return for treatment or follow-up, it does not necessarily mean they have recovered.

There is some evidence that some patients are left with morphologic changes following an episode of back pain that may produce problems at a later date. Hides et al.[52] demonstrated wasting of the multifidus in patients who recovered from an initial episode of back pain. The changes were seen in the muscle on the side of back pain, at the level of back pain and included fatty infiltration of the muscle. According to the authors, the muscle wasting did not improve following symptom resolution. They suggest these muscle changes alter the overall stability of the lumbar spine and sets the stage for future problems. This was discussed in greater detail in Chapter 5.

Clinical Pearl: Hides et al. demonstrated wasting of the multifidus in patients who recovered from an initial episode of back pain.

Finally, statistics regarding success rates based on return to work may be misleading and simplistic. Lost workdays are routinely measured because of obvious concerns of lost productivity. While absenteeism measures have been a staple determinant of successful outcomes, little thought has been given to the lost productivity of workers who report to work at a very limited capacity. The term for workers' lost productivity due to illness while remaining on the job is *presenteeism*. Although this term is not new,[53] the concept of presenteeism appears to have gained sufficient notice to gain the attention of researchers and industry over the past decade.[54] While the loss of productivity of this group of workers is thought to be significant, finding reliable measures to determine the degree of loss have not been established. As such, the losses suffered by industry in term of dollars due to reduced employee productivity remain speculative. Nevertheless, research to better understand and reliably determine the impact of this apparently overlooked aspect of industrial productivity is currently underway.[55,56]

Recovery Predictors One question worth discussing is: Can the clinician identify those patients who are likely to recover quickly and move on with their life versus those who will likely develop chronic problems? In this regard, the following factors have been identified that influence the likelihood of recovery:

1. Severity of pain: Within the first few days, the severity of symptoms is probably the best predictor of symptomatic recovery. However, within the first 3 weeks, psychosocial factors appear to become more important.[3]
2. Social interactions: Social interactions also have an important influence on clinical progress. It has been stated that it is very difficult to become a patient with chronic pain without a "partner in pain."[57,58]
3. Return to work: For obvious reasons, patients who are unemployed or who lose their jobs have much greater difficulty returning to work.
4. Compensation and litigation: Patients on compensation or in an adversarial legal situation have slower and poorer outcomes for return to work.[7,59]

Clinical Flags As mentioned earlier, red flags are signs and symptoms that represent the potential for serious physical illness. Also mentioned earlier, "yellow flags" are said to represent the potential for psychosocial concerns and are discussed in detail in Chapter 19. In addition to these two flags, **there have recently been identified blue and black flags.** These are related to concerns in the workplace and will be discussed in the section on *Chronic Disability Syndromes*. These new categories can be considered subsets of the yellow flags and will be discussed later in the chapter (see Table 11–3).

Suggested Questions The following questions may provide useful information for the patient suspected of a potentially poor recovery:

1. Have you had time off work in the past with back pain?
2. What do you understand is the cause of your back pain?
3. What are you expecting will help you?
4. How is your employer responding to your back pain? Your coworkers? Your family?
5. What are you doing to cope with your back pain?
6. Do you think that you will return to work? When?
7. What are the good and bad parts of your job?

TABLE 11–3. **Clinical Flags as indicators**

Red Flags: Signs of Serious Disease	Yellow Flags: Psychosocial Indicators	Blue Flags: Workers' Perception of the Workplace	Black Flags: Organizational and Structural Context of the Workplace
Age of onset <20 or >55	Externalizing responsibility or blame	High demand/low control	Conditions of employment
Significant trauma	Emotional constriction	Unhelpful management style	Sickness policy
Thoracic pain	Tearfulness or weeping during interview	Poor social support from coworkers	Return to work policy
Nonmechanical pain	A verbalized fear of ongoing disability	Poor supervisor support	
Past Medical Hx Carcinoma Systemic steroids Drug abuse, HIV	Denial that the physical problem is in any way related to life events and circumstances	Safety climate	
Systemically unwell	Dissatisfaction or frustration with job or anger at a boss or doctors		
Weight loss	A verbalized resentment at the way the claim is being handled		
Lumbar flexion <5 cm	Failure of a variety of reasonable treatments with worsening of symptoms		
Widespread neurology	Doctor becomes irritated at the patient		
Structural deformity ESR >25 X-ray			

Treatment Methods

In developing a comprehensive understanding of any disease, the final part of the equation involves treatment. Treatment is based, in part, on the current understanding of the etiology and the natural history of the condition. For example, for the patient with a common cold, since the etiology is viral and the natural history is typically self-limiting with few, if any, residual problems, treatment is commonly focused on reducing symptoms while the patient recovers. For someone with viral pneumonia, however, where the outcome is less optimistic, treatment focuses on supportive measures and on preventing secondary infections. Treatment is therefore, by necessity, more invasive and aggressive.

With regard to low back syndromes, treatment is also heavily influenced by the training and background of the practitioner. The patient who sees a general practitioner will probably get some form of medication and advice to restrict activities. The same patient who visits a physical therapist will likely receive some form of modality and exercise advice. If the advice of a chiropractor is sought, or perhaps a psychotherapist, treatment may take a much different course.

FROM "SIMPLE BACKACHE" TO PATHOLOGY

The Degenerative Process

It is generally taught that there is no clear correlation between the presence of degenerative changes in the spine, as seen on plain film radiographs, and the incidence of back pain and/or other symptoms. In fact, the routine use of plain film radiographs is typically discouraged, largely because of this lack of association.[60] Even when there are obvious pathologic changes, such as a herniation of an intervertebral disc, these pathoanatomic changes may not necessarily be linked to the presence of low back pain. This is evidenced by the fact that some 30%–40% of pain-free adults have disc herniations demonstrated by MRI.[61] Interestingly, while the degenerative process of the spine continues throughout life, the incidence of back pain tends to peak at somewhere around 50–55 years of age, after which a decline in the incidence occurs.[1] If degeneration were closely linked with the development of back pain, symptoms would continue to accelerate with advancing age.

Clinical Pearl: ...while the degenerative process of the spine continues throughout life, the incidence of back pain tends to peak at somewhere around 50–55 years of age, after which a decline in the incidence occurs.

CHRONIC DISABILITY SYNDROMES

While most individuals who suffer from an episode of back pain recover quickly, usually within the first few weeks, a small percentage remains symptomatic for prolonged periods and a few fail to recover and eventually become disabled. The impact of this small group is significant. It has been estimated that 10%–15% of those who fail to recover account for nearly 80%–90% of the total costs of back pain.[62] Frank et al.[63] stated that 7.4% of the claimants who were absent from work for more than 6 months were responsible for 73% of medical costs, and 76% of compensation and indemnity payments.

Clinical Pearl: It has been estimated that 10%–15% of those who fail to recover account for nearly 80%–90% of the total costs of back pain.

Injuries in the workplace confound the risks of chronicity. It is generally agreed that the primary causes of disability in back-injured workers have little to do with the nature and/or severity of the injury. Rather, the causes have more to do with a variety of psychosocial factors including such issues as life and job satisfaction, the presence of compensation and/or litigation, and the efficacy of social support mechanisms. These yellow flags for disability, as previously discussed, may be recognized as early as 3–4 weeks following the onset of back pain[64] (see Chapter 19).

Disability vs. Impairment

In an effort to understand the back-injured individual who becomes disabled, a different perspective must be used than has been done in the past. It is no longer adequate to equate the impact of an injury with the "seriousness" of the physical damage or ailment. Instead, it might be helpful to differentiate between the disease of back pain and the illness associated with the disease.

The process of disease may be defined as a biological disturbance. In the case of back pain, disease may be seen as the degenerative changes in the spine or the bulging of an intervertebral disc. The illness, on the other hand, is the subjective experience of the disease by the person in his or her environment. This may be represented by Waddell's nonorganic signs (e.g., exaggerated self-reports of pain that complicate the problem of back pain).[9] To put it simply, disease is the "stuff" that humans get and illness is how humans are affected by that "stuff." As such, an understanding of the behavior of an individual with a disease, in the context of his or her environment becomes crucial. Two individuals with similar diseases will often respond in very different ways. One person may be disabled by the condition while the second is merely inconvenienced. Understanding the factors that influence the individual response to disease is therefore imperative.

There is evidence that the disease of low back pain has not increased during the past decades.[65,66] The illness, however, has increased considerably. In fact, some estimate that while the overall lifetime incidence of back pain remains essentially the same, the number of people disabled by back pain has increased dramatically.[67] Therefore, a portion of the efforts in preventing or managing back pain should be directed at identifying those individuals who are at risk, not only for developing back problems but also for developing chronic problems that may ultimately lead to disability.

Clinical Pearl: There is evidence that the incidence of low back pain has not increased during the past decades. The illness, however, has increased considerably.

There are a number of factors that have been identified as predictors of back pain. Some of these "injury predictors" provide the means to foresee who is most likely to have a back injury on the job. Other factors, "chronicity predictors," enable clinicians to identify those individuals who, once injured, are less likely to recover quickly. Finally, there are a group of factors, or "disability predictors," that help clinicians to identify those individuals in whom back pain is likely to lead to disability.[68] Ideally, once these individuals have been identified, appropriate steps may be taken to address their situations.

Why Do Some Individuals Become Disabled?

With the numbers reported in the previous section, one question that must be asked is: Why is this small group so different? In other words, why does this small group of individuals become disabled, while the majority of back pain sufferers recover? Is it that they were injured more severely, suffered more serious damage to their spines, or were the recipients of poor treatment? Or, are other factors involved?

Injury Predictors Let us begin by looking at those factors that may serve to differentiate those individuals who are at risk for a back injury. Interestingly, the single-most important predictor for developing back pain is a prior history of back pain.[69] In other words, if you have had back problems before, you are more than likely going to have them again. Another injury predictor is weak trunk musculature. For those involved in material handling activities, the probability of injury is three times greater when the lifting requirements of the job approach or exceed the individual's functional capacity.[70] Also, we know that back pain is more common in those workers who are involved in heavy manual labor, as well as those who are exposed to vibration, to driving, and to prolonged sitting.[71] Poor general health and smoking have also been shown to increase the risk of back injury.[72,73]

In addition to the physical factors listed above, there are a number of nonphysical aspects that contribute to the likelihood of developing future back problems. These include such things as a short length of time on the job. Workers on the job less than 2 years tend to have more back problems than those with longer employment.[67] The reasons for this are not clear but it may be associated with more seasoned workers having a better understanding of workplace safety. It has also been suggested that workers with more seniority have more invested in their jobs and are therefore less likely to complain of problems. Other psychosocial issues include high levels of stress at work and a poor supervisor's rating within the past 6 months.[74–76] In addition, there has been some suggestion that injury rates are impacted by the economy and insurance benefits.[7] For example, injury rates are higher in seasonal work and during difficult economic times. It is worth noting that while heavy manual work is a known risk factor for developing back problems, many of the injury predictors have more to do with the work environment than with the type of work being performed.

Clinical Pearl: Workers on the job less than 2 years tend to have more back problems than those with longer employment.

Chronicity Predictors If one looks at those individuals who, once injured, take longer than normal to recover, it would appear that several factors involved in the clinical presentation may point the way to the development of chronicity. Certain aspects seen in the clinical presentation of a patient over the initial weeks after injury may serve as a valuable guide. For instance, it is clear that those patients presenting with low back pain that is complicated or accompanied by leg pain are likely to take longer to recover. While most individuals' low back pain recovers within the first few weeks, the outlook for those with accompanying leg pain is less optimistic. Approximately 50% of these individuals continue to suffer at 3 months.[77,78]

Clinical Pearl: While most individuals' low back pain recovers within the first few weeks, the outlook for those with accompanying leg pain is less optimistic.

In addition to leg pain, the presence of various nonorganic signs complicates the low back pain picture and may be associated with symptom magnification and/or malingering.[79] However, Main and Waddell later clarified their position regarding these nonorganic signs, stating that multiple signs suggest that the patient does not have a straightforward physical problem. Instead, they recommended that these findings mean that the patient may require treatment directed at physical, psychosocial, and behavioral aspects of their illness.[80] Later research by Fritz et al. found none of Waddell's signs to be effective as screening tools for patients with acute back pain.[81] More recently, Fishbain et al.[82] performed an evidence-based review of the nonorganic signs and concluded that they do not correlate with psychological distress or secondary gain, do not discriminate between organic and nonorganic problems, but that they are associated with poorer treatment outcomes and greater pain levels. Exaggerations on the patient's self-report of pain, or pain that does not conform to known physiologic patterns coupled with an abnormal pain drawing, should alert clinicians. Interestingly, while many claim that the actual cause of low back pain is often unknown, a nonspecific diagnosis is seen as a risk factor for patients developing chronic problems.[83] Perhaps patients react negatively when they are told that their doctor is not really sure what is causing their problems.

Clinical Pearl: While younger individuals (i.e., those under the age of 25) are at greater risk of injury, older workers tend to take longer to return to work.

Other factors such as age, sex, and the level of education are also considerations in predicting a lengthy recovery. While younger individuals (i.e., those under the age of 25) are at greater risk of injury, older workers tend to take longer to return to work.[67] Those injured workers between the ages of 30–55 tend to have a higher incidence of chronicity and disability.[84] In addition to age, gender also plays a role. Men file 80% of back injury compensation claims.[85] However, an occupationally injured woman is more likely to remain disabled and typically takes longer to recover.[86] It has also been shown that there is an inverse relationship between the level of education, low back pain, and disability with the most pronounced incidence in the least educated workers.[87–89] The reasons for this probably have to do with a number of factors including life and job satisfaction, control over their situations, and the number of choices available. Clearly, those with higher education levels have more opportunities for changing jobs and for adapting to their situations than do those with menial jobs requiring heavy exertion. The context of the injury also appears to be a particularly important factor.[90,91] An acute event related to lifting, bending, or twisting, or an accident such as a slip or fall has a predictive value for chronicity. When an injury occurs as the result of an everyday event such as bending or lifting, the impact is often reduced. In these days of managed care, inconsistency of medical care also has a negative impact on recovery,[92] as does a lack of availability of interim light duty work or work modification.[90]

Disability Predictors Another set of predictors is helpful in identifying those individuals for whom treatment or intervention is likely to fail and who are likely to progress to disability. It is this small group of patients who contribute most to the tremendously high cost of industrial back problems. These factors include compensation, litigation,[93] and lag time (i.e., the longer it takes for an injured worker to receive care, for a referral to a specialist to occur, and/or for special procedures such as surgery, the greater the likelihood of a negative outcome).[84] Also, when surgery is suggested but not performed, the outcome is less favorable. It may be that patients who are anticipating surgery feel that it is the only thing that will offer any final assistance. In their mind, recovery cannot occur until surgery is performed. As before, a lack of available work to return to plays an important role in the likelihood of future disability.[90]

Of particular importance, several studies have shown that the manner in which a supervisor, company doctor, or employer responds to the injured worker may have a significant impact on the seriousness of the injury. As stated earlier, these factors are referred to as "blue flags" and "black flags."[94]

Blue Flags

Blue flags are used to illustrate the workers' perceptions of the workplace and include the following factors:

1. High demand/low control (see Fig. 11–1): When the demands of a job are high and the control

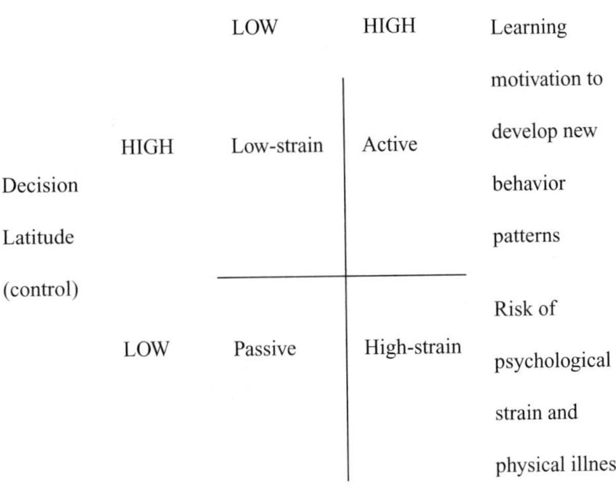

FIGURE 11–1. Demand/control. (*Adapted from Karasek et al.*[95])

an individual has on the way he or she accomplishes the job are low, the likelihood of disability is increased.[95]
2. Unhelpful management style: Several studies have shown that the support of managers and supervisors may play a significant role in return to work and/or the development of disability.[96]
3. Poor social support from colleagues: As with the support of supervisors and managers, the support and encouragement from coworkers may play a role in return to work and/or the development of disability.[97]

Black Flags

Black flags represent the structural and organizational context of the workplace and include the following factors:

1. Conditions of employment: Temporary and/or seasonal workers have a greater likelihood of developing chronic problems.
2. Sickness policy: Companies with liberal sickness policies may encourage a protracted return to work.

Burton[98] states that some managers, through their attitudes and management methods, may encourage a culture of coping and staying at work in the face of low back pain. Others may emphasize the attribution of back pain to work and encourage negative beliefs and attitudes about back pain. According to Burton, these attitudes may result in elevated levels of back pain reporting and related disability. It is also suggested that the presence of such factors may adversely affect the success of various interventions in the workplace.

Chronic back pain and disability are obviously not solely a result of physical injury. It is rather associated with a complex interaction of factors, including a number of psychosocial issues. Efforts must be made by management and by clinicians to understand the impact of the injury on the individual. It is only when the injury is considered in its full context that one can hope to reduce the impact of back pain and other musculoskeletal problems.

SUMMARY

1. This discussion has reviewed the multifactorial nature of low back syndromes, integrating topics from previous chapters while emphasizing the most common of spinal complaints called nonspecific back pain.
2. The role of both physical and psychosocial factors in the development of disability was also discussed. Each plays a part in determining the impact of an injury on the individual.
3. The "four flags" were addressed, which highlight key factors that can influence both the assessment and treatment of the condition.
4. When an injury does occur, whatever the reasons for delayed or incomplete recovery, it should be clear that the longer an individual remains off work, and the greater the incentives to remain disabled, the less likely he or she is to return to a productive life.
5. A clear understanding of these topics allows the clinician to establish a sound diagnostic impression, which is a necessary step toward the reasonable initiation of a corrective treatment program.
6. The reader is directed to ensuing chapters, which provide an overview of common diagnostic and therapeutic options in the conservative management of low back syndromes.

REFERENCES

1. Papageorgiou AC, Croft PR, Ferry S, Jayson MI, Silman AJ. Estimating the prevalence of low back pain in the general population. Evidence from the South Manchester Back Pain Survey. *Spine* September 1, 1995;20(17):1880–1894.
2. Cassidy JD, Carroll LJ, Cote P. The Saskatchewan health and back pain survey. The prevalence of low back pain and related disability in Saskatchewan adults. *Spine* September 1,1998 ;23(17):1860–1866.
3. Coste J, Delecoeuillierie G, Cohen de Lara A, Le Parc JM, Paolaggi JB. Clinical course and prognostic factors in acute low back pain: An inception cohort study in primary care practice. *BMJ* 1994;308:577–580.
4. Nachemson A. Ont i ryggen. Back pain—Causes, diagnosis, treatment. SBU Report. Stockholm: Swedish Council on Technology Assessment in Health Care, 1991:19.
5. Hooper PD. *Physical modalities: A primer for chiropractic.* Baltimore: Williams & Wilkins, 1996.
6. Carroll L, Mercade AC, Cassidy JD, Cote P. A population-based study of factors associated with combinations of active and passive coping with neck and low back pain. *J Rehabil Med* March 2002;34(2): 67–72.
7. Cassidy JD, Carroll L, Cote P, Berglund A, Nygren A. Low back pain after traffic collisions: A population-based cohort study. *Spine* May 15, 2003;28(10):1002–1009.
8. Lindena G, Diener HC, Hildebrandt J, et al. Committee for quality assurance of the German chapter (DGSS). Guidelines in pain treatment—Methodical quality of guidelines for treatment of pain patients *Schmerz* June 2002;16(3):194–204.
9. Waddell G. *The back pain revolution.* Edinburgh: Churchill Livingstone, 1998:11.
10. Burton AK, Waddell G, Tillotson KM, Summerton N. Information and advice to patients with back pain can have a positive effect. A controlled trial of a novel educational booklet in primary care. *Spine* December 1, 1999;24(23):2484–2491.
11. Snook SH, Work-related back pain: Secondary intervention. *J Electromyogr Kinesiol* February 2004; 14(1):153–160.
12. Cedraschi C, Nordin M, Nachemson AL, Vischer TL. 1998 health care providers should use a common language in relation to low back pain patients. *Baillieres Clin Rheumatol* February 2004;12(1):1–15.
13. Spitzer WO. Scientific approach to the assessment and management of activity-related spinal disorders. A monograph for clinicians. Report of the Quebec Task Force on Spinal Disorders. *Spine* September 1987;12(7, Suppl):S1–S59.
14. Lewit K. *Manipulative therapy in rehabilitation of the locomotor system.* Butterworth-Heinemann, 1984.
15. McGlynn EA , Asch SM, Adams J, et al. The quality of health care delivered to adults in the United States. *NEJM* 2003;348:2635–2645.
16. Bogduk N. In defense of radiofrequency neurotomy. *Reg Anesth Pain Med* 2002;27(4):439–441.
17. McGuirk B, King W, Govind J, Lowry J, Bogduk N. Safety, efficacy, and cost effectiveness of evidence-based guidelines for the management of acute low back pain in primary care. *Spine* December 1, 2001;26(23):2615–2622.
18. Deyo RA, Rainville J, Kent DL. What can the history and physical examination tell us about low back pain? *JAMA* August 12, 1992;268(6):760–765.
19. Jackson RP. The facet syndrome. Myth or reality? *Clin Orthop* June 1992;(279):110–121.
20. Dreyer SJ, Dreyfuss PH. Low back pain and the zygapophyseal (facet) joints. *Arch Phys Med Rehabil* March 1996;77(3):290–300.
21. Bogduk N. Management of chronic low back pain. *Med J Aust* January 19, 2004;180(2):79–83.
22. Riddle DL, Freburger DK. Evaluation of the presence of sacroiliac joint region dysfunction using a

combination of tests: A multicenter intertester reliability study. *Phys Ther* August 2002;82(8):772–781.

23. Saal SJ. General principles of diagnostic testing as related to painful lumbar spine disorders: A critical appraisal of current diagnostic techniques. *Spine* November 15, 2002;27(22):2538–2545.
24. Fahrni WH, Trueman GE Comparative radiological study of the spines of a primitive population with North Americans and Northern Europeans. *J Bone Joint Surg Br* August 1965;47:552–555.
25. Williams P. *Low back and neck pain: Causes and conservative treatment*. Springfield, Ill: Thomas, 1971:13–19.
26. McKenzie R. Low back pain. *N Z Med J* July 8, 1987;100(827):428–429.
27. Janda V. Muscles as a pathogenic factor in back pain. In: *Proceedings of the International Federation of Manual Therapists*. Christchurch, NZ, 1982.
28. McKenzie RA. *Lumbar spine: Mechanical diagnosis and therapy*. Waikanae, NZ, 1981:4–8.
29. O'Sullivan PB. Lumbaar segmental "instability": Clinical presentation and specific stabilizing exercise management. *Man Ther* February 2000;5(1):2–12.
30. Kovacs FM, Gestoso M, Gil del Real MT, Lopez J, Mufraggi N, Mendez JL. Risk factors for nonspecific low back pain in schoolchildren and their parents: A population based study. *Pain* June 2003;103: 259–268.
31. Weinstein SL, Dolan LA, Spratt KF, Peterson KK, Spoonamore JJMJ, Ponseti IV. Health and function of patients with untreated idiopathic scolisis: A 50-year natural history study. *JAMA* February 5, 2003;289(5):559–567.
32. ten Brinke A, van der Aa HE, van der Palen J, Oosterveld F. Is leg length discrepancy associated with the side of radiating pain in patients with a lumbar herniated disc? *Spine* April 1, 1999;24(7):684–686.
33. Soukka A, Alaranta H, Tallroth K, Heliovaara M. Leg-length inequality in people of working age. The association between mild inequality and low back pain is questionable. *Spine* April 1991;16(4):429–431.
34. Grundy PF, Roberts CJ. Does unequal leg length cause back pain? A case-control study.*Lancet* August 4, 1984;2(8397):256–258.
35. Bono CM. Low back pain in athletes. *J Bone Joint Surg Am* February 2004;86A(2):382–396.
36. Beutler WJ, Frederickson BE, Murtland A, Sweeney CA, Grant WD, Baker D The natural history of spondylolysis and spondylolisthesis: A 45-year follow-up evaluation. *Spine* May 15, 2003;28(10):1027–1035.
37. Gaber TA, McGlashan KA, Love S, Jenner JR, Crisp AJ. Bone density in chronic low back pain: A pilot study. *Clin Rehabil*. December 2002;16(8):867–870.
38. Bener A, Alwash R, Gaber T, Lovasz G. Obesity and low back pain. *Coll Antropol* June 2003;27(1):95–104.
39. Deyo RA, Bass JE. Lifestyle and low back pain. The influence of smoking and obesity. *Spine* May 1989;14(5):501–506.
40. Bernard TN Jr. Repeat lumbar spine surgery. Factors influencing outcome. *Spine* November 1993;18(15): 2196–2200.
41. Frank JW, Pulcins IR, Kerr MS, Shannon HS, Stansfeld SA. Occupational back pain—An unhelpful polemic. *Scand J Work Environ Health* February 1995;21(1): 2–14.
42. Carroll LJ, Cassidy JD, Cote P. Depression as a risk factor for onset of an episode of troublesome neck and low back pain. *Pain* January 2004;107(1–2): 134–139.
43. McGill S. *Low back disorders: Evidence-based prevention and rehabilitation*. Champaign, IL: Human Kinetics, 2002.
44. McGill S, Grenier S, Bluhm M, Preuss R, Brown S, Russell C. Previous history of LBP with work loss is related to lingering deficits in biomechanical, physiological, personal, psychosocial and motor control characteristics. *Ergonomics* June 10, 2003;46(7):731–746.
45. Wood DD, Fisher DL, Adnres RA. Minimizing fatigue during repetitive jobs: Optimal work–rest cycles. *Hum Factors* March 1997;39(1):83–101.
46. van den Hoogen HJ, Koes BW, van Eijkt JT, Bouter LM, Deville W. On the course of low back pain in general practice: A one year follow up study. *Ann Rheum Dis* January 1998;57(1):13–19.
47. Schiottz-Christensen B, Nielsen GL, Hansen VK, Schodt T, Sorensen HT, Olesen F. Long-term prognosis of acute low back pain in patients seen in general practice: A 1-year prospective follow-up study. *Fam Pract* June 1999;16(3):223–232.
48. Croft PR, Macfarlane GJ, Papageorgiou AC, Thomas E, Silman AJ. Outcome of low back pain in general practice: A prospective study. *BMJ* May 2, 1998; 316(7141):1356–1359.
49. von Korff M, Saunders K. The course of back pain in primary care. *Spine* December 15, 1996;21(24):2833–2837.
50. Hestbaek L, Leboeuf-Yde C, Manniche C. Low back pain: What is the long-term course? A review of studies of general patient populations [Review]. *Eur J Spine* April 2003;12(2):149–165.
51. Pengel LH, Herbert RD, Maher CG, Refshauge KM. Acute low back pain: Systematic review of its prognosis [Review]. *BMJ* August 9, 2003;327(7410): 323–328.
52. Hides JA, Stokes MJ, Saide M, Jull GA, Cooper DA. Evidence of lumbar multifidus wasting ipsilateral to symptoms in patients with acute/subacute low back pain. *Spine* January 15, 1994;19(2):165–172.
53. Canfield G, Soash D. Presenteeism—A constructive view. *Ind Med Surg* September 1955;24(9):417–418.
54. Aronsson G, Gustafson K, Daliner M. Sick but yet at work. An empirical study of sickness presenteeism. *J Epidemiol Community Health* July 2000;54(7):502–507.
55. Wang P, Beck A, Berglund P, et al. Chronic medical conditions and work performance in the health and work performance questionnaire calibration surveys. *J Occup Environ Med* December 2003;45(12):1301–1311.
56. Prasad M, Wahlqvist P, Shikiar R, Shih T. Self-report instruments measuring health-related work

productivity: A patient-reported outcomes perspective. *Pharmacoeconomics* 2004;22(4):225–244.

57. Engel GL. Psychogenic pain and the pain prone patient. *Am J Med* 1959;26:899–918.
58. Szasz TS. The painful person. *Lancet* 1968;88:18–22.
59. Fayad F, Lefevre-Colau MM, Poiraudeau S, et al. Chronicity, recurrence, and return to work in low back pain: Common prognostic factors. *Ann Readapt Med Phys* May 2004;47(4):179–189.
60. Deyo RA, Diehl AK. Lumbar spine films in primary care: Current use and effects of selective ordering criteria. *J Gen Intern Med* January–February 1986;1(1): 20–25.
61. van Tulder MW, Assendelft WJJ, Loes BW, Bouter LM. Spinal radiographic findings and non-specific low back pain. *Spine* 1997;22:427–434.
62. Spengler DM, Bigos SJ, Martin NA, Zeh J, Fisher L, Nachemson A. Back injuries and industry: A retrospective study. I. Overview and cost analysis. *Spine* 1986;11:241–245.
63. Frank JW, Brooker AS, DeMaio SE, et al. Disability resulting from occupational low back pain. Part II. What do we know about secondary prevention? A review of the scientific evidence on prevention after disability begins [Review]. *Spine*. December 15, 1996; 21(24):2918–2929.
64. Kendall NAS, Linton SJ, Main CJ. *Guide to assessing psychosocial yellow flags in acute low back pain: Risk factors for long term disability and work loss*. Wellington, NZ: Accident Rehabilitation and Compensation Insurance Corporation of New Zealand and the National Health Committee, 1997.
65. Hashemi L, Webster BS, Clancy EA. Trends in disability duration and cost of workers compensation low back pain claims (1988–1996). *J Occup Environ Med* 1998 40:1110–1119.
66. Leboeuf-Yde C, Lauritsen JM. The prevalence of low back pain in the literature: A structured review of 26 Nordic studies from 1954 to 1993. *Spine* 1995;20:2112–2118.
67. Allan DB, Waddell G. An historical perspective on low back pain and disability. *Orthop Scand* 1989;60(Suppl 234):10–23.
68. Hooper PD. Factors influencing disability. *DC Tracts* [audiotape]. Washington, DC, 1999.
69. Bigos SJ, Spengler DM, Martin NA, et al. Back injuries in industry: A retrospective study. III. Employee-related factors. *Spine* 1986;11:252–256.
70. Chaffin DB, Park KS. A longitudinal study of low-back pain as associated with occupational weight lifting factors. *Am Ind Hyg Assoc J* 1973;34:513–525.
71. Hildebrandt VH, Bongers PM, Gul J, van Dijk FJ, Kemper HC. The relationship between leisure time, physical activities and musculoskeletal symptoms and disability in worker populations. *Int Arch Occup Environ Health* 2000;73:507–518.
72. Cady LD, Thomas PC, Karwasky RJ. Program for increasing health and physical fitness of firefighters. *J Occup Med* 1985;2:111–114.
73. Battie MC, Bigos SJ, Fisher LD, et al. A prospective study of the role of cardiovascular risk factors and fitness in industrial back pain complaints. *Spine* 1989;14:141–147.
74. Magora A. Investigation of the relationship between low back pain and occupation. *Scand J Rehab Med* 1973;5:191–195.
75. Niemcryk S, Jenkins CD, Rose RM, Hurst MW. The prospective impact of psychosocial variables on rates of illness and injury in professional employees. *J Occup Med* 1987;29(8):645–652.
76. Magora A. Investigation of the relation between low back pain and occupation: Neurologic and orthopaedic conditions. *Scand J Rehabil Med* 1975;7:146–151.
77. Biering-Sörensen F. A prospective study of low back pain in a general population. I. Occurrence, recurrence and aetiology. *Scand J Rehabil Med* 1983;15: 77–79.
78. Troup JDG, Martin JW, Lloyd DCEF. Back pain in industry: A prospective study. *Spine* 1981;6:61–69.
79. Waddell G. A new clinical model for the treatment of low back pain. *Spine* 1987;12(7):632–644.
80. Main C, Waddell G. Behavioral responses to examination. A reappraisal of the interpretation of "nonorganic" signs. *Spine* November 1, 1998;23(21):2367–2371.
81. Fritz J, Wainner R, Hicks G. The use of nonorganic signs and symptoms as a screening tool for return-to-work in patients with acute low back pain. *Spine* August 1, 2000;25(15):1925–1931.
82. Fishbain D, Cole B, Cutler R, Lewis J, Rosomoff H, Steel Rosomoff R. A structured evidence-based review on the meaning of nonorganic physical signs: Waddell's signs. *Pain Med* June 2003;4(2): 141–181.
83. Cats-Baril WL, Frymoyer JW. Demographic factors associated with the prevalence of disability in the general population. *Spine* 1991;16:671–674.
84. Polatin PB. Predictors of low back disability. In: White AH, Anderson R, EDS. *Conservative care of low back pain.* Baltimore: Williams & Wilkins, 1991.
85. Klein BP, Jensen RC, Sanderson LM. Assessment of worker's compensation claims for back strains/sprains. *J Occup Med* 1984;26(6):443–448.
86. Dzioba RB, Doxey NC. A prospective investigation into the orthopedic and psychological predictors of outcome of first lumbar surgery following industrial injury. *Spine* 1984;9(6):614–623.
87. Deyo RA, Tsui-Wu YJ. Descriptive epidemiology of low back pain and its related medical care in the United States. *Spine* 1987;12:264–268.
88. Magora A, Taustein I. An investigation of the problem of sick leave in the patient suffering from low back pain. *Ind Med* 1969;38(11):80–90.
89. Astrand NE. Medical, psychological, and social factors associated with back abnormalities and self-reported back pain. *Br J Ind Med* 1987;44:327–336.
90. White AWM. Low back pain in men receiving workmen's compensation. *Can Med Assoc J* 1966;95:50–56.
91. Venning PJ, Walter SD, Sitt LW. Personal and job-related factors as determinants of incidence of back injuries among nursing personnel. *J Occup Med* 1987; 29:820–825.

92. Longstein M, Weisel SW. Standardized approaches to the evaluation and treatment of industrial low back pain. *Occup Med* 1988;3(1):147–156.
93. Fishbain DA, Goldbergy M, Labbe E, Steele R, Rosomoff H. Compensation and non-compensation chronic pain patients compared for DSM-III operational diagnosis. *Pain* 1988;32:197–206.
94. Main CJ, Burton AK. Economic and occupational influences on pain and disability. In: Main CJ, Spanwick CC, eds. *Pain management: An interdisciplinary approach*. Edinburgh: Churchill Livingstone, 2000:63–88.
95. Karasek R, Theorell T. *Healthy work: Stress, productivity, and the reconstruction of working life*. Basic Books, New York, 1990.
96. Shrey DE. Disability management in industry: The new paradigm in injured worker rehabilitation. *Disabil Rehabil* 1996;18(8):408–414.
97. Leroux I, Dionne CE, Bourbonnais R. Psychosocial job factors and the one-year evolution of back-related functional limitations. *Scand J Work Environ Health* February 2004;30(1):47–55.
98. Burton AK. Have researchers overlooked a major influence on disabling back pain? In: *The back letter.* Baltimore: Lippincott Williams & Wilkins, September 2001.

PART

III

ASSESSMENT OF THE LOW BACK

CHAPTER

12

HISTORY AND PHYSICAL EXAMINATION FOR LOW BACK SYNDROMES

Diane N. Resnick and Craig E. Morris

OUTLINE

OBJECTIVES

1. Provide a summary of physical examination procedures for patients with low back syndromes.
2. Demonstrate on an organized patient history, with explanation of its clinical relevence.
3. Describe the various components of the physical examination.
4. Describe strategies for quantitatively determining a patient's functional capacity.
5. Discuss strategies to differentiate organic from non-organic positive findings.
6. Discuss the importance of avoiding over-reliance on examination findings with poor validity or reliability.

PATIENT HISTORY

Introduction

It is a common maxim that the patient's history provides 80% of the information used to determine a diagnosis. The time devoted to obtaining a complete historical picture of the patient will reduce subsequent time spent in the performance of uncomfortable examination procedures and increase the likelihood of reaching an accurate diagnosis. The clinician should realize, however, that pathoanatomical diagnostic accuracy with respect to low back syndromes is often elusive because of the use of traditional but often unsubstantiated physical examination procedures, poor correlation between symptoms and imaging results,[1] and frequent use of nonspecific terms such as strain, sprain, and degenerative processes[2] as a catch-all for conditions of uncertain pathoanatomical origin.

A report issued by the Agency for Health Care Policy and Research,[3] now known as the Agency for Healthcare Research and Quality, suggests grouping back pain into five broad categories:

1. Potentially serious spinal conditions such as spinal tumor, infection, fracture, and cauda equina syndrome
2. Nonspinal causes secondary to abdominal involvement (gallbladder, liver, renal, pelvic inflammatory disease, prostatic carcinoma, ovarian cyst, uterine fibroids, aortic aneurysm, or thoracic disease)
3. Sciatica and dural tissue compromise
4. Nonspecific back symptoms, the majority of which are mechanical in nature
5. Psychological causes such as stress and work environment (disability, workers' compensation, secondary gain)

By using this guideline, information can be gathered from the patient in a timely, organized fashion. After screening for conditions that require immediate follow-up with advanced imaging, laboratory work, and/or referral, the clinician should complete the patient's historical picture using an acronym or clinically relevant pattern that covers all the historical bases.

Screening Questions for Potentially Serious Spinal Conditions ("Red Flags")

While the likelihood of a low back syndrome due to a serious condition is low, the consequences of a missed diagnosis or delayed treatment can be quite costly in terms of prolonged morbidity and, in the extreme, mortality. This topic was addressed in detail in Chapter 10, but is briefly reviewed here. Deyo and colleagues[4] evaluated data from the patient history and its correlation with a subsequent diagnosis of significant spinal disease. The most valuable positive responses were age over 70, history of cancer, recent unexplained weight gain/loss, duration of pain greater than 1 month, and unresponsiveness to previous conservative therapy. Table 12–1 offers a list of some of the most common causes of low back pain due to serious pathology and the more common findings elicited from the medical history.

Most of these historical questions are typically contained within the general health questionnaire given to new patients. However, if these screening questions are not grouped together, it is easy to overlook their combined significance. The clinician should make a habit of soliciting this information from each patient before continuing with the remainder of the historical query. For patients with chronic conditions who require treatment either regularly or periodically, effort should be made to update the historical information on a yearly basis, including screens for red flags.

Screening Questions for Nerve Root and Dural Tissue Compromise

After the probability of tumor, infection, fracture, and the like is reduced, the clinician should determine whether a radicular compromise is present. Conditions that may result in radicular symptoms include inflammatory irritation due to tissue injury, disc herniation, arthrosis involving the facet joints or vertebral body–disc interface, spinal hematoma, and congenital or acquired central or lateral canal stenosis.[8,9]

Pertinent questions for this category of lumbar pain focus on the quality and pattern of symptoms the patient experiences. While pain is suggestive of mechanical or chemical irritation, paresthesia, anesthesia, and weakness are attributed to decreased nerve or arterial function due to compression, constriction, or other blockage. The pattern of symptom radiation may give the examiner an indication of the origin of pathology. For instance, a dermatomal distribution of paresthesia or numbness suggests that the insult originates at the root level rather than within a more peripheral structure. The clinician should also ask the

TABLE 12–1. **Conditions and Pertinent Historical Screening Questions[4–7]**

Condition	Historical Information
Cancer	Age > 50 years History of cancer Persistent night pain Unexplained weight loss or gain (10–15 lb in 2 weeks or less) Failure to improve with 1 month conservative therapy No relief with bed rest Unwarranted fatigue Duration of pain > 1 month
Infection Osteomyelitis Diskitis Spinal abscess/infection (acute = bacterial; chronic = fungal, tuberculosis) Meningitis	Age > 50 or < 20 years Fever, chills, night sweats Unexplained weight loss or gain Recent infection, including urinary tract and skin Intravenous drug use Catheterization Prolonged corticosteroid use Transplant recipient
Fracture	Age > 50 years Major trauma Minor trauma or strenuous lifting in osteoporotic patient History of cancer Prolonged use of corticosteroids
Cauda equina syndrome Severe disc herniation or sequestration Epidural hematoma (recent spinal procedure, anticoagulant therapy, or trauma)	Saddle anesthesia Bowel or bladder dysfunction Severe or progressive neurological deficit in lower extremities

patient about any difficulty with coughing, sneezing, or abdominal straining (Dejerine's triad), each of which causes an increase in intrathecal pressure that may provoke radicular symptoms.

General Questions for All Patients with Low Back Pain

After focusing the interview on information that may rule out nonmechanical low back pain, the clinician should concentrate on illuminating the historical picture of the patient. A useful organizational acronym for this purpose is LOP_4QRST, which represents the following descriptors:

- Location
- Onset
- Prior history/treatment
- Palliative measures (including medications)
- Provocative factors (including movement/positional factors)
- Progression/course
- Quality of symptoms
- Referral patterns
- Severity
- Temporal factors

The purpose of these topics is to search for patterns that match with the various stereotypical syndromes in order to form the earliest clinical hunches. Each topic and hunch has value for the clinician by contributing to portions of the examination in order to emphasize appropriate diagnostic testing, the formation of differential and working diagnoses, appropriate treatment regimens, and/or overall prognosis. Keep in mind that some of the following information is elicited while screening for serious pathology and dural compromise, and so redundancy should be avoided for the sake of time management.

Also, as often follows an acute injury, for example during a sporting event, only a focused history is initially obtained; the clinician should complete the detailed history after the immediate complaint is addressed in order to uncover any unassociated problems or injury predisposition.[10]

Location The majority of patients with low back pain report nonspecific back symptoms localized to the lumbar region with symptom referral to the buttock or posterior thigh as a common secondary feature.[11] When interviewing a patient regarding the location of his or her pain/symptoms, it is important to discern whether the sensation is focal or diffuse and whether it is superficial or deep. Generally, if the paravertebral soft tissues are at fault, the presentation is one of somewhat diffuse, superficial to mid-depth pain, more pronounced on one side of the spine but often bilateral in deconditioned patients, with possible referral either laterally or inferiorly.[12] If the disc (without a radicular component) or bony elements are involved, symptoms tend to be more focal in distribution and are often described as originating from deep within the back.[12–14]

Onset There are several factors to assess when questioning a patient about the onset of his or her condition. The patient's age, while not directly related to the specific timing of symptoms, is important with respect to determining the likely presence of a particular condition and, in some cases, the overall prognosis. For example, symptoms of recent onset of low back stiffness in a 20-year-old patient would not likely be attributed to diffuse idiopathic skeletal hyperostosis or osteoarthritis. Similarly, acute onset of lumbar stiffness in a 60-year-old patient is not typically due to ankylosing spondylitis. There are a variety of primary neoplasms that may cause low back pain; osteochondroma, osteoblastoma, and giant cell tumor tend to present much earlier in life than colon cancer, prostatic cancer, or multiple myeloma.[9]

The clinician should be familiar with age ranges for conditions that may present with low back pain. To facilitate the diagnostic process, Table 12–2 lists the most common conditions that may cause low back pain, age ranges associated with those conditions, and gender specifics. Gender is included here as there are many conditions that are either gender-specific or demonstrate a higher prevalence for one gender over the other.

Typically, patients are able to classify their symptoms as sudden or insidious with respect to onset. Keep in mind that while most patients who experience a sudden onset of acute low back pain seek evaluation and treatment within the acute phase, some patients may not seek treatment until several months after the initial appearance of symptoms or may wait until several episodes establish the condition as one that can no longer be ignored any longer. This can be the case for patients experiencing low back pain resulting from tumors or infection in which the symptoms may start gradually unless there is associated pathological fracture. The clinician must take care to determine whether a condition is truly insidious in nature or reflective of the patient's incomplete recollection of events.

With respect to chemically mediated inflammation, the acute response by platelets, mast cells, basophils, and the like lasts up to 3 days and may be characterized by pain, swelling, warmth, erythema, and/or impairment of movement or function.[16] Provided that the source or mechanism of injury is eliminated, the proliferation of granulation tissue commences and continues for 3–7 days following the initial injury. Should the source of injury remain, chronic inflammation develops.[17] Repair of damaged tissue may last several weeks and remodeling may last several months. Depending on the tissue involved, healing may take 12 months or longer following the injury.[18] These time lines will help stage the condition, which in turn will help determine treatment and influence prognosis. Additionally, the time frame between injury (if known) and onset of symptoms provides important information concerning the likely structures involved as well as potential severity. Compare, for example, a patient who presents with the immediate onset of moderate low back pain the day after lifting heavy machinery with a patient who gradually develops moderate low back pain 2 weeks into a physical fitness regimen. While the mechanism of injury may be mechanical in nature for both patients, the degree of injury from a sudden macrotrauma versus a gradual onset is vastly different. Additionally, the potential for noncontractile tissue involvement may be greater in the first case.

Regarding acute, subacute, and chronic classifications, definitions vary.[5,14,19–21] A widely accepted time line proposed by the Quebec Task Force and Frymoyer[21] categorizes low back pain as acute if symptoms are of 6 weeks duration or less, subacute if back pain has a 6- to 12-week duration, and chronic if back pain exists for longer than 12 weeks.

Acute low back pain of a mechanical nature often has an identifiable mechanism of injury that should be elucidated in detail. Keep in mind that the degree of pain and disability experienced by the patient

TABLE 12-2. **Age and Gender Specifics for Some Conditions Causing Low Back Pain**[13,15]

Condition	Age Ranges	Gender Dominance	Incidence/ Prevalence
Abdominal aneurysm	50 to 70	M	
Aneurysmal bone cyst	Late teens to mid-30s	F	
Ankylosing spondylitis	Late teens to late 40s	M	0.50–5 per 1000 white males
Chordoma	Late 30s to 70s	M	
Colon cancer	Mid-50s to late 70s	Equal	155,000 new cases per year
Diffuse idiopathic skeletal hyperostosis	Late 30s to early 50s	M	
Endometriosis	Late teens to late 40s	F	8–30/100,000
Fibromyalgia	30 to early 50s	F	3/100
Giant cell tumor	20 to 45	F	
Hemangioma	Mid 30s to early 50s	Equal	
Herniated nucleus pulposus	Mid 20s to mid 50s	Equal	Lifetime prevalence: 60%–90%
Herpes zoster	No peak incidence	Equal	2–3/1000: ages 20–50 years 10/1000: >70 years
Hodgkin's lymphoma	Peaks at 20 and 70	M	3.5/100,000
Inflammatory bowel disease	Late teens to 50	F	50–75/100,000
Intraspinal neoplasms	30 to early 50s	Equal	
Metastasis	Early 40s to mid 70s	Equal	
Microcrystalline disease	Mid 30s to early 50s	M	100/100,000
Multiple myeloma	50 to early 70s	M	1% of all malignant disease
Muscle strain	Mid 20s to late 40s	Equal	
Osteitis condensans ilii	30 to early 50s	F	
Osteoarthritis	Late 30s to 60	Equal	
Osteoblastoma	20 to 45	M	
Osteochondroma	20 to 40	M	
Osteoid osteoma	Late teens to mid-30s	M	
Osteomyelitis	Late 30s to early 70s	M	Uncommon
Osteoporosis	40 to early 70s	F	30%–40% in females 5%–15% in males
Ovarian cancer	30 to 75	F	12,000 deaths/year
Paget's disease	Late 30s to 50	M	
Pancreatitis	30 to early 50s	Equal	10–22/100,000
Peptic ulcer	Early 40s to mid-70s	M (Duodenal) F (Gastric)	Duodenal: 200,000 to 400,000 cases annually Gastric: 87,500 new cases annually
Polymyalgia rheumatica	Mid-40s to mid-70s	F	50/100,000
Prostatic cancer	Mid-40s to mid-60s	M	69/100,000
Psoriatic spondylitis	Early 30s to mid-50s	Equal	
Reiter's syndrome	20 to 40	M	
Rheumatoid arthritis	20 to 60	F	
Scoliosis (adult)	Teens to 40	F	
Sickle cell anemia	Late teens to mid-30s	Equal	
Spinal stenosis	Mid-40s to 70	Equal	
Spondylolisthesis (isthmic)	Mid-20s to mid-50s	Equal	

often does not correlate with the specific forces incurred during the mechanism of injury. The patient should be queried whether he or she remembers performing any task in a biomechanically disadvantaged position. He or she may also recall an episode or episodes of eccentric or concentric repetitive loading, perhaps related to sporting, leisure, or work activities. Also, question the patient regarding sustained postures such as those required when gardening, playing a musical instrument, or driving for long distances.

Clinical Pearl: For acute low back pain syndromes of a mechanical nature, the degree of pain and disability experienced by the patient often does not correlate with the specific forces incurred during the mechanism of injury.

Prior History/Treatment Considering that the vast majority of the population experiences low back pain at some point in their lives,[22] it is not surprising that patients with a prior history of low back pain are likely to experience future episodes. Patients should be asked if they have experienced similar complaints or problems within the same region, even if the current complaint feels differently. If so, it is helpful to determine what treatment was provided, whether self-administered or by a health-care provider, over what length of time, and whether that treatment was effective. It is also advisable to note any prior provider's name and contact information for future reference.

Palliative Measures Most patients attempt to alleviate their suffering in some manner. It is important to determine what was attempted and what effect, if any, was achieved. Depending upon the nature of the pathology, certain body positions may bring relief. Lying supine with knees flexed decreases pressure on the spinal column and tension of neural elements. Similar relief may be felt in the side-lying position; however, patients with a neurocompressive disc herniation may find this position unsustainable on one side and tolerable on the other side. Standing or extension may be less provoking than seated or flexed positions in patients with disc pathology whereas the opposite is typically true of patients with spinal stenosis. A classic example of positional relief involves the patient with stenosis who leans on a shopping cart while walking to alleviate back and lower extremity symptoms. Disc and stenotic syndromes were covered in detail in Chapters 6 and 7 respectively. Bear in mind that patients often present with symptoms more complex than classic textbook examples allow.

With respect to degenerative conditions in the early phase of development, active motion and stretching are often palliative. Overuse syndromes are typically responsive to rest.[23,24] Pathology of nonmechanical origin is usually nonresponsive to provocative movement and may be negatively responsive to positional changes as in the case of sepsis within the abdominal cavity and neoplastic activity.[24]

Many patients are unaware of the mechanisms of inflammation and apply heat to the area of pain. Upon questioning, the common response from patients in the acute phase is that the pain initially subsided following application of heat but returned a few hours later with greater intensity. A brief interlude of patient education at this point is warranted. Patients may also apply ice, particularly if swelling is present. If the patient indicates that ice was not effective, determine if appropriate cryotherapy protocols were followed.

Should the patient indicate that over-the-counter pain relievers or anti-inflammatory medications, prescription medications, herbal supplements, or topical creams were used, determine the dosage, frequency, effect, and health-care provider's name, if appropriate.

Provocative Factors As mentioned above, movement may be tolerated to a greater or lesser degree depending on the condition. The same is true for various body positions. Determine what factors increase the patient's symptoms, paying attention to how long an activity must be performed or position sustained before symptoms become apparent. This type of quantification assists in determining the diagnosis, prognosis, and also serves as an outcome measure with which to monitor treatment effectiveness.

Progression/Course The progression or course of a patient's condition can be viewed on several levels. Specific to a current event, determine if symptoms are better, worse, or the same since onset. If the condition seems to be chronic, determine whether symptoms are fairly constant over time or whether they demonstrate periodicity in association with environmental, psychosocial, or biological changes. Ascertain the estimated duration of each episode as well as in which direction the patient's symptoms are trending.

Quality of Symptoms Pain is the most common initial complaint involving the low back. Descriptors used by the patient to characterize his or her pain can provide valuable clues to the origin of the problem. For example, pain associated with pathology of the bony tissues is often described as deep and boring. Pathology within the muscle, tendon, fascia, and similar soft tissues may produce dull, achy, or burning pain. Depending on the type of nerve tissue involved and the extent of pathology, symptoms originating from these tissues may be described as lancinating, shock-like, "pins and needles," numbness, burning, weakness, or cramping. Listed below are a few of the most common descriptors.

Origin	Common Descriptors
Bone	Deep ache, boring, "bone" pain
Muscle/Fascia	Dull, achy, sore, burning, cramping
Nerve	Sharp, knife-like, shooting, lancinating, "pins and needles," tingling, burning, numbness, weakness
Vascular	Burning, stabbing, throbbing, tingling, cold
Organ	Deep pain, cramping, stabbing

It is important to let the patient use his or her own set of descriptors. Placing adjectives in the patient's mouth is likely to prove frustrating for the patient and may be diagnostically misleading for the doctor. Only when the patient seems unable to express his or her experience, or the clinician is unable to interpret the patient's adjectives, should descriptors be offered to assist the process.

Radiation/Referral Patterns Low back pain that emanates from the bony structures, soft tissues, or neural elements often demonstrates an associated pattern of referral or radiation. At a given spinal level, the similar pain patterns of dermatomal, myotomal, and sclerotomal pain represent the distributions of a single nerve root. Fortunately, each type of tissue has a different quality of pain with which it is associated. Unfortunately, owing to the unique neurological development of each individual, pattern overlap is the norm.[25,26] Based on the pattern alone, it is difficult to determine the offending structure involved.

Radicular pain and dermatomal pain are often used interchangeably though their meanings are distinct. *Radicular pain* refers to pain initiated by nerve root irritation and presents itself along the pathway of the root. *Dermatomal pain* is defined as pain within the distribution of a single sensory nerve root that innervates the skin and presents itself at the surface. Two additional definitions are pertinent. A *myotome* consists of groups of muscles supplied by a single spinal segment whereas a *sclerotome* is an area of bone or fascia supplied by a single spinal segment. Given the variability of human anatomy, both of these entities can demonstrate differing patterns between patients.

Referred pain is thought to be due to spillover of neural signals in the dorsal horn, the origin of which the brain misinterprets, though it typically misinterprets these signals consistently. For instance, flank pain may be a manifestation of kidney pathology and myofascial trigger points in the quadratus lumborum manifest pain in the ipsilateral buttock and posterior thigh. Recognizing these patterns will reduce the potentially serious consequences of a missed diagnosis.

Severity Since the perception of pain, or other symptom such as paresthesia, is a subjective experience, it is difficult to quantify. There are several tools that attempt to bridge the gap between patient symptoms and doctor properly interpreting those symptoms. The most frequently used tool is a numerical rating scale, with 0 representing the absence of pain and either 10 or 100 representing the most extreme intensity of pain that the patient has experienced or can imagine. It is mandatory that the doctor determine what experience patient rates as his or her most severe intensity of pain in order to give the scale meaning.

There are several other tools that provide quantification of the patient's symptoms to greater or lesser degree. The visual analog scale is frequently used, particularly with new patients and during reexaminations. The scale consists of a 10-cm unmarked line with indicators of "no pain" at the left end of the line and "extreme pain" at the right end of the line. Patients are asked to mark the line at the point corresponding to their pain level. Color charts are useful for young patients and patients who have difficulty communicating information due to language barriers. The colors extend from red to violet, with red representing extreme pain and violet representing the absence of pain. Verbal descriptors, such as minimal, slight, moderate, and severe, may also be used to categorize pain levels, although they can be subject to misinterpretation.

It is important to quantify a patient's pain intensity at its current level, when it is at its lowest and highest points and an average estimate over a selected period of time, for example 1 week. This information may then be used as outcome measures for subsequent treatment.

Temporal Factors Determining the connection between time of day and onset of symptoms may help differentiate between mechanical and inflammatory disorders. For example, muscle strains may feel slightly sore in the morning upon waking but typically result in greatest intensity of pain at the end of the day following activity. A patient with an inflammatory arthropathy such as ankylosing spondylitis would experience greatest symptoms in the morning after the joints and surrounding tissues have had ample time to stiffen. Additionally, patients with mechanically based pain often report an increase in symptoms during the evening hours when their attention is not diverted by work or daily activities. This may also be true when looking at pain patterns during the week when much activity occurs at home and work versus during the weekends when rest is more likely. Night pain that wakes a patient may be an indicator of

TABLE 12–3. Overview of Key Information Elicited during the Historical Query

Heading	Key Information
Location	Focal vs. diffuse; superficial vs. deep; referral vs. radiation
Onset	Current age, age at onset, gender, mechanism of injury, acute vs. subacute vs. chronic, sudden vs. insidious
Palliative	Movement vs. rest, positions, medications
Provocative	Movement vs. rest, positions
Prior	Frequency and duration
Progression	Constant vs. episodic; better, worse, no change
Quality	Key adjectives for pain (bone, muscle, nerve) and sensory disturbances
Radiation/referral	Nerve vs. myofascial elements
Severity	Quantification with current, highest and lowest intensity
Temporal	Environmental and timing correlations

neoplastic activity or infection ("red flags") and should be addressed immediately. In contrast, a patient who awakens *following movement*, such as changing positions while sleeping, would be less of a risk for "red flags." The same is true of the patient who has difficulty returning to sleep after getting up, for example, to visit the restroom. For women, back pain may show a monthly periodicity related to the menstrual cycle.

Table 12–3 lists the key questions used during the historical query. Keep in mind that not all questions are equally pertinent for each patient.

Activities of Daily Living

In addition to this list of basic questions, the doctor should also query the patient regarding affected activities of daily living. It is important to determine what the patient is capable of outside the confines of an examination room, which activities provoke pain and which activities require assistance, and which are intolerable. With this information, the clinician can set a baseline with which to measure progress that is meaningful to the patient. Additionally, the clinician can determine whether the need for assistive devices is warranted. There are several useful tools such as the Roland and Morris Disability Questionnaire, the Modified Oswestry Low Back Pain Disability Questionnaire, and the SF-36. Further information on appropriate measures of daily activities is available in Chapter 14.

Psychosocial Factors and Nonorganic Signs

During the initial history, it is important to document any psychosocial factors or nonorganic signs and symptoms as these may directly affect the clinician's ability to accurately and completely diagnose the patient. The patient's response to treatment and prognosis will be impacted as well. The clinician should determine if there are any work stressors that may either physically or emotionally delay recovery or increase the likelihood of chronicity. This necessitates a full understanding of the patient's job description and workplace environment. Depending on the circumstances, lifestyle factors either may be a source of physical or psychosocial irritation for the patient or can be used as a motivational force during treatment. Additionally, the patient's participation in hobbies may be negatively impacted by back pain. Recovery and return to these activities can also be used as a motivational device.

As with activities of daily living, there are several resources available to assess psychosocial factors and nonorganic signs. The reader is referred to Chapter 19 for a detailed presentation of these issues.

Pertinent Health History

When collecting information about the patient's health history, a useful acronym is FAOMASHL: family health history, accidents, other associated/unassociated complaints, medications, allergies, surgeries, hospitalizations, and lifestyle factors. The clinician should solicit information from the patient regarding the presence or past existence of any major illnesses, including but not limited to diabetes, heart disease, cancer, and hypertension. Any allergies should be documented, as well as the use, including dosage and frequency, of over-the-counter preparations; prescription medications, particularly corticosteroids and anticoagulants; vitamins; and herbal supplements. The dates, provider contact information, and outcomes of hospitalizations and surgical procedures should be noted.

Clinical Pearl: A useful acronym is FAOMASHL: family health history, accidents, other associated/unassociated complaints, medications, allergies, surgeries, hospitalizations, and lifestyle factors.

The patient should be given the opportunity to discuss any symptoms that seem associated with the current complaint. As low back pathology may result in symptoms distal to the lumbar spine, the patient should also be encouraged to report any other symptoms, even if they seem unrelated. For example, rheumatic or inflammatory arthritic pain often presents in the appendicular skeleton prior to spinal symptoms. Additionally, a patient's complaint of low back pain may be the key he or she uses to open the door to address other worrisome health issues. Always ask each patient if he or she has any health concerns unrelated to the chief complaint.

Family history of major illnesses as well as lifestyle factors should be documented. A review of systems completes the patient history. It is recommended that the clinician take a few moments to review the historical information, particularly the contributory findings, with the patient to assure accuracy. This time also allows the doctor to formulate a list of differential diagnoses based on historical information and develops an appropriate list of examination procedures.

It is also vital, from a diagnostic as well as treatment viewpoint, to determine the patient's level of conditioning. Information regarding the patient's job description should include the estimated level of activity, from sedentary to strenuous. Also, elements such as lifestyle factors, hobbies, and exercise routine can contribute to the clinician's impression.

Clinical Pearl: A patient's complaint of low back pain may be the key he or she uses to open the door to address other worrisome health issues. Always ask each patient if he or she has any health concerns unrelated to the chief complaint.

PHYSICAL EXAMINATION

Based on information gathered from the patient's history, a focused physical examination is designed to rule in one of the differential diagnoses and rule out the others. The order of examination procedures should reflect awareness of the patient's potential discomfort and proceed from least to most invasive. It is also a matter of common sense to perform procedures in some sort of logical positional order. For instance, a patient who reports difficulty when lying on his or her stomach should be examined in the prone position only if necessary, saving this position for the end of the examination. A patient who has pain in the seated position will appreciate the clinician's efforts to minimize examinations performed in this position. For patients who are able to attain all positions without significant distress, it is most convenient for the clinician to perform procedures as gravity suggests, moving from the standing position to seated, supine, side-lying, and then prone.

Appropriate documentation is critical to provide an accurate clinical picture of the patient. Additionally, memorizing a specific examination routine can reduce the likelihood of committing performance and charting errors. Often, clinicians move through an examination noting positive or significant negative findings only at the end of the examination. This practice is discouraged as information that contributes to the diagnosis or prospective treatment plan may be forgotten. A discussion of this issue is found further in this chapter.

Clinical Pearl: Memorizing a specific examination routine can reduce the likelihood of committing performance and charting errors.

Inspection

Whether the clinician chooses to greet patients personally in the waiting room or in the examination room, the examination should begin with the initial contact. Note the patient's seated position and ability to rise from that position. A patient who attempts to decrease pain by pushing off from the chair arms or uses the thighs for support is considered to have a positive Minor's sign. Notice his or her gait pattern and any antalgia. Once in the examination room, the patient should be gowned appropriately to allow complete inspection of the lumbar spine and lower extremities. Postural alignment should be assessed, including pelvic tilt. Muscle hypertonicity, splinting, and atrophy are more easily viewed with an indirect light source that highlights asymmetry. Document the presence of any deformities, scars, skin lesions, pigmentation, erythema, and midline hair growth. The location and extent of any edema should be recorded as well. Edema extending to the lumbar region, a potential sign of cardiovascular, kidney, or lung dysfunction, should be noted and graded as described below.

Palpation

Palpation of the lumbar region is best performed with the patient in a prone position but may also be performed on a seated patient. The examiner should begin by assessing the soft tissues for an increase in focal temperature. Pressing a finger into the involved area for several seconds should assess edema involving the lumbar region as well as the lower extremities. When the skin swells so much that the fluid cannot be digitally displaced, it is termed *brawny edema*. In contrast, swollen tissue that remains imprinted following the removal of a finger is called *pitting edema*. A four-point scale is used to qualify the degree of pitting edema and is graded as follows[27]:

1+ Slight pitting (0″ to 1/4″) without visible distortion of the extremity. Indentation disappears rapidly.
2+ Somewhat deeper (1/4″ to 1/2″) than grade 1+, without distortion. Indentation disappears in 10–15 seconds.
3+ Noticeable depression (1/2″ to 1″) that may last 1–2 minutes. Contour of dependent extremity appears distorted.
4+ Very deep pit (>1″), lasting 2–5 minutes. Extremity is noticeably distorted.

The patient using descriptors listed previously, and subjectively graded using a numerical rating scale, should characterize tenderness to palpation. To objectively grade the pain response, a categorical scale is used as follows[28]:

0 No tenderness
+1 Mild tenderness; verbal response only
+2 Moderate tenderness; patient complains and winces
+3 Moderate to severe tenderness; patient complains, winces, and withdraws
+4 Severe tenderness; withdrawal response and inability to tolerate further testing

This scale is subject to the patient's input and the clinician's biases. Studies using a pressure algometer to quantify pain have shown promise. With this method, the clinician can grade the pain response in terms of pounds or kilograms of pressure applied. Drawbacks to this method include the lack of consistency when attempting to locate the target landmark and the patient's inconsistency when reporting pressure versus pain sensation.[29]

The presence of muscle atrophy, hypertonicity, active (Grade I) and latent (Grade II) trigger points, and crepitus in either the superficial tissues or bony structures is noted. Skin rolling may be performed if the history warrants. Beginning either at the base of the lumbar spine or at the T12 spinal level, the clinician grasps the skin on either side of the spine between his or her fingers and rolls it back and forth. Hypersensitivity may indicate the presence of Maigne's syndrome, an irritation of the cluneal nerves at the thoracolumbar junction.[30]

After assessing the surrounding soft tissues, the clinician should pursue palpation of the bony landmarks and spinal joints to include passive joint play. This procedure is detailed in the following sections.

Evaluation of the abdominal, inguinal, popliteal arteries and distal pedal pulses is dependent on the patient's profile and presentation. As a general rule, the abdominal aorta should be assessed for possible enlargement via auscultation and palpation in any patient over the age of 50 with acute onset of low back pain. Peripheral pulses should be routinely assessed for strength and symmetry, particularly in patients with potential for arterial or venous compromise. Pulses are graded on a five-point scale as follows[31]: 0 = absent; 1 = diminished; 2 = normal; 3 = increased; and 4 = bounding. Diminished pulses suggest lumenal compromise, decreased total volume, or loss of vessel tone. Bounding pulses may result from atherosclerosis, hyperthyroidism, or arteriovenus fistulas. Additional indications for this assessment include the presence of ischemic pain distal to a compromised artery, vascular disease, and diabetes.

Clinical Pearl: As a general rule, the abdominal aorta should be assessed for possible enlargement via auscultation and palpation in any patient over the age of 50 with acute onset of low back pain.

Percussion

Percussion of the spinous processes, typically performed with a hard-rubber reflex hammer, to rule out fracture is an often-performed procedure of questionable efficacy. Historically, distal percussion combined with auscultation proximal to the site of fracture was used to assess sound conduction and thereby determine the presence of fracture in long bones such as the femur, humerus, and clavicle.[32–35] A pain response elicited on spinous process percussion is not specific for the presence of fracture, and lack of response does not guarantee absence of fracture.[36] However, it is a quick and simple procedure and percussion may be used to narrow the level of spinal involvement.

Range of Motion

Range of motion assessment is used perhaps more than any other examination procedure to evaluate a patient's functional status. It is also used extensively as an outcome measure and therapy modulator. There are several sources of reference data concerning the measurement and proper notation of joint motion,[37–40] most concerning the measurement of appendicular joint motion. This section will describe the evaluation of active, passive, and resisted motions as well as joint play and end feel.

When assessing range of motion, the examiner should note symptom location, quality, severity, and end feel. When applicable, as in side bending and rotation, the noninvolved side should be evaluated before stressing the symptomatic side. The examiner should also take into consideration the patient's age, general physical condition, and any structural abnormalities that often affect voluntary motion.[41] Gender also influences the available range of motion, with women typically demonstrating greater mobility.[41,42] Always ask the patient to describe the symptoms elicited and rate pain or other sensory aberration on either a numerical or categorical scale.

A brief word concerning normal values is in order. The majority of published data concerning normal ranges of motion exist without concomitant data on the subjects' demographic background, specifically with respect to age, gender, and occupation. Knowing that these and several other factors can alter the potential limits of joint motion, it is questionable whether

TABLE 12–4. **Goniometric Landmarks, Normal Motion Values, and End Feel Descriptors for the Lumbar Spine**

Motion	Axis of Rotation	Arm Landmarks	Normal Values	Normal End Feel
Flexion	Coronal/axillary line at L5 level	Stationary arm: along thigh Active arm: axial line to L1 spinous process	70–90 degrees	Tissue stretch (firm elastic resistance)
Extension	Coronal/axillary line at L5 level	Stationary arm: along thigh Active arm: axial line to L1 spinous process	30–50 degrees	Bone to bone (hard, painless) or tissue stretch
Lateral flexion	Midline at S1 spinous process	Stationary arm: midline inferiorly Active arm: L1 spinous process	30 degrees	Tissue stretch
Rotation	Visual estimation only		35 degrees	Tissue stretch

existing reference data are valid for all patients. As Rothstein asserts,[43] it is unlikely that one set of values can describe what is normal for both sexes throughout a lifetime. In fact, the most widely used reference values are not the product of rigorous research but exist as a matter of tradition.

Most clinicians measure range of motion visually, a method referred to commonly as "eyeballing." In fact, this method is endorsed by the American Academy of Orthopedic Surgeons.[37] While this seems to be the fastest and easiest method, its validity is questionable.[44,45] There are a variety of tools available to enhance the validity of measuring active motion of the lumbar spine. The goniometer, also known as the universal goniometer, is the most accessible and least costly device. Various authors provide detailed instruction in placement of the instrument and follow through movement of the arms.[37,39,46] It should be noted that goniometric measurement of the lumbar spine often incorporates some thoracolumbar motion. It should also be noted that in a recent study, researchers found poor intra- and interrater reliability for all goniometric measurements of the thoracolumbar spine.[47] Table 12–4 lists the suggested landmarks used when assessing lumbar ranges of motion with a goniometer.

The ability of the examiner to mimic joint motion by accurately placing the goniometer's axis of rotation in line with the joint axis of rotation is highly questionable for several reasons. First, the goniometer operates as a simple hinge mechanism whereas joints of the body are complex structures that exhibit a continually changing axis of rotation throughout the arc of movement. Second, the examiner must rely on bony landmarks that are often unreliable, particularly when the structure lies deep to several layers of soft tissue. Last, alignment of the axis does not always allow proper alignment of the arms and vice versa. Robson,[45] among other authors, suggested aligning the arms prior to movement and foregoing placement of the goniometer's axis altogether.

The fluid goniometer,[48] also known as the bubble goniometer, consists of a fluid-filled circular tube attached to or embedded in a flat platform with 360-degree scale. With the joint in a neutral position, the device is either strapped to the distal aspect of an extremity or manually held in place on the patient, as can be the case when measuring trunk movement. While many clinicians appreciate the ease of use and elimination of landmark estimation required by the universal goniometer, this device still exhibits problems with reliable positioning, particularly if attached with a strap or when used on obese patients. Landmarks used are similar to those of the goniometer's active arm.

Inclinometers, initially called electrogoniometers, have advanced greatly since their introduction in 1959.[49] The device typically seen in the clinic is small, portable, and moderately priced. The original models, and current larger research models, require harnesses, a plethora of connecting wires and computer terminal. The typical office version consists of one (inclinometer) or two (dual inclinometer) elements and relies on a potentiometer to calculate joint motion. The device can be calibrated to allow for starting angles of other than zero degrees. If using a single device, it is positioned similar to the bubble goniometer. If using the dual inclinometer, one element is positioned at the axis of rotation and the other is placed at the distal motion segment.

While normative data do not exist for arcs of motion that occur between the vertical (X), horizontal (Y), and transverse (Z) planes (see Chapter 3), most injuries do not occur following movement in just one plane. The evaluator should feel free to subjectively evaluate combined, or coupled, motions between these strictly defined planes. For example, the clinician may choose to evaluate a patient's ability to simultaneously flex forward and rotate in a particular direction. The subjective information gathered during such an evaluation often assists in directing further treatment.

Clinical Pearl: As most injuries do not occur following movement in just one plane, evaluation of the patient should incorporate movement between planes of motion.

There are a few general considerations when assessing motion of the lumbar spine. The clinician should observe the patient in a standing position when evaluating active motion and with the patient in a seated position to better control body weight when assessing passive or resisted motion. Flexion and extension should be measured from the lateral aspect of the patient but viewed from the dorsal aspect as well to note any deviations from the midline. Lateral bending and rotation should be viewed and measured from the dorsal aspect. The clinician should instruct the patient to perform each motion fully, stopping only in the event of notable discomfort. If the patient reports mild discomfort but is able to continue with the motion, he or she should be encouraged to do so. The 0–180 system of notation, wherein all movements begin at 0 degree and move toward 180 degree, is the most widely used method of recording joint range of motion.[37,50,51]

Any symptom should be noted as to location, quality, presence of referral pain or radiation, and quantified on a numerical (preferable) or categorical scale. If full active range of motion is attained without the production of symptoms, the clinician need not assess passive motions. However, resisted motions may produce further clinical findings. If a particular active range of motion is symptom provoking, the clinician must log this finding, but may choose to defer the corresponding assessment of resisted motion to avoid unnecessarily exacerbating the patient's symptoms. Passive range of motion, however, should be assessed in this case. Regarding end feel, the clinician should lightly apply overpressure at the end range of active motion if the patient attains a full and pain-free end range or at the end range of passive assessment with or without pain. Table 12–4 lists the normal range of motion values for lumbar motion and corresponding appropriate end feel descriptors.

Clinical Pearl: A capsular pattern of restricted motion in the lumbar spine, wherein noncontractile tissues are chiefly responsible for limitation, is (in order of most restriction) lateral flexion and rotation followed by extension.

Pain induced by active range of motion may implicate a number of tissues including muscle and tendon, ligament and capsule, bone and nerve. Keeping in mind earlier comments regarding the challenge of achieving a specific diagnosis, the key to deciphering which offending structure is involved lies in determining the type of pain produced and whether active, passive, and/or resisted motions are provoking. Of course, in the chronic condition or with significant trauma multiple pain generators are not uncommon. Nevertheless, tissue-specific provocative tests may be invaluable in ruling in and ruling out key symptom generators. Furthermore, positive findings have been shown to yield poor inter-examiner reliability and the results must be integrated with the rest of the clinical findings. Classically, lumbar muscle and tendon injuries are provoked by either stretching the injured tissue through active or passive motion or forcing it to contract as occurs in resisted motions. Injuries involving noncontractile tissues such as ligaments, facet capsules, and intervertebral discs are provoked by loading the structure actively or passively whereas resisted isometric muscle contraction is typically nonprovoking, unless, in the case of disc herniation, "abdominal canister" (i.e., transversus, obliques, rectus, multifidi, pelvic floor, and diaphragm) contraction increases intrathecal pressure. A capsular pattern of restricted motion in the lumbar spine, wherein noncontractile tissues are chiefly responsible for limitation, is (in order of most restriction) lateral flexion and rotation followed by extension.

Active Ranges of Motion

Flexion The patient is instructed to tuck the chin toward the chest and bend forward at the waist, keeping the knees extended while attempting to touch the toes. The clinician should note any change in an existing scoliotic curve, deviation away from the midline which may suggest guarding due to disc pathology,[52] patient apprehension or assistance (use of hands on knees) lack of motion between spinal segments, and whether the normal lordosis decreases as expected.

Extension The patient is instructed to place his or her hands on the posterior iliac crests to provide support and then extend backward from the waist, keeping the knees extended and the gaze toward the ceiling. The clinician notes if the arc of extension is even throughout the lumbar spine or more pronounced at a specific spinal segment.

Lateral Flexion The patient is instructed to lean to the side without flexing forward or extending backward, sliding keeping the hands on the lateral thigh or hip. The clinician notes if the arc of bending is even or more pronounced at a specific spinal segment as well as whether the patient unintentionally rotates the torso to accommodate motion.

Rotation With the clinician stabilizing the patient's pelvis to limit distal movement, the patient is instructed to cross the arms over the chest and twist the torso. Patients frequently tend to laterally flex or extend the torso, and so the examiner must take care in avoiding such motion. The clinician notes whether combined motions are used and any asymmetry in muscle mass or skin folds produced at terminal rotation.

Passive Ranges of Motion

Flexion With the patient seated on the examination table, he or she is instructed to keep the arms to the side while the clinician grasps his or her shoulders and flexes the patient forward at the waist, keeping the pelvis firmly on the table. The clinician should note end feel and any change in an existing scoliotic curve, lack of motion between spinal segments, and whether the normal lordosis decreases as expected.

Extension While seated, the patient is instructed to place his or her hands across the chest. The clinician supports the upper back with one arm, the sacrum with the other hand, and then extends the patient backward in an arching motion rather than a leaning motion. The clinician notes end feel or any altered symptoms.

Lateral Flexion In the seated position, the patient is instructed to cross the arms across the chest. The clinician places one arm across the upper back and the other hand on the contralateral iliac crest. The clinician then bends the patient to each side, keeping the opposite crest from rising off the table. As with extension, an arching motion rather than a leaning motion is desired. End feel is noted or any altered symptoms.

Rotation In the seated, arms crossed position, the clinician grasps the shoulders and rotates the patient's torso. Alternately, the clinician may use a shoulder–scapula contact. End feel is noted or any altered symptoms.

Resisted Ranges of Motion

While typically thought of as an extremity assessment, resisted motions can provide valuable information regarding the origin of lumbar pathology as well as indicate basic strength parameters. The motions are assessed with the patient in a seated position. The clinician applies a resisting force by stabilizing the patient's upper back during resisted extension, and the shoulders during flexion, lateral bending, and rotation. The clinician notes the presence and type of pain produced and the degree of effort exerted.

End Feel

The end feel of a joint describes what the clinician manually feels at or just beyond the voluntary range of motion. The adjectives used refer to the quality of motion and to the structures that may contribute to cessation of motion. For instance, the clinician adding overpressure at end range lumbar flexion on a patient of average weight may perceive a soft tissue stretch end feel, representing the limits of soft tissue extensibility. The same overpressure assessment on an obese patient may result in a soft tissue approximation end feel, indicating that the end range of joint motion was not assessed. Tissue stretch is the normal end feel when applying overpressure at end range lumbar flexion, lateral flexion, and rotation. However, the clinician may perceive soft tissue approximation when attempting flexion overpressure on an obese individual.

Joint Play

The assessment of joint play may be static or active in nature and provides information regarding the passive flexibility of the motion segment. For static assessment, the patient should be in the lying position to reduce tension on the joints assessed. Active palpation should be evaluated with the patient seated. Using a hand contact, the clinician assesses each facet joint by applying direct pressure to various contact points. When assessing anterior movement, the clinician places the proximal palm over each spinous process and compresses in a posterior to anterior vector, taking into consideration the angle of the lumbar spine. For instance, when compressing the L1 spinous process, a slight inferior to superior vector is added while a slight superior to inferior vector is added during L5 assessment. Placing the thumb of one hand lateral to the spinous process and contacting over the contralateral mamillary process with the opposite thumb assesses rotational movements in the transverse plane. The spinous process is pushed laterally while the mamillary process is compressed ventrally. Assessing rotation in the coronal plane requires lateral thumb pressure against the spinous while the ipsilateral lower extremity is brought into abduction.

Neurological Testing

Any indication of neural dysfunction, whether obtained during the patient's history or discovered during any part of the physical examination, necessitates a thorough neurological evaluation. Even if the patient's history and physical examination do not suggest nerve involvement, a basic evaluation, consisting of sensory perception, voluntary motor control, and reflex assessment, should be performed to document baseline information as the patient's condition may progress beyond the current status.

Reflexes

There are three categories of reflex testing pertinent to the lumbar spine evaluation. The most commonly assessed reflex by far is the muscle stretch reflex, formerly known as the deep tendon reflex.[53–55] In the lower extremity, this test is most successfully applied to the superficial tendons of the quadriceps muscle group below the patella, the semitendinosus muscle, and the gastrocnemius/soleus group. The corresponding nerve levels are L4, L5, and S1, respectively.

With the muscle and tendon placed in a slightly tensioned position, typically midway between full flexion and full extension of the involved joint, the clinician applies a quick, deliberate strike to the tendon. Muscle response is either visually noted, as in joint movement or muscle twitch, or palpated. A diminished response should prompt the clinician to employ some form of distraction, termed a Jendrassik maneuver,[56] to divert the patient's attention away from the area of impending impact. If the patient's response is still diminished or absent following a Jendrassik maneuver, the addition of mental distraction such as solving a simple math equation or repeating a list of objects is often effective. The patient's response is graded using the Wexler scale as follows[28]:

0 No response
1+ Somewhat diminished
2+ Normal
3+ Somewhat brisk, hyperactive
4+ Very brisk; markedly hyperactive, often with clonus

Clinical Pearl: If the patient's response is still diminished or absent following a Jendrassik maneuver, the addition of mental distraction such as solving a simple math equation or repeating a list of objects is often effective.

Testing should be performed bilaterally to determine whether responses are asymmetrical. Responses other than normal (2+), specifically somewhat diminished or brisk responses, should be compared to findings of the opposite side and correlated with the patient's history as well as the remainder of the neurological examination. For example, a decreased reflex on the symptomatic radicular side is very different from bilaterally diminished reflexes in a patient without any leg symptoms. Findings of either clonus, markedly brisk activity or absent response mandate a thorough neurological evaluation, as significant pathology within the upper (hyperreflexive) or lower (hyporeflexive) motor neurons may exist.

Beacuse of the qualitative nature of reflex assessment, both in terms of the clinician's subjective judgment concerning the response elicited as well as the choice of reflex hammers used to elicit the response, inter-examiner reliability is low.[57–60] Additionally, there are a variety of factors, including age, gender, altitude, conditions such as hypoglycemia or hypothyroidism, and hip position that can affect the patient's response to tendon tap.[61–65]

There are a number of reflexes that occur in response to stimulation of the skin, known as the *superficial reflexes*. Three of these, the cremasteric (L1–L2), Geigel (L1–L2), and anal (S2–S5), are pertinent to nerves exiting the lumbar spine. Performance of these superficial reflex tests involves either stroking or pricking the skin of the upper inner thigh (cremasteric and Geigel) or perianal tissue and noting the presence of muscle contraction by the cremasteric (elevation of the testicles), iliopuepartal (elevation of the clitoral prepuce), or external sphincter muscles (also known as anal wink), respectively.[66]

In the event of an upper motor neuron lesion or neurological insult to the level involved, the superficial reflexes are lost. However, a patient without upper motor neuron involvement may also demonstrate lack of response to one or more of these reflexes. Again, without correlation from the history and physical examination findings, absence of a superficial reflex may not ultimately be clinically significant. If this evaluation is necessary, given the sensitive nature of the areas examined, it is important that the clinician be completely competent and comfortable examining these reflexes. Absent this prerequisite, the patient should be referred to a neurologist for further examination.

Pathological reflexes occur in the presence of motor cortex, brainstem, or corticospinal tract lesions (upper motor neuron lesions) wherein the motor response to a sensory stimulus is not modulated.[55] In a normally functioning patient, the expected response to invasive stimulus around the foot and ankle is either attempted withdrawal of the foot or no reaction. If pathology exists within the system described above, the classic pathological response is the Babinski sign, consisting of dorsiflexion of the first toe, possible dorsiflexion of the remaining toes, and fanning of the toes. Should the clinician elicit such response, an evaluation for hyperreflexia of the upper extremity is required to determine the level of involvement. The presence of pathological reflexes in the lower extremities while normal in the upper extremities suggests a lesion below the C6 level.[55]

A variety of maneuvers exist that may elicit the Babinski sign in the presence of a lesion to the pyramidal tract. The Babinski reflex is performed by using a blunt instrument to stroke along the lateral aspect of the footpad, beginning at the heel and then crossing the metatarsal heads. The plantar reflex is similar, except that the stimulus is applied to the center of the footpad. Other maneuvers that may produce a Babinski sign include stroking a blunt instrument around the lateral malleolus and across the dorsum of the foot (Chaddock), simultaneously stroking down both sides of the tibia from proximal to distal aspect (Oppenheim), squeezing the calf muscle (Gordon), squeezing the Achilles tendon (Schaefer), and plantar flexing the fourth distal phalanx (Gonda).[14]

Mensuration

Circumferential mensuration of the lower extremities can provide useful information regarding the presence of muscle atrophy that may occur with volitional disuse as a result of pain avoidance behaviors, issues of secondary gain, or frank motor nerve dysfunction. The clinician may also find these values useful as outcome measurements. Outside the focus of the lumbar examination, mensuration may also provide useful information regarding the presence of edema.

Clinical Pearl: To eliminate false-positive findings, remember to ask the patient about participation in one-sided activities either at work, at home, or during participation in sports or hobbies.

Using the femoral condyle and tibial plateau as bony landmarks, the clinician measures a determined distance away from each landmark and then ascertains the circumferential measurement at that distance. When measuring the lower leg, the greatest circumference of the calf is commonly utilized as the distal measurement. The amount of adipose tissue is often increased from the mid to proximal portion of the thigh as compared to the distal half, particularly in female patients. The clinician should therefore measure proximally from the femoral condyle, being certain to measure the more reliable distal half of the thigh. For convenience, the same distance measured from the tibial plateau to the calf muscle belly may be used to measure proximally from the femoral condyle. Do not neglect to chart the landmarks and distances used so that the same future measurements can again be utilized for consistency in order to ascertain clinical validity.

Asymmetry of an inch (2.5 cm) or more in circumference may be used to strengthen the significance of other physical examination findings.[67] Nonetheless, the human body is rarely symmetrical and discrepancies may exist for a number of reasons, none of which may involve pathology. To reduce the risk of false-positive findings, remember to ask the patient about participation in one-sided activities either at work, at home, or during participation in sports or hobbies. Also, the clinician should expect to see differences favoring the dominant side. To determine which leg is dominant, ask the patient with which leg he or she would kick a ball.

Sensory Perception

A thorough evaluation of the sensory system is quite an involved process because of the number of ascending pathways carrying information to the brain. This section will review the more common procedures used in primary care. As descriptions of the clinical testing of temperature sensation and the majority of posterior column perceptions (vibration, position and movement awareness, two-point discrimination, etc.) are outside the intent of this chapter, the reader is directed to the appropriate neurology texts. Neurodiagnostic testing is addressed in detail in Chapter 18.

As stated earlier, the majority of patients with low back pathology present with pain or some other aberrant sensory involvement (dysesthesias). Determining the type and pattern of involvement is essential if the clinician hopes to arrive at a correct diagnosis. In the general practice setting, a sensory examination consists of evaluating whether sensory stimulus is equally perceived in both lower extremities and whether any abnormal sensory findings follow a nerve root (dermatomal) or peripheral nerve distribution.

Evaluation of sensory perception is most commonly performed using a pinwheel, which provokes a mildly painful, or pricking, sensation. The patient is asked to close his or her eyes and note whether the sensation feels the same at each point on the right and left extremity. In the event of sensory loss, the clinician should assess the patient's ability to perceive light touch, such as with a cotton ball, as well since this information travels along different pathways within the spinothalamic tract. In addition to sensory evaluation of the lower extremities, the clinician should assess the trunk as well to determine the presence of any areas of focal irritation such as occurs with cluneal nerve irritation.

To perform the evaluation, the clinician lightly draws the pinwheel over the patient's skin along dermatomal or peripheral nerve patterns depending on the patient's presentation. If either loss or hypersensitivity is noted, the area should be mapped by drawing the pinwheel circumferentially around the extremity, moving in small increments to capture changes in perception. To differentiate between hypersensitivity over one area versus hyposensitivity of the opposite area, compare same side findings above and below the areas in question as well as drawing from physical and historical correlates. The most reliable areas for sensory testing include the medial calf (L4), the dorsum of the foot (L5), and the lateral side and sole of the foot (S1).[53]

Clinical Pearl: To differentiate between hypersensitivity over one area versus hyposensitivity of the opposite area, compare same side findings above and

below the areas in question as well as drawing from physical and historical correlates.

Motor Response

Clinical data elicited from testing lower extremity muscle response are less informative than one would anticipate. Often, a patient with low back pain is understandably hesitant to give full effort, knowing that such effort will cause increased pain. Any noted decrease in strength or hesitation to perform requires further questioning to determine if the loss is due to avoidance behavior. The general physical fitness of the patient should be considered as well as the strength of the patient as compared to the strength of the clinician.

As quantitative strength evaluation is unavailable in most clinical settings because of equipment size and cost, subjective assessment continues to be the favored method. While quick to perform, this type of assessment contributes little to the description of the patient's current status, is poor at determining changes in status, and is not a valid outcome measurement.[68,69] The clinician should note the findings but realize that the information may be representative of many potential factors such as the patient's deconditioned state, pain mediation response, inappropriate pain behavior, or other psychological inhibitions.

For patients with potential low back pathology, assessment of the following myotomes is appropriate.[70–72] Keep in mind that, in general, nerves from two adjoining spinal segments control the movement of a given joint.[72]

L1/L2/L3	Hip flexion	Hip flexion
L2/L3/L4	Knee extension	Quadriceps
L4/L5	Foot dorsiflexion/inversion	Tibialis anterior, extensor digitorum longus, extensor hallucis longus
L5/S1	Knee flexion and eversion	Hamstrings, peroneus longus/brevis
L5/S1/S2	Hip extension	Gluteus maximus
S1/S2	Foot plantarflexion	Gastrocnemius, soleus, tibialis Posterior, flexor digitorum longus Flexor hallucis longus

The evaluation is performed by instructing the patient to contract the target muscle against resistance, using the noninvolved side for comparison and keeping in mind that concentric muscle contraction is inhibited at the end ranges of motion. The clinician should apply resistance for 3–5 seconds to determine if the contraction is sustainable and use hand placements that provide a mechanical advantage while avoiding contacting immediately over the joints. The size and strength of the muscles tested should steer the examiner toward the application of appropriate force. Muscle strength is graded on a zero- to five-point numerical scale as follows, with 5 representing the normal muscle response:[73,74]

0	Zero	No contraction palpated
1	Trace	Evidence of slight contractibility but no joint motion
2−	Poor (−)	Initiates motion if gravity is eliminated
2	Poor (25%)	Complete range of motion with gravity eliminated
2+	Poor (+)	Initiates motion against gravity
3−	Fair (−)	Some but not complete range of motion against gravity
3	Fair (50%)	Complete range of motion against gravity
3+	Fair (+)	Complete range of motion against gravity with minimal resistance
4	Good (75%)	Complete range of motion against gravity with some/moderate resistance
5	Normal (100%)	Complete range of motion against gravity with maximal resistance

In addition or as a supplement to static testing, the clinician may choose to assess L3–L4, L4–L5, and S1 myotomes or the pertinent peripheral nerves by having the patient perform squatting, toe, and heel walking, respectively. If the clinician is uncertain whether myotomal involvement exists, repetitive muscle contraction may be used to clarify an ambiguous finding. In fact, repeated one-legged calf raises have higher value than static muscle testing when attempting to expose dysfunction in an otherwise subclinical patient. Bouncing on the toes of each foot (maintaining balance by touching, but not bearing weight, on a stable surface) incorporates a more dynamic concentric and eccentric loading to pick up the subtle differences bilaterally (C.E. Morris, personal communication, 2003). Should repeated calf raises or bouncing on the toes elicit an abnormal response, the clinician should determine whether the finding is due to the patient's general balance and coordination by performing Romberg's and/or Stein's (similar to Romberg's test but performed on one leg) test. If positive, further tests of the cerebellar tracts are warranted.

Orthopedic Testing

The following mechanically based tests are designed to elicit a positive response by stretching the neural, dural, and discal tissues or applying pressure to those same structures. Often, a confirming maneuver is involved wherein tension is decreased in some manner and then reapplied to elicit a second response. While none of the following tests are intended to diagnose muscle injury, there is one test that is used frequently to assess facet joint involvement.

With a few notable exceptions such as the straight-leg raising and well-leg raising tests, the reliability of most orthopedic testing is either poor or unproven. Therefore, the clinician is wise to avoid overreliance on labeling a specific test as positive or negative. Rather, the patient's response to provocative maneuvers should be carefully charted and be used to provide a framework within which the clinician builds a complete picture of the clinical entity.

The location, quality, and severity of symptoms for the tests described below should be recorded as well as the degree of hip flexion or extension that elicits the symptom. Charting that an orthopedic test is positive or negative is no longer sufficient because of differing descriptions of testing and interpretations in positive results. Therefore, one must describe the results of the test. For example, muscle stretch during straight-leg raising testing with or without foot dorsiflexion may result in posterior thigh, popliteal, or calf discomfort. The patient may, depending on their level of credibility, be quite helpful in explaining whether the symptoms provoked seem to be from tight muscles or from noncontractile tissues. Palpate the muscles and tendons to evaluate their status. Compression of the calf muscles (Homan's test) may be useful to differentiate vascular claudication from neurogenic claudication or radicular pain.

Clinical Pearl: Charting that an orthopedic test is positive or negative is no longer sufficient because of differing descriptions of testing and interpretations in positive results. Therefore, one must describe the results of the test.

Supine Tests

The straight-leg raising test (SLR) is designed to tension the dura and nerve roots of the lumbar spine by flexing the lower extremity. However, it can provoke secondary findings due to loading of the lumbar spine, sacroiliac joints, ipsilateral hip, ipsilateral knee, and regional myofascial tissues. Also, it can provoke a neurocompressive disc lesion affecting the contralateral side, which is known as the well-leg raising test (see below). Depending on age and physical condition, hip flexion with full knee extension should be well tolerated to ranges of 60–120 degrees in normal patients.[75] Hamstring tightness may be an associated finding but is not considered a positive response. A detailed discussion of the anatomy and mechanics involved in this test is found within Chapter 6.

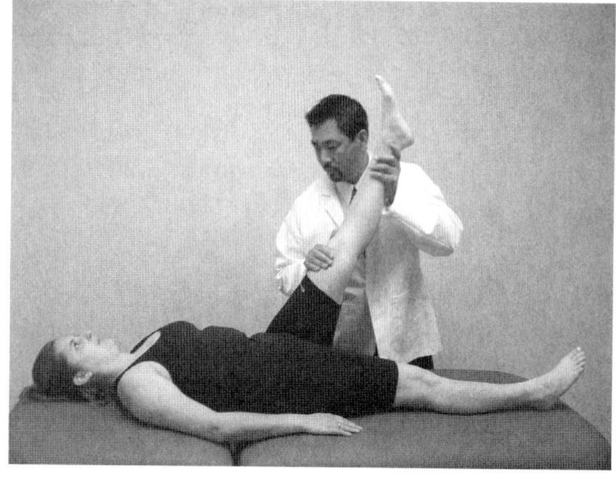

FIGURE 12–1. Straight-leg raising test (SLR). Assure that the patient is completely relaxed and the knee is held in full extension during the performance of this test.

With the patient supine, the examiner places one hand over the knee to maintain leg extension and the other hand under the heel. It must be emphasized that the SLR is a passive test on the patient's part. All too often, patients try to either assist the examiner or protect themselves by partially elevating the leg, which necessarily requires a bracing of the lumbopelvic region. This oftentimes accidental maneuver on the patients part can confound the clinical results and cloud the clinical picture. The clinician must therefore be on guard to avoid this subtlety and be certain to lift the entire weight of the leg during this test. The lower extremity is slowly flexed at the hip to 90 degrees (Fig. 12–1). A variety of patient responses are possible. Pain elicited between 0 and 30 degrees is typically focal to the lumbar region and attributed to the ipsilateral hip joint, either sacroiliac joint, or lumbopelvic soft tissues as the dura, nerve roots, and associated structures have not yet been tensioned. Pain radiating down the leg, elicited between 30 and 70 degrees and extending beyond the knee, may implicate some form of dural mobility compromise. This may include disc herniation, stenotic and osteophytic processes, tumor or hematoma, or other mechanical or chemical irritation of the dura or nerve root(s). Approximately 95% of patients with a proven disc herniation report radicular symptoms on straight-leg raising (high sensitivity), but it is also positive in 80%–90% of patients without any form of disc protrusion at surgery (low specificity).[76] Therefore, other pain generators, such as those mentioned earlier in this paragraph, must be considered and other discerning findings utilized in order to better differentiate the diagnosis.

A positive response in between 30 and 70 degrees coupled with resistance to further elevation is termed Lasegue's sign. Pain elicited beyond 70 degrees may stem from the sacroiliac joints, posterior thigh, or paraspinal musculature. The examiner should note if leg raising provokes ipsilateral or contralateral symptoms as well as if there is asymmetry of movement.

Modified SLR Tests

There are several modifications to the SLR that may increase the test's specificity,[77] help differentiate nerve involvement from other pathology, or simply provide options in patient positioning. Several of these variations involve the application of increased neural and dural tissue tension, using levers such as the head, torso, foot, and great toe. As with the physical examination in general, these more invasive tests should be performed only if less invasive tests are not sufficiently sensitive and specific.

The well-leg raising test, also referred to as the crossed leg raising test, is simply an SLR performed on the unaffected side. A positive response suggests pathology involving the central to medial posterior aspect of the intervertebral disc. In contrast to the SLR, crossed straight-leg raising is less sensitive but much more specific for disc herniation.[78–82] The interrater reliability of this test is moderate and the sensitivity in patients with lumbar spinal stenosis is about 50%.[83]

Braggard's test begins as with an SLR. At the point of pain, the leg is lowered approximately 5 degrees or until the pain response ceases and the foot is dorsiflexed. A return of leg pain indicates nerve root involvement. Fajersztajn's test is merely Braggard's test performed on the uninvolved side. In the Bowstring test, also referred to as the Cram test or popliteal pressure test, the examiner performs an SLR. At the point of pain, the patient's elevated thigh is stabilized and his or her leg is lowered to rest on the examiner's shoulder. Tension is applied to the popliteal fossa in an attempt to traction the sciatic nerve. While this test was designed for use on patients with radicular symptoms, it is difficult to perform if the initial point of pain is elicited at 30–40 degrees, as a clinician would have difficulty maneuvering in the small arc of space between the patient's extremity and the table.

In Lasegue's test, the examiner performs an SLR. At the point of pain the knee is flexed to decrease tension and continued hip flexion is attempted. A positive response is one of radicular pain during the SLR but decreased pain following knee flexion with continued hip flexion. Kernig's test is useful for patients who have difficulty achieving a completely supine position. With the patient recumbent and the thigh and knee each flexed to 90 degree, the knee is then extended upward. Radicular pain, resistance to further extension of the knee (Lasegue's sign), or contraction of the hamstring muscles is considered a positive response. Lindner's test (Fig. 12–2) is the most aggressive of the supine tension tests. In this test, the examiner passively flexes the patient's chin to his or her chest and then raises the straightened leg. An attempt by the patient to decrease neural tension by flexing both thighs and knees in an effort to prevent pain is considered a positive Brudzinski's sign. The presence of meningeal irritation or infection will also result in a positive Lindner's test and Brudzinski's sign.

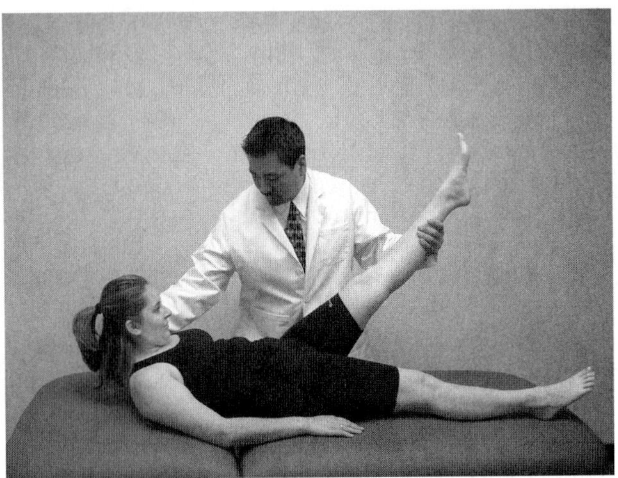

FIGURE 12–2. Lindner's test. More invasive than the SLR, this test will also provoke meningeal irritation in the presence of viral or bacterial meningitis.

Seated Tests

There are also variations of the SLR that may be performed with the patient in a seated position. Seated tests add an inherent element of axial compression in addition to tractioning potentially irritable structures. For this reason, these tests may be more provocative than their supine or prone counterparts. Bechterew's test is performed by asking the seated patient to actively extend his or her uninvolved leg, to lower that leg, and then subsequently extend the involved leg. If symptoms are not produced, the patient is asked to raise both legs simultaneously. A positive finding includes radicular pain below the knee, inability to attain full knee extension, leaning backward and bracing oneself on the table (tripod sign), or any combination thereof. The sciatic tension test, also referred to as the Deyerle and May test, reproduces the mechanics of the bowstring test in a seated position. The involved extremity is extended to the point of pain, and then lowered slightly to decrease pain. The clinician supports the patient's leg between his or her knees and then applies finger pressure to the popliteal fossa in an attempt to tension the sciatic nerve.

The sitting root test (Fig. 12–3) is similar to Lindner's test. With the patient seated and his or her neck flexed to the chest, the clinician places one hand on the patient's distal thigh to prevent knee flexion and uses the other hand to extend the lower leg. Any of the typical SLR responses is considered a positive finding. If

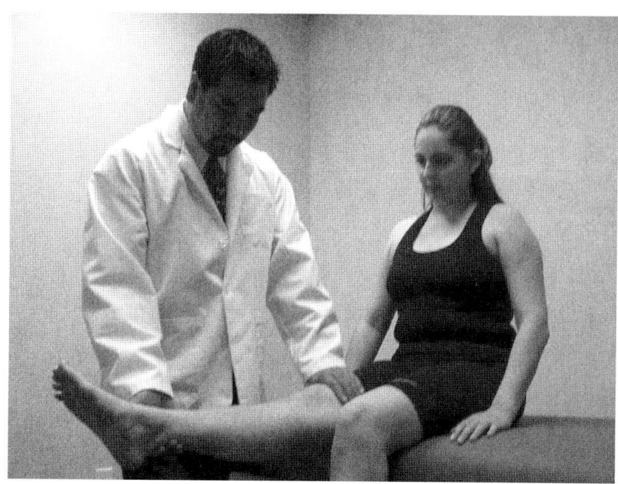

FIGURE 12–3. Sitting root test. This test is particularly appropriate for acute patients who demonstrate difficulty transitioning from a seated position to either prone or supine position.

the test is negative, the clinician may increase tension placed on neural elements by adding trunk flexion. This aggressive maneuver developed by Maitland is known as the slump test.[84]

Kemp's test (Fig. 12–4) uses the patient's trunk both as a lever to induce tension and as a compressive force. The test may be performed with the patient in either the seated or standing position. With the patient seated and arms crossed over the chest, the examiner uses one hand to stabilize the patient's lumbosacral region on the side to be tested and the other arm to control the patient's upper body movement. The patient is passively directed into flexion, rotation, lateral flexion, and finally extension. Depending on the patient's response, axial compression may be applied in the fully extended and rotated position to increase stress on the posterior joints. Radiating pain down the leg provoked anywhere along the arc of movement should be noted and the test should be discontinued at that point. Often, patients will report dull or achy pain stemming from the lumbar spine that may be due to facet or extraspinal soft tissue irritation.

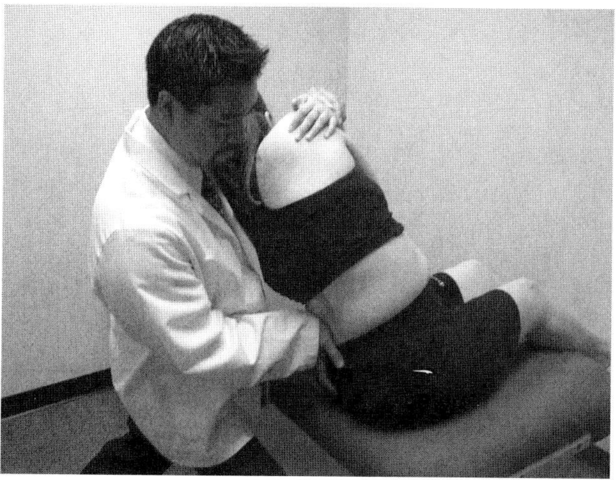

FIGURE 12–4. Seated Kemp's test. This maneuver may elicit symptoms from a variety of structures. As with all testing procedures, make sure to ask the appropriate follow-up questions to determine type and origin of pain.

The standing version of Kemp's test is performed by asking the patient to place the back of his or her hand on the ipsilateral gluteal region and then slide the hand distally down the posterior thigh. Axial compression may be applied by pressing downward on the patient's shoulders. For clinicians desiring either more control over patient positioning or less muscle activation, the seated version of Kemp's test may be preferable.

Clinical Pearl: Seated tests add an inherent element of axial compression in addition to tractioning potentially irritable structures. For this reason, these tests may be more provocative than their supine or prone counterparts.

Prone and Side-Lying Tests

Most of the tension tests performed in prone or side-lying positions are designed to stress the superior lumbar nerve roots and femoral nerve. However, patients with pathology affecting the lower roots may also demonstrate a positive reaction to these procedures. The clinician should pay particular attention to the distribution of symptoms. As with the SLR and its alternates, these tests do not demonstrate a high degree of specificity.

In Ely's test, the examiner passively flexes the patient's knee, approximating the heel to the ipsilateral buttock. A shortened rectus femoris muscle or pathology within the knee joint may hinder the performance of this test. The prone nnee bending test, also known as Nachlas test (Fig. 12–5), mimics Ely's test but adds pelvic stabilization via contact over the ipsilateral ilium to prevent lumbar extension. The femoral nerve traction test (Fig. 12–6) requires some coordination on the clinician's part. With the patient side-lying and the involved side up, the clinician stands behind the patient and stabilizes the pelvis with one hand while extending the hip 15 degrees. If leg symptoms are not provoked, the clinician then flexes the leg toward the ipsilateral buttock.

Standing Tests

If the following test is performed, it is usually during the assessment of active ranges of motion. As the patient attempts to flex forward at the waist and touch the toes, the knee on the affected side bends forward to relieve tension placed on the sciatic nerve. This is termed Neri's Bowing sign. If a patient exhibits this

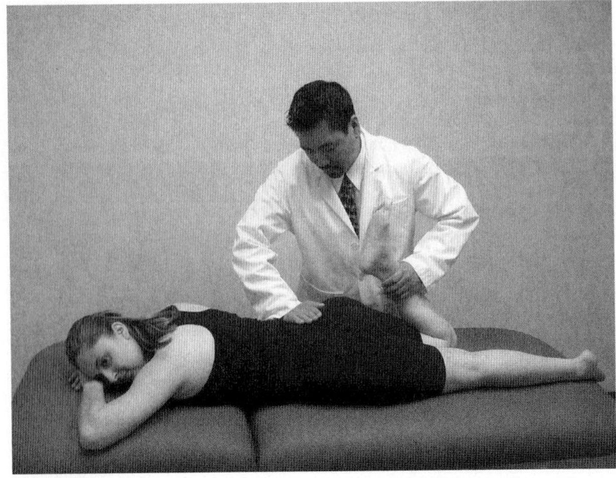

FIGURE 12–5. Prone knee bending test. The patient's pelvis should be braced with the clinician's hand to reduce the risk of symptoms arising from lumbar extension.

sign, Lewin's test is performed by passively extending the knee with the patient in the forward flexed position. The reproduction of radicular pain is considered a positive finding.

Intrathecal Pressure Tests

Valsalva's maneuver attempts to elicit a radicular pain response by forcefully increasing intra-abdominal pressure, which directly compresses the thecal sac and structures within. The maneuver consists of asking the patient to hold his or her breath and bear down as in moving the bowels or when attempting to inflate a resistant balloon. Often, patients with extraspinal complaints such as sprains and strains will report pain with this maneuver. The location, intensity, and quality of pain should be noted but only pain of a radicular nature is considered truly positive.

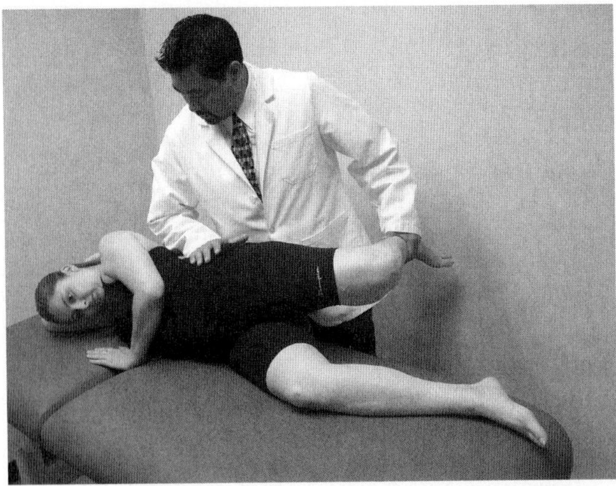

FIGURE 12–6. Femoral nerve traction test. It is important to keep the patient's pelvis stabilized perpendicular to the table while extending the thigh and leg.

Milgram's test is as much an assessment of abdominal muscle strength as it is intrathecal irritability. With legs fully extended, the supine patient is asked to actively raise both feet approximately 2 in off the table and maintain this position for at least 10 seconds and up to 30 seconds. The inability to perform this test owing to muscle weakness is not considered a positive finding within the context of this test, but should nevertheless still be charted.

Miscellaneous Tests

If the patient's history is noncontributory in differentiating between vascular intermittent claudication, including Leriche's syndrome (stenosis or occlusion at the junction of the abdominal aorta and the common iliac arteries), and neurogenic claudication, there are several tests that attempt to discriminate between the two conditions. Such tests include Deweese's test, claudication test, and the stoop test. In Deweese's test, the clinician first palpates the dorsalis pedis or posterior tibial pulse bilaterally to establish vascular integrity and symmetry. The clinician then releases the patient's leg and the patient is instructed to perform some form of cardiovascular exercise appropriate to the patient and setting until the symptoms are reproduced. The clinician then reassesses the pulses bilaterally to determine if a diminution of strength exists, indicating arterial insufficiency. Claudication test[85] is similar to the Deweese's test and may be used for patients who demonstrate the ability to walk at a rate of 2 steps per second and whose pain presents in less than 1 minute following exercise. This test may be modified for use as an outcome measure with increases in speed and time monitored as treatment objectives. Performance of the test consists of having the patient walk at a rate of 120 steps per minute for 60 seconds, either on a treadmill or along a long corridor. The clinician notes the location of pain and the time elapsed between the start of the test and the onset of leg cramping. Should claudication symptoms occur in less than 60 seconds, chronic arterial occlusion is probable. For patients complaining of either unilateral or bilateral pain in the buttock, thigh, leg, or foot after walking a certain distance or length of time, the stoop test may be used to differentiate between arterial and neurogenic claudication. The clinician asks the patient to walk around the office or on a treadmill until the symptoms begin. Once symptoms are provoked, the patient is instructed to flex forward from the trunk and continue walking. If symptoms persist, the patient is instructed to rest. Relief of symptoms with rest but not with trunk flexion indicates possible arterial claudication. If the symptoms are relieved with trunk flexion, neurogenic claudication (central canal stenosis) is indicated. The second part of this test can be completed using a stationary bicycle that induces trunk flexion during exercise.

Regional Examinations

Abdomen In a patient with hypertension, asymmetrical or decreased distal pulse strengths, or visual signs suggestive of arterial compromise such as pallid skin color, coldness, or trophic changes or the lower extremities, auscultate for bruits over the abdomen, femoral triangle, anteromedial thigh, and popliteal fossa in the lower extremities. The abdominal aorta may be palpated in the supine patient by pressing the medial edge of each hand, held in knife-like fashion, into the abdomen on either side of the vessel. The examiner should begin with a wide contact of 10 cm, moving the hands closer together until the pulse is distinguished. He or she should then assess the length of the abdominal aorta from its proximal end at the rib margin to its approximately at the level of L3-4. The approximate distance between the hands and the presence of pain on palpation should be noted. Keeping the patient's knees flexed eases tension on the abdominal muscles and facilitates palpation. However, the lumbar lordosis is also reduced with the knees flexed, so this factor should be taken into account.

Abdominal aneurysms are most common in males over 50 years of age. Greater than 90% of abdominal aneurysms occur distal to the renal arteries.[86] Patients may describe a mild to severe pain in the mid-abdominal or lower back region, becoming lancinating or knife-like upon rupture. However, most patients may be completely asymptomatic. The mortality rate following acute rupture is approximately 80%–90% with 25%–50% of these patients expiring before they reach the hospital.[86] Listed below are the generally accepted guidelines for addressing abdominal aneurysms when visualized on plain film radiography:

2 cm = normal
4 cm = aneurysm
5–6 cm = referral to a vascular surgeon
7 cm = impending rupture/death (emergency situation)

Thoracic Spine While pathology originating in the thoracic spine region does not commonly present as lower back pain, the competent practitioner will dutifully consider sources proximal and distal to the area of chief complaint. Useful examination procedures typically include evaluation of overall thoracolumbar motion, spinal percussion in cases of suspected fracture, determination of the presence and degree of scoliotic curve, and assessment of increased or decreased kyphosis. In the case of these last two evaluations, it is common to find compensation and concomitant symptoms occurring in the lumbar spine as a result of structural changes above.

Pelvis/Hip Conditions affecting the pelvis and hip may refer pain to the lumbar spine, posterior and lateral gluteal region, and posterior thigh. Likewise, lumbar spine pathology is often associated with symptoms referred to distal sites. Therefore, it is important to screen the pelvis and hip joints as well as the gluteal and thigh muscles for possible pathology. Orthopedically, there are several tests used to determine dysfunction in these areas. The clinician should always confirm whether a positive response to any of the test described below produces symptoms similar to the patient's chief complaint.

Beginning with the sacroiliac joint, the clinician should assess palpatory tenderness along the joint line and distally at the sacral notch. Little motion occurs at this joint and it cannot be measured with either a goniometer or an inclinometer. The clinician must rely on subjective assessments such as Gillet's test, assessing the overtake phenomenon and joint play evaluation. It is important to note that many authors find sacroiliac joint assessment frustrating owing to low inter-examiner reliability.[87–91] To perform Gillet's test, the examiner palpates the posterior superior iliac spine (PSIS) and the spinous process of L5 while the patient slowly raises one leg keeping the knee flexed. The examiner notes the amount of translation between thumb contacts and then asks the patient to raise the opposite leg in similar fashion. The examiner then switches the PSIS contact to the opposite side, maintaining the spinous process contact at L5 and the patient raises each leg in turn. The same procedure is followed with thumb contacts on the S1, S2, and S3 spinous processes. In each instance, the lateral thumb contact is made level to the spinous process contact. Movement is assessed at each point bilaterally.[92] Lewit and Rosina suggested a variation of this maneuver, known as the *spine sign*.[93] This is performed by allowing the hip to drop rather than asking the patient to raise the leg, thereby requiring decreased pelvic muscle contraction and stabilization. Decreased stabilization strategy allows the sacroiliac joint to be more consistently assessed. More about this will be discussed in the next chapter.[93]

To assess the overtake phenomenon, the clinician palpates each PSIS while the patient bends forward at the waist. The PSIS on the side of restriction should move further in a cranial direction than does the normal side.[94] To assess joint play, the examiner should load the joint with the patient in a prone position.

Orthopedically, the clinician can determine sacroiliac irritability by using a variety of tests. Gaenslen's test is performed with the patient supine. The clinician positions the patient at the edge of the table with the buttock over the edge. The patient is instructed to lower the thigh and leg off the side of the table while grasping the flexed knee of the opposite leg. The clinician may then apply overpressure to either the lowered thigh, the flexed knee, or to both contacts to stress the sacroiliac joint. Yeoman's test is performed with the patient prone. The clinician contacts the sacrum to stabilize against accessory lumbosacral movement, grasps the patient's bent knee, and then hyperextends the thigh off the table. Iliac compression is easiest to perform with the patient side-lying. The clinician uses either a hand or forearm contact over the ilium and applies pressure to stress the joint closest to the clinician's contact.

Owing to the infrequent presentation of coccygeal involvement in the general practitioner's office, some clinicians may fall into the habit of overlooking this region during the examination. And while pain resulting from coccygeal pathology seems to remain local to the area, there are conditions in which symptoms may refer to the low back region. The clinician should inspect the region for surface lesions, particularly the presence of pilonidal cysts or a potentially more serious sinus. The clinician should palpate the superficial tissues overlying the coccyx for tenderness as well as apply external traction in both cephalad and caudal directions to assess the quality of movement that exists at the sacrococcygeal junction. Keep in mind that the multifidus as well as the pelvic floor muscles may refer pain to the coccygeal region.[95] In appropriate cases, internal palpation of the coccyx and pelvic floor muscles may be achieved via access through the anal opening.

The clinician should also screen the more assessment-friendly hip joint, to include palpation of the trochanter, active and passive ranges of motion, resisted ranges of motion if indicated, performance of combined hip *f*lexion, *ab*duction, *e*xternal *r*otation, and *e*xtension, commonly referred to as Patrick's test, Patrick's Fabere test and the Sign of 4, and a weight-bearing peripheral joint clearance test (deep knee squat). If the clinician suspects muscle involvement, either from the iliopsoas, tensor fascia lata, iliotibial band, or the long muscles of the thigh, appropriate testing should follow, such as modified Thomas test, Ober's and modified Ober's tests, and Noble compression test of the iliotibial band.

Another source of lumbar pain, often overlooked and frequently inappropriately assessed, results from leg length asymmetry or insufficiency. In addition to discomfort, discrepancies of 1 cm or greater may result in visual signs of iliac crest unleveling and functional scoliosis. The presence of these findings warrants further therapeutic investigation.

Functional Capacity Testing

If asked, most patients would not place a great deal of value on the ability to achieve 80–90 degrees of pain-free hip flexion during the performance of SLR or give considerable thought to whether or not passive great toe dorsiflexion causes an increase in their back pain. Many of the tests performed on our patients provide valuable information that never translates to the everyday world in which the patient lives. Therein lies the impetus for the development of functional capacity testing. This paradigm of assessment provides a wealth of information regarding the soundness of the structures tested, the ability of the patient to perform activities of daily living and contribute appropriately to his or her own rehabilitation, and the propensity for future dysfunction in the absence of therapeutic intervention. The patient is intimately involved in this type of testing, can easily relate to its performance, and understand the implications of any results.

Given the myriad activities that involve the lumbar spine, there are relatively few categories of functional tests available. In general, muscle strength is assessed by determining static endurance, repetitive loading capacity and maximal force output of the lumbar extensor muscles.[96,97] The same assessments of the abdominal muscles may be determined. The specific performance of these tests depends on the devices available, with MedEx® machines providing the more quantitative data. Alternatively, Kraus–Weber tests can be used to determine the degree of decompensation.[98] Patients are required to perform one sit-up, one hook lying sit-up, a 30-degree leg lift in the supine position for 10 seconds, a prone torso lift for 10 seconds, a prone leg lift for 10 seconds, and one slow toe touch from the standing position. Inability to perform two or more of these functions indicates the probability of deconditioning.

Simmonds and colleagues found a timed 50 foot walk, loaded reach test from the standing position, repeated sit-to-stand and repeated trunk flexion clinically usefulness assessments of physical performance.[99] Other functional assessment tools include the Functional Capacity Evaluation,[100] the Functional Status test,[101] and the Physical Performance test.[102] More information regarding functional capacity testing is covered in both Chapters 14 and 35.

Nonorganic Signs

In the quest for a clear diagnosis, inconsistencies occurring during the history and examination that confound this clinical goal can indeed be disconcerting. For example, the patient who twists an ankle and subsequently complains of severe headaches will incite most clinicians to question the patient's credibility because of a seemingly inconsistent causal relationship. In a similar fashion, the patient who claims excruciating ipsilateral, radicular-type leg pain during the supine SLR maneuver who then makes no note of any discomfort during a seated SLR maneuver reasonably must be questioned for reliability. Such inconsistencies in subjective complaints and objective findings, which seem to be lacking in any somatic or organic base, have become known as *nonorganic* findings. For many clinicians, the assessment of nonorganic signs in a patient with physical complaints compounded by psychosocial factors provides an organized means to better define the inconsistencies involved. The tests themselves are fairly straightforward in their application. Additionally, interpretation of the results is straightforward, as positive findings simply indicate the presence of processes that appropriately belong, to some degree, in the biopsychosocial category. Nonorganic findings do not necessarily imply a nonexistent or fictitious condition. The astute clinician acknowledges that each patient carries with them more than just the sum of their physical parts.

Clinical Pearl: Nonorganic findings do not necessarily imply a nonexistent or fictitious condition. The astute clinician acknowledges that each patient carries with them more than just the sum of their physical parts.

Several questionnaires, including the Minnesota Multiphasic Personality Inventory,[103] the Beck Depression Inventory,[104] and the Pain Drawing,[105] are designed to evaluate the degree of psychological dysfunction that may compound the evaluation of patients with low back pain. In addition to recording initial levels of psychological dysfunction, they can also be used to monitor progress and contribute to determining overall prognosis. Further discussion of these and other outcome measures appears in Chapter 14, while biopsychosocial issues and assessment is addressed in Chapter 19.

Presented in 1961, Johnson's signs of hysterical or malingering weakness[106] suggest five characteristics that indicate psychological overlay. They are slowed motions; exaggeration; inconsistency; ratchety response to muscle testing; and either "la belle indifference" for hysterical weakness or the appearance of great worry, concern, or anger for malingering. Keefe and Block developed a similar list of overt pain behavior signs that includes guarded movement, bracing, rubbing the injured area, grimacing, and sighing.[107] Keeping these types of indicators in mind, Waddell et al. developed a series of tests designed to elicit nonorganic responses from patients in which psychosocial factors are present.[108] Following their initial presentation, Waddell's tests were often misused to label patients as malingerers. As stated earlier, it is important not to overinterpret positive nonorganic findings, as these tests cannot differentiate between patients who respond inappropriately owing to test anxiety, fear of pain, lack of coping skills, or learned pain behaviors from those with secondary gain issues.[109] When performing these tests, the clinician should keep in mind the subjective nature of pain and the reality that it is a rare patient who does not interact on a psychological level with their own physiological dysfunction.

There are four categories of assessments represented by Waddell's test for nonorganic physical signs, each with corresponding inappropriate responses, also known as Waddell signs. This is addressed in detail in Chapter 14. While tenderness, simulation, distraction, and regional disturbances are assessed during various portions of the physical examination, overreaction can be noted during both the history and physical examination (see Table 12–5).

Three or more inappropriate responses suggest the presence of confounding psychosocial or socioeconomic factors.

Hoover's sign is another often used predictor of nonorganic involvement. With the patient supine, the clinician places his or her hands underneath the patient's heels. The patient is then instructed to raise first one leg, lower it, and then raise the other leg several inches off the table. Lack of a downward force produced by the stabilizing (i.e., nonelevated) leg is termed Hoover's sign. In the presence of paralysis,

TABLE 12–5. Waddell's Test for Nonorganic Physical Signs[108]

Test	Inappropriate Response
Tenderness	Superficial, nonanatomical to light touch
Simulation	
Axial loading	Axial loading on standing patient's skull produces low back pain
Rotation	Passive, simultaneous rotation of shoulders and pelvis produces low back pain
Distraction	Discrepancy between findings on supine and seated straight-leg raising
Regional disturbances	
Weakness	Giving way (cogwheel) weakness
Sensory	Nondermatomal sensory loss
Overreaction	Disproportionate facial expression, verbalization, or tremor during examination

patients typically accentuate the downward pressure in an attempt to lift the paretic limb.[110]

Record Keeping

Charting a patient's information accurately and thoroughly is often the last subject that a busy health-care provider wishes to discuss. It can be a time-consuming endeavor, frequently left for later and then forgotten. Yet without this information, the patient's experience within the health-care setting is diminished. The ability to render a correct diagnosis, predict outcomes, and moderate a treatment plan to meet the patient's changing capabilities all depend on recording information so that it is not lost from the clinician's overtaxed memory.

Clinical Pearl: Avoid using (+) and (−) notations with reference to physical examination tests. A description of the patient's response to provocative testing is significantly more valuable to the diagnostic process.

While indicating that a test result is simply positive or negative is quick to write in the patient's chart and review later, it limits the clinical picture significantly. Positive SLR says something different from an SLR producing slight low back pain at 90 degrees, which indicates yet another difference from an SLR that produces radiating pain to the 5th toe at 40 degrees. The same holds true for a negative finding. For instance, one clinician may consider an SLR negative in the absence of root (radicular) findings, while another may consider it positive because it provoked back pain. Without clarifying the result, the result may provide more clinical confusion than was present preceding the test. Avoid using (+) and (−) notations with reference to physical examination tests. A description of the patient's response to provocative testing is significantly more valuable to the diagnostic process.

There are a variety of tools to assist the practitioner. Preprinted questionnaires and examination forms are useful provided they are filled out correctly and completely. These tools can be great assets to streamline the history and physical examination. The clinician should take the time to develop a set of core examination procedures, with associated secondary and tertiary tests used to either confirm or differentiate diagnoses, for the most common patient presentations.

Tape recorders reduce the amount of time spent taking notes in the examination room but this may be viewed negatively by many patients. While inappropriate for the initial examination because of the extent of information elicited, the clinician may choose to spend a few moments after a treatment encounter dictating notes. Hand-held electronic devices are a new addition to the charting experience. These devices allow information to be transmitted to a computer file but it can also be lost or deleted. Additionally, it can take more time to input data than when written in a chart. Whatever method is chosen, the clinician should establish a routine system of note-taking that is easily followed and understood by support personnel and third-party reviewers.

SUMMARY

1. Eliciting the history from a patient with a low back syndrome should progress in a logical fashion, beginning with screening questions to determine the presence of potentially serious conditions ("red flags"). In the absence of these pathologies, the clinician can move toward more common and less destructive possibilities.
2. By far the most common category of low back complaint is non-specific back pain.
3. While the majority of assessments used to differentiate between possible diagnoses have either not been critically assessed or lack inter-examiner, and in some cases, intra-examiner reliability, the clinician must make an effort to be as consistent as possible in the performance of each procedure.
4. Clinicians should avoid the tendency to hold steadfast to one diagnosis based on the outcome of one or two tests, as this is clinically presumptions.
5. The patient's global presentation, including data elicited from the history and impressions from the physical and functional examination, should culminate into a complete picture of the individual.
6. The following chapter will address the functional examination, another portion of the assessment that can provide significant insight into the patient's condition. Along with the information contained in this chapter, the next chapter provides a solid base for appropriate ensuing clinical strategies, including further diagnostic testing, treatment options, or referral to another clinician.

REFERENCES

1. White AA III, Gordon SL. Synopsis: Workshop on idiopathic low-back pain. *Spine* 1982;7:141–149.
2. Deyo RA, Weinstein JN. Low back pain. *N Engl J Med* 2001;344:363–370.
3. Bigos S, Bowyer O, Braen G, et al. Acute low back problems in adults. Clinical Practice Guideline No. 14. Rockville, MD: Agency for Health Care Policy and Research, Public Health Service, US Department of Health and Human Services, December 1994.
4. Deyo RA, Rainville J, Kent DL. What can the history and physical examination tell us about low back pain? *JAMA* 1992;268:760–765.

5. DeyoRA, Diehl AK. Cancer as a cause of back pain; frequency, clinical presentation, and diagnostic strategies. *J. Gen Intern Med* 1988;3:230–238.
6. Stith JS, Sahrmann SA, Dixon KK, Norton BJ. Curriculum to prepare diagnosticians in physical therapy. *J Phys Ther Educ* 1995;9:50.
7. Lew DP, Waldvogel FA. Osteomyelitis. *N Engl J Med* 1997;336:999–1007.
8. Reily B. *Practical trategies in outpatient medicine.* Philadelphia: WB Saunders, 1991:904–909.
9. Bouchier IAD, Ellis H, Fleming PR. *French's index of differential diagnosis*, 13th ed. Oxford: Butterworth Heinmann, 1996:44–45.
10. Walsh WM, Mellion MB. The team physician. In: DeLee JC, Drez D Jr, eds. *Orthopaedic sports medicine: Principles and practice.* Philadelphia: WB Saunders, 1994:346–355.
11. Murtagh J. Low back pain. *Aust Fam Phys* 1991;20:320–323.
12. Mackenzie I. *Tenderness of the spine.* In: Bouchier IAD, Ellis H, Fleming PR, ed. *French's index of differential diagnosis*, 12th ed. Oxford: Butterworth, 1996:72–80.
13. Borenstein DG, Wiesel SW, Boden SD. *Low back pain. Medical diagnosis and comprehensive management.* Philadelphia: WB Saunders, 1995:42–46.
14. Magee DJ. *Orthopedic physical assessment*, 4th ed. Philadelphia: WB Saunders, 2002:473–479.
15. Dambro MR. *Griffith's 5 minute clinical consult.* Baltimore: Williams & Wilkins, 1997.
16. Fantone JC, Ward PA. Inflammation. In: Rubin E, Farber JL, eds. *Pathology*, 2nd ed. Philadelphia: JB Lippincott, 1995:24–46.
17. Kumar V, Cotran RS, Robbins SL. *Basic pathology*, 6th ed. Philadelphia: WB Saunders, 1992:39.
18. van der Meulen JCH. Present state of knowledge and processes of healing in collagen structures. *Int J Sports Med* 1982;3:4–8.
19. Nachemson AL, Andersson GB. Classification of low-back pain. *Scand J Work Environ Health* 1982;8(2):134–136.
20. Ciol MA, Deyo RA, Kreuter W, Bigos SJ. Characteristics in Medicare beneficiaries associated with reoperation after lumbar spine surgery. *Spine* 1994;19:1329–1334.
21. Frymoyer J. Back pain and sciatica. *N Engl J Med* 1998;318:291–300.
22. Praemer A, Furner S, Rice DP. *Musculoskeletal conditions in the United States.* Chicago: American Academy of Orthopaedic Surgeons, 1999:24–26.
23. Samiy AH, Douglas RG Jr, Barondess JA. *Textbook of diagnostic medicine.* Philadelphia: Lea & Febiger, 1987: 608–637.
24. Dains JE, Ciofu Baumann L, Scheibel P. *Advanced health assessment and clinical diagnosis in primary care*, 2nd ed. St. Louis: Mosby-Year Book,Inc., 2003:357–369.
25. Wigh R. The thoracolumbar and lumbosacral transitional junctions. *Spine* 1980;5:215–222.
26. Jinkins JR. The pathoanatomic basis of somatic and autonomic syndromes originating in the lumbosacral spine. *Neuroimaging Clin North Am* 1993;3:443–463.
27. Johnson PH, ed. *Physical therapist's clinical companion.* Springhouse, PA: Springhouse Corp., 2000:10–11.
28. Greenberger NJ, Hinthorn DR. *History taking and physical examination: Essentials and clinical correlates.* St. Louis: Mosby-Year Book, Inc., 1993:203.
29. Hsieh CY, Hong CZ, Adams AH, et al. Interexaminer reliability of the palpation of trigger points in the trunk and lower limb muscles. *Arch Phys Med Rehabil* 2000;81(3):258–264.
30. Souza TA. *Differential diagnosis and management for the chiropractor: Protocols and algorithms*, 2nd ed. Gaithersburg, MD: Aspen Publishers, 2001:271.
31. Swartz MH. *Textbook of physical diagnosis: History and examination.* Philadelphia: WB Saunders, 1994:279.
32. Carter MC. A reliable sign of fractures of the hip or pelvis. *N Engl J Med* 1981;305(20):1220.
33. Siffert RS, Kaufman JJ. Acoustic assessment of fracture healing. Capabilities and limitations of "a lost art." *Am J Orthop* 1996;25(9):614–618.
34. Adams SL, Yarnold PR. Clinical use of the patellar-pubic percussion sign in hip trauma. *Am J Emerg Med* 1997;15:173–175.
35. File P, Wood JP, Kreplick LW. Diagnosis of hip fracture by the auscultatory percussion technique. *Am J Emerg Med* 1998;16:173–176.
36. Cipriano JJ. *Photographic manual of regional orthopedic and neurological tests*, 2nd ed. Baltimore: Williams & Wilkins, 1991:55.
37. *Joint motion: Method of measuring and recording.* Chicago: American Academy of Orthopaedic Surgeons, 1965.
38. Thurber P. *Evaluation of industrial disability*, 2nd ed. New York: Oxford University Press, 1960.
39. Gerhardt JJ, Russe OA.*International SFTR method of measuring and recording joint motion.* Bern, Germany: Huber, 1975.
40. White AA, Panjabi MM. *Clinical biomechanics of the spine*, 2nd ed. Philadelphia: JB Lippincott, 1990:86–118.
41. Bell BD, Hoshizaki TB. Relationships of age and sex with range of motion of seventeen joint actions in humans. *Can J Appl Sports Sci* 1981;6:202.
42. Clarke CR, Bonfiglio M. *Orthopedics: Essentials of diagnosis and treatment.* New York: Churchill Livingstone, 1994:20–21.
43. Rothstein JM. *Measurement in physical therapy.* New York: Churchill Livingstone, 1985:105.
44. Defibaugh JJ. Measurement of head motion. *J Am Phys Ther Assoc* 1964;44:157.
45. Robson P. A method to reduce the variable error in joint range measurement. *Ann Phys Med* 1966;8: 262.
46. Esch D, Lepley M. *Evaluation of joint motion: Methods of measurement and recording.* Minneapolis: University of Minnesota Press, 1974:3–13.
47. Nitschke JE, Nattrass CL, Disler PB, et al. Reliability of the American Medical Association Guides' model for measuring spinal range of motion. *Spine* 1999;24(3):262–268.

48. Schenker WW. Improved method of joint motion measurement. *N Y J Med* 1956;56:539.
49. Karpovich PV, Karpovich GP. Electrogoniometer. A new device for study of joints in action. *Fed Proc* 1959;18:79.
50. Silver D. Measurement of the range of motion in joints. *J Bone Joint Surg* 1923;21:569.
51. Moore ML. The measurement of joint motion. Part II. The technic of goniometry. *Phys Ther Rev* 1949;29:256.
52. Geraci MC, Alleva JT. *Examination of the spine and its functional kinetic chain.* In: Cole AJ, Herring SA, eds. *The low back pain handbook: A practical guide for the primary care clinician*. Philadelphia: Hanley & Belfus, Inc., 1997:49.
53. Braddom RL. Perils and pointers in the evaluation and management of back pain. *Semin Neurol* 1998;18(2):197–210.
54. Gilroy J. *Basic neurology*, 2nd ed. New York: McGraw-Hill, 1990:42–45.
55. Gilman S, Winans Newman S. *Manter and Gatz's essentials of clinical neuroanatomy and neurophysiology*, 8th ed. Philadelphia: FA Davis Co., 1992:84–95.
56. Hagbarth KE, Wallen G, Burke D, Lofstedt L. Effects of the Jendrassik maneuver on muscle spindle activity in man. *J Neurol Neurosurg Psych* 1975;38:1143–1153.
57. Stam J, Tan KM. Tendon reflex variability and method of stimulation. *Electroencephalogr Clin Neurophysiol* 1987;67(5):463–467.
58. Stam J, van Crevel H. Reliability of the clinical and electromyographic examination of tendon reflexes. *J Neurol* 1990;237(7):427–431.
59. Uysal H, Mogyoros I, Burke D. Reproducibility of tendon jerk reflexes during a voluntary contraction. *Clin Neurophysiol* 1999;110(8):1481–1487.
60. Marshall GL, Little JW. Deep tendon reflexes: A study of quantitative methods. *J Spinal Cord Med* 2002;25(2):94–99.
61. Carel RS, Korczyn AD, Hochberg Y. Age and sex dependency of the Achilles tendon reflex. *Am J Med Sci* 1979;278(1):57–63.
62. Koceja DM. Influence of quadricept conditioning on soleus motoneuron excitability in young and old adults. *Med Sci Sports Exerc* 1993;25(2):245–250.
63. Schmeling WT, Forster HV, Hosko MJ. Effect of sojourn at 3200-m altitude on spinal reflexes in young adult males. *Aviat Space Environ Med* 1977;48(11): 1039–1045.
64. Ballantyne GH, Crozson MS. The effect of exercise, thyroid status and insulin-induced hypoglycaemia on the Achilles tendon reflex time in man. *Eur J Appl Physiol Occup Physiol* 1981;46(1):77–83.
65. Chapman CE, Sullivan SJ, Pompura J, Arsenault AB. Changes in hip position modulate soleus H-reflex excitability in man. *Electromyogr Clin Neurophysiol* 1991;31(3):131–143.
66. Weisberg L, Strub RL, Garcia CA. *Essentials of clinical neurology*, 2nd ed. Rockville, MD: Aspen Publications, 1989:26.
67. McCombe PF, Fairbank JCT, Pynsent PB. Reproducibility of physical signs in low-back pain. *Spine* 1989;14:908–918.
68. Beasley WC. Quantitative muscle testing: Principles and applications to research and clinical services. *Arch Phys Med Rehabil* 1961;42:398–425.
69. Lamb RL. Manual muscle testing. In: Rothstein JM, ed. *Measurement in physical therapy*. New York: Churchill Livingstone, 1985:47–54.
70. Hoppenfeld S. *Orthopaedic neurology: A diagnostic guide to neurologic levels*. Philadelphia: JB Lippincott, 1977:65–70.
71. Keim HA, Kirkaldy-Willis WH. Low back pain. In: *Clinical Symposia 39*. New Jersey: Ciba-Geigy Corp., 1987:6–18.
72. Moore KL. *Clinically oriented anatomy*, 3rd ed. Baltimore: Williams & Wilkins, 1992:373–460.
73. Daniels L, Worthingham C. *Muscle testing: Technique of manual examination*, 4th ed. Philadelphia: WB Saunders, 1986:2–4.
74. Sapega AA. Muscle performance evaluation in orthopedic practice. *J Bone Joint Surg Am* 1990;72:1562–1574.
75. Gillette RD. Waddell signs in the evaluation of back pain. *Am Fam Physician* 1999;60:1666.
76. Brody M. Low back pain. *Ann Emerg Med* 1996;27:454–456.
77. Giles LGF, Singer KP. *Clinical anatomy and management of low back pain*. Oxford: Butterworth Heinemann, 1997:347.
78. Spangfort EV. Lumbar disc herniation: A computer aided analysis of 2504 operations. *Acta Orthop Scand Suppl* 1972;142:1–93.
79. Hakelius A, Hindmarsh J. The comparative reliability of preoperative diagnostic methods in lumbar disc surgery. *Acta Orthop Scand* 1972;43:234–238.
80. Hakelius A, Hindmarsh J. The significance of neurological signs and myelographic findings in the diagnosis of lumbar root compression. *Acta Orthop Scand* 1972;43:239–246.
81. Hudgins RW. The crossed straight leg raising test: A diagnostic sign of herniated disc. *J Occup Med* 1979;21:407–408.
82. Shiqing X, Quanzhi Z, Dehao F. Significance of straight-leg-raising test in the diagnosis and clinical evaluation of lower lumbar intervertebral disc protrusion. *J Bone Joint Surg* 1987;69:517.
83. Troyanovich SJ, Harrison DD, Harrison DE. Low back pain and the lumbar intervertebral disc: Clinical considerations for the doctor of chiropractic. *J Manipulative Physiol Ther* 1999;22:96–104.
84. Maitland GD. Negative disc exploration and positive canal signs. *Aust J Physiother* 1979;29:129–134.
85. Evans RC. *Illustrated essentials in orthopedic physical assessment.* St. Louis: Mosby-Year Book, Inc., 1994: 852–855.
86. Tierney LM Jr, McPhee SJ, Papadakis MA, eds. *Current medical diagnosis and treatment*, 36th ed. Norwalk, CT,: Appleton & Lange, 1997:391.
87. Potter NA, Rothstein JM. Intertester reliability for selected clinical tests of the sacroiliac joint. *Phys Ther* 1985;65:1671–1675.
88. Gemmell HA, Jacobson BH. Incidence of sacroiliac joint dysfunction and low back pain in fit college students. *J Manipulative Physiol Ther* 1990;13:63–67.

89. Laslett M, Williams M. The reliability of selected pain provocation tests for sacroiliac joint pathology. *Spine* 1994;19:1243–1249.
90. Meijne W, van Neerbos K, Aufdemkampe G, et al. Intraexaminer and interexaminer reliability of the Gillet test. *J Manipulative Physiol Ther* 1999;22:4–9.
91. Toussaint R, Gawlik CS, Rehder U, Ruther W. Sacroiliac joint diagnostics in the Hamburg Constructions Workers' study. *J Manipulative Physiol Ther* 1999;22:139–143.
92. Dreyfuss P, Dreyer S, Griffen J, et al. Positive sacroiliac screening tests in asymptomatic adults. *Spine* 1994;19:1138–1143.
93. Lewit K, Rosina A. Why yet another diagnostic sign of sacroiliac movement restriction? *J Manipulative Physiol Ther* 1999;22:154–160.
94. Heinking K, Jones JM, Kappler RE. Pelvis and sacrum. In: Ward RC, ed. *Foundations for osteopathic medicine*. Baltimore: Williams & Wilkins, 1997:612–613.
95. Travell JG, Simons DG. *Myofascial pain and dysfunction: The trigger point manual*, Vols. 1 and 2. Baltimore: Williams & Wilkins, 1992:110–127.
96. Moffroid MT. Endurance of trunk muscles in persons with chronic low back pain: Assessment, performance and training. *J Rehabil Res Train* 1997;34:440–447.
97. Moreland J, Finch E, Stratford P, et al. Interrater reliability of six tests of trunk muscle function and endurance. *J Orthop Sports Phys Ther* 1997;26:200–208.
98. Kraus H. *Diagnosis and treatment of muscle pain*. Chicago: Quintessence Publishing, 1988:29–30.
99. Simmonds MJ, Olson SL, Jones S, et al. Psychometric characteristics and clinical usefulness of physical performance tests in patients with low back pain. *Spine* 1998;23:2412–2421.
100. Goldstein TS. *Functional rehabilitation in orthopedics*. Gaithersburg, MD: Aspen Publishers, 1995:199–201.
101. Jette AM. Functional status index: Reliability of a chronic disease evaluation instrument. *Arch Phys Med Rehabil* 1980;61:395–401.
102. Rueben DB, Siu AL. An objective measure of physical function of elderly outpatients. The physical performance test. *J Am Geriatr Soc* 1990;38:1105–1112.
103. Hathaway SR, McKinley JC. *MMPI manual*, Rev ed. Psychological Corp., 1967.
104. Beck AT, Rush AJ, Shaw BF, Emery G. *Cognitive therapy and depression*. New York: Guilford Press, New York, N.Y., 1979:398–399.
105. Ransford HV, Cairns D, Mooney V. The pain drawing as an aid to psychological evaluation of patients with low back pain. *Spine* 1976;1:127.
106. Johnson EW, Worden RE, Burk RD. Diagnosis of hysterical weakness. Scientific exhibit, American Academy of General Practice, Miami Beach, FL, April 17–20, 1961.
107. Keefe FJ, Block AR. Development of an observation method for assessing pain behavior in chronic low back pain patients. *Behav Ther* 1982;13:363–375.
108. Waddell G, McCulloch JA, Kummel E, Venner RM. Nonorganic physical signs in low-back pain. *Spine* 1980;5:117–125.
109. Main CJ, Waddell G. Behavioral responses to examination. A reappraisal of the interpretation of "nonorganic signs." *Spine* 1998;23(21):2367–2371.
110. Post M. *Physical examination of the musculoskeletal system*. Chicago: Year Book Medical Publishers, Inc., 1987:155.

CHAPTER

13

FUNCTIONAL EXAMINATION FOR LOW BACK SYNDROMES

Craig E. Morris, Leon Chaitow, and Vladimir Janda

OUTLINE

OBJECTIVES

1. Provide the reader with the clinical rationale for utilizing the "functional examination" in the assessment of low back syndromes.
2. Describe the locomotor system, including an explanation of its development, mature stage, and decline.
3. Describe stereotypical postural syndromes commonly observed during the functional assessment.
4. Describe the still, upright postural assessment.
5. Describe postural tests associated with the still, upright postural assessment.
6. Describe gait assessment.
7. Describe functional test associated with quit assessment.

8. Describe additional functional in stability tests, including the movement patterns of Janda.
9. Describe the palpatory functional assessment of muscles and joints.
10. Describe how the functional examination can be practically utilized in its clinical application, while warning the reader of avoiding the pitfalls of "clinical presumptuousness."

INTRODUCTION

Low back syndromes comprise a group of multivariate disorders that, alone or in combination, are associated with a significant degree of disability in the industrialized world. These syndromes can be divided into three subgroups: those that cause local (i.e., low back region) symptoms, those that cause symptoms to extend into the pelvis and/or lower extremities, and those that cause both. While the etiology of such syndromes may at times stem from *pathoanatomy*, such as an intervertebral disc herniation compressing an adjacent nerve root, these findings are in reality merely a clinical curiosity in the absence of dysfunction. It is therefore the *pathophysiological sequelae* that alarm the patient that something is amiss. Whether from motor loss, sensory disturbance, altered posture, faulty gait, altered tissue tone, dysesthesia, or pain, significant levels of one or more of these expressions of dysfunction prompt their recipient to seek out the aid of the clinician.

Chapter 5 discussed the coordinated locomotor system, function, emphasizing the concerted program that defines functional lumbopelvic stability, of which much remains to be learned. Despite a poor understanding of the physiological and pathological complexities of such mechanisms, there are nevertheless clusters of findings present that are associated with the dysfunction of low back syndromes.

The previous chapter discussed in detail the physical examination for the lumbopelvic region. It entailed those aspects of assessment that are commonly employed in the clinical setting. It also discussed the strengths and weaknesses of reliability and validity of various aspects of the examination, warning the reader to build their conclusions on a number of findings instead of only on a few.

This chapter will emphasize visual and palpatory assessment skills designed to provide the clinician with the ability to critically appraise and organize locomotor faults in a manner that can establish a clinical basis, or at least supporting information, for the diagnosis of various low back syndromes as well as for the evaluation of change over time. This approach to assessment can be called the *functional examination or assessment* for want of a better term. The skills required to practically integrate this evaluation are among the most challenging in all of health care, requiring years to gain and decades to hone. The depth and breadth of the topic at hand is indeed immense, far exceeding the parameters of this chapter. The reader will be referred to other texts throughout the chapter in order to access greater depth and deeper understanding of the functional examination.

It should be noted that great technical advances are occurring in the posture and gait assessment. Indeed research laboratories continue to produce exciting new insights into locomotor system function, while proving or disproving prior empirical observations and conclusions upon which much of this subject was and is based. What is clear is that whatever the interpretations made in relation to palpation and/or visual observation, for example, during postural or gait analysis, functional evaluation provides evidence of the current degree of adaptation, compensation and/or decompensation of the individual, or the anatomical region.

Finally, it is important to understand that the functional examination is a science-based clinical art. Therefore multivariate factors abound at every turn due in these processes because of the human factor. Artistry, regardless of the form, is a skill that requires practical training. This chapter is designed to provide a didactic framework for the clinical artistry of functional assessment.

Clinical Pearl: While the etiology of such syndromes may at times stem from *pathoanatomy*, such as an intervertebral disc herniation compressing an adjacent nerve root, these findings are in reality merely a clinical curiosity in the absence of dysfunction.

FUNCTIONAL ASSESSMENT: A CLINICAL PARADOX

In an age of increasing emphasis on evidence-based health-care, clinical methods using relatively well-validated and reliable approaches are embraced, while those less so must be met with greater skepticism. As with all other aspects of health care, locomotor system functional assessment must be honestly evaluated to appreciate its true value. Little quality research has been brought forward to demonstrate adequate levels of inter-rater reliability regarding functional assessment methods, leading clinicians to question its proper place in patient assessment. Nevertheless, the visual assessment of posture, gait, and movement and palpatory assessment remain a staple of the orthopedic evaluation. This has spawned a paradoxical scenario in the clinical world that requires some explanation.

A ritual experienced by most, if not all, healthcare interns involves their amazement at their clinical instructor's ability to discern subtle yet important findings regarding a challenging patient's diagnosis. This typically occurs after the standard assessment has been performed and the clinical response is found unsatisfactory. While the evidence-based clinical approach to diagnosis is becoming the global standard, it is the ability to note the less obvious, yet significant, findings that defines the expert. Therefore, the exact value of the skills involved in the functional evaluation must for the time being be placed in the interesting position of skeptical envy, questioning the value while aspiring to gain such admirable expertise.

Clinical Pearl: While the evidence-based clinical approach to diagnosis is becoming the global standard, it is the ability to note the less obvious, yet significant, findings that defines the expert.

Clinical Shortcuts

Unfortunately, gaining expertise in these new skills can be rather frustrating for the experienced clinician. This can be likened to the youth who must learn to write in cursive after becoming proficient in printing. Although the second style may be quicker and more professional, the youth can reasonably question the necessity since he or she can already write!

Those who take up this challenge of functional assessment expertise find that the skills gained tend to provide *clinical shortcuts* in assessment and treatment strategies and a deeper understanding of the factors that tend to promote chronicity. It is the success of this functional approach, from symptom resolution and functional restoration at best, to reduced symptomatology and/or reduced activity restrictions, and improved management of previously recalcitrant cases, which motivates clinicians to use functional assessment methods. Finally, clinicians who use functional assessment methods often do so for those patients who have failed to benefit from more common evidence-based approaches. After all, if a cure for chronic, disabling back syndromes were validated, there would be no need for this book.

The functional assessment uses information derived from the patient's history and current complaints, in addition to visual and palpatory observations. The functional assessment capitalizes on the "significant subtleties" of faulty still, upright postures and movements, and palpated alterations in tissue tone, correlated with other findings, in order to arrive at patterns that ultimately reveal global patterns of dysfunction.

The "Elementary" Nature of the Functional Approach

The functional approach to clinical assessment requires a great deal of detective work. It involves gathering pieces of information that may individually seem trivial, but become significant when arranged with a series of other apparently minor findings. The functional approach to assessment is analogous to the renowned methods of the famous fictional sleuth, Sherlock Holmes. The author of this series of mysteries, Sir Arthur Conan Doyle, presented scenarios in which detective Holmes would arrive at astounding conclusions after being presented with the briefest of histories and only moments to survey the scene of a crime. The incredulous Dr. Watson, utilizing skepticism no doubt defined by his medical training, would question Holmes' summary, only to be shown a logical sequence of trivial findings that provided a reasonable history of what actually transpired. Once explained, the good doctor would be duly impressed by the brilliance of the insights and the obviousness of the conclusions, leading Holmes to his infamous retort, "Elementary, my dear Watson."

The functional approach to assessment is nothing less than the approach taken by Sherlock Holmes. It involves understanding the facts of the case and organizing seemingly insignificant findings into a logical clinical scenario. The functional assessment is not performed in place of other assessment methods, but rather *in addition to* other methods, providing a more comprehensive symbiotic approach.

Functional Assessment Categories

Lumbopelvic functional assessment is divided into the following categories:

1. Visual assessment—This includes the initial contact assessment, still, upright, or seated postural assessment and gait assessment.
2. Manual assessment—This includes hands-on methods to assess soft tissues and joints.

Clinical Pearl: The functional approach to assessment is nothing less than the approach taken by Sherlock Holmes. It involves understanding the facts of the case and organizing seemingly insignificant findings into a logical clinical scenario.

Prerequisite Skills

Functional evaluation requires a variety of skills and a deep practical understanding of topics discussed in earlier chapters. A clear understanding of functional anatomy and topographical landmarks is vital. So too is knowledge of human kinesiology and also of normal variants. Epidemiological, biomechanical, and physiological aspects of the locomotor system in general, and the lumbopelvic region in particular, are important. The pathological sequelae that can be cumulatively labeled low back syndromes must be understood, with skills that allow one to notice the presenting subtle changes that occur in each case.

Mitchell Jr[1] coined the term "sensory literacy" to describe a clinician's development of sensation for improved clinical excellence. Chaitow[2], inspired by this model and the manual practitioner's use of the all-important sense of touch, introduced the term "palpatory literacy." Palpatory excellence provides a greater ability to differentiate subtle alterations within tissues and to more effectively determine physiological versus pathological processes. The lead author expands this line of thinking to introduce "visual clinical literacy" to emphasize the importance of vital visual changes in morphology, posture, and movement that provide invaluable insights in clinical assessment. The key point here is that such skills provide information that allows the clinician to effectively assess the situation and determine a corrective course, in addition to dynamically monitoring the manual techniques as they are performed while assessing the patient's response.

Palpatory and visual clinical literacy provide the clinician *immediate feedback* that allows for instant assessment, with the fingers and eyes being the conduits of information. The palpating hands act as optimal therapeutic tools, dynamically performing fine alterations in manual techniques based upon such afferentation. The development of superior palpation and visual skills requires much practice and is accrued over time. Skills need to be developed so as to link tactile and visual senses to the intellectual interpretation of the transmitted data. Also, the patient's response elicited, by palpation and visual observation, can provide confirmatory support for findings made in other ways. For example, the patient whose breathing pattern changes during light palpation of the pelvic area may be demonstrating a deep emotional concern. This is very similar to what Nixon,[3] an eminent British cardiovascular expert, described as a "think test" following observation of altered respiratory patterns in patients when discussing, for example, domestic or relationship issues. In many instances, returning to these topics subsequently, and asking the patient to "think about what we were talking about" led to full-blown hyperventilation episodes. Observation of altered breathing rhythms can be a useful clinical tool during palpation, especially when such changes occur in the absence of any provoked discomfort.

Palpatory literacy requires the clinician to possess the skills to probe the tissues to differentiate variations in tone and detect the significant subtleties. This is called "layer palpation" (see Fig. 13–1). Expertise

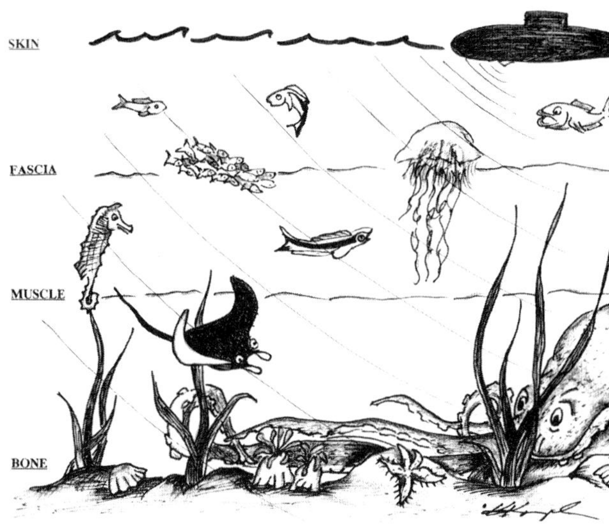

FIGURE 13–1. Layer palpation: Illustration depicts the analogous nature of layers of human tissue with that of the ocean and sea life. Layer palpation requires a careful probing of the various tissue depths for optimal palpatory assessment.

allows the clinician to more effectively determine the appropriate therapeutic measure based upon the mechanical properties of isolated pathological or dysfunctional tissue. Janda [4] stated, "The best and most frequently used means of evaluating muscle tone is still palpation, and in particular layer-by-layer palpation. There is no instrumental technique that could replace it in any aspect." As learning to read requires a common visual experience, *palpatory literacy is a learned skill that requires a common touch experience.* As Hyman[5] teaches during palpation training, "Don't do what I do; feel what I feel."

A novice to palpation may find it helpful to compare the same body region on the contralateral side, although the expert may use this trick during exceptional palpatory challenges. Of course, all clinicians can teach the patients to appreciate their own "abnormal" region by then palpating their "normal" contralateral side. This can be a powerful learning tool for the patient, helping to both confirm the dysfunctional area while gaining confidence in the practitioner's ability to localize the problem through touch. Hands-on practitioners tend to have a close "doctor–patient" relationships, which can be further strengthened by the patient's confidence in the clinician's palpatory literacy skills.

Acute, Subacute, and Chronic Cases

The functional approach is a strategy that can be successfully applied to the acute, subacute and chronic cases. However, because the acute and subacute cases are typically simpler in their nature, the history more clear-cut, and the findings more dramatic (i.e., marked hypertonicity, antalgia, inflammation, edema, etc.), subtle findings described in this chapter may be less important. After all, the experienced clinician has seen many dramatic acute pain presentations resolve in equally dramatic fashion, despite a less complex assessment and more generic treatment protocol. Therefore, the functional approach described in this chapter addresses in particular the patient with chronic pain syndrome.

There are, of course, exceptions to the above scenario, for example, involving the recurrent, acute pain episode in which the patient repeatedly experiences the same general symptom complex following similar activities. While the patient may explain the provoking activities and demonstrate dramatic (as opposed to subtle) findings, treatment of such cases has typically failed to prevent recurrences, despite the symptoms responding to conservative methods. Despite their acute nature, by definition such cases represent a chronic dysfunction. Ironically, they expose the weakness of the classification of acute, subacute, and chronic stages, which somewhat simplistically are based on chronology of symptom onset.

The chronic stage, in which adaptation potential is close to exhaustion, is the one in which clinicians come to truly appreciate functional approaches.[6] It is in this stage that a patient undergoes complex biopsychosocial changes (outlined in Chapter 19). Such changes include the multifaceted complex of ineffective illness behavior and deconditioning. The patient is coming, or has come, to the realization that he or she has a significant problem that cannot be fully controlled by conservative methods, considered conventional by that individual. It is therefore time to take the matter more seriously and invest the time and costs to either resolve or at least reduce the problem that is impacting his or her life.

Clinical Pearl: The chronic stage, in which adaptation potential is close to exhaustion, is the one in which clinicians come to truly appreciate functional approaches.

The chronic stage can also be a time, depending on their degree of pain, when the patient's postural, gait, and palpatory findings may better demonstrate the underlying dysfunction instead of short-term locomotor system response to a recent and significant nociceptive event.

Postural Age

The aging process can be described in several ways. The most routine measure is based on chronology starting at one's date of birth. However, other measures may be used to emphasize specific areas of interest. For example, gestational age is used to measure maturation from the time of conception. Skeletal age is used to quantify levels of osseous maturity, such as apophyseal assessment to determine growth activity. It is therefore proposed that a *postural age* may be used to determine the degree of the functional state of the postural system. This seems a logical approach, as chronological age and postural function do not consistently correlate. For example, a study of geriatric ex-Olympians demonstrated greater motor control and postural stability than their chronological peers, suggesting a more youthful postural age.[7]

The Functional Approach and Adaptation

A combination of inherited and acquired features and experiences will have merged in the individual to create whatever it is that is being palpated or observed. The structures and functions being evaluated represent the unique characteristics of a person's genetic inheritance, involving the biochemical, psychosocial, and biomechanical make-up, onto which has been overlaid all the developmental and maturational experiences of life, including acquired habits of use, work and leisure stresses, and injuries, surgeries, emotional burdens, etc.

From the first controlled movement of elevating the head, requiring the coordinated contraction of antagonistic muscles, the newborn, infant, and toddler mature in their locomotion, as neural pathways become established and kinetic chains engrained. This process continues through developmental stages, with habits of use being superimposed on postural habits and breathing patterns.[8]

A simplistic summary might state that genetics and maturation (or aging), together with overuse, misuse, abuse, and disuse, lead inevitably to adaptation, exhaustion, decompensation, and ultimately symptoms. Tissues gradually change from a state of *normotonicity* to a palpably dysfunctional state, at times involving hypertonicity, and at others hypotonicity, along with altered firing sequences, modified motor control, abnormal postural and/or movement patterns, and ultimately dysfunctional chain reactions.

Clinical Pearl: From the first controlled movement of elevating the head, requiring the coordinated contraction of antagonistic muscles, the newborn, infant, and toddler mature in their locomotion, as neural pathways become established and kinetic chains engrained.

For example, Janda[9] described a theoretical chain of events that may be associated with temporomandibular joint (TMJ) problems. On a local level TMJ dysfunction is likely to involve hyperactivity and tension in the temporal and masseter muscles with, because of this hypertonicity, reciprocal inhibition occurring in the suprahyoid, digastric, and mylohyoid muscles. This imbalance between mandibular elevators and mandibular depressors alters the condylar motion, a consequent redistribution of stress on the joint, and contributes to degenerative changes.

On a more global scale, Janda described a typical pattern of musculoskeletal dysfunction in an individual with TMJ problems. This may involve upper trapezii, levator scapulae, scaleni, sternocleidomastoidii, suprahyoids, lateral and medial pterygoids, and masseter and temporalis muscles, demonstrating a tendency to tighten and shorten. He noted that the scalenes may become atrophied and weak while also developing spasm, tenderness, and myofascial trigger points (TrPs).

Janda also suggested that the postural pattern associated with TMJ dysfunction might involve:

1. hyperextension of the knee joints,
2. increased anterior tilt of the pelvis,
3. pronounced flexion of the hip joints,
4. hyperlordosis of the lumbar spine,
5. rounded shoulders and winged (rotated and abducted) scapulae,
6. cervical hyperlordosis,
7. compensatory overactivity of the upper trapezius and levator scapulae muscles, and
8. forward thrust of the head resulting in opening of the mouth and retraction of the mandible.

This series of changes provokes increased activity of the mandibular elevator and protractor muscles, creating a vicious cycle of dysfunctional activity, and intervertebral joint stress in the cervical spine follows.

The message which can be drawn from this example is that patterns first need to be identified before they can be assessed for the role they might be playing in the person's apparently local pain and restriction conditions, and then can be successfully and appropriately treated.

The task of the practitioner is therefore to attempt to make sense of the background influences that lead to such changes and to then identify strategies that will reduce adaptive load, while enhancing adaptive capacity. Functional assessment and palpation skills offer insights into how efficiently the individual is adapting to the demands of life. Of course, the clinician must be able to effectively determine normal, or physiological, patterns before abnormal, or pathological, patterns can be determined.

Clinical Pearl: Functional assessment and palpation skills offer insights into how efficiently the individual is adapting to the demands of life.

Adaptive modifications can occur in a number of ways, such as compromises in optimal posture, gait, joint loading, neural function, muscle coordination, respiratory function, endurance, strength, and balance. Such widespread functional changes commonly lead to painful conditions, and may well interfere with the expected resolution of seemingly localized conditions, such as a might be seen with a mechanical back pain. Functional assessment aims to evaluate these changes and to suggest possible clinical solutions. Therapeutic options emerge as the nature and scale of the adaptive "load," together with inadequacies in adaptation potential, are identified. What these options might be, once an understanding of the nature and degree of decompensation (locally or globally) has been acquired, depends on the training and skill of the practitioner.

Integrating the Functional Assessment with the History and Physical Examination

Information deriving from the initial patient history and physical examination, as discussed in the previous chapter, should be integrated with data gathered during functional assessment, as described here.

Patient Attire

Standard protocols for patient attire vary with respect to, among other factors, regional, societal, religious, legal, health-care specialty, gender, and age-related issues. Clinicians should remain respectful of such issues, while remembering the reason for the patient presenting in the first place: amelioration of symptoms. Patients, on the other hand, must understand that the clinician must be able to reasonably perform a thorough examination, that any less is not in their best interest, and that they should feel as comfortable wearing as little in the examining room as they would at the public beach or swimming pool. The doctor–patient relationship is a sacred one and open communication and trust must remain a cornerstone of this relationship.

The simple rule for functional assessment is that the patient should wear as little clothing as appropriately possible, given the above-stated issues, in order to allow a comprehensive evaluation.

The clothing should be form-fitting to reveal body contours. As stated above, the functional approach integrates a strategy that extends beyond the periphery of the region of pain or symptomatology, often requiring assessment at anatomically distant sites. Therefore, the clinician must have access to these regions in order to hunt for the key links of dysfunction. Clothing compromises the quality of visual and palpatory assessment findings, so the clinical importance for varying degrees of disrobing must not be ignored. As Lewit stated, "One cannot properly palpate through textiles."[10]

One issue that should not be compromised is foot attire. The patient must be barefooted for the functional examination. Foot function has been insufficiently stressed in locomotor system assessment, and this is particularly true for assessment of low back syndromes. Shoes, compared with the patient being barefoot, have been shown to alter sensory input and to modify kinematic function.[11] In addition, the floor on which the patient stands and is assessed for gait, should be a level, hard surface. A slight degree of padded carpeting is acceptable, although a hard floor is preferable.

Clinical Pearl: The patient must be barefooted for the functional examination. Foot function has been insufficiently stressed in locomotor system assessment, and this is particularly true for assessment of low back syndromes.

Chapter 36 discusses ethical approaches to patient communication, examination, and informed consent. The reader is referred to that chapter for greater detail on this vitally important topic.

LOCOMOTOR SYSTEM DEVELOPMENT, MATURITY, AND DECLINE

In order to appreciate the functional approach to assessment, a brief overview of the locomotor system is presented. Although cursory in nature, it is hoped that these concepts assist in providing a foundation for understanding functional pathology of this system.

From birth, the locomotor system undergoes a maturation process that is poorly understood despite a plethora of research. The sheer complexity of the locomotor system boggles the mind. With estimated tens of millions of neural connections per second[12] an adequate understanding demands a deep knowledge of anatomy, kinesiology, biomechanics, pathology, and psychology.

With the passage of time, optimal mature function becomes established and then subsequently undergoes a gradual state of decline. For purposes of clarity, the declining locomotor system will be called the geriatric locomotor system, although this is not necessarily associated with chronology. Even in the geriatric state, the locomotor system is capable of remarkable adaptive compensation, as individuals in their tenth decade of life have been shown to acquire significant strength gains with a resistance exercise program.[13] Another study demonstrated that vestibulo-ocular reflex function was enhanced among a group of geriatric retirees who initiated a physical activity program.[14]

Clinical Pearl: From birth, the locomotor system undergoes a maturation process that is poorly understood despite a plethora of research. The sheer complexity of the locomotor system boggles the mind.

A brief summary of the emerging, mature, and declining locomotor system will be described to form a base for better understanding of the functional assessments described later.

The Developing Locomotor System

Locomotor system maturation occurs with the newborn, and so begins a contentious lifelong relationship with gravity with which functional battles and alliances occur. Stressing the individual nature of this battle, Janda stated, "As far as the locomotor system is concerned, each person is a self-made man or women."[15]

The coordinated actions of muscular cocontraction during locomotor maturation provide the initial opportunity for controlled head motion. This occurs as an extension of so-called hard-wired movements, those that are present at birth, in concert with incoming neural information. For example, a newborn will reflexively turn the eyes in the same direction (ipsiversive) as the rotating head (cervico-ocular reflex).[16] With ensuing maturation, visuomotor function and head/neck motion become more established and complex, largely due to incoming visual stimulation. However, the blind-from-birth infant will perform only the cervico-ocular reflex for a few weeks before discontinuing it in the absence of the visual afferentation necessary to promote visuomotor maturation.[17] Furthermore, according to Scott,[18] congenitally blind children never spontaneously attempt to stand or walk, but must be carefully taught to do so. However, whether the congenitally blind human develops as a biped or quadruped, the maturation of their autonomic postural reflexes occurs with the same degree of efficiency, demonstrating that the locomotor system develops with whatever afferent resources are available.[19]

Neuromaturation involves the extension and integration of neural components with other regions and types of sensory input as the requisite complexity increases for improving and increased locomotor control.[20]

Four types of input provide the majority of neural information. These are proprioceptive, mechanoreceptive, visual, and labarynthine sensory input.[21,22] At 1 month of age, newborns already have established a basic level of postural adjustments. Hedburg et al.[23] demonstrated that seated infants had the capacity to perform agonist activation or antagonist inhibition in response to forward or backward perturbations Visual input appears to heavily influence early neuromuscular control in the early phase of maturation, becoming less dominant after about 3 years of age.[22]

Sensory input helps to oversee coordinated movements and establish anticipatory strategies for various locomotor tasks. These include the establishment of kinetic chains of motion, of neural integration of ipsilateral and contralateral body regions, of proximal (i.e., core) stabilization in preparation for extremity activities, and of anticipatory actions for learned movements.[24,25]

The locomotor system undergoes a maturation process that can be considered goal oriented, including such controlled motions as rolling over, crawling, assisted standing, walking, and still, upright bipedal posture. Although it may seem contrary, unassisted still, upright postural stance requires greater stability than unassisted walking, which is why in a toddler walking occurs first. (Which parent has not observed their child beginning to walk, the child starts walking, comes to a stop, briefly wiggles the pelvis in the sagittal plane before promptly plopping down on the buttocks once equilibrium is lost?) Furthermore, lateral stability is the most important factor in gait in infants, since A–P stability is achieved with forward motion and also with the long lever effects of the feet.[26]

Clinical Pearl: Although it may seem contrary, unassisted still, upright postural stance requires greater stability than unassisted walking, which is why in a toddler walking occurs first.

Locomotor maturation is a multifaceted and complex series of events. As the infant starts to activate the postural system, skeletal muscles are tested to determine their specific uses in various movement strategies. With repetition, muscles and muscle groups are used for recurrent functions, as active participants of a variety of functions. Janda[27] organized the musculature by this function into two groups: those that are designed to counter gravitational loading and those that are not. These antigravity muscles, the so-called "postural muscles," tend to be relatively strong due to their ongoing battle with this attractive force. It has also been speculated that their older phylogenetic age reduces their tendency to atrophy. The second muscle group are named "phasic muscles," which tend to function in a dynamically antagonistic manner to the postural muscles. Phasic muscles tend to become relatively weak compared to the postural muscles and are more prone to atrophy. Table 13–1 provides a list of key lumbopelvic postural and phasic muscles. This model serves an important function by establishing a functional kinesiological model of motor control, while later forming a practical model in the etiology of chronic pain syndromes.

This model has gained support among a variety of authorities in a variety of specialties. Waddell, in his book *The Back Pain Revolution*[28] stated,

TABLE 13–1. Lower Half Postural and Phasic Muscles

	Postural Muscles	Phasic Muscles
Agonist/ Antagonist	Thoracolumbar erector spinae	Abdominal rectus
	Quadratus lumborum	
	Iliopsoas	Gluteus maximus
	Single joint Hip adductors	Gluteus medius/ minimus
	Piriformis	
	Hamstrings	Vastus medialis/ lateralis
	Rectus femoris	
	Tensor fascia latae	
	Tibialis posterior	Tibialis anterior
	Gastroc/soleus	

> Postural and phasic muscles are often antagonistic. Increased activity or contracture of the more postural muscle may not only mechanically limit the range of movement of its antagonist, but also inhibit that more phasic muscle. This produces an imbalance between antagonists.

In recent years other models have emerged. Norris[29] has noted,

> By categorizing muscles into stabilizer and mobilizer groups (equated to some extent with Janda's phasic and postural categorizations) the clinician can focus attention on the type of management likely to be required. Stabilizer muscles are likely to be poorly recruited, lax in appearance, show an inability to perform inner range contractions over time, and as a result alter body alignment by failing to provide a stable base for other muscles to work from. Mobilizer muscles on the other hand are likely to the tight, and show preferential recruitment in synergistic activities. These muscles will tend to dominate movements and may alter posture by restricting movement and preventing optimal segmental alignment. The combination of muscle laxity and poor holding ability on the one hand, with muscle tightness and dominance on the other hand, within an antagonistic muscle pairing, will alter the equilibrium point of the joint, tending to pull the joint towards the tight muscle.

A further categorization of muscles has been described by Bergmark[30] and expanded by Richardson et al.[31] They use the nomenclature of local (central) and global ("guy rope") muscles. The central muscles are those that are deep or have deep portions attaching to the lumbar spine. These muscles are seen as capable of controlling the stiffness (resistance to bending) of the spine and of influencing intervertebral alignment. The global category includes larger more superficial muscles. Global muscles include the anterior portion of the internal oblique, the external oblique, the rectus abdominis, the lateral fibers of the quadratus lumborum, and the more lateral portions of the erector spinae.[32] The local categorization includes the multifidus, intertransversarii, interspinales, transversus abdominis, the posterior portion of the internal oblique, the medial fibers of quadratus lumborum, and the more central portion of the erector spinae. The global system moves the lumbar spine, and also balances/accommodates the forces imposed by an object acting on the spine.

Irrespective of the categorization model used, what is clear is that some muscles (postural, mobilizer) respond to adaptation demands by shortening and tightening, while others (phasic, stabilizer) have a tendency to becoming inhibited and lax.

Even when an indiviual is able to independently walk and stand, human locomotor maturation continues as the individual grows, adapting to longer bones, greater girth, a heavier frame, and increasing strength. Early gait strategies demonstrated a heavy emphasis on anterior hip motion and knee flexion from 10 to 24 months of age, with a longer stride that integrates hip and knee extension developing later. Interlimb asymmetries were also noted for knee angle pattern and for stance and swing phase time.[33] The efficiency of this maturation can be mediated by a number of factors. For example, Gould[34] found that toddlers' ambulatory capabilities, including stance, gait, cadence, and stability, were jeopardized when wearing sneakers (i.e., soft-soled shoes) instead of hard-soled shoes.

Upright stance is heavily dependent on the hip for lateral stability, which is poorly controlled by the toddler. Indeed, Roncesvalles et al.[35] found that active hip responses to unexpected perturbations, which included quadriceps and abdominal recruitment and increased hip flexor torque, occurred in children several years after the initiation of walking. During this maturation period, the ambulatory "step factor" (i.e., step length divided by leg length) increases until age 4 and thereafter remains relatively constant. Children in this age group also tend to use their hip muscles more than their ankle plantar flexors for power generation, a strategy that later reverses.[36]

The locomotor system remains quite labile during childhood, improving motor control while adapting to the biomechanical effects of the evolving anthropomorphic environment associated with growth and gravity.[37] Indeed, gravity appears to be a major factor in morphological development, even primary and secondary spinal curves, as women who routinely carry weighted items such as baskets and vases on top of their heads demonstrated straighter spines in the thoracolumbar regions (average of 17 degrees in both regions combined) compared to controls.[38]

Clinical Pearl: The locomotor system remains quite labile during childhood, improving motor control while adapting to the biomechanical effects of the evolving anthropomorphic environment associated with growth and gravity.

After age 4, development of feedback (responsive) and feed-forward (anticipatory) control of upright stance begins. This central transmission maturation continues to develop until adolescence.[39] Malouin and Richards[40] reported that 4- to 6-year-olds, when compared with adults, demonstrated decreased tibialis anterior activity (i.e., decreased forward velocity), increased lateral motion, and a wider stance. This suggests that the maturing locomotor system continues to learn anticipatory behavior of gait initiation in the frontal plane, before the sagittal plane.

In addition to anticipatory activity, another central and peripheral processing strategy that involves locomotor response to unanticipated perturbations also enters a critical maturation stage at this age. This involves the transition of response synergies, motor coordination of proximal and distal musculature, which is relatively immature in 4- to 6-year-olds. As maturation occurs, the locomotor system becomes less vision-dependent and more posture-dependent. Afferents from the ankle mortise initially work alongside visual and vestibular input, but this relationship changes as ankle proprioception takes a greater role in postural maturation, while the vestibulo-visual sensation gradually takes on the secondary role of fine-tuning posture. In so doing, the vestibulo-visual system becomes free to focus on other motor skills, such as developing hand–eye coordination and scouting the environment. By 7–10 years of age, children demonstrate far more structured organization of response synergies, indicating the importance of this critical period of postural development between approximately 4 and 10 years of age.[41]

Reaching patterns with the hand, a complex accumulation of motor skills, continues to mature through age 8. Thereafter, older children tend to demonstrate stereotypical reaching patterns similar to those of adults.[42] However, this does not mean that the entire locomotor system is yet mature. While 7-year-old children visually appear to demonstrate gait dynamics similar to adults, quantitative measurements prove otherwise.[43] Ganley and Powers[44] found that 7-year-olds lack neuromuscular control, especially at the ankle, when compared with adults. Furthermore, McFayden et al.[45] reported that 7- to 9-year-olds anticipatory postural responses were not yet mature when challenged by obstacles. Stride dynamics of 11- to 14-year-olds approach the values observed in adults, proving that further maturation continues into adolescence.[43]

Indeed, neuromaturation is a very dynamic process, which occurs in an integrative versus a graded or linear manner.[41,42] This suggests that learning occurs based on prior motor skills obtained and the types of current challenges confronted. Of course, variations in locomotor system maturation rates and capacity do occur. While a number of factors may be influential, Falk et al.[46] demonstrated decreased physical capacity (i.e., decreased intermuscular coordination) among healthy 5- to 8-year-old children born prematurely.

Clinical Pearl: Neuromaturation is a very dynamic process, which occurs in an integrative versus a graded or linear manner. This suggests that learning occurs based on prior motor skills obtained and the types of current challenges confronted.

By age 11, locomotor system maturation has progressed considerably. However, one study demonstrated that children at this age have not yet fully matured in visuomotor coordination, as reflected with their slower movement times and slower modification in temporal accuracy when compared with adults.[47]

Interestingly, childhood low back pain prevalence is similar to that of adults: 75% of population by age 20. A psychosocial factor link has been identified in adults, but has yet not been determined in children. However, a "high difficulties" score, indicating high levels of adverse psychosocial exposure, was associated with increased risk of developing low back pain among 11- to 14-year-old children.[48]

The Mature Locomotor System

The mature locomotor system is in its prime, its functional peak. While there is no exact beginning or end date to this period, this era will last for a number of decades. This is when the daily challenges of posture, balance, coordination, endurance, and strength demands seem the least demanding, allowing the individual to focus on other issues.

The locomotor system reaches maturation at around 14 years of age, which allows for sufficient long bone growth, weight increase, and muscular gains to integrate with the learning process of neuromaturation. An increasing number of neural motor patterns move with repetition from short-term memory to become established in long-term memory, known as engram consolidation.[49] Motor control is composed to great degree of compiled motor engrams, while coordination develops in proportion to engram repetitions performed at near maximum capacity. All motor activity is based on inherent reflexes and modification of those reflexes by higher centers. A motor engram is formed by the repetition of a precise pattern. The precise pattern of inhibited muscles that should not be in that engram seems to be as important as the excitation of the correct muscles. Thousands of repetitions are required to begin the engram formation and millions to perfect it. Coordination is developed in proportion to the number of repetitions of an engram practiced just below the maximal level of ability to perform.[50] Optimal coordination requires that specific muscles be inhibited to avoid interference with agonistic and synergistic muscles. Sherrington first described this reduction as neuromotor noise or recurrent inhibition, at the beginning of last century.[51] Janda[27] coined the term "parasitic muscles" for "those muscles that should not be activated during a particular movement." The establishment of engram consolidation becomes an important aspect of both physiological and pathological locomotor system changes, as will be discussed later.

While in this stage the mature locomotor system is less dependent on sight for postural stability than in the immature stage, vision still holds a significant influence from a neurophysiological perspective.[52] This holds important clinical implications, forming the basis for visual synkinesis techniques that will be covered in mobilization techniques discussed in Chapter 23.

Chapter 5 discussed the complex nature of lumbopelvic functional stability. That summary covered the so-called feed-forward mechanism of core stability—a local-motor strategy designed to provide axial rigidity to accomplish a variety of loading mechanisms with reduced spinal buckling, shear, or torsion. Interestingly, Hodges et al.[53] also demonstrated that anticipatory spinal stabilization is a dynamic process dependent on the pending locomotor system challenge rather than simple spinal rigidification. This includes optimization of motor skills, strength, endurance, multitasking abilities, anticipatory (i.e., feed-forward) actions, and adaptive responses to expected and unexpected challenges (i.e., perturbations). The dampening capacity of the mature locomotor system to overcome forces is quite efficient, from grand-scale extrinsic perturbations, as occurring in contact sports, to the seemingly trivial intrinsic perturbations of the heartbeat.[54]

The mature locomotor system becomes, for the most part, an automated vehicle for typical activities of daily living, although specific motor learning tasks continue to be integrated as transient and perhaps consolidated engrams as the motor skill base expands. Such motor skills can include participation of new sports, learning to speak new languages, learning to drive an automobile, learning to play a musical instrument, etc. With increasingly automated movement, the individual also becomes capable of devoting greater attention to other aspects of existence.

Clinical Pearl: The mature locomotor system becomes, for the most part, an automated vehicle for typical activities of daily living, although specific motor learning tasks continue to be integrated as transient and perhaps consolidated engrams as the motor skill base expands.

The mature locomotor system efficiency continues to improve by adapting to the continued challenge of various physical demands. However, the improvements occurring might be considered fine-tuning, as the major skills necessary for human locomotion have been established. For example, long-distance runners have been found to demonstrate smoother gait and running patterns than nonathletes.[55] In another study, athletes participating in judo demonstrated better balance than dancers, demonstrating how motor control improves when challenged by unanticipated perturbations.[56] An interesting measure, that may prove to be of value, is that of sacral vertical motion during gait, with less motion suggesting a more efficient movement pattern.[57]

Gait has been divided into two phases: stance phase and swing phase, with each of these having subdivisions.[18] Stance phase, that aspect where the foot encounters the ground, includes heel strike, flat foot, midstance, heel raise, and toe-off. Swing phase can be divided into acceleration, midswing, and deceleration.[58] The swing phase was thought to be a passive movement, but it appears to instead be an actively controlled maneuver.[59]

The importance of the foot at heel strike as a shock absorber, as a stabilizer during gait, and as a propulsive device at toe-off cannot be overemphasized.[60,61] Furthermore, the incoming sensation from the foot cutaneous exteroceptors and intrinsic proprioceptors is also of vital importance.[62]

Clinical Pearl: The importance of the foot at heel strike as a shock absorber, as a stabilizer during gait, and as a propulsive device at toe-off cannot be overemphasized.

Another source of afferentation to control regulation of ambulation and stance involves the load receptor capacity of the leg muscles, primarily extensors, which is probably initiated in the Golgi tendon organs.[63]

Alterations in any of these mechanisms compromise the efficiency of ambulation. Mature gait tends to allow for an efficient, long stride as sufficient foot, ankle, knee, hip, and lumbopelvic stability makes this possible.

Clinical assessment of posture and gait is based on "soft signs" rather than firm findings because of a plethora of variable factors that can confound the clinician who places too great a weight on such observations. For example, even during its most stable period, mature gait varies on a daily basis. El-Sayyad[64] found significant daily variability in three aspects of gait (knee angle half-way through gait cycle; vertical reaction force and time spent in stance phase) during slow, medium, and fast walking. Hunter et al.[65] further demonstrated another variable, noting eye movement influences postural control.

Clinical Pearl: Clinical assessment of posture and gait is based upon soft signs rather than firm findings due to a plethora of variable factors that can confound the clinician who places too great a weight on such observations.

Other confounding possibilities include alteration during swallowing and respiration.[66–68] Balaban and Theyer[69] demonstrated that a tendency to an altered, more rapid, respiratory rate, in anxious individuals, affects balance control, and even healthy individuals exhibit a substantial increase in sway following voluntary hyperventilation. It is thought that this postural instability may be linked to peripheral and central changes in somatosensory function.[70]

The push-off, or toe-off, phase increases gait efficiency as a forward propellant along with ipsilateral forward arm swing, contralateral forward leg swing, forward body sway, and forward momentum. Another factor influencing forward propulsion may be soft tissue tensile resistance. As opposing arm and leg move in unison forward, a tension is created in a diagonal pattern across the dorsal aspect of the torso, which provides for balance and may assist in the propulsive force production as the body unwinds.

Gait and movement patterns have been assumed to be symmetrical,[18] although this concept has been challenged.[71] It appears to be a relative issue, depending on the patient's degree of morphological symmetry and past history of activities and injuries that may affect such symmetry.

The Declining Locomotor System

Locomotor system decline typically begins in a benign manner. It can occur following microtrauma, such as involving prolonged constrained postures like sitting, or it can occur with macrotrauma. Although there may be considerable synergistic interaction, alterations in motor control may be due to the following:

(a) *Nociception:* The locomotor system tends to prioritize its response in relation to incoming sensory information or demands placed upon it. Nociception, appears to occupy high priority in this relative system. For example, Moseley et al.[72] demonstrated delayed motor (transversus abdominis) reaction times compared with attention demanding tasks. Manetta et al.[73] measured altered hip and knee moments among patients with knee pain compared to controls.

It should be noted that subthreshold nociception is painless and it remains unclear as to what degree of reflexive response occur with subthreshold nociception. In any case, painful stimuli responses have been explored, and the locomotor responses to a few subtopics include the following:

1. *Acute low back pain:* Nociception alters motor control and feed-forward mechanism, delaying transversus abdominis activation, due to hypertonic saline of the longissimus at L4.[74]
2. *Chronic low back pain:* Low back pain affects motor control, trunk coordination, as well as kinetic chain reactions to perturbations, compared to controls, with absent or delayed firing patterns observed in, for example, erector spinae and rectus abdominis.[75–77]
3. *Sacroiliac pain:* Sacroiliac pain has been shown to modify ipsilateral motor control, for example, by delaying activation of the ipsilateral multifidus, gluteus maximus, and biceps femoris muscles.[78]

(b) *Sedentary Lifestyle:* Gait speed has been shown to correlate with physical activity levels and balance, and conversely a sedentary lifestyle results in a more cautious walking style involving shorter steps and slower step velocity.[79]

(c) *Single Muscle Dysfunction:* Pain or dysfunction of individual lower limb muscles, such as tibialis anterior, leads to modified motor control and function of other lower limb muscles and joints.[80,81]

(d) *Degenerative Joint Changes:* Unilateral osteoarthritis of the knee results in poorer performance in both limbs in partial weight-bearing tests, compared with controls.[82] Patients with a unilateral OA knee (compared with elderly controls) demonstrated decreased quadriceps activity, reduced knee and ankle function, as well as abnormal hip loading[83]; Patients with early OA hip demonstrated significant contralateral drop of the pelvis during the swing phase, as well as increased pelvic motion, excessive, and uneconomical, muscle power generation, and/or absorption modifications of the lower limb joints.[84]

(e) *Reduced Balance:* Geriatric gait–sway coordination and amplitude both change with age, with increased sway during platform sway and during visual sway referencing.[85,86]

(f) *Psychopathology:* Balance, and therefore posture and gait, may be modified in many people with mental illness, such as schizophrenia.[87]

(g) *Cognitive Alterations:* Posture and gait are frequently modified in individuals with special needs, such as ADHD and Down syndrome.[88] Children with Down syndrome exhibit gait patterns that deviate from the normal population.[89] Their awkward and inefficient movement patterns frequently result in the appearance of orthopedic problems in later life.[90]

(h) *Distant Trauma.* Significant deficits have been demonstrated in measured variables such as vibratory sensation and one-legged standing, in limbs in which a severe ankle sprain has occurred previously.[91,92]

(i) *Cerebral Vascular Accident* Gait instability may result from weakness in particular leg muscles, and consequent compensatory strategies, following a stroke.[93]

(j) *Spinal Stenosis* Elderly individuals with lumbar stenosis have been shown to lose functional mobility more markedly than healthy people of the same age.[94]

(k) *Weakness:* As an individual loses strength, compromises occur in movement patterns to accommodate the weakness. This typically occurs as part of the aging process. Riley et al.[95] measured age-related decreases in power transfer from the legs to the upper body of geriatric individuals compared to younger subjects. These decreases negatively affected gait speed.

(l) *Fatigue:* Muscular endurance is an important factor in locomotor function. As muscular fatigue occurs, compromises in locomotor stability, varying from minor to significant depending on the degree of fatigue, take place.[96]

(m) *Altered Breathing Pattern and/or Anxiety State:* Normal motor control is modified, and balance compromised,[97] when breathing pattern disorders, which commonly engender anxiety, are evident.[98,99]

(n) *Foot Dysfunction, Including Functional Hallux Limitus:* Dananberg[100] suggests that many cases of acute or chronic low back pain are related to gait anomalies, and that foot function and therefore gait mechanics alter when normal dorsiflexion of the first metatarsophalangeal joint is compromised, as in the case of functional hallux limitus and/or hallux rigidus.

> The ability of the joints proximal to the first MTP joint to undergo extension are directly related to the physical capacity of the first MTP joint to provide its normal range of motion ... movement will occur 180° opposed to the motion that should be taking place. For example, the thigh must extend on the hip, but failure to pivot sagittally at the foot negates the responsive hip joint motion. Flexion must replace extension as the accommodation to the power input for forward motion is now peaking.[101]

(o) *Leg Length Discrepancy:* Janda[102] emphasized the importance of a true leg length difference, stressing the importance of such anatomic asymmetry during functional assessment. He noted that altered postural and gait strategies, such as pelvic torsion, lateral pelvic shift, altered knee flexion, and foot positional changes occurred in order to allow the spine to rest on a more level base. However, each of these strategies compromise biomechanics, reduce economic locomotor function, and cause increased spinal loading, a factor in chronic pain syndromes. Liu et al.[103] and Young et al.[104] later supported these concepts. Boone and Hammans[105] demonstrated that acute leg length discrepancy increased Vo_2 demands, supporting the concept of diminished locomotor system economics.

(p) *Attention-Demanding Tasks:* Attention-demanding tasks were found to delay extrinsic muscular control and joint motion, although intrinsic (i.e., core) muscle function was unaffected.[72]

(q) *Limbic System Disturbance:* Janda[4] noted that a central source of muscular imbalance can be the result of limbic system dysfunction. This finding was supported when Moseley et al.[72] noted that stressful situations caused global motor control compromises following delays caused by pain and attention-demanding tasks.

Adaptation Alterations of the optimal motor engrams occur through life as the locomotor system constantly adapts to specific responses to imposed demands. Selye[106] described this process as the general adaptation syndrome, whose causes are multivariate. These can stem from repetitive movements or prolonged postures, from recurrent microtrauma, macrotrauma, or a combination of each. Alterations in the coordinated postural and movement pattern ensues, which is less economical than the original pattern. This can include, for example, a slight increase in pelvic tilt due to muscular imbalance with prolonged sitting, a compromise in joint mobility, a slight change in weight distribution to maintain balance, or an alteration in coordination to avoid pain. Once these alterations occur, the same mechanisms that allowed for improved motor control via repetitious engram consolidation turn against the individual, as the locomotor system learns a new compromised movement or postural strategy. One of the problems in explaining this process is that, as Janda stated, "there is no exact distinction between 'normal' and 'abnormal' status of the motor system."[107] With time, adaptive engram consolidations expand along the kinetic chain, resulting in altered movement patterns. In so doing a cavalcade of altered patterns may then ensue, adaptively reacting to the newly established compromise and creating subsequent strategies that become automated, habitual, with time and repetition. Because of their reduced efficiency and increased load to joint and myofascial tissue, these detrimental engram consolidation patterns ultimately lead to chronic pain syndromes.[75–77,107] And so this model of locomotor system degradation must in the end be considered the ultimate irony, in that the same mechanisms that promote improved motor control may indeed lead to its decline.

Clinical Pearl: Alterations of the optimal motor engrams occur through life as the locomotor system constantly adapts to specific responses to imposed demands. Selye described this process as the general adaptation syndrome, whose causes are multivariate.

Of course, locomotor decline can be facilitated by a host of other factors, including deconditioning and systemic factors such as cardiovascular compromise, diminished function of other organ systems, and decreasing muscle mass and strength, such as in the quadriceps muscles.[108] These factors integrate to form a synergistic degradation of motor control in addition to other organ system compromise.

Janda[15] observed that such changes lead to compromises in somatosensory input, which causes the locomotor system to increasingly depend on alternate sources of afferentation, such as incoming visual and vestibular information. However, these systems do not fully make up for compromised somatosensory input[109] with proprioception being the key mode of afferentation for mature postural control, especially stemming from the hip and trunk.[110]

Despite being a strategy doomed to fail, the geriatric locomotor system becomes increasingly dependent on visual input. Important compromises in the elderly include the swing phase of gate, which increases the risk of tripping as the foot travels forward without appropriate ground clearance, and diminished push-off forces at the toe-off phase of gait.[7]

As the individual loses confidence in their postural stability, additional sensory information is sought from other sensorimotor system sources to remain confidently upright. The person routinely uses the hand as a supplementary sensory device, which provides information by, for example, touching stable surfaces such as walls, or uses a cane.[111] While many assume that cane usage is to reduce weight bearing due to pain, the proprioceptive aspects are often overlooked.[112] Although this haptic strategy, recruiting exteroceptor input as proprioceptive input, becomes inadequate, it has been proven to reduce sway and increase stability,[113] a significant and unfortunate transition point occurs. That is, for the first time since learning to independently stand and walk as a toddler, the locomotor system has once again become dependent. In so doing, the efficiency of gait and a host of other motor patterns have become significantly and often permanently compromised.

As the locomotor system declines, certain predictable and stereotypical changes tend to occur.[114] These include increased lumbar lordosis and thoracic kyphosis,[115] decreased hip extension, decreased medial–lateral stability,[116] increased hip flexed posture due to muscle imbalance, decreased anterior–posterior stability, decreased stride length, greater weight placed on the forefoot,[117–119] increased double-foot stance time,[120] decreased joint position sense (proprioception), and harder heal strike.[121] Several of these changes that occur are similar to those of a person who ambulates on a slippery surface[122] walking with increased care. With decreased postural stability, the geriatric must confront a new postural threat, a fear of falling associated during independent gait, a process that had been taken for granted for decades.

Clinical Pearl: With decreased postural stability, the geriatric must confront a new postural threat, a fear of falling associated during independent gait, a process that had been taken for granted for decades.

As the decline progresses, the locomotor system becomes less adaptable to its environment, with regular movements and postures becoming less automated and requiring the person to give greater attention to use more sensory information in order to maintain postural control.[123] As such, they are less capable of performing multiple tasks and their response times to sudden challenges become slower.[124,125] This age-related decreased postural stability has been coined "presbivertigo," a misnomer in many cases where there is no dizziness, but nevertheless emphasizes the decreasing motor control and classical increasing fear of injury-related falls of the elderly.[126] Indeed, the lead author suggests a more correct term for this degradation in the absence of dizziness would be "presbydysequilibrium." Decreased balance and fear of falling leads to altered kinematics, such as increased enforcement of center of mass as the people becomes more conservative in their postural movement patterns to avoid risky imbalances.[127] When questioned, the second author has observed that such an individual may report hesitation in placement of the foot when taking the first step down, when at the top of a staircase. This observation is supported by Hamel and Cavanagh,[128] Christina and Cavanagh,[129] and Cavanagh et al.[130]

And so it is that many of the changes that occur in the developing locomotor system interestingly recur in some sort of reverse order in the degrading locomotor system. These changes include a transition from an ankle strategy during gait, back to a hip strategy; a broadened stance to combat increased medial lateral instability; a shortened stride length to better maintain center of gravity; decreased integration of upper body counter rotation; increased visual sensory input; recruitment of additional afferentation for postural equilibrium, such as the use of a cane, the aid of a more posturally stable person, or both (see Fig. 13–2).

The layman can identify the stereotypical geriatric posture and gait, including a stooped posture, rounded shoulders, shortened stride, slowed speed, and guarded motion. However, the early locomotor system changes are subtle, requiring special clinical skills. Some of the skills, designed to identify these subtleties, will be elaborated below. Although learning these skills is difficult, the real challenge lies in determining which subtleties are clinically significant. This requires the clinician to integrate these findings into the clinical history, symptom constellation, body mechanics, level of conditioning and emotional stability, etc. In this manner, the *significant subtleties* provide supporting clinical rationale for the diagnosis and treatment strategy.

POSTURAL SYNDROMES

Postural syndromes offer a practical method of describing commonly found postures outside physiological posture. While there are others, three that are found in the lumbosacral region will be addressed here.

Lower (aka Pelvic or Distal) Crossed Syndrome

The lower crossed syndrome (LCS) is one of Janda's[131] observations, a scenario that seems to occur frequently in industrialized societies due to inactivity and prolonged sitting. It consists of lumbopelvic muscle imbalances in which postural muscles become *relatively* shortened and strong with overactivity compared with their antagonistic phasic muscles, which become relatively weakened[27] due to reflex inhibition, decreased activity,[27] and stretch weakness.[132] The key

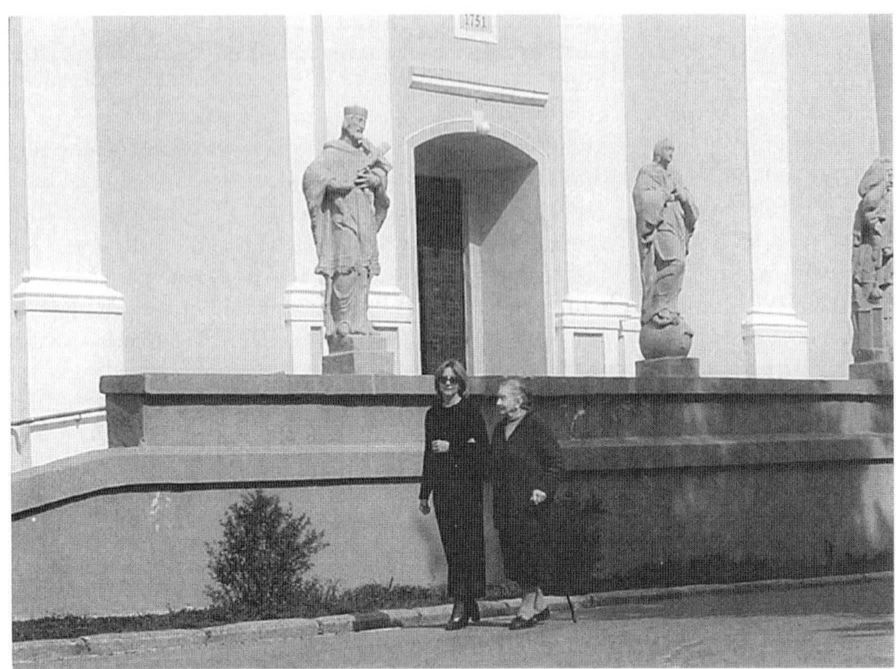

FIGURE 13–2. Geriatric gait: This can include a shortened stride, diminished propulsion at toe off, a slightly stooped posture, and a gait that has been compared to one who is walking on ice. Decreases in proprioceptive input, especially from the lower extremities, are typical, and it is common to see the unsure geriatric gait using additional sensory input, such as a cane and/or the arm of another person, to maintain postural equilibrium.

postural muscles of the LCS include the hamstrings, the hip adductors, the iliopsoas, and the thoracolumbar erector spinae. The key phasic muscles of the LCS include the gluteus maximus, the Gluteus medius and minimus, the lumbosacral erector spinae, and the rectus abdominis. When observed from a lateral aspect, an "X" forms the cross of muscle imbalance (see Fig. 13–3). The hypertonic muscles from the adductors, iliopsoas, and thoracolumbar erector spinae form one line of the "X." The relatively weak, phasic muscles from the gluteals and abdominis rectus form the other line.

This muscle imbalance results in an anterior pelvic tilt and increased lumbar lordosis. The patient appears to have a more rounded abdomen than would seem appropriate for his or her body mass index. There is a decrease in true hip extension due to the shortened iliopsoas, resulting in a shortened stride and toe-off. The body counters this loss of function by increasing toe-off with an anterior pelvic tilt and a *false hip extension*.[15] False hip extension occurs when the pelvis rotates in the sagittal plane, with the lumbosacral junction becoming a pivot point instead of the hip joint. This lumbosacral motion increases the stresses at that junction and is believed to be a factor in increasing the risk of chronic pain syndromes.[131] As such, the LCS presents a functional paradox: restricting the push-off phase of gait on one hand, while adaptively increasing it through two other functional mechanisms. Unfortunately, the replacement strategies are less desirable than the initial one because they require additional lumbosacral motion or decreased functional stability.[131,133]

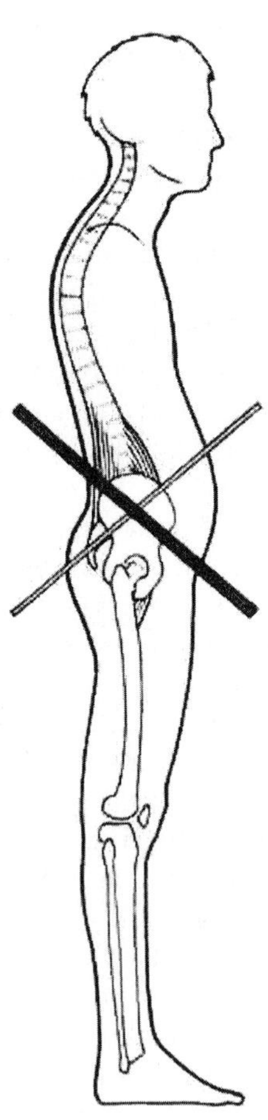

FIGURE 13–3. The lower (aka pelvic, aka distal) crossed syndrome: Janda's description of lumbopelvic muscle imbalance leading to altered posture, movement patterns, and believed to be associated with chronic pain syndromes.

Clinical Pearl: The LCS is one of Janda's observations, a scenario that seems to occur frequently in industrialized societies due to inactivity and prolonged sitting.

Sterno-Symphyseal Syndrome

The sterno-symphyseal syndrome (SSS) was observed by Brügger.[134,135] The SSS is the reverse of the LCS, in that the pelvis is posteriorly tilted and the lumbar lordosis is reduced or reversed. Logically, it can be remembered because the sternum and symphesis pubes become closer with this posture than with an erect posture. Individuals display a thoracolumbar kyphosis, rounded shoulders, and forward head carriage. These individuals tend to have postures that appear to be decades older than their chronological age.

In the case of SSS, the gluteus maximi tend to be more deconditioned and weak than with the LCS, because of the absence of hip extension caused as the acetabulum rotates anteriorly. These patients tend to have very tight hamstrings because they "pull" themselves along during gait because they are not able to propel forward the toe-off phase of gait. The abdominal muscles of such individuals are deconditioned and weak, while the thoracolumbar spine is remarkably stiff due to spinal osseous-visco-elastic resistance. Finally, a compromise of respiration is common due to reduced diaphragm activity as abdominal excursion is altered by the proximity of the anterior ribs and pubes.

Forward Drawn Syndrome

The forward drawn syndrome (FDS) is a rather simple posture in which the patients place their center of mass anteriorly, over the forefoot. These individuals tend to have tight rectus abdominis muscles and also tight gastroc-soleus muscles that must remain so to keep the individual from falling forward. They often tend to have chronic back pain, which may be associated with standing or sitting in prolonged, constrained postures.[135]

VISUAL EVALUATION

The visual appraisal entails a vital and early part of the assessment. It actually precedes the history, continues throughout all continuing patient contact, and also includes any candid visual aspects of the patient from a distance.

For practical purposes, however, the visual contact of the initial visit will be stressed here. *One of the most important functional assessment rules is that formal visual assessment should occur before the palpatory examination.* Janda[114] emphasized the importance of this issue, reminding all that the immediate, reflexive aspects of sensorimotor stimulation from palpation of the patient compromise the visual assessment. Following inspection, hands-on examination such as muscle length tests, palpation, and tests of basic movement patterns can be carried out for confirmatory purposes.

The Initial Patient Contact

The initial patient contact is when the functional assessment begins. It actually precedes the first spoken words. It involves the manner in which the patient presents themselves and their movement patterns. The image presented by the patient represents the way he or she wishes to be seen ("image posture"; see Fig. 13–4), and may bear little relationship to what is discovered once a degree of relaxation occurs ("residual posture") or when tissues are later palpated.[136]

A number of questions should arise at this time, some examples of which are presented here. How does he or she arise from a seated position to greet the clinician, easily or in a guarded manner? Does the patient look directly into the eyes of the clinician or look away? Is there a nervousness or fear present? Is there an exaggerated pain response, as demonstrated by facial expression and/or voiced complains? Does he or she sit to the side with the majority of weight on one buttock while the opposite leg is extended, a position associated with a root syndrome?[137,138] (See Fig. 13–5.) In the case of an adult, is a spouse, or significant other, in attendance, and does such a presence seem appropriate? For example, does the patient require assistance in ambulation, translation, or changing of clothing? Does the patient answer his or her own questions or have an overly attentive assistant (i.e., spouse, friend, or relative)? It is these pieces of observational information that forms the basis of the

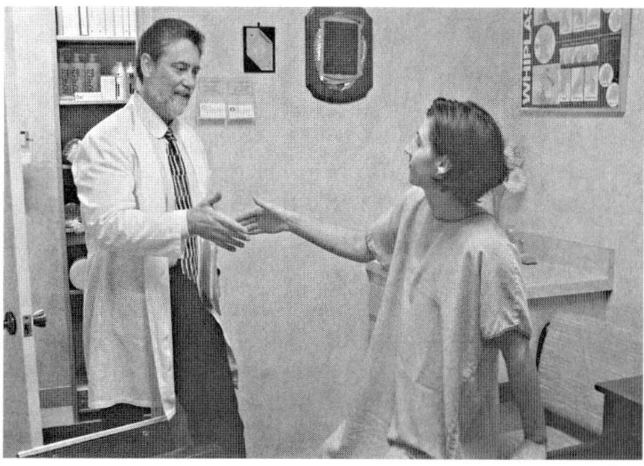

FIGURE 13–4. Image posture: The posture the patient wants the clinician to see at the first impression can provide important information from a physical and psychosocial perspective. This should later be compared to the "residual posture" once the patient has relaxed and returned to a more typical postural presentation. (*Reprinted with permission. From Chaitow L. Muscle Energy Techniques 2nd Ed. London. Elsevier 1996.*)

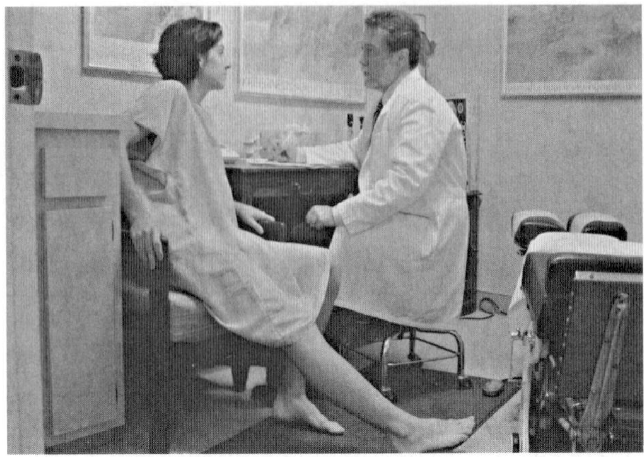

FIGURE 13–5. Sitting posture: The history provides an opportunity to observe the patient's seated posture while he or she focuses on explaining the case history.

early clinical impression. It is, in essence, the beginning of the clinical search for patient consistency and reliability. The questions that are raised, and the answers that are gleaned, can be vital in creating clinical shortcuts.

Still, Upright Postural Visual Assessment

Postural assessment typically begins with observation of the patient during simple, quiet, static standing. However, research over the past decade has proven that this description is problematic because it is not simple, quiet, or static[74,139,140] (see Fig. 13–6). This misnomer has occurred because of the lack of apparent gross motion coupled with a poor understanding of the challenges that the static stance places on the postural system. In an effort to avoid such misstatements, the lead author therefore recommends *still, upright posture* as an acceptable term for this activity. As previously noted, the motor control demands for stability are greater during standing than during gait, just as the stabilizing action of forward momentum on a bicycle is less demanding than remaining still on two wheels. Conversely, however, visual *assessment* of still, upright posture is less difficult than during gait because of the absence of gross limb and torso motion. As such, still, upright postural assessment should precede gait assessment, while learning visual assessment skills. The skills learned from still, upright posture could then be used while learning to assess gait.

Clinical Pearl: Postural assessment typically begins with observation of the patient during simple, quiet, static standing. However, research over the past decade has proven that this description is problematic because it is not simple, quiet, or static.

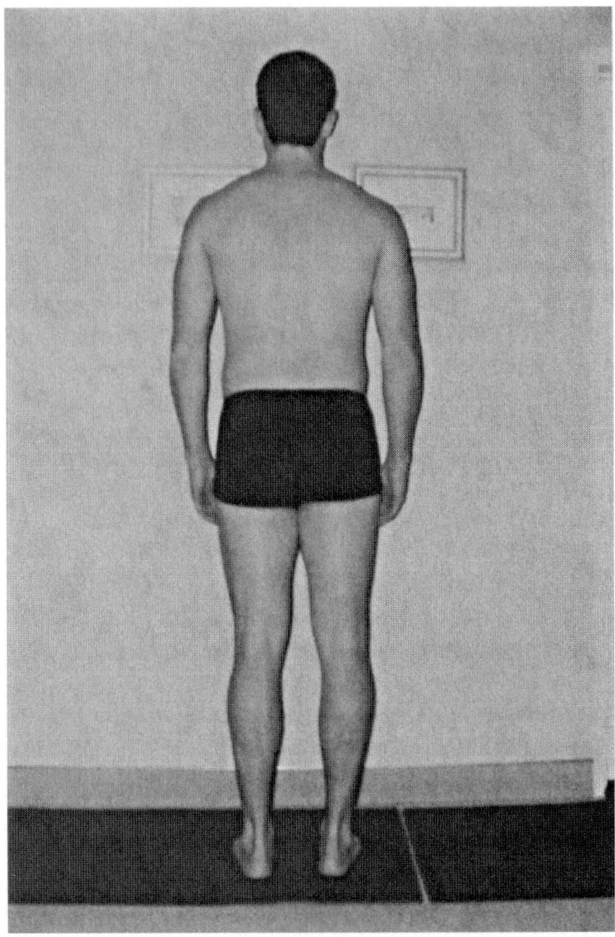

FIGURE 13–6. "Triaging" the still upright posture: This is a key part of "clinical visual literacy", and should begin from the posterior view. The initial global perspective should be perfomed before focusing on the pelvis. The opportunity for the greatest amount of relevant information begins there before moving to the feet.

During mature still, upright stance, the hip joints account for the majority of medial lateral stability while the ankle joints account for a great deal of anterior–posterior stability.[141] Two independent postural subsystems, reciprocally integrated, dynamically counter sway to create the facade of static standing.[142]

Interexaminer reliability for visual assessment of still, upright posture has been found to be poor, although intrarater reliability, a far more practical measure for the clinician, has been fair.[143]

As stated earlier, the still, upright postural assessment can be used as a clinical assessment shortcut. However, in the early stages of learning postural assessment skills, the extra time taken can seem long and at times frustrating. The lead author maintains that with experience, however, the still, upright assessment can demonstrate a virtual "visual chronology of dysfunction." That is, the natural consequence of faulty posture, such as microtrauma and macrotrauma, muscle imbalance, postural and gait compromise, and joint and connective tissue overload, along with psychosocial sequelae, may become apparent. In addition, these observations may help to contribute to significant insights into an otherwise confusing picture of chronicity.

The Dominant Eye

Mitchell,[1] writing on the topic of training to become accurate in observation, has noted that when attempting to observe anatomical landmarks and deviations from the norm, it is important to encourage visual accuracy by attention to the position of the dominant eye.

Identifying the dominant eye:

- Having made a circle with the first finger and thumb and holding the arm out in front of the face observe an object across the room, through that circle, with both eyes open.
- Close one eye.
- If the object is still in the circle, the dominant eye is open.
- If, however, the image shifts out of the circle when only one eye is open, open the closed eye and close the open eye, and the image should shift back into clear view, inside the circle.
- The eye that sees the same view when both eyes were open is the one to use in close observation of the body.
- When attempting to assess by observation a position should be adopted that allows the dominant eye to be closest to the center of what is being viewed.[144]

Rules for Still, Upright Postural Assessment

There are several general rules for still, upright postural assessment, which can help to assist in the learning process. These include the following:

1. As previously noted, the visual static assessment should be an initial part of the examination and prior to the palpatory examination. In this way the initial evaluation is "uncontaminated" by any physical contacts that might modify tone or influence holding patterns.
2. The patient must be barefoot.
3. The patient should be carrying or holding nothing. Carrying an object requires an adjustment of the locomotor system, compromising the assessment.
4. The patient should be wearing as little clothing as is professionally appropriate for the situation, including bare legs, abdomen, and back. Because of the importance of the pelvic, assesment, the overlying clothing should be form-fitting. (This has been discussed earlier in this chapter.)
5. "Generally, three views provide a far more accurate picture of a three-dimensional being."[100] The examination should be performed in the following order: posterior view, which provides the greatest postural information; the lateral view, which provides a second dimensional aspect; the anterior view, which provides additional observations and is used to confirm or refute prior observations.
6. Findings can be placed into three categories: positive, negative, and equivocal.
   (a) The positive signs are obviously present and potentially very important when combined with other findings.
   (b) The negative findings are obviously absent and assist in ruling out conditions in order to allow one to focus on those topics that would appear to be more clinically fruitful.
   (c) Equivocal findings are those that may or may not be positive. As such, it is recommended that such findings be placed in this undetermined category, in the hopes that further evaluation will help to either rule them in or out as significant findings.
7. The still, upright postural assessment can of course be performed on the acute and subacute patient. However, it is the chronic patient whose visual assessment falls under the category of the functional examination. In addition, it is the skills associated with assessing these types of cases that can dramatically expand the clinician's skills and clinical insights.
8. An important rule is that of the "soft" signs of visual assessment. The findings of visual assessment in the chronic patient are by no means pathognomonic. The presence of a postural fault may itself be questionable and the etiology of such findings multivariate. Perhaps more than any other aspect of clinical assessment, visual assessments must therefore not be overly relied upon, but instead integrated with other findings to clarify a clinical picture.
9. One of the key issues to assess for is that of body symmetry. That is symmetry bilaterally, comparing the left and right halves of the body. In addition, one should also assess for symmetry from a cephalic to caudal perspective. While assessment for bilateral symmetry is typical, cephalad to caudal symmetrical assessment is less so. Nevertheless, many patients tend to have a heavily developed upper body while having a relatively poorly developed lower half, and vice versa. In order to gain a proper picture, it is important to understand the congenital build of the patient.

10. In some cases, a patient may require assessment comparing their initial still, upright posture versus that of prolonged standing. This is particularly appropriate for the patient who complains of increased symptomatology with prolonged standing. In such cases, the clinician may observe dramatic postural changes occurring in the patient who initially appears to stand with significant stability and then gradually transitions to a relatively unstable posture. The patient may start to shift his or her weight in order to relieve symptoms or fatigue of postural muscles.

Still Upright Assessment: Posterior View

As previously stated, visual still, upright assessment begins from the posterior view. The goal is to assess the patient as if he or she were standing in as natural a stance as possible. To do this, the patient is instructed to march in place with high steps for 5–10 and then, when instructed, come to a sudden and abrupt halt. The purpose for this is that many patients with chronic pain syndrome and faulty postures are already aware of some of these faults. As such, they will tend to self-consciously correct their posture from their typical imbalance or asymmetry to one that would appear to be more aesthetically correct. If successful, the patient will finish the marching with the feet several inches apart and alongside each other (approximately 4–8 in (10–20 cm) apart, as too close together or too far apart affect lateral stability). The clinician must be sensitive to the patient's level of anxiety. Instruction should be provided in a calming manner, so that the patient is relaxed to avoid limbic system overactivation and any ensuing postural compromise.[4]

Still Upright Assessment: Global View

Janda[15,102] noted that a brief global assessment to determine the general state of the locomotor system should always initiate each view during visual assessment. This allows the clinician to take note of general clinical assessment topics also of specific regions that will require additional focus. This should include a general perspective of the postural age, the general degree of conditioning, muscular bulk and tone, erect stature, symmetry of motion, and smoothness of movement. During this period, the integration of prior findings during the history start to integrate with still, upright stance findings.

PELVIC VISUAL ASSESSMENT

Janda[15] stated that greatest immediate information from the static postural assessment comes from the pelvis, the transitional region between torso and lower extremities. Because of its unique morphology, it is capable of adapting in a variety of positions in order to optimize the transfer of loads and maintain functional stability in this strategic region. Specifically, there are six different positions of the pelvis that can be assessed:

1. *Anterior/posterior pelvic tilt:* This describes the rotation of the pelvis in the sagittal plane. Posterior tilting describes the posterior movement of the anterior superior iliac spine (ASIS) in relation to the pubes. Anterior pelvic tilting is the reverse. A neutral pelvic tilt is essentially half way between these two, and is considered physiological. The pelvic tilt can be assessed from the rear view, observing for a prominent buttocks and increased lumbar lordosis in the case of an anterior tilt and a somewhat flattened buttocks and lumbar spine when a posterior tilt is noted. The pelvic tilt is more effectively observed from the side view, which can help to confirm the findings.
2. *Lateral pelvic shift:* This describes the lateral translation of the pelvis. When present, the pelvis may be shifted over one foot or the torso will appear to be laterally shifted above the pelvis. It is often present in conjunction with pelvic obliquity, which is discussed next.
3. *Oblique pelvic tilt:* This describes one pelvic crest being higher on one side than the other. It is often found with a short leg syndrome, which can be either anatomical or functional.[145] This is best observed from the posterior view. It is often found in conjunction with a lateral pelvic tilt.
4. *Pelvic rotation:* This describes the anterior position of one side of the pelvis with the relative posterior position of the other side. This can be difficult to envision, so the following analogy may be of assistance. Imagine looking down on an axial view of the pelvic ring and relate that ring to the face of a clock. In the case of the left hemipelvis being relatively anterior and the right side being posterior, the pelvic ring would have moved from neutral position of the symphesis pubes at 12 o'clock toward 1 o'clock position. Because this is the same direction of movement that the hands of a clock follow, this would be considered *clockwise pelvic rotation*. In contrast, if the right hemipelvis is positioned anteriorly and the left posteriorly, then the symphesis would move toward 11 o'clock position or in a *counterclockwise pelvic rotation*.
5. *Pelvic torsion:* This describes hemipelvic rotation in the sagittal plane in one direction with the contralateral hemipelvic rotation in the opposite direction. The pivot point for this is the symphysis anteriorly, with sacro-iliac joints also being involved. Therefore, the relative position of one

posterior superior iliac crest (PSIS) may be quite different compared with its counterpart. Pelvic torsion is similar to pelvic tilting described above, in that it involves pelvic rotation in the sagittal plane. However, pelvic tilting involves the entire pelvis rotating as one unit, while pelvic torsion involves each innominate rotating in the opposite direction. Because of restrictions due to the symphysis and sacro-iliac joints, pelvic torsion is typically quite subtle and considered the most difficult pelvic observation. In addition to noting asymmetrical levels of the dimples that commonly approximate the SI joints, the clinician can also look for a relatively prominent buttock on one side versus a flattened buttock on the other side. As with all observations, assessment of the regional muscle bulk and past history can assist in determining how much weight to place on this finding.

6. *Anterior/posterior shift:* This describes the anterior or posterior translation of the pelvis along the sagittal plane. In contrast to pelvic tilting, pelvic shifting does not address rotation, but rather the simple movement of forward in relation to the feet and/or torso. Pelvic tilting can be observed from the posterior view, as the patient is slightly flexed at the waist with a posterior shift and slightly extended at the waist with an anterior shift. Like the pelvic tilt, the pelvic shift is more effectively assessed from the side view, which can help to confirm the findings.

Pelvic Visual Assessment Summary

Visual assessment of the pelvis provides a great deal of information regarding the postural system, including asymmetries, functional instability, and prior injuries. It is important to note that the six pelvic positions are for learning and descriptive purposes, but that pelvic distortion rarely, if ever, occurs in only one dimension. Therefore, a pelvis can demonstrate counterclockwise rotation, anterior tilting, lateral shifting, and obliquity.

Clinical Pearl: It is important to note that the six pelvic positions are for learning and descriptive purposes, but that pelvic distortion rarely, if ever, occurs in only one dimension.

FOOT/ANKLE VISUAL ASSESSMENT

There are four key points to assess for the feet and ankles:

1. *Internal/external rotation:* The feet should be slightly externally rotated, perhaps 5–10 degrees under physiological circumstances. The clinician, if positioned directly behind the patient can usually see the fifth and perhaps the fourth digits from this perspective. This vantage point makes it easy to determine external rotation, as more toes are in view, whereas no toes are visible during internal rotation.
2. *Pronation versus supination:* The neutral position of the foot is physiological. With pronation, the foot rolls medially, which can be seen with the superior aspect of the heel angled medially. This is an important point, as pronation affects foot loading and the ability to effectively propel forward during gait.[146,147] Another sign is the navicular bone, located slightly anterior and inferior to the medial malleolus, becomes prominent as it flares out with pronation. Foot supination is noted when the superior aspect of the heel is angled laterally.

   Foot pronation also tends to cause a functional shortening of the leg.[15] Asymmetrical pronation can occur in conjunction with the low side of an oblique pelvic tilt. Conversely, a pronation may balance the pelvis if the leg on that side is anatomically longer than the other. To clarify whether an asymmetrical pronation is affecting pelvic leveling, Janda devised a very practical test. The patient is instructed to stand on the outside, or fifth ray, of each foot. This maneuver removes the plantar arches from the equation, providing a truer picture of the leg length and degree of pelvic obliquity (see Fig. 13–7). Of course, the knees must be assessed for symmetrical positioning also.
3. *Medial versus lateral deviation of the ankle:* Neutral position of the ankle is physiological. Medial ankle deviation is typically associated with the foot pronation, whereas lateral ankle deviation is with foot supination.
4. *Relative tension of the Achilles tendon:* Achilles tendon tension, determined by its shape, can provide information regarding the posture in the sagittal plane. Relatively speaking, the shape under it in physiological circumstances is that of a "U." When the patient's posture is "forward drawn," that is when the center of mass is anterior to the midfoot, there is increased tension on the Achilles tendon as the gastroc/soleus complex must maintain compensatory equilibrium. In this event, the Achilles shape slightly alters in its contour, taking on a "V" shape. Conversely, the patient who is "posteriorly drawn," that is with the center of mass behind the midfoot ("on their heels"), requires less gastroc/soleus activity. As such, the Achilles tendon in this instance slightly alters in its contour with a block ("LI") shape.

Is Weight Bearing Symmetrical? The clinician can typically determine visually whether there is greater

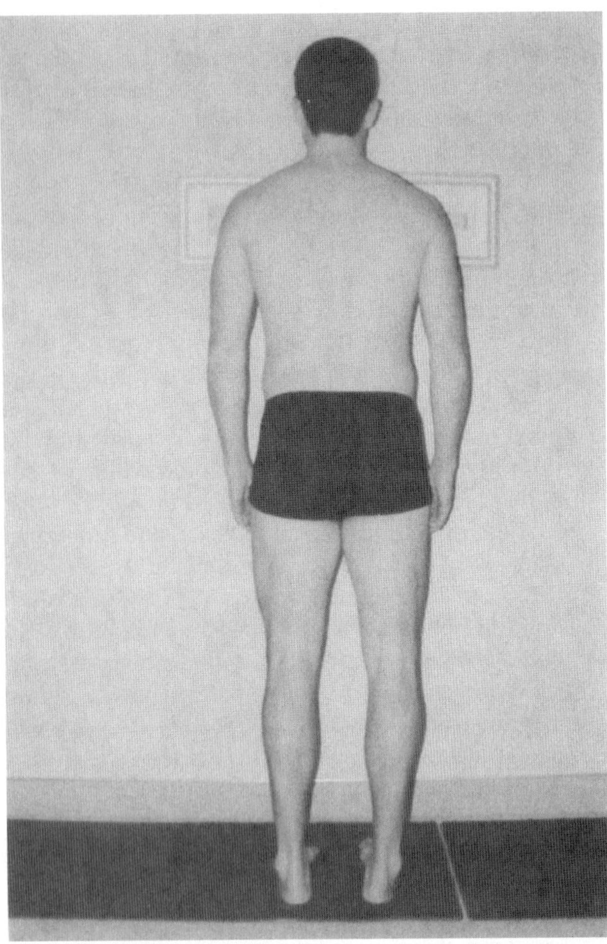

FIGURE 13–7. Fifth ray maneuver: This helps to rule out a functional short leg caused by an asymmetrical foot pronation. Secondarily, the degree of internal rotation of the feet is a quick test for hyper- or hypomobility.

weight bearing on one leg, if the difference is significant. However, it is good to confirm suspected weight imbalance withith objective measures, which also helps to improve observational reliability. Standing on two sets of calibrated scales can offer evidence of excessive one-sided stance. Lewit[135] suggests that if there is uneven weight distribution (more than 8 lb/4 kg) and if there is a leg length inequality, a heel wedge should be used on the short-leg side to evaluate whether this allows better weight distribution to be achieved.

CALF VISUAL ASSESSMENT

There are two topics of assessment with regard to the calf:

1. *The soleus muscle:* A muscle that spans only the ankle joint, the soleus is assessed one third of the way up the calf between the heel and knee. It should be assessed for tone and bulk in relation with the contralateral soleus. Asymmetrical soleus hypertrophy suggests overuse of the muscle, which can be found when additional foot dorsiflexion is used *with the knee flexed* to aid in forward propulsion during gait. This can occur when gastrocnemius function is decreased (see Fig. 13–8).

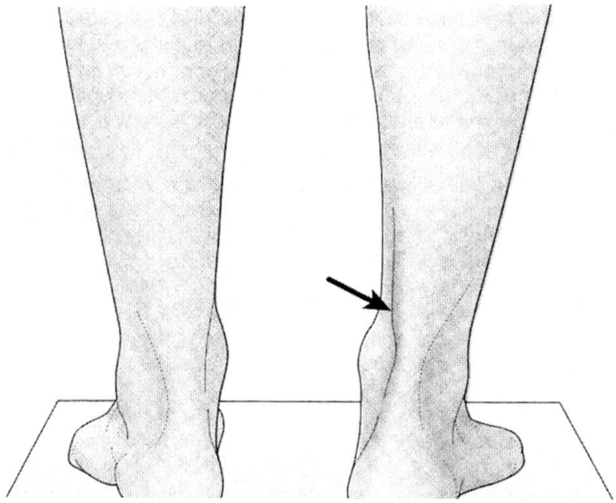

FIGURE 13–8. Hypertonic soleus: The Achilles tendons present with a more hour-glass shape and the soleus belly typically is more developed than its mate. (*Reprinted with permission from Tunnell*[153].)

2. *The gastrocnemius muscle:* A two-joint muscle that crosses the ankle and knee, the gastrocnemius should be assessed two third of the way up the calf between the heel and knee. It should be assessed for tone and bulk in relation with the contralateral gastrocnemius. Asymmetrical gastrocnemius hypertrophy suggests overuse of the muscle, which can be found when additional foot dorsiflexion is used to aid in forward propulsion *with the knee extended* during gait. This can occur when soleus function is decreased. A rare finding of medial gastrocnemius atrophy strongly suggests an S1 root lesion (see Fig. 13–9).

Knee Visual Assessment

The knee should be assessed for the following:

1. *Flexion and extension:* The knee should be slightly flexed, perhaps 1–2 degrees. This allows the knee to flex and the quadriceps to be reactive to sudden postural changes and loads, while directing the majority of load down through the adjacent long bones. Increased flexion requires additional quadriceps energy expenditures, which is uneconomic. An extended knee places increased axial loading on the knee joint and also provides end-range loading. Furthermore, the knee locked in

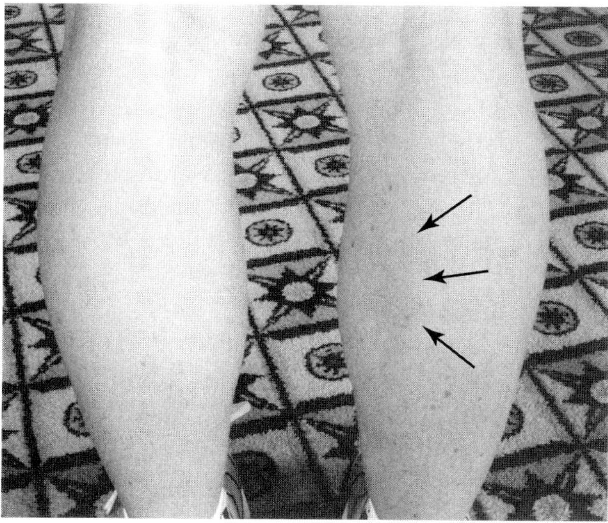

FIGURE 13–9. Significant subtleties: Atrophy of the medial gastrocnemius, as noted on the right side, may indicate a latent radiculopathy. Such findings should be investigated.

extension is poorly prepared for sudden loading, which leaves the end-range-loaded joint at risk of injury.

2. *Varus and valgus deformity:* The knee should be straight. Medial deviation of the knee is called valgus deformity, while lateral deviation is called varus. With a valgus deformity weight bearing is displaced laterally and there is greater stress on the medial collateral ligament, the lateral meniscus, and the joint surface of the lateral tibial and fibular condyles. With varus deformity there is medial weight-bearing deviation and stresses increase on the lateral collateral ligaments, and the medial meniscus and the joint surface of the medial tibial and fibular condyles[148] (see Fig. 13–10).

Thigh Assessment

There are two key aspects to assess with regard to the thigh:

1. *Hamstrings:* The hamstrings should be assessed one third of the way up from the knee to the buttocks. Bulk, contour, and relative tone should be assessed and compared with the opposite thigh.
2. *Adductors:* A slight indentation at one point along the adductors is commonly found bilaterally. This is typically a point of insertion of hypertonic tissue, which is tender on later palpation. Adductor notches are rarely observed at the same level, or are generally found to be more pronounced (i.e., a deeper notch) and more superiorly located (i.e., closer to the torso). This notch suggests a greater degree of hypertonicity.

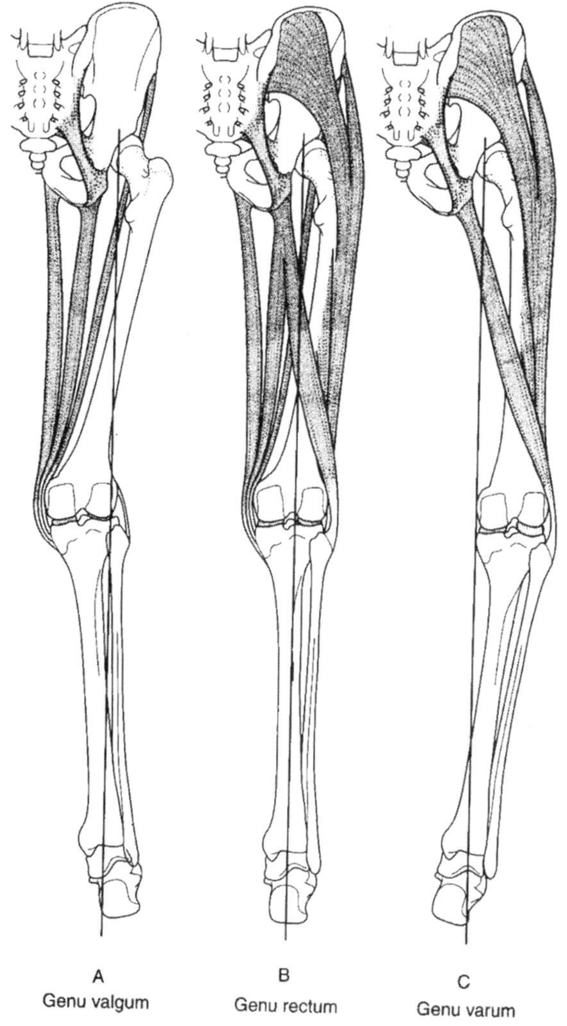

FIGURE 13–10. Knee: *A.* In genu valgus, or knock-kneed, the weight-bearing line is displaced (see plumb lines) laterally, placing additional stress on the medial collateral ligament and the lateral meniscus. *B.* A normal leg/knee alignment. *C.* genu varum (bow-legged). Genu varum causes the weight bearing line to be displaced medially, loading the lateral collateral ligament and also the medial meniscus. (*Reprinted with permission, from Chaitow L. Clinical Applications of Neuromuscular Therapy. Vol 2 (lower body). Churchill Livingstone 2002.*)

Pelvic Assessment

There are four topics of observation with regard to the pelvis, in addition to those issues previously discussed regarding pelvic positioning:

1. *Pelvic motion:* No obvious motion of the pelvis during still stance should be present. However, Mok et al.[149] found poor hip strategy control among patients with chronic low back pain compared with an asymptomatic control group, suggesting pelvic motion may be a significant finding.
2. *The upper outer quadrant of the buttocks:* Janda[15] considered this the most reliable region to assess

the gluteus maximus. A muscular, rounded buttock is considered physiological, while a flattened contour suggests relative weakness and atrophy. It should be compared with the contralateral buttock.

3. *The inferior aspect of the buttocks:* The inferior aspect of the buttock should be assessed. A relatively flabby buttock that hangs lower than its counterpart suggests gluteus maximus relative weakness and atrophy. The findings of the upper outer quadrant and the inferior aspect of the buttocks should be consistent. Additionally any asymmetry in regard to the relative depth and height of the gluteal folds (lower margins of buttocks) may relate to iliac (pelvic) distortion. Clinical experience suggests that an anteriorly rotated ilium elevates and reduces the depth of the ipsilateral fold, whereas a posteriorly rotated ilium increases the depth of the fold. Finally, a unilateral hypotonic or atrophied buttock suggests an ipsilateral sacro-iliac dysfunction due to arthrogenic inhibition of that joint.[78,150]
4. *Coccygeal alignment:* Does the contour of the coccyx continue that of the sacrum? And does it align with the rest of the spine? Deviations are suggestive of local trauma.

Lower Lumbar Spine Visual Assessment

The lower lumbar region should be observed for the following:

1. *Paraspinal muscular development:* The lumbopelvic paraspinal musculature should be bilaterally well developed, with appropriate bulk on each side of the spine, forming a longitudinal crease. The degree of bulk and the depth of the crease should be relatively uniform as it continues superiorly toward the thoracic region.
2. *Horizontal grooves:* A lateral groove that interrupts the continuum of paraspinal muscle bulk is considered a pathological finding. This may be unilateral or bilateral, often noted at slightly different segmental levels when bilateral. Janda noted that this finding suggested atrophy of the multifidus.[15] This was supported decades later by electromyographic findings that demonstrated decreased multifidus activity among patients with low back pain.[151]
3. *Lordosis*: The lumbar lordosis should be relatively uniform throughout the region. A sudden hollowing of the lordosis at one segmental level suggests poor antagonistic activity of the stabilizing abdominals.
   (a) A loss of lordosis is suggestive of a functional pathology.
   (b) The degree of lordosis will typically be consistent with the degree of pelvic tilting, with an anterior pelvic tilt found with an increased lumbar lordosis and a posterior pelvic tilt with a decreased lordosis. If this *lumbopelvic relationship* is not present, then it is a strong indication of a lumbar *or* pelvic region functional pathology. For example, a patient with a neutral pelvis and lumbar hyperlordosis suggests a muscle imbalance, with increased activity of the lumbar erector spinae and decreased activity of the abdominals.

Clinical Pearl: If this *lumbopelvic relationship* is not present, then it is a strong indication of a lumbar *or*pelvic region functional pathology.

4. *Lateral curvature:* Lateral deviation is suggestive of curvature. The side of deviation, when present, will typically be toward the low iliac crest. If this is not the case, then either there is a structural deformity with asymmetry causing the spine to deviate toward the high ilium, or there has been an error in the assessment.
5. *Flank contour:* The relative degree of obesity should be assessed in relation to the contour of the flank or lateral aspects of the abdomen. A lean person should have bilaterally linear flanks. Increased rounding suggests poor activation of the intrinsic or core musculature, especially the transversus abdominis. In the presence of scoliosis or pelvic distortion, the flank may be asymmetrical. This can be magnified in the presence of obesity as horizontal folds may be asymmetrically present at differing levels.

Thoracolumbar Region Visual Assessment

In the thoracolumbar region, it is important to visually assess the following:

1. *Paraspinal musculature:* The development should be bilaterally equal and comparable with the lower lumbar region. Asymmetrical bilateral development or significantly greater bulk compared to lumbar paraspinal musculature suggests functional pathology. According to Janda[15] relative overdevelopment of the thoracolumbar erecter spinae suggests compensatory overload due to functional instability, typically in the lumbopelvic region. Janda[150] noted that excessive development of the thoracolumbar erector spinae musculature is likely to be associated with gluteus maximus inhibition, which was later described by others[152,153] (see Fig. 13–11).

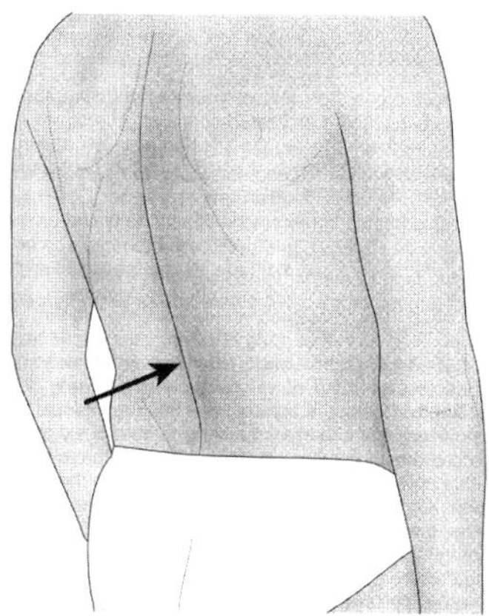

FIGURE 13–11. Thoracolumbar crease: Should be relatively deep, with well-developed paraspinal musculature evenly placed bilaterally and extending up from the lumbosacral region. Paraspinal hypertrophy suggests overload, possibly due to lumbosacral functional instability. (*Reprinted with permission from Tunnell*[153].)

2. *Lordosis or kyphosis:* There should be little, if any lordosis or kyphosis in this transitional area.
3. *Lateral curvature:* Lateral deviation of the crease formed by the paraspinal musculature is suggestive of lateral curvature. If present, it should be noted whether this continues to deviate laterally from the lumbar spine below or toward the midline, as a compensatory curve.
4. *Lower rib position:* The distance between the lower ribs and the crests of the pelvis should be symmetrical. If not this may indicate altered rib positioning, pes excavatum, scoliosis, ipsilateral shortness of quadratus lumborum and/or latissimus dorsi, and/or pelvic obliquity or inequality of leg length.
5. *Symmetry of rib excursion on inhalation:* There should be an even degree of rib excursion observable on inhalation. If no rib restrictions are present, soft tissue changes may be impeding free movement.

Middle Thoracic Spine Visual Assessment

While not part of the lower half visual assessment, there are key findings in the upper half that either affect or support lower half observations. These are as follows:

1. *Shoulder level:* Uneven shoulder levels suggest spinal curvature, asymmetry, and/or increased postural loading. It supports earlier findings of a pelvic asymmetry, in addition to lateral curvature in the thoracic and/or lumbar regions.
2. *Scapula position:* Uni-or bilateral elevation of the scapula(e) may result from excessive tone in upper trapezius and/or levator scapula, and/or weakness of the lower fixators of the shoulder, as in the upper crossed syndrome discussed earlier. Scapula winging may also be evident.
3. *Arm position:* The arm should ideally fall to the sides with the elbows pointing posteriorly and the palms medially. Internal (i.e., medial) arm rotation suggests hypertonicity of the latissimus dorsi, suggestive of low back functional instability. When present, the elbows typically point outward and the palms posteriorly. The clinician must be careful, however, to look for a significant valgus deviation at the elbow, which has been observed more often in women than in men. Patients with valgus elbows often pronate their forearms to keep them closer to the body. This posterior palm position presents a false-positive finding for hypertonic latissimus dorsi. Other reasons for excessive pronation may include hypertonicity of pectoralis major, teres major, or subscapularis. Conversely if there is excessive supination (i.e., external or lateral rotation of the arm) the supinator muscles and biceps brachii may have shortened. Again, these can be confirmed with additional observational viewpoints (i.e., side view or front view) and/or palpation.

STILL, UPRIGHT VISUAL ASSESSMENT: (CORONAL) SIDE VIEW

The lateral view provides new assessment information from the added dimension, while also supplying confirmatory observations that were not fully determined from the posterior view. Key points to assess for are as follows:

1. *The plumb line:* In a patient with a neutral posture, the external auditory meatus should be over the summit of the shoulder, which should be over the middle of the hip joint and over the mid foot.
2. *Stability:* There should be no visible sway in the A–P plane from the lateral perspective.

Feet

Key points to look for with regard to the feet in the lateral view:

1. *Weight over midfoot:* Under physiological conditions, the center of body mass should be over the mid-foot.
2. *Weight over forefoot:* The center of mass shifts forward-when there is a physiologically stressful forward drawn posture. The gastrocnemius and/or soleus are typically tight and hypertrophic because of the overactivity associated with maintaining equilibrium when the center of mass has shifted forward. The gastrocnemius will be more

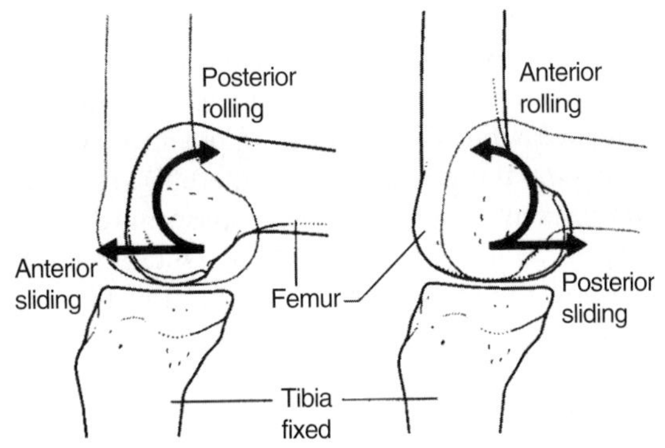

FIGURE 13–12. Tibiofibular sliding: The rolling motion of the femoral condyles during knee flexion and knee extension. (*From Levangie and Norkin*[154].)

affected when the patient's knees are straight, with the soleus more involved when the knees are flexed. The degree of forward sway is greater than posterior sway due to the relatively long levers of the feet.

3. *Weight over rear foot:* As the center of mass shifts posteriorly, the weight shifts to the rear foot. There is less musculature activity with this strategy, as the body weight extends down through the talus and calcaneus. However, postural stability will be compromised, partly because of reduced proprioceptive input, and the individual is at an increased risk of falling backward if perturbed. The knees are usually hyperextended with this posture, creating increased stress for the knee joints and soft tissues, particularly the menisci[154] (see Fig. 13–12).

Knees

Key points to visually assess for in the side view for the knees:

1. *Position:* The knees should be in a neutral position, neither flexed nor locked in hyperextension. This allows for optimal muscular control and balance, utilizing an economical strategy that allows the majority of upper body weight to transfer down the shafts of the femurs to the lower extremities.
2. *Flexion:* Increased knee flexion can occur bilaterally or unilaterally. It is usually noteworthy because this postural strategy is not economical, requiring additional muscular exertion to maintain equilibrium. Therefore, there should be a logical reason why the body has chosen this postural compromise despite its faults. Unilateral knee flexion can occur due to a short leg syndrome, as the knee of the longer leg flexes to level the pelvis. Flexion can suggest a strategy for unloading a painful knee joint, which can occur unilaterally or bilaterally. It can also occur due to a unilateral painful condition elsewhere in the lower extremity, hip or pelvis, as knee flexion reduces the loading on that side and transfers it to the opposite limb. Knee flexion will typically coincide with hypertrophy of the ipsilateral quadriceps and, to a lesser degree, hamstring.
3. *Hyperextension:* Hyperextension, or locking of the knee, suggests many possible scenarios. In contrast with knee flexion, this strategy can reduce the muscular exertion required in still, upright posture, as body weight can be transferred down through the locked knee via an osteo-ligamentous strategy ("i.e., resting on their ligaments"). Unfortunately, this locked maneuver tends to place the knee joint at risk for sudden perturbations, as there is no adaptive joint play to counter sudden changes in center of body mass. Also, the shock absorbing capacity of the limb, hip, and pelvis is compromised, as the flexible knee is lost in the hyperextended position, increasing risk of ground force-related trauma. This is also present with weakness due to a host of etiologies, such as neurological disease, muscle-wasting disease, deconditioning, hypermobility, and aging. Unilaterally, it can suggest a painless knee condition that left the knee weakened.

Thighs

There are three key points to visually assess for the thighs:

1. *Position of the thigh:* The thighs should be vertical. If they are not, then this is often due to dysfunction from the regions below (i.e., feet, ankles, knees) or above (i.e., hips and pelvis).
2. *Iliotibial band (ITB) groove (or crease):* The ITB should not be typically prominent in women because of a relatively greater subdermal adipose layer and lesser degree of muscular development compared to men. Of course, the above statement is generic, so body type and degree of conditioning are mediating factors for both sexes. With men, a more prominent ITB is not unusual, although it should not be too deeply entrenched either.
3. *Muscular development:* The relative muscular development of the thigh musculature can provide vital information to determine the relative strength and symmetry anterior to posterior and inferior to superior.

Pelvis

Two of the six pelvic alterations can be well visualized from the side: the pelvic tilt and the pelvic shift.

1. *Anterior versus posterior pelvic tilt:* This was previously described as the rotation of the pelvis in the sagittal plane. A posterior pelvic tilt involves the PSIS in relatively close proximity to the lower

lumbar spine and posterior to the pubis. The relative position of the PSIS with an anterior pelvic tilt is just the opposite. From the side, a posterior pelvic tilt has a decreased contour of the buttock and flattened lumbar lordosis and abdomen. Conversely, the anterior pelvic tilt demonstrates a more prominent buttocks, increased lumbar lordosis, and rounded abdomen. This combination of findings for the anterior pelvic tilt is consistent with the lower crossed syndrome described before in this chapter. Schafer[155] reported that an anterior pelvic tilt may involve, or be the result of, a combination of weak hamstrings, weak abdominal muscles, or both, combined with excessive tone in the hip flexors, rectus femoris, and lumbar extensors.

2. *Anterior versus posterior pelvic shift:* This was previously described as the forward or backward translation of the pelvis in the sagittal plane and in relation to the rest of the body. The anterior pelvic shift is more common than the posterior shift because it can provide added postural stability with decreased muscular exertion and also provide additional proprioceptive information as the anterior thigh/hip tissues are tensioned. From the lateral perspective, the patient with an anteriorly shifted pelvis will present with locked knees, a forward pelvis, a rounded lower abdomen, and a receding upper abdomen as the thorax is relatively posterior to maintain postural equilibrium.

Lumbar Spine

Key point to visually assess for in the lumbar spine:

1. *The relative lordosis:* The lumbopelvic relationship described earlier comes into play here. The degree of pelvic tilt or shift should be consistent with the degree of lumbar lordosis. Therefore, an anterior pelvic tilt and a pronounced lumbar lordosis would be consistent. A neutral pelvic tilt and a moderate lordosis would be both consistent and physiological. A sharp angle at the apex of the lordosis would be faulty, as the contours should be gradual. Finally, the bulk of the buttocks should be assessed, as greater bulk can create the illusion of increased lordosis.

Abdomen

Key point to visually assess for in the abdomen:

1. *The degree of rounding versus flattening of the abdomen:* The abdomen should be relatively flat along the anterior and lateral surfaces in the lean patient under physiological circumstances. Janda[131] observed that the rectus abdominis and transversus abdominis can become compromised with the lower crossed syndrome, with the abdomen appearing relatively rounded in appearance.

Thoracic Spine

Key issue to visually assess for in the thoracic spine:

1. *The degree of kyphosis:* Like the lumbopelvic relationship, the thoracolumbar relationship is believed to determine the degree of thoracic kyphosis.

STILL, UPRIGHT VISUAL ASSESSMENT: ANTERIOR VIEW

The anterior still, upright postural visual assessment is often largely a matter of confirmation of findings from the previous perspectives. As should be obvious, a great deal of information can be gleaned from the posterior still, upright postural assessment with the anterior view offering confirmation and a few additional clues. The key areas that should be visually assessed from the anterior perspective are discussed below:

Clinical Pearl: The anterior still, upright postural visual assessment is often largely a matter of confirmation of findings from the previous perspectives.

Feet

Key issues to visually assess for in the feet and ankles:

1. *Internal versus external rotation:* This has been discussed above. It is more easily seen from the front, as the posterior foot and ankle block the rear view. Marked toeing out of the foot (external rotation) is commonly associated with hypertonic external hip rotators, gluteus maximus, and, to a lesser extent, the iliopsoas, and usually implies relative weakness of the medial hip rotators. Marked toeing in (internal rotation) of the foot suggests the possibility of excessive tone in tensor fascia latae, or the anterior fibers of gluteus medius and minimus, together with weakness of the lateral hip rotators.
2. *Pronation versus supination:* This was also discussed above, although the anterior view of the medial arches and medial translation of the navicular bone can at times be better visualized from the front, especially when the feet are externally rotated.
3. *Great toe position:* The hallux should be straight, with the weight loaded evenly across the pad that forms the distal plantar surface. A valgus deformity is often seen in relation to pronation of the ipsilateral foot as the medial portion of the hallux is forced to bear increased loading to maintain equilibrium. However, high-heeled shoes with a small, pointed toe box can provoke valgus deformity.

4. *Position of second through fifth toes:* The four toes should be slightly flexed as they meet the floor in a balanced manner. Increased toe flexion, or clawed toes, provides a greater mechanical advantage for weight bearing when foot mechanics are faulty and additional loading is applied to the lateral forefoot.

Shins

Key aspects to observe with regard to the lower leg:

1. *Tibial bowing:* The tibial shaft should be relatively straight, which aids in maintaining equilibrium. Tibial bowing is typically associated with a varus deformity of the knee, which can be either unilateral or bilateral. Because the tibia rotates internally and externally during the various phases of gait, the torsional forces of tibial bowing represent an additional locomotor challenge.
2. *Atrophy of the anterior tibialis:* The tibialis anterior muscle is strongly innervated by the L5 root. As such, neural compromise at that level can profoundly affect gait due to the classic loss of dorsiflexion during the swing phase of gait called "foot drop." In such a case, tibialis anterior atrophy will occur, bringing a hollowed appearance of the anterior lower leg just lateral to the tibial shaft.
3. *The angle at which the tibia meets the femur:* A line drawn from the ASIS to the middle of the patella and another line drawn from the tibial tuberosity, extending through the patella, bisect each other. An angle (*Q* angle) of 10–15 degrees is considered normal. Women frequently have an increased *Q* angle due to greater width of pelvic structures. If the angle is greater than 15 degrees there is an increased danger of patella dysfunction[156] (see Fig. 13–13).

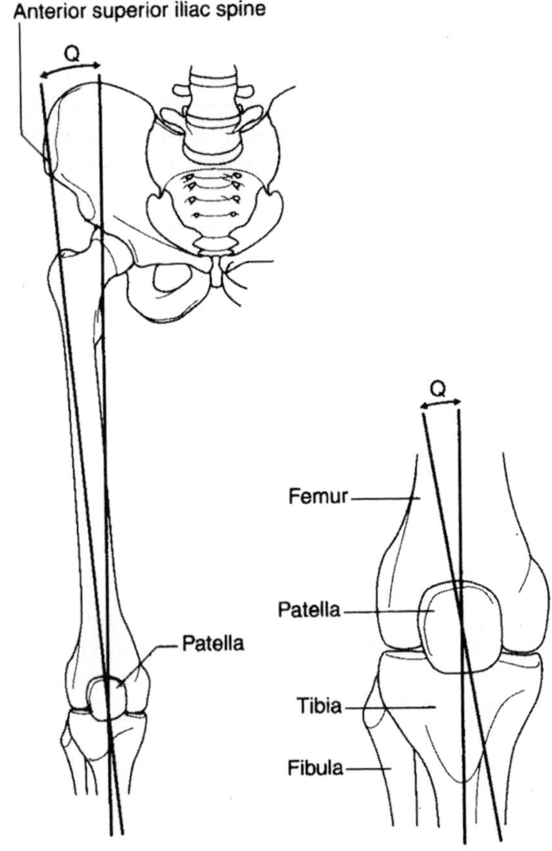

FIGURE 13–13. Quadriceps angle (*Q* angle): This describes the angle of the thigh as it extends from the hip joint. It is determined by measuring the angle of the intersection of lines bisecting at the center of the patella, one of which continues up through the ASIS, while the other continues down through the tibial tuberosity. An angle of 10–15 degrees is considered normal. (*After Cailliet*[156].)

Knees

We have already discussed the visual assessment of the knees from the posterior and lateral view. The anterior view is therefore largely, although not exclusively, confirmatory. Key aspects to observe from the front should include the following:

1. *Sagittal plane position:* The position of the knees has already been discussed. A locked knee is hyperextended, while a flexed knee demonstrated a prominent patella.
2. *Transverse plane position:* This has already been discussed from the posterior view, and a rectus, varus, or valgus position should be confirmed from the front.
3. *Patellar position:* The patella should be centered in the patellar groove, which cannot be visualized from behind or the side. Medial translation is called "patellar squinting," which suggests overactivity of the thigh muscles that insert in the medial aspect of the patella. The patella is housed within the fibrous patellar pouch, which can shorten in the medial portion, drawing the patella medially. The patella can also translate laterally, with overactivity of the lateral muscles of the thigh. Excess tone in the quadriceps can pull a patella cephalad. Any of these patella deviations may involve altered patella tracking on movement, and this may lead to erosion of the patellofemoral surface, instability of the patello-femoral joint, and pain.[157]
4. *Definition/development of the vastus medialis oblique:* The vastus medialis oblique (VMO) is a comprised of the vastus medialis, the gracilis and the sartorius, in addition to the fascia that blends the

muscles together. The quadriceps, specially the VMO, is known to atrophy following trauma to the neighboring knee joint, especially of the anterior cruciate ligament, because of reflex inhibition.[158–160] Kapandji[161] observed that relative imbalance between the more powerful vastus lateralis and the prone-to-atrophy medialis allows the patella to "escape" laterally, a possible mechanism involved in recurrent dislocation.

Thighs

Visual assessment of the thighs from the anterior perspective should include the following:

1. *Development of the quadriceps:* Muscle development of the quadriceps should be assessed bilaterally. It should be compared with the relative degree of development with other regional muscle groups. It can also be assessed in relation to the knee position, in that a flexed knee tends to increase quadriceps activity and cause a relative hypertrophy. Conversely, the routinely locked knee in still, upright stance will lead to decreased quadriceps development.
2. *Adductor notching:* Adductor notching, a sign of overactivity of the single joint muscles of this group, was previously described from the posterior view. It can also be confirmed from the front perspective.

Pelvis

Assessment of the pelvis from the anterior perspective should include the following:

1. *Confirmation of pelvic findings observed from previous views:* For example, is there symmetry between left and right, and are the iliac crests, and the ASIS level?
2. *Pelvic tilt:* As stated earlier, a relationship exists between the contour of the lumbar region and also the abdomen. This was referred to as the *pelvic–torso relationship*. A patient with an anterior pelvic tilt tends to have a slightly creased and hollowed contour at the junction of the torso and thighs. A relatively rounded abdomen is also noted, which is somewhat of an illusion because it is makes the patient appear more obese than is the case. This façade occurs as the torso arises from the pelvis anteriorly.

Abdominals

Anterior view of the abdominals is important and can provide important information. Important assessment findings can include the following:

1. *Physiological features:* The abdomen should be relatively flat under physiological circumstances. In a lean patient, shallow longitudinal creases along the either side of the rectus abdominis demonstrate the underlying morphology, which can be less prominent with a mild degree of overlying adipose tissue. The abdomen should protrude with inspiration as the diaphragm lowers and abdominal contents are in turn displaced. Conversely, the abdominal contour withdraws with expiration as the diaphragm retreats superiorly and the abdominal contents are directed to pre-inspiration position by the tone of the musculature of the abdominal wall and pelvic floor.
2. *Rounded abdomen:* A rounded abdominal contour suggests poor muscle tone of key abdominal muscles, excessive adipose tissue, or a combination of each. Anteriorly, the rectus abdominis, obliques, and transversus abdominis musculature affect this contour, with the rectus having the greatest mechanical advantage in retaining the anterior wall of the group and the transversus on the lateral contours or flank. If present, the degree of obesity versus degree of anterior convexity should be relatively assessed for consistency.

   There are conditions that affect abdominal tone. For example, postsurgical adhesive scar tissue (see Fig. 13–14) and umbilical hernia (in which the bulging umbilicus looks like the yolk of a poached egg) can interfere with abdominal tone and lead to a rounded appearance. It is believed that a diastasis recti can lead to the same result, and that all of these scenarios compromise the normal function of the pressurized canister, or core, for lumbopelvic stability.[162]
3. *Grooves bilateral to the rectus abdominis muscle:* Theses creases should be present, but shallow, in a lean patient under physiological conditions. Janda[131] observed that this indicates overactivity of the external obliques—a sign of poor lumbopelvic stability. Ng et al.[151] provided electromyographic support for these observations decades later (see Fig. 13–15).
4. *Contour of the flank:* The lateral aspects of the abdomen should be observed. There should be a slight concavity at the midpoint between rib cage and pelvis because of the muscular activity of the abdominal wall. This concave contour is considered to be an important sign of transversus abdominis activity, as this deep muscle is the only one of the abdominal wall muscles that has the mechanical advantage to hollow the flank. (The oblique musculature can of course draw in a convex contoured abdomen, but only to a point of being in line with the ribs and pelvis since these points represent their origin and insertion.) If present, the

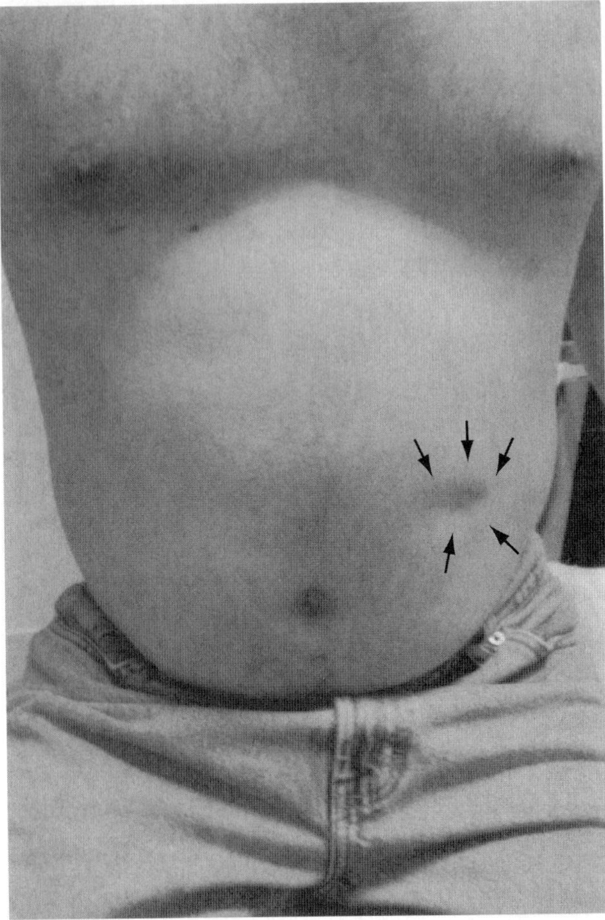

FIGURE 13–14. Rounded abdomen: In a relatively lean individual, this suggests inhibition of the transversus abdominis and a compromise of the "inner unit" of lumbopelvic stability. In this case, adhesive postsurgical scar from a gastric tube is believed to be the culprit. Other causes are believed to include diastasis recti, abdominal hernia, umbilical hernia, and inguinal hernia. (The patient in this photo developed a diastasis recti several months after this photo was taken.)

degree of obesity versus degree of flank convexity should be relatively assessed for consistency.

5. *Abdominal versus thoracic respiration:* The absence of abdominal excursion and incursion during respiration suggests decreased diaphragmatic activity. The mechanism of such altered function remains poorly understood, although emerging research supports this finding and correlates this with poor core function.[74] (The topic of diaphragmatic activity in lumbopelvic functional stability was addressed more thoroughly in Chapter 5.) Because of the body's ongoing demand for oxygen, a secondary locomotor strategy must arise to allow for pulmonary expansion. In the absence of sufficient diaphragm activity, thoracic respiration must then predominate. This requires a recurrent increase in thoracic circumferential caliber, thoracic elevation, or a combination of each. Respiratory rate is also likely to increase[3,163] with significant effects on global pH because of respiratory alkalosis,[164,165] altered balance efficiency,[166] modification of motor control,[167] and less efficient core stability.[65,168] Therefore, the lack of respiratory abdominal motion and increased thoracic respiration is a significant, positive finding, and should be keenly investigated.

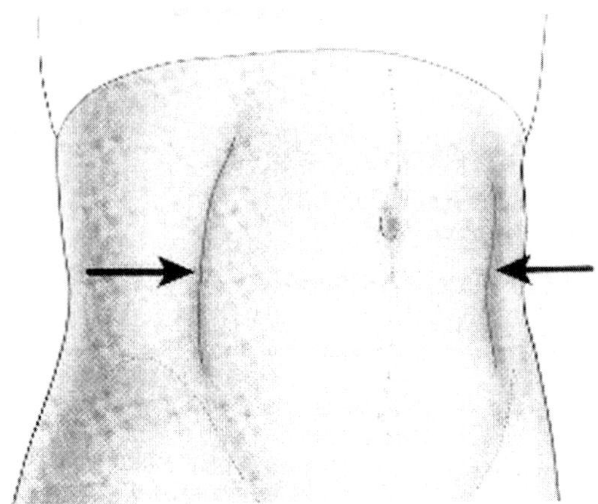

FIGURE 13–15. Abdominal oblique groove: A shallow groove on each side of the rectus abdominis is considered normal, while a deep groove is considered a sign of abdominis oblique overactivity and abdominis rectus weakness. (*Reprinted with permission from Tunnell*[153].)

Thorax

Thoracic assessment is technically beyond the scope of this chapter. Nevertheless, some brief points regarding this anatomically neighboring region will be addressed in order to provide a more complete summary of the lower region.

1. *Symmetrical breast development in women:* The importance of the assessment of morphological symmetry has already been discussed in the assessment process. Asymmetrical breast development among women can provide an important support in this process.
2. *Symmetrical pectoral development:* Pectoral development can also assist in determining the degree of morphological asymmetry, although the lead author considered this as less reliable than breast asymmetry because of a number of events that can influence the muscular hypertrophy or atrophy of these scapular protractors. A slight degree of increased development is typical for the dominant hand, or of habitual overuse patterns.

3. *Clavicular elevation during respiration:* Clavicular elevation during inspiration is a sign of thoracic respiration ("upper chest breathing") and suggestive of faulty diaphragmatic respiration. Increased clavicular elevation suggests overactivity of the secondary respiratory muscles, such as the scaleni, which should assist in respiration during times of increased oxygen demand as with exercise. As such, a synergistic substitution occurs with faulty diaphragmatic respiration and the scaleni become activated and clavicles elevate during regular respiration in the absence of increased oxygen demand. This is considered to be a significant visual finding.
4. *Unequal excursion of rib cage during respiration:* Observation of asymmetrical rib excursion may relate to pleural adhesions or rib restrictions.
5. *Internal versus external rotation of the arms:* This was previously discussed from the posterior view. The anterior view can nevertheless provide a confirmatory perspective.

By the time still, upright assessment is completed, the clinician should have confirmed the significantly positive findings. This information, along with the negative findings, should then be integrated within the existing body of information from the history in order to further clarify the clinical picture. In so doing, the differential diagnosis receives greater support, as the march toward the clinical impression proceeds.

Table 13–2 provides a check-off sheet for still, upright assessment. While some clinicians may wish to use this in the clinic for charting their findings, it is suggested that this simply be used until the clinician becomes familiar with each key point. In so doing, time is saved and the clinician gains valuable skills in observing posture in a more global manner.

FUNCTIONAL TESTS ASSOCIATED WITH STILL, UPRIGHT POSTURAL ASSESSMENT

ONE-LEGGED STANCE

Janda[169] stated that assessment of the patient standing on one foot is very logical, since only about 15% of the gait cycle occurs on two feet. The one-legged stance is a practical test that can be performed as part of the visual assessment. It is used to assess the stability of the postural system. It is a challenge of the proprioceptive and labyrinthine systems, with additional information deriving from visual input. With the eyes closed, the visuomotor system function is withdrawn so that balance can be assessed without this aid.[102]

Clinical Pearl: The one-legged stance is a practical test that can be performed as part of the visual assessment. It is used to assess the stability of the postural system.

Bullock-Saxton[92] demonstrated that lower limb function remained compromised in individuals with a prior history of ankle sprain versus a control group. The measured variables of this study included the one-legged stance test, which was compromised in the ankle sprain group, suggesting faults in the afferent feedback. Various adaptive strategies occur as the unstable patient attempts to maintain equilibrium on one leg. The most common of these being use of the ankle mortise so that a positive test often occurs with marked foot and ankle motion.[170]

One-Legged Stance with Eyes Open The one-legged stance with eyes open provides a safe screening test for the patient. The practicality and popularity of this test are evident by the fact that several authors have evaluated it and determined a variety of "normal" results. Unfortunately, this variety can lead the clinician to be more confused as to what constitutes a true, positive finding. In addition to the recommendations below, more is given about the one-foot standing test in Chapter 14.

- Purpose: To practically assess the patient's functional ability to maintain a stable posture, especially in the transverse plane, while standing on one foot with the eyes open. Also, this test serves as baseline measure for functional stability of the next sequential test, the one-legged stance with eyes closed. Finally, this is a screening test to determine whether the patient can *safely* perform more demanding balance testing or sensorimotor training (see Chapter 28).
- *Patient's position:* The patient stands with the arms resting at the side.
- *Clinician's position:* Standing behind the patient with both hands prepared to catch the patient in case he or she loses balance and starts to fall.
- *Clinician's instruction:* The patient is instructed to simply lift one leg so that the elevated ankle approximates the knee of the stance leg. However, the flexed limb must not touch the stance limb, as this would provide exteroceptive input in functional stability and compromises the test reliability.
- *A negative test:* The patient is able to stand without additional motion for a prescribed length of time. The length of time for maintaining balance is a matter of differing opinions (see below), although

TABLE 13–2. Visual Assessment: Still, Upright Postural Examination

Posterior View			
Foot pronation (P)/supination (S)	Left P ( ) S ( )	Right P ( ) S ( )	
Foot rotation internal (I)/external (E)	Left I ( ) E ( )	Right I ( ) E ( )	
Achilles squared (S)/pointed	Left S ( ) R ( )	Right S ( ) R ( )	
Soleus shape hypertrophy (H)/atrophy (A)	Left H ( ) A ( )	Right H ( ) A ( )	
Gastrocnemius hypertrophy (H)/atrophy (A)	Left H ( ) A ( )	Right H ( ) A ( )	
Knee position hyperextended (H)/flexed (F)	Left H ( ) F ( )	Right H ( ) F ( )	
Hamstrings hypertrophy (H)/atrophy (A)	Left H ( ) A ( )	Right H ( ) A ( )	
Adductor notching	Left ( )	Right ( )	
Glut max hypotrophy (upper outer quadrant)	Left ( )	Right ( )	
Pelvis			
Lateral shift	Left ( )	Right ( )	
Anterior (A)/posterior (P) shift	anterior ( )	Posterior ( )	
Anterior (A)/posterior tilt	Anterior ( )	Posterior ( )	
Oblique (elevated iliac crest)	Left ( )	Right ( )	
Torsion	Present ( )		
Rotation	Clockwise ( )	Counter-Clockwise ( )	
Short leg/pronation—niliac crests	Level ( )	Unchanged ( )	Worse ( )
L/S erector hypertrophy (H)/atrophy (A)	Left H ( ) A ( )	Right H ( ) A ( )	
Multifidus sign	Left ( )	Right ( )	
T/L erector hypertrophy (H)/atrophy (A)	Left H ( ) A ( )	Right H ( ) A ( )	
Mid-thoracic erector atrophy	Left A ( )	Right A ( )	
Scapular winging	Left ( )	Right ( )	
Internal rotation of arms	Left ( )	Right ( )	
Gothic shoulders	Left ( )	Right ( )	
Upper trap notching	Left ( )	Right ( )	
Head carriage anterior	Present ( )		
Lateral View			
Posture posterior (P)/neutral (N)/forward (F)	P ( )	N ( )	F ( )
TFL/ITB tight	Left ( )	Right ( )	
Lower crossed–lower (L)/upper (U)/full (F)	L ( )	U ( )	F ( )
Upper crossed–lower (L)/upper (U)/full (F)	L ( )	U ( )	F ( )
Anterior View			
Toe positions curled	Left ( )	Right ( )	
Tibialis anterior hypertrophy (H)/atrophy (A)	Left H ( ) A ( )	Right H ( ) A ( )	
VMO hypertrophy (H)/atrophy (A)	Left H ( ) A ( )	Right H ( ) A ( )	
Patellar "squinting" lateral (L)/medial (M)	Left L ( ) M ( )	Right L ( ) L ( )	
Quadriceps hypertrophy (H)/atrophy (A)	Left H ( ) A ( )	Right H ( ) A ( )	
Flank-TA inhibition/bulging	Present ( )		
Abdominal oblique notching	Left ( )	Right ( )	
Pectoral hypertrophy (H)/atrophy (A)	Left H ( ) A ( )	Right H ( ) A ( )	
SCM notching	Left ( )	Right ( )	
Respiration: scaleni activation	Present ( )		

10 seconds is considered a practical screening time for the practicing clinician.

- *A positive finding:* The test is considered negative if the patient is able to stand with little or no motion body motion. Inability to stand quietly for less than 10 seconds, without squirming is considered a positive test.

Bohannon et al.[171] suggest that between the age of 20 and 49 a maintained balance time of between approximately 25 and 29 seconds is normal. Between ages 49 and 59, 21 seconds is normal, while between 60 and 69 just over 10 seconds is acceptable. After 70 years of age 4 seconds is normal.

Downes[172] suggests:

	Time (seconds)	
Age (years)	Eyes Open	Eyes Closed
20–59	±30	21–28
60–69	±22	10
≥70	±14	4

It is up to the clinician to determine which timing method is best. However, it is recommended to take into account the *relative postural age* of the patient, a topic discussed earlier in this chapter. The lead author prefers the 10-second measure as a simple screening device, while the more strongly referenced measures are effective as true outcomes measures tools.

Once the results are logged, the patient is instructed to perform the same maneuver on the opposite leg.

The One-Legged Stance with Eyes Closed Once the patient has demonstrated sufficient postural stability on one leg, he or she can then be safely assessed with the eyes closed to better determine function that must rely more heavily on the proprioceptive and labyrinthine systems in the absence of visual afferentation. (see Fig. 13–16).

- Purpose: To practically assess the patient's functional ability to maintain a stable posture, especially in the transverse plane, while standing on one foot with the eyes closed.
- *Patient's position:* The patient stands with the arms resting at the side.
- *Clinician's position:* Standing behind the patient with both hands prepared to catch the patient in case he or she loses balance and starts to fall.
- *Clinician's instruction:* The patient is instructed to close his or her eyes and repeat the prior maneuver by lifting one leg so that the elevated ankle approximates the knee of the stance leg. However, the flexed limb must not touch the stance limb, as this would provide exteroceptive input in functional stability and compromises the test reliability.
- *A negative test:* The patient is able to stand without additional motion for a prescribed length of time. The length of time varies among authors, although 10 seconds is considered a practical screening time for the practicing clinician.

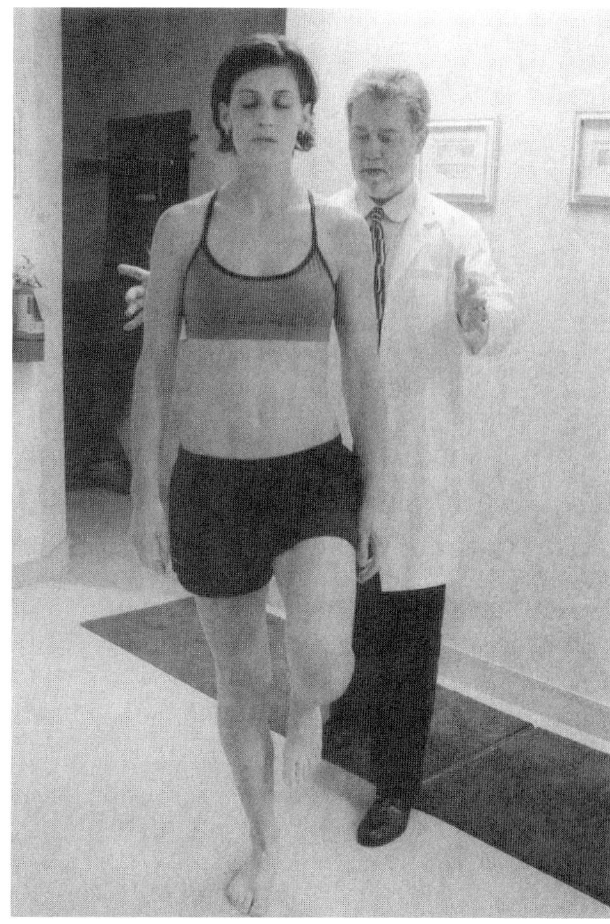

FIGURE 13–16. One-legged stance: After the patient has demonstrated satisfactory stability with the eyes open, the test is continued with the eyes closed to remove additional exteroceptive input. The clinician, as demonstrated, should always spot the patient, to avoid the risk of injury from falling.

- *A positive finding:* The test is considered positive if the patient is unable to stand with little or no motion body motion. Inability in standing quietly for less than 10 seconds without squirming is considered a positive test.

Once the results are logged, the patient is instructed to perform the same maneuver on the opposite leg.

Toes-Up Test

The lead author devised this test to confirm whether the patient is bearing weight on the forefoot during the quiet stance. Because the body's center-of-mass should be over the midfoot in the transverse plane, forefoot weight bearing is generally associated with the forward-drawn posture (see Fig. 13–17).

- Purpose: To assess for forward drawn posture.
- *Patient's position:* The patient stands with the arms resting at the side.

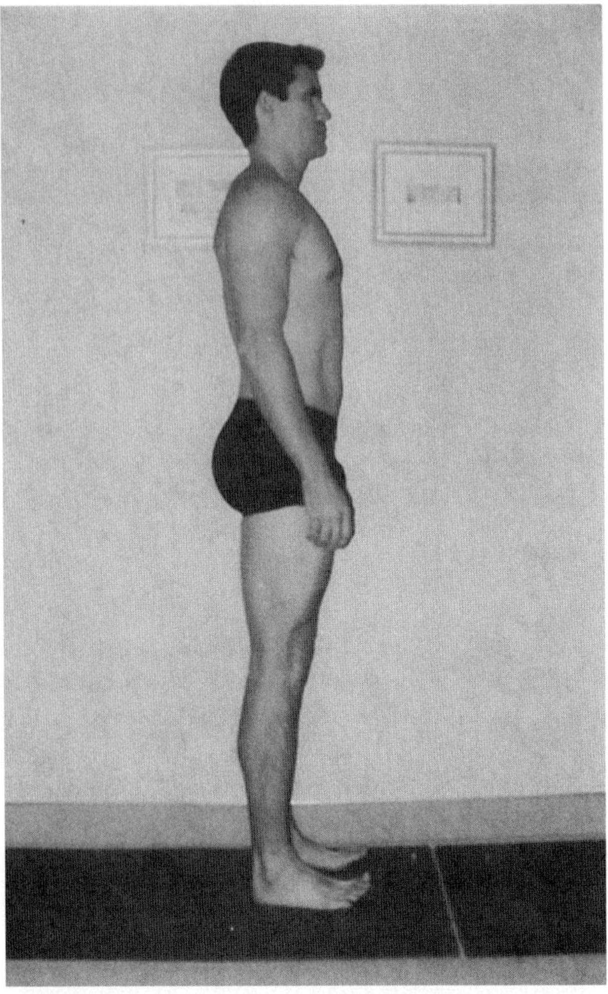

FIGURE 13–17. Toes-up test: This is a quick test to assess for the forward drawn posture, which is positive when the patient sways posteriorly as the toes are elevated and unloaded. (Note the abdominal oblique groove)

- *Clinician's position:* The clinician stands at the side of the patient in order to gain a lateral view and optimally assess any antero-posterior body motion.
- *Clinician's instruction:* The patient is instructed to keep the feet on the floor while elevating or lifting all ten toes off the floor.
- *A negative test:* The patient does not sway posteriorly, a sign that the center-of-mass was not on the forefoot.
- *A positive finding:* The patient sways backward, a sign that the center-of-mass was on the forefoot. In order to comply with the instruction, the patient had to shift the center-of-mass posteriorly in order to unload the toes before elevating them.

Heel Stance Test

The heel stance test is the lead author's offshoot of the classic neurological screening test. Heel walking is an accepted and practical test for motor function of the L5 root level. In addition to testing muscles like the extensor hallucis longus and anterior tibialis, additional stresses are placed on the postural system because many of the functional (biomechanical and neurological) benefits derived from plantar function are removed and replaced by two single-point calcaneal-floor contacts. Because the center of gravity should be over the mid-foot, there is additional provocation to the postural system by forcing the load-bearing point posteriorly to the rear foot. As, previously mentioned, the lumbopelvic region is often the site of postural convections in the saggital plane. Therefore, this maneuver can be used in the functional assessment to isolate individuals with poor lumbopelvic control. One group of such individuals is those with low back pain.[173]

Placing weight on the heels requires additional motor control to adapt to a posteriorly shifted center-of-mass. The strategic response to this challenge provides the basis for this quick and practical screen. The lead author has observed that patients with poor lumbopelvic stability in the sagittal plane generally assume a hip-flexed posture. The test appears to be consistent with the findings of Mok et al.,[149] who found that patients with low back pain compared to a control group demonstrated compromised trunk and hip control. This test does not need to be performed as a stand-alone test, but can be noted while the patient performed the classic motor tests of the lumbosacral plexuses of squatting and heel and toe walking.

- Purpose: To assess lumbopelvic stability, especially in the sagittal plane.
- *Patient's position:* The patient stands with the arms resting at the side.
- *Clinician's position:* The clinician stands at the side of the patient in order to gain a lateral view and optimally assess the patient's antero-posterior body motion.
- *Clinician's instruction:* The patient is instructed to stand on his or her heels.
- *A negative test:* The patient maintains an upright, neutral posture without a hip-flexed strategy.
- *A positive finding:* The patient assumes a hip-flexed posture while attempting to maintain the heel stance.

One-Foot Hopping Test

The one-foot hopping test is an excellent plyometric test designed to compare dynamic stability of each lower limb with the other. While the test seems quite simple, the demands on the locomotor system are not. This test stresses proprioception, balance, coordination, and strength of each lower leg and provides insight into the functional capacity of each limb.

Clinical Pearl: The one-foot hopping test is an excellent plyometric test designed to compare dynamic stability of each lower limb with the other. While the test seems quite simple, the demands on the locomotor system are not.

A brief overview of the mechanics of this maneuver may be of assistance. The hopping maneuver requires the descending forefoot, as it contacts the approaching floor, to adaptively find a balance point, to eccentrically contract musculature (especially the plantar flexors and ankle flexors), and to decelerate and halt downward motion. Simultaneous co-contraction of antagonists for appropriate intrinsic joint stability of the limb, pelvis, and spine is also required, as is integration with labyrinthine, proprioceptive, and exteroceptive input for balance and coordination. Finally, a coordinated, ballistic concentric contraction, primarily (although not solely) involving the flexors of the toes, foot, and ankle completes the motor task as the patient hops and elevates from the floor.

The patient should instinctively remain on the forefoot during the activity, although a severely dysfunctional limb may force the patient to be incapable of successful, early deceleration. In this instance, the patient will only be capable of halting downward motion by landing on the rear foot, after the forefoot contact. Knee flexion and hip flexion then becomes necessary to perform the maneuver, a sign of greater functional compromise. As with other functional tests, the law of relativity comes into play here. The patient's relative degree of global conditioning and functional capacity allows the clinician to determine the expected results, or even whether the patient can safely perform the test.

This test is best performed on a hard floor, with hardwood being optimal because of the added benefit of acoustics.

- Purpose: To assess the patient's dynamic functional stability in performing the plyometric challenge of hopping on one leg and to then compare this function with the opposite lower limb.
- *Patient's position:* Standing on one foot with the arms at the side.
- *Clinician's position:* Behind the patient with arms outstretched in order to assist the patient if he or she loses balance.
- *Clinician's instruction:* The patient is instructed to keep his or her knee as extended (i.e., straight) as possible during the test, since this is a test for the foot and ankle. The patient is instructed to hop on one foot as rapidly and lightly as possible for 30 seconds. The speed and agility of the hopping is assessed, as is the sound of the foot as it lands each time. The patient is then instructed to switch legs and repeat the maneuver.
- *A negative test:* The patient will demonstrate bilateral agility and speed while hopping.
- *A positive test:* A less functional limb will be appear clumsy in relation to its' pair, and clearly slower, while appearing to strike the ground with greater weight.
- *Commentary:* The one-legged hopping test is another quick and practical test. The clinician requires very little training to spot the positive test, either unilaterally or bilaterally. Perhaps the greatest strength lies in the fact that the patient can easily notice a slight difference in function between each leg.

Observation of Altered Contours During Standing Extension, Flexion, and Side Bending[135]

Note: None of these observations are in themselves diagnostic, but as with all other observations discussed earlier in this chapter, these should be added to the findings of direct assessment that follow, to allow diagnostic findings to emerge. These observations also offer points of reference so that when repeated subsequent to, or during, a course of treatment, functional changes can be noted.

Extension The clinician stands back and slightly to the side of the standing patient, and observes as the patient slowly extends the spine, within limits of comfort.

Questions to be asked during this observation exercise include the following:

- Is the movement smooth or restricted?
- Is it possible to note movement from the thoracolumbar junction to, and including, the sacrum?
- Is there excessive mobility between L5 and S1?
- Is the angle formed by extension of the spine smooth or sharp?
- Is any pain reported during extension or during the return to neutral?

Flexion Following this, the patient is asked to bend forward at the waist toward the toes. The clinician observes range of motion, and looks for evidence of rotoscoliosis (e.g., "rib hump"), as the patient reaches the end of range.

Rotoscoliotic deviations, and greater fullness in one group of paraspinal muscles as opposed to the other side when flexing, compared with when standing upright, suggests functional or structural rotational changes. If such rotations are slight they may only become evident when spinal flexion is introduced.

Observation from an anterior position, viewing down the flexed spine, offers an additional opportunity to evaluate such changes. Observation of the distance of the fingertips from the feet provides further evidence of symmetry or asymmetry. If flexion ability is excessive (hands flat on the floor), a tendency to hypermobility (or excessive application of yoga exercises) should be considered. A side view of the flexed spine allows visual evaluation of areas of relative "flatness," where flexion is restricted. Flatness is normal in the area of the lumbodorsal (thoracolumbar) junction and between L5 and S1.

Questions to be asked during this observation exercise include the following:

- Is there excessive kyphosis in the thoracic spine during flexion?

Observation is also made of the relationship between the lumbar spine and the pelvis.

- Does the pelvis remain in posterior rotation during full spinal flexion?
- Does this change if, while the spine is flexed, the knees are relaxed to reduce hamstring influence? Retesting flexion from a seated position allows the lumbar spine alone to be evaluated, without hamstring influence.[174]

More generalized pain noted on flexion may relate to the presence of myofascial trigger points (TrPs) in muscles being lengthened during the exercise.[175]

Side Flexion *Note:* It is important to ensure that the patient remains in the midline, not flexing or extending, when side flexing. The arms should remain at the side, and the feet should be close together.

Asking the patient to side flex from the erect position allows observation of the range of movement. How close to the knees do the fingertips reach?

Spinal and/or (contralateral) quadratus lumborum restriction may be implicated if side-flexion is obviously reduced. Additionally it is useful to observe the relative smoothness of the arc formed by the spinous processes. Sudden "breaks" in what should be a smooth contour suggests the presence of dysfunctional spinal segments.

It is also useful to observe the degree of rotation that accompanies side-flexion of any vertebrae as a result of coupling. Is rotation symmetrically present on side-flexion? Does the pelvis rotate toward the convexity of the curve, as is physiological (i.e., side-flexion to the left should be accompanied by pelvic rotation to the right)? SI joint or lumbar joint dysfunction may relate to a failure of such movement to occur.

Leg Length Assessment Test

Assessment for leg length discrepancy is a controversial issue. Several clinical approaches have been proposed, and the clinical relevance of such assessment remains debatable. Nevertheless, the presence of pelvic obliquity on posterior inspection, or a level pelvis in the presence of pelvic or leg asymmetry, is cause for suspicion. Janda[15,102] separated leg length differences into two categories: a true leg length deficiency in which there is an anatomical shortening and a functional short leg in which alterations of the pelvis (i.e., torsion, rotation, lateral shift), knees (flexion, extension), and the feet (pronation, supination) altered the level of the pelvis.

Janda[15,131] demonstrated a practical method for assessing leg length inequality. It has not been validated and is quite subjective; however, the lead author recommends this approach because of a significant degree of success in personal clinical experience.

- *Patient's position:* The patient maintains still, upright standing.
- *Clinician's position:* Standing or sitting behind the patient.
- *Clinician's actions:* The clinician, already suspecting a leg length deficiency, places a series of thin (approximately 1–2 mm) spacers underneath the foot of the patient's suspected *long leg* until such time as he or she notes a sensation that that leg has been elevated. This is generally felt in the ipsilateral hip region mainly due to increased joint loading of the elevated limb. Now the patient knows what the sensation of an elevated leg is and can reference it again when the other leg is tested. Once noted, the clinician withdraws the spacers from beneath the suspected long leg and then proceeds to elevate the short leg with the spacers. If the patient feels the same sensation in the hip of the short leg with the same spacer height, then this would be considered a negative test and a heel lift would not be recommended. If, however, the patient does not feel the ipsilateral hip pressure until several millimeters of additional spacers are added, then this would be a positive test and a trial course of a heel lift would be performed for a few days to see if there is a difference in symptomatology.

Sitting Assessment

Transition from upright standing to sitting changes the postural strategy from one in which the feet contact the ground forces to one in which the ischia and thighs provide the contact. Functional assessment in the sitting position is a practical strategy for several reasons. First, it can provide clinical insights by recreating the physical factors that provoke a recurrent pain syndrome with sitting position. It seems like a rather elementary approach, but it is surprising to learn of how many patients have presented to the authors for assessment of this complaint, yet have never been assessed for sitting posture! Therefore, if the patient finds back pain with 5 or 10 minutes of sitting, then have him or her sit for this period of time and observe the postural changes that occur. Take note of the type of chair that brings on the symptoms and also note whether the patient uses the backrest for support or sits forward in the chair instead.

Second, the change of postural strategy can relieve back pain, and this finding can suggest that the patient is poorly adapting to a bipedal stance. The stand-to-sit test discussed below describes utilization of strategies along these lines that can add invaluable insights into the variable scenarios involved in this transition.

Third, the lead author notes that pain can originate from an asymmetrical pelvis, leaving the spine resting on a sacral base that is not level. This can occur from pelvic torsion, such as occurs with sacro-iliac dysfunction, which would cause one ischium to be inferior in relation to the other.[176] It may also occur in the instance of anatomic pelvic asymmetry or hemipelvis. Badii et al.[177] found pelvic asymmetry in approximately 5% of the population. Assessment of hemipelvis is best performed on a firm, flat stool, as this surface provides a true plane that avoids the potential confounding variables of sinking unevenly into an upholstered cushion. In some cases, especially in lean individuals where the pelvic anatomy can be well visualized, pelvic asymmetry can be quite obvious. A wedge should be available to be placed under one ischium, typically for the requisite period necessary to reproduce pain, in order to learn if this increases or reduces pain.

Fourth, the patient who typically sits forward in the chair and soon experiences a backache should be assessed for sitting posture. If the patient observes pain while seated far sooner than while standing, the sitting posture will demonstrate increased lumbar kyphosis or hyperlordosis while seated.

Fifth, the seated position allows for tests that require less activation of the postural system, which can provide tissue-specific loading once co-contraction strategies associated with standing are removed. The slump test, described below, is one such set of tests that incorporate this approach.

Stand-to-Sit Test

The stand-to-sit test tries to answer the following question: "How does the lumbopelvic region change when the patient sits, compared with when he or she stands?" This test is designed to assess postural stability when the base upon which body bears weight changes from feet on the floor to buttocks on a stool. It should be differentiated from the sit-to-stand test, which is performed in the reverse order and which addresses the functional stability as the body transitions from sitting to standing. Because the act of sitting down and standing up are complex maneuvers, many different findings can be observed.[178] However, for the purposes of this chapter, only the comparative postural aspects of the lumbopelvic region in each static position will be discussed.

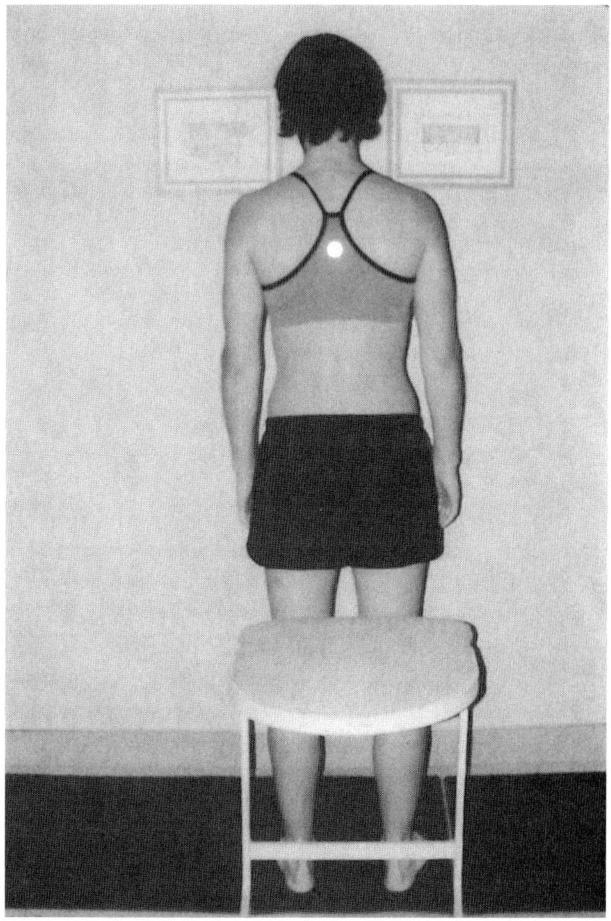

FIGURE 13–18. Stand-to-sit test: Part one of the test is designed to observe the patient's still upright stance, paying particular attention to pelvic levelness, degree of primary and secondary spinal curves, the degree of the muscular activity, elevation of the shoulders, and position of the head. A mental picture of the key observations is made in preparation for part two of this test.

- *Patient's position:* The patient stands with the arms resting at the side. A stool is placed directly behind the patient so that he or she is able to sit down on it from the current standing position (see Fig. 13–18).
- *Clinician's position:* The clinician stands directly behind the patient and the stool.
- *Clinician's instruction:* After the clinician briefly observes the patient's still, upright posture with an emphasis on the lumbopelvic region, the patient is instructed to sit down on the stool. The patient's arms should hang along both sides, as they were

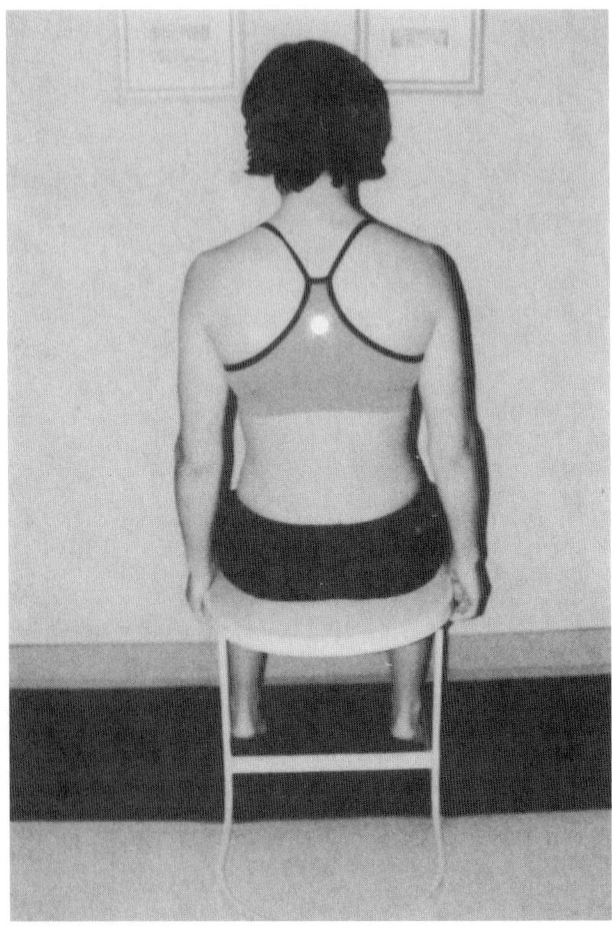

FIGURE 13–19. Stand-To-Sit Test: Part two is designed for comparison once the weight-bearing base has shifted from the tarsals to the ischia and, to a lesser degree, thighs. The key issue is to compare the seated postural findings with those of the standing posture.

while standing, rather than resting on the stool or lap (see Fig. 13–19).

- *A negative test:* The lumbopelvic contours, such as lordosis, pelvic obliquity, lateral spinal deviation, and degree of muscle activation remain relatively unchanged.
- *A positive finding:* The lumbopelvic contours, such as lordosis, pelvic obliquity, lateral spinal deviation, or degree of muscle activation change significantly. A significant finding should cause the clinician to look further to determine the reasons for changes in upright postural stability strategies, when the base of stability changed.

Slump Test

The slump test[179,180] is a popular and practical maneuver designed to assess for mobility and sensitivity of neural tissues along the neuraxis and contiguous peripheral neural tissues (see Fig. 13–20). It is helpful to envision the neuraxis descending from the brain through the spinal canal and on to the lower extremities as a bicycle break cable passes through the surrounding tubing. Like the passive supine straight leg raise (SLR) test, the slump test is designed to tension nervous, vascular, and connective structures within and beyond the neural canal. The SLR, as discussed in the previous chapter, by means of mechanically loading, has been found to produce up to 5 mm of caudal migration of the exiting nerve roots from L4–S1.[181] Brieg and Troup[182] demonstrated that medial hip rotation increased the caudal neural tensioning. Kobayashi et al.[183] surgically demonstrated that lumbar disc herniations adhere to the dura mater and that there was a subsequent marked disturbance of nerve root gliding to only a few millimeters. Also, a significant reduction of intraradicular blood flow was noted at the site of the herniation during SLR, with blood flow reduced from 40% before SLR to 98% during SLR. Following removal of the herniation, nerve root gliding was restored and there was no marked decrease in the intraradicular blood flow.

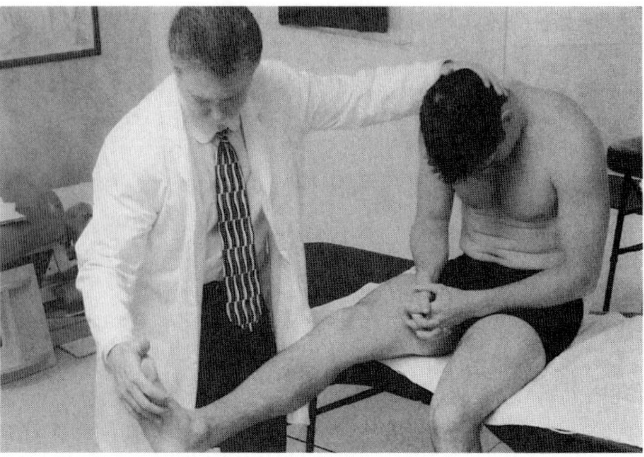

FIGURE 13–20. Slump test: This is a practical test to determine the mobility of the structures of the neuraxis and lower extremity. Care must be taken to avoid provoking a patient's condition who may not be able to tolerate the test.

The slump test can be used for differential diagnosis following a positive SLR test for radicular pain, although it is recommended that it be used with all patients. In comparison to SLR, the slump test provides additional information, in that it incorporates the upper lumbar, thoracic, and cervical region into the neural gliding scheme, whereas the SLR focuses only on the lumbar region and lower extremities. This allows for a strategy to diagnostically differentiate between a local lumbar neurocompressive condition (i.e., disc herniation) and an adhesive restriction (i.e., a "tethered" nerve) in the canal that causes similar symptoms. This differential diagnosis is very important, as it can make the difference between an appropriate and inappropriate disk surgery.

Clinical Pearl: The slump test can provide additional information to the SLR, in that it incorporates the upper lumbar, thoracic, and cervical region into the neural gliding scheme, whereas the SLR focuses only on the lumbar region and lower extremities.

To understand the slump test, one must appreciate exactly which maneuvers promote a superior, or cephalad, neural migration versus those that promote an inferior, or caudal migration. Cephalad migration motions include cervical flexion, lumbar flexion, anterior pelvic tilting, hip extension, hip abduction, external hip rotation, knee flexion, ankle/foot plantar flexion, and toe flexion. Conversely, movements that cause neural caudal migration are cervical extension, lumbar extension, posterior pelvic tilting, hip flexion, medial knee rotation, hip adduction, knee extension, ankle dorsiflexion, and toe extension. Therefore, one can selectively tension various neural regions by simply combining joint maneuvers to tension the neural tissues of a target region. The ultimate neural tension would be to flex the spine, the hip, medially rotate and adduct the hip, while extending the knee, ankle/foot, and toes. The first part of this position, in which the spine is flexed, or slumped, provides the name for this test.

Warning: This test can provide significant mechanical advantages and can irritate neural tissues or mechanical instabilities. One must be careful to determine that the patient can safely tolerate the positions of the slump test by carefully positioning the patient without any preloading. If the patient experiences a significant increase in symptoms, or becomes dizzy or light-headed, the test should be discontinued. This should not be used on patients who had recently undergone surgery or those with worsening neurological or cauda equina signs.

- *Patient's position:* The patient is seated on a table or chair.
- *Clinician's position:* The clinician stands next to the patient, on the side of the body to be tested.
- *Clinician's actions:* The patient is directed into a slumped position, with the head and chest brought toward the thighs. After confirming that this is tolerable for the patient, a slight overpressure is applied to hold the upper body in this position. The clinician then grasps the patient's distal foot and brings the knee into extension, the foot into dorsiflexion, and the toes into extension. The clinician may wish to increase the neural tensioning by adding hip adduction and medial hip rotation, although this is often unnecessary as the neural tensioning has typically been established with the slump position. The symptoms that were provoked by the SLR should have now been recreated. The clinician now releases the caudal tension of the upper neuraxis by *extending* the patient's neck while maintaining the lower body tension with the knee, ankle, and toes extended.
- *Test results:* If the radiating pain remained unchanged once the neck was moved into extension, then this suggests a local neurocompressive lesion, such as a disc herniation. If the leg pain was relieved with the neck extension, then this reduces the likelihood of a local herniation creating the symptoms. The clinician can then alter combinations that isolate neural tensions along the neuraxis or periphery to isolate from where the symptom generator is coming. The ability to isolate each region makes the slump test a very practical test for isolation of neural sensitivity.

GAIT ASSESSMENT

Gait assessment, like posture, occupies a paradoxical position in the world of spine care. It has historically been taught as a part of the physical examination, although its clinical value remained elusive. In addition to the authors, some believe that the full value of gait assessment for practical clinical applications has not yet been fully tapped.[184] While elaborate equipment is now available for such assessment, such as force plate devices, electronic goniometry and optoelectric recorders, less expensive devices, such as tape measures and stopwatches are available to provide a variety of quantitative measures.[185] This chapter will discuss the qualitative aspects of gait assessment, utilizing visual observation as a part of the clinician's physical examination, which can provide the initial information used to determine whether more intricate measures are appropriate.

Clinical Pearl: Gait assessment, like posture, occupies a paradoxical position in the world of spine care. It has historically been taught as a part of the physical examination, although its clinical value remained elusive.

Many, including the authors, believe gait assessment to be the most challenging functional assessment skill. The difficulty lies in being able to isolate significant subtleties while the patient is in motion, which requires a series of mental snapshots be taken to determine normal from abnormal function. Nevertheless, an in-depth understanding of this complex motor skill, including the coordinated kinematics and biomechanics, is essential for optimal rehabilitation of gait, and can also be used for evaluating running.[186]

For the novice, the constant motion of gait provides insufficient time to observe key alterations compared with a postural still, upright assessment. As such, the involved motion magnifies the challenge of gait assessment significantly. Training and achieving an experienced eye for gait assessment requires time and determination.

The soft findings noted in still, upright postural assessment become magnified during gait assessment, requiring the clinician to consider the observed movement patterns of the patient in relation to the patient's body type, weight, degree of conditioning, past history of injuries, past history of sports participation, past work history, and body symmetry, all or any of which might have caused alterations in gait. For example, if the patient has a history of involvement in sports, such as hockey or ballet, movement patterns associated with these activities are likely to have become integrated in their gait, and these subtleties and influences would need to be factored into the gait assessment.

As with other aspects of assessment described in this chapter, gait assessment findings are considered to be "soft" findings due to, among other things, high levels of variability among individuals. For example, 25 (62.5%) of 40 individuals demonstrated ≥5 degrees of maximal knee flexion difference.[187] Despite the fact that the findings of gait assessment are considered soft findings, it does not mean that they are without any clinical benefit nor does it mean that these findings can be relied upon to form a diagnosis. In fact, clinicians are clearly not the first ones to make assessments by movement patterns. It is after all the skilled eye of the predator that detects the slightest fault in movement patterns of a potential prey in a herd—a decision that determines survival. A different form of survival involves scouts hunting for skilled athletes in a particular sport, who routinely assess movement patterns.

There are sufficient stereotypical aspects of an individuals gait pattern to allow the clinician to access important information. This is best accomplished by having the patient walk at his or her freely chosen step rate, or so-called "free walk."[188]

From a practical clinical standpoint, learning gait assessment skills is eased by the skills learned while assessing the still, upright standing posture. However, this is a strategy for learning purposes only, as gait is considered a more basic movement and still, upright posture should be derived from it.[189] Indeed, parents routinely observe that their toddler, while learning to walk, remain upright longer while moving than while standing still. Later, the child's ability to maintain a bipedal still, upright posture marks the maturation of another level of locomotor function. Sherrington[51] stated "posture follows gait like a shadow."

Some clinicians use a treadmill to observe gait. This method was not recommended by Janda [15], as the additional postural control challenge caused by this labile surface alters the normal gait cycle, thereby compromising the validity of the evaluation. A variety of studies have substantiated this view.[190–193] In fact, Janda considered treadmill walking for exercise to be detrimental to gait patterns, as he felt the labile surface recruited increased hamstring during heel strike and midstance, while decreasing the propulsive phase at push-off.[15] These observations are supported by Yack et al.,[191] who measured a treadmill increase of midstance vertical forces of 9.7% and a decrease of 5.1% at push-off when compared with over ground gait.

In order to develop skill in gait analysis, a great deal of prior assessment ability needs to be acquired. Ironically, many of these abilities tend to become superfluous once gait can be evaluated accurately and swiftly, since this particular skill can provide so much clinical information. A master of this form of assessment, Janda demonstrated to practitioners around the world that a remarkable amount of clinical information could be gleaned by close observation of patients after just a few steps.[194]

There are several general guidelines relating to gait assessment that can assist in the learning process:

1. Gait assessment should be a part of an initial examination, prior to any palpatory assessment.
2. The patient must be barefoot.
3. The patient must be carrying or holding nothing.
4. The patient should be wearing as little clothing as professionally appropriate for the situation. (This has already been discussed in this chapter.)
5. The patient should be as relaxed as possible, as increased tension or anxiety will compromise the findings.[114]
6. The free-walk strategy should be observed to allow for the greatest consistency. As previously noted, this means the patient should walk at his or her own "natural" stride length and speed.[188]
7. Findings can be placed into three categories: positive, negative, and equivocal. (These rules have been discussed under *Rules for Still, Upright Postural Assessment*.
8. Still, upright postural assessment can be performed on the acute patient. These tend to be more gross observations, which tend to changes rapidly as the patient recovers from the acute episode. However, the significant subtleties discussed in this chapter are for the chronic patient.
9. Although it is very difficult to gain initial skills, persistence in use of gait assessment leads to proficiency and ultimately to a level of expertise.
10. It is important to observe for body type. The classical division of ectomorph (relatively thin, long torso, and extremities), endomorph

(relatively thick, short torso, and extremities), or mesomorph (moderate torso and extremities) can be used as a practical, general standard.

11. It is helpful in gait assessment to observe for morphological symmetry, both bilaterally and superior to inferior. Are the extremities and torso equal in length, girth, and contour? Is the upper and lower half of the body equal in dimension, or is the lower half less well developed? If postural assessment was previously performed, then this assessment should have already been performed.
12. Kinetic symmetry should be evaluated, noting equality of bilateral movement in addition to smoothness of movement along the kinetic chain. Efficient gait is very fluid and the person seems to almost effortlessly glide forward.
13. Observation of relative mobility includes looking at features such as length of stride, arm swing, and relaxed gait speed (as opposed to hurried or cautiously delayed gait speed). Is the patient moving with a stride length, arm swing, and relaxed speed that commensurate with his or her body type, age, and postural age? Greenman[195] suggests that the clinician should look for the "functional capacity of the gait," not just for pathological conditions.
14. Because gait assessment is commonly preceded by still, upright postural assessment, the findings of still, upright postural assessment should be correlated with gait assessment findings. It is possible that findings that were positive and equivocal among the still, upright assessment findings may be either confirmed or ruled out during gait assessment.

For most patients, the most revealing period of gait involves the first three steps. Janda[15] stated that the expert in gait assessment should be capable of arriving at a clinical conclusion after three steps. The most important step is the initial step, as it demonstrates how the person initiates forward propulsion and stable one leg standing without the assistance of forward momentum. The greatest energy drain, interestingly, occurs on the second step with the push-off of the foundation leg.[196] The amount of lateral sway during the initial step suggests a great deal about the hip abductor function of the foundation leg. A significant degree of lateral sway (i.e., the patient sways to the right as the left leg swings forward while the right leg is weight-bearing) suggests poor abductor function.[197]

Gait Overview

As previously mentioned, gait can be divided into four phases: heel strike, midstance, toe-off, and the swing phase (see Figs. 13–21 to 13–24).

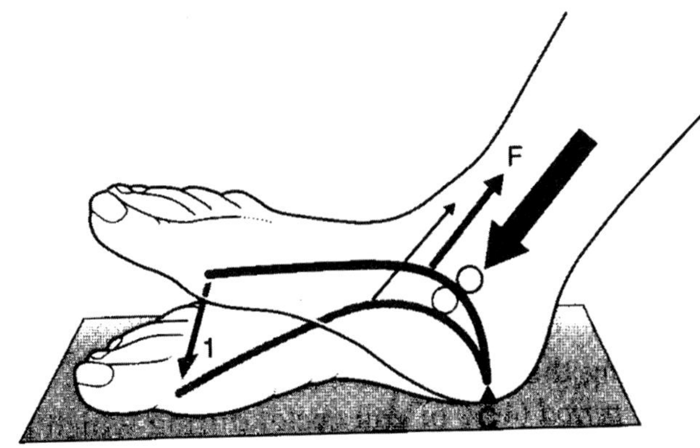

FIGURE 13–21. The heel strike and rocker: F = Foot flexors, 1 = the thrust of the leg flattens the foot, and C = posterior support of the plantar vault. (*After Kapandji* [161].)

The gait assessment should initially occur from the posterior view, followed by a front view as the patient turns around and returns toward the clinician. After sufficient information is obtained from these views, the clinician should observe the patient from the side view, walking back and forth to see both sides.

Gait Observation: Posterior View

Global View Janda[15,102] noted that a brief global assessment to determine the general state of the locomotor system should precede the rest of the gait assessment in order to make note of specific areas requiring additional focus. This should include a general perspective of the postural age, the general degree of conditioning, muscular bulk and tone, erect stature, symmetry of motion, and smoothness of movement. During this period, the integration of prior findings during the history and still, upright postural assessment start to integrate with gait findings. For example, a slight limp may be spotted that might correlate with a previously noted soleus hypertrophy during

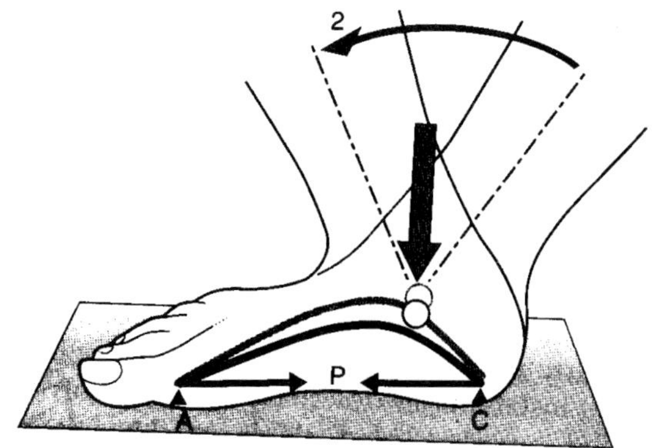

FIGURE 13–22. The ankle rocker: 2 = Tibeal motion from extension to flexion, P = plantar tighteners, and A and C = anterior and posterior support of the plantar vault. (*After Kapandji* [161].)

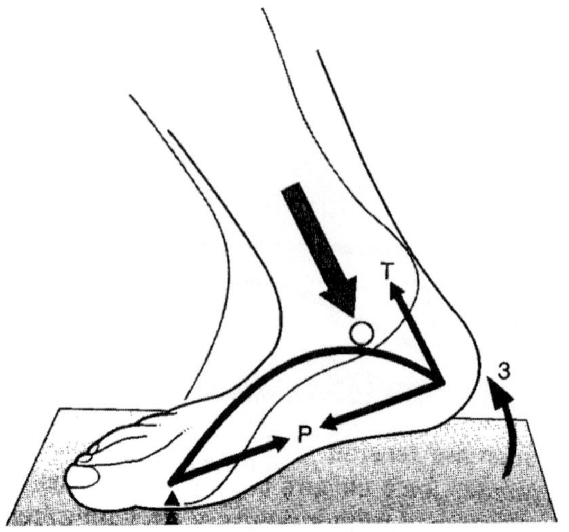

FIGURE 13–23. The metatarsal (i.e., forefoot) rocker: 3 = Heel rises, P = plantar tighteners, A = anterior support of the plantar vault, and T = pull of the triceps surae. The combined tensioning of the myofascial components of the planta and triceps surae produces the windlass mechanism of gait. (*After Kapandji*[161].)

the still, upright stance assessment and history of prior knee injury.

Heel Strike The foot performs several vital aspects of human locomotion. But first of all, it must interact with the impending ground, with the first interaction being that of the heel strike. As such, this initial contact can provide important information on how the individual interacts with the ground. Optimally, the heel strike should be relatively soft, with the initial contact being dampened by the fat of the heel pad. The heel is initially slightly inverted at this point.[198] At heel-strike the knee is fully extended and the hip is flexed. The ankle is at 90 degrees, being maintained there by the dorsiflexors of the foot. This contact also begins initial double limb stance since the second leg is still in contact with the floor, though there is not yet equal sharing of body weight by both legs.[199]

In extreme cases of a hard heel strike, a "shutter wave" will continue up into the torso from the force.

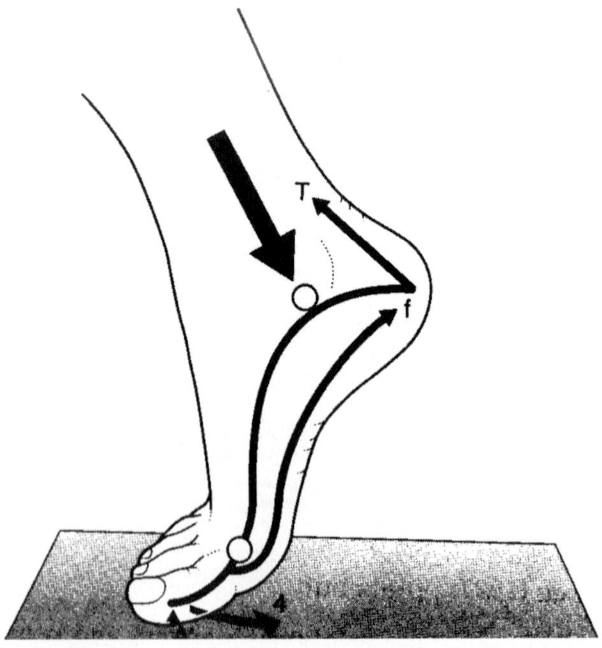

FIGURE 13–24. Preparation for toe-off. 4 = Propulsive force provided by flexors (f) of the toes and A^1 = anterior support moves to the great toe. (*After Kapandji* [161].)

Plantar Stability As the patient extends from rear foot contact to a single leg midstance, the clinician should watch to see if the patient maintains a rectus position of the foot, or whether there is excessive supination or pronation. In one study, maximum Pronation occurred at 39.7% of the stance-phase duration.[198] Excessive pronation is more common, which can also be considered an increase of valgus angle for the ankle. A very high medial longitudinal arch is also dysfunctional, as the tarsal bones take on a more "close-packed" formation, a rigid formation that allows for decreased dampening capacity of ground forces. Increased shock absorption alters the functional capacity of the lower extremities and spine with time. For example, Williams et al.[200] found that high-arched runners demonstrated increased leg stiffness compared to low-arched runnersand greater vertical loading rates and increased activation of knee extensor musculature.

It should also be noted whether the patient's foot is internally or externally rotated. Medially rotated, or "toe-in," feet tend to increase hip adductor activity.[201]

To assist the acceptance of body weight, the heel functions as a rocker. The posterior portion of the calcaneus contacts the surface and the body "rocks" over the rounded bony surface as the remainder of the foot simultaneously falls to the floor in loading response (foot flat). This rapid fall of the foot is decelerated by the dorsiflexors, which also restrain ankle motion and act as shock absorbers.[199]

Once the forefoot contacts the floor, joint motion shifts to the ankle as the movement of the tibia begins to rock over the talus (ankle rocker) at which time the knee slightly flexes. This period of midstance is the introduction of single limb support, which requires not only the acceptance of full body weight, but also the repositioning (laterally) of the body as a whole to align over the weight-bearing foot.

Heel Lift and Forefoot Push-Off As the heel starts to elevate at the end of stance phase, a tensioning of a contiguous plantar fascial band occurs when the first metacarpophalangeal joint moves into extension. The tension increases as the heel rises, forefoot weight bearing is boosted, and foot dorsiflexion increases. The fascial band continues over the calcaneus and superiorly as part of the Achilles tendon. This fascial band provides a pivotal role in the propulsive aspect of gait, using the viscoelastic properties to generate forward momentum instead of relying solely on muscular activation. This fascial band in essence acts as a type of winch, parlaying a mechanical advantage to accomplish work efficiently and is called the *windlass mechanism of the foot.*[202] The windlass mechanism also assists in providing additional medial and lateral rear foot stability during heel strike and the early stance phase.[203] The windlass mechanism transfers forces generated by the gastrocnemius and soleus, via the Achilles tendon, to be transported along the long lever of the foot. Hopson et al.[204] reported that approximately 65 degrees of first metatarsophalangeal joint extension are necessary for normal walking. Without the windlass mechanism, the efficiently propulsive aspect of gait would be lost, and the biped would plod forward by essentially pulling him or herself along by the heels, instead of springing forward off the toes. The vigorous action of gastrocnemius and soleus to decelerate the tibial advancement contributes to the beginning of rapid knee flexion as well as plantar flexion.[199]

Approximately 80% of the forefoot loading should be on the first ray. Thus, it is important to know whether the patient is pushing off with the forefoot or whether there is excessive internal or external rotation at the point of push-off. The postural assessment findings may come into play here, and consistencies help to establish clear patterns. For example, the valgus position of the hallux at the first metatarsophalangeal joint may coincide with a functional pronation, a functionally short leg and a toe-off position over the medial aspect of the hallux, rather than over the middle of the digit. This provides an excellent example of a dysfunctional kinetic chain, one that is consistent and logical, bringing increased clinician confidence of the findings because of the significant subtleties from various vantage points.

Knee Motion Perry[199] describes three phases in limb advancement; these being initial swing, mid swing, and terminal swing. Cailliet[205] and Hoppenfeld[58] note a similar division, using different nomenclature (acceleration, midswing, deceleration). During the swing phase, the knee should increase in flexion so as to allow the foot to swing free with sufficient space to avoid contacting the ground. However, at the point of rear foot heel strike, the knee should be starting to extend, although not be fully extended. As the patient moves to a single leg midstance, the knee should be continuing toward extension but still not be fully extended. As the patient moves toward forefoot push-off, the knee should continue toward full extension, although still not be fully extended at the point of push-off.

Terminal swing provides full knee extension, neutral positioning of the ankle, and preparation for initial floor contact (heel strike). Terminal swing phase ends the gait cycle and, with surface contact, a new gait cycle begins.

Hip Motion The hip joint in gait should be assessed for two main issues. The first is for lateral deviation during ipsilateral, single leg midstance. A mild degree of lateral deviation is considered physiological. However, it is important to determine the breadth of the pelvis, length of the legs, and the quadriceps angle[206] (*Q* angle) of the hips, because the degree of lateral deviation is significantly dependent on these factors. Therefore, a patient with a broad pelvis and long limbs and higher *Q* angle would have a greater mechanical challenge to reduce medial to lateral deviation on single leg during standing and also during gait.[207] Therefore, a greater degree of ipsilateral, lateral deviation on single-leg stance would be considered acceptable. Conversely, a patient with shorter and thicker limbs and a relatively narrow pelvis and a lower *Q* angle would be expected to have far less lateral deviation.

The second aspect of hip assessment during gait entails hip extension at the forefoot push-off phase. This is where one can determine whether there is a true hip extension at push-off, with approximately 10 degrees of hip extension. Under physiological circumstances, a 10-degree hip extension would fit the description of a "true hip extension." This would be in contrast to a "false hip extension," discussed briefly earlier, in which there is little or no extension of the hip joint and instead one finds a "hinging" type of extension at the lumbosacral junction above. With the true hip extension, there should be an activation of the gluteus maximus, which is the agonist involved from 0° to 10° of hip extension.

Clinical Pearl: A 10-degree hip extension would fit the description of a "true hip extension." This would be in contrast to a "false hip extension," in which there is little or no extension of the hip joint and instead one finds a "hinging" type of extension occurring at the lumbosacral junction above.

Hip, Knee, and Ankle Mortise Timing In addition to localizing each joint for inspection, it is also important to look at the whole movement complex of the lower extremity for timing. As the lower extremity transitions from midstance toward forefoot toe-off, there is an optimal timing that should occur with hip extension, knee extension, and plantar flexion that should be smooth and coordinated.

Pelvis During gait, the pelvis becomes slightly more anteriorly tilted. In one study[208] it was found to be tilted by an average of 1.4 degrees. Pelvic rotation should occur smoothly and bilaterally with each step, without jerky or jarring movement. As one leg swings forward, the ipsilateral ilium should slightly elevate due to contralateral gluteus medius contraction so that the swinging foot clears the ground. In case of a faulty gluteus medius function, the contralateral quadratus lumborum often becomes the key agonist, which is generally noted as the patient's torso laterally flexes contralaterally to allow the ipsilateral leg to swing through without tripping. Minimal pelvic rotation should occur during regular gait, although this is once again relative to the breadth of the pelvis and the *Q* angle. Generally speaking, the greater the *Q* angle, the greater is the degree of pelvic rotation. Also, the greater the stiffness of the hip joints, the greater the degree of pelvic rotation that will occur to assist in the anterior and posterior motion of the lower extremities during gait. The pelvis should rotate about an axis located in the lumbar spine in order for the hip of the advancing limb to prepare to move forward. If it were not for a mixture of such compensating motions (gait determinants), the vertical and horizontal displacements of the trunk as a whole would be presented jerkily, in an inefficient and muscularly taxing manner.

Perry[199] notes

> Vertical lift of the [upper body] during single limb support is lessened by lateral and anterior tilt of the pelvis, combined with stance limb ankle plantar flexion and knee flexion. Lowering of the body center by double limb support is reduced by terminal stance heel rise, initial heel contact combined with full knee extension, and horizontal rotation the pelvis. Lateral displacement is similarly minimized by the pelvic rotators, medial femoral angulation, and the substitution of inertia for complete coronal balance. As a result, the body's center of gravity follows a smooth three-dimensional sinusoidal path that intermingles vertical and horizontal deviations.

The Sacroiliac Joint As the right leg swings forward, the right ilium rotates backward in relation to the sacrum.[195] Simultaneously, sacrotuberous and interosseous ligamentous tension increases to brace the sacroiliac (SI) joint in preparation for heel strike.

Just before heel strike, the ipsilateral hamstrings are activated, thereby tightening the sacro-tuberous ligament (into which they merge) to further stabilize the SI joint. Vleeming et al.[209] have demonstrated that as the foot approaches heel strike there is a downward movement of the fibula, increasing (via biceps femoris) the tension on the sacrotuberous ligament, while simultaneously tibialis anterior (i.e., anterior) fires, in order to dorsiflex the foot in preparation for heel strike.

Tibialis anterior links via fascia to peroneus longus under the foot thus completing this elegant sling mechanism (the "anatomical stirrup"), which both braces the SI joint and engages the entire lower limb in that process.

Biceps femoris, peroneus longus, and tibialis anticus together form this longitudinal muscle-tendon-fascial sling, which is loaded to create an energy store to be used during the next part of the gait cycle. As Lee[210] points out, "Together, gluteus maximus and latissimus dorsi tense the thoracolumbar fascia and facilitate the force closure mechanism through the SIJ" (Form and Force Closure is discussed in Chapter 8 of this text; see Fig. 13–25).

During the latter stage of single support period of the gait cycle, biceps femoris activity eases, as compression of the SI joint reduces and the ipsilateral iliac bone rotates anteriorly.

As the right heel strikes, the left arm swings forward and the right gluteus maximus activates to compress and stabilize the SI joint.

There is a simultaneous coupling of this gluteal force with the contralateral latissimus dorsi by means of thoracolumbar fascia in order to assist in counter-rotation of the trunk on the pelvis. In this way, an oblique muscle–tendon–fascial sling is created across the torso, providing a mechanism for further energy storage to be utilized in the next phase of the gait cycle. As the single support phase ends and the double support phase initiates, there is a lessened loading of the SI joints and gluteus maximus reduces its activity, and as the next step starts, the leg swings forward and nutation at the SI joint starts again.

Lumbar Spine During gait, the lumbar spine becomes slightly less lordotic as the torso leans forward.[208] In addition, there should be relatively little anterior and posterior motion during the gait cycle. If there is increased anterior and posterior excursion, this suggests lumbopelvic instability and should generally be investigated. One should also watch for lateral excursion during gait. As previously noted, this may suggest overactivity of the quadratus lumborum in a synergistic substitution for ilium and hip elevation during the swing phase.

Thoracic Region Thoracic counter-rotation is an important part of maintaining a smooth and balanced gait. This should be a natural and smooth movement to maintain balance in the sagittal plane as the lower extremities are transitioning in weight bearing and

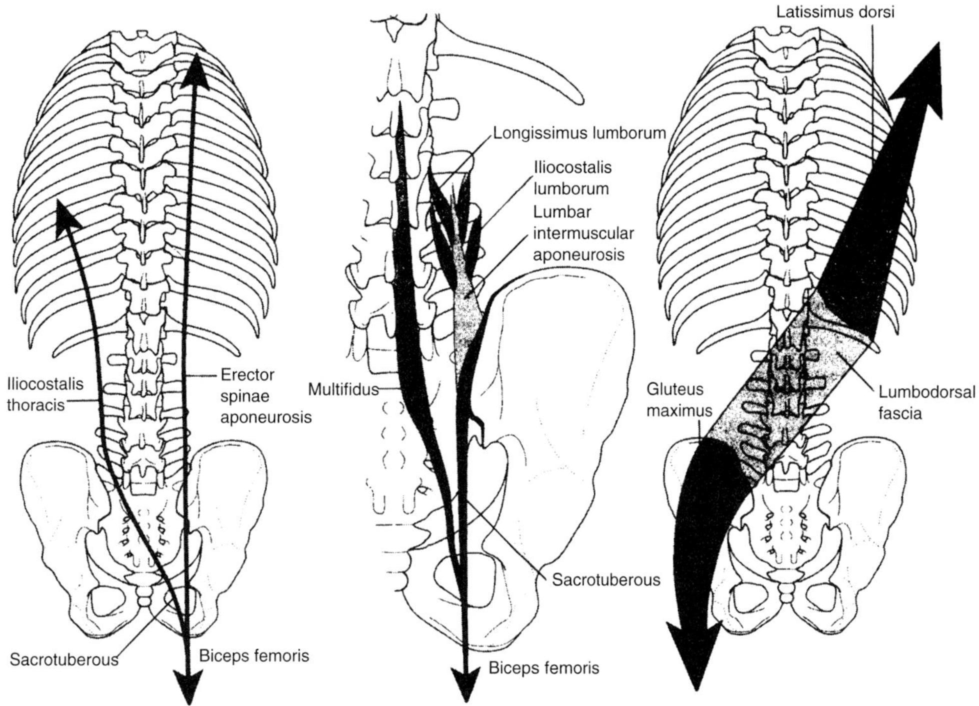

FIGURE 13–25. The posterior unit: Loads are transferred longitudinally and obliquely from the upper torso, down through the pelvis and to each lower extremity during gait. *A*. The biceps femoris is directly connected to the trunk via the contiguous sacrotuberous ligament, the erector spinae aponeurosis, and iliocostalis thoracis. *B*. Enlarged view of the lumbar spine demonstrating the functional continuity of the biceps femoris, the lumbar intermuscular aponeurosis, longissimus lumborum, iliocostalis lumborum, and multifidus. *C*. This demonstrates the functional relationship between the gluteus maximus, lumbodorsal fascia, and latissimus dorsi. [*Reprinted with permission from: Movement stability and Low Back Pain. (The Essential Role of the pelvis.) Vleeming A, et al. New York, Churchill Livingstone 1997.*]

alternate movements. Two relatively obscure muscles, the serratus posterior superior and inferior, recently gained notice when their theoretical role as respiratory synergists was discredited and they are now thought to largely offer proprioceptive in function.[211] Their role, along with other muscles that perform functions that facilitate coordination of gait and upper torso counterrotation, may provide greater insights into locomotor function. The motion should extend into a natural and smooth arm swing, which is in opposition to the ipsilateral lower extremity motion.

The importance of the latissimus dorsi on upper torso motion[212] in functional spinal stability[213] and as part of a contiguous transition of load transfer to the pelvis and legs via the thoracolumbar fascia and erector spinae[214–216] has gained increased notice over the past decade.

The pivot point for the arm during gait should be at the glenohumeral and scapulocostal junctions, as opposed to at the elbow joint, which Janda[15] considered pathological. In addition, the upper extremities should be assessed for the position of the palms. The palms should, under physiological circumstances, be "facing inward" or should be facing medially, in opposition to the thighs. In case of chronic lumbopelvic instability, chronic latissimus dorsi tightness has been observed, which at least tends to increase internal rotation of the arms with the palms facing posteriorly. In the case of posterior facing palms, it is important to check the angle of the upper arm at the elbow joint, for a valgus elbow will very often prompt the self-conscious person to pronate the forearms to keep the forearms and wrists closer to the body during gait. In such an instance, this would be a false-positive finding and not associated with lumbopelvic instability.

Stereotypical Gait Patterns

The following gait patterns have been adapted from Chaitow and DeLany[217], with two noted exceptions. These movements typically demonstrate significant gait alterations, although the findings may instead be subtle in the presence of a less severe condition. Therefore, the clinician should be careful to incorporate these patterns into the assessment, as each pattern can lead the clinician to significant findings.

- *Antalgic gait:* A characteristic gait resulting from pain on weight bearing in which the stance phase of gait is shortened on the affected side.

- *Ataxic gait:* Wide-based gait characterized by staggering, lateral veering, unsteadiness, and irregularity of steps, often with a tendency to fall to forward, backward, or to one side.
- *Calcaneal gait:* Characterized by walking on heel as aresult of paralysis of the calf muscles (poliomyelitis, neurological diseases).
- *Cerebellar gait:* Same as ataxic gait; this is due to cerebellar disease.
- *Charcot gait:* The gait of hereditary ataxia.
- *Circumduction gait:* See hemiplegic gait.
- *Equine gait:* See high-steppage gait.
- *Festinating gait:* Gait in which patient walks on toes (as though pushed) with flexed trunk, legs flexed at the knees and hips (but stiff) with short and progressively more rapid steps (parkinsonism and other neurological diseases).
- *Gluteus maximus gait:* Compensatory backward propulsion of trunk to maintain center of gravity over the supporting lower extremity when the gluteus maximus is significantly weak and incapable of weight bearing.
- *Gluteus medius gait (early stage):* There is an increased lateral sway of the ipsilateral pelvis during the single-leg phase of gait. This is due to gluteus medius/minimus inhibition and Janda noted this is often the first sign of an ipsilateral hip arthrosis,[15] due to arthrogenic inhibition, preceding pain or positive radiographic findings.
- *Gluteus medius gait (painful hip stage):* Compensatory leaning of the body to the painful and weak gluteal side, with increased hip flexion, to dampen ground forces that otherwise transfer through the hip joint and place the center of gravity over the supporting lower extremity.
- *Gluteus medius gait (middle stage):* This is the same as the early stage, except that there is a more pronounced degree of lateral pelvis sway during the single-leg stance phase of gait. However, gait motion still remains relatively smooth and fluid. It should be noted that the painful and middle stages may be integrated, depending on a variety of provoking factors. For example, patient's may have days in which they must walk quite a lot, which subsequently increases their pain and increases compensatory learning.
- *Gluteus medius gait (late stage):* This occurs with a severely degenerated hip joint. The hip joint is maintained by the capsule and surrounding ligaments, but supporting hip musculature is significantly diminished. The key finding in this stage is that there is now a "hitch" in the patients gait during the ipsilateral single-leg stance phase of gait. Gait is no longer smooth, but is literally disjointed as the joint appears to subluxate with weight bearing and return to the joint during the swing phase. Despite walking with a catch in their hip, patients often appear to be unaware of the unusual gait because it is not relatively or completely painless and the onset is insidious, occurring over many years.

  It should be noted that there is no distinct delineation between the early, middle, and late stage of gluteus medius gait, but rather a gradual transition that is relatively determined with an experienced eye.
- *"Helicopod" gait:* A gait in which the feet (or foot) describe half circles with each step (hysteria and in some conversion reactions).
- *Hemiplegic gait (circumduction or spastic gait):* Gait in which the leg is held stiffly and abducted with each step and swung around to the ground in front, forming a semicircle.
- *High-steppage gait (equine gait):* Gait characterized by high steps to avoid catching a drooping foot and brought down suddenly in a flapping manner (peroneal nerve palsy, tabes).
- *Hysterical gait:* A variety of bizarre gaits in which the foot is frequently held dorsiflexed and inverted and is usually dragged or pushed ahead, instead of lifted (hysteria-conversion reaction).
- *Minimal circumduction gait:* This is the lead author's description of the subtle manner in which individuals with uneven leg lengths swing the "long leg" around and forward to avoid tripping. One must remember that the long leg must somehow maintain sufficient clearance for the swinging foot. The minimal circumduction gait is one strategy.
- *Skater's gait:* This is the lead author's description of the gait often found with Janda's lower crossed syndrome. Because of tight hip flexors and inhibited/weak gluteus maximus, the patient employs an alternate strategy for the toe-off phase of gait by externally rotating the hip, posteriorly rotation the ipsilateral pelvis, and using false hip extension. This altered movement pattern will allow for some propulsive force at toe-off, although the altered movement pattern tends to cause secondary postural and gait dysfunction and pain syndromes with time and repetition. The "skater's gait" may be unilateral or bilateral.
- *Scissor gait:* Gait in which each leg swings medially as well as forward to cross during walking (cerebral palsy).
- *Spastic gait:* See hemiplegic gait.
- *Steppage gait:* Because it cannot dorsiflex, the advancing foot is lifted higher than usual to clear the ground (peroneal neuropathies, dorsiflexion weakness, peripheral neuritis, diabetes, alcoholism, chronic arsenical poisoning).
- *Toppling gait:* Patient displays uncertain and hesitant steps, totters, and sometimes falls (balance disorder, in elderly patients poststroke).
- *Trendelenburg gait:* Pelvis sags on the side opposite the affected side during single leg stance on

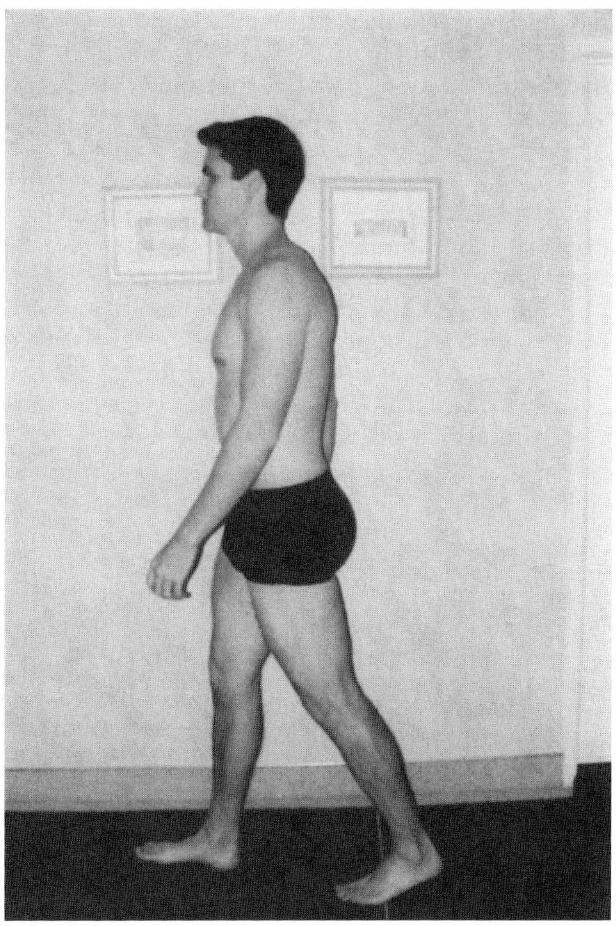

FIGURE 13–26. The side view: This presents a second dimension for the inspector, supporting earlier observations, excluding other possibilities, while adding new findings that can either gain support or be discarded with subsequent evaluation.

the affected side; compensation occurs during gait by leaning the torso toward the involved side during the affected extremity's stance phase (congenital dislocation, hip abductor weakness, rheumatic arthritis, osteoarthritis).

- *Waddling gait:* Rolling gait in which the weight-bearing hip is not stabilized and feet are placed widely apart, while the opposite side of the pelvis drops, resulting in alternating lateral trunk movements, which resemble the waddle of a duck (gluteus medius muscle weakness, muscular dystrophies, coxa vara).

Gait Assessment: Lateral View

Lateral view (see Fig. 13–26) during gait is generally confirmatory for the still, upright assessment and posterior gait assessment.

Feet The lateral view can be very helpful in determining the function of the feet. Specifically, it helps to confirm a hard heel strike and also the degree of pronation, as one looks at the opposite foot during midstance. That is, if the clinician is observing from the left of the patient, this will provide an optimal view of the right foot during midstance to check for pronation or supination. When the patient turns around so that the medial perspective of the left foot is made available, this can then be checked for pronation or supination.

The lateral view also helps to provide additional information regarding the efficiency of the patient's swing phase of gait. One significant subtle finding will be toe hyperextension during the swing phase of gait, which suggests a faulty mechanism in the swing phase requiring the patient to add the extreme measure of toe extension in order to avoid and to reduce the risk of tripping, as the leg swings forward. In such an instance, the clinician may look for functional short leg or a faulty hip elevation program, as would be expected with gluteus medius dysfunction, and perhaps early hip arthrosis.

During the forefoot toe-off phase, it is also important to look to see if the patient is propelling himself or herself with the entire leg at push-off, or if the knee has not sufficiently extended. In such an instance, the patient may then over utilize the single joint plantar flexor, the soleus muscle, to "flick" their toe off phase in order to gain additional propulsion in the absence of a coordinated lower leg propulsion strategy. In this instance, the patient will generally demonstrate a hypertrophic soleus muscle in the lower portion of the calf.

Clinical Pearl: One significant subtle finding will be toe hyperextension during the swing phase of gait, which suggests a faulty mechanism in the swing phase requiring the patient to add the extreme measure of toe extension in order to avoid and to reduce the risk of tripping, as the leg swings forward.

Hips The lateral view provides confirmatory information regarding the presence of a true or false hip extension during gait. The lateral view may also demonstrate that in the absence of a true hip extension strategy, there may be additional pelvic posterior rotation during the forefoot push-off phase of gait. In this event, one should look for an ipsilaterally tight iliopsoas muscle, which is inhibiting true hip extension resulting in the compromise of posterior pelvic rotation in order to compensate for the dysfunctional hip.

Lumbopelvic Region The lateral view provides supporting information for the position of the lumbar spine and pelvis. Is the patient in a rectus position or perhaps are the hips flexed during gait? Is there excessive anterior/posterior excursion during gait?

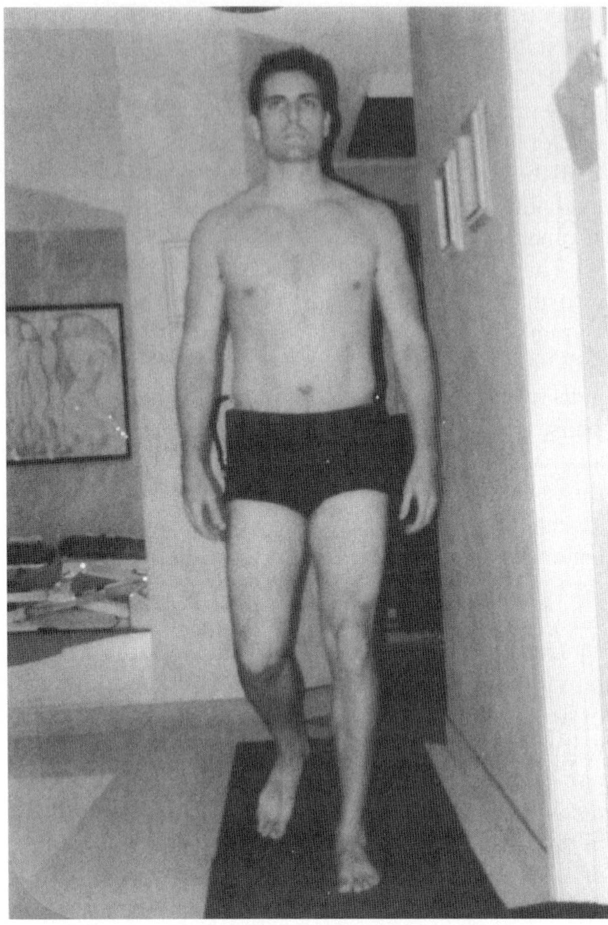

FIGURE 13–27. Front view: This represents a third dimension for the clinical observer, cementing several findings as the clinical picture becomes clarified with a consistent string of observations, coupled with the patient's history.

Gait Assessment: Anterior View

The anterior view (see Fig. 13–27) once again provides confirmatory information for the previous visual assessment findings, to be integrated with the patient's history, to help establish a stronger degree of clinical suspicion.

From the anterior view, the clinician is able to view whether the patient is swinging straight through on the leg swing, or whether there is a tendency to move in a roundabout fashion on one leg compared to the other. In this case, a functional short leg is suggested. One can also again confirm whether the toes are hyperextending during the swing phase, which suggests the same finding. The activation of the anterior tibialis during gait should be noted bilaterally, as should the degree of knee flexion during the swing phase and a gradual change toward knee extension as the patient transitions to midstance, and then forefoot toe off.

The lateral pelvic excursion and abdominal stability should be noted. In addition, the transition of the thorax and the upper extremities during gait as a counterrotational measure can then be confirmed as additional features of gait. It is suggested that gait assessment be performed on a hard floor or on a carpet that is minimally padded.

Table 13–3 provides a summary check-off sheet for gait assessment. While this can be utilized in the clinic to chart patient findings, the authors suggest that it be used until each key observation point is remembered in order to save time and allow the clinician to establish a more global clinical picture instead of performing continual assessments in a "piecemeal" fashion. Once these skills are learned, the clinician can then simply record the relevant positive findings.

TABLE 13–3. Visual Assessment: Gait Examination

Pelvis		
Anterior/posterior tilt	Anterior ( )	Posterior ( )
Lateral shift/stance phase	Left ( )	Right ( )
Lateral "catch"/stance phase	Left ( )	Right ( )
Rotation	Left ( )	Right ( )
Feet		
Hyperpronation	Left ( )	Right ( )
External rotation	Left ( )	Right ( )
Hard heel strike	Left ( )	Right ( )
Tight gastroc/soleus	Left ( )	Right ( )
Legs		
Lateral deviation/swing phase	Left ( )	Right ( )
Knees		
Early syperextension	Left ( )	Right ( )
Failure to extend at push off	Left ( )	Right ( )
Low back		
False hip extension	Present ( )	
Shoulder/arm swing		
Arm swing w/o trunk rotation	Left ( )	Right ( )
Arm swing from shoulders	Left ( )	Right ( )
Arm swing from elbows	Left ( )	Right ( )
Arm swing asymmetry/medial	Left ( )	Right ( )
Side view		
Forward drawn posture	Present ( )	
Posterior drawn posture	Present ( )	

Notes: ____________________

Gait Facilitation Methods

After gait has been assessed from the posterior, lateral, and anterior views, some additional strategies can be included to provide extra information. The first two maneuvers are designed to challenge and therefore facilitate the postural system. If these methods do indeed improve the movement patterns, it suggests that the patient may benefit from a sensorimotor training program.

Walking Backward (Aka Retro Walking) Instructing the patient to walk backward can provide valuable insight into the true state of function of their locomotor system. Walking backward creates new strategies and challenges for the locomotor system. Specifically, visuomotor strategies are reduced and hip elevation for leg swing becomes altered.

"Retro walking" is indeed complicated. It requires a specific facilitation of the gluteus maximus, which now becomes an initiator of backward gait. In a sort of reversed role from its antagonist, the iliopsoas, the facilitated gluteus maximus should increase its contractibility and establish a relatively smooth backward walking maneuver. However, in a truly weakened gluteus maximus, the muscle is incapable of such a maneuver and as a result, there will be additional pelvic rotation and knee flexion as the locomotor system attempts to move backward without the requisite gluteus maximus function. In the case of an asymmetrical dysfunction, the difference between the dysfunctional extremity and gluteus maximus and the physiological side can be striking.[218–220]

Walking with Tray Over Head A second strategy to challenge the locomotor system during gait is to have the patients reach as high as possible with both hands and hold a tray at the fingertips (see Fig. 13–28). Such a strategy facilitates the entire locomotor system. If the patients' faulty gait strategies dramatically improve, that is, if their movement pattern improves, their toe-off extension pattern becomes much smoother. This is a strong sign of an inhibited locomotor system, which may respond well to facilitory methods. Such a sign is very positive and strongly suggests that a sensory motor training program will be highly beneficial to the patient.

Tandem Arm–Leg Gait The importance of upper torso counterrotation (UTCR) cannot be overemphasized in the economics of gait. The counterrotation uses the active and passive myofascial tissues of the so-called posterior oblique system—a key component of the outer unit of lumbopelvic stability.[221] The posterior oblique system utilizes the muscle–fascia–muscle regions of the hamstrings/gluteals-lumbodorsal

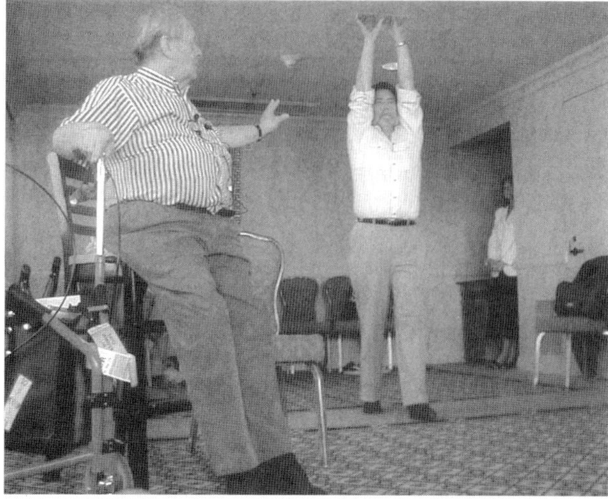

FIGURE 13–28. Walking with a tray overhead: With the fingers outstretched, balancing a tray challenges and facilitates the locomotor system. An improvement in gait suggests a sensorimotor training program would be beneficial because inhibitory actions were overcome. If there is no improvement, then a sensorimotor training program would be less promising, as facilitating the locomotor system did not overcome the gait difficulties.

fascia-contralateral latissimus dorsi to form a functional kinetic chain. The lead author has observed that this mechanism provides propulsive assistance as these stretched passive tissues return to normal length as opposite leg and arm move posteriorly, improved balance with the coordinated counterforces, reduced pelvic rotation, and reduced tibial rotation. This may then result in a less economic and efficient gait, in addition to placing additional torsional stresses on the knees and ankle/foot complex. Therefore, the lead author designed the *tandem arm-leg gait* (TALG) for two reasons: to have the clinician test it on himself or herself to practically appreciate the importance of this maneuver and then to assess the patient for appropriate UTCR. Although there is no known research on this maneuver, it is a simple learning and assessment tool.

The first part of the TALG involves the clinician performing the maneuver to appreciate the importance of torso counterrotation during gait. The TALG involves walking while the ipsilateral arm and leg move *together*, instead of in opposition as is normal.This is difficult for most individuals to accomplish because it is contrary to long-established motor engrams. Once the TALG becomes coordinated, the patient and clinician will find that their forward propulsion is compromised and that there is increased torso and leg rotation with each step. Increased rotational torsion is often noted in the knees, as is increased foot pronation. The added challenges in gait control and diminished efficiency of the TALG help to clarify the importance of upper torso counterrotation during gait for the clinician.

Once the clinician has learned to perform and appreciate the TALG, it is time to assess patients. There are different scenarios that arise when the UTCR mechanism of gait is faulty. Typically, the patient fails to rotate the upper body and appears to walk with the torso in a rigid manner. Two other scenarios are mentioned here. These include the patient who is very tight in the latissimus dorsi and/or hamstrings and also the patient with a marked kyphosis. The first situation involves overly tense myofascial components reducing motion, while the second involves compromised torso rotation due to kyphosing and perhaps decreased tensioning of the latissimus dorsi due to postural compromise. The interesting thing about the TALG is that patients with poor torso counterrotation generally learn to perform it easier than those with a normal UTCR pattern because the faulty patterned patients do not rely on it.

A final word on the TALG: the most important part of this test is the first part in which the clinician self tests to understand the importance of UTCR. After some practice of observing patients, the test becomes less necessary because the clinician has learned to appreciate UTCR importance and then routinely integrates this component into the gait assessment.

Three Movement Pattern Tests of Janda[107,152,222]

Because faulty movement patterns have been found to be associated with chronic pain syndromes, Janda noted six stereotypical faulty movement patterns associated with chronicity. Three of these test lumbopelvic movement patterns and will be described here. It is important to note that Janda's movement pattern tests should be performed prior to the palpatory portion of the examination, in order to avoid additional sensory motor stimulation that might reduce the reliability of such findings. As with other functional tests, these findings should be correlated with other observations to establish a consistent line of clinical assessment and reasoning.

Clinical Pearl: It is important to note that Janda's movement pattern tests should be performed prior to the palpatory portion of the examination, in order to avoid additional sensory motor stimulation that might reduce the reliability of such findings.

Test 1: Hip Extension Altered hip extension has been discussed earlier in this chapter as one of the factors noted in the declining locomotor system. Vogt et al.[223] noted altered gait activation patterns among patients with chronic low back pain compared to asymptomatic controls and it is with this in mind that the hip extension test is considered (Fig. 13–29).

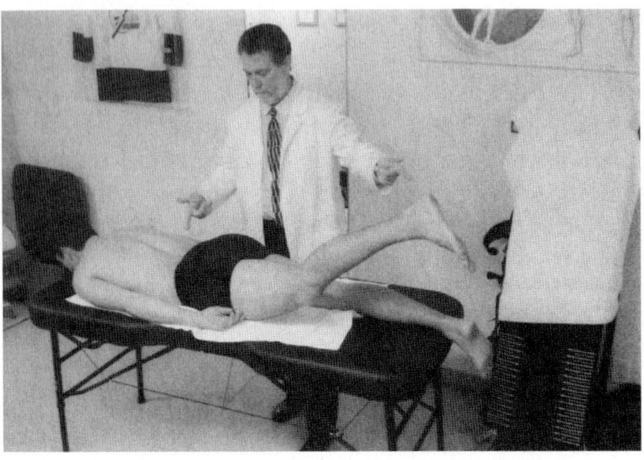

FIGURE 13–29. The hip extension test: This is a practical test for coordinated and stable hip extension. The clinician must observe knee flexion, timing of the posterior muscular contraction, pelvic lateral stability, and false hip extension.

This test is performed to assess for the presence of true or false hip extension, in addition to check for coordinated firing patterns during the hip extension maneuver.

Jull and Janda[152] observed that the firing order of the key muscles for this test would be as follows:

1. Ipsilateral hamstring
2. Ipsilateral gluteus maximus
3. Contralateral lumbosacral erector spinae
4. Ipsilateral lumbosacral erector spinae
5. Contralateral thoracolumbar erector spinae
6. Ipsilateral thoracolumbar erector spinae

Janda also stated that the hamstrings and gluteus maximus serve as prime movers, while the erector spinae stabilize the spine and pelvis.[152] However, Vogt and Banzer[224] found the firing pattern of the musculature to be different based on their EMG studies. They found the firing pattern for prone hip extension to be as follows:

1. Ipsilateral erector spinae
2. Ipsilateral hamstring
3. Contralateral erector spinae
4. Tensor fascia latae
5. Gluteus maximus

While some controversy remains regarding the timing of contraction of muscles for this movement pattern, there are key points that should be emphasized that allow this test to be of practical value regardless of controversy. For example, Bullock-Saxton et al.[225] found consistent uncoordinated hip extension patterns among patients with a history of chronic ankle sprain when compared with controls, demonstrating the practicality of the test while providing information regarding the global functional alterations that can occur following a localized trauma.

- *Primary purpose:* To assess for dynamic stability of instability during a unilateral hip extension maneuver.
- *Patient's position:* The patient is placed in a prone position with the arms resting at the side and the feet hanging freely beyond the end of the table.
- *Clinician's position:* The clinician stands at the side of the table at the level of the patient's pelvis and does not touch the patient during this test. (Some authors recommend that fingers be placed on the hamstrings and pelvis to feel the timing of the muscular contraction. Janda was specifically against this approach, as it compromised the results due to sensory motor stimulation from the tactile contact, while interfering with the clinician's potential for improvement of visual assessment skills.)
- *Clinician's instructions:* The instructions to the patient for this test must be concise without being too specific in order for the patient to move in his or her own way. For example, the instruction for the right hip extension test would be as follows: "Please lift your right leg up toward the ceiling."
- *Negative test:* An initial isometric contraction of the thoracolumbar erector spinae is considered to be normal to stabilize the torso prior to limb elevation. Contraction of the ipsilateral hamstring, gluteus maximus, stability of the trunk
- *Positive test:* Several pathological movement patterns can occur. These include the following:
  1. Significant knee flexion of the ipsilateral leg suggests overactivation of the hamstring.
  2. Delayed or absent ipsilateral gluteus maximus contraction. This is considered a very important finding.
  3. The presence of false hip extension. This is demonstrated when the pivot point of the leg extension during the initial 10 degrees occurs totally or in part at the sacro-iliac region instead of totally at the hip joint.
  4. Lowering of the flank on either side suggests rotation due to poor lumbopelvic functional stability.
  5. Early contraction of the periscapular musculature strongly suggests a chronic functional low back instability. It is most frequently observed to occur on the contralateral side. This finding suggests that recruitment of the upper torso musculature has occurred during the hip extension movement pattern in order to expedite the process.

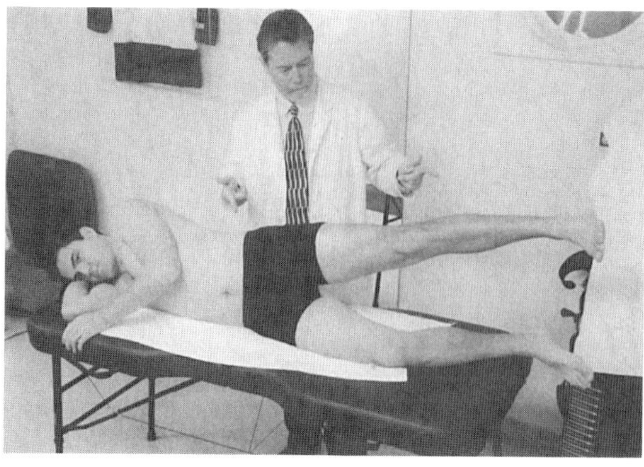

FIGURE 13–30. The hip abduction test: This is a practical test for coordinated and stable hip abduction. One must watch for hip flexion, external rotation, and hip "hiking."

Test 2: Hip Abduction Test

- *Primary purpose:* To screen for the dynamic stability or instability of the lumbopelvic region during hip abduction (Fig. 13–30).
- *Agonist:* Gluteus medius/minimus.
- *Antagonist:* Ipsilateral hip adductors.
- *Synergist:* Quadratus lumborum.
- *Patient's position:* The patient lies in side with superior leg resting in a crook formed by the lower leg, which is hip flexed at 45 degrees and knee flexed at 60 degrees. It is very important that the patient's upper superior leg is in line with his or her torso.
- *Clinician's position:* Standing at the side of the table at the level of the patient's pelvis.
- *Clinician's instruction:* The patient is instructed to slowly lift his or her leg toward the ceiling.
- *Normal test:* The leg should abduct to 20 degrees without any internal or external rotation, without any hip flexion, or without any ipsilateral pelvic cephalad elevation. The clinician may notice a slight initial contraction of the lumbar erector spinae or quadratus lumborum, which is considered physiologically an isometric stabilizing contraction in the absence of cephalad hip elevation.
- *Positive test:* Several pathological movement patterns can occur. These include the following:
  1. Ipsilateral external hip/leg rotation suggesting overactivity and possible shortening of piriformis.
  2. Ipsilateral external pelvic rotation, suggesting overactivation of the piriformis and other external hip rotators.

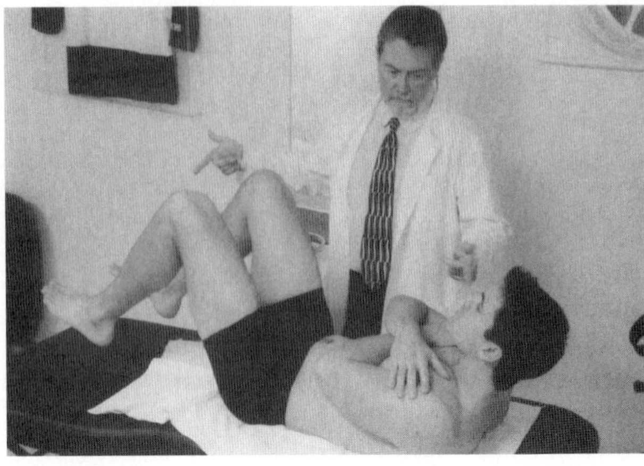

FIGURE 13–31. The curl-up test: This is a practical test for coordinated and stable elevation of the upper torso while rounding of the spine occurs.

3. Ipsilateral hip flexion, suggesting overactivity and probable shortening of hip flexors, including tensor fascia latae.
4. Cephalad elevation of the ipsilateral pelvis prior to 20 degrees of hip abduction, suggesting overactivity and shortening of quadratus lumborum.
5. Combination of any of the above.

Test 3: Trunk Curl Up Test

- *Primary purpose:* To screen for lumbopelvic dynamic instability during trunk flexion. (Fig. 13–31)
- *Secondary purpose:* To establish possible etiology of faulty trunk flexion.
- *Agonist:* Rectus abdominis.
- *Antagonist:* Thoracolumbar erector spinae.
- *Synergist:* Iliopsoas.
- *Patient's position:* The patient should lie in a supine position with the hips and knees as close to the buttocks as possible with the arms flexed across his or her chest.
- *Clinician's position:* Standing at the side of the table at the level of the patient's pelvis.
- *Clinician's instruction:* Instruct the patient to elevate the head and shoulders away from the floor or table.
- *Negative test:* Contraction of the abdominis rectus and rounding of the thoracolumbar spine. The feet should remain planted on the resting surface. The movement pattern should begin with elevation and the rounding should begin superiorly.
- *Positive test:* There are several pathological findings. These include the following:
  1. The feet elevate off the supporting surface. This suggests recruitment of the hip flexors in order to provide adequate leverage to perform the maneuver. Janda[107,152] initially suggested that this finding indicated synergistic substitution of the iliopsoas; however, Juker et al. later challenged this assumption.[226]
  2. The thoracolumbar spine remains rigidly straight and elevates in a rod-like manner instead of a curling manner. This suggests incoordination of the torso flexors and extensors, where they act as synergists to isometrically co-contract instead of synergists in which the rectus abdomus (the main torso flexor) concentrically contracts as the erector spinae eccentrically contracts.
  3. Shaking of the rectus abdominis muscle, which indicates significant weakness.
  4. A combination of any of the above.

Prone Instability Test

McGill,[227] a leading spinal biomechanist, designed "manual testing for prone lumbar joint shear stability." This has become known as the prone instability test (PTS), a screen for patients with poor lumbopelvic stability in the form of ligamentous laxity and aberrant motion. While issues regarding reliability and validity remain, Hicks et al.[228] found the PTS was more reliable than segmental mobility testing.

- *Primary purpose:* To assess for dynamic lumbopelvic stability or instability.
- *Patient's position:* The patient lies prone with his or her torso resting on the lower end of the table. The legs are off the table, with the hips flexed and both feet resting on the floor. Both arms are holding on to the table to maintain this position throughout the test.
- *Clinician's position:* The clinician stands at the side of the table next to and facing the patient, approximating the level of the patient's low back.
- *Clinician's actions:* With the patient relaxing the torso musculature, the clinician applies an anterior-superior load, beginning at the sacrum, and continuing with each successive spinous process superiorly. Complaints of pain by the patient or a sensation of actual joint shear displacement are logged for each loaded joint, with the pain response being considered more important. If there is no pain or palpable joint shearing, the test is discontinued.

  The patient is then instructed to slightly elevate both legs off the floor and maintain this position, while also contracting the low back extensor musculature, which activates the lumbopelvic stabilizers. The clinician again loads each spinal joint in the same order and manner as before.
- *Test results:* If the pain is diminished or erased once lumbopelvic stabilizers are activated, the test is positive, which suggests functional lumbar instability.

THE PALPATORY EVALUATION

Clinical palpation has been one of the cornerstones of patient assessment. It provides clinical information that can be vital in the determination of the diagnosis. Despite being a cornerstone of the physical examination, an increasingly important question has arisen regarding this diagnostic tool. The question is that of reliability. Can palpation findings be reproduced in order to be of any clinical value? Although there are many methods to determine reliability, research on this topic has, to a great degree, centered on two approaches. These reliability approaches compare findings between evaluators, *interexaminer* reliability, and between the same evaluator, *intraexaminer* reliability, with the former being more scientifically regarded than the later.

Clinical Pearl: Clinical palpation has been one of the cornerstones of patient assessment. It provides clinical information that can be vital in the determination of the diagnosis.

Several studies on palpation have demonstrated unacceptable interexaminer reliability with regard to cranial rhythm palpation,[229] trigger point (TrP) location,[230,231] thoracic segmental mobility,[232] thoracolumbar segmental mobility,[233] lumbar segmental mobility,[228,234,235] and sacroiliac mobility.[235,236]

There are four important studies of note demonstrating palpation reliability. One study demonstrated high single-examiner reliability of cervical spine zygapophyseal joint assessment when confirmed by radiographically controlled facet blocks.[237] A second study demonstrated improved levels of interexaminer reliability for the detection of myofascial trigger points (TrPs) among a group of experts, once they established unified assessment protocols.[238] Third study, which demonstrated interexaminer acceptable levels of reliability, was accomplished by Sciotti et al.[239] when assessing for TrPs in the trapezius musculature. Most recently, Humphreys et al.[240] introduced a "gold standard" for joint hypomobility (i.e., congenital block vertebra) assessment to demonstrate that relatively inexperienced examiners could reach substantial agreement to correctly identify cervical spine intersegmental fixations. While each of these studies includes small patient numbers, the findings suggest that acceptable levels of interexaminer reliability can be achieved if the current barriers to improved outcomes can be identified and corrected.

Although interexaminer reliability is a benchmark for the scientific method, palpatory intraexaminer reliability has been found to be significantly better in a number of studies.[232–234,241–243] *The importance of this point cannot be overstated, as intraexaminer reliability practically relates to what is performed in the typical clinical setting.* After all, it is what the clinician palpates before, during, and after treatment, and also during succeeding visits, that helps to determine comparative changes in patient status. Therefore, the importance of acceptable intrarater reliability remains a key reason for continuing to integrate palpatory findings in the evaluation of musculoskeletal disorders.

Clinical Pearl: Although interexaminer reliability is a benchmark for the scientific method, palpatory intraexaminer reliability has been significantly better in a number of studies. The importance of this point cannot be overstated, as intra-examiner reliability practically relates to what is performed in the typical clinical setting.

Finally, the literature also provides some insights into achieving better interexaminer reliability outcomes. First, palpatory expertise does not appear to be guaranteed simply by years of experience of manual assessment and treatment,[238,241–243] suggesting that such skills require a consistent focused strategy rather than just working in the field. Second, differences in the abilities to isolate key anatomical landmarks by palpation may confound better results.[236] Third, clinicians may with time come to rely on their own method of palpatory assessment, which may be quite different from that of other clinicians.[241] This may explain why the previously mentioned Gerwin study[238] results improved significantly after the examiners established agreed-upon assessment criteria.

Palpatory Literacy

Palpation is to touch what reading is to sight. Chaitow[2,244] brought forth the concept of "palpatory literacy" to emphasize the importance of developing high levels of clinical skill for health-care providers. Leaders in the professions that rely heavily on manual clinical techniques have stressed the importance of developing these skills,[10,15,135] with the understanding that expertise comes with decades of diligent training. How does one go about gaining such expertise? While an in-depth discussion of palpatory training exceeds the parameters of this chapter, a basic overview of palpatory principles will be addressed. However, palpatory literacy, like all clinical arts, cannot be truly taught in a text, but merely explained. Such skills must be practically taught.

Clinical Pearl: Palpation is to touch what reading is to sight. Chaitow [2,244] brought forth the concept of palpatory literacy to emphasize the importance of developing high levels of clinical skill for health care providers.

Basic Principles of Palpation

Tissue Tone *The hand as an instrument:* Lewit has called the hand the greatest diagnostic and therapeutic tool that ever has been, or ever will be, invented.[10] Because of the capacity to accept a multitude of palpatory sensations (i.e., texture, tone, temperature, skin resistance, etc.), it almost immediately dynamically adapts to these sensations, and then performs a multitude of maneuvers, the clinical applications are only limited by the imagination of their operator.

"Carpal multiplicity": This is the lead author's term to overcome a common palpatory misperception. Many techniques are taught to use each hand as a one-dimensional tool during diagnostic or therapeutic manual procedures. For example, one hand will be considered the contact hand, while the other one the stabilizing hand. However, this strategy fails to appreciate the multitasking capacity of the hand, limiting its clinical applications. Indeed, one hand can stabilize with the first and fifth digits, provide a therapeutic contact with the third digit, and simultaneously palpate for resulting tissue changes as the thenar and hypothenar eminences provide additional stabilizing and sensory duties. All of these activities are well within the locomotor system's capacity to functionally integrate.

In addition to being capable of several tasks at once, the hand is a multidimensional tool. One can use the finger pads for fine palpation, the finger tips for deeper probing, the dorsum of the hand for temperature assessment, the opposing thumb and fingers for grasping or for pincer palpation, a soft or relaxed palm and fingers to gently stabilize a sensitive region, or a tense palm or fingers to more forcefully stabilize a less sensitive region. Contacts utilizing different parts of the hand are commonly used for various assessment and treatment methods, such as pisiform contact, thenar contact, relaxed (soft) hypothenar contact, firm ("knife-edge") hypothenar contact, and a knuckle contact. The clinician can be taught how to employ the hand in this manner for use in various manual skills, but the manual dexterity, strength, sensibility, and mobility of the hand vary greatly among individuals. Therefore, it is ultimately up to the clinician to experiment and practice diligently to acquire the most effective manner in which to clinically use his or her hands (see Fig. 13–32).

Distal palpability requires proximal stability and mobility. Optimal palpation occurs with the minimum of extraneous motion, and the maximum of stability of the palpating limb. Therefore, the palpating hand should remain close to the clinician's body and the joints of the upper extremity should be within their neutral range of motion. Extending the arm or moving joints near their end-range requires additional locomotor control, which is distracting in terms of attention and neuromotor control. The same holds true for more distal instability, as would occur if the clinician were standing on an unstable surface.

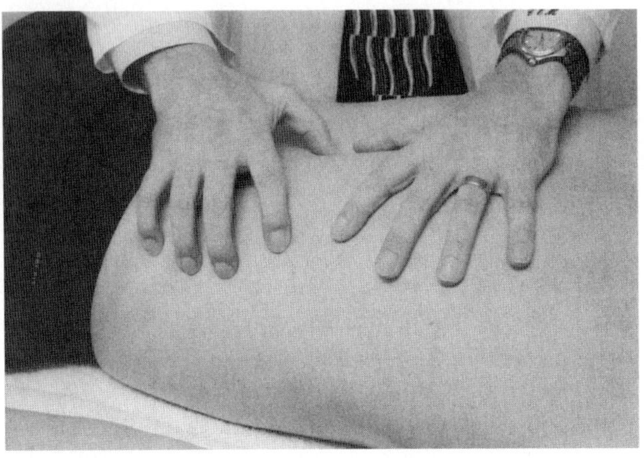

FIGURE 13–32. Palpatory multiplicity and literacy: Excellence requires a prolonged and concerted effort to learn to use the hands as optimal, multifunctional, diagnostic, and therapeutic tools. Here the clinician's hands maintain two very different assessment and or diagnostic positions, demonstrating the wide variety of options available once properly trained.

Mechanical Advantages The clinician should be aware of the mechanical advantages available when planning for a manual procedure. In keeping with the previous paragraph, the less the strain required, the more the relaxed palpating hand can focus on the dynamic alterations necessary for optimal results. Would it be more efficient to draw the target body region closer, or to move it away? Should the fingers extend and the wrist pronated for a specific technique, or should the hand and wrist remain firm while the elbow extends? Should the finger pads be used for optimal palpation, or should the fingertips be used for better mechanical advantage? These types of questions should be asked as the clinician finds the optimal means of achieving the clinical goal.

Clinical Pearl: The clinician should be aware of the mechanical advantages available when planning for a manual procedure. The less the strain required, the more the relaxed palpating hand can focus on the dynamic alterations necessary for optimal results.

Patient Relaxation Although a plethora of scenarios can lead to increased muscle tone,[4] it is incumbent upon the clinician to have the patient as relaxed as possible in preparation for palpatory assessment in order to gain the highest level of reliability. With increased relaxation, the clinician can more effectively probe in order to differentiate physiological from pathological tissue tone, and to isolate localized areas of dysfunction.

Janda stated that the most efficient locomotor relaxation occurs while the patient is supine.[15] He stated that the supine position inhibits the gamma system, which provides optimal palpation of soft tissues and joints. This notion is probably based on the work of Freeman and Wyke,[245] which was later supported by Johansson et al.[246]

For optimal relaxation, palpation should also be achieved while the patient's body, or at least target region, is placed in an anatomically neutral position. The neutral position of each joint is generally considered to be that which places the least tension on the intrinsic joint structures or surrounding tissues. Deviation from the anatomical position increases tension in both joints and regional soft tissues, stimulating proprioceptors and exteroceptors and reflexively increasing the regional tone (i.e., decreased relaxation).[247,248]

Primum Non Nocere Because the palpatory examination described here is performed on the relaxed patient, the clinician must be aware that some risk is involved with various assessment maneuvers. In essence, the patient has agreed to let his or her guard down in allowing the clinician to perform an evaluation. Whenever this occurs in health care, the clinician must take pause and determine the risk–benefit ratio before proceeding. There is no specific rule for making a determination, but a negligible risk should require no specific prior communication, while greater levels of risk should require greater levels of prior communication and informed consent.

Clinical Pearl: Because the palpatory examination described here is performed on the relaxed patient, the clinician must be aware that some risk is involved with various assessment maneuvers. In essence, the patient has agreed to let his or her guard down in allowing the clinician to perform an evaluation.

Tissue Layers Tissue types can be divided into skin, subdermal, fascial, muscle, visceral, and bone/joint. Palpation of each requires an appreciation of the unique properties of the tissues in order to differentiate and assess each (see Fig. 13–1).

Lightness of Touch A common error in palpation occurs with pressing too hard. The individual tries to gain greater information with additional loading, only to further compress the tissues of the patient and his or her own fingers. The secret of optimal palpation comes with applying the lightest of pressure and allowing the subtle tissue differences to become more clearly delineated with repetition. Lewit[10] states, "In palpation, your fingers are your eyes, so don't press on them!" and "If you press too hard, the only thing you will feel is your own fingers!"

The Barrier Phenomenon All soft tissues have a degree of elasticity. As the probing finger carefully loads a tissue, an initial barrier of resistance will be encountered. This first point where the mechanical properties of a given tissue reache the first endpoint is called *the barrier phenomenon*,[135] while the initial resistance point is known as *the barrier*. It is often very subtle and easily missed as one searches for more dramatically resistant barriers. This barrier represents the basis of clinical palpation, as it alerts the clinician to the degree of resistance of the target tissue. The barrier is present in the skin, subdermal tissue, fascia, muscle, and joints. Under physiological circumstances there will be a gradual increase in resistance leading to the barrier, whereas an abrupt barrier will occur under pathological circumstances.

Clinical Pearl: This first point where the mechanical properties of a given tissue reach the first endpoint is called *the barrier phenomenon*, while the initial resistance point is known as *the barrier*.

Once the barrier has been identified, the clinician then slightly releases the pressure, palpating as the tissue length returns to normal. This has been likened to pressing on a spring and then feeling the spring return to its normal length, while measuring the degree of tension and length of motion. This analogy led to the term *"springing the barrier"* as an accepted means of assessing a target tissue's function. The clinician familiar with "springing" a joint in order to evaluate its end-feel should easily recognize that this is what is being done when skin, muscle, fascia, or other soft tissue structures are being "sprung." It is their end-of-range "feel" that is being evaluated.

The barrier of a tissue can vary significantly, depending on its structure, as well as its degree of physiological or pathological function. The barriers of the same tissues, in different body regions, can also be quite different. The barriers of different tissues can also have quite unique palpatory properties, for example, there are major differences between the feel of the end-of-range barriers of skin, muscle, tendon, ligament, and joint capsule. There are also wide variations in tissue tone relative to genetically acquired traits, with hypermobility being an easily comprehended example.

Learning to differentiate physiological from pathological barriers is considered to be the most important skill in palpation, and in fact in all manual techniques, since it forms the basis of assessment and treatment. Unfortunately, acquiring expertise in palpation of the barrier requires perseverance that few appreciate and even fewer undertake.

Hypermobility Benign hypermobility has been recognized as a normal variant of elasticity of connective tissue, or less commonly a manifestation of a definitive disease process such as Ehlers-Danlos syndrome. A possible reason for recurrent joint trauma in hypermobile persons may be the recently demonstrated impairment of proprioception noted in both small and large joints.[249]

There appears to be a link between hypermobility and increased risk of musculoskeletal pain in general[250–252] and low back pain in particular. Muller et al.[253] examined over 330 patients with back pain, using among other methods Janda's functional tests. They found that 33% (112 patients, predominantly female) demonstrated constitutional hypermobility compared with 13% of normal controls. They conclude: "Hypermobility proved to be an independent factor in the genesis of chronic back pain. Therefore hypermobility should be considered in the clinical examination of each back pain patient."

Clinical Pearl: There appears to be a link between hypermobility and increased risk of musculoskeletal pain in general[250–252] and low back pain in particular.

Hypermobility is more common in females, with rates ranging from 5% in Caucasian adults to rates as high as 38% in younger Middle Eastern women.[254] Prevalence in African populations is also higher than in Caucasians.[255,256] It is worth noting that breathing pattern disorders, such as hyperventilation, are more common in hypermobile individuals, particularly where hypermobility is associated with chronic pain syndromes.[257,258]

Greenman[195] discusses three types of hypermobility:

1. Hypermobility due to diagnosable conditions such as Marfan and Ehlers-Danlos syndromes. In these syndromes there is an altered biochemistry of the connective tissue, which often reflects an extremely loose skin, a tendency for cutaneous scarring ("stretch marks"). There may also be vascular symptoms such as mitral valve prolapse and dilatation of the ascending aorta.
2. Physiological hypermobility as noted in particular body types (e.g., ectomorphs) and in ballet dancers, gymnasts, and ice hockey goalies. Joints such as fingers, knees, elbows, and the spine may be able to demonstrate greater than normal degrees of range of motion. This can be further subdivided into individuals with global versus local hypermobility.
3. Compensatory hypermobility may result from hypomobility, with patients presenting with painful joint and spinal symptoms. Greenman points out that, "Segments of compensatory hypermobility may be either adjacent to, or some distance from, the area(s) of joint hypomobility. Clinically there also seems to be relative hypermobility on the opposite side of a segment that is restricted."

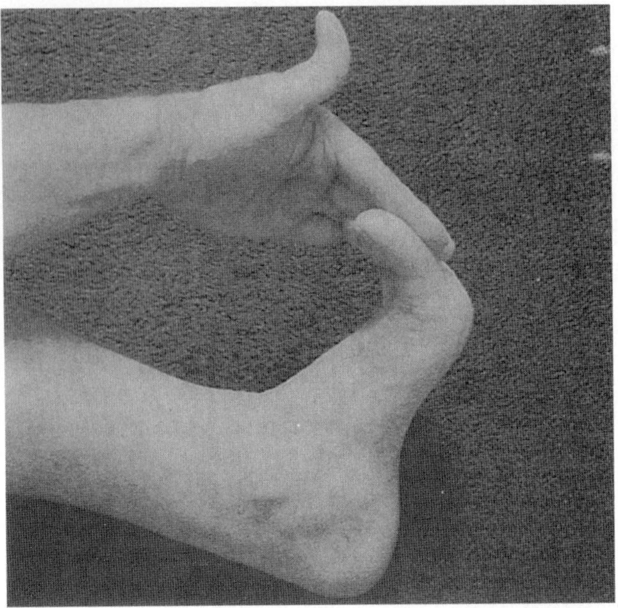

FIGURE 13–33. Hypermobility syndrome: This can be quickly assessed by extending either the patient's great toe (beyond 60 degrees is generally considered hypermobile) and/or the thumb (beyond 180 degrees is hypermobile).

A quick and practical screen for hypermobility can be performed by bringing the patient's relaxed great toe or thumb to end-range extension (see Fig. 13–33).

Skin Assessment The skin overlying areas of dysfunction (what Lewit[135] calls "hyperalgesic skin zones"—HAZ), including inflamed tissue, areas of excessive hypertonicity, spasm, or trigger point (TrP) activity, is characterized by a series of pathophysiological changes, most of which are readily palpable.

The skin overlying such zones[135]:

(a) adheres to the underlying fascia more efficiently, and is therefore more resistant to movements such as sliding (on underlying fascia), lifting, or rolling.
(b) displays increased sympathetic activity, resulting in increased hydrosis (sweat). This sudomotor activity brings about a noticeable resistance during light stroking movements of (say) a finger less easy. This resistance is known in clinical shorthand, as "skin drag."
(c) appears to be more "compacted," resisting effective separation, stretching methods.
(d) displays altered thermal qualities, allowing for some discrimination between such areas and normal surrounding tissue.

Skin Palpation Tests The three methods described below do not need to be used during the same treatment session, although they can be. Usual clinical application involves one or the other being employed, once sufficient skill levels have been achieved. The three methods described support or replace each other, with some clinicians having a preference for one or the other. The second author of this chapter primarily uses the drag palpation approach (method b); however, at times the other two methods are also employed. More detailed descriptions, and palpation exercises, can be found in *Palpation and Assessment Skills: Assessment and Diagnosis Through Touch.*[2]

(a) *Skin on fascia assessment method:* This assessment approach is based on methods derived from German Bindegewbsmassage (connective tissue massage).[259–261]

Note: It is easier to displace skin against underlying tissue in slim individuals, with little fatty tissue. Obese individuals have a higher fat and water content subcutaneously, making displacement more difficult.

- The patient is prone and practitioner stands to the side, at hip level.
- The clinician applies both hands (or the pads of several fingers of each hand) flat against the skin bilaterally, at sacral level.
- Only sufficient pressure should be used to produce adherence between the fingertips and the skin.
- The skin and subcutaneous tissues should be displaced simultaneously on each side, against the fascia in a cephalad direction, with a small pushing action, to the elastic barrier.
- The degree of displacement possible should be symmetrical if the deeper tissues are physiologically normal and are not hypertonic.
- It is important that symmetrical areas be examined simultaneously.
- The pattern of testing should be performed from inferior to superior, either moving the tissues superiorly, or bilaterally in an obliquely diagonal direction, toward the spine.
- The two sides should be compared for symmetry of range of movement of the skin and subcutaneous tissue, to its elastic barrier.
- It should be possible to identify local areas where the skin adherence to underlying connective tissue reveals restriction, as compared to the opposite side.
- This is likely to be an area housing active myofascial trigger points (TrPs) or tissue that is dysfunctional or hypertonic.

It is often possible to visualize these reflex areas. They are characterized by being retracted or elevated, most commonly close to the lower thoracic border of the scapula and over the pelvic and gluteal areas, and are considered to be the result of viscerocutaneous reflex activity involving altered blood supply leading to colloidal changes in the cells and tissues.

The findings noted from this method can be compared with the following two methods.

(b) *Drag palpation assessment:* Atrichial sweat glands, controlled by the sympathetic division of the autonomic nervous system, empty directly on the skin, creating increased hydrosis (sweat) presence, and in the process the mechanical, electrical, and heat transfer properties, and characteristics, of the skin are altered.[262]

Lewit[135] suggests that clinicians should be able to identify active reflex activity (such as are involved with TrPS) simply by assessing the degree of elasticity in the overlying skin, and comparing it with surrounding tissue, one of the mechanical changes resulting from increased sympathetic activity. The simultaneously occurring hydrosis phenomenon explains why, prior to the introduction of methods of electrical detection of acupuncture points, any skilled acupuncturist could quickly locate "active" points by palpation, and also why measurement of the electrical resistance of the skin can now do this even more rapidly (i.e., when skin is moist it conducts electricity more efficiently than when dry).

Note: There should be no oil or lubricant on the patient's skin or clinician's hands for this method to be efficient.

(h) *Drag palpation method*

- Using an extremely light touch ("skin on skin"), without any pressure, the digit (finger, thumb) is stroked across the skin overlaying areas suspected of housing dysfunctional changes (such as TrPS).
- The areas chosen are commonly those where skin on fascia movement (see previous test) was reduced compared with surrounding skin.
- When the stroking digit passes over areas where a sense of hesitation, or "drag," is noted, increased hydrosis will have been identified.
- A degree of searching pressure, into such tissues, precisely under the area of drag, may locate a taut band of tissue, and when this is compressed a pained response is commonly elicited.
- If pressure is maintained for 2–3 seconds a report of a radiating or referred sensation may be forthcoming.
- If this sensation replicates symptoms previously noted by the patient, the point located is an active TrP.[175]

Skin Stretch Method[135] *Note:* At first, it is necessary to practice this method slowly. Eventually, it should be possible to move fairly rapidly over an area that is being searched for evidence of reflex activity (or acupuncture points). Choose an area to be assessed, where abnormal degrees of skin on fascia adherence, and/or drag sensations, were previously noted.

- To examine the back region, the patient should be lying prone.
- Place two index fingers adjacent to each other, on the skin, side by side or pointing toward each other, with no pressure at all onto the skin, just a contact touch.
- Lightly and slowly separate the fingers, feeling the skin stretch to its "easy" limit, to the point where resistance is first noted.
- It should be possible in normal tissue to "spring" the skin further apart, to its elastic limit.
- Release this stretch and move both fingers 0.5 cm (between 1.4 and 1/2 in) to one side of this first test site, and test again in the same way, and in the same direction of pull, separating the fingers, and adding a spring assessment once the barrier is reached.
- Perform exactly the same sequence over and over again until the entire area of tissue has been searched, ensuring that the rhythm adopted is neither too slow nor too rapid. Ideally one stretch per second should be performed.
- When skin being stretched is not as elastic as it was on the previous stretch a potential HAZ will have been identified.
- This should be marked with a skin pencil for future attention.

  Light digital pressure to the center of that small zone would almost always locate a sensitive contracture, which on sustained pressure may radiate or refer sensations to a distant site. If such sensations are familiar to the patient, the point being pressed is an active trigger point.

Modification and often normalization of the reduced elastic status of the skin, as identified in the previous assessments, is possible by various methods, including sustained light stretching (mini-myofascial releases), or by means of positional release techniques or introduction of isometric contractions into the underlying tissues, or via sustained compression, or by acupuncture.[2]

Scar Assessment Lewit[135] advises that where conditions are resistant to conventional treatment, or where symptoms do not seem to be explained by findings, scar tissue should be evaluated. He suggests deep palpation for pain spots near scars, assessing for increased resistance ("adhesions") as well as for HAZs, by skin stretching (as described above). If release of the skin by stretching fails to resolve the situation (simple skin stretching is usually very successful with scars, according to Lewit), needling (into tender spots), or local infiltration injections may be called for.

Trigger points often develop in scar tissue[263] and may perpetuate the original pain pattern, even after the original cause of the pain has been removed. Scar tissue might also block normal lymphatic drainage and may in this way encourage trigger point formation or recurrence.[264]

Apart from a possible association with trigger points, Braggins[265] notes that one cause of disturbed neural dynamics ("adverse mechanical or neural tension") involves the presence of scar tissue.

To take Braggins' point a step further, the adverse tension from scar tissue (dermal or adhesive) appears to affect the fusimotor, or gamma, system that determines regional muscle tone, as was discussed in Chapter 9. The lead author has observed that acute and subacute scarring tends to be locally facilitory, while chronic scarring tends to be inhibitory. In other words, the gamma system that regulates tone becomes compromised by the presence of increased local tension from scar tissue, which stimulates local mechanoreceptors, causing increased regional inhibition and decreased muscle tone. However, this remains observational and the mechanism, while reasonable, is also theoretical.

Clinical Pearl: Apart from a possible association with trigger points, Braggins notes that one cause of disturbed neural dynamics (adverse mechanical or neural tension) involves the presence of scar tissue.

Scar sites are examined by pinching, compressing, and rolling the scar tissue between the thumb and finger to examine for evidence of trigger points (see Fig. 13–34). Upledger and Vredevoogd[266], discussing scar tissue, illustrate its importance with the example of a patient with chronic migraine headaches, which appeared to result from chronic fascial drag, produced by an appendectomy scar. Deep pressure medially, on the scar, produced the headache, while deep pressure laterally caused relief. Mobilization of the scar was performed by sustained and deep, but gentle, pressure.

Trigger Point (TrP) Review and Assessment The topic of myofascial trigger points is covered thoroughly in Chapter 9 and the reader must refer Chapter 9 to establish a clear understanding of its etiological aspects. In addition to the underlying physiologic basis, key stereotypical trigger point patterns were provided among key muscles in which myofascial pain can be

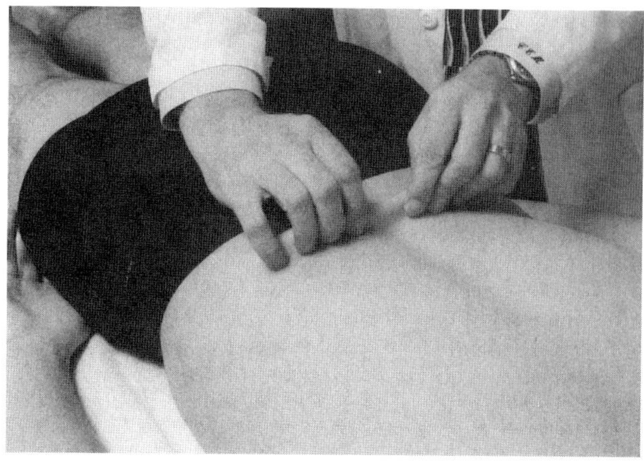

FIGURE 13–34. Skin assessment: This can be performed in many ways. Here, a skin rolling technique is employed.

associated with low back syndromes. It was also explained that the proper abbreviation for the trigger point is "TrP," in order to avoid confusion with the term tender point, which is used for myofascial pain and employs the abbreviation "TP." In addition to that complete summary, a brief overview of trigger points is presented in this chapter.

Myofascial pain syndrome, or myofascial syndrome, is defined by Simons et al.[175] as "Pain, tenderness, and autonomic phenomena referred from active myofascial trigger points (TrPs), with associated dysfunction." They define the TrP as

> A focus of hyperirritability in a tissue that, when compressed, is locally tender and, if sufficiently hypersensitive, gives rise to referred pain and tenderness, and sometimes to referred autonomic phenomena and distortion of proprioception. Types include myofascial cutaneous, fascial, ligamentous and periosteal trigger points.

While these definitions are not new, few clinicians appreciate that myofascial pain necessarily requires the presence of a TrP. Furthermore, the fact that TrPs exist in other tissues besides myofascial tissue seems often overlooked.

To identify a TrP requires a systematic palpation of muscles, across the direction of the fibers. Target tissues can be identified using any of the skin palpation methods outlined above. By then palpating perpendicularly to the fiber direction a clinician may be able to locate a taut band. This string-like structure feels like a bundle of contracted fibers.[175]

Clinical Pearl: Few clinicians appreciate that myofascial pain necessarily requires the presence of a TrP. Furthermore, the fact that TrPs exist in other tissues besides myofascial tissue seems often overlooked.

Palpation along a taut band may reveal an exquisitely tender nodule that, when stimulated, produces typical patterns of referred pain. Recognition of pain as familiar by the patient is now considered to be a major diagnostic criterion for an active TrP (in addition to the presence of a taut band).[238]

Taut bands and TrPs are only considered clinically relevant when the patient recognizes the elicited pain, or when the functional limitations imposed by the taut band contribute to mechanical dysfunction, secondary to muscle shortening.[267,268]

Dommerholt and Issa[269] note, "The taut band, trigger point and local twitch response are objective criteria, identified solely by palpation, that do not require a verbal response from the patient. A local twitch response is an indication of the presence of an active trigger point." It is a brief involuntary contraction of the taut band, which can be recorded electromyographically, be felt with the needle during trigger point injection or needling, observed visually or by diagnostic ultrasound. It is mediated primarily through the spinal cord without supraspinal influence.[270,271] High resolution sonography was not sensitive enough to visualize the actual TrP, but allowed researchers to visualize the twitch response of the taut band following stimulation of the trigger point by insertion of a hypodermic needle.[272,273]

Several studies have considered the interrater reliability of the TrP examination; however, reproducible protocols have recently been established by Gerwin et al.[238] and by Sciotti et al.[239] In Gerwin's study, a team of recognized experts could initially not agree until they developed consensus regarding the criteria, indicating that training is essential for the accurate identification of active TrPs.

Dommerholt[269] reports,

> The International Myopain Society (IMS) is currently conducting a worldwide multicenter study to establish reliable methods for the diagnosis of MPS, determine the interrater reliability of trigger point examination, and the sensitivity and specificity with which classification criteria can distinguish patients with MPS from healthy control subjects.[274]

TrP Assessment Methods Palpatory confirmation of TrPs comprises a set of skills that are often overlooked. Learning requires supervised practice to gain true proficiency, but the authors considered expertise to be a necessity in optimal locomotor system assessment and a description of the typical methods is therefore provided. Because such palpatory exploration can be somewhat painful for the patient, prior patient explanation and consent to proceed is warranted.

Clinical Pearl: Palpatory confirmation of TrPs comprises a set of skills that are often overlooked. Learning requires supervised practice to gain true proficiency, but the authors considered expertise to be a necessity in optimal locomotor system assessment.

It was previously noted that skin drag palpation might be used to locate underlying TrPs because of an overlying HAZ. However, specific confirmation requires a more specific palpatory strategy. Palpatory confirmation also utilizes the "local twitch response" (LTR). The LTR is a reflexive rather than cognitive response of a TrP to painful stimuli (i.e., palpation or needling), provoking a sudden contraction of a portion of the muscle surrounding the TrP. This may at times be followed by, and confused with, a contraction of the entire muscle or region, a so-called "jump sign." The jump sign, however, is a supraspinal response to pain sensation and must be separated from the LTR, since the LTR is a spinal reflexive response. A LTR is considered to be specific, or pathognomonic, for the presence of a TrP, assuming the clinician can properly differentiate the response from other similar palpatory findings.

According Simons et al.,[175] there are three key palpation techniques that may be employed, each of which is designed for assessment of different morphological challenges. It should be noted that, although these methods are differentiated for purposes of teaching and clarity, the lead author states that overlap of these methods is typically employed once expertise is established. The three TrP palpatory assessment methods are as follows:

(a) *Flat palpation:* This is digital palpation, typically using the pads of the fingertips transversely across, or at a right angle to, the alignment of the muscle fibers, while compressing over a firm or bony underlying structure. One can "trap" the TrP in this manner and palpate the nodule. Direct compression will provoke a pain response from the patient, and often a stereotypical referral pattern.

The muscle should be as relaxed as possible for flat palpation. Logically, flat palpation is typically used for broad, flat muscles, such as the gluteals. It can also be used for muscles that are not broad and flat, but have underlying bony or firm surfaces such as the piriformis, or muscles with difficult anatomical access such as the diaphragm or middle portion of the psoas.

(i) *Snapping palpation:* This skill technique is also called "snapping the TrP" because it uses the brisk snapping motion of a rigid finger across the muscle fibers housing the TrP. As the TrP is provoked, the LTR is elicited. The motion is similar to snapping a guitar string, so the muscle should be at a neutral or slightly lengthened state to allow for optimal assessment. A shortened, flaccid muscle would be like trying to pluck a loose guitar string, while an overly stretched muscle would interfere with the ability to isolate and provoke the TrP.

Snapping palpation is quite effective and convenient (i.e., timesaving) for long muscles with superficial access. Typical lumbopelvic muscles that are assessed with snapping palpation include the rectus abdominis and erector spinae. It is important to learn to differentiate between a LTR and a muscle that simply rolls under one's fingertip once the myofascial components are sufficiently tensioned.

(ii) *Pincer palpation:* This strategy uses rigid fingers and opposable thumb in a "C-shape" manner to pinch target tissues in search of the TrP. The muscle should be as relaxed as possible for pincer palpation. The target tissues typically are contoured in a manner so that the thumb and fingers can reach sufficiently around and beyond the suspected TrP. The clinician then pinches the tissue between thumb and fingers, while allowing tissue to roll between the digits while slowly withdrawing the hand. The clinician assesses for local taut bands of fibers, to identify TrPs, and assess for an LTR.

Pincer palpation is quite effective and practical. A typical lumbopelvic muscle that is assessed by pincer palpation is the transversus abdominis. As with snapping palpation, it is important to learn to differentiate between a LTR and a muscle that simply rolls under one's fingertip once the myofascial components are sufficiently tensioned.

Muscle Length Assessment Assessment of muscle tone allows for additional confirmatory information. Muscle imbalance has been previously discussed in this chapter, and muscle tone forms the basis of this phenomenon. Janda considered muscle length an important assessment tool, but stressed that clinicians must strive to be as specific as possible to isolate target muscles in order to maintain optimal levels of reliability,[131,222] while always warning against over-reliance of any specific finding.

Specific testing requires a solid understanding of functional anatomy and kinesiology. It is also important to remember that many muscles change their function when the angle of the joint(s) they span is significantly altered. Janda described this phenomenon as muscle paradox.[15] For example, does the piriformis remain an external hip rotator when the femur is fully flexed upon the torso, or does it become an internal rotator? Therefore, it is best to try to evaluate muscle length while these joints are as close to their neutral anatomic position and/or along the arc of motion accomplished by the target muscle as possible. A clear understanding of the barrier phenomenon is also imperative.

The Modified Thomas Position The modified Thomas position (MTP)[222] is considered the most practical position for isolating and assessing several key lumbopelvic muscles in succession. When properly performed, it is a position that requires minimal physical demand on the clinician because of the mechanical advantages provided. However, a strong mechanical advantage has its disadvantages. A painful condition can be easily provoked unless the clinician is careful to apply loads in a judicious manner. As a rule, the MTP should never be used for the patient in the acute or subacute stage following injury.

While the MTP is well established, the manner in which one positions the patient and establishes stabilizing and loading strategies varies among authors and clinicians. The variety of methods for the MTP is dependent on the size and physical capacity of both clinician and patient. It may also be dependent on the gender of the clinician. Therefore, the following explanation will provide an example of establishing the MTP with the understanding that the reader should then adapt his or her specific situation. Because of the importance of the MTP, additional detail will be provided describing this maneuver.

Clinical Pearl: The modified Thomas position (MTP) is considered the most practical position for isolating and assessing several key lumbopelvic muscles in succession. When properly performed, it is a position that requires minimal physical demand on the clinician because of the mechanical advantages provided.

Equipment: The MTP should be performed on a relatively high table, approximating the height of the hip as one stands alongside it, which is also quite stable.

Goal 1: Place the patient safely in a supine position with his or her coccyx at the edge of the table, with one leg flexed and the other extended off the end of the table. Because the patient is typically one with chronic pain, extra care is necessary to establish this initial position without provoking an exacerbation.

- *Patient's position:* The patient stands with his or her back to the end of the table, with the buttocks touching the table. The patient is instructed to flex the contralateral (i.e., nontested) knee and hip, grasping the limb to bring it to the torso. This position allows for increased lumbopelvic stability in the neutral position in preparation for the upcoming maneuver.
- *Clinician's position:* The clinician stands alongside the patient.
- *Clinician's action:* Assuming the clinician has the physical capacity to do so, the patient is grasped with both arms, one around the patient's back and the other around the flexed leg. The patient then is rocked backward onto the table by the clinician. The clinician must perform this procedure in a manner that the patient can feel secure, able to allow him or herself to be lowered without incident.

Goal 2: Establish the MTP in preparation for muscle assessment. This requires that the patient's lumbopelvic region be optimally immobilized, while the target leg mobility is unrestricted.

- *Patient's position:* The patient is now supine, with the nontested leg flexed at the hip and knee, tightly grasped to the chest with both arms. The target leg is extended, hanging off the end of the table. The coccyx should be at the edge of the table to allow for target limb motion unencumbered by the table. Conversely, the patient must not be positioned too low on the table, as when the sacrum is placed at the table edge, or the pelvis will not be sufficiently stabilized by the table.
- *Clinician's position:* The clinician should be positioned at the end of the table, facing the patient's target leg. For example, the clinician's left side should approximate the patient's right leg, while facing the extended left leg. The clinician must be close, preferably in contact with the patient's nontarget ischial region in order to establish the necessary mechanical advantages.
- *Clinician's action:* The plantar surface of the patient's nontarget foot is placed on the clinician's lateral chest, just below the axilla. The clinician leans into the table, with the additional loading added to the flexed nontarget leg in order to remove any remaining lumbar lordosis and secure the region tightly against the table. The clinician must maintain this pressure for the rest of the assessment, as any lumbar motion will compromise the reliability of all muscles evaluated in the MTP. With this placement of the foot on the chest and the patient "locked" into position, the clinician is then able to use both free hands to focus on muscle assessment. The proximal hand (i.e., the one closer to the table) is generally used to assess and add necessary stability to the pelvic region, while the distal

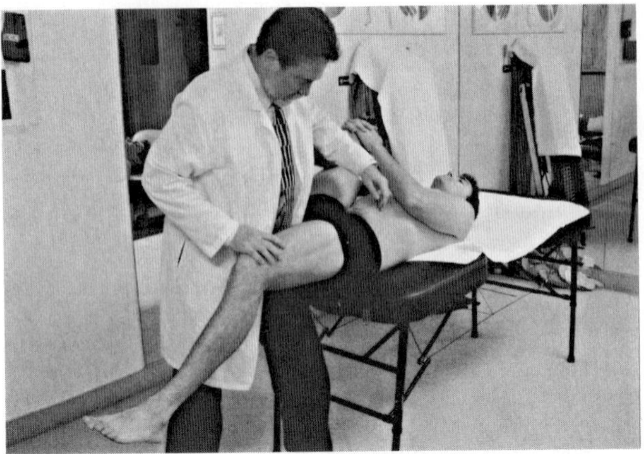

FIGURE 13–35. Iliopsoas assessment: The modified Thomas position is quite convenient for this assessment. Note that the patient's right foot is placed against the clinician's left rib cage and that the clinician bears weight against that foot to flatten the low back against the table. Since gravity takes the extended limb to the first barrier of resistance, a light springing palpation is used at the distal femur.

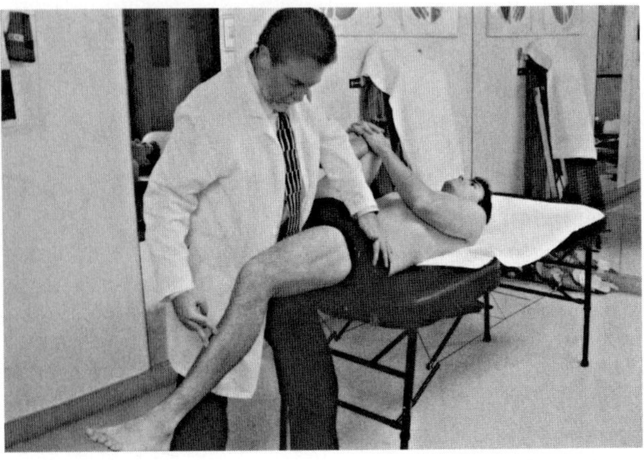

FIGURE 13–36. Rectus femoris assessment: Springing palpation of the lower leg is employed, while ensuring that the thigh does not elevate, which would give a false negative finding.

hand provides specific loading and assessment of the target muscle.

Finally, the clinician places a firm proximal hand at the target side ASIS. This will serve as a third measure (The first is the patient's arms grasping the nontarget thigh and pulling it tightly to the torso to flatten the low back against the table. The second involves the previously noted clinician's lateral chest pressure.) to guard against extraneous lumbopelvic motion.

The patient is now placed in the MTP and is ready for muscle length assessment of several muscles.

Assessment of the Iliopsoas[222] *(see Fig. 13–35)* It should be remembered that the first barrier of iliopsoas resistance has already been established by gravity. Therefore, the assessment of the muscle occurs prior to any clinician loading simply by proper MTP. Because hip extension should be about 10 degrees, the thigh should be at horizontal or perhaps the knee a little lower than the hip under physiological circumstances.

- *Clinician's action:* The fingertips of the clinician's distal hand are placed on the distal target thigh, just proximal to the patella. The clinician should then lightly spring the muscle, assessing for any abrupt barrier and the nature of the rebound.

Assessment of the Rectus Femoris[222] *(see Fig. 13–36)* It should be remembered that the first barrier of rectus femoris resistance has already been established by gravity. Therefore the assessment of the muscle occurs prior to any clinician loading simply by proper MTP. Because knee flexion should be about 90 degrees, the lower leg should approximate vertical under physiological circumstances.

- *Clinician's action:* With the patient in the MTP, the fingertips of the clinician's distal hand are placed on the distal shin, just proximal to the ankle. The clinician should then lightly spring the muscle, assessing for an abrupt barrier and the nature of the rebound.

Note: the clinician must monitor for elevation of the target knee during this maneuver, which can occur with a tight rectus femoris. This could present a false-negative finding in that springing the muscle would be free of a pathological barrier because the resistance was reduced with the extraneous knee motion. In this event, the clinician's stabilizing proximal hand should be placed on the patient's distal thigh, just proximal to the patella in order to avoid extraneous knee motion.

Because expertise comes with repetition, the novice should notice that the rectus femoris would typically have a more gradual springing than the shorter iliopsoas. The relative length and resistance of each muscle to springing varies with each muscle and among individuals. Nevertheless, an expected range of motion and springing with each muscle comes with experience, allowing the clinician to assess with increased speed and, hopefully, reliability.

Assessment of the Hip Abductors[222] *(see Fig. 13–37)* Because of the regional morphology, hip adduction is limited to approximately 10 degrees.

- *Clinician's action:* With the patient in the MTP, the clinician places the fingertips of the distal hand on the patient's lateral distal thigh, just proximal to the knee joint, and draws the knee medially, abducting the hip to the first barrier of resistance.

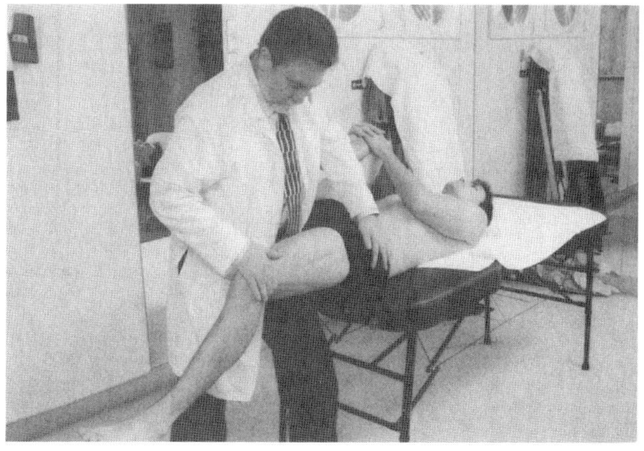

FIGURE 13–37. Hip abductor assessment: Notice the ITB groove at the lateral thigh, which is mildly increased and abnormal in this case.

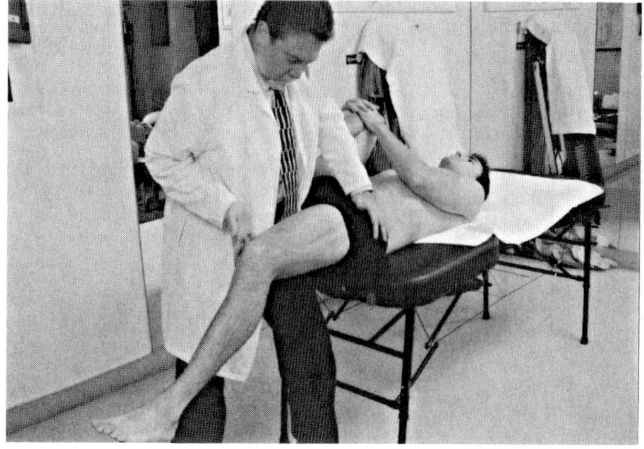

FIGURE 13–38. Single-joint hip adductors: Note the lateral springing direction of assessment.

The clinician then springs the muscle to further assess the resistance and rebound of the tissue.

Janda[222] stated that the modified Thomas position, especially during the abductor assessment, was an ideal time to evaluate the iliotibeal band (ITB). The degree of tightness will generally coincide with that of the hip abductors when one performs springing palpation. However, there is another observational shortcut that can be utilized. This involves the ITB crease along the lateral thigh. In men, who *generally* to have less subdermal adipose tissue, the crease can be shallow and considered to be normal. A relatively deep crease would suggest a tight ITB. In women, the generally increased level of subdermal adipose tissue tends to fill in the lateral thigh crease, so the presence of any crease would suggest a tight ITB band.

Assessment of the Single Joint Hip Adductors[222] (see Fig. 13–38) The single joint adductors are those whose origin is at the pubic ramus and insertion is at the femur, meaning that they only span the acetabulum. Therefore, the knee bent position of the MTP allows these single-joint adductors to be easily localized and assessed.

- *Clinician's action:* With the patient in the MTP, the clinician places the fingertips the distal hand on the patient's distal thigh, just proximal to the knee joint, and lightly pushes it laterally, abducting the hip to the first barrier of resistance. The clinician then springs the muscle to further assess the resistance and rebound of the tissue.

Assessment of the Two-Joint Hip Adductor[222] (see Fig. 13–39) The gracilis is a two-joint hip adductor whose origin is at the pubic ramus and insertion is at the tibia, meaning that it spans both the acetabulum and knee. Therefore, an extended knee strategy is required to lengthen this muscle to be localized and assessed. As such, the MTP would not be appropriate to evaluate the gracilis. Janda[15] emphasized the importance of maintaining as little hip flexion as possible for this assessment, noting that more than about 4 degrees of flexion tended to be inhibitory and compromised the findings.

- *Clinician's action:* With the patient in a supine position and both legs extended and resting on the table, the clinician places the heel of the patient's target leg in the crook of the clinicain's elbow of the caudal arm. The clinician's upper arm is placed against the lateral foot and the clinician's forearm and hand wrap around the anterior potion of the lower leg, distal to the knee joint. The clinician places the cephalad hand firmly on the patient's ipsilateral pelvis at the region of the ASIS in order to stabilize it and avoid unwanted pelvic motion. The clinician then, remaining low with leg to avoid hip flexion, draws the leg away from the midline,

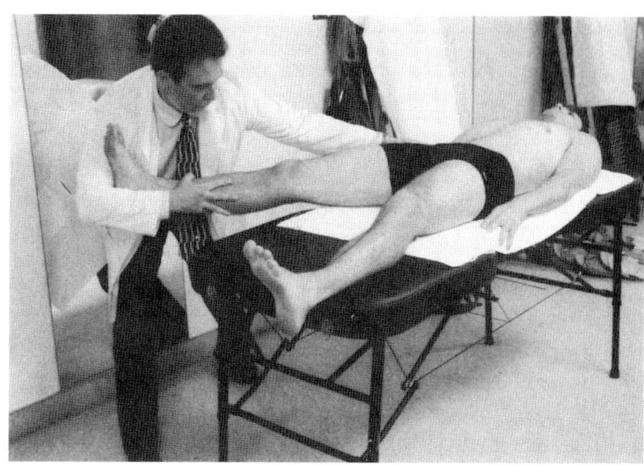

FIGURE 13–39. Two-joint hip adductors: Avoiding hip flexion, internal or external rotation is mandatory for this maneuver.

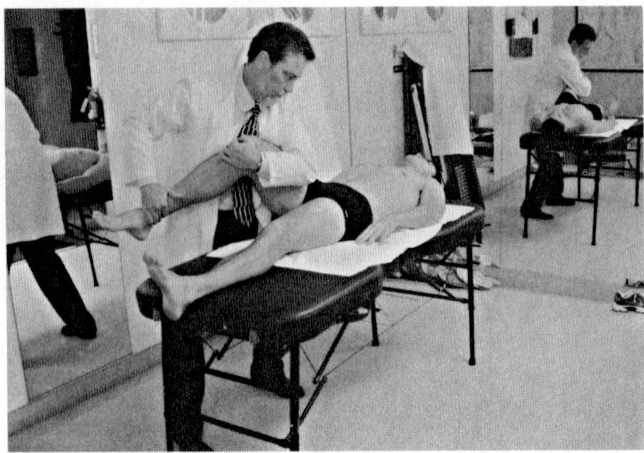

FIGURE 13–40. The piriformis assessment: This is a challenging test. The key to this test is maintaining the pressure from the knee down the axis of the femur, anchoring the hip to the table in order for hip rotation to be localized to the hip joint alone.

abducting it to the first barrier of resistance. The clinician then springs the muscle to further assess the resistance and rebound of the tissue.

Assessment of the Piriformis[222] *(see Fig. 13–40)* An external rotator of the hip, this muscle is quite challenging to isolate. Janda stressed that this muscle be assessed with a minimum of hip flexion.

- *Patient's position:* The patient is placed supine on the table, closer to the edge on the side of the target leg.
- *Clinician's position:* Standing at and facing the side of the table at the level of the patient's pelvis.
- *Clinician's action:* The patient's target hip is flexed to 10 degrees. The clinician grasps the patient's knee with the cephalad hand and draws it to the clinician's chest. The clinician then loads the thigh from the knee down the shaft of the thigh to stabilize the hip joint. This pressure must be maintained during the entire test or the reliability is compromised, as the hip is not well stabilized. The clinician then contacts the patient's target ankle and draws it toward him or herself. This motion internally rotates the hip, which is taken to the barrier and then sprung. This is a relatively short muscle, so the barrier is attained with little motion and the springing is rather shallow.

Assessment of the Hamstrings (see Fig. 13–41) Because it is classically tight and often strained, the hamstring is probably the most commonly assessed muscle. Janda emphasized and demonstrated a specific maneuver to ensure optimal reliability. The challenges include avoiding hip rotation and knee flexion while attempting to elevate a long lever.

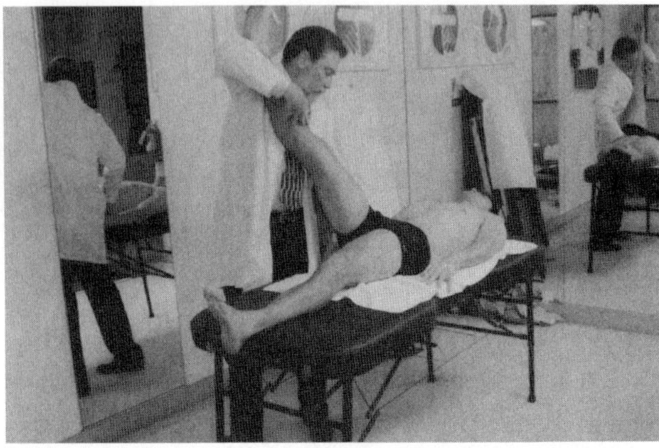

FIGURE 13–41. The hamstring assessment: The key to this test is to avoid Hip external, internal, medial, or lateral deviation.

- *Patient's position:* The patient is placed supine on the table, closer to the edge on the side of the target leg.
- *Clinician's position:* Standing at and facing the side of the table at the level of the patient's knee.
- *Clinician's action:* The clinician places the patient's target heel in the crook of his or her caudal arm, wrapping that forearm and hand around the anterior shin. This hand on the shin helps to control the knee from flexing, while the crook of the elbow and wrapping forearm avoids internal or external hip rotation. The clinician's cephalad arm can then be used to assist in controlling the elevating leg, ensuring against any aberrant motion.

The clinician then elevates the straightened leg to the first barrier of resistance. The normal range of flexion is 70–80 degrees. When the nontarget hip and knee is flexed at 30–45 degrees, then one can anticipate 10 degrees more hip flexion of the target leg.

Assessment of the Thoracolumbar Erector Spinae This is a physically demanding maneuver that entails lifting the patient's pelvis and legs. Because of the bulk of the musculature, the increased diameter of the trunk, and added resistance of the skeletal, ligamentous, and fascial structures, attempting to manually assess the erector spinae length in the same manner as the other muscles described in this section is different. Nevertheless, it can be accomplished and it can provide important clinical insights, so it is considered another valuable skill in the functional examination.

- *Patient's position:* The patient is placed supine on the table, close to the side in order to optimize clinician access.
- *Clinician's position:* The clinician is positioned alongside the table approximating the level of the patient's pelvis.

- *Clinician's action:* The clinician draws both of the patient's knees toward the patient's chest. The hips and knees should both be flexed for this. As the patient's hips and knees approximate 90 degrees of flexion, the clinician stabilizes the flexed legs with the cephalad forearm placed across the patient's lower legs, just distal to the knees, in a manner that allows for optimal mechanical advantage of controlling the patient's legs in this position. The clinician then draws the patient slightly toward him or herself, away from the neutral position, so that the contralateral pelvis elevates slightly off the table. This allows the clinician to then slide the caudal hand, with fingers aligned in a manner pointing up along the patient's spine, so that the palm is placed over the sacral base and lower lumbar segments. The patient is then returned back to the neutral position and the arm of the caudal hand is aligned with the patient's spine to ensure loading along the sagittal plane.

Once the initial patient and clinician positions are established, the erector spinae can be evaluated. The clinician then, using safe lifting mechanic, uses both arm contacts in synchrony to continue to draw the patient's knees closer to the chest. The clinician's cephalad hand has the greater mechanical advantage as it loads the lower legs, while the caudal hand slightly distracts and elevates the lumbosacral region. The clinician must be sensitive to the first barrier of resistance and then perform springing to further evaluate the tissues. The clinician should

1. Tightness of the thoracolumbar erector spinae can practically be determined on direct palpation on visual inspection.
2. There is second, less physically demanding position for this maneuver that is performed with the patient lying on his or her side. There are two problems with that method, which include having to factor in resistance from the table when springing the muscle and using only single-arm strength to perform the springing without the added benefit of the using lifting mechanics as with the patient supine.
3. The topic of patient risk was addressed under *Primum non nocere* earlier in this chapter. Erector spinae assessment provides an excellent example of this topic. If the patient has an *extension bias,* meaning that forward bending as in a typical disc syndrome provokes their pain, then placing him or her in a passively flexed posture with loading can indeed cause harm.
4. Another option for the thoracolumbar and lumbar erector spinae assessment include snapping palpation, which was described earlier in the chapter (see Fig. 13–42).

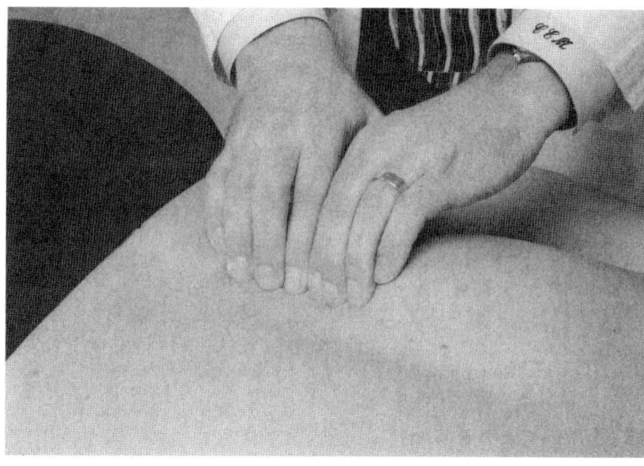

FIGURE 13–42. Erector spinae assessment: This demonstrates snapping palpation of this muscle group.

5. There is a third method of assessing this region. The patient is seated on the side of the examining table with the apart and instructed to flex as far forward as possible. There are real strengths and weaknesses to this method. On the positive side, there is little physical demand placed upon the clinician. On the other hand, this is a somewhat active maneuver on the patients part, which means the erector spinae are not assesed in a fully relaxed state.

Additional Muscle Assessment There are a variety of approaches to assess the musculature. Additional assessment skills of unique muscles are presented below to demonstrate TrP evaluation.

Assessment of the Diaphragm The diaphragm is a clinically overlooked muscle because of its unique morphology. Hidden away by the thoracic cage and also by the neighboring abdominal viscera, relatively little attention has been paid to this, the most important of all skeletal muscles. This has been complicated by the fact that it resides in a transitional region of the body that historically left it outside discussions involving the lumbosacral spine. Because of its unique characteristics, it is discussed separately in this chapter. This topic has already been covered in Chapter 5, and herein some additional commentary is provided.

While the overall understanding of respiratory control is relatively poor,[275] advances over the past decade have occurred regarding the understanding of the diaphragm's role, direct and indirect, in lumbopelvic function, which now requires the inclusion when discussing this region. The diaphragm has been linked to trunk control,[53] postural adjustments,[276] intra-abdominal pressure,[277] in a feed-forward manner (i.e., anticipatory motor pattern),[278] and functioning in concert with muscles of the abdomen the pelvic floor.[279] In addition, spinal stiffness was recently found to be affected throughout the respiratory

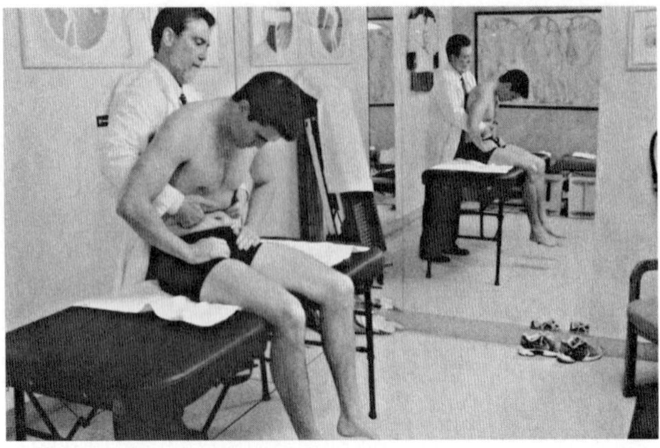

FIGURE 13–43. Diaphragm assessment: The patient must be relaxed and forewarned that this maneuver may be unpleasant or painful. Relaxation of the abdominals is mandatory in order for the fingertips to probe the diaphragm.

cycle[280] and increased when the ribcage was constrained,[281] leaving one to wonder how else the diaphragm affects these mechanisms.

The entire diaphragm cannot be palpated due to morphological constraints. The fact that this dome-shaped muscle travels medially and superiorly from the lower ribs restricts palpatory possibilities. Nevertheless, a practical and significant assessment can be performed. The assessment of myofascial trigger points (TrPs) was briefly discussed earlier in the chapter. Palpatory assessment of the diaphragm is essentially a search for TrPs in the sternal and lateral, or costal aspects of the muscle, where digital access is practical although challenging.[175]

Diaphragm assessment (see Fig. 13–43)

- *Patient's position:* The patient should be seated in a slumped posture with his or her arms resting at the side. There can be no clothing over the contact regions, so appropriate professional decorum must be in place. Also, palpation of the diaphragm can be unpleasant and even painful, so the patient should be forewarned of this possibility and agree to proceed before the clinician begins.
- *Clinician's position:* The clinician stands behind the patient with both arms reaching around and contacting the patient's lower ribs.
- *Clinician's activities:* With the patient is seated in a slumped posture, the clinician curls his or her fingertips under the patient's lower ribs, searching for the areas of increased tone that suggest TrPs. This can be unpleasant for the patient, so a protective tensing of the abdomen is not uncommon. The clinician must instruct the patient to remain relaxed in order for the assessment to continue.

Once the clinician finds one or more points of resistance, then he or she can snap the TrP by running the fingertips over the point of increased tone. This should elicit a TrP "twitch response" causing the patient to retract and tense the abdomen reflexively. The clinician can palpate as deeply into the diaphragm as the abdominal tissues will allow before working the way around under the lateral lower ribs of the flank region. Finally, a deeper palpation can be performed on one side when the patient's torso rotates the contralateral direction. For example, left rotation of the torso allows for deeper palpation of the right diaphragm.

As with many assessment techniques, the diaphragm evaluation and treatment procedures are essentially a continuation of the same maneuvers. This is because the mechanics that allow for isolated assessment provide the same strategy for therapeutic access. This is true for the diaphragm, in that mobilization techniques, as discussed in Chapter 23, require the same patient and clinician positioning and palpation.

Assessment of Abdominis Rectus[222,282] (see Fig. 13–44)

- *Patient's position:* The patient lies supine with his or her legs extended and resting on the table.
- *Clinician's position:* Standing alongside the patient approximating the abdomen.
- *Clinician's actions:* The clinician palpates for tenderness at the origin at the lower ribs and zyphoid, in addition to the insertion at the symphysis. The clinician then applies a snapping palpation for TrPs, as described earlier in the chapter under TrP assessment. This is performed bilaterally and compared, and the clinician can remain on one side to evaluate both recti.

Assessment of the Transversus Abdominis[222] (see Fig. 13–45)

- *Patient's position:* The patient lies supine with both legs extended and resting on the table.

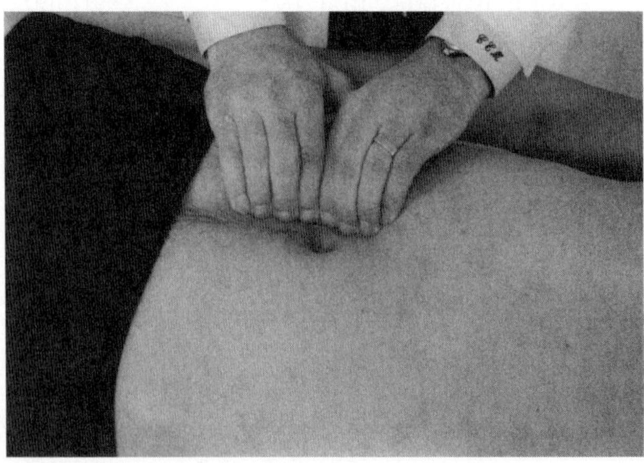

FIGURE 13–44. The rectus femoris assessment: Flat or snapping palpation can be used here.

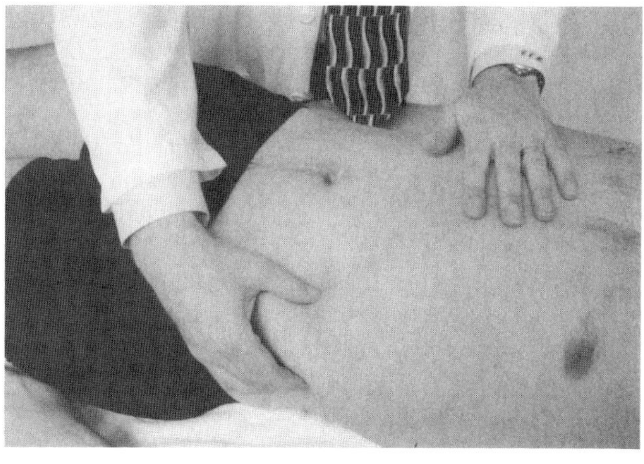

FIGURE 13–45. The transversus abdominis assessment: Pincer palpation is recommended for this muscle.

- *Clinician's position:* Standing alongside the patient approximating the abdomen.
- *Clinician's actions:* The clinician can assess the ipsilateral, contralateral or both sides of the taransversus from the same position, depending on preference. The clinician employs a pincer palpation for TrPs on each side at the flank, as described earlier in the chapter under TrP assessment.

Assessment of the Iliacus (see Fig. 13–46)

- *Patient's position:* The patient lies supine with both legs extended, slightly abducted, and resting on the table.
- *Clinician's position:* Standing alongside the patient approximating the abdomen.
- *Clinician's actions:* The iliacus is an interesting muscle in that it is a relatively flat muscle at its origin where it attaches to the upper two thirds of the inner surface of the iliac fossa and anchors to the internal lip of the iliac crest.[282] Therefore, this portion of the muscle can be assessed with palpation as one would assess a flat muscle, except that the clinician must gently probe through the tissues of the lateral aspect of the lower abdomen to reach the target muscle. The clinician's probing fingers should wrap around the region of the ASIS, compressing the tissue against the inner surface of the ilium. A flat palpation for TrPs, as described in the TrP assessment earlier, is then performed, with clinician's fingers probing as deeply along the wall of the iliac fossa as comfortably possible.

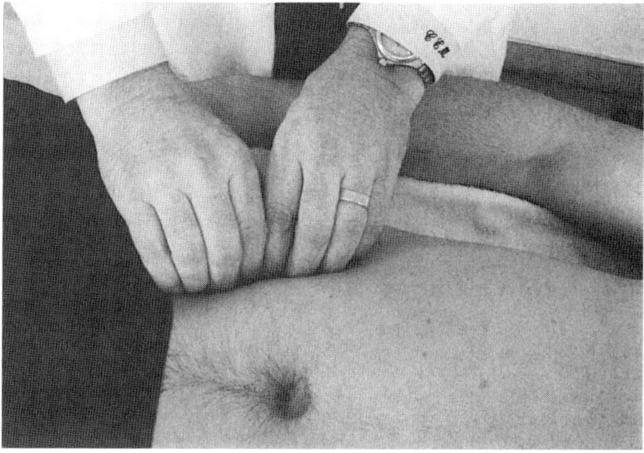

FIGURE 13–46. The iliacus assessment: Like the diaphragm, this muscle is challenging to reach, so abdominal relaxation is important.

Assessment of the Psoas[222]

- *Patient's position:* The patient lies supine with both legs extended and resting on the table. It is very important that the legs be extended for this specific muscle, as this allows the lumbar spine to assume a greater lordosis than if the patient's hips were flexed. The increased lordosis tends to allow for a more effective palpation.
- *Clinician's position:* Standing alongside the patient approximating the abdomen.
- *Clinician's actions:* The clinician palpates for the lateral border of the rectus abdominis, inferior to the umbilicus and superior to a line connecting the two ASIS prominences. Once this point is established, the clinician gently depresses the fingers down, posteriorly and medially, into the abdomen and toward the lumbar spine. The pressure of the fingers and underlying abdominal contents will compress the psoas against the spine. Utilizing this technique, Travel and Simons[282] state,

> It is amazing how little pressure elicits so much pain when the psoas harbors active TrPs. One cannot usually palpate the tension of the muscle itself, but in thin patients with loose skin, one may be able to palpate its tension.

The active psoas TrP tends to refer pain to the low back.

Assessment of the Distal Iliopsoas The iliacus and psoas integrate into one myotatic unit distally, which is an important site for assessment.

- *Patient's position:* The patient lies supine with both legs extended, slightly abducted and externally rotated, while resting on the table.
- *Clinician's position:* Standing alongside the patient approximating the hip.
- *Clinician's actions:* In comparison to the proximal iliacus and psoas, the distal iliopsoas is relatively superficial. Point palpation for TrP tenderness is

performed by pressing the fingers against the lateral wall of the femoral triangle. The lateral wall of the femoral triangle is formed by the sartorius superficially and then the insertion of the iliopsoas at the lesser trochanter is deep to that. Hip abduction and external rotation assists in allowing access to the iliopsoas insertion without pressing on the femoral nerve, which is located medially.

Assessment of the Hip Adductors[222] This is a practical assessment for TrP activity of three hip adductors, the adductors magnus, brevis, and longus.

- *Patient's position:* The patient lies supine with both legs extended, slightly abducted resting on the table.
- *Clinician's position:* Standing alongside the patient approximating the hip.
- *Clinician's actions:* The clinician places the fingers on the posteromedial thigh, approximately 2–3 in (5–8 cm) inferior to the pubic ramus, to find the adductor magnus. It is well named, a relatively large muscle, and this, the middle third of the muscle is most accessible for palpation. One can use flat, pincer, or snapping palpation, although there is rarely a brisk local twitch response. To locate the adductors brevis and longus, the hand moves toward the anteromedial aspect of the thigh at the same distance from the pubic ramus. These muscles tend to overlap in this region and can be assessed together. To differentiate one from the other, simply move proximally to isolate the adductor brevis, or distally to isolate the adductor longus. Again, one can use flat, pincer, or snapping palpation, with similar results as with the adductor magnus.

Assessment of the Piriformis[222] The piriformis is an extremely sensitive muscle; therefore, provocative trigger point assessment can exacerbate the patient's symptomatology. Janda therefore, recommended the following assessment method:

- *Patient's position:* The patient lies prone on the table.
- *Clinician's position:* Standing alongside the patient approximating the hip.
- *Clinician's actions:* The clinician can find the piriformis by simply finding the bisection of a line between the greater trochanter and the ipsilateral posterior, superior iliac spine (PSIS). The clinician then places the cephalad hand (i.e., the hand closer to the patient's head) flat on the posterolateral buttocks, with the fingertips just superior to the piriformis. The clinician's caudal hand is then placed over and parallel with the other hand. The two hands, working together as one, then slide inferiorly toward the piriformis. Janda emphasized the importance of using the hand on top to apply the proper load, while the fingers of the hand underneath were then free to palpate. Janda[15] noted that a positive finding was evident when the piriformis was hypertonic and felt like a small wiener or sausage. He stated that this indicated the presence of one or more active TrPs, but recommended against further palpatory assessment. He emphasized the importance of avoiding repeated palpation to this muscle, since this could provoke a painful episode of an otherwise healthy muscle.

Assessment of the Pelvic Floor (see Fig. 9–8 in Chapter 9) The pelvic floor has received a great deal of clinical attention during the past two decades among researchers and clinicians interested in low back syndromes. This is because it has been shown to be intricately involved in lumbopelvic stability. This occurs in two stages: the first involving myofascial TrPs in association with pelvic organic conditions and the second integrating that information with the pressurized canister that contributes to lumbopelvic stability. This has also been called the "inner unit,"[221] which also includes the transversus abdominis, the diaphragm, and the multifidus. Neurophysiological mechanisms of lumbopelvic stability, including function of the local and global systems, and of intra-abdominal pressure, has been described in detail in Chapter 5.

Clinical Pearl: The pelvic floor has received a great deal of clinical attention during the past two decades among researchers and clinicians interested in low back syndromes. This is because it has been shown to be intricately involved in lumbopelvic stability.

In addition to its growing importance in the etiology of lumbopelvic instability, there are a number of other conditions for which the pelvic floor should be assessed. The pelvic floor muscles should be examined when the patient presents with pain in the anal, vaginal, perineal or retroscrotal regions, pain during intercourse, defecation or when sitting, or with lower back pain.[282]

Slocumb[283] described trigger points that were causing chronic pelvic pain, many of which were located in the abdominal wall. Slocumb found that deactivation of such triggers frequently removed symptoms that had been present for years and had at times resulted in abortive surgical investigation. He noted an overlap of referral patterns from a variety of locations,

> The same pain sensation was reproduced by pressure over localized points in several tissues

seemingly anatomically unrelated ... for example, 1) pinching the skin over the lower abdominal wall; 2) single-finger pressure in one reproducible abdominal wall location [trigger point]; 3) single-finger pressure on tissue overlying the pubic bone; 4) lateral pressure with one finger over one or both levator muscles; 5) single-finger or cotton tip applicator pressure lateral to the cervix; 6) single-finger or cotton tip applicator pressure over vaginal cuff scar tissue, more than 3 months after hysterectomy; 7) single-finger pressure on tissue over the dorsal sacrum.

The results of treating a series of patients with symptoms of chronic pelvic pain by means of trigger point deactivation, using anesthetic injections, were successful response in 89.3% of 131 patients with nearly 70% followed up for 6 months or more.

The work of Weiss[284] confirmed Slocumb's findings and demonstrates that interstitial cystitis may also result from trigger point activity. This study involved 42 people with chronic cystitis, whose main symptoms were painful urgency and frequency. Following manual treatment of myofascial trigger points in the pelvic muscles, 35 of these people (83%) reported moderate to marked improvement, with some being completely relieved, after up to 14 years of suffering these symptoms. Seven of the 10 (70%) people who had been diagnosed with interstitial cystitis had moderate to marked improvements.[284]

In 1989, Silverstolpe[285] correlated a reflexive activation of "snapping palpation" (see trigger point section above) of the lower thoracic erector spinae with mechanical pelvic dysfunction. This erector spinae response, later named the Silverstolpe reflex (or S-reflex), was completely erased by digital massage of the sacrotuberous ligament, located lateral to the coccyx and inferomedial to the gluteus maximus near the insertion of the ischial tuberosity. Lewit[10] later opined that Silverstolpe's contact point would have more effect on the pelvic floor musculature than the sacrotuberous ligament. He noted that a contact between the ischial tuberosity and coccyx, medial to the gluteus maximus and lateral to the anus, would be at the levator ani. He considered this to be a strategically practical palpatory location to assess pelvic floor function. Although this was not the anatomical landmark that Silverstope explained in his paper, as noted above, this altered contact has become to be known as the Sylverstolpe contact.

Travell and Simons[282] provided ample support for the complex clinical integration of pelvic floor myofascial pain and other conditions including coccygodynia, levator ani syndrome, proctalgia fugax, and tension myalgia of the pelvic floor. They emphasized the importance of proper examination methods that included both external and internal assessment via the rectum and vagina.

Gurel and Atar Gurel[286] correlated chronic pelvic pain with dyspareunia and back pain among 235 females, providing additional support for the clinical integration of pelvic organic and lumbopelvic dysfunction.

Maclennan et al.[287] noted that pelvic floor disorders are very common and strongly associated with female gender, aging, pregnancy, parity, and instrumental delivery.

In contrast to other skeletal muscles, pelvic floor muscles demonstrate resting myoelectric activity due to smooth muscle fibers detected in the levator ani.[288] This development is theoretical terms due to the adaptation to intra-abdominal pressure and reaction to gravitational loading from the viscera.

Sapsford et al.[279] demonstrated that the muscles surrounding the abdominal cavity, including the pelvic floor and abdominal musculature, co-contract during voluntary exercise among healthy female volunteers. They found that the abdominals co-contract with pelvic floor exercises and preliminary evidence that the pelvic floor contracted during abdominal exercise. This research helped to clarify the participation of the pelvic floor in the pressurized canister model for lumbopelvic stability.

Critchley[289] added important information by demonstrating facilitation of abdominis transversus activation by adding pelvic floor exercises to low-abdominal hollowing exercises.

More recently, Pool-Goudzwaard et al.,[290] utilizing a simulated tensioning model on 18 cadavers, determined that the pelvic floor musculature increased pelvic ring stiffness. They further found that the pelvic floor influenced SI joint stiffness (i.e., force closure, see Chapter 8) in females, while producing backward rotation of the sacrum in both genders.

In a recent development, Bo et al.[291] found that diagnostic ultrasound was a more valid assessment tool that palpation for pelvic floor evaluation. These results demonstrate that technological advances must be continually integrated into various aspects of health care.

(a) External palpatory pelvic floor assessment

- *Patient's position:* The patient is placed in a prone position.
- *Clinician's position:* Standing at the side of the table approximating the patient's pelvis.
- *Clinician's actions:* The clinician isolates the inferior tip of the coccyx with the caudal hand and also the ischial tuberosity. Following the medial border of the gluteus maximus muscle, the clinician palpates with the tip of the

forefinger into the pelvic floor. The superficial pelvic muscle at this point is the iliac portion of the levator ani muscle, which has become known as the Silverstolpe contact (or "S" contact). This contact should not be tender with moderate pressure, although it can be exceedingly tender with pelvic floor dysfunction. The patient can cough to demonstrate the activation of the musculature under the clinician's fingertip, or can also draw up the pelvic floor if he or she has the motor control to do so. There are verbal cues to assist in this process. For women, an effective cue is to have them imagine they are suddenly interrupting the flow of urine, while men are instructed to elevate their scrotum. While myofascial trigger points are quite common at the "S" contact, so is the patient's inability to control the pelvic floor at this point.

(b) Internal palpatory pelvic floor assessment (assessment of intrarectal region)

- *Patient's position:* The patient is in the sidelying position with the uppermost hip fully flexed and supported on a cushion or lying directly on the table if stretch of the piriformis and obturator internus are required.

  The side being described is the internal aspect of the pelvis of the uppermost side, when sidelying. The patient is asked to lie on the opposite side, for the other half to be treated.
- *Clinician's position:* The practitioner stands behind the patient at the level of the upper thigh and wears protective gloves throughout the assessment and/or treatment. (The gloves should be disposed of immediately after the assessment because of contact with potentially hazardous waste products present in the body.)
- *Clinician's actions:* The practitioner's cephalad hand is placed on the uppermost hip and used to palpate externally. The index finger of the caudad hand (with fingernails well trimmed) is used to gently assess and/or treat. A gel can be used as a lubricant on both the glove and the orifice.

Note: If latex gloves are worn, all forms of oil are to be avoided and any residue of oil on the practitioner's hands should be scrupulously removed before donning the gloves as it dissolves latex upon contact and would compromise the protective barrier provided by the gloves.

The lubricated index finger of the caudad hand is placed at the anal orifice with the fingerpad facing posteriorly and gently slid into the anus, past the anal sphincter, which should be examined for both external and internal hemorrhoids.

Gentle pressure applied toward the sphincter muscle usually produces relaxation response of the muscle; however, Travell and Simons[282] note that trigger points in these tissues might respond adversely to this type of pressure, producing moderate discomfort, and suggest that the patient might instead bear down on the rectum to relax the muscle as the practitioner inserts the finger.

Gentle pressure (or mild pincer compression against the externally placed thumb) is applied first to the sphincter muscles at fingertip widths around the inside of the sphincter while searching for taut bands and trigger points. If found, the trigger points in the sphincter muscles may be treated (usually with gently applied pincer compression) before further entry can be made.

The index finger is then gently inserted further with the pad of the finger facing posteriorly and moving cephalad at the midline. As it approaches the coccyx, caution should be exercised to avoid impacting the distal tip of the coccyx. Instead, the finger should be slid onto the anterior surface of the coccyx, if possible. Sometimes the coccyx may be found to have formed a near 90-degree angle to the sacrum, in which case the index finger will need to be flexed and hooked around it in order to contact the anterior surface.

Gentle, exploring, short gliding strokes, or gentle sustained pressure, can be applied to the anterior surface of the coccyx to assess the muscles, fascia, and ligaments attaching to these bony surfaces. A gentle flexing of the finger can assess for motion of the coccyx, which should offer approximately 30 degrees of flexion/extension movement.

The practitioner's entire hand and forearm is now smoothly supinated as the straight index finger sweeps laterally across the surface of levator ani and coccygeus muscles. This sweeping action is repeated several times while pressure is applied into the anterior surface of the muscles. The palm of the external hand can offer a supporting surface against which to compress the tissues.

The index finger is then gently inserted further until the pad of the index finger contacts the anterior surface of the sacrum. The finger is slid along the anterolateral aspect of the sacrum until contact with the piriformis tendon is made. The location of the tendon attachment can be confirmed by having the person lift the ipsilateral (flexed) knee toward the ceiling, which will cause the muscle to contract and, therefore, its tendon to move. Gentle sustained pressure can be applied to the attachment if it is found to be tender or to cause referred pain.

The practitioner's hand and forearm again supinates repeatedly as the index finger sweeps laterally along the surface of the piriformis muscle. Pressure can be supplied by the external hand to offer a broad surface against which the tissue can be compressed.

The Muscles of the Pelvic Diaphragm The pelvic diaphragm is composed of the levator ani and coccygeus muscles. These muscles support the viscera, contract with the abdominal muscles and the abdominothoracic diaphragm and multifidus, raise intra-abdominal pressure, are instrumental in pelvic ring stability, and are active during the inspiratory phase of respiration.[278,279,282,290]

- Levator ani, a broad muscular sheet with varying thickness, is divisible into three portions.[148,292]
  1. *Puborectalis muscle:* Inseparable from pubococcygeus at its origin, these fibers form the crura of the levator, which encloses the genital hiatus, some blend with the sphincter ani externus, and some form the retrorectal sling behind the rectum (anal canal). Anterior to the puborectalis fibers lie the urethra and the genital canal.
  2. *Pubococcygeus:* These fibers course from the back of the body of the pubis to the sphincter urethrae, to levator prostatae in males or walls of the vagina in females, to the perineal body and rectum, and to the anterior surface of the coccyx.
  3. *Iliococcygeus:* Arising from obturator fascia between the obturator canal and the ischial spine to contribute to the anococcygeal ligament and to attach to the last two segments of the coccyx.

  The levator ani supports and elevates the pelvic floor. By compressing the visceral canals and reinforcing the sphincter muscles, some fibers contribute to continence and must relax for evacuation to occur,[292] while others can help to eject a bolus of feces or help empty the urethra at the end of urination.[282] Loss of tone of these tissues or injuries incurred during childbirth may contribute to uterovaginal prolapse.[292]
- The coccygeus (ischiococcygeus) muscle is a triangular musculotendinous sheet arising from the pelvic surface, tip of the ischial spine, and the sacrospinous ligament to attach to the lateral margins of the coccyx and the fifth sacral segment. Coccygeus acts with the levator ani as noted above and to also pull the coccyx forward. Travell and Simons[282] report, "It also stabilizes the sacroiliac joint and has powerful leverage for rotating that joint. Therefore, abnormal tension of the coccygeus muscle could easily hold the sacroiliac joint in a displaced position."
- In addition the pelvic diaphragm musculature, there is the more superficial urogenital diaphragm musculature. This group includes the bulbospongiosus, the ischiocavernosus and transverse perinii. The urogenital diaphragm is stabilized posteriorly the coccyx via the perineal body, the sphincter ani, the anococcygeal body, and the coccygeal fascia.[282]

Joint Assessment

Joint assessment for dysfunction has been the subject of a great deal of research. Although assessment and subsequent correction formed a key part of several schools of thought, reliability issues have arisen. Interexaminer reliability, the capacity to consistently arrive at the same conclusion, between different clinicians, has been consistently poor.[293,294]

The following section will describe several practical palpatory assessment skills for key joints lumbopelvic joints. The methods described here are similar to several techniques explained in the Chapter 23. The reader is directed to a number of illustrations there that demonstrate patient and clinician positioning.

Assessment Key: The following icons are designed to assist the reader in following the assessment description skills listed below:

HOW TO
Patient's position
Clinician's position
Clinician contacts
Key to assessment

Sacroiliac Joint The SI joint was discussed in detail in Chapter 8. A recent study by Hungerford et al.[78] is, however, noteworthy. Fourteen men diagnosed clinically with SI joint pain demonstrated ipsilateral delays in activation of the obliquus internus, multifidus, and gluteus maximus muscle, whereas the contralateral musculature was comparable to the earlier onset of the age-matched control group. These findings strongly suggest that SI dysfunction compromises the motor strategy of weight transference through the pelvis to the ipsilateral leg, disrupting lumbopelvic stability. Also, the finding of the gluteus maximus inhibition due to ipsilateral SI dysfunction supports findings by Janda[150] almost 40 years earlier.

The SI joint can be practically separated into a superior and inferior portion for assessment purposes.

HOW TO
(A) Upper SI assessment
Patient's position

The patient is placed in a side-lying, hook-lying position, ensuring that he or she is well balanced (i.e., neither swaying forward or backward) in order to avoid activation of pelvic stabilizing muscles. For patients with a broad pelvis and narrow legs, a pillow placed between the knees will reduce unwanted regional tension caused by hip adduction.

Clinician's position

The clinician sits on the table in the space provided by the patient's side lying, crook-lying (hip-flexed at 45 degrees and knee-flexed at 90 degrees) legs. The clinician faces toward the patient's head.

Clinician's hand contacts

One of the clinician's hands contacts the patient's lateral and *superior* aspect of sacral base, just medial to the PSIS and the SI joint. There are two recommended options for contacts: Lewit recommends the dorsum of the second and third proximal phalanges, while the volar portion of the distal phalanx of the first digit (i.e. pad of the thumb) traverses the target SI to contact the PSIS[10]. This allows for improved differentiation of SI motion during mobilization. A second option is to make the sacral contact with the hypothenar pad (see Chapter 23, Fig. 23–15).

The other hand contacts the patient's ipsilateral ASIS. This should be a soft palmar contact, as a hard contact on the bony ASIS is uncomfortable and will cause the patient to become protective and tense.

The clinician then lowers his or her arms so that the forearms are horizontally opposing each other.

Key to assessment

The clinician then lightly compresses the hands together in a scissor-like motion, feeling for the first barrier of resistance. Once obtained, the clinician springs the joint in search of a pathological barrier (see Chapter 23, Fig. 23–17).

(B) Inferior or lower SI assessment

Patient's position

The patient is placed in a side-lying, hook-lying position, ensuring that he or she is well balanced (i.e., neither swaying forward or backward) in order to avoid activation of pelvic stabilizing muscles. For patients with a broad pelvis and narrow legs, a pillow placed between the knees will reduce unwanted regional tension caused by hip adduction.

Clinician's position

The clinician sits on the table in the space provided by the patient's side lying, crook-lying (hip-flexed at 45 degrees and knee-flexed at 90 degrees) legs. The clinician faces toward the patient's head.

Clinician's hand contacts

One of the clinician's hands contacts the patient's lateral sacrum, just medial to the *inferior* aspect of SI joint. There are two recommended options for contacts: The first is to make the contact with the thenar pad. A second option is to make the inferior sacral contact with the hypothenar pad.

The other hand contacts the patient's ipsilateral ASIS. This should be a soft palmar contact, as a hard contact on the bony ASIS is uncomfortable and will cause the patient to become tense.

The clinician then lowers his or her arms so that the forearms are horizontally opposing each other.

Key to assessment

The clinician then lightly compresses the hands together in a scissor-like motion, which loads the inferior SI joint, feeling for the first barrier of resistance. Once obtained, the clinician springs the joint in search of a pathological barrier **(**see Chapter 23, Fig. 23–17**).**

(C) Supine functional sacroiliac assessments (form/force closure)[210,221]

The patient is supine and is instructed to raise one leg. If there is evidence of compensatory rotation of the pelvis toward the side of the raised leg, during performance of the movement, dysfunction is suggested.

The same leg should then be raised as the practitioner imparts compressive medially directed force across the pelvis with a hand on the lateral aspect of each innominate at the level of the ASIS (this augments form closure of the SI joint). If this *form* closure strategy, applied by the practitioner, enhances the ability to easily raise the leg this suggests that structural factors within the joint may require externally enhanced support, such as a trochanter belt.

To test for the influence of *force* closure, the same leg is raised with the patient simultaneously attempting to slightly flex and rotate the trunk toward the side being tested, against the practitioner's resistance, which is applied to the contralateral shoulder. This increases oblique muscular activity and force-closes the ipsilateral SI joint (which is being assessed). If initial leg raising suggests SI dysfunction, and this is markedly reduced or absent by means of force-closure, the prognosis is good if the patient engages in appropriate rehabilitation exercise.

(D) Prone functional SI joint assessment (form/force closure)[210,221]

The prone patient is asked to extend the leg at the hip by approximately 10 degrees. Hinging should occur at the hip joint and the pelvis should remain in contact with the table throughout.

Excessive degrees of pelvic rotation in the transverse plane (anterior pelvic rotation) indicates possible SI joint dysfunction.

If *form* features (structural) of the SI joint are at fault, the prone straight leg raise will be more normal when medial compression of the joint is introduced by the practitioner applying firm bilateral medial pressure toward the SI joints, with hands on the innominates.

Force (active) closure may be enhanced during the assessment if latissimus dorsi can be recruited to increase tension on the thoracolumbar fascia. Lee[221] states, "This is done by [the practitioner] resisting extension of the medially rotated [contralateral] arm prior to lifting the leg."

As in the supine straight leg raising (SLR) test, if force closure enhances more normal SI joint function, the prognosis for improvement is good; which can be achieved by means of rehabilitation exercises and reformed use patterns.

Coccyx The coccyx presents a unique challenge due to is regional morphology. An osseous, segmented peninsula surrounded by soft tissue, embedded within the gluteal crease and in proximity to the anus, efficacious coccygeal assessment is often overlooked. In the presence of pain of the coccyx, functional locomotor alterations have been observed. For example, Vacek et al. noted coccygodynia was associated with altered hip extension.[295] It is important to remember that the pericoccygeal tissue encompasses the posterior pelvic floor myofascia.

Ⓟ Patient's position

Prone on the table with a roll placed underneath the pelvis to flex the hips and elevate the coccygeal region.

Clinician's position

Standing alongside the table at the level of the patient's mid-thighs and the clinician's torso faces toward the head of the table.

Ⓘ Clinician's hand contacts

The palms are placed on the buttocks, with the proximal hand positioned along each side of the coccyx. The fingers of each hand are parallel with and in opposition with the other, and the arms are placed in a scissor-like position. Although a broad palmar contact is established, the greatest load is placed on "heels" of the palms (proximal thenar and hypothenar eminences), just lateral to the coccyx (see Fig. 23–18).

Key to assessment

The clinician tensions the pericoccygeal tissues by drawing the tissues on each side of the coccyx laterally. The clinician must focus on lowering his or her elbows to provide a greater lateral loading instead of a posterior to anterior load. Increasing the posterior to anterior load tends to stabilize the coccyx, locking the joints, and reducing the reliability of the assessment. Once the pericoccygeal tissue is taken to the barrier of resistance, this contact is established and the joint is gently loaded, feeling for the first barrier of resistance. Once obtained, the clinician lightly springs the joint in search of a pathological barrier.

Once assessed, the joint is evaluated in the same manner on the opposite side.

Lumbar Spine Rotational Assessment As described in Chapter 4, lumbar rotation is actually a coupled motion due to anatomical restrictions from the zygapophyseal joints. However, the low back practically rotates bilaterally on its axis and segmental restrictions can be assessed using a simple rotational strategy.

HOW TO

Assessment of lumbar segmental rotation.

Ⓟ Patient's position

The patient is placed in a prone position on the table.

Clinician's position

The clinician stands at the side of the table at the level of the patient's waist.

Ⓘ Clinician contacts

The clinician reaches across the patient's body and places his or her caudal hand along the lateral and anterior aspect of the contralateral iliac crest, grasping that ilium. This is performed in a manner that allows for rotation of the lumbar spine as the clinician draws the prone patient's grasped ilium up and away from the table. The clinician's cephalad hand then makes a thumb pad contact along the lateral aspect of the ipsilateral spinous process of the lowest mobile lumbar segment, typically L5 (see Chapter 23, Fig. 23–19).

Key to assessment

The assessment is performed as the clinician rotates the contralateral pelvis posteriorly while holding a firm contact of the spinous process (i.e., interfering with its rotation while the pelvis continues to rotate). The clinician once again assesses for the first barrier of resistance using the thumb pad contact against the spinous process as the main sensory tool to assess the barrier. Once obtained, the clinician springs the joint in search of a pathological barrier.

Once the SI joint is assessed, the clinician can then move to the adjoining superior segment and repeats the assessment procedure. Of course, with each succeeding level, there will be additional joint play due to the additional joints between the target spinous process and ASIS contact.

Once the lumbar joints are corrected on one side, the clinician then switches sides and repeats the procedures for contralateral joint rotational assessment.

Lumbar Spine A–P Assessment

Ⓟ Patient's position

The patient is placed in a side-lying, hook-lying position on the table. Both knees are just off the side of the table, while the lower legs remain on the table. The patient's lumbar spine should be in a relaxed neutral or slightly lordotic (i.e., as opposed to a rounded or kyphotic) position. A high table, preferably one that approximates the clinician's waist level is preferable.

Clinician's position

The clinician stands, facing the table and next to the patient's flexed knees.

Clinician contacts

The clinician places the patient's knees into his or her lower abdomen. The clinician then reaches across the table and contacts the patient's lowest mobile lumbar spinous process with the finger pad of the third digit. The other finger pads are placed alongside the third digit, but with a less firm contact. The finger pads of the other hand are placed on top of the fingers of the contact hand for increased digital stability (see Chapter 23, Fig. 23–20).

Key to assessment

The clinician then simultaneously moves his or her abdomen forward (i.e., driving the patient's knees, thigh, and pelvis posteriorly) while drawing the target spinous process closer (i.e., anteriorly) with the contact hands. The clinician palpates for a resistant pathological barrier as he or she springs the joint.

This maneuver is then repeated at each successive, superior joint.

Pubic Symphysis Assessment The symphysis pubis is, clinically speaking, a largely ignored joint. Relatively little is written about this joint in the absence of trauma, although Greenman[195] states that joint dysfunction is quite common. It is the pivot point for the recurrent rotational motion of the innominates during gait. It is a powerful joint, held in place by strong superior and inferior ligaments.

Interestingly, Bierma-Zeinstra et al.[296] positively correlated degeneration of the symphysis with mononeuropathy of the lateral femoral cutaneous nerve, also known as *meralgia paresthetica*. This relationship was found among both men and women. While the correlation is interesting, the etiology of the relationship is unknown.

The symphesis is not easily assessed due to

1. difficulty in establishing fine assessment of a strong joint with little motion.
2. a small and sensitive contact area.
3. complication of the proximity of the genitalia.

Therefore, additional care should be observed regarding proper professional decorum and patient communication regarding pubic assessment.

Greenman[195] states that the symphesis pubes tend toward a shearing type of dysfuction because of the vertical joint alignment. Therefore, one should assess for a superior versus inferior disrelationship at this joint.

HOW TO

Assessment of the pubic symphesis

The assessment steps given below are recommended by Greenman.[195]

Patient's position

The patient is placed supine on the table with the legs slightly apart.

Clinician's position

The clinician stands at the side of the table approximating the patient's pelvis.

Clinician contacts

The clinician places a flat palm of the caudal hand on the lower abdomen.

Key to assessment

The hand slides inferiorly until it contacts the pubic symphysis. Once this anatomic landmark is established, the clinician places palpating index finger pads on each side of the superior aspect of the symphysis. Each of the fingers then move laterally approximately 2 cm, palpating for the superior aspect of the pubic tubercles. One tubercle superior to the other is a positive finding.

Hip Assessment The hip joint is a clinically deceiving joint because referred pain from it can extend to the low back, SI joint, groin, thigh, and knee. Assessment techniques must be carefully planned because of the size of the joint, the weight of the local tissues, and challenges involved in gaining a mechanical advantage because of the torso and involved limb. The clinician must therefore strategize to use his or her body in a manner that can neutralize these mechanical disadvantages, while utilizing a contact that allows for fine palpation to monitor subtle changes in the hip joint during assessment.

Clinical Pearl: The hip joint is a clinically deceiving joint because referred pain from it can extend to the low back, SI joint, groin, thigh, and knee. It is often overlooked as the clinician bypasses it on the way to evaluate the knee after assessing the low back.

HOW TO

Assessment of the hip joint.

Patient's position

The patient is supine for this procedure, lying close to the same side of the table as the target hip (i.e., left edge of table for left hip joint). The target hip is positioned in the hook-lying position.

Clinician's position

The clinician typically kneels alongside the table, next to the target hip, facing toward the head of the table.

Clinician contacts

The clinician then elevates the target leg and places it to rest on his or her shoulder. The clinician then places both hands around the proximal thigh, firmly interlacing the fingers along the anterior aspect to form one functional unit.

Key to assessment

The clinician then elevates his or her torso slightly, bringing the foot of the target leg off the table and then maneuvering the target hip to approximately 90 degrees of flexion. The assessment entails the coupled movements of the bent leg on the clinician's shoulder and the interlaced hands at the anteromedial thigh. The clinician should then lightly distract the hip joint by moving his or her body away from the target hip (Fig. 23–24).

With the hip in this relaxed, distracted position, the clinician can then spring the joint in an A–P direction, a medial to lateral motion, in circumduction, in varying degrees of hip abduction or adduction, or any combination of these.

FUNCTIONAL REASSESSMENT

So far, the functional assessment has only been described with regard to the initial patient visit. It is therefore important to dispel any notion that it is a one-time endeavor. *The initial functional assessment establishes a baseline from which the clinician can later compare.* There are only four aspects of the clinical assessment that can be practically used on a regular basis. These include the updated history, outcomes measures, physical examination procedures such as those described in the previous chapter, and the functional assessment. Other assessment tools are either time consuming, costly, invasive, or some combination of these.

Of the reassessment tools, two of these should be used at the beginning of each patient encounter and at the end of each patient encounter, where some sort of treatment was provided: the updated history and the functional assessment. All too often, clinicians perform procedures without rechecking the patient's subjective and objective response. Was there a change in symptomatology? Was there a corresponding change in tenderness? Were there changes in posture, gait, movement patterns, or palpation? These are vital topics because they, to a great degree, justify the treatment. In a time of heavy emphasis on instant gratification, the wise practitioner should remember to appreciate the patient's perspective. Finally, immediate results and those encountered at the next visit, if necessary, should greatly influence the methods of treatment that will be subsequently be employed.

Clinical Pearl: All too often, clinicians perform procedures without rechecking the patient's subjective and objective response. Was there a change in symptomatology? Was there a corresponding change in tenderness? Were there changes in posture, gait, movement patterns or palpation?

Later chapters will address various treatment and rehabilitative methods commonly employed for the treatment of low back syndromes. No visit that uses manual treatment methods should be considered complete without a reassessment at the end of that visit.

PATIENT CONFIDENCE

Clinicians who integrate functional assessment protocols in their practice realize that these skills can help top build a strong relationship with the patient. When the patient realizes the clinician can palpate the painful spot, can observe subtle alteration in gait or the slight improvement in posture, a close relationship is often established based on a deep degree of trust.

THE PRACTICAL FUNCTIONAL APPROACH

The functional approach is not a structured set of tests, but rather a strategy to better understand the etiology of the patient's presenting condition and provide practical comparisons before, after, and between treatments. If this is a chronic condition, then it must be accepted that the current complaints may stem from a prolonged chronology of dysfunction elsewhere in the body. When discussing chronic pain syndromes, Lewit stated, "The clinician who only searches at the site of pain is lost."[15] Although this text is devoted to conditions of the lumbopelvic region, one must not assume that the evaluation skills and strategies described in this chapter mean that assessment of distant regions, including the feet, head, and neck, are unnecessary.

Clinical Pearl: The functional assessment for low back syndromes demonstrates the complexity of the subject and a plethora of clinical pitfalls that can occur to clinicians who places an overreliance on individual or subsets of positive findings. Such *clinical presumptuousness* must be avoided, while consistent strings of observations, the *significant subtleties,* must be investigated.

The functional evaluation is based upon clinical "common sense," which can be defined as the practical application of reason to decision making. Therefore, the functional approach will have a patient, who experiences low back pain after 10 or 15 minutes of standing, stand for 10 or 15 minutes and observe the changes that occur in the still upright posture to better understand the mechanism of pain. The functional approach can be used to determine why a patient might flare-up with one type of treatment, such as a compressing-type of manipulation, yet improve with a distraction manipulation maneuver. Once one understands the basic functional strategy, then it can be applied to every patient to glean additional information beyond that from the more classical physical examination and history. In the end, the depth and variety of functional evaluation strategies are only limited by one's imagination.

SUMMARY

1. This chapter provided an overview of the clinical functional assessment for the lumbopelvic region. As has been demonstrated, it is indeed a science-based art.
2. The functional assessment for low back syndromes demonstrates the complexity of the subject and a plethora of potential clinical pitfalls that can occur to clinicians who place an overreliance on individual or subsets of positive findings. Such *clinical presumptuousness* must be avoided, while consistent strings of observations, the *significant subtleties*, must be investigated.
3. With time, proper training, and experience, the clinical methods explained here can nevertheless provide significant diagnostic insights and confirmatory findings that can provide clinical shortcuts and increased confidence to the clinician.
4. It is the *coupled findings*, the grouping of observations that follow a common clinical pathway to the diagnostic impression, which allow the clinician to transition from the beginner to the master.
5. As with all other diagnostic approaches, the main risks involved are performing tests that are poorly tolerated poorly performed, and overly reliant on insufficient clinical observations.
6. All aspects of the twenty-first-century health-care world must be prepared to justify their existence. This reigns true for the examination procedures described in this chapter. The placement of the functional assessment in the world of neuromusculoskeletal treatment remains uncertain. The complexity of the topic in comparison to the relative dearth of knowledge is indeed daunting.
7. The methods described here encompass a number of assessment skills employed by those who practice manual functional restoration of the locomotor. It is therefore up to the teaching institutions, researchers, instructors, clinicians, and students to establish and maintain increasingly higher levels of excellence and standardization of the functional assessment in order to appreciate the value of this difficult and challenging method of evaluation.
8. The information gleaned from the functional assessment can be integrated with the physical examination findings from the prior chapter and with the ensuing diagnostic chapters to provide a stronger, more cogent, diagnostic impression, which will then pave the way for a variety of treatment options described in later chapters.

REFERENCES

1. Mitchell F. Training and measurements of sensory literacy. *J Am Osteopath Assoc* 1976;75(6):874–884.
2. Chaitow L. Palpation and assessment skills, 2nd ed. Edinburgh: Churchill Livingstone, 2003.
3. Nixon PGF, Freeman, LJ. The 'think test': A further technique to elicit hyperventilation. *J R Soc Med* 1988;81:277–279.
4. Janda V. Muscle spasm—A proposed procedure for differential diagnosis. *J Manual Med* 1991;6:136–139.
5. Hyman J. *Spinal rehabilitation course workshop.* Whittier, CA: Los Angeles College of Chiropractic, 1997.
6. Grieve G. *Modern manual therapy.* London: Churchill Livingstone, 1986.
7. Wooley S, Sigg J, Commager J. Comparison of change in level walking activities in three groups of elderly individuals. *Posture Gait* June 1995;3(2):81.
8. Lum L. Editorial: Hyperventilation and anxiety state. *J R Soc Med* January 1981;74:1–4.
9. Janda V. Extracranial causes of facial pain. *J Prosthet Dent* 1986;56(4):484–487.
10. Lewit K. Personal communication with the lead author. *Manual Medicine Workshop*, Tucany, Italy, March 1998.
11. Kurz M, Stergiou N. The spanning set indicates that variability during the stance period of running is affected by footwear. *Posture Gait* April 2002;17(2):132–135.
12. Hastings H. Sixty million connections per second. *Biosystems* 1989;23(2/3):171–173.
13. Hruda K, Hicks A, McCartney N. Training for muscle power in older adults: Effects on functional abilities. *Can J Appl Physiol* April 2003;28(2):178–189.
14. Gauchard G, Vancon G, Gentine A, Jeandel C, Perrin P. Physical activity after retirement enhances vestibulo-ocular reflex in elderly humans. *Neurosci Lett* April 22, 2004;360(1/2):17–20.
15. Janda V. *Sensory motor system assessment & treatment workshop.* Redondo Beach, CA: Functional Action, Inc.,. June 2001.
16. Reisman J, Anderson J. Compensatory eye movements during head and body rotation in nfants. *Brain Res* April 10, 1989;484(1/2):119–129.
17. Prechi H, Cioni G, Einspieler C, Bos A, Ferrari F. Role of vision on early development: Lessons from the blind. *Dev Med Child Neurol* March 2001;43(3):198–201.

18. Inman V, Ralston H, Todd F. *Human walking*. Baltimore, MD: Williams & Wilkins, 1981.
19. Nakata H, Yabe K. Autonomic postural response systems in individuals with congenital total blindness. *Posture Gait* July 2001;14(1):36–43.
20. Okamoto T, Okamoto T, Andrew P. Electromyographic developmental changes in one individual from newborn stepping to mature walking. *Posture Gait* February 2003;17(1):18–27.
21. Yasuda T, Nakagawa T, Inoue H, Iwamoto M, Inokuchi A. The role of the labyrinth, proprioception and plantar mechanoreceptors in the maintenance of an upright posture. *Eur Arch Otorhinolaryngol* 1999;256(Suppl I):S27–S32.
22. Woolacott M, Debu B, Mowatt M. Neuromuscular control of posture in the infant and child: Is vision dominant? *J Mot Behav* June 1987;19(2):167–196.
23. Hedberg A, Forssberg H, Hadders-Algra M. Postural adjustments due to external perturbations during sitting in 1-month-old infants: Evidence for the innate origin of direction specificity. *Exp Brain Res* March 13, 2004;157(1):10–17.
24. Hortobagyi T, Taylor J, Peterson N, Russell G, Gandevia S. Changes in segmental and motor cortical output with contralateral muscle contractions and altered sensory inputs in humans. *J Neurophysiol* October 2003;90(4):2451–2459.
25. Miyahara T. Modulation of soleus H-reflex by teeth clenching. (Article in Japanese.) *Kokubyo Gakkai Zasshi* December 1991;58(4):670–686.
26. Yaguramaki N, Kimura T. Acquirement of stability and mobility in infant gait. *Posture Gait* August 2002;16(1):69–77.
27. Janda V. Postural and phasic muscles in the pathogenesis of low back pain. In: *Proceedings of the XIth Congress International Society of Rehabilitation and Disability*, Dublin, Ireland,1968:553–554.
28. Waddell, G. *The back pain revolution*. Edinburgh: Churchill Livingstone, 1998:144–148.
29. Norris C. (in Bullock-Saxton J, Murphy D, Norris C, Richardson C, Tunnell P) The Muscle Designation Debate *Journal of Bodywork and Movement Therapies* 2000;4(4):225–241.
30. Bergmark, A. Stability of the lumbar spine. A study in mechanical engineering. *Acta Orthop Scand* 1989;230(Suppl):20–24.
31. Richardson C, Jull G, Hodges P, Hides J. *Therapeutic exercise for spinal segmental stabilisation in low back pain*. Edinburgh: Churchill Livingstone, 1999.
32. Bogduk N, Twomey L. *Clinical anatomy of the lumbar spine,* 2nd ed. Edinburgh: Churchill Livingstone, 1991.
33. Grimshaw P, Marques-Bruna P, Salo A, Messenger N. The 3-dimensional kinematics of the walking gait cycle of children aged between 10 and 24 months: Cross sectional and repeated measures. *Gait Posture* January 1998;7(1):7–15.
34. Gould N. Shoes versus sneakers in toddler ambulation. *Foot Ankle* October 1985;6(2):105–107.
35. Roncesvalles M, Woolacott M, Brown N, Jensen J. An emerging postural response: Is control of the hip possible in the newly walking child? *J Mot Behav* June 2004;36(2):147–159.
36. Sutherland D. The development of mature gait. *Posture Gait* October 1997;6(2):163–170.
37. Breniere Y. How locomotor parameters adapt to gravity and body structure changes during development in children. *Mot Control* April 1999;3(2): 186–204.
38. Makin M, Glanem J. Reduction of dorsolumbar angulation by headloading. *Posture Gait* June 1995;3(2):66–71.
39. Haas G, Diener H, Rapp H, Dichgans J. Development of feedback and feedforward control of upright stance. *Dev Med Child Neurol* August 1989; 31(4): 481–488.
40. Malouin F, Richards C. Preparatory adjustments during gait initiation in 4-6 year-old children. *Posture Gait* June 2000;11(3):239–253.
41. Shumway-Cook A, Woolacott MH. The growth of the stability: Postural control from a developmental perspective. *J Mot Behav* June 1985; 17(2):131–147.
42. Schneiberg S, Sveistrup H, McFadyen B, McKinley P, Levin M. The development of coordination for reach-to-grasp movements in children. *Exp Brain Res* September 2002;146(2):142–154.
43. Hausdorff J, Zemany L, Peng C, Goldberger A. Maturation of gait: Stride-to-stride variability and its temporal organization in children. *J App Physiol* March 1999;86(3):1040–1047.
44. Ganley K, Powers C. Gait kinematics and kinetics of 7-year-old children: A comparison to adults using age-specific anthropometric data. *Posture Gait,* 2005 Feb; 21(2):141–145.
45. McFadyen B, Malouin F, Dumas F. Anticipatory locomotor control for obstacle avoidance in mid-childhood aged children. *Posture Gait* February 2001;13(1):7–16.
46. Falk B, Eliakim A, Dotan R, Liebermann D, Regev R, Bar-Or O. Birth weight and physical ability in 5–8-yr-old healthy children born prematurely. *Med Sci Sports Exerc* September 1997;29(9):1124–1130.
47. Ferrel C, Bard C, Fleury M. Coordination in childhood: Modifications of visuomotor representations in 6–11-year-old children. *Exp Brain Res* June 2001; 138(3):313–321.
48. Jones G, Watson K, Silman A, Symmons D, McFarlane G. Predictors of low back pain in British schoolchildren: A population based prospective cohort study. *Pediatrics* April 2003;111(4):822–828.
49. Agnati L, Franzen O, Ferre S, Leo G, Franco R, Fuxe K. Possible role of intramembrane receptor-receptor interactions in memory and learning via formation of long-lived heteromeric complexes: Focus on motor learning in the basal ganglia. *J Neural Transm Suppl* 2003;(65):1–28.
50. Kottke F, Halpern D, Easton J, Ozel A, Burrill C. The training of coordination. *Arch Phys Med Rehabil* December 1978;59(12):567–572.
51. Sherrington CS. *The integrative action of the nervous system*. London, Archibald Constable & Co., Ltd., 1906.

52. Lisberger S, Pavelko T, Broussard D. Responses during eye movement of brain stem neurons that receive monosynaptic inhibition fro the flocculus and ventral paraflocculus in monkeys. *J Neurophysiol* August 1994;72(2):909–927.
53. Hodges P, Cresswell A, Daggefeldt K, Thorstensson A. Three dimensional preparatory trunk motion precedes asymmetrical upper limb movement. *Posture Gait* April 2000;11(2):92–101.
54. Onell A. The vertical ground reaction force for analysis of balance? *Posture Gait* September 2000;12(1) 7–13.
55. Hreljac A. Stride smoothness evaluation of runners and non-athletes. *Gait Posture* June 2000;11(3):199–206.
56. Perrin P, Deviterne D, Hugel F, Perrot C. Judo, better than dance, develops sensorimotor adaptabilities involved in balance control. *Gait Posture* April 2002;15(2):187–194.
57. Kerrigan D, Viramontes B, Corcoran P, LARaisa P. Measured versus predicted vertical displacement of the sacrum during gait as a tool to measure biomechanical gait performance. *Am J Med Rehabil* 1995;74(1):3–8.
58. Hoppenfled S. *Physical examination of the spine and extremities*. New York, Appleton-Century-Crofts, 1976: P134–P141.
59. Whittlesey S, van Emmerik R, Hamill J. The swing phase of walking is not a passive movement. *Mot Control* July 2000;4(3):273–292.
60. Wakeling J, Liphart A, Nigg B. Muscle activity reduces soft-tissue resonance at heel-strike during walking. *J Biomech* December 2003;36(12):1761–1769.
61. Winters J, Crago P., eds. *Biomechanics and neural control of posture and movement*. New York: Springer, 2000.
62. Kavounoudias A, Roll R, Roll J. Foot sole muscle inputs contribute jointly to human erect posture regulation. *J Physiol* May 1, 2001;532(Pt 3):869–878.
63. Dietz V, Duysens J. Significance of load receptor input during locomotion: A review. *Posture Gait* April 2000; 11(2):102–110.
64. El-Sayyad M. Effect of walking speed on gait measurements of young men. *Posture Gait* September 1995;3(3):174–176.
65. Hunter M, Hoffman M. Postural control: Visual and cognitive manipulation. *Posture Gait* December 2001;13(1):41–48.
66. McFarland DH, Lund JP, Gagner M. Effects of posture on the coordination of respiration and swallowing. *J Neurophysiol* November 1994;72(5):2431–2437.
67. Shirley D, Hodges P, Eriksson A, Gandevia S. Spinal stiffness changes throughout the respiratory cycle. *J Appl Physiol* October 2003;95(4):1467–1475.
68. Grimstone S, Hodges P. Impaired compensation for respiration in people with recurrent low back pain. *Exp Brain Res* July 2003;151(2):218–224.
69. Balaban C, Thayer J. Neurological bases for balance–anxiety links. *J Anxiety Disord* 2001;15(1/2):53–79.
70. Yardley L, Redfern M. Psychological factors influencing recovery from balance disorders. *J Anxiety Disord* 2001;15(1/2):107–119.
71. Sadeghi H, Allard P, Prince F, Labelle H. Symmetry and limb dominance in able-bodied gait: A review. *Posture Gait* September 2000;12(1):34–45.
72. Moseley GL, Nicholas M, Hodges P. Pain differs from non-painful attention-demanding or stressful tasks in its effect on postural control patterns of trunk muscles. *Exp Brain Res* May 2004;156(1):64–71.
73. Manetta J, Franz L, Moon C, Perell K, Fang M. Comparison of hip and knee muscle moments in subjects with and without knee pain. *Posture Gait* December 2002;16(3):249–254.
74. Hodges P, Gurfinkel V, Brumagne S, Smith T, Cordo P. Coexistance of stability and mobility in postural control: Evidence from postural compensation for respiration. *Exp Brain Res* June 2002;144(3):293–302.
75. Newcomer K, Jacobson T, Gabriel D, Larson D, Brey R, An K. Muscle activation patterns in subjects with and without low back pain. *Arch Phys Med Rehabil* June 2002;83(6):816–821.
76. McGregor A, Anderton L, Gedroye W. The assessment of intersegmental motion and pelvic tilt in elite oarsmen. *Med Sci Sports Exerc* July 2002;34(7):1143–1149.
77. Chen W, Chiou W, Lee Y, Lee M, Chen M. Myo-electric behavior of the trunk muscles during static load holding in healthy subjects and low back pain patients. *Clin Biomechan (Bristol, Avon)* 1998;13(1, Suppl 1):S9–S15.
78. Hungerford B, Gilleard W, Hodges P. Evidence of altered lumbopelvic muscle recruitment in the presence of sacroiliac joint pain. *Spine* July 15, 2003;28(14):1593–1600.
79. Rosengren K, McAuley E, Mihalko S. Gait adjustments in older adults: Activity and efficacy influences. *Psychol Aging* September 1998;13(3):375–386.
80. Jonkers I, Stewert C, Spaepen A. The complimentary role of the plantar flexors, hamstrings and gluteus maximus in the control of stance limb stability during gait. *Posture Gait* June 2003;17(3):264–272.
81. Madelaine P, Voigt M, Arendt-Nielsen L. Reorganization of human step initiation during acute experimental muscle pain. *Posture Gait* December 1999; 10(3):240–247.
82. Garsden L, Bullock-Saxton J. Joint reposition sense in subjects with unilateral osteoarthritis of the knee. *Clin Rehabil* April 1999;13(2):148–155.
83. McGibbon C, Krebs D. Compensatory gait mechanics in patients with unilateral knee arthritis. *J Rheumatol* November 2002;29(11):2410–2419.
84. Watelain E, Dujardin F, Babier F. Dubois D, Allard P. Pelvic and lower limb compensatory actions of subjects in an early stage of hip osteoarthritis. *Arch Phys Med Rehabil* December 2001;81(12):1705–1711.
85. Hobeika C. Equilibrium and balance in the elderly. *Ear Nose Throat J*. August 1999;78(8):558–562, 565–566.
86. Speers R, Kuo A, Horak F. Contributions of altered sensation and feedback responses to changes in coordination of postural control due to aging. *Posture Gait* August 2002;16(1):20–30.
87. Marvel B, Schwartz B, Rosse R. A quantitative measure of postural sway deficits in schizophrenia. *Schizophr Res* June 1, 2004;68(2/3):363–372.

88. Woollacott M, Shumway-Cook A. Attention and control of posture and gait: A review of an emerging area of research. *Posture Gait* August 2002;16(1):1–14.
89. Hernandez-Reif M, Field TM, Thimas E. Attention deficit hyperactivity disorder: Benefits from Tai Chi. *J Bodywork Movement Ther* 2001;5(2):120–123.
90. Parker AW, Bronks R. Gait of children with Down's syndrome. *Arch Phy Med Rehabil* 1980;61:345–351.
91. Harris DE. A review of joint pathologies in individuals with Down's syndrome: Implications for the practitioner. *Clin Kinesiol* 1992; 46(1):10–13.
92. Bullock-Saxton J. Sensory changes associated with severe ankle sprain. *Scand J Rehabil Med* September 1995;27(3):161–167.
93. Siegel K. Preventing limb collapse during gait: Control strategies in the severely weak lower extremity. *Posture Gait* April 1996;4(2):202–203.
94. Whitehurst M, Brown L, Eidelson S, D'angelo A. Functional mobility performance in an elderly population with lumbar spinal Stenosis. *Arch Phys Med Rehabil.* April 2001;82(4):464–467.
95. Riley P, DellaCroce U, Kerrigan D. Effect of age on lower extremity joint moment contributions to gait speed. *Posture Gait* December 2001;14(3):264–270.
96. Verkerke G, Ament W, Wierenga R, Rakhorst G. Measuring changes in step parameters during an exhausting running exercise. *Posture Gait* August 1998;8(1):37–42.
97. Aust G, Fischer K. Changes in body equilibrium response caused by breathing. A posturographic study with visual feedback. *Laryngorhinootologie* 1997;76(10):577–582.
98. Balaban C, Thayer J. Neurological bases for balance–anxiety links. *J Anxiety Disord* 2001;15(1/2):53–79.
99. Chaitow L. Breathing pattern disorders, motor control, and low back pain. *J Osteopath Med* 2004;7(1):34–41.
100. Dananberg H. 1997 Lower back pain as a gait-related repetitive motion injury. In: Vleeming A, Mooney V, Dorman T, Snijders C, Stoekart R, eds. *Movement, stability and low back pain.* New York: Churchill Livingstone,.1997.
101. Dananberg H. Functional hallux limitus and its relationship to gait efficiency. *J Am Podiatr Med Assoc* 1986;76(11):648–652.
102. Janda V. Muscles, central nervous motor regulation and back problems. In: Korr I, ed. *The neurobiological mechanism in manipulative therapy.* New York: Plenum Press, 1978:27–41.
103. Liu X, Fabry G, Molenears G, Van Auderkercke L, Moens P. Functional analysis of patients with leg length discrepancies. *Posture Gait* December 1995;3(4): 286–287.
104. Young R, Andrew P, Cummings G. Effect of simulating leg length inequality on pelvic torsion and trunk mobility. *Posture Gait* June 2000;11(3):217–223.
105. Boone T, Hammans R. Acute leg length causes increased Vo2. *Posture Gait* April 1996;4(2):108–111.
106. Selye H. *The stress of life.* New York: McGraw Hill, 1956.
107. Janda V. Low back pain: Trends, controversies, community-based rehabilitation approach. In: Proceedings from the *Consultation on disability prevention and rehabilitation*, Turku, Finland, 1984.
108. Gross M, Stevenson P, Charette S, Pyka G, Marcus R. Effect of muscle strength and movement speed on the biomechanics of rising from a chair in healthy elderly and young women. *Posture Gait* December 1998;8(3):175–185.
109. Simoneau G, Ulbrecht J, Derr J, Cavanagh P. Role of somatosensory input in the control of human posture. *Posture Gait* September 1995;3(3):115–122.
110. Allum J, Bloem B, Carpenter M, Hullinger M, Hadders-Algra M. Proprioceptive control of posture: A review of new concepts. *Posture Gait* December 1998;8(3):214–242.
111. Dickstein R, Shupert C, Horak F. Fingertip touch improves postural stability in patients with peripheral neuropathy.*Posture Gait* December 2001;14(3):238–247.
112. Jeka J. Light touch as a balance aid. *Phys Ther* May 1997;77(5):476–87.
113. Jeka J, Easton R, Benzen B, Lackner J. Haptic cues for orientation and postural control in sighted and blind individuals. *Percept Psychophys* April 1996;58(3):409–423.
114. Janda V. Pain in the locomotor system. In: *Proceeding of the Second Annual Interdisciplinary Symposium on rehabilitation in chronic low back disorders.* Los Angeles, CA: Los Angeles College of Chiropractic Postgraduate Division, 1988.
115. Tuzin C, Yorulmaz I, Cindas A, Vatan S. Low back pain and posture. *Clin Rheumatol* 1999;18(4):308–312.
116. NcClenaghan B, Williams H, Dickerson J, Dowda M, Thombs L, Eleazer P. Spectral characteristics of aging postural control. *Posture Gait* September 1995;3(3):123–131.
117. Kernozek T, LaMott E. Comparison of plantar pressures between the elderly and young adults. *Posture Gait* September 1995;3(3):143–148.
118. Kerrigan D, Lee L, Collins J, Riley P, Lipsitz L. Reduced hip extension during walking: Healthy elderly and fallers versus young adults.*Arch Phys Med Rehabil* January 2001;82(1):26–30.
119. Balzini L, Vannuchi L, Benvenuti F, Benucci M, Cappozzo A, Stanhope S. Clinical characteristics of flexed posture in elderly women. *J Am Geriatr Soc* Oct 2003;51(10):1419–1426.
120. Indge J, Davis R, Ounpuu S. Age-associated reduction in step length: Testing the importance of hip and ankle kinetics.*Posture Gait* June 1995;3(2):81–83.
121. Bullock-Saxton J, Wong W, Hogan N. The influence of age on weight bearing joint reposition sense of the knee.*Exp Brain Res* February 2001;136(3):400–406.
122. Cham R, Redfern M. Changes in gait when anticipating slippery floors. *Posture Gait* April 2002;15(2):159–171.
123. Teasdale N, Simoneau M. Attention demands for postural control: The effects of aging and sensory regulation. *Posture Gait* December 2001;14(3):203–210.

124. Cao C, Schultz A, Ashton-Miller J, Alexander N. Sudden turns and stops while walking: Kinematic sources of age and gender differences. Gait Posture January 1998;7(1):45–52.
125. Cao C, Ashton-Miller J, Schultz A, Alexander N. Effects of age, available response time and gender on ability to stop suddenly when walking. *Posture Gait* October 1998;8(2):103–109.
126. Bracchi E, Rizzo S, Longari F, Bernadini M, Bizzotti C, Frenguelli A. Balance disorders in the elderly. *Acta Otorhinolaryngol Ital* October 2002;22(5):263–267.
127. Brown L, Frank J. Postural compensation to the potential consequences of instability: Kinematics. *Posture Gait* October 1997;6(2):89–97.
128. Hamel K, Cavanagh P. Stair performance in people aged 75 and older. *J Am Geriatr Soc* April 2004;52(4):563–567.
129. Christina K, Cavanagh P. Ground reaction forces and frictional demands during stair descent: Effects of age and illumination. *Gait Posture* April 2002 ;15(2):1530–1538.
130. Cavanagh P, Mulfinger L, Owens. How do elderly negotiate stairs? *Muscle Nerve Suppl* 1997;5:S52–S55.
131. Janda V, Schmidt H. Muscles as a pathogenic factor in back pain. In: *Proceedings of the International Federation of Orthopaedic Manual Therapists,* New Zealand, 1980.
132. Kendall F, McCreary E, Provance P. *Muscles: Testing and function,* 4th ed. Baltimore, MD: Lippincott, Williams & Wilkins, 1993:334.
133. Janda V. Muscle weakness and inhibition (pseudoparesis) in back pain syndromes. In: Grieve G, ed. *Modern manual therapy of the vertebral column.* Edinburgh: Churchill Livingstone, 1986:197–201.
134. Brügger A. Lehrbuch der Funktionellen Storungen des Bewegungssystems. Brugger-Verlag, Zollikon, Benglen, 2000.
135. Lewit K. *Manipulation in rehabilitation of the locomotor system*, 3rd ed. London: Butterworths, 1999.
136. Latey P. Feelings muscles and movement. *J Bodywork Movement Ther* 1996;1(1):44–52.
137. Puranen J, Orava S. The hamstring syndrome. A new diagnosis of gluteal sciatic pain. *Am J Sports Med* 1988;16(5):517–521.
138. Christie HJ, Kumar S, Warren SA. Postural aberrations in low back pain. *Arch Phys Med Rehabil* March 1995;76(3):218–224.
139. Prince F, Winter A, Archer E. Assessment of postural control during quiet stance with different foot configurations. *Posture Gait* June 1995;3(2):110–111.
140. Winter D. Balance control: An overriding challenge in standing and walking. *Posture Gait* September 1995;3(3):170.
141. Winter D, MacKinnon C, Ruder G, Weiman C. An integrated EMG/biomechanical model of upper body balance and posture during human gait. *Prog Brain Res* 1993;97:359–367.
142. Balasubramaniam R, Riley M, Turvey M. Speificity of postural sway to the demands of a precision task. *Posture Gait* February 2000;11(1):12–24.
143. Fedorak C, Ashworth N, Marshall J, Paull H. Reliability of the visual assessment of cervical and lumbar lordosis: How good are we? *Spine* August 15, 2003;28(16):1857–1859.
144. Dinnar U, Beal M, Goodridge J, et al. An osteopathic method of history taking and physical examination. *J Am Osteopath Assoc* January 1982;81(5):314–321.
145. Vogel F. 1984 Short-leg syndrome. *Clin Podiatr* December 1 19841(3):581–599.
146. Ledoux W, Hillstrom H. The distributed plantar vertical force of neutrally aligned and pes planus feet. *Posture Gait* February 2002;15(1):1–9.
147. Catani F, Benedetti M, Montanari P, et al.Functional evaluation of gait in children with flat feet. *Posture Gait* December 1995;3(4):287.
148. Platzer W. *Color atlas/text of human anatomy. Vol 1. Locomotor system*, 4th edn. Stuttgart: Georg Thieme, 1992.
149. Mok N, Brauer S, Hodges P. Hip strategy for balance control in quiet standing is reduced in people with low back pain. *Spine* March 11 2004; 29(6):E107–E112.
150. Janda V. *Movement patterns in the pelvis and hip region with special reference to pathogenesis of vertebrogenic disturbances*. PhD Thesis, Charles University, Prague, 1964.
151. Ng J, Richardson C, Parnianpar M, Kippers V. Fatigue-related changes in torque output and electromyographic parameters of trunk muscles during isometric axial rotation exertion: An investigation in patients with back pain and in healthy subjects. *Spine* March 15, 2002;27(6):637–646.
152. Jull G, Janda V. Muscles and motor control in low back pain: Assessment and management. In: Twomey L, Grieve G, eds. *Physical therapy of the low back.* Edinburgh: Churchill Livingstone, 1987:253–278.
153. Tunnell P. Protocol for visual assessment. *J Bodywork Movement Ther* 1996;1(1):22–27.
154. Levangie C, Norkin P. *Joint structure and function: A comprehensive analysis*, 3rd ed. Philadelphia: F A Davis, 2001.
155. Schafer R. *Clinical biomechanics,* 2nd ed. Baltimore, MD: Williams & Wilkins, 1987.
156. Cailliet R. *Soft tissue pain and disability,* 3rd ed. Philadelphia: FA Davis, 1996.
157. Levangie C, Norkin P. *Joint structure and function: A comprehensive analysis*, 3rd ed. Philadelphia: F A Davis, 2001.
158. Spencer J, Hayes K, Alexander I. Knee joint effusion and quadriceps reflex inhibition in man. *Arch Phys Med Rehabil* April 1984;65(4):171–177.
159. Gerber C, Hoppeler H, Claases H, Robotti G, Zehnder R, Jakob R. The lower-extremity musculature in chronic symptomatic instability of the anterior cruciate ligament. *J Bone Joint Surg Am.* September 1985;67(7):1034–1043.
160. Morrisey M. Reflex inhibition of thigh muscles in knee injury. *Sports Med* April 1989;7(4):263–276.
161. Kapandji I. *The physiology of the joints. Vol. 2. Lower limb*, 5th ed. Edinburgh: Churchill Livingstone, 1987.
162. Hodges P. Personal communication with lead editor-2004.
163. Nixon P. A study of anaerobic threshold in chronic fatigue syndrome (CFS). *Biol Psychol* 1996;43(3): 246–247.

164. George S. Changes in serum calcium, serum phosphate and red cell phosphate during hyperventilation. *New Engl J Med* 1964;270:726–728.
165. Pryor J, Prasad S. *Physiotherapy for respiratory and cardiac problems*, 3rd ed. Edinburgh: Churchill Livingstone, 2002.
166. Aust G, Fischer K. Changes in body equilibrium response caused by breathing. A posturographic study with visual feedback. *Laryngorhinootologie* 1997;76(10): 577–582.
167. Winters J, Crago P, eds. *Biomechanics and neural control of posture and movement*. New York: Springer, 2000.
168. McGill S, Sharratt M, Seguin J. Loads on spinal tissues during simultaneous lifting and ventilatory challenge. *Ergonomics* 1995;38(9):1772–1792.
169. Janda V. On the concept of postural muscles and posture in man. *Aus J Physiother* 1983;29:83–84.
170. King D, Zatsiorsky V. Periods of extreme ankle displacement during one-legged standing. *Posture Gait* April 2002;15(2):172–179.
171. Bohannon R, Larkin P, Cook A, Gear J, Singer J. Decrease in timed balance test scores with aging. *Phys Ther* 1984;64:1067–1070.
172. Downes J. 2004 Hyperpronation and reciprocal limb syndromes as precipitators of low back and pelvic pain. Presentation. In: *Journal of Bodywork & Movement Therapies Multidisciplinary Conference*, Safety Harbour Resort, Tampa Bay, June 11–13, 2004.
173. Hodges P, Moseley G. Pain and motor control of the lumbopelvic region: Effect and possible mechanisms. *J Electromyogr Kinesiol* August 2003;13(4):361–370.
174. Cyriax J. *Textbook of orthopaedic medicine*. London: Cassell, 1977.
175. Simons D, Travell J, Simons L. Myofascial pain and dysfunction. *The trigger point manual,* 2nd ed, *Upper Body*. Baltimore, MD: Williams & Wilkins, 1999.
176. Chaitow L. *Palpation and assessment skills* 2nd ed. Edinburgh: Churchill Livingstone, 2003.
177. Badii M, Shin S, Torreggiani W, et al. Pelvic bone asymmetry in 323 study participants receiving abdominal CT scans. *Spine* June 15, 2003;28(12):1335–1339.
178. Linda T, O'Brien S, White H, Yack J. Kinetic analysis of the sit-to-stand movement used by elderly females. *Posture Gait* April 1996;4(2):207–208.
179. Maitland G. The slump test: Examination and treatment. *Aust J Physiother* 1985;32:215–219.
180. Butler DS. *Mobilisation of the nervous system*. Melbourne: Churchill Livingstone, 1991.
181. Smith S, Massie J, Chesnut R, Garfin S. Straight leg raising. Anatomincal effects on the spinal nerve root without and with fusion. *Spine* June 15, 1993; 18(8):992–999.
182. Breig A, Troup J. Biomechanical considerations in the straight-leg-raising test. Cadaveric and clinical studies of the effects of medial hip rotation. *Spine* 1979;4(3):242–250.
183. Kobayasi S, Shizu N, Suzuki Y, Asai T, Yoshizawa H. Changes in nerve motion and intraradicular blood flow during an intraoperative straight-leg raise test. *Spine* July 1, 2003;28(13):1427–1434.
184. Chao E. Clinical application of gait in orthopedics. *Posture Gait* September 1995;3(3):175.
185. Edelstein J. Low cost gait documentation. *Posture Gait* September 1995;3(3):170.
186. Schachse A, Bennell K, Blanch P, Wrigley T. The coordinated movement of the lumbo-pelvic-hip complex during running: A literature review. *Posture Gait* September 1999;10(1):30–47.
187. Maupas E, Paysant J, Datie A, Martinet N, Andre J. Functional asymmetries of the lower limbs. A comparison between clinical assessment of laterality, isokinetic evaluation and electrogoniometric monitoring of knees during walking. *Posture Gait* December 2002;16(3):304–312.
188. Nagasaki H. Walking patterns in human free gait. *Posture Gait* December 1995;3(4):268–270.
189. Janda V. Pain in the locomotor system – A broad approach. In: Glascow EF, Twomey LT, Scoll ER, Kleynhans AM, Idczak RM, eds. *Aspects of manipulative therapy.* Melbourne: Churchill Livingstone, 1985:148–151.
190. McAnelly R, Walden J, Chahande A, Walsh N. Principle and component analysis of kinematic overground and treadmill gait: A pilot study. *Posture Gait* June 1995;3(2):109.
191. Arseneault A, Winter D, Martenuik R. Treadmill versus walkway locomotion in humans: An EMG study. *Ergonomics* May 1986;29(5):665–676.
192. Yack H, Scott C, White C, Collins H. Comparison of overground and treadmill vertical ground reaction forces. *Posture Gait* June 1995;3(2):86–94.
193. Savelberg H, Vorstenbosch M, Kamman E, van de Weijer J, Schambardt H. Intra-stride belt-speed variation affects treadmill locomotion. *Posture Gait* January 1998;7(1):26–34.
194. Morris C, Greenman P, Bullock M, Basmajian J, Kobesova A. Professor Vladimir Janda: *A tribute. Spine,* in process.
195. Greenman P. *1996 Principles of Manual medicine* (second edition). Williams and Wilkins, Baltimore.
196. Miller C, Verstraete M. A mechanical energy analysis of gait initiation. *Posture Gait* July 1999 ;9(3):158–166.
197. Brunt D, Liu S, Trimble M, Gauer J, Short M. Principles underlying the organization of movement initiation from quiet stance. *Posture Gait* October 1999;10(2):121–128.
198. McPoil T, Cornwall M. Relationship between neutral subtalar joint position and patterns of rearfoot motion during walking. *Foot Ankle Int* March 1994;15(3):141–145.
199. Perry J. Gait analysis: Normal and Pathological Function. Slack, 1992. Thorofare New York.
200. Williams D, Davis I, Scholz J, Hamill J, Buchanan T. High-arched runners exhibit increased leg stiffness compared to low-arched runners. *Gait Posture* June 2004;19(3):263–269.
201. Lin C, Lai K, Chou Y, Ho C. The effect of changing the foot progression angle on the knee adduction moment in normal teenagers. *Gait Posture* October 2001;14(2):85–91.

202. Fuller E. The windlass mechanism of the foot. A mechanical model to explain pathology. *J Am Col Podiatr Med Assoc.* January 2000;90(1):35–46.
203. Kappel-Bargas A, Woolf R, Cornwall M, McPoil T. The windlass mechanism during normal walking and passive extension. *Clin Biomech (Bristol, Avon)* April 1998;13(3):190–194.
204. Hopson M, McPoil T, Cornwall M. Motion of the first metatarsophalangeal joint. Reliability and validity of four measurement techniques. *J Am Podiatr Med Assoc* April 1995;85(4):198–204.
205. Cailliet R. *Foot and ankle pain.* Philadelphia: F A Davis, 1997.
206. Kernozek T, Greer N. Quadriceps angle and rearfoot motion: Relationships in walking. *Arch Phys Med Rehabil* April 1993;74(4):407–410.
207. Messier S, Davies A, Moore D, Davis S, Pack R, Kazmar S. Severe obesity: Effects of foot mechanics during walking. *Foot Ankle Int* January 1994;15(1):29–34.
208. Whittle M, Levine D. Sagittal plane motion of the lumbar spine during normal gait. *Gait Posture* June 1995;3(2):82–85.
209. Vleeming A, Snijders C, Stoeckart R, Mens J. The role of the sacroiliac joints in coupling between spine, pelvis, legs and arms. In: Vleeming A, Mooney V, Dorman T, Snijders C, Stoekart R, eds. *Movement, stability and low back pain.* New York: Churchill Livingstone, 1997.
210. Lee D. Treatment of pelvic instability. In: Vleeming A, Mooney V, Dorman T, Snijders C, Stoekart R, eds. *Movement, stability and low back pain.* New York: Churchill Livingstone, 1997.
211. Vilensky J, Baltes M, Weilel L, Fortin J, Fourie L. Serratus posterior muscles; anatomy, clinical relevance, and function. *Clin Anat* July 2001;14(4):237–241.
212. Davis J, Mirka G. Transverse-contour modeling of trunk muscle-distributed forces and spinal loads during lifting and twisting. *Spine* January 15, 2000; 25(2):180–189.
213. Kim D, Glazer P. Progression of idiopathic thoracolumbar scoliosis after breast reconstruction with a latissimus dorsi flap: A case report. *Spine* March 1, 2000;25(22):622–625.
214. Vleeming A, Pool-Goudzwaard A, Stoeckart R, van Wingerden J, Snijders C. The posterior layer of the thoracolumbar fascia. Its function in load transfer from spine to legs. *Spine* April 1, 1995 ;20(7);753–758.
215. Vleeming A, Pool-Goudzwaard A, Hammudoghlu D, Stoeckart R, SnijdersC, Mens J. The function of the long dorsal sacroiliac ligament: Its implication for understanding low back pain. *Spine* March 1, 1996;21(5):556–562.
216. Barker P, Briggs C, Bogeski G. Tensile transmission across the lumbar fasciae in unembalmed cadavers: Effects of tension to various muscular attachments. *Spine* January 15, 2004;29(2):129–138.
217. Chaitow L, Delany J. *Clinical application of neuromuscular techniques. Volume 2: The lower body.* Edinburgh: Churchill Livingstone, 2002.
218. Duysens J, Tax A, Murrer L, Dietz V. Backward and forward walking use different patterns of phase-dependent modulation of cutaneous reflexes in humans. *J Neurophysiol* July 1996;76(1):301–310.
219. Van Duersen R, Flynn T, McCrory J, Morag E. Does a single control mechanism exist for both forward and backward walking? *Posture Gait* May 1, 1998;7(3):214–224.
220. Nadeau S, Amblard B, Mesure S, Bourbonnais D. Head and trunk stabilization strategies during forward and backward walking in healthy adults. *Gait Posture* December 2003;18(3):134–142.
221. Lee D. *The pelvic girdle. An approach to the examination and treatment of the lumbo-pelvic-hip region,* 2nd ed. Edinburgh: Churchill Livingstone, 2000.
222. Janda V. *Muscle function testing.* London: Butterworth, 1983.
223. Vogt L, Pfeifer K, Banzer W. Neuromuscular control of walking with chronic low back pain patients. *Man Ther* February 2003;8(1):21–28.
224. Vogt L, Banzer W. Dynamic testing of the motor stereotype in prone hip extension from the neutral position. *Clin Biomech* March 1997;12(2):122–127.
225. Bullock-Saxton M, Janda V, Bullock M. The influence of ankle sprain injury on muscle activation during hip extension. *Int J Sports Med* August 1994;15(6):330–334.
226. Juker D, McGill S, Kropf P, Steffen T. Quantitative intramuscular myoelectric activity of lumbar portions of psoas and the abdominal wall during a wide variety of tasks. *Med Sci Sports Exerc* February 1998;30(2):301–310.
227. McGill S. *Low back disorders: Evidence-based prevention and rehabilitation.* Champagne, IL: Human Kinetics, 2002.
228. Hicks GE, Fritz JM, Delitto A, Mishock J. Interrater reliability of clinical examination measures for identification of lumbar segmental stability. *Arch Phys Med Rehabil* December 2003;84(12):1858–1864.
229. Moran R, Gibbons P. Intraexaminer and interexaminer reliability for palpation of the cranial rhythmic impulse at the head and sacrum. *J Manipulative Physiol Ther* 2001;24(3):183–190.
230. Nice D, Riddle D, Lamb R, Wayhew T, Rucker K. Intertester reliability of judgements of the presence of trigger points in patients with low back pain. *Arch Phys Med Rehabil* October 1992;73(10):893–898.
231. Lew P, Lewis J, Story I. Inter-rater reliability in locating latent trigger points using palpation. *Man Ther.* May 1997;2(2):87–90.
232. Christenson H, Vach W, Vach K, et al. Palpation of the upper thoracic spine: An observer reliability study. *J Manipulative Physiol Ther* June 2002;25(6):425.
233. Love R, Brodeur R. Inter-and intra-examiner reliability of motion palpation for the thoracolumbar spine. *J Manipulative Physiol Ther* February 1987;10(1):1–4.
234. Mootz R, Keating J, Kontz H, Milus T, Jacobs G. Intra- and interobserver reliability of passive motion of the lumbar spine. *J Manipulative Physiol Ther* December 1989;12(6):440–445.

235. French S, Green S, Forbes A. Reliability of chiropractic methods used to detect manipulable lesions in patients with chronic low-back pain. *J Manipulative Physiol Ther* May 2000;23(4):231–238.
236. O'Haire C, Gibbons P. Inter-examiner and Intra-examiner agreement for assessing sacroiliac anatomical landmarks using palpation and observation: Pilot study. *Man Ther* February 2000;5(1):13–20.
237. Jull G, Bogduk N, Marsland A. The accuracy of manual diagnosis for cervical zygapophysial joint pain syndromes. *Med J Aust* March 7, 1988;148(6):233–236.
238. Gerwin RD, Shannon S, Hong CZ, et al. Interrater reliability in myofascial trigger point examination. *Pain* 1997;69(1/2):65–73.
239. Sciotti VM, Mittak VL, DiMarco L, et al. Clinical precision of myofascial trigger point location in the trapezius muscle. *Pain* 2001;93(3):259–266.
240. Humphreys B, Delaye M, Peterson C. An investigation into the validity of cervical spine motion palpation using subjects with congenital block vertebrae as a 'gold standard'. *BMC Musculoskelet Disord* June 15, 2004;15(1):19.
241. Mior S, McGregor M, Schut B. The role of experience in clinical accuracy. *J Manipulative Physiol Ther* February 1990;13(2):68–71.
242. Panzer D. The reliability of lumbar motion palpation. *J Manipulative Physiol Ther* October 1992;15(8):518–524.
243. Herzog W, Read L, Conway P, Shaw L, McEwen M. Reliability of motion palpation procedures to detect sacroiliac joint fixations. *J Manipulative Physiol Ther* April 1989:12(2):86–92.
244. Chaitow L. *Palpation skills*. Wellingborough, UK: Thorsons/HarperCollins, 1991.
245. Freeman M, Wyke B. The innervation of the ankle joint. An anatomical and histological study in the cat. *Acta Anat (Basel)* 1967;68(3):321–333.
246. Johansson H, Sjolander P, Sojka P. Actions on gamma motoneurons elicited by electrical stimulation of joint afferent fibres in the hind limb of the cat. *J Physiol* June 1986;375:137–152.
247. Grigg P, Hoffman A. Stretch-sensitive afferent neurons in cat knee joint capsule: Sensitivity to axial and compression stresses and strains. *J Neurophysiol* May 1996;75(5):1871–1877.
248. Khalsa P, Hoffman A, Grigg P. Mechanical states encoded by stretch-sensitive neurons in feline joint capsules. *J Neurophysiol* July 1996;76(1):175–187.
249. Mallik AK, Ferrell WR, McDonald AG, Sturrock RD. Impaired proprioceptive acuity at the proximal interphalangeal joint in patients with the hypermobility syndrome. *Br J Rheumatol* 1994;33:631–637.
250. Karaaslan Y, Haznedaroglu S, Ozturk M. Joint hypermobility and primary fibromyalgia. *J Rheumatol* 2000;27:1774–1776.
251. Acasuso-Diaz M, Collantes-Estevez E. Joint hypermobility in patients with fibromyalgia syndrome. *Arthritis Care Res* 1998;11:39–42.
252. Russek LN. Hypermobility syndrome. *Phys Ther* 1999;79(6):591–599.
253. Müller K, Kreutzfeldt A, Schwesig R, et al. *(Hypermobilität und chronischer Rückenschmerz) Manuelle Medizin* 2003;41(2):105–109.
254. Al-Rawi ZS, Adnan J, Al-Aszawi AJ, Al-Chalabi T. Joint mobility among university students in Iraq. *Br J Rheumatol* 1985;24:326–331.
255. Birrell EN, Adebajo AO, Hazleman BL, Silman AJ. High prevalence of joint laxity in West Africans. *Br J Rheumatol* 1994;33:56–59.
256. Bridges AJ, Smith E, Reid J. Joint hypermobility in adults referred to rheumatology clinics. *Ann Rheum Dis* 1992;51:793–796.
257. Bulbena A, Duro J, Porta M, et al. Anxiety disorders in the joint hypermobility syndrome. *Psychiatry Res* January 1993;46(1):59–68.
258. Martin-Santos R, Bulbena A, Porta M, Gago J, Molina L, Duro J. Association between joint hypermobility syndrome and panic disorder. *Am J Psychiarty* November 1998;155(11):1578–1583.
259. Dicke E. *Meine Bindegewebsmassage (My Connective Tissue Massage)*. Stuttgart, 1954.
260. Bischof I, Elmiger G. Connective tissue massage. In: Licht S, ed. *Massage, manipulation and traction*. New Haven, CT: Licht, 1960.
261. Reed B, Held J. Effects of sequential connective tissue massage on autonomic nervous system of middle-aged and elderly adults. *Phys Ther* August 1988;68(8):1231–1234.
262. Adams T, Steinmetz M, Heisey S, Holmes K, Greenman P. Physiologic basis for skin properties in palpatory physical diagnosis. *J Am Osteopath Assoc* February 1982;81(6):366–377.
263. Defalque R. Painful trigger points in surgical scars. *Anesth Analg* June 1982;61(6):518–520.
264. Chikly B. *Lymph drainage therapy study guide level I*. Palm Beach Gardens, FL: UI Publishing, 1996.
265. Braggins S. *Back care: A clinical approach*. Edinburgh: Churchill Livingstone, 2000:116.
266. Upledger J, Vredevoogd W. *Craniosacral therapy*. Seattle, WA: Eastland Press, 1983.
267. Scudds RA, Landry M, Birmingham T, et al. The frequency of referred signs from muscle pressure in normal healthy subjects (abstract). *J Musculoskeletal Pain* 1995;3(Suppl 1):99.
268. Gerwin RD, Dommerholt J. Treatment of myofascial pain syndromes. In: Weiner R, ed. *Pain management; a practical guide for clinicians*. Boca Raton, FL: CRC Press, 2002:235–249.
269. Dommerholt J, Issa T. Differential diagnosis: Myofascial pain syndrome. In: Chaitow L, ed. *Fibromyalgia syndrome: A practitioner's guide to treatment*. Edinburgh: Churchill Livingstone, 2003.
270. Hong C-Z, Torigoe Y. Electrophysiological characteristics of localized twitch responses in responsive taut bands of rabbit skeletal muscle. *J Musculoskeletal Pain* 1994;2:17–43.
271. Hong C-Z. Current research on myofascial trigger points—Pathophysiological studies. *J Musculoskeletal Pain* 1999;7(1/2):121–129.

272. Gerwin RD, Duranleau D. Ultrasound identification of the myofacial trigger point. *Muscle Nerve* 1997;20(6):767–768.
273. Lewis J, Tehan P. A blinded pilot study investigating the use of diagnostic ultrasound for detecting active myofascial trigger points. *Pain* 1999;79(1): 39–44.
274. Russell IJ. Reliability of clinical assessment measures for the classification of myofascial pain syndrome. *J Musculoskeletal Pain* 1999;7(1/2):309–324.
275. Devieger H. The respiratory pump: Past and present understanding. *Acta Paediatr* November 2003;92(11):1245–1247.
276. Hodges P, Gandevia S. Changes in intra-abdominal pressure during postural and respiratory activation of the human diaphragm. *J Appl Physiol* September 2000;89(3):967–976.
277. Hodges P, Gandevia S. Activation of the human diaphragm during a repetitive postural task. *J Physiol* January 1, 2000;522(Pt 1):165–175.
278. Hodges P, Butler J, McKenzie D, Gandevia S. Contraction of the human diaphragm during rapid postural adjustments. *J Physiol* December 1, 1997;505(Pt 2):539–548.
279. Sapsford R, Hodges, Richardson C, Cooper D, Markwell S, Jull G. Co-activation of the abdominal and pelvic floor muscles during voluntary exercises. *Neurourol Urodyn* 2001;20(1):31–42.
280. Shirley D, Hodges P, Eriksson A, Gandevia S. Spinal stiffness changes throughout the respiratory cycle. *J Appl Physiol* October 2003;95(4):1467–1475.
281. Chansirinukor W, Lee M, Latimir J. Contribution of ribcage movement to thoracolumbar posteroanterior stiffness. *J Manipulative Physiol Ther* 2003;26(3):176–183.
282. Travell J, Simons D. Myofascial pain and dysfunction. In: *The Trigger point manual: The lower extremities*, Vol 2. Baltimore, MD: Williams and Wilkins, 1992.
283. Slocumb J. Neurological factors in chronic pelvic pain: Trigger points and the abdominal pelvic pain syndrome. *Am J Obstetr Gynecol* 1984 July 1;149(5):536–543.
284. Weiss J. Pelvic floor myofascial trigger points : Manual therapy for interstitial cystitis and the urgency-frequency syndrome. *J Urol* 2001;166: 2226–2231.
285. Silverstolpe L. A pathological erector spinae reflex—A new sign of mechanical pelvic dysfunction. *Man Med* 1989;4(1):4–28.
286. Gurel H, Atar Gurel S. Dyspareunia, back pain and chronic pelvic pain: The importance of this pain complex in gynecolgical practice and its relation with grandmultiparity and pelvic relaxation. *Gynecol Invest* 1999;48(2):119–122.
287. MacLennan A, Taylor A, Wilson D, Wilson D. The prevalence of pelvic floor disorders and their relationship to gender, age, parity and mode of delivery. *BJOG* December 2000;107(12):1460–1470.
288. Sapsford R, Hodges, Richardson C, Cooper D, Markwell S, Jull G. Co-activation of the abdominal and pelvic floor muscles during voluntary exercises. *Neurourol Urodyn* 2001;20(1):31–42.
289. Critchley D. Instructing pelvic floor contraction facilitates transversus abdominis thickness increase during low-abdominal hollowing. *Physiother Res Int* 2002;7(2):65–75.
290. Pool-Goudzward A, Hock Van Dyjke G, Van Gurp M, Mulder P, Snijders C, Stoeckjart R. Contribution of the pelvic floor muscles to stiffness of the pelvic ring. *Clin Biomech (Bristol, Avon)* July 2003;19(6): 564–571.
291. Bo K, Sherburn M, Allen T. Transabdominal ultrasound measurement of pelvic floor muscle activity when activated directly or via transversus abdominis muscle contraction. *Neurolog Urodyn* 2003;22(6): 582–588.
292. *Gray's anatomy,* 38th edn. Edinburgh: Churchill Livingstone, 1995.
293. Christensen H, Vach W, Manniche C, Haghfelt T, Hartvigsen L, Hollund-Carlsen P. Palpation for muscular tenderness in the anterior chest wall: An observer reliability study. *J Manipulative Physiol Ther* October 2003;26(8):469–475.
294. Billis E, Foster N, Wright C. Reproducibility and repeatability: Errors of three groups of physiotherapists in locating spinal levels by palpation. *Man Ther* November 2003;8(4):223–232.
295. Vacek J, Veverkova M, Janda V, Besvodova V, Dvorakova P. The painful coccyx and its influence on the movement pattern for hip extension. *J Orth Med* 2000;22(2):42–44.
296. Bierma-Ziestra S, Ginai A, Prins A, et al. Meralgia paresthetica is related to degenerative pubic symphysis. *J Rheuatol* September 2000;27(9):2242–2245.

CHAPTER

14

SUBJECTIVE AND OBJECTIVE OUTCOMES ASSESSMENT OF LOW BACK SYNDROMES

Mark S Edinger, Steven G Yeomans, and Alan C Breen

OUTLINE

OBJECTIVES

1. To introduce health care providers to common outcomes assessment tools used with low back pain patients.
2. Discussion of several subjective questionnaires is covered allowing the practitioner to make appropriate decisions regarding choice and utilization of outcomes assessments. This will result in improved delivery and assessment of care to patients.
3. The Quantitative Functional Capacity Evaluation (QFCE) will also be presented, which allows the practitioner to obtain objective outcomes data to support and determine exercise rehabilitation needs of the patient.
4. Case studies are presented throughout this chapter to help the reader understand utilization of outcomes assessment tools in both simple and complicated low back pain presentations.

INTRODUCTION

Previous chapters have addressed the low back in historical, anatomical, and physiological terms. Subsequently, the pathological aspects of low back syndromes were covered in terms of etiology, clinical manifestations, and biopsychosocial sequelae. In an attempt to resolve the complex and critical issue of low back syndromes, various strategies to clinical management, both assessment and treatment, are addressed in this text. One aspect of such management that is growing in importance interestingly supports all the other methods by comparing and supporting their efficacy. This topic can be grouped under the generic heading of outcomes assessment (OA) measures.

WHY HEALTH OUTCOMES ARE MEASURED: PAST AND PRESENT

Like a population census, the measurement of health outcomes is based essentially on need; specifically, the need to communicate between clinicians, to estimate health impacts, to plan services, and to satisfy customers (patients, family, friends, and insurers). In the past, instruments for measuring health outcomes were mainly focused on the elderly and infirm residing in hospitals and care homes, and were mainly targeted at situations where pathological change was at the root of the problem. Inability to care for oneself because of incontinence, spasticity, musculoskeletal trauma, and other pathologies drove the need for outcome measures. In the 1960s and 70s, for example, functional incapacity and independence were measured by instruments such as the Index of Independence of Daily Living and the Barthel Index,[1,2] which were designed mainly to help to determine when hospital discharge or admission were appropriate.

Attitudes to the need to measure health at that time were reflected in the World Health Organization (WHO) definition of health as simply "the absence of disease."[3] This, however, was to change as a result of the need to communicate and plan services in community and practice settings with an increasing variety of clinical specialties. "Health" became defined as "complete mental, physical, and social well-being" and the focus shifted toward general populations and well beyond the traditional biomedical model of "etiology, pathology, and manifestations".[4] In 1980, WHO published a new conceptual scheme in which any intrinsic disturbance was also considered in terms of its linked impairment, disability, and social handicap (Table 14–1).

In search of outcome measures that would provide a more comprehensive assessment of functional status, researchers at the RAND Corporation in California launched "Health Insurance Experiment"

TABLE 14–1. The WHO Conceptual Scheme

Intrinsic situation	Disease or disorder
Situation exteriorized	Impairment
Experience objectified	Disability
Experience socialized	Handicap

1. Managed Care: the Quality Wheel (9)

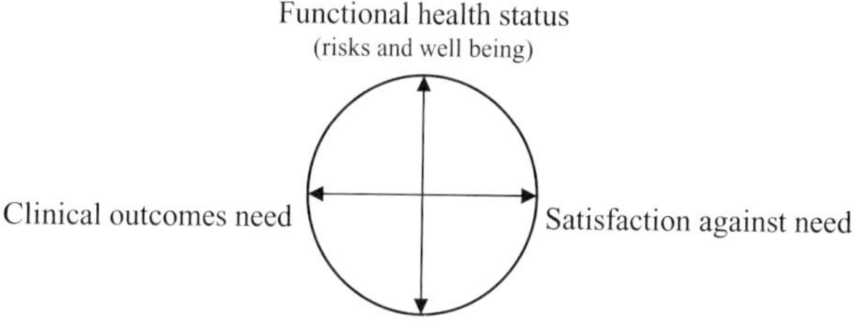

Costs
(direct, indirect, health and social care)

2. Total Quality Improvement (10)

- Listen to the voice of the consumer
- Management by data
- Analysis of the process of care

3. Needs Assessment (11)

- Incidence, Prevalence, Natural history without intervention
- Cost without intervention
- Local culture on importance of: impact, measures, and existing services

4. Health Technology Assessment (12)

- Effectiveness
- Cost
- Broader Societal Impact

FIGURE 14–1. Outcome measures and the organization of care.

in six large US populations. This research identified five basic categories of outcome: (1) self-care activities, (2) mobility, (3) physical activities, (4) role activities, and (5) leisure activities.[5] It coincided with the dawn of the age of "evidence-based practice," where a swell of research into the effectiveness of treatments was being frustrated by the lack of reliable outcome measures. In order to be able to compare the outcomes of different approaches, RAND built on its previous work with the "Medical Outcomes Study" developing a 149-item comprehensive survey instrument (35 scales and 8 summary indices).[6] At a similar point in time Bergner et al. developed a measure of behavioral dysfunction in terms of the patient's perception of the impact of sickness on daily activities and called it the Sickness Impact Profile.[7] These were more rigorously validated for their psychometric properties than most previous instruments. Their key feature was multidimensionality, and some of the instruments, which will be discussed in this chapter, arose from those measures (e.g., Roland–Morris Low Back Disability Questionnaire).

With the proliferation of evidence and its synthesis using the methods of systematic review, outcomes were increasingly being measured against claims of clinical effectiveness, as well as to inform need, and by the time the "guidelines" age dawned in the early 1990s, a major issue in the evidence for effectiveness of a treatment, or the natural course of a condition, was the quality of the instrument by which it was measured.[8] Outcome measures were also in demand for the monitoring required by managed care organizations, measuring total quality improvement, needs assessment, and for health technology assessment[9–12] (see Fig. 14–1).

The scope of outcome measures is as wide as the methods utilized are varied. They encompass the whole range of human experience from biology to the environment. They can be used to describe or predict outcomes, to address impairment, disability, or handicap, with or without interventions, for general or special needs, to assess against a set standard, or to research effects. This chapter will address subjective and objective outcomes for the patient with low back syndrome in the setting of clinical practice. The essential distinction between this usage and that of research is the requirement to fulfill societal expectations rather than meeting the measurement criteria required by a specific research question or design. These expectations are generally for evidence-based practice and accountability for outcomes and not for the practitioner to "do research." Instead, the emphasis is on *basing care decisions on evidence about one's patients and in line with standards of care, which clinicians are expected to meet.* To assist in this process, the authors will suggest criteria for using some common questionnaire instruments, and offer a quantitative functional capacity evaluation (QFCE) that can be used to monitor function, plus options for more specialized assessment and monitoring of patients who are at risk of becoming, or have already become, chronic. For readers who might wish to construct their own questionnaire battery, the authors recommend keeping in mind the following seven factors identified by Deyo et al[13]:

1. Breadth of coverage
2. Validity and reproducibility
3. Responsiveness

4. Practicality (brevity and cost)
5. Compatibility with widely promoted instruments
6. Importance to patient
7. Importance to society

OUTCOMES UTILIZATION IN AN EVIDENCE-BASED PRACTICE

The concept of implementing evidence-based methods into the clinical setting is becoming the standard as many peer-reviewed outcomes assessment (OA) methods now exist and insurers are demanding their use. When considering all the information commonly reported in a clinical record, there is a strong argument for eliminating softer, less useful, qualitative methods in both the subjective and objective areas of clinical practice and adopting harder, evidenced-based methods. By doing so, changes over time can be quantitatively appreciated and plateaus in care easily identified. This leads to prompt critical clinical decision making and thus eliminates wasted time and the associated costs.

The reward of incorporating OA into practice is the benefit that results for all personnel involved in the clinical management of a patient, which includes the provider, insurer, and patient. The provider benefits from having valid, reliable, and practical approaches to be followed on a consistent basis to help guide clinical decision making when designing a treatment plan. This results in an increased level of provider confidence and awareness that the care being rendered is accomplishing a patient-satisfying goal. If not, a change in the treatment plan can be implemented in a timely manner. Similarly, this approach can help to reduce much of the guesswork often encountered when clinical decisions are not clear, such as when managing a chronic, nonresponsive patient. The insurer benefits by being able to follow the progress of a case over time, because the scores of both subjective questionnaires as well as the objective functional tests can be reviewed to determine if "medical necessity" criteria of the treatment approach are being met. This allows for increased confidence by the insurer that both cost-effectiveness and quality assurance controls are in place in the care being rendered. The patient benefits from outcomes management as sometimes slow improvement is not appreciated and reviewing the OA data with the patient confirms their actual progress and therefore to the most appropriate treatment plan. This encounter often includes a discussion of other treatment options and ultimately, increased patient participation and confidence in the chosen method of care. It may also help the patient to establish more realistic goals, should resolution of their condition, despite prior expectations, not be attainable.

In summary, the overall concept of implementing OA into a clinical setting is as follows:

1. Evidence-based subjective and objective measures are used initially and on follow-up.
2. Clinical decisions are more transparently made to continue, modify, or discontinue care in a timely fashion based on the information derived from the tools.
3. Collection and collation of interprovider OA data, including functional improvement, patient satisfaction, cost, and treatment duration, allows for more effective quality control. Furthermore, it simplifies the comparison of the care rendered to what is acknowledged to be "best practice" in similar circumstances.
4. These "best practice" approaches are then shared with the provider groups to enhance provider panel quality

Professional Liability

Another health-care provider benefit of incorporating OA approaches is the malpractice buffer that OA can provide. Specifically, malpractice cases in which OA approaches were employed tend to be more defensible than those without OA. In many cases, demonstrating clearly that appropriate care was rendered can be greatly facilitated by reviewing the results of the different tools utilized. In one specific case reviewed by the lead author, the use of a pain drawing and numerical rating pain scale easily proved that a treatment benefit was achieved in a patient who had filed a suit against a clinician. In addition, the patient satisfaction score regarding the provider's care rendered was high. This particular claim was easily defended, ending without a settlement or even court proceedings. This significantly reduced the costs, shortened the duration of the claim, as well as the psychological discord that these cases typically create. The outlook is often more ominous in cases where outcomes-oriented information is absent and the use of character witnesses dominate the defense's strategy.

OUTCOMES AND THE MANAGEMENT OF THE PATIENT WITH CHRONIC BACK PAIN

Most patients with a first ever episode of back pain of less than 6-weeks duration will recover unassisted from the episode within a month. However, some will persist, proceeding to subacute and chronic stages or to multiple recurrent episodes.[14,15] A plethora of research led to multidisciplinary and international consensus regarding assessment and treatment of acute back pain, which is briefly summarized in Table 14–2.[16] Because the vast majority of back pain

TABLE 14–2. Evidence-Based Assessment and Management of the Patient with Acute Back Pain

Assessment
- Diagnostic triage: serious spinal pathology, nonspecific back pain, root pain
- Psychosocial assessment
- Avoidance of imaging unless pathology suspected

Management of nonspecific back pain
- Information from assessment and reassurance
- Effective pain control: acetaminophen and simple NSAIDs if necessary and at regular intervals preferred, avoiding benzodiazepines and strong opioids
- Avoidance of bedrest
- Maintenance of normal activity and work as much as possible
- Monitoring time course and assessment for:
  - manipulation if not on course to recover by 5–6 wk
  - active overall physical reconditioning exercise if not recovered at 6 wk
  - avoidance of specific back exercises

disability and health-care costs are attributable to those sufferers who have been troubled the longest coupled with the fact that the evaluation of treatments for chronic back pain is methodologically difficult, much of the evidence-based guidance has addressed the resolution of the acute episode to avoid this chronicity.[17]

Given that chronic back pain commonly takes the form of recurring episodes over time, the previous triage category cannot be taken for granted. When applying diagnostic triage, the first, most important element is to rule out serious underlying pathology, commonly referred to as "red flags." For low back pain, there are four major types of disorder that are consistently included in the various guidelines.[18,19]

(a) Cauda equina syndrome
- Subjective
  1. Urinary retention or incontinence
  2. Anal sphincter tone loss/sensation
  3. Sciatica (uni- or bilateral)
  4. Progressive motor/sensory loss
  5. Saddle anesthesia
  6. Nerve root tension signs (sometimes absent)
- Objective
  1. Ortho/neurological physical exam
  2. MRI/CT

(b) Cancer
- Subjective
  1. Older than 50 years old[20]
  2. Past history of cancer[20]
  3. Unexplained weight loss[20]
  4. Pain > 1 month[20]
  5. No improvement with conservative Tx[20]
  6. Low back pain
  7. Positive neurological losses[21]
  8. X-ray: 99% were identified on initial x-ray
  9. Pain at rest/awakens patient at night
- Objective
  1. Special testing (MRI, CT scan, bone scan, ESR, liver function tests, CBC)

(c) Fracture
- Subjective
  1. History of osteoporosis
  2. Mild trauma age > 50 years old
  3. Low back pain > 70 years old
  4. Significant trauma (any age)
  5. Prolonged use of corticosteriods
- Objective
  1. X-ray

(d) Infection
- Subjective
  1. Urinary tract infection history
  2. Skin infection
  3. Respiratory tract infection
  4. Intravenous drug use
  5. Elderly or debilitated patient
- Objective
  1. Vital signs: febrile (>100°)
  2. Blood tests: ESR, CBC with differential
  3. Blood culture
  4. Bone scan

The assessment for these requires the use of case history data as well as examination information. See Chapter 10 for a more detailed discussion of red flags.

Once the prospect of serious pathology is ruled out, diagnostic triage turns to differentiating between mechanical low back pain and nerve root pain. A careful neurological examination along with the assessment of nerve root tension signs will facilitate this.

Chronic back pain is generally a problem of greater complexity. It is also the greatest cause of persistent pain and in some settings, of work loss.[22] Outcomes assessment starts with the acute patient who may not be acute at all, but actually acute recurrent, and detecting hidden chronicity can be done using the Chronic Pain Grade.[23] This is a short (7 item) scale divided into pain intensity and disability items assessed over the previous 6 months. A patient who appears to catastrophize about his or her pain could signal poor prospect of recovery from a single episode. This can be measured and monitored in the longer term with the Back Beliefs Questionnaire.[24] The detection of psychosocial factors, commonly called "yellow flags," suggests the

TABLE 14–3. Psychological Predictors of Poor Outcomes in Back Pain[25]

Outcome	Predictor	Instruments
Chronicity (males only)[26]	Distress/ depression	GHQ-12
Disability/cost[27,28]	Somatization/ depression	MSPQ, Zung, Beck
Disability[29]	Distress	DRAM
	Poor coping	CSQ
	Somatization	MSPQ
	Fear avoidance (possibly)	FABQ
Satisfaction[30]	Depression	Zung, Beck

need to go further to evaluate the risk of chronicity, future disability, and the prospect of high future healthcare costs. Pincus et al. have reviewed the evidence and recommended instruments suitable for assessing these issues (see Table 14–3).[25]

There are several other instruments or OA tools that can help identify patients with yellow flags. For example, the depression screening questions included in the HSQ-12 or -36 as well as the mental health scale and/or emotional scale can be used to determine those patients that should complete a more thorough questionnaire such as the severity index, the New Zealand Questionnaire, the symptom checklist 90-revised (SCL 90-R), the Beck Depression Inventory (BDI), and others.[31–34]

Items under the "Examination" heading and the Waddell Signs are captured by physical examination, while all others are captured by the Severity Index Questionnaire.[35]

Symptoms

1. Duration of symptoms >12 weeks[36,37]
2. Duration of symptoms 4–12 weeks[37]
3. Sciatica[29,36,38–41]
4. Past history of previous episodes of back pain requiring treatment[29,36,38]
5. Severe pain intensity (at 3 weeks, 4 weeks, 6 weeks, 8 weeks)[27,29,42,43]
6. Delaying treatment at least 7 days[39,44]
7. Clinical course (improving, worsening, fluctuating, static)

Examination

8. Positive straight leg raise test[29,45–47]
9. Positive neurological examination (motor, sensory, reflex)[46,48]
10. Positive range of motion (ROM) or orthopedic findings[46,48,49]
11. Lack of centralization of peripheral symptoms with repetitive ROM testing[50]

Psychosocial

12. Three or more Waddell signs of illness behavior[39]
13. Self-rated health as poor[27]
14. Distress[25]
15. Fear-avoidance beliefs (three questions)[13,27,32,51]:
    (a) Belief that physical activity makes pain worse
    (b) Belief that if a person has pain with activity he or she should cease the activity
    (c) Belief that person with pain should not perform normal activities with pain
16. Depression[13,27,32,38,46,51]
17. Poor locus of control (inability of the patient to control pain on their own)[29,32,48,51]
18. Low expectation of recovery[32,51]
19. Blaming others[39]
20. Negative family and/or workplace social situation[39]
21. Increased number of dependent children[48]

Work Related

22. Receiving compensation[39]
23. Litigation[39]
24. Physically demanding job (or perception of)[48,52]
25. Job dissatisfaction[32,38,47,51,53–55]
26. Subjective work-related ability[48]
27. Prior disability in the past 12 months[32,51]

Functional

29. Light work tolerance[32,51]
30. Sleep interruption[32,39,51]

Once a patient is classified as chronic, either by virtue of having continuous pain for more than 3 months or recurrent pain, which interfered with normal activities on at least half of the days of the previous year, it is likely that a major manifestation of his or her condition will be depression.[23] However, of patients who are off work, 60% of them fear going back, 30% believe that normal activity will cause damage (fear-avoidance beliefs), and 20% have some kind of job dissatisfaction.[28] This is consistent with the finding that the longer a patient is off work, the less the chance of ever returning.[22] This includes the risks associated with increased workloads, unemployment, early retirement, multiple pain sites, and the gradual onset of disability.

Given these risk factors for poorer outcomes, the treatments chosen should reflect both the current evidence and the individual needs of patients[56] (Table 14–4). Management strategies can then reflect a

TABLE 14–4. Summary of Evidence for Effectiveness of Treatments for Subacute or Chronic Nonspecific Low Back Pain

	Evidence for	Evidence Against	Evidence of No Effect
Active treatments			
Back schools[57]	++		
Behavioral treatment[58]	++		
Multidisciplinary biopsychosocial rehabilitation[59]	++		
Exercise therapy [60–63]	+		
Physical reconditioning and aerobic exercise[57,60–62]			Conflicting evidence
Passive treatments[62,64–67]			
Massage[68]			+
Acupuncture[69]			+
Lumbar supports[70]			+
Bedrest[62,71]		++	
Antidepressants[62,65,72–74]			++

Note: +, weak; ++, moderate; + + +, strong.

sequence that builds on reassurance and information-giving about the key perpetuators of the problem. This can lead to new understanding and the empowerment of patients to take an active and effective part in their care (Fig. 14–2).

Such care partnerships can be even more effective if discussions about progress are based on identifiable outcomes. Such partnerships may also be with

1. the patient (to promote commitment to long-term change).
2. family and partners (to obtain cooperation in addressing the redefined condition).
3. employers (to obtain agreement to interim activity modification at work).
4. other practitioners (e.g., to report progress, reassess, coordinate physical interventions, and advice)
5. social authorities (to facilitate lifestyle changes and graded independence).

1. Reassure

2. Identify key perpetuators

3. Redefine condition with patient

4. Establish care partnership(s)

5. Initiate active management

6. Monitor

7. Modify

8. Withdraw

FIGURE 14–2. A sequenced management strategy for chronic low back pain.

For chronic patients, it is necessary to *monitor* compliance and progress, perhaps over 1–2 years, readministering the outcome instruments that initially reflected the greatest barriers to recovery. It will always be necessary to *modify* daily activities and exercise intensity as tolerance increases and to reset personal targets to optimize progression. Ultimately, it is necessary to *withdraw* the frequency of assessments once a dependable pattern of improvement and independence has been clearly established. Paradoxically, a successful outcome of management to the chronic pain patient may not be the removal of all pain. Recovery from chronic pain states tends to have more to do with the restoration of self-efficacy, sense of coherence, and the reduction of disability and social handicap than the eradication of specific impairments.[4,75–77] Improvement is also linked to the nature of the presenting problem (Table 14–5).

What emerges from such reviews of the evidence is the need to track change so that the patient and the practitioner can monitor progress. Seen in this light, the quality of the outcome measures used and their relevance to the key clinical problem is important.

TABLE 14–5. Successful Recovery from Chronic Back Pain

	Main Outcome Measure Change		
Main Problem	Pain	Work Disability	Social Handicap
Deconditioning		↓	↓
Proxy pain		↓	↓
Sense of coherence		↓	↓
Overuse	↓		↓
Distress		↓	↓

Key: ↓ = Reduction in each category.

CRITERIA FOR A "GOOD TEST"

In order for the questionnaire or physical performance test to be considered "good," certain criteria must exist. Examples of these criteria include, among others, validity, reliability, responsiveness, practicality, and utility. In general, it is appropriate to use outcome measures that are tested by the criteria presented in the following section instead of those that have not been tested.

Validity

The validity of an instrument is the extent to which it has any systematic error. It is a particularly important concept to consider when choosing a questionnaire, *since its measured validity may only extend to the purpose for which it was originally developed.* Therefore, one must be aware that the same degree of validity reported with the instrument may not apply simply because it is put to a similar, yet unequivalent, use. There are several subcategories for validity.

- *Concurrent validity*: The comparison of two measures completed at the same time. This is of two types:
  i. Convergent, where the score from two measures increase or decrease together. An example of this would occur when a pain rating reduces from 4/10 to 2/10 and the Oswestry Low Back Pain Disability Questionnaire also reduces from 36/100 to 18/100. (These measures will be discussed later in the chapter.)
  ii. Divergent or discriminative, where the score between two or more measures that are totally unrelated to each other do not change together. Good discriminative validity occurs when the two unrelated measures do not correlate with each other. For example, if depression is independent of intelligence, then there should not be a strong correlation between the two.
- *Discriminative validity*: An instrument with good discriminative validity should *not* correlate with another unrelated measure. For example, if anxiety does not correlate with intelligence, then one should not find a strong correlation between the two.[78]
- *Content validity*: The extent to which the measurement incorporates the domain of the entity under study. For example, a tool that measures functional health status should include activities of daily living, occupational, family, and social functioning.
- *Construct validity*: This is assessed by hypothesizing the relationship between the measure and another measure.[56]In other words, are the results of its use those that you would expect, given the theory the questionnaire is based upon? Once this is established, the hypothesized relationship can be tested statistically. For example, if a new disability measure is hypothesized to be relevant for patients with hip disorders, its construct validity can be tested by looking for a positive correlation between the new disability measure and an existing, previously validated measure such as range of motion or isometric strength.
- *Criterion validity*: This refers to the comparison of some type of a gold standard against another measure. However, there are no true gold standards for health status measures because health is a latent (or nonobservable) trait, so health status can never be quantified with certainty. It is preferable, therefore, to try to compare the instrument with a superior measure for each of its constructs. One type of criterion validity that is used is called "predictive validity." Here, the baseline measures are compared to a future event/state (i.e., readmission rates to a hospital) to see if the measure could in fact predict that future event/state.

Reliability

The definition of reliability is "the degree of stability exhibited when a measurement is repeated under identical conditions."[79] There are several subcategories for reliability.

- *Test–retest reliability* refers to score stability, or repeatability over time as long as patients in the sample and the conditions of administering the questionnaire have not changed between tests. The interval between tests is crucial to this assessment: too little and it will suffer from recall bias (i.e., they remember their previous answer); too much and the instrument will actually be measuring change.

- *Intraobserver reliability* is a specific type of test–retest reliability where the degree of repeatability within the same examiner is evaluated.
- *Interobserver reliability* is the repeatability of different observers measuring the exact same phenomenon. This relates to the clinician or observer asking the questions rather than the patient self-administered questionnaires, which would have little effect on the resultant scores.
- *Internal consistency* is a special type of reliability that tests the homogeneity of an instrument. It is important when one particular trait is being measured; therefore, all parts must correlate. For example, it is less important when the instrument is multidimensional, although it would be expected to examine each dimension for internal consistency.

Responsiveness

Responsiveness testing is defined as "the accurate detection of change when it has occurred."[80] If a tool is responsive to that change, a questionnaire score should improve as a patient's health status improves. It is closely related to validity since an instrument may be systematically unable to detect important changes (floor effect) or sensitive to unimportant change (ceiling effect). The measure of responsiveness is the "effect size," of which there are three main types reflecting the difference between baseline and follow-up scores in circumstances similar to those in which the instrument is to be used.[81] An effect size greater than 1 is generally desirable; however, there is debate about what level of change is clinically important.[82]

Response scale: "The response choices (numbers and their definitions) presented to a respondent with which to answer a particular question (e.g., 1 = yes; 2 = no)." This is also linked to "response bias," in which respondents may, for example, tend to answer "yes" to everything, and can be minimized by keeping questions short and avoiding monotony. Likewise, patients may feel threatened and be unwilling to answer yes to psychosocial questions, especially if the questionnaire is completed by interview. Providing the patients the opportunity to complete the questionnaire in private and assuring confidentiality can alleviate this.

Practicality

Practicality is more important for the busy clinician than for the researcher. An outcome tool that is practical is simple to administer, simple to understand, straightforward to score, and easy to interpret. It is also time- and cost-efficient, while meeting other criteria that includes validity, reliability, and responsiveness. Self-administered questionnaires are usually best for the clinical practice setting, where the whole team's enthusiasm and understanding is both necessary and worthy of continuous support and encouragement.

Utility

Utility is the usefulness of a procedure or questionnaire to the degree which it meets the needs of the patient, payer, researcher, practitioner, etc. Outcomes which measure cost containment is meaningful to a payor or purchaser, benefits perceived by patients is useful to outcomes experts, and clinical/health status is meaningful to healthcare providers. If the healthcare provider is to rely on measurements, they must be useful or meaningful. It is then that the practitioner can make decisions about the progress of a patient based on the measure selected.

SUBJECTIVE MEASURES

Outcomes assessment starts with the patient history. An outcomes-oriented history includes entries that are quantitative, that is, tagged with a measurement unit such as time, distance, frequency, and/or repetitions. A history that is only qualitative does not include a measurement unit and therefore is not responsive to change over time. A popular approach of taking a history includes the "O, P, Q, R, S, T" method, which stands for onset, palliative/provocative, quality, radiation, severity, timing, and past history, respectively. Using this method, Table 14–6 offers a comparison between histories taken in a qualitative vs. a quantitative manner.

TABLE 14–6. Quantitative versus Qualitative (Examples)

	Qualitative	Quantitative
O	"Patient presents with LBP"	Acute onset of LBP and below knee (BK) left leg pain 2-4-02 after lifting child
P↑	Sitting ↑ LBP	Sitting >5 min ↑ LBP and left leg pain
P↓	Lying ↓ LBP	Lying ↓ LBP and left leg pain after 30 min; 6× sleep interruption
Q	Both achy and sharp	Achy constant, sharp jabs ~6 × per h (10% awake h)
R	Pain radiates	Pain radiates BK to left lateral ankle/foot constantly
S	Pain is severe	Pain now is 6/10; on average 4/10; ranges 2–8/10
T	AMs are worst	First 2 h of the AM is worst

Note: An outcomes-oriented history is obtained by using a unit of measurement that is responsive to change over time.
(AM = morning hours)

Outcome Tools—An Overview

There are many OA tools that are available when managing patients with low back conditions. Popular tools for measuring a patient's pain perception include the *Visual Analog Scale (intensity)* and the *Pain Diagram (location)*. Functional measurements include both objective quantifiable tests of physical performance such as isolating muscles and/or joints as well as subjective questionnaires to determine the patient's perception of his or her disability or functional capacity.[83–85] Objective outcomes measures include *range of motion, strength, endurance, proprioception,* and *nonorganic signs* (see QFCE discussed later in this chapter). Examples of subjective outcomes tools include *the Oswestry Low Back Pain Disability Questionnaire, Neck Disability Index, Roland–Morris Disability Scale,* and the more recent *Functional Assessment Screening Questionnaire* and *the Bournemouth Questionnaire for both low back pain and neck pain.*[85–88] Work capacity can also be measured in tests that simulate whole body movements typically used in the work place.[89] Examples of functional capacity tests include (but are not limited to) *lifting, carrying, aerobic capacity, static positional tolerance, balancing,* and *hand function.*[90] These OA categories and specific outcomes will be broken down and discussed throughout the chapter. Outcomes-based case studies will be presented, which will help the practitioner understand and implement OA into practice.

Well-being or *quality of life* and how it relates to general health is commonly measured with tools such as the SF-36 questionnaire or the shorter version SF-12.[91,92] *Disability* can be measured in a variety of ways, but most important is the duration of time off work. *Satisfaction* includes measures that assess one's health care or one's job.[93–95] A measurement of satisfaction with care includes the assessment of symptom satisfaction.[31]

Psychosocial status can also be measured through questionnaires that assess fear-avoidance behavior, locus of control, self-efficacy, depression, anxiety, and satisfaction. These factors help predict the course of care and thus have been described as yellow flags.[29,32,38,51,52,96] While red flags require urgent attention, further testing, and possibly specialist referral, yellow flags usually require only a shift in the focus of care. Subjective psychological screening through standard history taking has both low sensitivity and predictive value for identifying distressed patients, thus formal screening of some sort such as with a questionnaire is recommended.[97]

General Health Tools

The use of general health tools (GHTs) in patients with low back pain is less specific then condition-specific tools and hence will only be briefly summarized as more in-depth information can be obtained elsewhere.[31] Generic health outcome measures include but are not limited to global ratings of health status as well as multidimensional measures of health-related quality of life, which include the Sickness Impact Profile (SIP), SF-36 Health Survey, Nottingham Health Profile (NHP), and the Dartmouth COOP Health Charts.[7,91,98,99]

Probably, the most used general health questionnaire is the SF-36, which is used in outcomes-based research, is translated into more than 40 languages as part of the International Quality of Life Assessment (IQOLA), and is used in clinical settings as well.[100] The fact that GHTs or questionnaires are not low back or condition specific is both a strength and a weakness. One of the strengths is that GHTs can be applied to all patients regardless of their presenting condition. This is useful if there are no condition-specific tools for the presenting condition, such as an ingrown toenail. Also, most GHTs include multiple domains or categories of assessment. For example, the SF-36 includes eight subscales or domains including (1) health perception, (2) physical function, (3) role limitations due to physical health, (4) role limitations due to emotional problems, (5) social function, (6) mental health, (7) bodily pain, and (8) energy/fatigue (vitality). A weakness is that GHTs are less responsive to change over time, previously defined as poor test–retest reliability, compared to condition-specific tools.[31] Another important strength of the SF-36 is that normative data exists for both healthy as well as nonhealthy populations. This allows for patient data comparisons to both health as well as nonhealthy patient data as well as against each other. Versions 1.0 and 2.0, published in 1988 and 1996, respectively, are broken down into eight scales where each represents different aspects of general health. By using the eight individual scales, two composite scores are derived from Version 2.0, which include physical health and mental health. The physical component summary (PCS) is made up of the following four scales: physical function, role physical, bodily pain, and general health. The mental health component (MHC) is made up of mental health, role emotional, social function, and vitality. Grouping all 36 questions into two rather than eight scales enhances reliability. The mean score for healthy adult population regarding both scales is 50 ± 10 points (combined), which carries a reliability level of 0.92 and 0.88 for the PCS and the MHC, respectively.

To improve the practicality, ergo broadening the utility, of the SF-36, the abbreviated SF-12 was subsequently introduced.[92] The SF-36 can also be used to form two distinct scales: the physical function and mental health scales. The advantage of the SF-12 over the SF-36 is the brevity of time needed to complete the form (typically 2–5 minutes). Standard and acute versions of the SF-12 and 36 are available in multiple languages.[100]

Measurement of Patients' Severity of Back Pain

The measurement of the severity of low back pain can be very crucial in determining the overall symptom severity as well as subsequent course of care. It is important that the health-care provider uses a valid and reliable scoring scaling method to report the patient's perceived pain. Typically, when evaluating pain using a pain scale, the person who is experiencing pain uses numbers or words to describe their pain intensity. Price states that measurement of pain is equal to assessment of vision, taste, smell, audition. As such the assessment depends on the accuracy of the efforts of the examining/interviewing health-care professional and the person experiencing pain.[101]

Pain Scales

Direct scaling methods of pain measurement can be done with two basic approaches.[102] The first of these two approaches is based on a rating scale method. With this method the patients rate their pain intensity on a scale that is defined by numerical intervals or on a verbal rating scale. The second is a direct scaling method that uses continuous scales and sensation intensity without constraints and categories or numbers. An example of this would be to allow a patient to adjust volume and/or sound where an unlimited number of intensities exist to represent their perceived pain level.

Visual Analogue Scales

A very popular assessment of pain severity in a clinical setting is the use of a visual analogue scale (VAS). The patient is given instructions to rate his or her perceived pain level by placing a mark on a 10 cm line. The 10 cm line is labeled with UNBEARABLE PAIN on the right-hand side of the line and with NO PAIN on the left-hand side. The examiner then overlays a transparent 10-cm ruler on the line and then scores the patient's response on a 0 to 10 scale. For example, 6.5 cm would equal 6.5/10 on a pain scale and so on.

There has been a reported reliability and validity with this approach.[103] There are several distinct advantages of this approach over other measurement methods that have been published and used.[101,104–107] Besides measuring pain severity the VAS can also be used to measure pain sensation intensity as well as pain unpleasantness and/or pain-related emotional disturbances, and has the ability to do each of these separately.[101,105,106,108]

The Quadruple Visual Analogue Scale

Von Korff et al. published this specific application of the VAS in 1992.[23] The quadruple VAS is based on the following factors:

1. Patient's pain level at time of presentation at the office.
2. The average pain since the last visit, or since the onset of the condition.
3. The maximum pain level the patient has experienced since last visit or since date of onset.
4. The lowest the pain level has been or the best pain level the patient has experienced since the onset, or since last patient visit (see Form 14–1 in the Appendix)

If using the quadruple VAS with a patient with chronic pain, it is important that the health-care provider ask the patient what the average pain has been over the last 6 months when first evaluating this pain scale. When analyzing the patient's results, the ratings are averaged and then multiplied by 10 to yield a score from 0 to 100.[23] From this point one can categorize the patient as either "low intensity" (pain graded less than 50) or "high intensity" (pain greater than 50). The use of this type of VAS may help to quantify a patient's improvement during the course of care. It is not uncommon for the patient to present to the office being relatively pain-free at presentation, while experiencing the majority of their pain outside the clinic, be it at home performing average daily activities or at work. Thus, using this tool helps quantify the levels of pain during the course of care. The utilization frequency of this tool can vary, from being used each visit to a minimum of once every 2 weeks to monitor the patient's progress. It has been reported that VAS should be performed every 2 weeks, as a failure to progress over a 2-week period may indicate the need for a change in therapeutic approaches.[109]

Numerical Pain Scale

Another popular pain scale that has been used in a clinical setting is the numerical pain scale (NPS), also known as the numerical rating scale (NRS).[110,111] There are two commonly used measures: the 11-point NPS and the 101-point NPS.

11-Point NPS This OA tool contains 11 numbers (0 to 10); the patient simply circles the appropriate number that represents his or her pain level for the condition from which he or she is suffering. When comparing this method to the VAS, various reports suggest that the NPS is not as reliable as the VAS; however, one study suggests that the VAS and the NPS are comparable.[112] Two other studies suggest that the

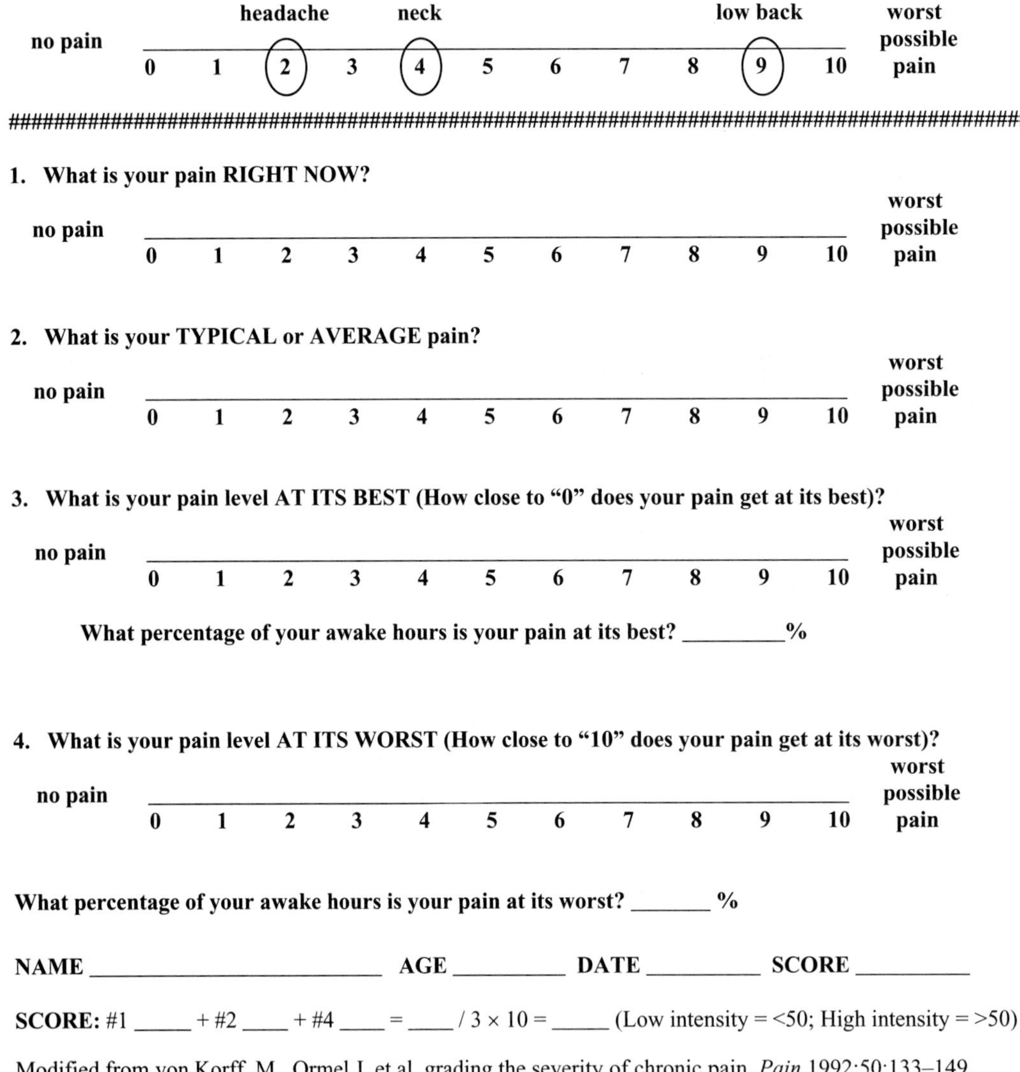

FORM 14–1.

QUADRUPLE VISUAL ANALOGUE SCALE

INSTRUCTIONS: Please circle the number that best describes the question being asked.
NOTE: If you have more than one complaint, please answer each question for each individual complaint and indicate the score is for each complaint. Please indicate your average pain levels and pain at minimum / maximum using the last 3 months as your reference.

EXAMPLE:

			headache		neck					low back		
no pain	0	1	(2)	3	(4)	5	6	7	8	(9)	10	**worst possible pain**

\##

1. What is your pain RIGHT NOW?

no pain	0	1	2	3	4	5	6	7	8	9	10	**worst possible pain**

2. What is your TYPICAL or AVERAGE pain?

no pain	0	1	2	3	4	5	6	7	8	9	10	**worst possible pain**

3. What is your pain level AT ITS BEST (How close to "0" does your pain get at its best)?

no pain	0	1	2	3	4	5	6	7	8	9	10	**worst possible pain**

What percentage of your awake hours is your pain at its best? _________%

4. What is your pain level AT ITS WORST (How close to "10" does your pain get at its worst)?

no pain	0	1	2	3	4	5	6	7	8	9	10	**worst possible pain**

What percentage of your awake hours is your pain at its worst? _______ %

NAME ________________________ **AGE** _________ **DATE** _________ **SCORE** _________

SCORE: #1 _____ + #2 ____ + #4 ____ = ____ / 3 × 10 = _____ (Low intensity = <50; High intensity = >50)

Modified from von Korff, M., Ormel J, et al. grading the severity of chronic pain. *Pain* 1992;50:133–149.

NPS is superior to that of the VAS.[110,113] Bolton and Wilkinson concluded that the ease of use of completing the score on the 11-point NPS involves the method of asking the patient to report their usual pain versus their current pain level and appears to enhance the responsiveness of the measures and thus becomes more representative of the patient's pain experience.[110]

101-Point NPS This OA tool contains 101 numbers (0 to 100); the patient simply circles the appropriate number that represents his or her pain level for the condition from which he or she is suffering. The 101-point NPS was found to be more responsive and sensitive than the 11-point NPS.[114] The ease of utilization makes the NPS a favorable tool in a clinical setting. However, there are arguments that have been presented regarding the patient's ability to memorize prior pain levels that could skew the results. Both the NPS and the VAS are commonly used to track the outcomes of certain treatments in regards to therapy programs and protocols. The Mercy Center Conference quality assurance guidelines state that severe pain intensity greater than 6 on a scale from 0 to 10 is one of four factors that can be used to document that a patient's care may be more complicated than usual. As such, the management of acute low back pain may be appropriate for a longer period of treatment, such as 12–16 weeks as opposed to 6–8 weeks.[109] Thus, utilizing this type of pain severity tool is an important factor in case management, allocating resources and assessing prognosis of an individual case.

In general, numerical scales can affect several different clinical factors, such as psychosocial (i.e., fear of pain, fear of injury, coping) and estimates of returning to work.[87,115]

Measurement of Pain Location Using the Pain Diagram

The pain diagram typically consists of front and back outline of the human body in the anatomical position in which the patient draws, using different symbols for different qualities of pain, such as sharp, ache, pins and needles, numbness, etc. This information helps capture a representation of the patient's verbal pain. The pain diagram can also reveal information in regards to the patient's interpretation of his or her pain as well as mood and/or psychological state. This is helpful in determining whether the patient's pain behavior is appropriate or consistent with the verbal complaint and objective findings.[116]

The pain diagram is primarily a qualitative tool. However, several scoring methods have described pain.[116–120] Unfortunately, none of these popular scoring methods have shown any reliability when measuring psychological distress from a pain drawing.

In summary, the pain diagram is one of the most clinically useful outcomes tools because of its utility and practicality as it allows the health-care provider to quickly triage a patient "at first glance." An illustration of a pain diagram may be found in Chapter 12.

Measurement of Activity Intolerance in Patients with Low Back Pain: Condition- or Region-Specific Questionnaires

There are many condition-specific OA tools that can be used to assess outcomes in patients that present with low back pain. Two very popular tools include the Oswestry Low Back Disability Questionnaire and the Roland–Morris Questionnaire.

Roland–Morris Questionnaire The Roland–Morris Questionnaire is one of the most commonly used tools for measuring spinal disability.[121,122] This questionnaire was developed by shortening the 136-item Sickness Index Profile (SIP). Roland and Morris extracted 24 items, which they felt were relevant to low back pain. It was this version that became the Roland–Morris Questionnaire (RMQ). In 1986, Deyo helped establish the reliability of the RMQ by comparing it to the SIP and its major subscales, which include physical and psychosocial dimension.[123] This study revealed that the RMQ correlated better (.89) than the overall SIP (.85) to the physical dimension. However the RMQ did not compare well with the psychosocial dimension (.59) to the SIP (.88). Reproducibility was shown when studying two groups of patients. The first group had reported no clinical changes and second group stated they had not resumed full activities. Test–retest results showed correlations above .80 for the first group and .76 for the second group. These results showed that the RMQ was comparable and in some cases was a stronger outcomes tool than the SIP. Deyo concluded that the RMQ was as valid as the lengthier SIP.[123] The condition-specific RMQ's advantages over the general health SIP discussed in this study included its brevity (24 vs. 136 items), correlation to physical dimension of the SIP, and less susceptible change to psychosocial function than physical function. *These attributes favor this outcome tool when evaluating the low back pain population. Von Korff referred to the Roland–Morris study as the best single study of assessing short-term outcomes of patients with back pain.*[124]

The RMQ is relatively easy to use in a clinical setting. The patient simply answers yes or no to 24 questions, which refer to the effect of their low back pain on daily activities. To score the RMQ simply add all the yes answers. Each affirmative answer is worth 1 point. When assessing clinical changes with the RMQ, a range of 2.5 to 5 points is considered clinically significant but depends on the initial score. In 1998, Stratford et al. reported the following in regards to clinical significant changes related to the level of initial score[125]:

- If the initial RMQ score showed little disability, 1–2 points would be accepted as change.
- If the initial RMQ score showed high levels of disability, 7–8 points would be indicative of changes.
- Unselected patients = 5 points.

A revised version of the RMQ containing only 18 items has been shown to meet accepted reliability and validity criteria.[126] The sensitivity and specificity was found to be identical to the 24-item questionnaire. Currently there are no validated values to determine the level of the patient's disability based on the RM-18 score alone. As with all outcomes an initial and follow-up questionnaire must be administered to truly become an OA. Because of its validity, in addition to relative brevity, the RM-18 has become a popular measure among clinicians (see Form 14–2).

FORM 14–2.

MODIFIED ROLAND–MORRIS (RM-18) QUESTIONNAIRE

When your back or leg hurts, you may find it difficult to do some of the things you normally do. This list contains some sentences that people have used to describe themselves when they have back pain or sciatica. When you read them, you may find that some stand out because they describe you today. As you read the list, think of yourself **today**. When you read a **sentence that describes you today**, *circle* the letter **"Y"** for **YES**. If the sentence **does not describe you today**, *circle* the letter **"N"** for **NO**.

Y **N** 1. I stay at home most of the time because of my back.

Y **N** 2. I walk more slowly than usual because of my back.

Y **N** 3. Because of my back, I am not doing any of the jobs that I usually do around the house.

Y **N** 4. Because of my back problem, I use a handrail to get upstairs.

Y **N** 5. Because of my back, I lie down to rest more often.

Y **N** 6. Because of my back problem, I have to hold onto something to get out of an easy chair.

Y **N** 7. Because of my back, I try to get other people to do things for me.

Y **N** 8. I get dressed more slowly than usual because of my back.

Y **N** 9. I only stand for short periods of time because of my back.

Y **N** 10. Because of my back problem, I try not to bend or kneel down.

Y **N** 11. I find it difficult to get out of a chair because of my back.

Y **N** 12. My back or leg is painful almost all the time.

Y **N** 13. I find it difficult to turn over in bed because of my back.

Y **N** 14. I have trouble putting on my socks (or stockings) because of my back.

Y **N** 15. I sleep less well because of my back.

Y **N** 16. I avoid heavy jobs around the house because of my back.

Y **N** 17. Because of my back, I am more irritable and bad tempered with people then usual.

Y **N** 18. Because of my back problem, I go upstairs more slowly than usual.

Name____________________________ File # ______________ Score ______________

Signature **X** _________________________ Date **X** ______________ Staff Initials ________

Stratford PW, Binkley JM. Measurement properties pf the RM18: A modified version of the Roland-Roland-Morris Disability Scale. *Spine* 1997;22:2416–2421.

Oswestry Low Back Pain Disability Questionnaire Another OA tool that is popular for assessing low back pain is the Oswestry Low Back Pain Disability Questionnaire.[85] This tool can be quickly completed by the patient and is easy to score. The questionnaire consists of 10 categories with six possible responses per category. The patient marks the response that best fits his or her level of disability for each category. The patient can score from 0 to 5 in each category for a maximum possible score of 50 points. To convert the point value into a percentage take the patients total points and divide by the total points possible and multiply by 100. If a section is omitted, divide the patient's total score by the number of sections completed times five.

Using this scoring format, 100% would represent the highest disability possible, while 0% would represent no apparent disability. In 1994, Erhard et al. stated that a score of 11% is an appropriate cut-off score for practitioners to use when addressing return to work and/or discharge issues for patients with uncomplicated low back pain.[127]

The ability of the Oswestry and the Roland–Morris questionnaires to discriminate between patients without nerve root signs or mechanical low back pain and patients with nerve root signs and confirmed evidence of radiculopathy with electromyography was studied by Leclaire and colleagues in 1997.[128] They concluded that both scales were able to discriminate functional disability and diagnosis between the two groups. A study in 1989 found the RMQ to be more sensitive to functional change with patients with mild disability, while the Oswestry Questionnaire was more sensitive to functional status change with patients with more severe disability.[129] Moderate correlation between the Oswestry and RMQ was revealed in a study of 162 patients with low back pain.[130]

The original version of the Oswestry included a category identified as "sex life." This category was often left blank by responders. A "revised" version was introduced, which replaced this category with "changing degree of pain."[131] This version was more responsive in practice settings and was completed more often than the original 1980 version. In 1999, it was revised again and validated in order to increase its responsiveness further to that of the Roland–Morris Questionnaire, and as an alternative choice for primary care users.[132] In deference to the authors of the original Oswestry Questionnaire, it has been renamed as the Primary Care Low Back Disability Questionniare.

Other Outcome Assessment Tools Used for the Lumbar Spine

In addition to the Roland–Morris and the Oswestry Low Back Disability questionnaires, there are many other low back specific OA tools having strong attributes that can be used. These outcome tools have been validated and one (the NASS) incorporated the Oswestry Low Back Disability Questionnaire into the tool. The following will be briefly described as a more complete description of these OA tools and the tool itself can be found elsewhere[31]:

- The Quebec Pain Disability Scale[133]
- The North American Spine Society (NASS) Instrument[134]
- Curtin Back Screening Questionnaire (CBSQ)[135]
- Activities Discomfort Scale[136]
- Low Back Outcome Score (LBOS) [137]
- Clinical Back Pain Questionnaire (CBPQ) [138]
- Spinal Stenosis Questionnaire[139]
- Bournemouth Questionnaire (low back pain specific)[87,88]

Quebec Back Pain Disability Index This questionnaire is a 20-question self-administered type instrument designed to evaluate functional disability in individuals with back pain.[133] This outcome tool was reported to be reliable, valid, and responsive in a group of 24 patients with back pain. Responsiveness was tested against the Global Index of Change and direct comparison to the SF-36, Oswestry, and Roland–Morris scales was made. Reliability was reported with a test–retest of .92 and the responsiveness to change in disability had a Cronbach's alpha coefficient of .96.

North American Spine Society Instrument The NASS instrument was developed to incorporate several various validated instruments, which included measures of symptoms, functional status, and role-functional. Medical history, comorbidity, and satisfaction are also evaluated in this questionnaire.[134] This version takes approximately 20 minutes to complete and is quite lengthy compared to most of the others.

Curtin Back Screening Questionnaire This outcome tool was developed to be a discriminate screening assessment to help evaluate early recognition of disability and the management of patients who have disabling occupational low back pain.[135] The Curtin Back Screening Questionnaire can be self-administered or completed by an interview.

Activities Discomfort Scale This OA tool has also been reported to be reliable in predicting the outcome in patients with chronic low back pain treated conservatively.[136] The questionnaire consists of 18 activities of daily living that include, but are not limited to, walking, bending, sitting, standing, driving, etc. The patients simply check the column that best describes how that activity affects their low back pain, and the responses are graded on a 0 to 5 point scale. Adding the total points scored and dividing by the total points possible times 100 can generate a percentage. Yellen had previously reported a high internal consistency and ability to differentiate between patients with low back pain and those without.[137]

Low Back Outcome Score In 1992, Greenough and Fraser introduced the low back outcome score (LBOS).[138] This questionnaire gathers information regarding the patient's prior abilities and also tracks both minimal reductions in performance as well as more severe disability. Outcomes from both surgical and nonsurgical patient populations can be tracked with the LBOS. The LBOS uses strictly subjective data

FORM 14–3.

PCLBDQ

Primary Care Low Back Pain Disability Questionnaire

Date .... Code ....

Name .... DOB .... M ☐ F ☐

THIS QUESTIONNAIRE IS DESIGNED TO HELP US TO UNDERSTAND HOW MUCH YOUR LOW BACK/LEG PAIN IS AFFECTING YOUR ABILITY TO MANAGE EVERYDAY ACTIVITIES. PLEASE ANSWER <u>EACH SECTION</u> BY MARKING ONLY THE <u>ONE</u> BOX THAT BEST APPLIES TO YOU <u>TODAY</u>.

SECTION 1 - PAIN INTENSITY

☐ I have no pain.
☐ The pain is mild.
☐ The pain comes and goes and is moderate.
☐ The pain does not vary much and is moderate.
☐ The pain comes and goes and is severe.
☐ The pain does not vary much and is severe.

SECTION 2 - PERSONAL CARE (Washing and Dressing)

☐ I do not get any pain when washing or dressing.
☐ Washing and dressing causes some pain but I do not normally change the way I do it.
☐ Washing and dressing causes some pain and I have to change my way of doing it <u>a little</u>.
☐ Washing and dressing causes some pain and I have to change my way of doing it <u>a lot</u>.
☐ Washing and dressing causes pain and I need help for <u>some</u> of it.
☐ Washing and dressing causes pain and I need help for <u>all</u> of it.

SECTION 3 - LIFTING

☐ I can lift heavy weights without extra pain.
☐ I can lift heavy weights but it causes extra pain.
☐ Pain prevents me from lifting heavy weights from any height.
☐ Pain prevents me from lifting heavy weights off the floor, but I can manage if they are conveniently positioned (e.g. on a table).
☐ Pain prevents me from lifting heavy weights off the floor, but I can manage medium weights if they are conveniently positioned.
☐ I can only lift only very light weights at the most.

SECTION 4 - WALKING

☐ I can walk as fast and as long as I want without getting pain.
☐ Walking fast gives me pain but it <u>does not</u> increase as I go.
☐ Walking fast gives me pain which <u>does</u> increase as I go.
☐ Walking slowly gives me pain but it <u>does not</u> increase as I go.
☐ Walking slowly gives me pain which <u>does</u> increase as I go.
☐ I cannot walk at all because of the pain.

SECTION 5 - SITTING

☐ I can sit in any chair as long as I like without pain.
☐ I can sit in some types of chair as long as I like without getting pain.
☐ I get pain only when I get out of some seats.
☐ I get pain after sitting in most seats.
☐ I get pain soon on sitting in most seats.
☐ Sitting in most seats gives me pain straightaway.

Breen AC, Preutu G. (2000) A Revised Oswestry Disability Index (RODQ2). Proceedings of the 4th International Forum for Primary Care Research on Low Back Pain. Eilat. Israel.

SECTION 6 - STANDING

- ☐ I can stand as long as I like without pain.
- ☐ Standing eventually causes some pain, but it does not increase with time.
- ☐ Standing eventually gives me pain, which I can relieve by shifting my weight.
- ☐ Standing eventually gives me pain, which I cannot relieve by shifting my weight.
- ☐ I get pain soon on standing.
- ☐ I avoid standing because I get pain straight away.

SECTION 7 - SLEEPING

- ☐ I get no pain in bed.
- ☐ I get some pain in bed but it does not disturb my sleep.
- ☐ I get some pain in bed which sometimes disturbs my sleep.
- ☐ I get pain in bed which often disturbs my sleep.
- ☐ I get pain in bed which always disturbs my sleep.
- ☐ Pain prevents me from sleeping at all.

SECTION 8 - SOCIAL LIFE

- ☐ My social life is normal and gives me no pain.
- ☐ My social life is normal but increases the pain.
- ☐ Pain has no significant effect on my social life apart from limiting more energetic activities (e.g. dancing).
- ☐ Pain has restricted my social life and I do not go out very often.
- ☐ Pain has restricted my social life to my home.
- ☐ I have hardly any social life because of the pain.

SECTION 9 - TRAVELLING

- ☐ I get no pain whilst traveling.
- ☐ I get some pain whilst travelling but none of my usual forms of travel make it any worse.
- ☐ I get extra pain whilst travelling but it does not compel me to seek alternative forms of travel.
- ☐ I get extra pain whilst travelling which compels me to seek alternative forms of travel.
- ☐ Pain restricts all forms of travel
- ☐ Pain prevents all forms of travel except that done lying down.

SECTION 10 - CHANGING DEGREE OF PAIN

- ☐ My pain has gone.
- ☐ My pain is rapidly getting better.
- ☐ My pain is slowly getting better.
- ☐ My pain is getting neither better nor worse.
- ☐ My pain is slowly worsening.
- ☐ My pain is rapidly worsening.

Scoring: Each Section is scored 0–5

Total all sections (maximum 50)

Questionnaire % score = Total score/50 × 100

Breen AC, Preutu G. (2000) A Revised Oswestry Disability Index (RODQ2). Proceedings of the 4th International Forum for Primary Care Research on Low Back Pain. Eilat. Israel.

to assess several factors such as pain via the VAS, physical demand characteristics of the employed versus unemployed, and sporting activity levels. Other activities that were evaluated include resting, past treatment frequency, sex life, and analgesia in relationship to low back pain. The 1992 study includes a comparison between the LBOS versus the Oswestry Low Back Disability Questionnaire and the Waddell Disability Index. In a study of nonsurgically treated patients with low back pain, the LBOS compared favorably with the results derived from the Oswestry Questionnaire and the Waddell Disability Index.

Clinical Back Pain Questionnaire Ruta et al. developed the Clinical Back Pain Questionnaire (CBPQ) in 1994.[139] The CBPQ was compared with the SF-36 in a population group with low back pain. They noted that the low back pain sufferers were less healthy than the general population. They also noted improved responsiveness and/or sensitivity to change over time compared to that with the SF-36. The authors go on to report the benefits of using a general health questionnaire, such as an SF-36, along with the CBPQ, as the general health questionnaire helps detect general measures as well as detecting comorbid factors.

Spinal Stenosis Questionnaire The Spinal Stenosis Questionnaire is an 18-item tool that consists of 7 symptom severity scales, 5 physical function scales, and 6 satisfaction scales. This tool has been reported to be reproducible, valid, internally consistent, and responsive to clinical change in geriatric patients who suffer from spinal stenosis both pre- and postsurgery.[140] The score range for the symptom severity scale is 1 to 5, and for the physical function and satisfaction scale, a 1 to 4 score is used. Scoring is completed by calculating the unweighted mean of all answered items. The score from a scale missing more than two items is considered invalid. It must be noted that this questionnaire does not stand by itself, but must be used in conjunction with other existing generic spine-related disability and health status questionnaire instruments. Tested–retested reliability was found to be .82 to .96 and internal consistency was .64 to .92. Responsiveness of this questionnaire was .96 to 1.07.[139]

The Bournemouth Questionnaire Most of the OA tools described thus far are domain specific, that is, they measure one aspect of the patient's presentation. The biopsychosocial model embraces the concept that low back pain crosses multiple domains and because of this it has been necessary to include several questionnaires when assessing the patient with low back pain.[141] Questionnaires that include domains such as pain intensity and activity intolerance are common, but separate questionnaires that address psychometric aspects such as fear-avoidance, depression, anxiety, and poor coping strategies are needed if the patient with low back pain is to be fully assessed. Bolton and Breen designed such a questionnaire that includes multiple domains.[87] This measure's strengths include its brevity (7 items), easy to score, research oriented, acceptable to patients, clinicians, and researchers, and reliability, validity, and responsiveness to clinically significant change. The 7 items of the Bournemouth score include (1) pain intensity, (2) effect of work on pain, (3) effect of pain on social activity, (4) anxiety, (5) depression, (6) ability to carry out normal activity, and (7) pain locus of control (ability to control the pain). Each question is answered on a 0–10 (11 item) NRS, a method previously validated for measuring pain intensity.[81] This type of questionnaire is referred to as "hybrid questionnaire" because it incorporates multiple domains in the same tool.

Validity, reliability, and responsiveness of the Bournemouth Questionnaire (BQ) have been demonstrated. The internal consistency is high (Cronbach's alpha = 0.9) as is the test–retest reliability (Intraclass correlation coefficient = 0.95). The effect size of the instrument is also high (1.29) and is comparable with other established measures. A change in scores greater than 4.5 between administrations are indicative of real change. Statistically significant results between all correlations to other tools utilized in the third phase of the study supporting good construct validity ($P < .05$). The most sensitive to change over time were the pain intensity and physical activity scales of the BQ and its counterpart measures compared to the items associated with cognitive and affective aspects of the back pain experience, which were moderate to weak. For comparison purposes, the initial pretreatment scores ($n = 55$), in percentage terms, were similar between the revised Oswestry Disability Questionnaire (RODQ) and the BQ (43.7% ± 20.0% and 50.3% ± 18.8%, respectively) as were the posttreatment scores (22.3% ± 18.4% and 26.0% ± 20.1%). In phase three, 55 patients (mean age 45.7 ± 12.5 years gender distribution of females 50.9%) with a mean pre- vs. posttreatment time of 32.2 (SD = 14.7) days were studied. Scoring was accomplished by dividing the patient's score by the highest score possible, or 70, multiplied by 100 to yield a percentage.[87]

In summary, the BQ appears to fulfill its goals of being a brief, valid, reliable, responsive instrument that fits the needs of both a busy clinical setting as well as a research center. It is unique in that it includes seven domains rather than a singular domain such as activity intolerance or pain intensity. Also, it includes psychometric issues. It therefore embraces the biopsychosocial model of back pain, a trend in current literature and back pain guidelines, while moving away from the disease or injury model[141,142] (see Form 14–4).

FORM 14–4.

The Bournemouth Questionnaire

NAME ______________________ DATE __________ AGE _______

The following scales have been designed to find out about your back pain and how it is affecting you. Please answer ALL the scales by circling ONE number on EACH scale that best describes how you feel:

1. Over the past week, on average, how would you rate your back pain?
   No pain ... Worst pain possible
   0 1 2 3 4 5 6 7 8 9 10

2. Over the past week, how much has your back pain interfered with your daily activities (housework, washing, dressing, walking, climbing stairs, getting in/out of bed/chair)?
   No interference ... Unable to carry out activity
   0 1 2 3 4 5 6 7 8 9 10

3. Over the past week, how much has your back pain interfered with your ability to take part in recreational, social, and family activities?
   No interference ... Unable to carry out activity
   0 1 2 3 4 5 6 7 8 9 10

4. Over the past week, how anxious (tense, uptight, irritable, difficulty in concentrating/relaxing) have your been feeling?
   Not at all anxious ... Extremely anxious
   0 1 2 3 4 5 6 7 8 9 10

5. Over the past week, how depressed (down-in-the-dumps, sad, in low spirits, pessimistic, unhappy) have you been feeling?
   Not at all depressed ... Extremely depressed
   0 1 2 3 4 5 6 7 8 9 10

6. Over the past week, how have you felt your work (both inside and outside the home) has affected (or would affect) your back pain?
   Have made it no worse ... Have made it much worse
   0 1 2 3 4 5 6 7 8 9 10

7. Over the past week, how much have you been able to control (reduce/help) your back pain on your own?
   Completely control it ... No control whatsoever
   0 1 2 3 4 5 6 7 8 9 10

Bolton JE, Breen AC. The Bournemouth Questionnaire: A short-form comprehensive outcome measure. I. Psychometric properties in back pain patients. *J Manipulative Physiol Ther* 1999;22:503–510

Measurement of Patient Satisfaction in Patients with Low Back Pain

The Patient Satisfaction Subscales Tracking patient satisfaction is perhaps one of the most important issues in assessing quality control of an individual practitioner, a specific office visit, and/or the practice environment. To address this issue, a study was performed involving 305 patients with mechanical low back pain, from a primary care clinic, to develop the patient satisfaction subscales (PSS).[143] From a total of 17 items, 10 reflect three distinct dimensions of care: information (3 items), caring (4 items), and effectiveness of treatment (3 items). The other 7 items address biographical information and other nonoutcomes-oriented information and therefore are not included in the scoring method. Each item in the PSS is scored on a response scale of 1 = strongly agree to a 5 = strongly disagree. Each of the three subscales are scored by calculating the unweighted mean of the items in each subscale and an overall, total scale score is obtained by adding the numerical value of the 10 subscale items (maximum score possible is 5 × 10 or 50).

Hudak discussed a multidimensional approach to assess patient satisfaction in patients with low back pain. Comparing the subscale scores with other items associated with patient satisfaction tested construct validity. The PSS was specifically recommended for use in outpatient settings because of its practicality of being short (10 items) and easy to score.[144]

Symptom Satisfaction A simple way of determining patient satisfaction is to ask just one question, "If you had to spend the rest of your life with your condition as it is right now, how would you feel about it?" In a sample of 219 patients where 82% presented for their first low back pain episode of less than 3 weeks from onset, Cherkin et al. asked this question and reported the following: at 1 week, one third were satisfied; at 3 weeks, one half were satisfied; at 7 weeks, two thirds were satisfied, and at 1 year, 85% were satisfied.[38] This one question, which uses a 0 to 10 scale anchored by the descriptors 0 = "delighted" and 10 = "terrible," can accurately give the health-care provider an index of satisfaction with high reliability and validity, not to mention the great practicality of accomplishing this through one question.

Workplace Specific Satisfaction Another method of obtaining information about satisfaction in patients with low back pain includes the assessment of satisfaction in the workplace. The 7-item tool called the modified Work APGAR was derived initially from the 6-item family APGAR.[95,145,146] Additional modifications were based on findings from the retrospective analysis of the Boeing company work force where two additional questions were added for this study increasing the total number of questions to seven.[95,147] A scoring formula includes the following: patient score/total possible × 100% = % risk. The response choices include "almost always," "some of the time," and "hardly ever" for which points are assigned at 0, 1, and 2, respectively. A score of 0 represents no risk, while a maximum score of 14 (7 × 2 = 14; divided by the highest score possible (for example, 14) equals 1. The 1 is then multiplied by 100% to equal 100%, which represents the highest risk possible.

When to Use Outcomes During the Course of Care

Table 14–7 represents the use of several outcomes tools that extend beyond the low back and pain scales discussed in this chapter. Information on the different categories has been briefly discussed previously in this

TABLE 14–7. Clinical Application of Outcomes Assessment

Test	First Visit	Each Office Visit	Reexam 2–4/wk	Exacerbations	End of Care	6 mo Postdischarge*
Pain Questionnaires	√		√	√	√	√
Pain drawing	a		a	a	a	a
VAS (QVAS)	b		b	b	b	b
NPS	c	√	c	c	c	c
General Health	√		Case specific		√	√
SF/HSQ-36 or 12	a				a	a
COOP	b				b	b
Condition-Specific	√		√	√	√	√
Oswestry LBPQ	a		a	a	a	a
Bournmouth Questionnaire	b		b	b	b	b
Roland–Morris	c		c	c	c	c
Patient Satisfaction			√		√	√
Chiro. Satisfaction			a		a	a
Visit-specific questionnaire			b		b	
Patient satisfaction questionnaire			c		c	b
Psychometric			Possibly		Possibly	
Waddell's			a		a	
SCL-90-R, Beck Depression Inventory			b		b	
Total	3	1	3 or 4	2	4 or 5	1 to 4*

Note: Options a, b, or c can be used for the main category listed (given in italics). It is necessary to stay with the original choice for follow-up evaluations, as the instruments are not interchangeable.

*To determine the long-term benefits of the treatment rendered, follow-up at a 6-month point is suggested.

chapter and a more complete discussion can be found elsewhere.[31]

INTERPRETATION OF DIFFERENT CASE OUTCOMES WITH THE USE OF SUBJECTIVE OUTCOME ASSESSMENT TOOLS

Case 1

A 42-year-old male presents with a chief complaint of localized low back pain without radiation to the lower extremities following a lifting injury that took place at his place of employment the previous day. The patient's present history and past history were collected, which revealed more than four previous episodes of low back pain, poor self-rated health, and a heavy job classification. Subjective OA tools included the use of the Oswestry Low Back Disability Questionnaire where the patient scored a 45% (0–100% scale). The patient rated his pain on the NPS at 7/10 "right now," 6/10 "on average," 5/10 "at best," and 9/10 "at worst."

Physical examination findings included the following: Observation revealed an antalgic gait pattern, poor proprioception, and elevation of the right hemipelvis and left shoulder. Moderate muscle hypertonicity of the lumbar paraspinal muscles and tenderness of L3–L5 facets were noted on palpation. Joint dysfunction in the lumbar and pelvic region was documented. Lumbar range of motion revealed limitations in both flexion and extension with pain at end range without peripheralization of symptoms (extension pain intensity was greater than flexion). Orthopedic tests performed included double leg-raise test that provoked low back pain without radiation with pain graded at 7/10 bilaterally (0 = no pain, 10 = extreme). Straight leg raise was limited by hamstring tension and failed to reproduce nerve root tension signs, measured at 47/54 degrees (left/right, respectively). Yeoman's hip extension test provoked low back pain without radiation. Neurological findings were symmetrically normal for muscle strength, reflexes, and sensation for the L4–S1 nerve roots. The initial diagnosis of acute lumbar sprain/strain with associated joint dysfunction and myofascial pain was made.

The treatment plan included spinal manipulative therapy of the lumbopelvic region with the objectives of improving mobility and reducing segmental fixation at a frequency of three times a week for a period of 2–4 weeks. Interferential electrical therapy was used to decrease inflammation and pain. Neuromuscular reeducation techniques to improve proprioception and gait pattern were introduced as tolerable. The patient was given instructions on home icing and was placed on light duty work restrictions. William's low back flexion exercises were issued 1 week into care. On the date of the first reexamination (2 weeks after the initial visit), the patient completed the Oswestry Low Back Disability Questionnaire, which was scored at 10%. NPS ratings were 1/10 "right now," 3/10 "on average," 1/10 "at best," and 6/10 "at worst," (0 = no pain, 10 = unbearable pain). Physical examination revealed improvement in range of motion and decreased provocative tests; however, limitation in range of motion and joint dysfunction were still present. Pelvic stabilization exercises were given after static back endurance testing revealed a 48%, or normal function, without provocation of symptoms. The patient returned to work at full duty 2 weeks after the injury and the frequency of care was decreased. On the third reexamination, the patient completed an Oswestry Low Back Disability Questionnaire and scored 0%. Pain was rated at 0/10 "right now," 1/10 "on average," 2/10 "at worst," and 0/10 "at best" on the NPS. Physical examination findings revealed normal range of motion without pain or hesitation. Orthopedic tests all failed to provoke any symptoms. The static back endurance test scored 89% of the normal function. The patient was rescheduled for a follow-up examination 3 weeks later and findings were 0/10 on the QVAS and 0% on the Oswestry Low Back Disability Questionnaire as well as normal physical examination findings. Assessment at that time was that the patient was at maximum therapeutic improvement and was discharged from care with instructions to continue home exercise protocols indefinitely.

In this case, the Oswestry Low Back Disability Questionnaire and NPS clearly indicate improvement during the course of care that was consistent with physical examination findings, which makes interpretation of subjective outcomes very easy. This quantitative approach of documentation during the course of care is beneficial for establishing "medical necessity" for patient, clinician, and third party reviewer for the care rendered as outcomes clearly identified need for treatment and exercise protocols as well as improvement with the approach used.

Case 2

A 22-year-old male presented with the chief complaint of low back and right leg pain. Patient's history was collected and the patient stated that his pain developed as a result of moving heavy furniture up a flight of stairs to his apartment. He stated he had sharp pain that "shot" down the right leg as well as numbness in the foot, affecting the first and second toes. He stated that his back and leg symptoms were provoked by coughing, sneezing, and straining ("Dejerine's triad"). Patient denied any changes in bowel and bladder function. He rated his pain at the time of presentation as a 9/10, "on average" 9/10, "at best" 9/10, and "at worst" 10/10. A RMQ was used and the patient scored 10 out of a possible 18. A pain drawing was utilized and revealed excessive use of pain descriptions, which were not necessarily consistent with that of his chief complaint, suggesting possible psychosocial or pain behavior issues. The past history revealed that the patient had received treatment for prior episodes of low back pain consisting of manipulation, modalities, and exercises. He had received treatment for sporadic episodes since high school for low back pain; however, he denied any history of leg pain. Physical examination revealed point tenderness at the level of L4–L5 of the lumbar spine. Joint dysfunction in the lumbar spine was noted with vertebral palpation and a decrease in flexion and extension movements of the lumbar spine was noted. Centralization of peripheral symptoms with lumbar spine extension was noted and peripheralization of his leg pain to the ankle was observed with lumbar spine flexion. The patient was resistant to the idea of flexing forward or sitting during the examination, suggesting fear-avoidance. Orthopedic testing revealed a positive supine straight leg raise test when performed on the right provoking sharp pain to the ankle at 42 degrees. Well leg raise provoked right lower extremity symptoms and increased low back pain at 55 degrees. Lasegue straight leg raise supported a diagnosis of radiculopathy in the right lower extremity. Neurological assessment revealed decreased sensation over the L5 dermatome and weakness was noted in the tibialis anterior (mild or 4/5 weakness was noted with foot dorsiflexion with resistance). Reflexes were equal bilaterally at 2/5 for L4–S1. The diagnosis was that of a lumbar intervertebral disc syndrome with L5 radiculopathy to the right lower extremity. Waddell nonorganic low back pain signs were scored at 3/5 suggesting pain behavior. Treatment consisted of manipulative therapy to improve joint mobility and ultrasound therapy in order to decrease myofascial pain and inflammation as well as increase blood flow. Extension-based exercises were given to the patient, both in the clinic and at home, at the onset of care because of the centralization of symptoms in extension vs. flexion. Two weeks into care the patient rated his pain on a NPS as a 4/10, on "average" 4/10, at "worst" 6/10, at "best" 1/10 (0 = no pain, 10 = unbearable pain). Centralization of leg pain was also noted with a reduction in frequency of radicular symptoms. The RMQ was given to fill out and the patient scored 15 out of a possible 18. The pain drawing continued to be consistent with that of his chief complaint. Physical exam findings revealed continued nerve root tension signs provoked at approximately 56 degrees. Lumbar range of motion had improved and no sensory deficits were noted. Continued tibialis anterior weakness was noted at 4+/5 muscle grade weakness.

Review of OA tools revealed a worsening of the RMQ score despite improvement in the NPS and improvement of objective findings. An inconsistency between OA measures and examination findings always requires further investigation by the clinician. Upon questioning, the patient admitted that his excruciating pain and the voluminous amount of paperwork caused him to hurry and inaccurately complete the initial RMQ. This admission was immediately logged into the patient's chart and he was then instructed to fill out another RM-18 Questionnaire based on how he felt during his initial presentation. *This type of retesting, using the same type of questionnaire, retrospectively, has been studied and found to be valid for as long as 3-months postinitial presentation.*[86,148] After the patient again completed the RM-18 based on his initial presentation, he scored a 17 out of a possible 18. In this case, because of the patient's pain, frustration, or poor attention span when initially completing the questionnaire, a misrepresentation of the patient's disability level resulted. By readministering the OA tool, asking the patient to complete the questionnaire a second time, as if it was the initial presentation, the increased effort on the part of the patient allowed for a more accurate representation of the true outcome over this time interval.

Case 3

A 63-year-old female presents with the chief complaint of pain in the right hip pain, aching into both buttocks. The patient stated the pain began after gardening for 2 hours roughly 3 weeks prior to the initial visit. She initially rated her pain on the QVAS as a 6/10, "on average" 4/10, "at worst" 9/10, and "at best" 3/10. The Bournmouth Questionnaire was filled out and the patient scored 39%. The pain drawing was consistent with the chief complaint. Past history and review of systems were unremarkable except for depression, which was clinically diagnosed and was being managed with prescription medication after the loss of her husband 2 years earlier. An SF-12 General Health Questionnaire was used and revealed scores below the mean for physical function, bodily pain, social functioning, and mental health. Physical examination revealed a provocation of right sacroiliac pain with Yeoman's hip extension test, and Gaenslen's test provoked low back and right sacroiliac region pain. Hip range of motion was normal and without pain. Lumbar range of motion was limited in right lateral flexion and extension with pain noted throughout movement. Joint dysfunction of the pelvis was observed with static palpation of the sacroiliac joint as well as abnormal findings with Gillet's motion palpation test. Standing x-rays suggested a left leg length deficiency with elevation of the right hemipelvis and mild spondylosis in the lumbar spine and right sacroiliac joint. The patient was diagnosed as having a right sacroiliac sprain/strain (grade 1) with osteoarthritis and associated joint dysfunction of the right sacroilliac joint. The patient received manipulation of the sacroiliac joint and reported gradual improvement through the initial 2 weeks of care. The patient was scheduled for reexamination on the second week of care when she stated that she had reinjured her low back the night before while working in her garden and her pain was now worse than when she initially presented (pain at that time was graded at a 9/10 on the NPS). The Bournmouth Questionnaire was used and the patient scored 62%. Lumbar range of motion was limited by localized pain in flexion, extension, and right lateral flexion, all provoking right sacroiliac joint pain. Lower extremity neurological functions were within normal limits. An exacerbation of right sacroiliac joint sprain/strain was reported. Electrical stimulation (interferential current) was added to the treatment plan to aid in modulating pain and decreasing inflammation. Frequency of care continued at three times per week for 2 weeks.

In the above case the patient suffered an exacerbation prior to the reexamination. Based on patient's exacerbation one day before the examination, one would believe that this patient had been worsening throughout the course of care, if only the physical examination portion and OA tools were reviewed. In cases such as this, where exacerbations occur shortly before a formal reexamination, it is recommended to have the patient fill out the previously used outcomes tools based on how the patient felt prior to the exacerbation. This may help substantiate that the patient was improving with the course of care rendered up until the point of exacerbation. In this case the patient was given the Bournmouth Questionnaire, VAS, and a pain drawing to fill out *on the basis of how she felt prior to the exacerbation*. In this case the patient scored a 13% on the Bournmouth Questionnaire and rated the VAS with a 1/10, "on average" 2/10, "at best" 0/10, and "at worst" 4/10. Utilizing pain scales such as a VAS or NPS as frequent as each visit is acceptable and would enable the health-care provider to monitor the patient's pain levels more closely. In this case such an approach would have confirmed subjective improvements during the visits leading up to the exacerbation.

OBJECTIVE MEASURES

There is a balance in documentation that must be maintained between reporting subjective and objective data. That is, when there are little to no objective findings reported to support ongoing subjective complaints, "medical necessity" for treatment is usually, and appropriately, challenged. Also, when charting a patient's progress, a strong case can be made for measuring a wider spectrum of health outcomes than just pain, as disability, activities of daily living intolerance, and other subjective or patient-generated information are vital to present a complete clinical picture. Probably the biggest challenge for the health-care provider is finding objective testing measures that are sensitive enough to support ongoing complaints after the initial 4–6 weeks of management, since most nociception or pain-generating tissue damage is controlled in that time frame. The classic physical examination approach used in patients presenting with neuromusculoskeletal conditions are based to a significant degree on pain provocation. This makes sense in the acute stage of a condition but as time passes and healing occurs, pain typically dissipates and other dysesthesias occur. Therefore the same tests used initially may not be supportive of ongoing complaints for those who are not satisfied with their progress after the acute stage. *Hence, there is a need for a different focus, away from tests that measure pain provocation to tests that measure loss of function.* In the biopsychosocial model, transitioning patients from passive to active care in a timely manner is the expectation and objective outcome measures are required to support the necessity for active care protocols to restore locomotor system function.

There are objective OA tools that are very helpful in providing information for disability evaluations, general physical abilities, as well as in identifying specific functional deficiencies to help develop a specific rehabilitation approach. Physical performance tests measure an individual's strength, endurance, aerobic capacity, coordination, as well as fear-avoidance (psychometric factors). Physical performance tests make up a system of testing called the Quantitative Functional Capacity Evaluation (QFCE), which includes the following:

- Strength and endurance (eight tests)
- Muscle length (six tests)
- Waddell nonorganic signs (five signs)
- Range of motion of the cervical and lumbar spine
- Aerobic function
- Proprioception

The tests that make up the QFCE have been previously validated (see specific references in the section where each test is described), and are reliable, practical, safe, and responsive to change over time. To date, the instrument as a whole has not been validated. Each test is supported by normative data and is performed using a low tech, low cost approach, making it a very user-friendly evaluation in a clinical setting. It is important that the tests be performed as described to assure valid and reliable results. More specifically, Ekstrand et al. observed that after using the tests for 2 months there was a CV (coefficient of variation) improvement from 7.5 ± 2.9 to 1.9 ± 0.7. He also stated that paying attention and detail to inclinometer placement, stiffening of the exam table, proper identification of anatomical landmarks, and the use of a standardized exam bench height were important.[149]

The Quantitative Functional Capacity Evaluation

Test 1: The Visual Analogue Scale The examiner has the patient evaluate the perception of his or her pain on a scale from 0 to 10, in which 10 equals unbearable pain and 0 equals no pain. This is done at both the beginning and the ending of the QFCE. Specifically, the patient is given instructions to answer by giving a pain level perceived as "right now." The examiner then overlays a transparent 10-cm ruler on the line and then scores the patient's response on a 0 to 10 scale. For example, 6.5 cm would equal 6.5/10 on a pain scale and so on.

Example: Pretest VAS

Please place a mark through the line below that most accurately represents the pain level that you are feeling *RIGHT NOW*. Please note that UNBEARABLE PAIN is located on the right-hand side of the line and NO PAIN is located on the left side.

No Pain ______________________________ Unbearable

Test 2: Three-Minute Step Test This test is performed to help determine the patient's cardiovascular state. The evaluator first asks the patient to sit while the radial pulse is taken for a full 1 minute. The patient is then asked to step up and down off a 12 in bench at a rate of 24 steps per minute for 3 minutes. A metronome at 96 beats per minute can be used to keep the patient on pace with the "up, up, down, down." After the patient has completed 3 minutes, the patient is then asked to sit and the practitioner then evaluates the radial pulse for a full 1 minute. Normative data is categorized based on male, female, and age group. (This test was adapted from the YMCA's *Y's Way of physical fitness* with permission from the YMCA of the USA, 101 North Wacker Drive, Chicago, IL 60606.)

Test 3: Lumbar Spine Range of Motion Lumbar range of motion helps the practitioner assess both articular structures and the muscle component of the lumbar spine.[31,149] Flexion and extension motion of the lumbar spine is assessed in the sagittal plane. The practitioner starts by centering one of the inclinometers at the T12 spinous process and placing the second inclinometer over the sacral base. The patient then flexes and extends noting the starting and end points on each inclinometer. To evaluate lateral flexion the practitioner then places the inclinometer horizontally at the bony landmarks so that the needle hangs freely to assess lateral flexion or frontal plane motion. True lumbar range of motion is then determined by taking the difference between the two inclinometer end points of movement, i.e., T12 minus S2 equals X degrees. A minimum of three consecutive readings must be taken and the three individual readings must fall within 10% of the average or 5 degrees of the average. The highest of the three readings is then recorded. This procedure may be repeated up to a maximum of six times in attempt to achieve consecutive readings within the 5 degrees, 10% rule in regards to maintaining a valid range of motion.[150] For normative data of the lumbar spine see Table 14–8.[151,152]

TABLE 14–8. Normative Data for Lumbar Range of Motion

Motion	Mean and SD*	Percent of Normal†
True flexion	58 ± 9.6	89.2 (65°)
True extension	22 ± 9.7	72.7 (30°)
Pelvic flexion	60 ± 13.8	109.1 (55°)
Straight leg raise		
Right	77 ± 12.5	102.9 (75°)
Left	77 ± 12.0	102.9 (75°)
Right lateral flexion	24 ± 7.4	96.9 (25°)
Left lateral flexion	25 ± 8.2	100.6 (25°)

*Data taken of 160 male railroad workers. Average age 35 (±8) years, average height 70 (±3) in, and average weight 187 (±29) lbs.[150]

†Values in parentheses indicate the normal range of lumbar motion.

Modified from Mayer et al.[151]

Waddell NonOrganic Low Back Pain Signs These nonorganic low back pain signs are measures for evaluating psychosocial issues that can be considered abnormal.[153] These tests are performed in an attempt to determine if patient may have pain behaviors. The purpose of the test is not to attempt to provoke pain, which is the opposite of typical orthopedic tests in which pain production is the goal of the test. These tests are reported as either positive or negative. There are five categories of nonorganic low back pain tests (see Table 14–9). The evaluator should determine if there is a psychological or organic explanation for the response and repeat the tests as many times as needed in order to determine evaluator objectivity. A final score is given based on the total number of positive signs out of the five categories. If three or more of the five categories are positive, nonorganic low back pain should be considered and thus, psychosocial issues should be addressed.

Test 4: (Waddell NonOrganic Back Pain Sign 1) The first Waddell test is called tenderness, which consists of two tests for both superficial and deep pain tenderness. Superficial tenderness is evaluated by applying very light touch over the lumbar skin in a manner that normally does not provoke pain. A nonorganic

TABLE 14–9. **Waddell's Low Back Pain Signs**

Signs	Examination Method	Reporting
1. Tenderness		
Superficial	Light pressure to skin	+ or −
Deep	Nonanatomical, widespread pain	+ or −
2. Simulation		
Axial compression	Light downward pressure on calvarium	+ or −
Trunk rotation	Minimal twisting of the pelvis without excess shoulder rotation	+ or −
3. Distraction	Sitting (distracted) SLR is nonpainful verses the nondistracted supine SLR	+ or −
4. Regional neurology		
Motor	Nonanatomical or inconsistent findings during a routine neurological exam	+ or −
Sensory	Nonanatomical or inconsistent findings during a routine neurological exam	+ or −
5. Exaggeration	Noted at any time during the physical examination	+ or −

pain response would be positive if there was a disproportionate or exaggerated reaction to this nonnoxious stimulus. Examples would be that of a positive jump sign or withdrawal by the patient. Deep tenderness, which is the second component of this test, is characterized by a nonanatomical area of pain that is not localized to one anatomical region.[153]

Test 5: (Waddell NonOrganic Back Pain Sign 2) This sign is called simulation and is the second of the Waddell signs. The results comprise two tests, which include axial compression and trunk rotation. While the patient is standing, axial compression is performed by placing pressure on the top of the head in the direction of the floor. It should be noted that the compression should not be great enough to provoke a pain response. If the patient reacts with exaggerated low back pain, a positive response would be observed. Any neck pain that occurs with axial loading is not considered a positive test for simulation. If the patient has a neck condition this test may be contraindicated, as described by Waddell in the original article.[153] This test can then be modified by performing pressure over the shoulders in a downward vector. Applying mild pressure should not normally provoke pain.

The second component of the simulation test consists of trunk rotation. During this test the patient is again standing while the health-care evaluator grasps onto the patient's wrists, pressing them against the hips and pelvis, and then manually rotates the trunk in a manner that should normally not provoke any pain. Again, if exaggerated pain is observed in the low back area, a positive test is documented. If a lumbar nerve root condition is present this test may be contraindicated, as a false positive response may occur. Thus, orthopedic and neurological exams should also be performed to correlate if one is to proceed with this test[153](for more information see Ref. 153). The remaining Waddell nonorganic low back pain sign tests will be discussed later in the QFCE evaluation.

Test 6: Horizontal Side Bridge This test is helpful in determining overall strength of the pelvic core stabilizing musculature. The patient lies in a left side lying position, knees extended with the upper (right) leg in front of the lower (left) leg, while resting on the lower (left) hip/thigh and left elbow/forearm. The upper (right) arm is placed against the chest with the hand touching the anterior lower (left) shoulder. The pelvis is then raised off the table or floor and held in line with the long axis of the body supporting the weight between the feet and the elbow/forearm. The patient is then asked to hold this position for as long as possible. The practitioner then notes the duration/time of the hold. This is repeated on the opposite side. Normative data is broken down for men and women (see Table 14–10).[154]

Test 7: Gastrocnemius/Ankle Dorsiflexion Test The ability to assess the gastroc and soleus (see test 8 given below) length is important, as these muscles play an important role in balance and coordination in relationship to the kinetic chain. The patient is instructed to stand upright with feet standing apart and knees straight.[149] To measure the length of the gastrocnemius muscle, the

TABLE 14–10. **Normative Data for the Horizontal Side Bridge**[152]

	Men			Women			All		
Task	*Mean*	*SD*	*Ratio*	*Mean*	*SD*	*Ratio*	*Mean*	*SD*	*Ratio*
Extensor	146	51	1.0	189	60	1.0	177	60	1.0
Flexor	144	76	0.99	149	99	0.79	147	90	0.86
Side bridge, right	94	34	0.64	72	31	0.38	81	34	0.47
Side bridge, left	97	35	0.66	77	35	0.40	85	36	0.5

knee is placed in maximum extension and the ankle is dorsiflexed. Evaluation of the gastronemius muscle in regards to muscle tension and tone is noted as well as the integrity of the ankle joint flexibility. The inclinometer is then positioned above the lateral malleolus and "zeroed" in the upright standing position, or neutral position. The angle of the lower leg is then measured with maximum ankle dorsiflexion maintained, or keeping the heel placed firmly on the floor. The patient then places the hands on the wall and leans on the wall while leaning forward for increased stability when this position is being obtained. This procedure is then repeated for the opposite lower extremity. Normative data reveals 22.5 degrees, standard deviation of .7, intra-assay CV of 2.2%, and inter-assay CV of 2.5%.[149]

Test 8: Soleus/Ankle Dorsiflexion Test This test is done in relatively the same manner as the gastrocnemius dorsiflexion test. However, with this test the knee is placed into flexion, which removes tension off the gastrocnemius muscle (remember, it is a two-joint muscle). The test starts with the patient standing upright, placing the inclinometer above the lateral malleolus and "zeroed." The patient then places the lower extremity foot, which is being measured on a stool, chair, or bench. The patient then rocks forward with knee bent while maintaining heel contact on the stool. This angle is then measured.[149] Normative data is 24.9 degrees and standard deviation .8, intra-assay CV of 2.2%, and inter-assay CV of 2.6%.[149,155]

Test 9a,b: One Leg Standing Test with Eyes Open/Eyes Closed One leg standing test helps determine the patient's level of proprioception. The test is best performed with patient being bare feet or in socks. The patient is instructed to stand on one foot with the eyes open and balance up to a maximum of 30 seconds. The patient should practice with eyes open twice for up to 10 seconds while fixing the eye on a spot on the wall ahead in order to gain confidence. The evaluator observes the quality of the patient's ability to balance as well as quantifies the time the patient maintained the position before losing balance. Test termination is determined by reaching out, hopping, putting the elevated foot down, and/or touching the foot to the weight-bearing leg. The patient should then attempt to balance as long as possible on one leg with eyes closed for up to 30 seconds and the best score with eyes closed for each leg should be recorded. If the subject maintains the position for 30 seconds on the first "eyes-closed" attempt, he or she does not need to perform it a second time

This is a very practical test and has been well validated.[156,157,158,159] Normative data has been published based on age, which allows the evaluator to calculate the percent of normal (see Table 14–11).[156,160]

Test 10: Exaggeration (Waddell NonOrganic Back Pain 5) This is not a specific test, but rather an observation throughout the entire examination. If the patient shows signs of exaggeration, overreaction, or response that is not traditional or expected, such as collapsing, an outcry, or excessive tremor, this can be considered an exaggeration. This test will then be reported as positive or negative as it relates to low back pain of nonorganic origin. An example of this would be when performing an orthopedic test and before normal provocation is noted, patient cries out or verbally responds before pain is normally induced.[153]

Test 11: The Repetitive Squat This test is used to assess joint mobility of the lower extremities including hip, knee, ankle, and foot as well as generalized strength, endurance, and coordination of the lower extremities.

TABLE 14–11. **Normative Data for One Leg Standing***

Age (y)	Eyes Open (s)	Eyes Closed (s)
20–59	29–30	21–28.8 (25 s average)
60–69	22.5 average	10
70–79	14.2	4.3

*Data for eyes open and eyes closed based on age group.[155,159]

TABLE 14–12. **Normative Data for Repetitive Squatting Test**

	Males (n = 242)						Females (n = 233)					
	Blue Collar		*White Collar*		*All*		*Blue Collar*		*White Collar*		*All*	
Age	Mean*	SD	Mean*	SD	Mean*	SD	Mean*	SD	Mean*	SD	Mean*	SD
35–39	39	13	46	8	42	12	24	11	27	12	26	12
40–44	34	14	45	9	38	13	22	13	18	8	20	12
45–49	30	12	40	11	33	13	19	12	26	13	22	13
50–54	28	14	41	11	33	14	13	10	18	14	14	11
35–54†	33	14	43	10	37	13	20	12	23	12	21	12

*The average or mean number of repetitions.

†Average of all subjects tested (35–54 years old). A maximum of 50 repetitions allowed.

Reprinted with permission from Alaranta et al.[83]

The patient is instructed to stand with feet approximately 15 cm apart and then is to squat downward to a point in which the thighs are parallel to the floor. The patient then returns to the upright position. Each repetition should take approximately 2–3 seconds to complete. The patient is asked to continue squatting repetitively up to 50 repetitions. The patient continues to perform the maximum number of squats they can perform, or 50 squats, whichever is reached first. The examiner evaluates quality of the movement as well as the number of repetitions. This evaluation leads to the determination of an exercise prescription, and the number of repetitions is important for tracking the outcomes when a follow-up QFCE is performed. If during the task the patient is having difficulty and compensating with use of hands or is unable to perform a squat completely, it may be best to end the test and record the maximum number of repetitions up to that point. Normative data is given based on age, gender, and occupation[83] (see Table 14–12).

Test 12: Sitting Straight Leg Raise/Distraction (Waddell NonOrganic Back Pain 3-A) This test is traditionally a provocative orthopedic test that helps the examiner determine whether nerve root tension signs are present. This test also helps evaluate for abnormal psychological issues that may be present. The patient is takes a seated position while the evaluator performs a sitting straight leg raise test. The evaluator attempts to distract the patient by focusing the patient's attention away from the low back while performing such tasks as either a reflex at the knee or ankle or superficial plantar reflex, then rapidly extending the knee. This test is considered positive when little or no pain is noted during a distracted seated straight leg raise test *and* if the patient has a high level of pain observed during a nondistracted supine straight leg raise test. This is sometimes referred to as a positive "flip sign." If the patient has true nerve root tension signs, this test is contraindicated. The evaluator should be cautious in regards to the speed in which the seated straight leg raise test is performed if nerve root tension is suspected. This test is simply reported as either negative or positive, in which it relates to the low back pain, which is nonorganic in origin.[153] (See Test 18A for the supine straight leg raise portion of this test.)

Test 13: Regional Neurological Exam (Waddell NonOrganic Back Pain Test 4) This is the fourth of five Waddell signs and consists of two tests that include the evaluation of both motor and sensory divisions of the nerve roots in the lower extremities. The examiner evaluates standard neurological protocols such as deep tendon reflexes, muscle strength, and sensory perception. A positive test would be indicated by a neurological examination that does not follow an expected neurological pathway and/or is highly inconsistent.[153]

Test 14: Cervical Range of Motion Cervical range of motion evaluates muscular and articular components of the cervical spine. Flexion and extension of the cervical spine are measured in the sagittal plane with an inclinometer placed at the vertex of the calvarium while the other inclinometer is placed over the T1 spinous process. The neutral positions are zeroed at both inclinometers and the patient is asked to flex or extend and the end range points are then measured. Lateral flexion is measured by assessing the planes in the frontal plane by placing the base of the inclinometer horizontal over the same bony landmarks. Cervical rotation can be performed by having the patient lay supine, placing only one inclinometer over the forehead horizontally, and asking the patient to rotate their head to each side, recording the end point in degrees. While

TABLE 14–13. Normative Data for Cervical Spine Range of Motion

Motion	Mean and SD*	Percent of Normal†
Flexion	53 ± 12.1	105.6 (50°)
Extension	71 ± 14.1	112.6 (63°)
Right lateral flexion	49 ± 7.2	109.6 (45°)
Left lateral flexion	50 ± 7.8	112.0 (45°)
Right rotation	88 ± 10.6	103.3 (85°)
Left rotation	90 ± 9.6	105.5 (85°)

*Data taken of 160 male railroad workers: Average age 35 (±7.5) years, average height 64.9 (±2.6) in, and average weight 187 (±28.6) lbs.

†Values in parentheses indicate the normal range of lumbar motion.

Modified from Mayer et al.[151]

performing cervical spine rotation range of motion, make sure that the chest and back are stabilized so that rotation of the torso does not occur with the rotation of the cervical spine. It is appropriate to instruct the patient to stretch prior to taking the readings by performing three repetitions in each plane of motion. Range of motion is then calculated by taking the difference between the two inclinometers at the end points of movement while using the simple equation of occiput minus T1 = X degrees. An average of three consecutive readings must be calculated. If the three readings fall within 5 degrees or 10% of the average, the highest of three readings is then recorded. This can be repeated up to a maximum of six times in an attempt to achieve three consecutive readings within the 5 degree/10% rule.[150] Normative date for cervical spine range of motion is given in Table 14–13.[150,151,161]

Test 15: Cervical Strength (Two Methods)

1. *Cervical spine muscle strength assessment test:* This test has been originally described using a sphygmomanometer dynamometer that is no longer available. However, this was reported reliable.[161] The test was conducted on 40 normal subjects with an average age of 25 (±2) years and 24 symptomatic patients with an average age of 39 (±7) years. Isometric pressure levels produced by the individuals were measured in millimeters of mercury (mmHg) by this device. This was then converted into kilopascals (kPa). The first portion of the study included repeated period trials, using a standardized weight of 20 pounds. This produced a coefficient variation of .84% with virtually no difference between the two trials in regards to the mean. Test–retest correlation coefficients were high, .79 to .97 for all range of motion strength assessments. The ratio between flexion and extension was reported at .75–1. This indicates that flexion is approximately 40% weaker compared to extension in a normal symptomatic-free population. Symptomatic subjects were well below the normal cutoff values and flexion/extension ratios for whiplash type individuals was .25–1, which is about half in comparison to normative data for flexion and extension. The authors of this study concluded that the modified sphygmomanometer dynamometer was a very promising tool in evaluating neck injury patients.[162]

   To perform this test in a clinical setting one can use a Nexercisor ball dynamometer (Nexerciser, Bedford, NH). The Nexercisor can be modified by changing the LED indicator for strength with a sphygmomometer gauge and ball, allowing the pressure exerted against the ball to be read in millimeters of mercury. The Nexercisor is preset with a pressure of 15–30 mmHg. This test is performed with the patient standing facing the Nexercisor, which is placed between the forehead and the wall. The patient is standing upright, not leaning into or toward the wall. The patient is then asked to flex the head forward into the ball without using the body. This position is held for 5 seconds and the maximum reading is then recorded for flexion. This is repeated, changing the patient's position to evaluate lateral flexion and extension. There is no published normative data for the Nexercisor that the lead author is aware of. However, the ratio between the flexors and extensors can be calculated, as well as the quantity of strength in the sagittal and frontal planes, which can be used as an outcome tool for a follow-up reexamination. The strength differences between cervical spine flexors and extensors is significant as indicated in Table 14–14. These findings are consistent with trunk strength as noted by[163]
2. *Chin flexion test:* The chin flexion test (also called the chin tuck test) helps to identify the functional status of the deep neck flexors. The patient lies in a supine position and is instructed to flex the chin toward the sternal notch (i.e. head retraction) while lifting the head approximately 1 inch (2–3 cm) in off the examination table. The patient is then instructed to hold this position as long as tolerable. The practitioner observes for dropping of the head below 1 in, and notes patient's hold time in seconds. Placing a wooden stick, which is 1-in thick, underneath the patient's head will help properly set up patient position as well as indicate when the patient's head has fallen below the 1-in mark. Preliminary data gathered from 36 females and 20 males, and deleting the highest and lowest cases, revealed an average hold time of 59.94 seconds for females and 98.65 seconds for males.[164]

TABLE 14–14. **Normative Data for Cervical Spine Strength**

	Normal ± SD (kPa)	Norm ± SD (mmHg) (kPa × .0075)*	CV (%)	Lower Cutoff (mean −1) (kPa/mmHg)6†	Reliability Coefficient‡	Average % Difference, Trial 1 vs. 2	Intraclass Correlation Coefficient, Trial 1 vs. 2
Flexion	4615 ± 1317	34.61 ± 9.88	28	3300/24.75	.93	10.4	0.98
Extension	7927 ± 2128	59.45 ± 15.96	27	5800/43.5	.97	7.0	0.95
Right lateral flexion	7930 ± 1995	59.48 ± 14.96	25	6200/46.5	.87	6.4	0.99
Left lateral flexion	8512 ± 2261	63.84 ± 16.95	27	6200/46.5	.95	NA	NA
Right rotation	7315 ± 1862	54.86 ± 13.97	26	5200/39.0	.79	4.0	0.98
Left rotation	6783 ± 1859	46.37 ± 13.94	28	5200/39.0	.79	NA	NA
Total	NA	NA	NA	NA	NA	7.0	0.98

*The normative data and standard deviations of cervical spine strength are converted from kilopascals to mmHg by multiplying the kPa by a factor of 0.0075.

†The lower cutoff was computed by subtracting 1 SD from the mean.

‡The reliability coefficient values reveals moderate to high reliability was obtained by this testing approach.

Modified with permission from Vernon et al.[161]

Test 16: Repetitive Sit-Up Test This test evaluates strength and endurance of the rectus abdominis muscle. The patient lies supine with the knees flexed 90 degrees and the ankles secured either by the evaluator's hands or some type of strapping device. The patient is then asked to perform sit ups in which he or she approximates the thenar pads of the hands to the patella, then come back down to a supine position. The patient is asked to perform as many sit-ups as possible, up to a maximum of 50. Each repetition should take approximately 2 or 3 seconds to complete. Normative data for sit-ups, broken down by age, gender, and occupation, is presented in Table 14–15.[83]

Test 17: Hip Flexion Test/Modified Thomas Test The Modified Thomas Test evaluates range of motion of the hip and the length or tension of the psoas muscle. The patient lies in a supine position on a sturdy table and an inclinometer is zeroed out on the quadraceps femoris muscle or thigh. The patient is then repositioned at the end of the table so that the ischii approximate to the edge of the table and the nontested knee is brought to the chest and held by the patient. The patient is laid down or "rocked" onto the back into the supine position, keeping the knee held as tight as possible to chest by both the examiner as well as the patient. This must be performed carefully to eliminate any pelvic movement during the test once the patient is in the supine position. This can be done by having the examiner lean against the foot of the nontested leg. The leg being tested is then brought to 90-degrees hip flexion (allow knee flexion) from the starting point and then

TABLE 14–15. **Repetitive Sit-Up Test**

	Males ($n = 242$)						Females ($n = 233$)					
	Blue Collar		*White Collar*		*All*		*Blue Collar*		*White Collar*		*All*	
Age (y)	Mean*	SD	Mean*	SD	Mean*	SD	Mean*	SD	Mean*	SD	Mean*	SD
35–39	29	13	35	13	32	13	24	12	30	16	27	14
40–44	22	11	34	12	27	13	18	12	19	13	19	12
45–49	19	11	33	15	24	14	17	14	22	15	19	14
50–54	17	13	36	16	23	16	9	10	20	13	11	11
35–54†	23	13	35	13	27	14	17	13	24	15	19	14

*The average number of repetitions.

†Average of all subjects tested (35–54 years old). A maximum of 50 repetitions is allowed.

Reprinted with permission from Alaranta et al.[83]

"zeroed." The leg is then brought down and allowed to hang freely off the end of the table. This angle is then recorded. Normative data of this test is 83.5 degrees, SD 1.1, intra-assay CV .7%, and inter-assay CV 1.2%.[149,154]

Test #18: Hip Flexion/Supine Straight Leg Raise-(Waddell NonOrganic Pain Sign 3B) This test consists of two components. The first (Test 18A) is part of the third nonorganic low back pain sign, which is the nondistracted supine straight leg raise test compared against the sitting distracted straight leg raise test (see Test 12). The second (Test 18B) consists of supine straight leg raise test that measures hamstring length and/or hip range of motion. The evaluator may simply record whether a positive pain response was noted, which is usually consistent with the seated straight leg raise test. If these two tests do not provoke similar symptomatology, positive Waddell signs may be present. In the second portion in regards to the simple straight leg raise test, the examiner elevates the lower extremity to evaluate tension and flexibility of the hamstring. The examiner starts by zeroing out the inclinometer while the patient lies supine. With the caudal hand, the examiner holds the inclinometer at mid-tibia. The leg is then elevated to a point at which the knee begins to flex and/or posterior pelvic tilt is noted. This can be best evaluated by placing the opposite hand, or the cephalad hand, on the ASIS while lifting the lower extremity with the caudal hand, looking for knee flexion or feeling posterior pelvic tilt. This number is then recorded off the inclinometer at a point just prior to posterior pelvic tilt and/or knee flexion. Normative data for straight leg raise is 70 degrees to 90 degrees with an average of 80 degrees.[149]

Test 19: Double Leg Lowering The patient lies in a supine position and the inclinometer is zeroed on the mid-tibia. A ruler is then placed under the lordosis of the lumbar spine (approximately at the level of L2–3) and the patient is then asked to elevate both legs with the hips flexed to 90 degrees and the knees fully extended. The patient is then asked to maintain posterior pelvic tilt (PPT) while actively lowering the legs. As the patient lowers the legs, the doctor evaluates the angle of the inclinometer, at which the posterior pelvic tilt is lost, or when the ruler can be pulled from beneath the low back. This test is considered normal if the horizontal to leg angle is 65 degrees or less when PPT is lost. To determine the percent of normal, divide 65 degrees by the patient result.[167]

Test 20: Static Back Endurance The static back endurance test is performed by placing the patient in a prone position with the anterior–superior iliac spine on the edge of the table, the trunk off the end of the table, and the arms are at the side. The pelvis, thighs, and ankles are then fixed to the table with strapping. While setting the patient up, the patient may rest his or her upper extremities on a chair or stool to support his or her upper torso. The test begins by asking the patient to place the hands by the sides without grasping onto the strapping or table. The patient is then instructed to hold this horizontal position for as long as possible or 240 seconds, whichever comes first. Normative data for this test, broken down by age, gender, and occupation, is shown in Table 14–16.[83]

Test 21: Knee Flexion Test/Modified Nachlas Test The Nachlas knee flexion test evaluates the tension in the quadriceps femoris muscle group. The patient lies in a prone position with lower extremities extended and feet hanging down off the end of the table. An inclinometer is then placed on the lower portion of the leg with the knee fully extended. An inclinometer is then zeroed and the pelvis is then strapped down to

TABLE 14–16. Static Back Endurance Test

	Males ($n = 242$)						Females ($n = 233$)					
	Blue Collar		*White Collar*		*All*		*Blue Collar*		*White Collar*		*All*	
Age (y)	Mean*	SD	Mean*	SD	Mean*	SD	Mean*	SD	Mean*	SD	Mean*	SD
35–39	87	38	113	47	97	43	91	61	95	48	93	55
40–44	83	51	129	57	101	57	89	57	67	51	80	55
45–49	81	45	131	64	99	58	90	55	122	73	102	64
50–54	73	47	121	56	89	55	62	55	99	78	69	60
35–54†	82	45	123	55	97	53	82	58	94	62	87	59

*Average amount of time (seconds).

†Average of all subjects tested (35–54 years old). The maximum amount of time allowed is 240 seconds.

Reprinted with permission from Alaranta et al.[83]

a firm table and the knee is then passively flexed so that the heel is brought toward the buttocks. The end point is recorded at the point at which hip flexion or hip hiking occurs. The normal angle is 147.9 degrees, standard deviation 1.6, intra-assay CV .5%, and inter-assay CV1.1.[83]

Test 22: Hip Range of Motion The patient is asked to lie in the prone position so as to evaluate internal and external rotation of the hip. The inclinometer is then fixed to the distal third of the lower leg in the coronal plane with the knee flexed at 90 degrees. The pelvis should be stabilized with a strap to prevent rotation of the pelvis during evaluation. The hip is then passively rotated both internally and externally to a point of firm end feel without pelvic rotation. The maximum angle is then recorded for both internal and external rotation of the hip. Normative data has been established by Chesworth et al., with a mean of 45 degrees for internal rotation and 42 degrees for external rotation.[166] (For more information, see Refs. 150 and 167).

Test 23: Grip Strength Dynamometry This test is performed by using a Jamar hand dynamometer, with the handle placed in the optimum position, which is usually the second or third position depending upon the patient's hand size. Three readings are taken and the readings are then averaged. These tests can be taken at three different times throughout the examination and are considered reliable if there is less than a 20% variation among the three. Normative data for grip strength and pinch strength, broken down by occupation, age, and gender, is given in Table 14–17.[150,168]

Test 24: Repetitive Arch-Up Test This test is performed in the similar way as the static back endurance test in regards to placement and setup of the patient. However, in this test the patient is asked to flex the trunk approximately 45 degrees toward the floor and then extend back to the horizontal position, which equals one cycle. This is repeated up to a maximum of 50 repetitions. Each cycle should take approximately 2–3 seconds to complete. The number of repetitions are documented and then compared to the normative data to calculate the percent of normal (see Table 14–18).[83]

Posttest Using the Visual Analogue Scale

At the end of the examination, patient is again asked to complete a VAS. This helps to identify a patient whose pain has been aggravated by the examination, thus proper home-care instructions can be given to the patient, such as applications of heat or cold, stretched or rest, etc. Of all the physical performance tests included in the QFCE, the Alaranta strength and/or endurance tests tend to be the most difficult, which include the repetitive squat (Test 11), the repetitive sit-up (Test 16), the static back endurance test (Test 20), and the repetitive arch-up (Test 24. In 1994, Alaranta reported that no significant iatrogenic injury was observed in the patient sample with respect to back injuries associated with the performance of those tests.[83] These tests can also serve as a screening tool for fear-avoidance behavior, which can become quite apparent when a patient lacks the courage to perform a test. There may be times in which it is unsafe to perform some of these tests and this should be considered on a case-by-case basis. Fear-avoidance behaviors usually decrease following the successful completion of rehabilitation exercises.

TABLE 14–17. The Normative Data for Dominant ("Major Hand") and Nondominant ("Minor Hand") Grip Strength and Pinch Strength

	Males		Females	
	Major Hand	Minor Hand	Major Hand	Minor Hand
Grip strength (kg)				
Occupation				
Skilled	47.0	45.4	26.8	24.4
Sedentary	47.2	44.1	23.1	21.1
Manual	48.5	44.6	24.2	22.0
Average	47.6	45.0	24.6	22.4
Age group				
<20	45.2	42.6	23.8	22.8
20–29	48.5	46.2	24.6	22.7
30–39	49.2	44.5	30.8	28.0
40–49	49.0	47.3	23.4	21.5
50–59	45.9	43.5	22.3	18.2
Pinch strength (kg)				
Occupation				
Skilled	6.6	6.4	4.4	4.3
Sedentary	6.3	6.1	4.1	3.9
Manual	8.5	7.7	6.0	5.5
Average	7.5	7.1	4.9	4.7

Reprinted with permission from Swanson et al.[167]

ANALYZING QFCE DATA

During the QFCE, the examiner records the patient's data on an examination form (Form 14–5), which is then transferred to a QFCE summary form (Form 14–6). Once information is transferred, the percent of normal is calculated. If the test result is less than 85% of the published normative data, a rehabilitation approach specifically addressing the physical performance loss should be implemented in the patient's treatment plan.

Case Example

A 23-year-old female had been suffering from chronic low back pain as the result of a motor vehicle

TABLE 14-18. **Repetitive Arch-Up Test**

	Males (*n* = 242)						Females (*n* = 233)					
	Blue Collar		*White Collar*		*All*		*Blue Collar*		*White Collar*		*All*	
Age	Mean*	SD	Mean*	SD	Mean*	SD	Mean*	SD	Mean*	SD	Mean*	SD
35–39	26	11	34	14	29	13	28	13	27	11	27	12
40–44	23	12	36	14	28	14	25	14	20	11	23	13
45–49	24	13	34	16	28	15	25	15	31	16	27	15
50–54	21	11	35	17	26	15	18	14	26	14	19	14
35–54†	24	12	35	15	28	14	24	14	26	13	24	14

*Average number of repetitions.

†Average of all subjects tested (35–54 years old). A maximum of 50 repetitions is allowed.

Reprinted with permission from Alaranta et al.[83]

accident that occurred approximately 2 years earlier. Since the date of injury the patient had received prescription pain medication from her physician as well as two 1-month trials of modalities and exercise, which consisted of range of motion exercises, stationary bicycling, and ultrasound treatment. These active approaches improved her function and decreased her pain; however, her condition worsened after discontinuing therapy. She subsequently consulted a physiatrist who evaluated her history and presenting condition and determined that she may respond to manipulative therapy and thus the appropriate referral was made. Initial physical examination highlights included limited lumbar and thoracic range of motion with pain in all ranges. Abnormal gait patterns and postural weakness were noted with observation. Multiple levels of joint dysfunction and paraspinal muscle tenderness in the thoracic, lumbar, and pelvic regions were observed and palpated. Trigger points were palpated in the lower thoracic pararspinal musculature. Orthopedic testing provoked pain at the thoracic/lumbar, the lumbosacral, and sacroiliac regions. Neurological findings were normal for motor strength, reflexes, and sensation. Prior imaging studies, which included MRI and CT, were negative.

The patient received 2 weeks of conservative management that consisted of manipulation to improve joint motion and electrical stimulation to decrease pain. Myofascial release techniques were performed to normalize hypertonic myofascial tissue. Neuromuscular reeducation techniques were implemented to address muscle imbalances, faulty posture, and gait patterns. Outcomes assessment tools included a visual pain scale where levels improved approximately 50% over the 2-week period; however, the Oswestry Low Back Disability Questionnaire score showed little improvement. A QFCE was conducted to determine if rehabilitation was needed and if so, to help to determine which specific rehabilitation approaches were most appropriate.

Quantitative Functional Capacity Evaluation

The 23 physical performance tests that make up the QFCE were completed and the results scored (see Table 14–19). Any score below the 85% threshold of the published normal has been tagged and is supportive of deconditioning. The table indicates the test name in the first, or left, column, the published normative data in the second column, the patient's results in the third column, and the percentage of normal in the fourth, or far right, column. Tests given in bold fall at or below the 85% cutoff.

The QFCE summary (Table 14–19) reveals deficiencies, or scores below 85% for the following tests: 3-minute step test, lumbar extension range of motion, horizontal side bridge, one leg standing test with eyes closed, repetitive sit-up, repetitive arch-up, straight leg raise, bilateral leg and static back endurance, and internal and external rotation of the right hip. Based on this information, a rehabilitation regimen was implemented that included cardiovascular exercises (walking, stationary bike, and treadmill) 20 minutes a day, three times a week. Specific lumbar range of motion exercises emphasizing extension were prescribed. The horizontal side bridge exercise and proprioceptive gym ball exercises (superman, wall squats, and seesaw) addressing strengthening of the low back extensor muscles and lower extremities were included. In addition, hamstring stretching exercises and hip internal and external rotator stretches were also given to the patient. Other proprioceptive exercises included the use of a rockerboard, balance sandals, and a

FORM 14–5.

QUANTITATIVE FUNCTIONAL CAPACITY EVALUATION

NAME____________ **DATE**________ **DOB**________ **DOI**________ **TIME IN**________
Dx:________________________

TEST *Standing*	**INITIAL** Date:		**1st Re-exam** Date:		**2nd Re-exam** Date:		**3rd Re-exam** Date:	
1. Pre-Test VAS	____/10		____/10		____/10		____/10	
2. 3-minute Step Test (pulse)	___pre ___post-		___pre ___post-		___pre ___post-		___pre ___post-	
3. ROM: PAIN SCALE: LUMBAR EXTREMITY (L/R)								
FLEXION (FORW.FLEX)	FL ___ +2,1,0,-1,2		FL ___ +2,1,0,-1,2		FL ___ +2,1,0,-1,2		FL ___ +2,1,0,-1,2	
EXTENSION (BACKWARD EXT)	EXT___ +2,1,0,-1,2		EXT___ +2,1,0,-1,2		EXT___ +2,1,0,-1,2		EXT___ +2,1,0,-1,2	
RT. LAT. FLEX (ABDUCTION)	RLF___ +2,1,0,-1,2		RLF___ +2,1,0,-1,2		RLF___ +2,1,0,-1,2		RLF___ +2,1,0,-1,2	
LT. LAT. FLEX (ADDUCTION)	LLF___ +2,1,0,-1,2		LLF___ +2,1,0,-1,2		LLF___ +2,1,0,-1,2		LLF___ +2,1,0,-1,2	
4. PAIN (Superficial): Waddell #1	+ / -		+ / -		+ / -		+ / -	
5. SIMULATION: Waddell #2								
a. Trunk Rotation	+ / -		+ / -		+ / -		+ / -	
b. Axial Compression (5 kg)	+ / -		+ / -		+ / -		+ / -	
TESTS	**L**	**R**	**L**	**R**	**L**	**R**	**L**	**R**
6. Horizontal Side Bridge (record in seconds)	Time/sec ___	Time/sec ___	Time/sec ___	Time/sec ___	Time/sec ___	Time/sec ___	Time/sec ___	Time/sec ___
7. Gastroc/Ankle DF (Knee extd)	___ °	___ °	___ °	___ °	___ °	___ °	___ °	___ °
8. Soleus/Ankle DF (Knee flexed)	___ °	___ °	___ °	___ °	___ °	___ °	___ °	___ °
9a.* One-Leg Stand (eyes open)	___Sec.	___Sec.	___Sec.	___Sec.	___Sec.	___Sec.	___Sec.	___Sec.
9b.* One-Leg Stand (eyes closed)	___Sec.	___Sec.	___Sec.	___Sec.	___Sec.	___Sec.	___Sec.	___Sec.
10. Exaggeration (Waddell #5)	+ / -		+ / -		+ / -		+ / -	
11. Rep. Squat (feet 15cm apart) • Thigh horizontal, 1 rep/2-3 sec., note # of reps; max. reps 50;	___ # of reps.		___ # of reps.		___ # of reps.		___ # of reps.	

Seated **TESTS**	**L**	**R**	**L**	**R**	**L**	**R**	**L**	**R**

wobble board. The patient received 15–30 minutes of in-office rehabilitation covering the exercises discussed above at a frequency of three times a week for 1 month during which time the exercises were gradually transitioned for home use, when the patient could demonstrate the proper technique for each exercise. At the conclusion of a 4-week rehabilitation trial, a follow-up QFCE reexam was performed and compared to the initial/baseline QFCE results (Table 14–20). Please note that only those tests in which the patient was initially deficient were retested. In this case, improvement was noted in all categories; however, not all categories were above 85%. Thus, rehabilitation protocols were continued, primarily at home if proper technique was demonstrated by the patient. The patient was rescheduled 6 weeks later to retest these deficiencies and all were above 85%. An Oswestry and QVAS were filled out by the patient and revealed dramatic improvement in comparison to the previous outcome scores. The patient was discharged from active care and instructed to continue home exercise.

12. Sitting SLR / DISTRACTION (Waddell #3; see #13) ↑ LBP: (circle)	↑ LBP: yes / no	↑ LBP: yes / no	↑ LBP: yes / no	↑ LBP: yes / no	↑ LBP: yes / no	↑ LBP: yes / no	↑ LBP: yes / no	↑ LBP: yes / no
13. Regional Neuro. (Waddell #4)	+ / -	+ / -	+ / -	+ / -	+ / -	+ / -	+ / -	+ / -

14. ROM: PAIN SCALE: CERVICAL EXTREMITY (L/R)				
FLEXION (FORW.FLEX)	FL ______ +2,1,0,-1,2	FL ______ +2,1,0,-1,2	FL ______ +2,1,0,-1,2	FL ______ +2,1,0,-1,2
EXTENSION (BACKWARD EXT)	EXT____ +2,1,0,-1,2	EXT____ +2,1,0,-1,2	EXT____ +2,1,0,-1,2	EXT____ +2,1,0,-1,2
RT. LAT. FLEX (ABDUCTION)	RLF____ +2,1,0,-1,2	RLF____ +2,1,0,-1,2	RLF____ +2,1,0,-1,2	RLF____ +2,1,0,-1,2
LT. LAT. FLEX (ADDUCTION)	LLF____ +2,1,0,-1,2	LLF____ +2,1,0,-1,2	LLF____ +2,1,0,-1,2	LLF____ +2,1,0,-1,2
RT. ROTATION (EXT. ROT.)	RR ______ +2,1,0,-1,2	RR ______ +2,1,0,-1,2	RR ______ +2,1,0,-1,2	RR ______ +2,1,0,-1,2
LT. ROTATION (INT. ROT.)	LR ______ +2,1,0,-1,2	LR ______ +2,1,0,-1,2	LR ______ +2,1,0,-1,2	LR ______ +2,1,0,-1,2

ROM PAIN SCALE: -2 = centralization; -1 = decreased pain; 0 = no change in pain; +1 = increased pain; +2 = peripheralization

COMMENTS____

____

____

____

______________________________ **GO ONTO PAGE 2 ⇒ ⇒ ⇒ ⇒**

NAME______________________ **DATE**____________ **DOI**____________

Supine TESTS	L	R	L	R	L	R	L	R
15.* (2 methods) CERVICAL STRENGTH – mmHg (dynamometer) CHIN FLEXION TEST (timed) Time to the point of Shakes / Drops head	Fl____ RLF_____ Ext____ LLF_____ C-Flexion Test: ______/______ Sec.		Fl____ RLF_____ Ext____ LLF_____ C-Flexion Test: ______/______ Sec.		Fl____ RLF_____ Ext____ LLF_____ C-Flexion Test: ______/______ Sec.		Fl____ RLF_____ Ext____ LLF_____ C-Flexion Test: ______/______ Sec.	
16. Repetitive Sit-up Test Sit-up, knees 90°, feet anchored, 1 rep/2-3 sec, touch thenar to patella, curl back down; max. 50 reps	*Endurance* reps________/ 50		*Endurance* reps________/ 50		*Endurance* reps________/ 50		*Endurance* reps________/ 50	
17. Hip Flexion Test / Modified Thomas Measure: Passive Hip extension (psoas tension)	a. _____°	a. _____°	a. _____°	a. _____°	a. _____°	a. _____°	a. _____°	a. _____°

Benefits of the QFCE

Using a tool such as the QFCE can be of great benefit to the health-care provider, the patient, and any third party reviewer/payer. The results can help drive specific rehabilitation exercises, screen for pain behaviors, document effectiveness of prescribed rehabilitation protocols, reinforce patient compliance with rehabilitation and or therapy, provide information to third party payers to establish "medical necessity" for appropriate reimbursement, and to determine if there is a need for continued care.

Indications and Applications of the QFCE

The QFCE is a clinical tool that allows clinicians, patients and 3rd-party reviewers to determine the patient's functional capacity utilizing low-tech methods. Unlike other outcomes tools such as pain scales and activities of daily living measures, the QFCE is not

18. Hip Flexion/Supine SLR **a. Waddell #3: supine + vs. sit-SLR** **b. Measure angle:** at point of knee flexion	a. + / - b.___°	a. + / - b.___°	a. + / - b.___°	a. + / - b.___°	a. + / - b.___°	a. + / - b.___°	a. + / - b.___°	a. + / - b.___°
19. Double Leg Lowering (maintain lordosis < 65 degrees)	________ degrees		________ degrees		________ degrees		________ degrees	

***Prone* TESTS**	**L**	**R**	**L**	**R**	**L**	**R**	**L**	**R**
20. Static Back Endurance • Static Back Endurance: Pt holds trunk horizontal up to max. of 240 sec.	Static Time________/2 40 sec.		Static Time________/ 240 sec.		Static Time________/2 40 sec.		Static Time________/2 40 sec.	
21. Knee Flexion Test / Modified Nachlas Test	____°	____°	____°	____°	____°	____°	____°	____°
22. Hip ROM • Internal Rotation • External Rotation	IR ____° ER __°	IR ____° ER __°	IR ____° ER __°	IR ____° ER __°	IR ____° ER __°	IR ____° ER __°	IR ____° ER __°	IR ____° ER __°

TESTS	**L**	**R**	**L**	**R**	**L**	**R**	**L**	**R**
23. Grip Dynamometry **Dominant: Left / Right (circle)** • **Use Jamar** • **Use Position 1 or 2** • **Three trials (average)**	1.____ 2.____ 3.____ ave____	1.____ 2.____ 3.____ ave____	1.____ 2.____ 3.____ ave____	1.____ 2.____ 3.____ ave____	1.____ 2.____ 3.____ ave____	1.____ 2.____ 3.____ ave____	1.____ 2.____ 3.____ ave____	1.____ 2.____ 3.____ ave____
24. Repetitive Arch Up Test • Repetitive arch up: Waist at table's edge fixed at ankle flexed 45° raises up to horizontal; 1 rep/2-3 seconds; max. 50reps	Reps________/ 50		Reps________ /50		Reps________/5 0		Reps________/5 0	
25. Post-Test VAS	_____/10		_____/10		_____/10		_____/10	

SIGNED________________________ **DATE**____________ **TIME OUT**____________
SIGNED________________________ **DATE**____________ **TIME OUT**____________
SIGNED________________________ **DATE**____________ **TIME OUT**____________
SIGNED________________________ **DATE**____________ **TIME OUT**____________

to be utilized on all patients, but rather a very select subset of patients. Most patients with low back syndromes will recover with conservative measures and an introduction to independent home exercises. However, there are those uniquely difficult cases where the subacute patient is not progressing as anticipated, or demonstrates a past history of failed attempts at long-term recovery for their chronic back disorder, which is where the QFCE can provide important information. Because of the additional costs of the QFCE, clinicians must be ethical in their practices to ensure that this assessment is properly utilized.

The QFCE is ideal when the patient has reached a subacute status, as physical performance measurement is not appropriate to measure in an acute state. This is because acute pain promotes temporary compensatory defensive movements and postures that resolve as pain dissipates. When a patient has reached a 2–4 week point post-acute presentation, and an unsatisfactory outcome exists from both a patient and provider viewpoint, the transition from provocative testing to physical performance testing such as the QFCE is appropriate. It is not appropriate to perform QFCE tests in the following situations:

1. In the acute stage of an injury/illness
2. When a test may exacerbate a condition
3. More than once every 2–4 weeks, as it takes time to strengthen and rehabilitate dysfunction
4. After a plateau has been reached and good compliance with a rehab program does not result in further benefit (i.e., an end-point of rehab is reached with residual impairment, with or without disability exists)
5. When an underlying pathology, clinically reasonable for the presenting condition, hasn't been

FORM 14–6.

QUANTITATIVE FUNCTIONAL CAPACITY RESULTS

NAME: ______________________ **Occupation:** WC / BC*
DATE:_______ **BD:**_______ **AGE:**_______
Dx:____________________ **Test #:** 1, 2, 3, 4 **Symptom Duration:**_________ **Prior Episodes:** YES / NO

TEST NAME	NORMAL	PATIENT RESULT		PERCENT OF NORMAL	
1. Pre-test VAS	0/10	____/10			
2. 3-minute Step Test (pulse)	______/______yo F M	_____ Pre- ____Post-		%	
3. ROM / Lumbar Spine					
Flexion	65°	_____°		%	
Extension	30°	_____°		%	
Rt. Lateral Flexion	25°	_____°		%	
Lt. Lateral Flexion	25°	_____°		%	
4. Waddell #1: Pain	Negative	Positive / Negative		NA	
5. Waddell #2: Simulation	Negative	Positive / Negative		NA	
6. Horizontal Side Bridge	________ (max. 240 sec.)	________ sec.		%	
7. Gastrocnemius /Ankle DF	23°	Lt.:	Rt.:	%	%
8. Soleus / Ankle DF	25°	Lt.:	Rt.:	%	%
9a & b. One leg standing test	EO____sec. EC_____	L___/___ R___/___		L___/___ R___/___	
10. Waddell #5: Exaggeration	Negative	Positive / Negative		NA	
11. Repetitive Squat*	_____ / (max 50)	_____ / ( )		%	
12. Sitting SLR/ Distraction w/ #17a	LBP: YES / NO	LBP: YES / NO		NA	
13. Waddell #4: Regional Neuro	Negative	Positive / Negative		NA	
14. ROM / Cervical					
Flexion	50°	_____°		%	
Extension	63°	_____°		%	
Rt. Lateral Flexion	45°	_____°		%	
Lt. Lateral Flexion	45°	_____°		%	
Rt Rotation	85°	_____°		%	
Lt Rotation	85°	_____°		%	
15. Cervical spine strength 2 methods: 1) Sphyg; 2) C-Flex T.	NOT ESTABLISHED	Fl______ RLF______ Ext______ LLF______		C-Flexion Test: Shake/drop____/____Sec.	
16. Repetitive Sit-Up*	________ (max. 50)	_______/ ( )		%	
17. Hip flexion/Modified Thomas					

appropriately ruled out utilizing clinically accepted diagnostic methods.

6. When the patient is responding to conservative therapy and exercise programs with no perceived or anticipated disability, work intolerance, and/or minimal or no residual pain.
7. When the patient's pain level is at or below 6/10 on an 11-point scale, which indicates he or she should be able to tolerate the testing.

The indications for performing a QFCE include:

1. At a 2–4 week post-acute status presentation (i.e. 6–8 weeks after the onset of symptom) with an unsatisfying endpoint despite a combined trial of passive and active treatment methods and independent exercise.
2. When a patient has a chronic, recurrent history of spinal complaints.

Iliopsoas	84°	Lt.:	Rt.:	%	%
18a. Waddell #3: Distraction/SLR	Negative	Positive / Negative		NA	
18b. Straight Leg Raise*	80°	Lt.:	Rt.:	%	%
19. Double leg lowering	<65 degrees w/ pelvic tilt	________ degrees		________ %	
20. Static Back Endurance*	______ (max. 240 sec.)	______ seconds		%	
21. Knee Flexion	147 +/- 1.6	Lt.:	Rt.:	%	%
22. Hip Rotation ROM					
Internal Rotation ROM	41-45 (43)	Lt.:	Rt.:	%	%
External Rotation ROM	41-43 (42)	Lt.:	Rt.:	%	%
23. Grip Strength*	Lt.: Kg Rt.: Kg	Lt.: Kg	Rt.: Kg	%	%
24. Repetitive Arch-Up*	______ (max. 50)	______/ ( )		%	
25. Post-test VAS	0/10	____/10			

AGE years	EYES OPEN (seconds)	EYES CLOSED (seconds)
20-59	29-30	21-28.8 (25 Sec. ave.)
60-69	22.5 ave	10
70-79	14.2	4.3

*** Normative data is determined by age, sex and occupation (Blue vs. white collar: BC / WC)**

**** A positive test #13 (Supine SLR) and a negative sitting / distracted SLR (test #8)= +Waddell sign for Distraction**

3. When a plateau has been reached with passive care approaches and with independent exercises and the patient remains functionally restricted due to their back disorder.
4. When deconditioning is evident despite a trial of in-office and independent exercising and the patient's condition is considered sufficiently stable to tolerate the QFCE testing.

There are times when individual tests from the QFCE are appropriate to run prior to assessing strength and/or endurance. In these cases, unless at least 8 of the 15 minutes per unit of physical performance testing is performed, it is not appropriate to bill for a unit of physical performance testing. For example, placing an inclinometer on a tibia to measure hamstring length/SLR is not sufficient to support a 97750 i.e. United States CPT billing code. On the other hand, there are times when a modified or brief QFCE, such as eliminating some of the more difficult tests (eg., static back endurance, repetitive arch-up, repetitive sit-up tests, etc.) is appropriate. In those cases, billing should reflect the amount of time taken to perform the modified QFCE (eg., one or two units of 97750). Here again, it is not appropriate to evaluate a patient more than once every 2–4 weeks, as time for improvement is necessary, as is the case with all rehabilitation programs. Hence, over utilizing the QFCE is inappropriate and clinical documentation must support the level of testing to justify its necessity.

Finally, it is important to note that the QFCE is comprised of a number of validated tests, but it has not yet been validated.

Classic Patient Presentations to Utilize the QFCE

Example one

A patient received 1–3 weeks of care and subjectively feels 50–75% improvement. Home-based exercises have been prescribed and patient is compliant. Minimal risk factors are present for the development of chronicity. Provocative orthopedic tests no longer produce or provoke the patient's pain. The patient remains dissatisfied with current status of his or her condition.

A full or partial QFCE may be performed to help determine deficiencies in strength, range of motion, and proprioception. Exercises should then be prescribed based on the QFCE results.

TABLE 14–19. **QFCE Patient Results Compared to Normative Data**

Test Name	Normal	Patient Result	Percent of Normal
1. VAS	0/10	3/10	NA
2. 3-Minute step test (pulse)	See chart for 23-year-old female	Pre-Post-103	**65%**
3. ROM/lumbar spine			
Flexion	65°	64°	98%
Extension	30°	22°	**73%**
Right lateral flexion	25°	25°	100%
Left lateral flexion	25°	28°	112%
4. Waddell no. 1: Pain	Negative	Positive/**Negative**	NA
5. Waddell no. 2: Simulation	Negative	Positive/**Negative**	NA
6. Horizontal side bridge	96 M, 75 F (max 240 s)	L: 32 s; R: 28 s	**43%; 37%**
7. Gastrocnemius/ankle DF	23°	L: 26; R: 20	113%; 87%
8. Soleus/ankle DF	25°	L: 23; R: 30	132%; 120%
9a,b. One leg standing test	EO: 30 s; EC: 25 sec.	L: 30/6; R: 30/5	L: 100/**24;** R: 100/**20**
10. Waddell no. 5: exaggeration	Negative	Positive/**Negative**	NA
11. Repetitive squat*	24/(max 50)	23/(24)	96%
12. Sitting SLR/distraction with no. 18a	LBP: Yes/No	LBP: Yes/No	NA
13. Waddell no. 4: Regional neuro	Negative	Positive/**Negative**	NA
14. ROM/cervical			
Flexion	50°	63°	126%
Extension	63°	60°	95%
Right lateral flexion	45°	47°	104%
Left lateral flexion	45°	48°	107%
Right rotation	85°	85°	100%
Left rotation	85°	88°	104%
15. Cervical spine strength 2 methods: Sphyg; C-flex T	Not established	FL: RLF: EXT: LLF:	C-Flexion Test; Shake/drop 15/30 s
16. Repetitive sit-up*	24 (max 50)	19/(24)	**79%**
17. Hip flexion/modified Thomas Iliopsoas	84°	L: 73; R: 78	87%; 93%
18a. Waddell no. 3: distraction/SLR	Negative	Positive/**Negative**	NA
18b. Straight leg raise*	80°	L: 51; R: 51	**64%; 64%**
19. Double leg lowering	<65° with pelvic tilt	72°	90%
20. Static back endurance*	91 (max. 240 s)	42 s	**46%**
21. Knee flexion	147+/−1.6	L: 139; R: 138	95%; 94%
22. Hip rotation ROM			
Internal rotation ROM	41–45 (43)	L: 37; R: 36	86%; **84%**
External rotation ROM	41–43 (42)	L: 40; R: 35	95%; **83%**
23. Grip strength*	L: 23 kg; R: 25 kg	L: 27 kg; R: 31 kg	117%; 124%
24. Repetitive arch-up*	28 (max 50)	6/(28)	**21%**
25. Posttest VAS	0/10	6/10	NA
Normative data for test no. 9 (One-leg standing test*)	Age (y)	Eyes Open (s)	Eyes Closed (s)
	20–59	29–30	21–28 (25 s average)
	60–69	22.5 average	10
	70–79	14.2	4.3

*Normative data is determined by age, sex, and occupation (blue vs. white collar).

**A positive Test 18A (supine SLR) and a negative sitting/distracted SLR (Test 12) and negative/positive Waddell sign for distraction.

TABLE 14–20. Comparisons of Serial QFCE Results

Test Name	Percent of Normal (03-18-03)	Percent of Normal (04-22-03)	Percent of Normal (06-02-03)
1. VAS	NA	NA	NA
2. 3-Minute step test (pulse)	**65%**	**70%**	**85%**
3. Lumbar ROM			
Flexion	98%	102%	NA
Extension	**73%**	87%	NA
Right lateral flexion	100%	120%	NA
Left lateral flexion	112%	128%	NA
4. Waddell no. 1: pain	NA	NA	NA
5. Waddell no. 2: simulation	NA	NA	NA
6. Horizontal side bridge	**43%; 37%**	**67%; 73%**	91%; 88%
7. Gastrocnemius/ankle DF	113%; 87%	NA	NA
8. Soleus/ankle DF	132%; 120%	NA	NA
9a,b. One leg standing	Left: 100/**24;** Right: 100/**20**	Left: 100/**76;** Right: 100/**80**	Left: 100/96; Right: 100/88
10. Waddell no. 5: exaggerate	NA	NA	NA
11. Repetitive squat*	96%	NA	NA
12. Sitting SLR/distraction with no. 18a	NA	NA	NA
13. Waddell no. 4: regional neuro	NA	NA	NA
14. Cervical ROM			
Flexion	126%	NA	NA
Extension	95%	**NA**	**NA**
Right lateral flexion	104%	NA	NA
Left lateral flexion	107%	NA	NA
Right rotation	100%	NA	NA
Left rotation	104%	NA	NA
15. Cervical spine strength 2 methods: Sphyg; C-Flex T.	C-flexion test Shake/drop: 19/30 s	C-flexion test Shake/drop: 19/39 s	C-flexion test Shake/drop: 22/63 s
16. Repetitive sit-up*	**79%**	121%	121%
17. Hip Flexion/Modified Thomas Iliopsoas	87%; 93%	NA	NA
18a. Waddell no. 3: distraction/ SLR	NA	NA	NA
18b. Straight leg raise*	**64%; 64%**	**76%; 78%**	89%; 85%
19. Double leg lowering	90%	NA	NA
20. Static back endurance*	**46%**	92%	92%
21. Knee flexion	95%; 94%	NA	NA
22. Hip rotation ROM			
Internal rotation ROM	86%; **84%**	100%; 100%	NA
External rotation ROM	95%; **83%**	105%; 90%	NA
23. Grip strength*	117%; 124%	NA	NA
24. Repetitive arch-up*	**21%**	**43%**	87%
25. Posttest VAS	NA	NA	NA

Example two

The patient has been seen for 4–6 weeks of care and has failed to reach preinjury status. Risk factors for chronicity may or may not be present. A home-based exercise approach has been given and the patient states they are compliant. Provocative orthopedic tests continue to be present and the patient's chief complaints remain relatively unchanged since the initial presentation.

A full QFCE offers the opportunity to implement a specific rehabilitation approach. The goal is to prevent the development of chronicity in this type of presenting patient. A face-to-face rehabilitation approach may be the best approach to deter fear-avoidance or pain behaviors that can limit a self-directed home exercise regimen, especially since a home-based exercise program failed to obtain a patient-satisfying outcome. In this presentation, the results of the QFCE help to establish "medical necessity" required for third party payer reimbursement as the tests prove to the patient his or her need for rehabilitation, as well as provide an alternative therapy approach for the health-care provider to implement with the patient.

Example Three

A patient has experienced 6 or more weeks of care and has failed to reach preinjury status. Risk factors for chronicity are significant, which includes failing multiple previous therapies as well as other yellow flags including psychosocial problems, smoking, and poor job satisfaction. The patient remains frustrated and is disappointed with the progress of his or her current condition. Home-based exercises had been prescribed and the patient describes partial compliance with these exercises as a result of fear-avoidance, admitting that several exercises were not performed due to fear of pain provocation. Provocative orthopedic tests continue to be present during follow-up examinations and remain relatively the same since the initial presentation and examination.

An aggressive one-on-one active care approach to this type of patient is required. A full QFCE should be performed and the rehabilitation exercises should be prescribed based on the results. This type of patient must be encouraged to participate in rehabilitation exercises as fear-avoidance and pain behavior are present in this case. The QFCE will reinforce to the patient that they have functional weakness and if they address these issues, they should see improvement in function and symptoms. A follow-up QFCE is helpful in determining if the exercise regimen is successful and documented improvement gives the patient assurance that they are making progress. Without an aggressive approach, a successful outcome may be more difficult with this type of patient.

CONCLUSION: BACK PAIN OUTCOME MEASURES AND THE CLINICAL–SOCIAL INTERFACE—THE FUTURE

Much of the progress and change in outcomes measurement and care of people with low back syndromes has come in recognition of the importance of the biopsychosocial model. While this topic has been briefly addressed in this and other chapters, the reader may refer to Chapter 19 of this text for greater detail. This model recognizes that disability is "not always principally a problem of the person themselves, directly caused by a disease, trauma or other health condition, but is often a socially created problem basically related to the full integration of individuals into society."[169] The *International Classification of Function*, endorsed by the 54th WHO Assembly, has broadened the *Conceptual Scheme* presented at the beginning of this chapter in an attempt to integrate the opposing medical and social models of health.[4] Those who manage back pain in clinics at a community level are at the "sharp end" of this change in that they are forced to ponder whether their interventions could be, or should be, considered to be clinical, social, or both. Whichever view prevails, the need to document the outcomes of care for low back syndromes seems unlikely to diminish.

SUMMARY

1. This chapter has provided subjective and objective OA tools, which can be easily used in the clinical settings.
2. The subjective, self-administered OA tools allow providers to assess the patient's ADLs as well response to care.
3. Outcomes assessment tools can give insight regarding general health, depression, pain, patient satisfaction, job dissatisfaction, chronicity, and disability issues. It is this information that allows the practitioner to provide the most appropriate and effective care by tracking these subjective outcomes in series during the course of care.
4. The low-tech approach of the QFCE allows for evaluation of physical performance with the same validity and efficacy as high-tech approaches, along with a lower cost and flexibility of implementing in almost any clinical setting.
5. To achieve reliable and valid results, care must be taken to perform these tests exactly as described. The information generated is valuable in driving rehabilitative treatment plans, enforcing patient compliance, and providing objective information to establish medical necessity for third party reviewers.
6. When the subjective, self-administered OA tools, and the objective, QFCE, are combined with traditional history and examination findings, the clinician can feel confident that he or she is providing leading-edge, evidence-based, comprehensive, and effective assessment protocols.

REFERENCES

1. Katz et al. *Staff of Benjamen* Rose hospital, 1959.
2. Mahoney FI, Barthel DW. Functional evaluation:The Barthel Index. *Md State Med J*, 1965;14:61–65.
3. World Health Organisation. *International classification of diseases*, 7th rev. Geneva: WHO, 1966.
4. World Health Organisation. *International classification of impairments, disabilities and handicaps*. Geneva: WHO, 1980.
5. Stewart A, Ware JE, Brook RH, et al. *Conceptualization and measurement of health for adults in the health insurance study, Vol II: Physical health in terms of functioning*,Publication No. 1987/2-HEW. Santa Monica, CA: RAND Corp., 1978.
6. Stewart AL, Ware JE. *Measuring functioning and well-being: The medical outcomes study approach*. Durham, NC: Duke University Press, 1992.
7. Bergner M, Bobbitt RA, Carter WB, et al. The Sickness Impact Profile: Development and final revision of a health status measure. *Med Care* 1981;19:787–805.
8. Chalmers I, Altman D, eds. *Systematic reviews*. London: BMJ Publishing, 1995.
9. Nelson EC, Mohr JJ, Batalden PB, Plume SK. Improving health care, Part 1: The clinical value compass. *J Qual Improv* 1996;22(4):243–256.
10. Deyo RA, Schall M, Berwick DM, Nolan T, Carver P. Innovations in education and clinical practice: Continuous quality improvement for patients with back pain. *J Gen Intern Med* 2000;15:647–655.
11. Acton C, Newbronner E. Health Needs Assessment—Step by Step: A Practical Guide to Practice Based Health Needs Assessment for GPs and Primary Health Care Team Members. In: York Health Economics Consortium, 1997.
12. Granados, A. Health technology assessment and clinical decision making: Research notes. *Int J Technol Assess Health Care* 1999;15(3):585–614.
13. Deyo RA, Battie M, Beurskens AJ, et al. Outcome measures for low back pain research. *Spine* 1998;23:2003–2013
14. CSAG. *Back pain*. London: Department of Health, 1994.
15. Thomas E, Silman AJ, et al. Predicting who develops chronic low back pain in primary care: a prospective study. *Br Med J* 1999;318:1662–1667.
16. Koes BW, Van Tulder MW, et al. Clinical guidelines for the management of low back pain in primary care. *Spine* 2001;26(22):2504–2514.
17. Main C, Burton K, et al. *Evidence of psychological distress unrelated to chronicity in back pain patients attending osteopaths*. The Society for Back Pain Research, 1992.
18. Bigos S, Bowyer O, Braen G, et al. *Acute low back problems in adults. Clinical practice guideline* no. 14. Rockville, MD: U.S. Department of Health and Human Services, Public Health Service, Agency for Health Care Policy and Research, 1994.
19. Waddell G, Feder G, McIntosh A, Lewis M. *Hutchinson a low back pain evidence review*. London: Royal College of General Practitioners, 1996.
20. Deyo RA, Rainville J, Kent DL. What can the history and physical examination tell us about low back pain? *JAMA* August 12, 1992;268(6):760–765.
21. Weinstein JN, McLain F. Primary tumors of the spine. *Spine* 1987;12:843–851.
22. CSAG. *Epidemiology review: The epidemiology and cost of back pain*. London: Department of Health, 1994.
23. Von Korff M, Ormel J, et al. Grading the severity of chronic pain. *Pain* 1992;50:133–149.
24. Symonds TL, Burton AK, et al. Do attitudes and beliefs influence work loss due to low back trouble? *Occup Med* 1996;46:25–32.
25. Pincus T, Burton K, et al. A systematic review of psychological factors as predictors of chronicity/disability in prospective cohorts of low back pain. *Spine* 2002;27(5):E109–E120.
26. Macfarlane GJ. Fibromyalgia and chronic widespread pain. In: Crombie IK ed. *Epidemiology of pain*. Seattle: IASP Press, 1999:113–123.
27. Dionne CE, Koepsell TD, Von Korff M, et al. Predicting long-term functional limitations amount back pain patients in primary care settings. *J Clin Epidemiol* 1997;30:31–43.
28. Von Korff M, Deyo RA, Cherkin D, Barlow SF. Back pain in primary care: Outcomes at 1 year. *Spine* 1993;18:855–862.
29. Burton AK, Tillotson K, Main C, Hollis M. Psychosocial predictors of outcome in acute and sub-acute low back trouble. *Spine* 1995;20:722–728.
30. Cherkin DC, Deyo RA, et al. A comparison of physical therapy, chiropractic manipulation and provision of an educational booklet for the treatment of patients with low back pain. *N Engl J Med* 1998;339(15):1021–1029.
31. Yeomans, SG. *The clinical application of outcomes assessment*. Stamford, CT: Appleton & Lange, 2000.
32. Linton SJ, Hallden K. Risk factors and the natural course of acute and recurrent musculoskeletal pain: Developing a screening instrument. In: Jensen TS, Turner JA, Wiesenfeld-Hallin Z, eds. *Proceedings of the 8th World Congress on Pain, Progress in Pain Research and Management*, Vol 8. Seattle: IASP Press, 1997.
33. Bernstein IH, Jaremko ME, Hinkley BS. On the utility of the SCL-90-R with low-back pain patients. *Spine* 1994;19:42–48.
34. Beck A. *Depression: Clinical, experimental and theoretical aspects*. New York: Harper & Row, 1967.
35. Liebenson CS, Yeomans SG. Yellow Flags: Early identification of risk factors of chronicity in acute patients. *J Rehabil Outcomes Meas* 2000;4(2):31–40.
36. Frank JW, Kerr MS, Brooker AS, et al. Disability resulting from occupational low back pain, Part I: What do we know about primary prevention? a review of the scientific evidence on prevention before disability begins. *Spine* 1996;21:2908–2917.
37. Frank J, Sinclair S, Hogg-Johnson S, et al. Preventing disability from work-related low-back pain. New evidence gives new hope—if we can just get all the players onside. *Can Med Assoc J*1998;158:1625–1631.
38. Cherkin DC, Deyo RA, Street JH, Barlow W. Predicting poor outcomes for back pain seen in primary

care using patients' own criteria. *Spine* 1996;21:2900–2907.

39. McIntosh G, Frank J, Hogg-Johnson S, Bombardier C, Hall H. Prognostic factors for time receiving workers' compensation benefits in a cohort of patients with low back pain. *Spine* 2000;25:147–157.
40. Selim AJ, Xinhua SR, Graeme F, et al.. The importance of radiating leg pain in assessing health outcomes among patients with low back pain. *Spine* 1998:23:470–474.
41. Lancourt J, Ketteljut M. Predicting return to work for lower back pain patients receiving worker's compensation. *Spine* 1992;17:629–640.
42. Gatchel R, Polatin PB, Kinney RK. Predicting outcome of chronic back pain using clinical predictors of psychopathology: A prospective analysis. *Health Psychol* 1995;14:415–420.
43. Epping-Jordan JE, Wahlgren DR, Williams RA, et al. Transitionto chronic pain in men with low-back pain: Predictive relationships among pain intensity, disability, and depressive symptoms. *Health Psychol* 1998;17:421–427.
44. van den Hoogen HJM, Koes BW, Deville W, van Eijk JTM, Bouter LM. The prognosis of low back pain in general practice. *Spine* 1997;22:1515–1521
45. Lanier DC, Stockton P. Clinical predictors of outcome of actue episodes of low-back pain. *J Fam Pract* 1988;27:483–489.
46. Klenerman L, Slade P, Stanley I, et al. The prediction of chronicity in patients with an acute attack of low back pain in a general practice setting. *Spine* 1995;20:478–484.
47. Coste J, Delecoeuillerie G, Cohen De Lara A, Le Parc JM, Paolaggi J. Clinical course and prognositc factors in acute low back pain: An inception cohort study in primary care practice. *BMJ* 1994;308:577–580.
48. Haldorsen EMH, Inhalhl A, Ursin H. Patients with low-back pain not returning to work. A 12-month follow-up study. *Spine* 1998;23:1202–1208.
49. Takala EP, Vikari-Juntura E. Do functional tests predict low back pain. *Spine* 2000;25(16):2126–2132.
50. Werneke M, Hart DL. Centralization phenomenon as a prognostic factor for chronic low back pain and disability. *Spine* 2001;26:758–765.
51. Linton SJ, Hallden BH. Can we screen for problematic back pain? A screening questionnaire for predicting outcome in acute and subacute back pain. *Clin J Pain* 1998;14:1–7.
52. Hazard RG, Haugh LD, Reid S, Preble JB, MacDonald L. Early prediction of chronic disability after occupational low back injury. *Spine* 1996;21:945–951.
53. Cats-Baril WL, Frymoyer JW. Demographic factors associated with the prevalence of disability n the general population: Analysis of the NHANES I database. *Spine* 1991;16:671–674.
54. Williams RM, Myers AM. A new approach to measuring recovery in injured workers with acute low back pain: Resumption of activities of daily living scale. *Phys Ther* 1998;78:613–623.
55. Hoogendoorn WE, van Poppel MN, Bongers PM, et al. Systematic review of psychosocial factors at work and private life as risk factors for back pain. *Spine* 2000;25:2114–2125.
56. Breen AC. Effectiveness of common treatments for back pain. *Euro J Chiropractic* 2002;49:47–53.
57. van Tulder MW, Esmail R, Bombardier C, Koes BW. Back schools for non-specific low back pain (Cochrane review). In: The Cochrane Library, Issue 1. Oxford, Update Software, 2001:1.
58. van Tulder MW, Ostelo RWJG, Vlaeyen JWS, Linton SJ, Morley SJ, Assendelft WJJ. Behavioural treatment for chronic low back pain (Cochrane review). In: The Cochrane Library, Issue 1. Oxford: Update Software, 2001:2.
59. Karjalainen K, Malmivaara A, van Tulder M, et al. Multidisciplinary biopsychosocial rehabilitation for subacute low back pain among working age adults (Cochrane review). In: The Cochrane Library, Issue 1. Oxford: Update Software, 2001.
60. Evans G, Richards S. *Low back pain: An evaluation of therapeutic interventions*. Bristol: Health Care Evaluation Unit, University of Bristol; 1996.
61. Faas A. Exercises: Which ones are worth trying, for which patients and when? *Spine* 1996;21(24):2874–2879.
62. Waddell G, McIntosh A, et al. *Low back pain evidence review*. London, Royal College of General Practitioners, 1999.
63. van Tulder MW, Malmivaara A, Esmail R, Koes BW. Exercise therapy for low back pain (Cochrane review). In: The Cochrane Library, Issue 1. Oxford: Update Software, 2001:3.
64. Agency for Health Care Policy Research. . *Management guidelines for acute back pain*. Washington DC:AHCPR, US Department of Health and Human Services, 1994.
65. Koes BW, Scholten RJP, Mens JMA, Bouter LM. Efficacy of NSAIDs for low back pain: A systematic review of randomised controlled trials of 11 interventions. In: van Tulder MW, Koes BW, Bouter LM, eds. *Low back pain in primary care: Effectiveness of diagnostic and therapeutic interventions*. Amsterdam: Institute for Research in Extramural Medicine, 1996:pp 171–190.
66. Shekelle PG, Adams AH, Chassin MR, Hurwitz EL, Brook RH. Spinal manipulation for low back pain. *Ann Int Med* 1992;117(7):590–598.
67. Assendelft WJJ, Morton S, Yu E, Shekelle PG. The relative effectiveness of therapy that includes spinal manipulation compared to other therapies for patients with low back pain: A meta-regression analysis of randomised clinical trials. *Proceedings of the 5th International Forum for Primary Care Research on Low-Back Pain*, Montreal, Canada, May 2002.
68. Furlan AD, Brosseau L, Welch V, Wong J. Massage for low back pain (Cochrane review). In: The Cochrane Library, Issue 1. Oxford: Update Software, 2001.
69. van Tulder MW, Cherkin DC, Berman B, Lao L, Koes BW. Acupuncture for low back pain (Cochrane review). In: The Cochrane Library, Issue 1. Oxford: Update Software, 2001:4.
70. van Tulder MW, Jellema P, van Poppel MNM, Nachemson AL, Bouter LM. Lumbar supports for prevention and treatment of low back pain (Cochrane

review). In: The Cochrane Library, Issue 1. Oxford: Update Software, 2001:5.
71. Hagen K, Jamtvedt G, Hilde G, Winnem M. The updated cochrane review of bed rest for low back pain and sciatica. *Spine* Mar 1;30(5):542–546.
72. De Craen AJM et al. Analgesic efficacy and safety of paracetamol-codeine combinations versus paracetamol alone: A systematic review. *Br Med J* 1996;313: 321–325.
73. Henry D, Lim LLY, Rodriguez LAG, et al. Variability in risk of gastrointestinal complications with individual non-steroidal anti-inflammatory drugs: Results of a collaborative meta-analysis. *BMJ* 1996;312:1563–1566.
74. van Tulder MW, Koes BW, Bouter LM, eds. *Low back pain in primary care: Effectiveness of diagnostic and therapeutic interventions.* Amsterdam: Institute for Research in Extramural Medicine, 1996:171–190.
75. Aronoff GM, Feldman, JB. Preventing disability from chronic pain: A review and reappraisal. *Int Rev Psychiatry* 2000;12:157–169.
76. Melzack R. Pain and stress: A new perspective. In: Gatechel RJ, Turk DC eds. *Psychosocial factors in pain: Critical perspectives.* New York: Guildford Press, 1999: Chapt. 6, 89–106.
77. Antonovsky H, Sagy S. The development of a sense of coherence and its impact on responses to stress situations. *J Social Psychol* 1986;126(2):213–225.
78. Streiner DL, Norman GR. *Health measurement scales: A practical guide to their development and use*, 2nd ed. New York: Oxford University Press, 1995.
79. Last JM. *A dictionary of epidemiology*, 3rd ed. New York: Oxford University Press, 1995.
80. De Bruin AF, Diederiks JP, de Witte LP, et al. Assessing the responsiveness of a functional status measure: The Sickness Impact Profile versus the SIP68. *J Clin Epidemiol* 1997;50:529–540.
81. Bolton JE. On the responsiveness of evaluative measures. *Eur J Chiropractic* 1997;45:5–8.
82. Juniper EF, Guyatt GH, et al. Determining a minimal important change in a disease-specific quality of life questionnaire. *J Clinl Epidemiol* 1994;47(1):81–87.
83. Alaranta H, Hurri H, Heliovaara M, et al. Non-dynamometric trunk performance tests: Reliability and normative data. *Scand J Rehab Med* 1994;26:211–215.
84. Rissanen A, Allaranta H, Sainio P, Harkonen H. Isokinetic and Non-dynamometric tests in low back pain patients related to pain and disability index. *Spine* 1994;19:1963–1967.
85. Fairbank J, Davies J, et al. The Oswestry Low Back Pain Disability Questionnaire. *Physiotherapy* 1980; 66(18):271–273.
86. Roland M, Fairbank J. The Roland-Morris Disability Questionnaire and the Oswestry Disability Questionnaire. *Spine* 2000;25:3115–3124.
87. Bolton JE, Breen AC. The Bournemouth Questionnaire: A short-form comprehensive outcome measure. I. Psychometric properties in back pain patients. *J Manipulative Physiol Ther* 1999;22:503–510
88. Bolton JE, Humphreys BK. The Bournemouth Questionnaire: A short-form comprehensive outcome measure. II. Psychometric properties in neck pain patients. *J Manipulative Physiol Ther* 2002;25:141–148.
89. Fishbain DA, Khalil TM, Abdel-Moty A, et al. Physician limitation when assessing work capacity: A review. *J Back Musculoskelet Rehabil* 1995;5:107–113.
90. Mayer TG, Polatin P, Smith B, et al. Contemporary concepts in spine care: Spine rehabilitation—secondary and tertiary non-operative care. *Spine* 1995; 20:18:2060–2066.
91. Ware JE, Sherbourne CD. The MOS 36-item Short Form Health Survey (SF-36). *Med Care* 1992;30:473–483.
92. Ware JE Jr., Kosinski M, Keller SD. *SF-12: How to score the SF-12 physical the mental health summary scales*, 2nd ed. Boston: The Health Institute, New England Medical Center, 1995.
93. Deyo RA. Comparative validity of the Sickness Impact Profile. *Spine* 1986;11:951.
94. Cherkin D, MacCormack F. Patient evaluations of low-back pain are from family physicians and chiropractors, *Western J Med* 1989;150:351–355.
95. Bigos S, Battie M, Spengler DM, et al. A prospective study of work perceptions and psychosocial factors affecting the report of back injury. *Spine* 1991;16:1–6.
96. Kendall NAS, Linton SJ, Main CJ. *Guide to assessing psychosocial yellow flags in acute low back pain: risk factors for long-term disability and work loss.* Wellington, New Zealand: Accident Rehabilitation & Compensation Insurance Corporation of New Zealand and the National Health Committee, 1997.
97. Grevitt M, Pande K, O'dowd J, Webb J. Do first impressions count? A comparison of subjective and psychologic assessment of spinal patients. *Eur Spine J* 1998;7:218–223.
98. Hunt SM, McEwen J, McKenna SP. Measuring health status: A new tool for clinicians and epidemiologists. *J R Coll Gen Pract* 1985;35:185–188.
99. Nelson EC, Landgraf JM, Hays RD, et al. The COOP function charts: a system to measure patient function in physicians' offices. In: Lipkin M Jr, ed. *Functional status measurement in primary care: Frontiers of primary care.* New York: Springer-Verlag, 1990:97–131.
100. Ware JE Jr. SF-36 Health survey update. *Spine* 2000;23:3130–3139.
101. Price DD, Bush FM, Long S, Harkins SW. A comparison of pain measurement characteristics of mechanical visual analogue and simple numerical rating scales. *Pain* 1994;56:216–226.
102. Guilford JP. *Psychometric methods.* New York: McGraw-Hill, 1954:597.
103. Jensen MP, Karoly P. Self-report scales and procedures for assessing pain in adults. In: Turk DC, Melzack, eds. *Handbook of pain assessment.* New York: Guilford Press, 1993.
104. Scott J, Huskisson EC. Graphic representation of pain. *Pain* 1976;2:175–184.
105. Price DD, Harkins SW, Baker C. Sensory-affective relationships among different types of clinical and experimental pain. *Pain* 1986;28:297–307.
106. Price DD, Harkins SW, Rafii A, Price C. A simultaneous comparison of fentanyl's analgesic effects on experimental and clinical pain. *Pain* 1986;24:197–203.

107. Price DD, Harkins SW. The combined use of experimental pain and visual aalogue scales in providing standardized measurement of clinical pain. *Clin J Pain* 1987;3:1–8.
108. Price DD, McGrath PA, Rafii A, Buckingham B. The validation of visual analogue scales as ratio scale measures for chronic and experimental pain. *Pain* 1983;17:45–46.
109. Haldeman S, Chapman-Smith D, Peterson DM Jr. *Guidelines for chiropractic quality assurance and practice paramenters*. Gaithersburg, MD: Aspen, 1993.
110. Bolton JE, Wilkinson RC. Responsiveness of pain scales: A comparison of three pain intensity measures in chiropractic patients. *J Manipulative Physiol Ther* 1998;21:1–7.
111. Chapman-Smith D. Measuring results—The new importance of patient questionnaires. *Chiro Rep* 1992; 7(1):1–6.
112. McDowell I, Newell C. *Measuring health: A guide to rating scales and questionnaires*. Oxford: Oxford University Press, 1987.
113. Downie WW, Leatham PA, Rhind VA, et al. Studies with pain rating scales. *Anal Rheum Dis* 1978;37:378–381.
114. Jensen MP, Karoly P, Braver S. The measurement of clinical pain intensity: A comparison of six methods. *Pain* 1986;27:117–126.
115. Feuerstein M. Multidisciplinary rehabilitation of occupational musculoskeletal disorders: Rationale, assessment strategies and clinical interventions. In: LACC Chiropractic Rehabilitation, Chicago, Session 1, September 23–24, 1995: class notes, pp. 87.
116. Tait RC, Chibnall JT, Margolis RB. Pain extent: Relations with psychological state, pain severity, pain history and disability. *Pain* 1990;41:295–301.
117. Kirkaldy-Willis WH. *Managing low back pain*. New York: Churchill Livingstone, 1983:635.
118. Uden A, Astrom M, Bergenudd H. Pain drawings in chronic low back pain. *Spine* 1988;13:389–392.
119. Parker H, Wood PLR, Main CJ. The uses of the pain drawing as a screening measure to predict psychological distress in chronic low back pain. *Spine* 1995;20:236–243.
120. Ohlund C, Eek C, Palmblad S, Areskoug B, Nachemson A. Quantified pain drawing in subacute low back pain: Validation in a non-selected outpatient industrial sample. *Spine* 1996;21:1021–1031.
121. Roland M, Morris R. A study of the natural history of back pain: Part I: Development of a reliable and sensitive measure of disability in low-back pain. *Spine* 1983;8:141–144.
122. Roland M, Morris R. A study of the natural history of low back pain:Part II. *Spine* 1983;8(2):145–150.
123. Deyo RA. Comparative validity of the Sickness Impact Profile. *Spine* 1986;11:951.
124. Von Korff M, Saunders K. The course of back pain in primary care. *Spine* 1996;21:2833–2839.
125. Stratford PW, Binkely JM, Riddle DL, Guyatt GH. Sensitivity to change of the Roland-Morris Back Pain Questionnaire: Part 1. *Phys Ther* 1998;78:1186–1196.
126. Stratford PW, Binkley JM. Measurement properties of the RM18: A modified version of the Roland-Morris Disability Scale. *Spine* 1997;22:2416–2421.
127. Erhard RE, Delitto A, Cibulka MT. Relative effectiveness of an extension program and a combined program of manipulation and flexion and extension exercises in patients with acute low back syndrome. *Phys Ther* 1994;74:1093–1100.
128. Leclaire R, Blier F, Fortin L, Proulx R. A cross-sectional study comparing the Oswestry and Roland-Morris functional disability scales in two populations of patients with low back pain with different levels of severity. *Spine* 1997;22:68–71.
129. Baker DJ, Pynsent PB, Fairbank J, et al. The Oswestry disability index revisited: Its reliability, repeatability and validity, and a comparison with the St. Thomas's disability index. In: Roland M, Jenner JR, eds. *Back pain: New approaches to rehabilitation and education*. Manchester, UK: Manchester University Press, 1989:174–86.
130. Yang Y, Eaton S, Maxwell MW. The relationship between the St. Thomas and Oswestry Disability scores and the severity of low back pain. *J Manipulative Physiol Ther* 1983;16:14–18.
131. Hudson-Cook N, Times-Nicholson K, Breen AC. A revised Oswestry disability questionnaire. In: Roland M, Jenner J, eds. *Back pain. New approaches to rehabilitation and education*. Manchester, UK: Manchester University Press; 1989:187–204.
132. Breen AC, Preutu G. A revised Oswestry Disability Index (RODQ2). *Proceedings of the 4th International Forum for Primary Care Research on Low Back Pain*, Eilat, Israel, March 2000.
133. Kopec JA, Esdaile JM, Abrahamowicz M, Abenhaim L, Wood-Dauphinee S, Lamping DL. The Quebec Back Pain Disability Scale: Measurement properties. *Spine* 1995;20:341–352.
134. Deyo RA, Andersson G, Bombardier C, et al. Outcome measures for studying patients with low back pain. *Spine* 1994;19:2032S–2036S.
135. Harper AC, Harper DA, Lambert LJ, et al. Development and validation of the Curtin Back Screening Questionnaire (CBSQ). *Pain* 1995;6:73–81.
136. Turner JA, Robinson J, McCreary CP. Chronic low back pain: Predicting response to nonsurgical treatment. *Arch Phys Med Rehabil* 1983;64:560–563.
137. Yellen AN. Doctoral dissertation, California School of Professional Psychology, 1978.
138. Greenough CG, Fraser RD. Assessment of outcome in patients with low back pain. *Spine* 1992;17:36–41.
139. Ruta DA, Garratt AM, Wardlaw D, Russell IT. Developing a valid and reliable measure of health outcome for patients with low back pain. *Spine* 1994;19:1887–1896.
140. Stucki G, Daltroy L, Liang MH, Lipson SJ, Fossel AH, Katz JN. Measurement properties of a self-administered outcome measure in lumbar spinal stenosis. *Spine* 1996;21:796–803.
141. Waddell G. A new clinical model for the treatment of low back pain. *Spine* 1987;12:632–644.

142. Bolton JE. Future directions for outcomes research in back pain. *Eur J Chiropractic* 1997;45:57–64.
143. Cherkin D, Deyo RA, Berg AO. Evaluation of a physician education intervention to improve primary care for low-back pain: II. Impact on patients. *Spine* 1991;16:1173–1178.
144. Hudak PL, Wright JG. The characteristics of patient satisfaction measures. *Spine* 2000;25:3167–3177.
145. Good MD, Smilkstein G, Good BJ, Shaffer T, Aarons T. The family APGAR index: A study of construct validity. *J Fam Pract* 1979;8:577–582.
146. Smilkstein G. The family APGAR: A proposal for family function test and its use by physicians. *J Fam Pract* 1978;6:1231–1235.
147. Bigos SJ, Spengler DM, Martin NA, et al. Back injuries in industry: A retrospective study. II. Employee-related factors. *Spine* 1986;11:252–256.
148. Von Korff M, Jensen MP, Karoly P. Assessing global pain severity by self-report in clinical and health services research. *Spine* 2000;25:3140–51.
149. Ekstrand J, Wiktorsson M, Oberg B, Gillquist J. Lower extremity goniometric measurements: A study to determine their reliability. *Arch Phys Med Rehab* 1982;63:171–175.
150. American Medical Association. *Guides to the evaluation of permanent impairment*, 5th ed. Chicago, IL: AMA Press, 2001.
151. Mayor TG, Tencer A, Kristoferson S, Mooney V. Use of noninvasive techniques for quantification of spinal range-of-motion in normal subjects and chronic low-back dysfunction patients. *Spine* 1984;9:588–595.
152. Mayer TG, Gatchel RJ, Keeley J, Mayer H, Richling D. A male incumbent worker industrial database. *Spine* 1994;19:762–764.
153. Waddell G, McCulloch JA, Kummel E, Venner RM. Nonorganic physical signs in low-back pain. *Spine* 1980;5:117–125.
154. McGill SM, Childs A, Liebenson C. Endurance times for low back stabilization exercises: Clinical targets for testing and training from a normal database. *Arch Phys Med Rehabil* 1999;80:941–44.
155. Wang S, Whitney SL, Burdett RG, et al. Lower extremity muscular flexibility in long distance runners. *J Orthop Sports Phys Ther* 1993;2:102–107.
156. Bohannon RW, Larkin PA, Cook AC, Gear J, Singer J. Decrease in timed balance test scores with aging. *Phys Ther* 1984;64:1067–1070.
157. Stones M, Kozma A. Balance and age in the sighted and blind. *Arch Phys Med Rehabil* 1987;68:85–89.
158. Briggs RC, Gossman MR, Birch R, Drews J, Shaddeau S. Balance performance among noninstitutionalized elderly women. *Phys Ther* 1989;69:748–756.
159. Johansson G, Jarnlo G-B. Balance training in 70-year-old women. *Physiother Theory Pract* 1991;7:121–125.
160. Byl N, Sinnot PL. Variations in balance and body sway in middle-aged adults: Subjects with healthy backs compared with subjects with low-back dysfunction. *Spine* 1991;16:325–330.
161. Loebl W. Measurements of spinal posture and range in spinal movements *Ann Phys Med* 1967;9:103–110.
162. Vernon HT, Aker P, Aramenko M, et al. Evaluation of neck muscle strength with a modified sphygmomanometer dynamometer: Reliability and validity. *J Manipulative Physiol Ther* 1992;15:343–349.
163. Triano JJ, Schultz AB. Correlation of objective measures of trunk motion and muscle function with low back disability rating. *Spine* 1987;12:561–565.
164. Yeomans SG, Pomplin C. Normative data for the chin flexion test. Manuscript in preparation.
165. Basmajian JV, Nyberg R. *Rational manual therapies*. Baltimore, MD: Williams and Wilkins, 1993:47.
166. Chesworth BM, Padfield BJ, Helewa A, Stitt LW. A comparison of hip mobility in patients with low back pain and matched healthy subjects. *Physiother Canada* 1994;46:267–274.
167. Ellison JB, Rose SJ, Sahrmann SA. Patterns of hip rotation range of motion: A comparison between healthy subjects and patients with low back pain. *Phys Ther* 1990;70:537–541.
168. Swanson AB, Matev IB, de Groot Swanson G. The strength of the hand. *Bull Prosthet Res Fall* 1970;145–53.
169. World Health Organisation. *International classification of functioning, disability and health*. Geneva: WHO, 2001.

CHAPTER

15

McKENZIE PROTOCOLS FOR MECHANICAL ASSESSMENT OF THE LOW BACK

Steven Heffner, Robin McKenzie, and Ronald Donelson

OUTLINE

OBJECTIVES

1. Describe and differentiate the derangement, dysfunction and postural syndromes.
2. Describe and differentiate between the McKenzie syndromes and other spinal conditions.
3. Describe the epidemiological factors associated with low back pain.
4. Describe the risk and prognostic factors of low back pain.
5. Describe the components of the History section of the McKenzie Assessment form and the clinical relevance of each.
6. Discuss the aims of the physical examination.
7. Accurately complete the history and clinical examination sections of the Standard McKenzie assessment forms for the lumbar spine.

INTRODUCTION

This chapter concerns a musculoskeletal assessment protocol developed by Robin McKenzie for the purpose of diagnosing and treating spinal complaints based on the mechanical and symptomatic responses to loading. In its abbreviated form, this has been referred to as mechanical diagnosis and therapy (MDT) of the spine. In 1959 McKenzie had been treating a person with a 10-day episode of low back and leg pain, without any significant resolution of complaints. The patient had mistakenly laid down prone on a treatment table, which positioned his lumbar spine into hyperextension and, much to the surprise of both the patient and McKenzie, the predominant leg complaints had resolved with back complaints increasing somewhat. The patient felt that his change of symptoms was for the better. It took little time for McKenzie to put all patients within the clinic in such a position and, although many responded favorably to such positionings, some did not change. In fact, some were affected adversely.

This represented the beginning of a meticulous exploration of the use of repeated movements and sustained positionings for the purpose of examining and treating low back disorders[1] and, subsequently, the cervicothoracic spine[2] and extremities[3] as well.

Recognizable patterns (which predicated specific treatment protocols) and responses to movements and positionings gradually emerged. The most intriguing response was the *centralization* of symptoms in response to certain end-range loading strategies. McKenzie defined the term *centralization* to mean the reduction of symptoms such as pain and paresthesia from the periphery, or extremities, to the torso. This definition contrasts a second term, known as *peripheralization*, which means an increase in symptoms from the torso to the extremities or periphery. It was discovered that the phenomenon of centralization offered optimistic prognostication; so various strategies were developed subsequently to promote centralization. In most cases, the patient's self-treatment played a crucial role in the utilization and success of these strategies. Diligent investigation and classification on the part of McKenzie led to the delineation of three mechanical syndromes (i.e., three syndromes amenable to mechanical therapy). Furthermore, a supporting philosophy emphasizing self-treatment, both therapeutically and prophylactically, was introduced. The strategic activities of the patient for treatment increased while the role of the clinician diminished in this system. In a sense, it was a Copernican revolution in physical medicine wherein the patient no longer revolved around the practitioner. Rather, just the reverse came true.

The McKenzie approach has gained acceptance by clinicians of various degrees and specialties around the world. This method, like this textbook, is for all professionals in all countries.

LIFESTYLE FACTORS

In his personal research of low back pain (LBP), McKenzie noticed certain frequent predisposing lifestyle factors.

The first factor he noticed was *poor sitting posture*. "Slouched" sitting places the spine in flexion and duplicates the flexed standing posture, thus perpetuating at rest the strains present during work. In the sitting position, the more the lumbar spine approximates kyphosis, the higher the intradiscal pressure. The more the spine approximates lordosis, the lower the intradiscal pressure. The slouched position also causes end-range overstretch of the posterior spinal ligamentous structures. Some LBP is caused and almost all LBP is aggravated by poor sitting posture.

The second factor McKenzie noticed was the *frequency of lumbopelvic forward flexion in our lifestyle*. Between rising from bed in the morning until returning to bed in the night man is constantly flexed.

The third factor he noticed was *lack of lumbopelvic extension*. During the diurnal cycle man also rarely extends.

These three predisposing factors combined lead to loss of lumbopelvic extension.

McKenzie developed a system of classifications based on a pattern of responses for conditions amenable to mechanical (movement and positioning) therapies. These patterns are then assigned an *inferred* pathological process, not vice versa. Spinal complaints amenable to mechanical therapy are classified under one of three mechanical and symptomatic response patterns: the *postural syndrome*, *dysfunction syndrome*, and *derangement syndrome*.

POSTURAL SYNDROME

Patients with this syndrome suffer from symptoms secondary to maintaining end-range loading positioning for extended periods. This can be true in any end-range position but the vast majority of patients suffer with sitting postural syndrome. This is causal in nature to the sedentary vocations of most workers throughout the industrialized world.

The stereotypical complaints associated with the postural syndrome usually begin insidiously after long hours of sitting and progress to the point that it takes less and less time sitting to provoke the symptoms. These patients may go days without any complaints. The clinician will not usually see these patients in for treatment in the acute or subacute stages because they can abolish the symptoms themselves by aborting the end range that is precipitating their pain. They are generally not desperate patients because they can control their pain by changing their posture or getting up and moving around. However, because they are oblivious to the causal nature of their symptoms they cannot maintain the pain-free status. Therefore, these patients present to the clinician's office when they are tired of the chronic nature of their pain. Other reasons include unacceptable frequency of recurrences, more easily provoked recurrences as time passes, or because the symptoms are interfering with their life or work style in a manner that is no longer acceptable.

The subjective history will always indicate a central or symmetrical pain distribution that many times will be present in the thoracic and cervical areas also. There are never any radiating symptoms and the symptoms are never provoked by movement, but rather by the offensive, static position.

The pain associated with the postural syndrome is always intermittent. There will be no loss of movement present. No scoliotic deformity (relevant to pain) will be present and there will be no objective orthopedic or neurological signs or associated pathology present.

Examination does not reveal any altered mechanics (loss of motion, deviation from the intended movement plane) nor is there any pain during movement. When these patients are active (frequently changing positions, not remaining at any particular end range), there are no complaints. Most commonly, the culpable end ranges relate to poor sitting posture. With poor sitting posture, the end ranges assumed are extension of the upper cervical spine and flexion of lower cervical, thoracic, and lumbosacral articulations.

The McKenzie classification system follows strict assessment guidelines to determine this syndrome. As stated above, there are very few pure McKenzie postural syndrome classifications, but poor posture will almost universally be present in all mechanical patients evaluated with this protocol. As such, clinically relevant, secondary postural syndrome complications may arise that require appropriate interventions. Such interventions will be described in the McKenzie treatment chapter (Chapter 22) of this textbook.

DYSFUNCTION SYNDROME

The dysfunction syndrome is the second of the McKenzie method. The patients with this syndrome present a clinical picture demonstrating a loss of mobility in a specific movement plane. It is frequently a saggital direction, restricted in either flexion or extension, and secondary to a trauma and/or surgical intervention, producing significant scar tissue. Such adaptively shortened scar tissue tends to restrict mobility. There will be no pain or loss of mobility in any other direction except the compromised motion. End-range pain in the affected direction will always be present and will not rapidly change, neither improving nor worsening, with repetition of the movement to end-range pain.

The subjective history will be that of a condition that is greater than 6 weeks of duration. The pain will always be intermittent and unchanging. There will be no rapidly reversible deformity (i.e., antalgia, lordosis, kyphosis, scoliosis) present. The patient will usually be over 30 years of age, deconditioned, and demonstrate poor posture.

A true dysfunction syndrome is also infrequently treated because patients with this classification are frequently able to self-manage the problem. In the postural syndrome, the patients can control their symptoms by discontinuing or avoiding the provoking static posture, whereas in the dysfunction syndrome, the patients can control their symptoms by avoiding the provoking motion. They are fine as long as that avoidance does not affect daily function. Patients with dysfunction syndrome will be observed in a clinical setting, but this is frequently an incidental finding, secondary to a derangement syndrome (see below) being present.

As stated above, the dysfunction syndrome cause is *inferred* to be by mechanical deformation of short tissues that have undergone adaptive shortening. This is known by many terms such as shortening, scarring, contracture, fibrosis, myofascial shortening, hypertonicity, spasm, etc.

The concept of shortened tissue is not unique among those clinicians involved in the treatment of musculoskeletal conditions, although correctness of this determination is questionable. Tissues may be assumed shortened wherever patients localize complaints, whether or not the clinician confirmed the assumption on examination by palpation and/or motion testing. For example, low back muscles are often lengthened in individuals who can place their hands on the ground but have lost two thirds of their extension.

Within the McKenzie conceptual framework, one can see how the postural syndrome may lead to adaptive shortening of other regional tissues. On the basis of the postural distortion of sitting, one might expect a loss of upper cervical flexion and extension of all lower spinal areas.[4] Appropriate treatment protocols for the dysfunction syndrome will be addressed in detail in the McKenzie treatment chapter (Chapter 22) of this textbook.

DERANGEMENT SYNDROME

The patterns associated with the derangement syndrome are more complicated than those associated with the postural and dysfunction syndromes. In some patients, all the possible attributes of a derangement syndrome are displayed. In other patients, only partial patterns are noticed.

In patients with the derangement classification, one can see rapid changes in response to movement and positioning of the spine. The changes can be beneficial or detrimental depending on the loading direction evaluated.

It is *inferred* that this syndrome is due to the mechanical deformation of soft tissue as a result of derangement of internal joint structures. For the spine, the corresponding structure would be the semiviscous nucleus pulposis and its effect on the surrounding annulus and associated/neighboring neurological structures. Depending on the degree of this derangement, symptoms may be constant or intermittent, determined by the patient's movements and positions during the day as it affects nuclear positioning. When derangements are severe, fixed deformities or antalgias can result, known as acute kyphosis, acute scoliosis, or acute lumbar lordosis. In these cases, nuclear material is assumed to have migrated posteriorly, laterally, or anteriorly, respectively.

In regards to the subjective history, there is always mechanical loss of motion in one direction and frequently several directions. The pain can be constant or intermittent and may have been present for months or hours. The symptoms can be central, symmetrical, unilateral, radicular, and/or even cause scoliotic deformities. Because of the chameleon-like tendencies of this syndrome, McKenzie developed a subclassification of derangements secondary to the subjective complaints and/or the presence of a postural deformity. These have specific attributes and are treated separately.[5] These will be discussed in length in the treatment chapter.

Like the postural syndrome, the derangement syndrome cannot be resolved until deleterious end ranges are avoided. Like the dysfunction syndrome, resolution also involves challenging range of motion losses to recover motion. For the dysfunction syndrome, the challenge is to remodel shortened tissue; for the derangement syndrome it is to reposition displaced nuclear material.

Like the postural syndrome, the culpable or pain-provoking end range of the derangement syndrome is avoided. Contrary to the postural syndrome, loading at the culpable end range in the derangement syndrome would cause mechanical responses (there are none in the postural syndrome) and symptomatic responses, both of which may persist after the culpable end-range loading ceases. In other words, the derangement syndrome end-range loading is avoided in the direction that is *symptomatically impeded.* Like the dysfunction syndrome, end-range loading is pursued in the direction that is *mechanically impeded.*[1–3] For the derangement syndrome, movement is obstructed owing to intra-articular (intradiscal) displacement vs. the dysfunction syndrome where motion was *limited* by what is conceived to be *extra-articular* shortening of muscle, tendon, ligament, fascia, nerve root adherence, etc.

The Derangement Syndrome Subclassifications

The derangement syndrome has seven subclassifications. These subcategories will be discussed in greater detail in Chapter 22, which will also cover McKenzie treatment protocols in detail.

The seven subclassifications are briefly listed below[6]:

1. Derangement 1: Acentral symmetrical symptom pattern that does not extend to the extremities.
2. Derangement 2: This is the same as Derangement 1, but with a fixed kyphotic deformity.
3. Derangement 3: Unilateral symptoms extending to the knee.
4. Derangement 4: This is the same as Derangement 3, but with a fixed scoliotic deformity.
5. Derangement 5: Unilateral symptoms extending below the knee.
6. Derangement 6: This is the same as Derangement 5, but with a fixed scoliotic deformity.
7. Derangement 7: This is the same as Derangement 1, but with an accentuated lumbar lordosis.

COMMON MISCONCEPTIONS REGARDING McKENZIE THERAPY

There are five main misconceptions concerning McKenzie treatment.

Misconception #1: Extension is the only direction used in McKenzie protocols. Because typically people perform forward flexion hundreds of times per day, extension is more often the treatment direction applicable in this treatment. But there are many times when there is a derangement, where extension in loaded and unloaded positions is deleterious or at least of questionable benefit. It is at that time that frontal or transverse movements are the direction of choice. In fact, one of the derangement syndromes' subclassifications is an anterior derangement and flexion is the loading strategy of choice.[4]

Misconception #2: McKenzie protocol is a self-treatment program only. Robin McKenzie stresses the rationale for trying all potential of the patients' self-treatment options before any therapeutic intervention occurs. It comes as a great surprise to most of the clinicians who attend a McKenzie conference/seminar that instructors actually do touch the patient and even manipulate or mobilize the patient if necessary. But the progression of force is performed only when the self-treatment protocol is not enough to centralize or abolish the symptoms.[4]

Misconception #3: McKenzie protocol addresses only the disc. The primary goal of the McKenzie approach is to establish empirical, logical, observations regarding how mechanical and symptomatic responses relate to variable loading strategies. The nucleus is not assumed to be the key component in all these cases. It is *inferred* to be so only when appropriate. McKenzie protocols will also *infer* other short tissues or processes are culpable if and when a reasonable determination comes forth. McKenzie himself stated that at the time of his writing of the lumbar spine book the disc was the only logical tissue to explain the derangement syndrome. If a better explanation were made available he would embrace it, but as yet none has come forth.[4]

Misconception #4: McKenzie protocols are too simple. In contrast, it has been the authors' experience that many practitioners have difficulty with the manner in which McKenzie protocols attempt to simplify things. The McKenzie protocols cause one to take a stark, sober look at the phenomena of spinal complaints, challenging practitioners to strip themselves of theories lacking empirical substance. In this model, simple maneuvers should be tried first, attempted before more complex approaches are instituted.[4]

Misconception #5: McKenzie protocols are just an exercise program. The McKenzie approach is a program that does include exercise. However, there are profound psychological elements involved as well. In fact, if the patient's movements (exercises) reduce any mechanical or symptomatic findings, this is considered to be progress. Should this fail and these findings persist, the McKenzie approach includes hands-on applications by the clinician utilizing mobilization and manipulation as an intervention, with the hopes of returning the patient to that exercise program so that they may soon become independent in self-care.[5]

Clinicians who attend McKenzie courses are frequently surprised to hear that the McKenzie system has a progression of forces that even involves spinal manipulation. The progression of forces consist of:

1. Self-treatment
2. Self-treatment with overpressure
3. Self-treatment with clinician overpressure
4. Mobilization
5. Manipulation

Once manipulative forces are indicated the directional movement is already established, movement further along that end-range plane is indicated. Therefore, MDT has helped clarify the reason and direction of manipulative forces of a treatment protocol.

THE PRESENTING PATIENT

The McKenzie practitioner, in essence, initially evaluates which patients may be amenable to mechanical therapy. This is somewhat different from determining which patients have "mechanical back pain."[8] Mechanical *diagnosis* evaluates static and dynamic loading within different movement planes to end range by means of history taking, examination, and during course of treatment. Not only are movement plane directions explored to determine a preferred, or beneficial, loading strategy, but also to find which movement plane directions loading might be detrimental. It is the strategic combination of the pursuit and avoidance of end-range loadings that is the game plan.

Patients may have back pain due to mechanical, chemical (inflammation due to trauma, infection, systemic disease), psychological, and/or other pathological causes (such as neoplasm).[7]

The purpose of a mechanical evaluation is to determine which spinal complaints are mechanical in nature and, therefore, amenable to mechanical therapies.

A patient who reports no mechanical signs or symptoms during mid-range and end-range motions, performed statically and/or dynamically, must be considered for the evaluation of nonmechanical causes of spinal complaints. It may not be prudent for a practitioner of MDT to manage those complaints.

Patients who complain of symptoms that are "constant" may very well be nonmechanical in nature. Therefore, such patients constitute the most important group to rule out "red flags" before initiating mechanical treatment protocols.

Chemical and inflammatory pain syndrome symptoms are, typically, symptomatically improved in the morning, after a night's rest. They are also better when the patient is stationary and worse with any and all movements mid range or at end range.

Complaints amenable to mechanical therapy are, more often, better when patients move around, worse when static, and, in the case of derangements, worse upon awakening in the morning when intradiscal pressures may be the greatest.[8]

If a patient's constant complaints do not appear to be amenable to movement and positioning tactics, the presence of a chemical, inflammatory process or mechanical derangement not amenable to mechanical therapies must be considered. A trial of anti-inflammatory measures may be explored for a short period of time in the hope that inflammation resolves, permitting beneficial mechanical and symptomatic responses to a preferred loading strategy.

THE McKENZIE EVALUATION FORMS

The McKenzie evaluation forms are practical tools used to discover and organize complaints amenable to mechanical therapies, and what those mechanical therapies should be. Such assessments are of course obtained through the process of the meticulous history and examination.

Subjective History

1. Where is the present pain? "Present" in this case means the symptoms (pain, paresthesia, numbness) within the past couple days, extending up to a week.

2. Where were the symptoms at onset? Did the symptoms begin local to the spine and gradually begin to radiate, or did they begin in the periphery?
3. How long has the pain been present? When did this episode begin?

Clinical Pearl: A derangement syndrome can occur for any time length but a dysfunction syndrome must be 6 weeks or greater.

4. How did the pain commence? The clinician searches for no apparent versus an apparent causation or incident for the pain. If there was a reason, gather information regarding the mechanics of the event.
5. Is the pain constant or intermittent? Do the symptoms come and go (actually shut-off in certain positions, with certain movements, etc.) or are they present all the time (may vary in intensity)?

Clinical Pearl: Constant pain indicates a derangement (if not chemical). Intermittent pain indicates a mechanical disorder, which may be a dysfunction or posture but does not rule out a derangement.

6. Better/Worse: Ascertain whether the following activities and positions make the symptoms better or worse. Determine which symptoms are affected; i.e., is it the back or leg pain that is worsened, etc.?
   - Bending: The effect of sustained or *repeated flexion* in a loaded (weight-bearing) position.
   - Sitting: The effect of *sustained flexion* in a loaded position.
   - Rising from sitting: Is there pain and difficulty in obtaining *curve reversal* (kyphosis to lordosis) after sustained flexion?
   - Standing: The effect of *sustained extension* in a loaded position.
   - Walking: The effect of *repeated extension* in a loaded position.
   - Lying: The effect of *unloading* the spine. Determine which positions affect the symptoms.
   - Morning: What is the effect of resting during the night upon waking before getting out of bed, as well as rising from the bed?
   - Evening: What is the effect of the day's activities on the symptoms?
   - Sleep Disturbed: Does pain prevent the patient from falling asleep, or is the sleep interrupted due to pain?
   - Cough/Sneeze: Looking for dural signs often associated with derangement.

Clinical Pearl: A derangement syndrome produces lasting changes with the above movements/positions. Dysfunction syndrome changes will not last. Postural syndrome will not have any changes with movement, only static positions.

Clinical Pearl: Ask the patient if there are associated mechanical (i.e., pain or movement) changes with the symptoms. If so, this indicates a derangement.

Clinical Pearl: This is probably the most important section of the subjective history. Understanding the mechanical effects that repetitive movements and static positioning have on the patient's symptoms prior to actually performing the testing facilitates and speeds the ensuing physical examination.

7. Previous history and treatment: Identify the first episode of back pain, as well as the number of episodes between that initial episode and the current episode. Determine the length of time to recover during previous episodes, and whether this episode differs from the previous ones. Then, determine, generally, which previous treatments have been provided and their outcome.

Clinical Pearl: Several prior episodes could be indicative of a derangement. Derangements have a pattern of producing symptoms that are short-lived and self-limiting. But they also show a pattern of subsequent episodes becoming more severe and 35% of recurring episodes produce sciatica.

8. X-rays: Have X-rays been taken during the episode to rule out serious pathology. What were the findings? Have other tests been performed (computerized axial tomography, magnetic resonance imaging, etc.)? If so, what were the findings?

Clinical Pearl: This section is used for "red flag" incidences only. Otherwise, the focus is what effect repetitive movements and static positioning have on their symptoms and mechanics.

9. General Health: Is there any evidence of serious pathology (unexplained weight loss, etc.), or other conditions that could affect the examination and treatment procedures?
10. Recent Surgery: Has there been recent surgery that could influence the patient's condition? Is there any reason not to perform repetitive movements on the patient?
11. Medications: Analgesics, non-steroidal anti-inflammatories (NSAID's) and steroids alter pain sensation, which compromises the patient's response to the movements of the McKenzie assessment. In addition, prolonged use of steroids can increase the risk of osteoporosis, another "red flag" that must be considered.

12. Accidents: Have there been any injuries that could have precipitated the onset of back pain, or influenced the clinical findings during the examination, or affected the treatment?
13. Bowel/Bladder: Is there evidence of S3–S4 compression, or cauda equina syndrome, which contraindicates mechanical therapy?

See Figure 15–1 for reference.

Examination

Examination While taking the history, have the patient sit without back support on the treatment table in order to observe the patient's postural habits. The sitting posture will be generally assessed, based on whether the patient sits fully slouched (rated as poor), fully erect (rated as good) or somewhere in-between (rated as fair). The clinician should also note the degree of lordosis present in the sitting position. Standing posture will be examined in the same manner, and again described as good, fair, or poor. The clinician must differentiate the assessment of postural habits standing for the presence of deformity (see Fig. 15–2 for reference).

Lordosis In the standing position, the clinician examines the patient for the presence of the deformities of either a fixed lordosis, or kyphosis. If either were present, one would suspect a possible Derangement 2.

Lateral Shift The clinician examines the patient's posture in the standing position for the presence of a lateral shift, which is defined as follows: A lateral shift is said to be present in the spine. When observed from behind, this lateral flexion appears to occur at about the level of the waist. The impression is created that the patient has a list or tilt to one side. This usually occurs at about the level of the fourth and fifth lumbar segments. There is frequently a compensatory curve seen at a higher spinal level. A right lateral shift, for example, is said to exist when the patient's upper half is listing or tilting to the right. The pelvis, in this example, will be prominent on the left. If the lateral shift is present, one should suspect a Derangement 4 or 6.

A standing radiological examination usually reveals that lateral flexion has occurred at the affected segment, thus causing the trunk to appear off-center.

Clinical Pearl: If the lateral shift is present, one should suspect a Derangement 4 or 6.

Approximately 9 out of every 10 subjects exhibiting a shift do so away from the painful side (contralateral shift). One in 10 lists toward the painful side (ipsilateral shift).[1]

The incidence of sciatica, and the incidence of neurological deficit, is higher in those patients with an ipsilateral shift than in those exhibiting a contralateral shift.[1]

The ipsilateral shift is resistant to mechanical therapy and can take up to four times longer to resolve than a contralateral shift.[1]

Leg Length Examine the levels of the iliac crests for possible leg length discrepancy. However, remember the lack of reliability of this procedure. One must correlate any possible leg length difference to those activities that worsen the.patient's symptoms (i.e., if the patient states they are worse bending and sitting, when leg length issues are removed, and better standing and walking, leg length is not a factor).

Movement Loss This section of the examination examines the quality of movement in the lumbar spine in the standing position. The clinician asks the patient if his or her movement now is any different than before this episode and if so will be graded (subjectively) as a major, moderate, minimal loss, or no loss. The clinician must consider the tremendous range of normal flexibility and extensibility between individual patient in making this assessment. The clinician will also be looking for deviations from the mid-sagittal plane during flexion and extension, and the patient's general willingness to move. Pain is not assessed at this point in the examination. The intent of this portion of the examination is to obtain a baseline of information on the quality of movement, from which to compare change achieved during subsequent test movements following treatment.

Test Movements The effect of movement on the patient's symptoms will be determined in this portion of the examination, providing further support for the mechanical diagnosis. It is imperative to establish the symptoms present prior to starting each new test movement, especially after changing test positions. The effect of the movements on the patient's symptoms is defined and coded according to the following guidelines:

- Increases: Symptoms already present are increased in intensity. (I)
- Decreases: Symptoms already present are reduced in intensity. (D)
- Produced: There are no symptoms at rest. Movement creates symptoms. (P)
- Abolishes (A): Symptoms are present. Movement eliminates symptoms.
- Worsened (W): Symptoms present or produced are increased with each movement, and remain worse as a result.

The McKenzie Institute
Lumber Spine Assessment

Date ..../............./............

Name ______________________________
Address ______________________________
Date of Birth ______________________ Sex: *M / F*
Occupation ______________________________
Postures / Stresses ______________________________
Telephone ______________________________
Referral: *GP / Orth / Self / Other* ______________________
Off work because of current episode? *Yes / No Since* ..../........./.........

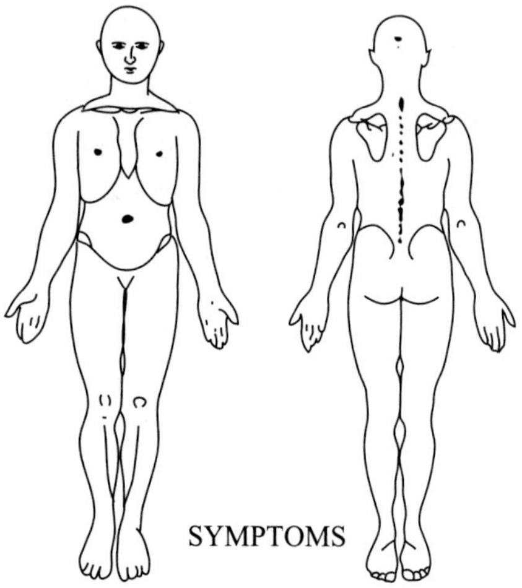

SYMPTOMS

Symptoms this episode to be marked on body diagram

HISTORY

Describe relevant symptoms ....

Present since .... /........... /.. *Improving / unchanging / worsening*

Commenced as a result of:.. or no apparent reason

Symptoms at onset *back / thigh/ leg* ....

Constant Symptoms: *back / thigh/ leg* Intermittent Symptoms: *back / thigh / leg*

Worse: *bending* *sitting / rising* *standing* *walking* *lying*
am / as day progresses / pm *when still / on the move*
other..

Better: *bending* *sitting* *standing* *walking* *lying*
am / as day progresses / pm *when still / on the move*
other..

Disturbed sleep? *Yes / No* Sleeping postures: *prone / sup / side* (R / L) Suface: *firm / soft / sag / w. bed*

Cough / sneeze / strain: *+ve / -ve* Bladder: *normal / abnormal* Gait: *normal / abnormal*..........................

Previous Episodes: *0 1-5 6-10 11+* Year of first episode: 19......................

Previous history:..

....

Previous treatments: ....

....

X-Rays: *Yes / No*..

Gen. Health: *Good / Fair / Poor* ....

Medications: *Nil / NSAID / Analg / Steroids / Anticoag / Other* ....

Recent or major surgery: *Yes / No* ....

Accidents: *Yes / No* .... Unexplained weight loss: *Yes / No*

BY PERMISSION OF THE McKENZIE INSTITUTE INTERNATIONAL
ORTHOPEDIC PHYSICAL THERAPY PRODUCTS, PO BOX 47009, MINNEAPOLIS, MN 55447 (612) 553-0452 ©1993, OPTP, Inc.

FIGURE 15–1. The McKenzie Assessment Sheet—Page 1. *(Reprinted with permission from The McKenzie Institute International.)*

EXAMINATION

POSTURE

Sitting: Good / Fair / Poor Standing: Good / Fair / Poor Lordosis: Red / Acc / Normal Lateral Shift: Right / Left / Nil

Other Observations: ....

MOVEMENT LOSS	maj	mod	min	nil
Flexion				
Extension				
Side Gliding (R)				
Side Gliding (L)				

Deviation in Flexion: Right / Left / Nil

Deviation in Extension: Right / Left / Nil

TEST MOVEMENTS: Describe effects on present pain - produces, abolishes, increases, decreases, centralises, peripheralises, better, worse, no better, no worse, no effect	PDM	ERP
Describe pretest pain standing		
FIS		
Rep FIS		
EIS		
Rep EIS		
Describe pretest pain lying:		
FIL		
Rep FIL		
EIL		
Rep EIL		
If required SGIS (R)		
Rep SGIS (R)		
SGIS (L)		
Rep SGIS (L)		

STATIC TESTS *If required*

Sitting Slouched .... Sitting erect ....

Standing Slouched .... Standing erect ....

Lying prone in extension .... Long sitting ....

NEUROLOGICAL

Motor Deficit: .... Reflexes: ....

Sensory Deficit: .... Dural sings: ....

OTHER

Hip Joints: ....

SI Joints: ....

CONCLUSION

Posture *Dysfunction* *Derangement No.* *Trauma*

Other ....

PRINCIPLE OF TREATMENT

Posture Correction ....

Extension ....

Flexion ....

Lateral ....

Other ....

FIGURE 15–2. The McKenzie Assessment Sheet—Page 2. *(Reprinted with permission from The McKenzie Institute International.)*

- Not worsened (NW): Symptoms present or produced are increased with each movement, but do not remain worse as a result.
- Better (B): Symptoms present or produced are decreased or abolished with movement, and remain better as a result.
- Pain during movement (PDM): Pain appears or increases as movement occurs. Pain disappears or reduces when movement stops.
- Pain at end range (ERP): Pain does not appear until end range is reached. Pain disappears when end range is released.
- No effect (NE): Movement has no effect on the subject's symptoms.
- No better (NB): Symptoms are decreased or abolished with each movement, but do not remain decreased or abolished.

Be certain to control the mechanics of the test movements, including the proper starting position. The stress should be intermittent (pressure on–pressure off).

Clinical Pearl: PDM (*p*ain *d*uring *m*ovement) indicates a derangement. ERP (*e*nd-*r*ange *p*ain) could be a derangement or dysfunction. If PDM or ERP is present then it rules out a postural syndrome.

Clinical Pearl: Repetitive test movements that produce lasting symptomatic changes [i.e. Better (B), Abolished (A), or Worsened (W)] indicates a derangement syndrome.

Lumbar Test Movements

1. Flexion in standing (FIS) (see Fig. 15–3)
2. Repeated flexion in standing (RFIS)
3. Extension in standing (EIS) (see Fig.15–4)
4. Repeated extension in standing (REIS)
5. Side gliding in standing (SGIS) (see Fig. 15–5)
6. Repeated side gliding in standing (RSGIS)
7. Flexion in lying (FIL) (see Fig. 15–6)
8. Repeated flexion in lying (RFIL)
9. Extension in lying (EIL) (see Fig. 15–7)
10. Repeated extension in lying (REIL)

Examination of the Effects of Movements on Pain Test movements in standing apply normal stress on normal or abnormal tissue.

Test movements in lying apply abnormal stress on normal or abnormal tissue.

Repeated movements—flexion

1. In posterior derangement:
    - progressive increase of derangement

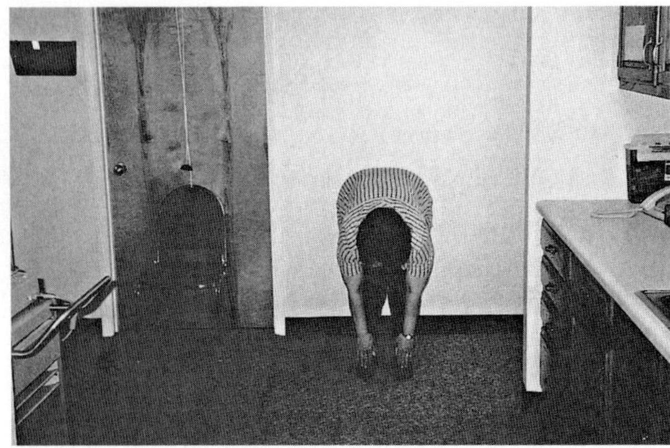

FIGURE 15–3. Mechanical test movement—Flexion in standing (FIS).

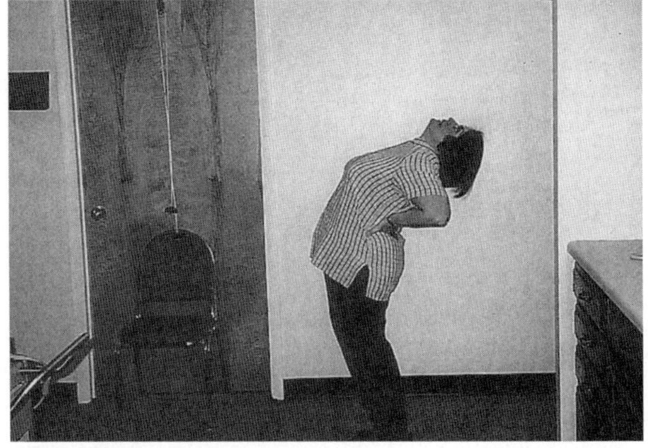

FIGURE 15–4. Mechanical test movement—Extension in standing (EIS).

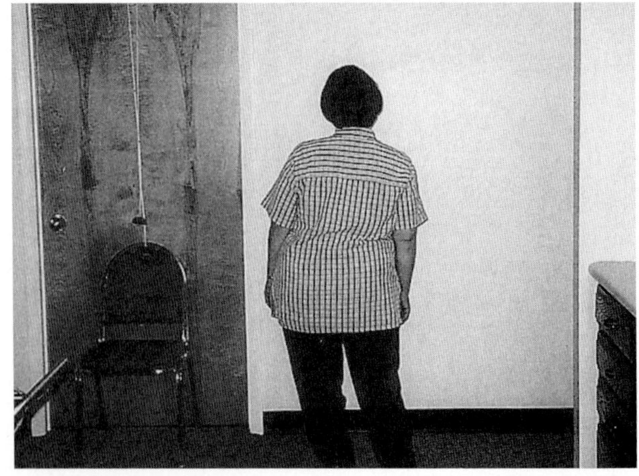

FIGURE 15–5. Mechanical test movement—Side gliding in standing (SGIS).

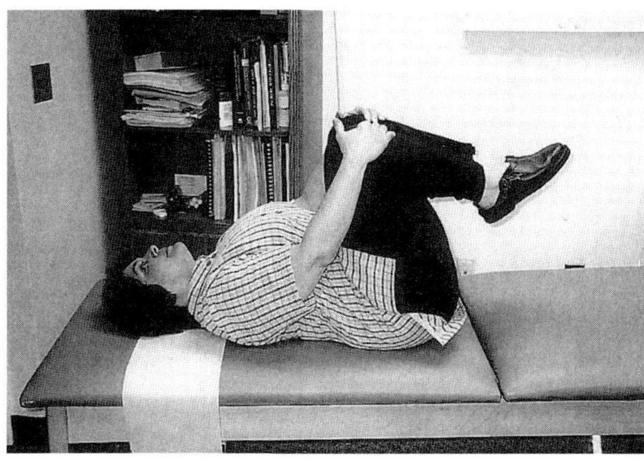

FIGURE 15–6. Mechanical test movement—Flexion in lying (FIL).

- increase and peripheralization of pain
- condition remains worse

2. In anterior derangement:
   - progressive decrease of derangement
   - centralization of pain
   - condition remains better

Repeated movements—extension

1. In posterior derangement:
   - progressive decrease of derangement
   - decrease and centralization of pain
   - condition remains better
2. In anterior derangement:
   - progressive increase in derangement
   - increase or peripheralization of pain
   - condition remains worse

In Presence of Irreducible Herniation of Intervertebral Disc

Repeated flexion or extension or both:

- increase of radiating pain on each movement
- condition does not improve
- condition may remain worse

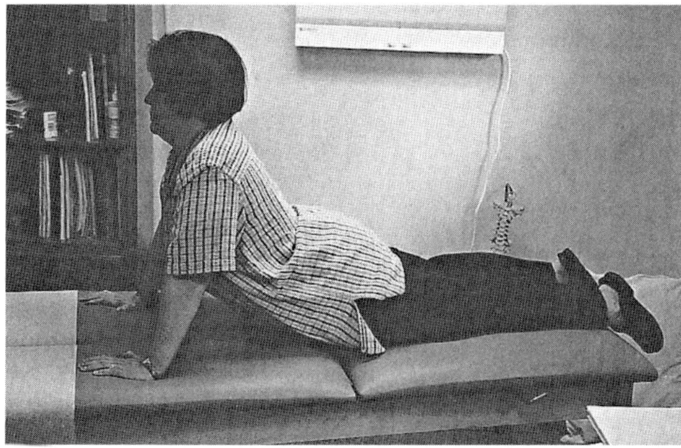

FIGURE 15–7. Mechanical test movement—Extension in lying (EIL).

Diagnosis and Repeated Movements

1. Postural syndrome
   - no effect
2. Dysfunction syndrome
   - pain at end range only
   - no pain during movement
   - no radiation
   - not progressively worse
   - pain stops shortly afterwards
   - no rapid changes occur
3. Derangement syndrome
   - pain during movement
   - may radiate or centralize
   - progressively worsens or improves
   - remains worse or better
   - rapid changes occur

REASONS FOR PROTOCOL FAILURE WHEN SUCCESS SHOULD BE REALIZED

Some patients for whom end-range loading strategies should be beneficial unfortunately do not realize that improvement. There are four main reasons that success is not realized, even if one assumes that the correct preferred end-range loading strategy was established.

Reason for Failure #1. The patient is not performing the prescribed number of movements throughout the day.

Reason for Failure #2. The patient is not achieving end-range loading, if needed, as part of the prescribed exercise program.

Reason for Failure #3. The patient is not maintaining vigilance regarding the avoidance of the culpable or provoking end-range loading. For most patients, this involves failure to maintain vigilance about spinal lordosis when reclining, sitting, standing, and making transitions between these postures. For a minority of patients, the prescription is for lordosis to be lost or avoided.

Reason for Failure #4. Inadequate overpressure on the part of the practitioner may be a reason for failure. For most patients, self-generated end-range loading, when needed, will suffice. For those patients who plateau as a result of self-generated end-range loading, clinician intervention is required. The appropriate movement plane direction end range, having been identified by self-generated end-range loading proven to be of benefit, is the movement plane direction within which the clinician applies overpressure. Logic and ethics require end-range loading be performed in a graded fashion. Therefore, the practitioner first applies manual mobilization therapies. If the therapeutic goals are realized, a greater force is not required. If only limited benefit results, the progression of forces would then explore manipulation in the same movement plane direction. Inadequate manual skills, on the part of the practitioner (including failure to explore an adequate number of manual overpressure strategies), may result in failure. Inability, on the part of the practitioner, to perform spinal manipulation may not permit the full exploration regarding the potentials of end-range loading strategies.

DISCOGENIC CLASSIFICATION VERSUS THE THREE SYNDROMES

At the McKenzie International Conference in Ottawa, Canada, in 2001, Jean-Yves Maigne, MD, gave a thought-provoking presentation, comparing the clinical classification of lumbar discogenic pain and its relationship with the McKenzie classification. To the author's knowledge it is the first incidence of comparison of discogenic pain and all three of the McKenzie syndromes.[9]

Dr. Maigne stated in his presentation that identifying all the patients whose pain arises from the disc appears to be an impossible task. But some clinical syndromes are frequent and could be linked with experimental observations. These syndromes could also interestingly be compared with the three McKenzie syndrome classifications. He describes the comparisons as follows.

Dehydration of the Nucleus—Postural Syndrome

If a slow (requiring years) dehydration process appears as a normal feature of the aging disc, dehydration appearing after a loading in certain position could not be so well tolerated. In fact, studies have illustrated that after creep (tissue deformation due to compressive forces) loading of 3 hours in the sitting posture, peaks of stress concentration appeared within the annulus, which could potentially aggravate the free nerve endings of the annulus and end plates and become a source of pain.[11]

This is a frequent situation, where patients experience LBP after remaining static for a long time in an end position, such as sitting in a bad seat or vacuuming (sustained lumbar flexion) or standing up and marking time (sustained lumbar extension). This situation was described by Troisier[11] and matches perfectly with the postural syndrome described by McKenzie, where pain is produced by position, not by movements, where activity relieves the pain and where the clinical examination is normal.

Inflammatory Lesion of the Disc—Dysfunction Syndrome

It is now well documented that the so-called mechanical back pain has an inflammatory component. Inflammatory cell and proinflammatory enzymes, or "breakdown products," have been found in the disc. Magnetic resonance imaging can reveal inflammatory changes in the vertebral end plates in certain cases and nonsteroidal anti-inflammatory drugs can improve the patients. Inflammation is more or less present in many cases of painful degenerated disc. Efficacy of nonsteroidal anti-inflammatory drugs may therefore be a convenient criterion for inflammation. There is a condition described by Revel as rapidly degrading discopathy.[12] It is defined by LBP related to a rapidly narrowing disc space (more than 50% in less than 2 years, a degradation not witnessed in controls). Revel noticed that NSAIDs were more effective in this condition than in other forms of LBP in that they reduced the symptoms but had no effect on the degenerative process. More recently, we have described a subgroup of patients with LBP who received a 10-day course of oral steroids. A significant number (70%) experienced markedly decreased signs and symptoms on the third day of treatment, strongly suggesting that inflammation here play a primary role. It should be underlined that oral steroids are deemed inefficient in LBP and thus contraindicated by the guidelines. The features of this syndrome are (1) pain occurring spontaneously (without any trauma), worse in the second half of the night (the patient being awakened at 3 a.m. to 5 a.m. by pain), with stiffness in the morning, and (2) pain worsened by lumbar extension (at the end range), while flexion was not pain provoking or restricted. Some minor criteria for rapidly degrading discopathy may also be commonly found: partial efficacy of NSAIDs (followed by a relapse following this course of care) and failure or impossibility of a manipulative therapy. Surprisingly, 90% of the patients are females between 30 and 60 years of age.

These conditions should parallel the McKenzie dysfunction syndrome. In this syndrome, pain often commences without any apparent provocation (which is believed to be characteristic of inflammation). McKenzie states that the pain is felt at the end range of certain ordinary movements. He notes that there is stiffness in the morning, with loosening as the day progresses. As time passes, flexion and extension become reduced and the morning stiffness does not recede. Patients often state that they feel better when they are active and moving about than while resting. All these features are typical of inflammation and resemble our own description. McKenzie, however, does not speak of inflammation, but of an adaptive shortening with a resultant loss of mobility causing "premature" pain (i.e., before reaching full, normal end-range movement). Perhaps this may be another way of describing the same phenomenon in some of these cases.

Mechanical Lesions of the Anulus—Derangement Syndrome

If, according to Bogduk, one considers the annulus as a ligament, a traumatic rupture of some its collagen fibers could be likened to a discal sprain.[13] Pathologic studies have identified three different types of annular fissures. Rim lesions, or transverse fissures, are a posttraumatic rupture of the fibers attaching to the vertebral rim. Radial fissures are most often located in the posterolateral region of the disc. They also are the result of a traumatic lesion (bending and axial torsion). A circumferential tear can result.

In case of a radial tear, the fissure provides a migratory track for nuclear material. If that material enters the fissure (depending upon its size, location, and mechanism of the migration), it may reach to or beyond the peripheral layers of the disc (disc hernia causing sciatica) or remain contained within the annulus, perhaps provoking nociceptive stimulation of the sinuvertebral nerve (lumbalgia characterized by a list without radicular pain or disc herniation). In both cases, the pressure applied on the walls of the fissure could account for the deviation in flexion (flexion bias) that is frequently observed.

This condition could correspond to the derangement syndrome described by McKenzie. This syndrome occurs most frequently in men between 20 and 55 years of age and is elicited by a single significant overload, a less significant overload applied frequently, or a sustained flexion or extension overload (which is most common). Interestingly, McKenzie notes that the reduction of the derangement often provides immediate and lasting relief from pain, logically indicating the presence of a purely mechanical condition with the absence of an inflammatory component.

SUMMARY

1. The collection of information from the history, examination, and mechanical evaluation will indicate whether the patient is suffering from the postural, dysfunction, or derangement syndrome, or a nonmechanical cause.
2. In teaching the McKenzie system, confusion typically arises regarding the placement of individual patient into one of the three syndromes. Clinicians become confused when the postural syndrome is used in the strictest sense. Or there is confusion as to the term dysfunction in the dysfunction syndrome because dysfunction in the medical sense can mean several things.
3. This differentiation of each syndrome is necessary, as the treatment of each will be completely different. McKenzie treatment protocols and practical case studies will be discussed and illustrated in detail in Chapter 22.
4. The initial prognosis may appear discouraging following the history and examination. However, it is a mistake to provide the patient with a dismal clinical impression before providing a fair trial course of mechanical treatment for a few days.
5. It is not always possible for a prognosis to be so certain. Therefore it is best to avoid giving an incorrect impression of the nature and extent of the problem before it is fully apparent.
6. Once it is clear that the nature of the problem is such that mechanical therapy will have little or no impact on the condition, it is important that a realistic picture be conveyed to the patient. This allows the patient to come to terms with a persistent problem in order to determine the necessary strategies for personally addressing their condition. Of course, referral to the appropriate specialist when necessary is important.
7. Prolonged manual care for intractable pain syndromes, without providing the patient other reasonable treatment options, can be a waste of resources and strains the boundaries of professional ethics. Conversely, patient education, the provision of various treatment options maintaining as active a lifestyle as possible, and a focus on self-dependence rather than clinician-dependence hallmarks the McKenzie approach.

REFERENCES

1. McKenzie RA. *The lumbar spine: Mechanical diagnosis and therapy*. Lower Hutt, New Zealand: Spinal Publications, 1981.
2. McKenzie RA. *The cervical and thoracic spine: Mechanical diagnosis and therapy*. Lower Hutt, New Zealand: Spinal Publications, 1990.
3. McKenzie RA, May S. *The human extremities: Mechanical diagnosis and therapy*. Lower Hutt, New Zealand: Spinal Publications, 2000.
4. Jacob G, Heffner S, Medcalf R, Barenberg D, Starler S. Evaluating the patient using the McKenzie approach. In: *Stude DE: Spinal rehabilitation*. Stamford: Appleton & Lange, 1999:147–178.
5. Heffner S. *McKenzie protocols in cervical spine rehabilitation*. In: Murphy D, ed. *Conservative Management of Cervical Spine Syndromes*. New York: McGraw-Hill, 2000:641–661.
6. Jacob G. Teaching syllabus: Mechanical diagnosis and therapy of the lumbar spine. Los Angeles College of Chiropractic Rehabilitation Diplomate course training, Whittier: California, October, 1996.
7. Bogduk N. The anatomy and physiology of nociception. IN: *Key Issues in Musculotskeletal Physiotherapy*. Crosbie J, McConnell J eds. Butterworth-Heinemann, Oxford, 1993.

8. Adams MA, Dolan P, Hutton WC. Diural stresses on the lumbar spine. *Spine* 1989;12(2):130–137.
9. Maigne JY. Classification des lesions discales lombires. *Rev Med Orthop* 1992;30:5–8.
10. Adams M, McMillan DW, Green TP, Dolan P. Sustained loading generates stress concentration in lumbar intervertebral discs. *Spine* 1996;21:434–438.
11. Troisier O. *Semiologie et traitement des lesions discales et ligamentaires du rachis*. Paris: Masson, 1973.
12. Revel M. La discopathie destructrice rapide. *Rev Med Orthop* 1990;20:19–22.
13. Bogduk N, Twomey LT. *Clinical anatomy of the lumbar spine*, 2nd ed. Melbourne: Churchill Livingstone, 1991.

CHAPTER

16

DIAGNOSTIC IMAGING APPROACHES TO THE EVALUATION OF LOW BACK SYNDROMES

Dennis R. Skogsbergh and Kendall M. Jones

OUTLINE

OBJECTIVES

1. Discuss the basic principles of, and indications for, conventional radiography, CT, MRI, bone scanning, and other diagnostic imaging techniques.
2. Familiarize the reader with the pathological entities that are best demonstrated by each of these modalities.

INTRODUCTION

Diagnostic imaging, in all of its various forms, is a fundamental resource in the investigational workup of a patient with low back pain. Imaging studies often provide strong direction for the decisions necessary for patient management. Furthermore, the findings discovered at imaging may heighten ones understanding

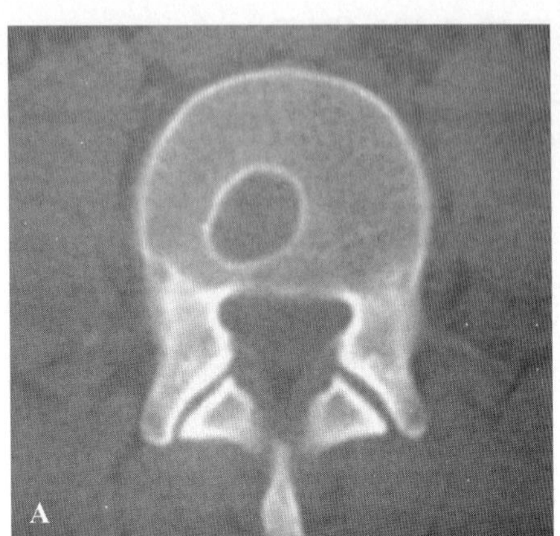

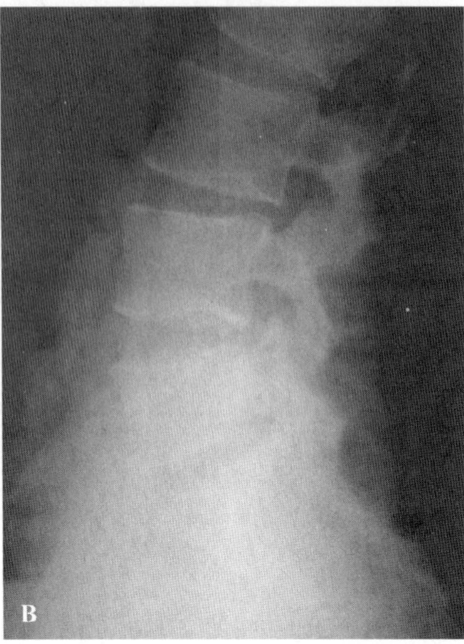

FIGURE 16–1. *A.* Axial CT through the L4 vertebra. There is a well-circumscribed lucency in the body of L4. Overall it measured 1.0 × 1.5 × 1.7 cm with a sharply defined sclerotic border. On MRI this same area was fluid-filled. *B.* The lateral plain film appears completely normal with no conspicuity of the cystic abnormality.

of issues that could limit certain types of conservative treatment or demand significant treatment modification. The vital role of diagnostic imaging has been expanding as new and improved imaging techniques have been developed.

In earlier years, clinical spine practice was conducted exclusively with conventional plain radiographic techniques, including myelography. Greatest attention in those days was paid to the technical issues of obtaining high image quality and there was concern for low exposure. Today, these same conventional techniques continue to be at the forefront of imaging approaches and the concern about radiation remains unchanged, as the radiation dose to skin, gonads, and bone marrow is high in lumbar spine imaging.

The use of standard techniques is practical for the initial appraisal of gross bony morphology, vertebral alignment, intervertebral spacing, intersegmental stability, significant patterns of osseous disease, and fracture. Furthermore, conventional radiography is readily available, simple, and inexpensive.

When therapeutically significant, conventional studies investigating lumbar spine trauma, degenerative disease, infection, neoplasia, inflammatory disease, and the postoperative situation have been shown to be up to 90% sensitive.[1] The actual film series necessary in a specific clinical situation is dictated by the specific goals of the study.

However, while routine imaging provides important information even when more advanced studies are planned, significant limitations do exist. With standard radiographic techniques some bony abnormalities and subtle bony processes may escape detection. For example, 30%–50% bone destruction may occur before a solitary vertebral lesion becomes conspicuous (Fig. 16–1). The spatial relationships of the central canal and lateral recesses are commonly inaccurately determined using osseous landmarks on lumbar plain films. Also, the intricate anatomical relationships of complex vertebral anomalies may not be well portrayed. Moreover, soft tissue abnormalities, for example, disc extrusion, ligament tear, cyst, and tumor, and bone marrow abnormality usually go unrecognized. In some cases, timely and proper treatment may be delayed. Advanced imaging studies allow clarification of these types of uncertainties.

For 70 years after Roentgen's discovery of x-rays (1895) there was only slow evolutionary change. Pneumoencephalography and ventriculography were in use in 1918, linear tomography in 1932, followed by polytomography (1954) and angiography in the 1950s and 1960s.[2] The institution of radiation safety measures did not occur until 1930. With the advent of the computer[3] there was a rapid change in the growth curve that heralded the development of computed tomography (CT) in 1972 and magnetic resonance imaging (MRI) in 1982.

Initially, CT and MRI were both used to image the brain, but today their use extends strongly into musculoskeletal investigations. This has occurred largely because of the huge improvement in soft tissue contrast, spatial resolution, and critical definition of anatomy. The manner in which diseases of the spine are diagnosed has been significantly affected as these two technologies have matured. The added insight into variations of the bone marrow, intervertebral disc, and para-articular soft tissues including ligaments and muscle often allow elegant portrayal of a problem, and both CT and MRI have become widely accepted in clinical practice.

Today with the potential for obtaining and storing digital images, filmless x-ray departments are now a reality and may shortly become the norm. Radiography is the last modality to enter the digital world. Even though the process has been slow, digital radiography (DR) systems are improving with larger image receptors and higher resolution. The obstacle to progress toward digitization in radiography at this point is the considerably greater cost of a DR system.

Subsequently, the imaging revolution has made the detection of earlier and subtler pathology almost routine. As it turns out, the new imaging modalities can partner together with the old to suggest crucial diagnostic considerations, the extent of injury or pathological abnormality, and sometimes the clinical significance of an abnormality. While all the modalities have some practical applicability, the utilization and sequencing of diagnostic examinations in a given clinical situation is important not only in the initial stages of diagnosis and treatment, but also later in case follow-up. Differences of opinion remain as to the most effective imaging strategy and choice of the optimal (and cost-effective) study.

STANDARD RADIOGRAPHIC IMAGING

The various contrasts between radiographic densities of air, fat, water (soft tissue structures), and bone produces the images that we rely onto portray spinal anatomy and pathology on conventional imaging. The finished image is the result of attenuation of x-rays passing through the body and being absorbed to varying degrees or scattering before they strike the film, receptor, or detector. The greater the number of x-rays reaching the film, the greater is the relative blackening of the image. Numerous technical factors are manipulated and equilibrated in order to produce a high-quality diagnostic image, while keeping the radiation dose as low as possible. The notions of long focal film distances, short object film distances, small focal spots, short exposure time, tight collimation, and optimal film/screen combinations are well known and are applied in general practice.

Reducing radiation exposure to the lowest levels may be addressed in several ways. Attention to the details of patient centering, shielding, and collimation, reducing repeat films, and the timely calibration of x-ray equipment all help to lower exposure.

The ability to recognize the early signs of a disease process requires thorough appreciation of normal radiographic anatomy as well as an understanding of the disease itself. This includes the characteristic and variant appearances. A systematic approach is always recommended. The basic concepts of a search for alignment, joint interspacing, bony mineralization, and soft tissue abnormalities, as in other musculoskeletal areas, are similar for the spine.

The usefulness and shortcomings of high-quality conventional imaging is illustrated in the following examples of lumbar spine and related pathology.

Pathology

Abdominal Soft Tissues In the lumbar region, presence of calcifications often reflect organ and other abnormalities. Calcification of the walls of the abdominal aorta provides some insight into the vessel's transverse dimension (Fig. 16–2). This is important for the recognition of aneurysmal dilatation, but CT and ultrasound are far better modalites to use for detection and measurement of these lesions. Bowel overlay and poor quality images often preclude the visualization of any calcification. Furthermore, dilatation may exist without concurrent calcification. In a study by Brown et al., the risk of rupture of abdominal aneurysms measuring 5–5.9 cm was found to be 1% in men, but 3.9% in women. And for those measuring greater than 6 cm, the rupture risk was found to be 14.1% (male) versus 22.3% (females).[4]

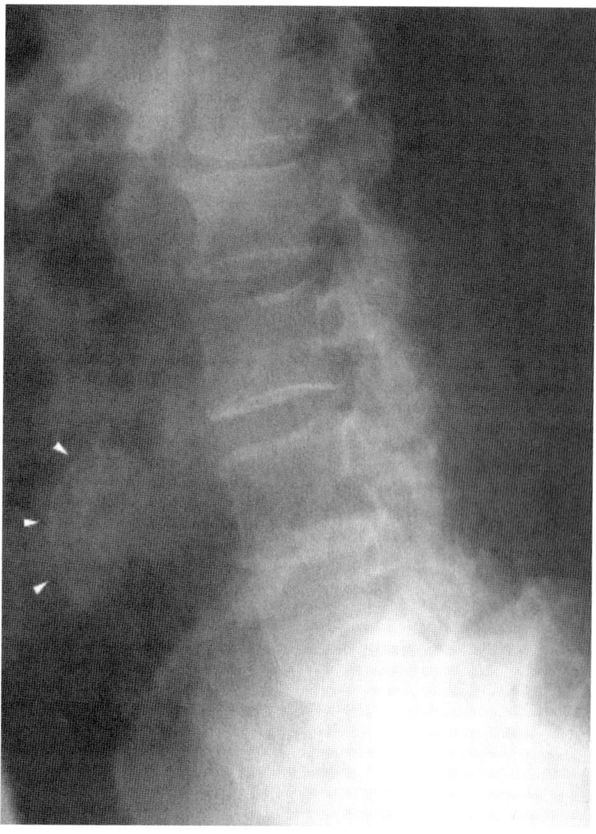

FIGURE 16–2. Abdominal aneurysm. A lateral lumbar spine projection shows a calcified outline of the abdominal aorta. It measured 6 cm transversely.

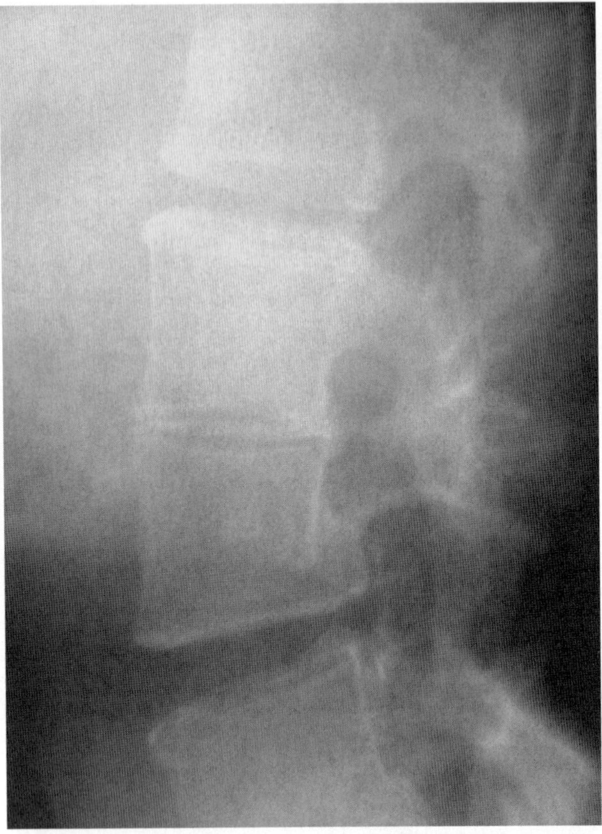

FIGURE 16–3. Lumbar nonsegmentation. A lateral lumbar projection demonstrates a congenital nonsegmentation pattern at L3–L4. There is a remnant disc interspace. Any subtle abnormality of the pedicles and posterior arch that may be present in these types of cases is not clearly evident on conventional images. Furthermore, the presence of any soft tissue abnormality (including neural) may remain undisclosed. Complex bony configurations are visualized much better on CT. Associated soft tissue abnormalities including neural malformation may be visualized best on MRI.

Developmental Malformations Many patterns of development and variant osseous anatomy are well visualized on standard radiographs. These include the initial appearance and progression of vertebral ossification centers, the anomalies of disordered segmentation, nonsegmentation (Fig. 16–3), spinal dysraphism, and agenesis or hypoplasia.

Lumbar Facet Disease Conventional imaging offers little for the differential diagnosis of the facet syndromes. Hypertrophic facet changes are indicators of advanced disease, but early to moderate disease usually is not well appreciated. When clarification is needed, both CT and MRI do provide good visualization of the facet anatomy.

Spondylolysis/Spondylolisthesis Anterior vertebral displacement of one segment upon the next caudad segment is readily graded on a lateral view according to the Meyerding classification.[5] The superior aspect of the subjacent segment is divided into four equal sectors and is used to calculate any degree of translation by using the placement of the posteroinferior margin of the displaced segment into the respective quadrants. Anterolisthesis also may be calculated as an exact percentage by using the following formula: distance of slip divided by the A–P diameter of subjacent segment × 100.

The oblique lumbar view (25–45 degrees) has traditionally been used to portray defective integrity of the pars interarticularis (isthmus), and while the popularized concept of the "scotty dog" configuration needs no further elucidation, the importance of this visualization cannot be denied. Unfortunately, oblique visualization may fail to reveal spondylolysis in as many as 13% of cases[6] (Fig. 16–4). In those cases where the index of suspicion is high, but visualization is inadequate, additional conventional imaging may be fruitful. Further clarification may come from a spot lateral, an AP 30–45 degrees caudal or cephalic tilt view,[6] or with oblique projections with varied angulation.[7] In some cases apparent bilateral spondylolysis can be purely projectional in nature. Bowel gas overlaying the osseous structure can also simulate a pars break, and hypoplasia of the L5 body can create a false impression of slippage.

Computed tomographic demonstration of a pars defect may be difficult on disc protocols as adjacent facet interfaces may simulate spondylolysis. However, when visualized on stacked CT images through the mid-vertebral body region, characterization of the status of the pars is superior, for example, narrowed, elongated, sclerotic, or interrupted.[8] Associated findings on CT with multiplanar reconstruction include disc protrusion and foraminal or spinal canal encroachment from soft tissue or bony callus formation.[9] Pars defects, pars marrow abnormality, and any degree of stenosis may be visualized on MRI (Fig. 16–24).

Bone scintigraphy is of value in determining whether the pars interarticularis exhibits tracer accumulation that suggests active stress reaction or healing. Single photon emission computed tomography (SPECT) visualization provides more specific localization in different planes (Fig. 16–4C).

Disorders of the Intervertebral Discs Disorders of the intervertebral disc may produce clues on the plain film examination, but routine radiography is limited and most soft tissue abnormalities can be virtually imperceptible. This includes the intrinsic morphological character of the disc. For clarification of these types of uncertainties, advanced imaging is needed.

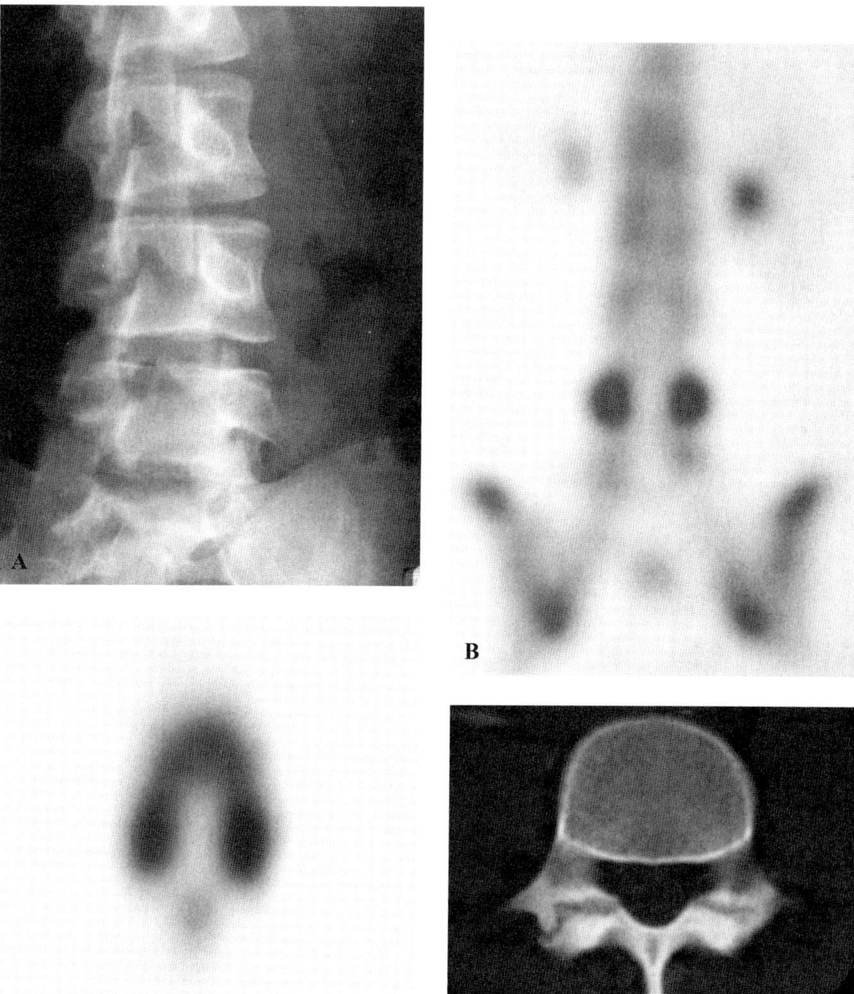

FIGURE 16–4. Spondylolysis. *A.* A standard oblique view shows a normal appearing pars interarticularis at L4 in this 14-year-old girl. The opposite side was equally negative. *B.* Posterior (coronal) planar image from the nuclear scan in the same case shows increased tracer uptake in the posterior arches of L4. *C.* SPECT shows location of the tracer in axial format. *D.* Axial CT demonstrates bilateral pars defects at L4 with a suggestion of bony callus and repair, greater on the right side.

Nevertheless, disc space thinning and marginal reactive changes at the discovertebral interface are indicators of degenerative disease. These changes are often limited to more advanced disease and early degenerative thinning may go unnoticed. Similarly, other important and potentially painful lesions related to the intervertebral discs (e.g., Schmorl's nodes, posterior rim fractures, and rim apophysis injury) may be seen, but smaller lesions may be overlooked.

Accurate measurements of disc height are problematical because of errors caused by lateral tilt or longitudinal axis rotation. A semiquantitative approach is more realistic, particularly when a comparison is attempted with serial examination. Saraste et al. demonstrated the mensuration of the degree of vertebral slip and lordotic angulation to be more accurate than that of vertical height.[10]

Osteophytes and traction spurs signal adjacent disc abnormality and sometimes, excessive intersegmental movement. Pitkanen et al. believe that segmental lumbar spine instability noted on flexion/extension (FE) radiography can be predicted by conventional imaging findings such as traction spurs.[11] In this study the authors suggested that FE radiography be limited to those cases when symptoms are not explained by the findings on the plain radiographs or when they are likely to alter the treatment plan. Unfortunately, in actual practice the presence of traction spurs and disc interspace thinning is present only in a smaller number of cases with actual instability. Flexion/extension views are necessary to demonstrate excessive degrees of translatory or angular movement (Fig. 16–5).

Spinal Stenosis In the stenotic spine, conventional radiographs allow only for the general quantification of significant bony abnormalities, disc interspace thinning, marginal spurring, and facet disease. Central and lateral recess changes are often missed or underestimated, and cutoff dimensional mensuration guidelines should not be strictly applied.

On the other hand, CT is well suited to exhibit the bony changes of stenosis at any site, flaval ligament thickening, incorporation of bone grafts, facet cysts,

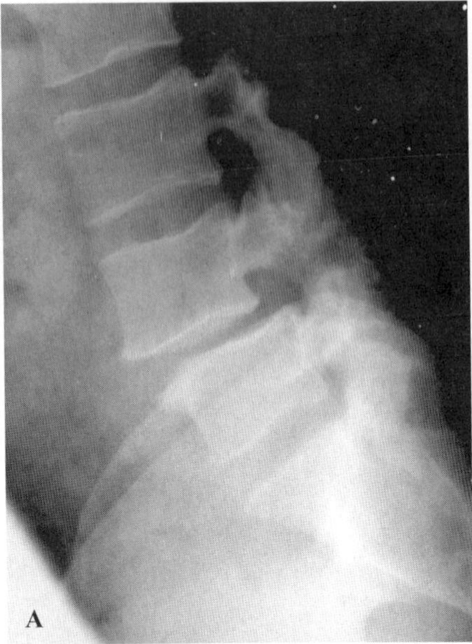

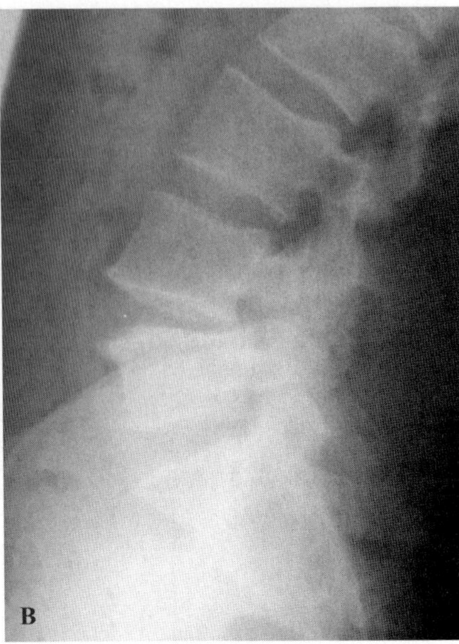

FIGURE 16–5. Lumbar intersegmental instability. This 40-year-old male had experienced chronic lower back pain for many years. In time he became resistant to conservative management including physical therapy, bracing, and manipulation. Nonstressed views demonstrated anterolisthesis of L4 and thinning of the intervertebral disc space at L4–L5 with marginal spurring including traction spur formation. *A.* Flexion; *B.* extension. Note the degree of angular displacement that occurs upon extension stressing.

and intrusion into the confines of the foramina and spinal canal. MRI shows similar findings (see Figs. 7–4, 7–5, 7–7*A*, 7–7*B*, and 7–8) and also often provides additional information about intrinsic changes within the spinal cord proper, nerve rootlets, and related soft tissues, including epidural fibrosis, infection, and tumors.

The goal of lumbar CT and MRI evaluation in patients with radiculopathy or myeloradiculopathy is to identify the presence of stenosis at entrance, mid, or exit zones, and to evaluate any adjacent nerve root or cord compression.

The diagnosis of well-developed cases of diffuse idiopathic skeletal hyperostosis (DISH) is usually clear on plain films, even in the stages before the classical criteria are met: four contiguous levels of vertebral ossification, disc height preservation, and no bony ankylosis of the posterior joints.[12] Reduction of the disc space height may occur in cases where disc degeneration has antedated the development of hyperostosis. The posterior facets often exhibit hyperostosis as well.

CT, and to a lesser degree MRI, is necessary only in those cases where posterior longitudinal ligament ossification is suspected, as it allows accurate identification of canal stenosis and abnormalities of the spinal cord. Scrutiny for occult injury in cases of DISH is important in posttrauma situations, and radionuclide scanning, CT, and MRI are helpful.

Lumbar Spine Trauma Plain radiography remains the initial examination in spine trauma cases. Careful attention must be directed to intervertebral alignment and interspacing, the posterior elements, and any paraspinal soft tissue swelling. Intervertebral malalignment in the setting of trauma must be considered traumatic until proven otherwise. Correlation with a known injury mechanism strengthens the search for abnormality.

Clinical Pearl: Intervertebral malalignment in the setting of trauma must be considered traumatic rather than degenerative until proven otherwise.

Spine fractures have been classified according to their morphological characteristics and by mechanisms of injury. Hyperflexion injury and anterior vertebral compression are the most common in the lumbar spine.

The management of fractures in the thoracolumbar region depends on stability and the risk for neurological injury. The three-column model helps predict acute fractures that may be unstable.[13] In this model, the anterior column comprises the anterior longitudinal ligament, anterior half of a vertebral body, and the related intervertebral disc. The middle column includes the posterior half of a vertebral body with its disc and the related posterior longitudinal ligament. The posterior column consists of the posterior elements with facet articulations and the restraining ligaments.

Fractures of the anterior column (e.g., simple compression fractures) that do not implicate the middle column are usually stable. Shearing and burst fractures often disrupt the middle column and these are commonly unstable. The integrity of the middle column and the posterior longitudinal ligament and anulus largely determines the mechanical stability of the spine.[14] Involvement of two columns usually results in instability (Fig. 16–6). In the common vertebral compression injury, slight buckling or overlap of the anterior vertebral cortex is frequently visible. However, many patterns of injury are not seen or are

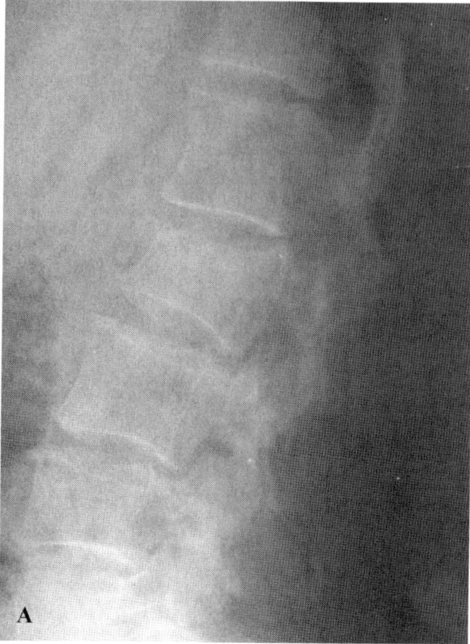
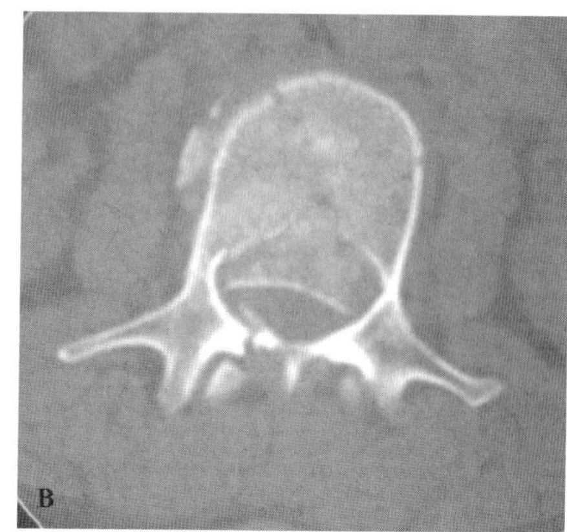

FIGURE 16–6. Unstable fracture. This patient fell onto his buttocks and experienced acute mid-lumbar pain. *A.* A lateral view reveals superior end plate depression and slight overlap of the anterior cortex at L2. The lumbar lordosis is regionally reversed. *B.* The axial CT through the level of the fracture demonstrates an unexpected degree of retropulsion with intrusion into the spinal canal, about 1.5 cm. Furthermore, there is disruption of the posterior arch on the right side. Both were inconspicuous on the plain film examination. This is an example of three-column involvement and instability.

poorly defined on conventional imaging studies. This in part may be due to poor image quality because of movement (pain), exaggerated bowel pattern, or the patient's weight. Similarly, subtle seat belt injuries and burst fractures may be underappreciated or overlooked. In a burst fracture, a posteriorly migrated fragment may readily be concealed (Fig. 16–6). Unexplained or unreasonable symptoms should provoke additional diagnostic investigation. Advanced imaging helps define subtle abnormalities, soft tissue damage, ligamentous restraint loss, and also allows for the estimation of neurological risk.

Transverse Process Fracture Transverse process fractures may occur vertically across the base or tip of the process. Local hematoma in the psoas muscle may efface its fascial plane. More than one segment may be involved, and bilateral fracture is possible. The fracture line is often subtle in appearance and when there is no displacement, detection can be difficult.

These injuries should serve as sentinel markers for other skeletal[15] or abdominal injury.[16] Miller et al. and Patten et al. showed that about 50% of those with transverse process fractures had concurrent abdominal injuries.[16,17] Computed tomography should follow the initial studies to rule out such associated injury.

Sacral Stress Fracture Visualization of abnormalities at the sacrum and sacroiliac joints is difficult. The degree of degenerative alteration and marginal hypertrophic change or bridging of the sacroiliac joint often go unrecognized (Fig. 16–7). Similar problems with the conspicuity of osseous abnormalities occur relative to the sacrum proper and pelvis.

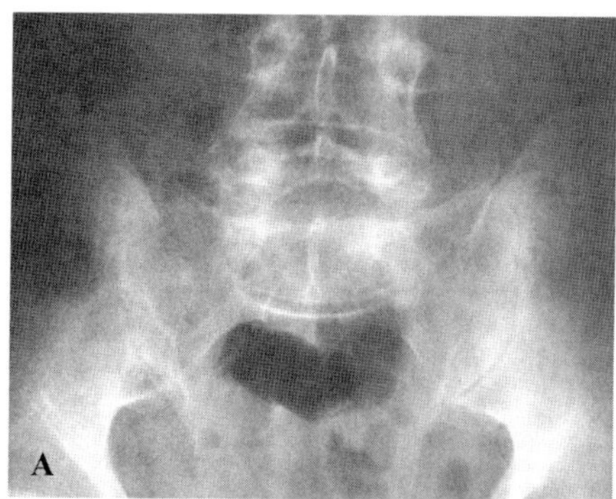
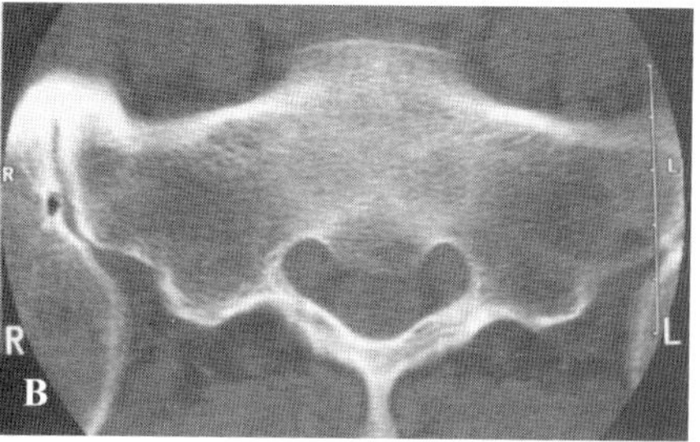

FIGURE 16–7. Sacroiliac joint arthrosis. *A.* The anteroposterior pelvic projection demonstrates some increased density in the region of the sacroiliac joints consistent with degenerative disease, but the joints are otherwise unremarkable. *B.* An axial CT at the level of the upper sacrum revels complete bony bridging across the right sacroiliac joint. This degree of change was not anticipated on the plain film examination. Such a finding may be of considerable importance in patients receiving manual and rehabilitative therapy.

Without imaging recognition, the diagnosis and proper treatment of a sacral stress fracture may be delayed. In these cases the clinical examination may not provide reliable findings. Pain due to sacral stress fractures may be felt in the lower back and groin mimicking sacroiliac joint or hip pathology, with pain radiating into the leg. Tenderness may be present over the sacrum and near the sacroiliac joint but this may be difficult to differentiate from primary joint inflammation.

Sacral and buttock pain that does not respond to treatment in a timely fashion should alert one to the potential of sacral stress reaction.[18] The suggestion of sacral fracture is most reasonable in elderly women with bone density loss who have sustained unknown or minimal trauma. In these situations there may be acute onset back pain,[19,20] and metastatic disease is often the clinical suspicion.[21] Their occurrence in clinical practice is more common than might be expected.[22] Parasymphyseal and pubic rami fractures may be concurrent.[23]

Not all patients with sacral stress injuries are elderly. Major et al. reported stress injuries in the pubic symphysis and sacroiliac joints of athletes. These patients may have back, leg, and groin symptoms that suggest other low back syndromes.[24] Sclerotic changes at the symphyseal interface, erosions, or pubic offset, and avulsion of the gracilis insertion should be sought.

When present, findings of cortical disruption and sclerosis along the sacral alae are usually difficult to identify on conventional radiographs because of the irregular and varied geometry of the sacrum and overlying bowel pattern. Improved visualization of the SI joint space and margins can be obtained using oblique or other SI projections.[25] However, in a given case they are rarely productive. In these cases, CT, MRI, and bone scintigraphy all provide crucial information.

Sacrococcygeal Trauma Radiography is used to search for evidence of fracture and sacrococcygeal displacement, although many false positives (misaligned coccygeal joints that are not pain provocative) are common. Maigne et al. described a radiographic technique and classification system, in which images obtained in a lateral sitting position (the painful position) are compared with standard lateral radiographs.[26,27]

Post-Lumbar Spine Surgery Assessment In the postsurgical setting there are a large number of important issues that arise and may exhibit findings on conventional imaging.

Concerns about infection emerge with all invasive procedures. Most infections of the intervertebral discs occur as an extension of osteomyelitis, or direct inoculation during diagnostic or surgical procedures. For instance, lumbar discography is complicated by infectious discitis in about 0.6% of cases.[28,29] The frequency of postsurgical spine-related infection is quite variable. There is an incidence of approximately 1% for both lumbar discectomy and iliac crest donor sites, and 3%–13% for posterior lumbar fusion.

Other causes of infection are much less common. In non-surgery-related instances of discitis/infection, the most common age group is children younger than 5 years of age and the greatest incidence is in the lumbar spine. Classically, the infection begins in the vertebral endplates, which are highly vascular in youth, and later spreads to the intervertebral discs. It may be viral or bacterial in origin. By the time the diagnosis is made, the disc and both end plates are often involved. *Staphylococcus aureus* is the most common organism found, but 50%–70% of cultures are negative.

Infection may involve the vertebra (osteomyelitis, spondylitis), intervertebral disc (discitis), or the pavertebral spaces (cellulitis, abscess). Anteriorly located infections in the thoracolumbar (TL) spine have the potential to cause subdiaphragmatic abscess, peritonitis, and psoas abscess. Posterior infections may involve the subcutaneous space (wound infection, infected seroma), subfascial space (deep wound infection, paraspinous abscess), or the posterior elements (osteomyelitis). Involvement of the spinal canal takes on several forms: the epidural space (epidural abscess), meninges (arachnoiditis, meningitis), subdural space (subdural abscess), or spinal cord proper (intramedullary abscess) (See Fig. 16–8).

In any case, conventional x-ray examination is usually normal in the early stage of infection. It may take as long as 5–12 weeks for definitive changes to become evident, and perhaps even longer in tuberculosis. Irregularity of the end plates, displacement of the paravertebral line, and visible bony sclerosis are the earliest signs (Fig. 16–9).

Clinical Pearl: The loss of intervertebral disc space height with destructive change of adjacent endplates, with or without vertebral sclerosis or adjacent soft tissue masses, is characteristic of vertebral osteomyelitis, especially in the appropriate clinical setting with appropriate risk factors.

The constellation of clinical, radiological, and pathological findings along with rapid progression over a short period is typical of hematogenous bacterial disc space infection. MRI is the gold standard for early detection of discitis and osteomyelitis, showing additional changes of abscess formation and other soft tissue abnormalities, in comparison to nuclear scans.

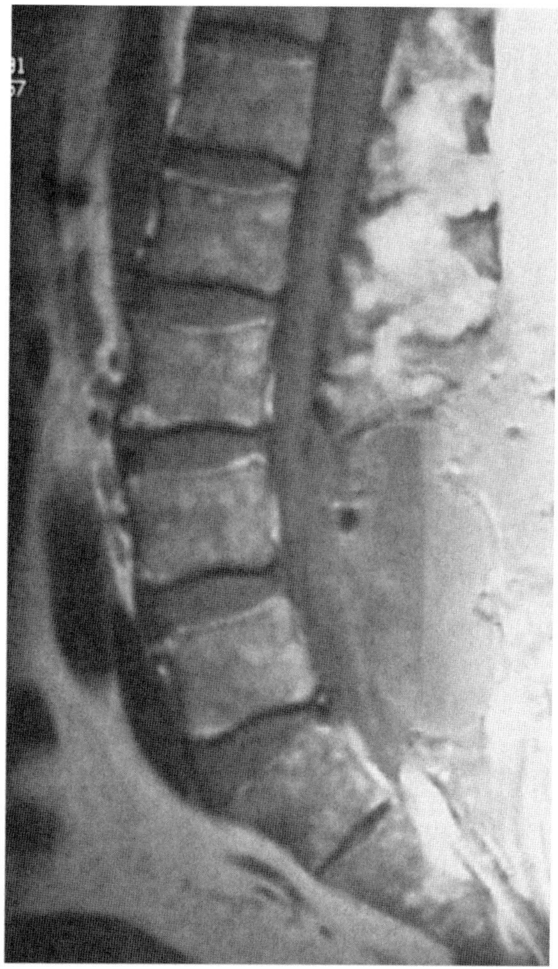

FIGURE 16–8. Abscess formation. Sagittal lumbar MRI in a patient 2 months post-decompression procedure at L4–S1. Note the large abscess posteriorly spanning two and a half levels and approximately 5 cm deep. There is cellular layering within the abscess.

In lumbar spine fusion cases there are a number of issues that arise besides infection. These include hardware placement; hardware breakage, shift, expulsion, subsidence, or loosening of a screw, graft, or cage; and pseudoarthrosis. Any may give rise to persistent or recurrent spine complaints. To varying degrees, all of these problems may be evaluated by the various imaging techniques. Whether or not a solid fusion has occurred, or has been lost, is a question of paramount concern, especially for those patients who are being considered for rehabilitation and/or manual therapy. And these same concerns arise in cases complicated by interim trauma.

Placement of Surgical Hardware The relationship of hardware to the neuroforamen is important. For example, excessive lateral placement of a pedicle screw may result in foraminal violation and nerve root abutment (Fig. 16–10). Similarly, fusion cages may violate a foraminal space, subside, or migrate (Fig. 16–11). Conventional radiographs are not reliable for determination of fusion cage or pedicle screw placement, and MRI often has metallic artifact that obscures the field of view. CT has shown ten times as many pedicle screws violating the medial cortex as plain film examination. The use of CT imaging is therefore important in cases of postoperative neurological deficit.[30,31]

Hardware breakage (rods, connectors, screws, etc) is likely to be visualized on plain films. Similarly, expulsion of a bone graft of fusion cage may be relatively straightforward (Fig. 16–12). Loosening, however, may not be so apparent. One should look for a halo of lucency around the interface between the screw/cage and adjacent bone (Fig. 16–13). Furthermore, there may be settling of the implant, cage, or graft with shift into or through the bony endplate.

Plain radiography is the most widely used initial method for determining intersegmental fusion. Continuous bridging adjacent to an interspace indicating osteosynthesis across a graft–host interface is the desired finding (Fig. 16–14). Often there only is vague increased density, which is inconclusive. At 6 months post-fusion surgery, Shah et al. noted trabeculation bridging the interspace in 95% of cases on CT examination, but could note only 4% of cases on conventional radiographs.[32] In their study radiographs failed to demonstrate all the loose cages. Within the first 3 months postsurgery, the degree of fusion is underestimated in up to 20% of cases.[33] This should not be unexpected as premineralized osteoid, while possibly functionally fused, is radiolucent on x-ray. X-ray alone is therefore unreliable, especially in cases with posterior instrumentation.[34]

CT affords a better assessment of the stages of arthrodesis[35] (Fig. 16–15). Thin cut 1-mm CT is the most efficacious method for identifying bone formation within and around fusion cages.[32,36,37] Ideally, both sagittal and coronal reformatted images should be obtained and carefully evaluated for bony fusion across the endplates or for characteristic halos of demineralization surrounding the graft plugs.

The question of a solid fusion often remains after conventional static imaging study. Flexion and extension lumbar radiographs have been used to determine intersegmental motion characteristics, intersegmental instability, and therefore the status of fusion.

Lumbar FE Study A larger body of experience exists for functional radiographs of the cervical spine versus the lumbar spine.[38–40]

Some studies have reported the value of determining segmental ranges of motion, translational movements, and other measurements as useful

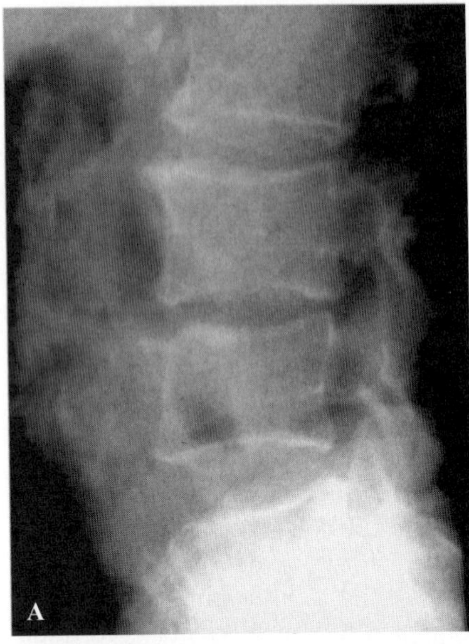
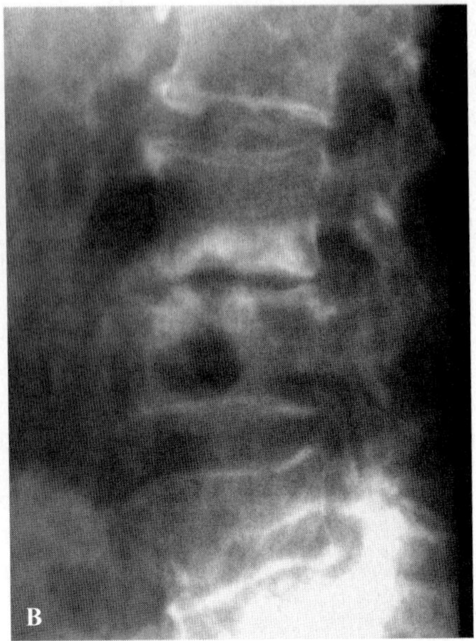
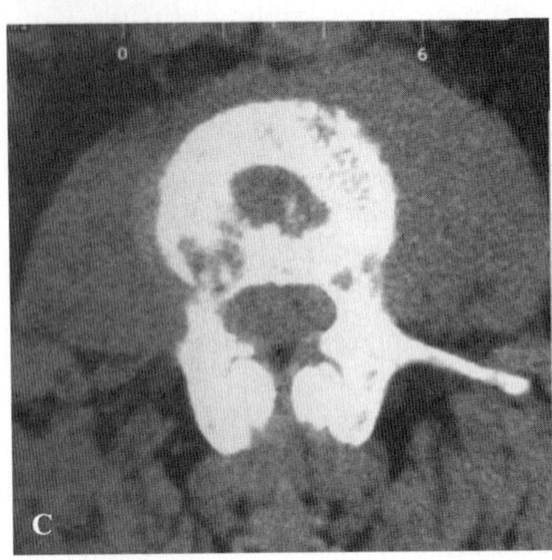

FIGURE 16–9. Infection. *A.* Conventional radiographic examination in a 58-year-old male patient with lower back pain and no history of injury. There are signs of disc interspace thinning at L3–L4 and, to a lesser degree, at L2–L3, with some modest marginal osteophytic development. This is most consistent with degenerative disc change. The end plates appear to be intact. There is a significant overlying obstructing bowel pattern. *B.* The same patient about 6 weeks later. The films now reveal progressive disc space loss and marginal irregularities. There also are areas of sclerosis at the end plates. Although the interval change is obvious and substantial, the bowel pattern again precludes clear definition of the status of the end plate region. *C.* Axial CT through the region of the end plate shows bony destruction including involvement of the vertebral body and its arch. There was no abscess formation.

parameters for assessing lumbar spine stability. Various radiographic imaging techniques have been used to study segmental lumbar spine stability. In 1944, Knutsson examined lateral FE plain films to determine instability.[41] Alternative methods such as biplanar x-ray photogrammetry and the determination of instantaneous axes of rotation have also been proposed. However, there remains no consensus as to the optimal method and FE examination of the lumbar spine remains controversial.

Frobin et al. identified factors of imprecision leading to inaccuracies in measurement from sagittal plane radiography, including distortion in central projection, off-center position, axial rotation, and lateral tilt

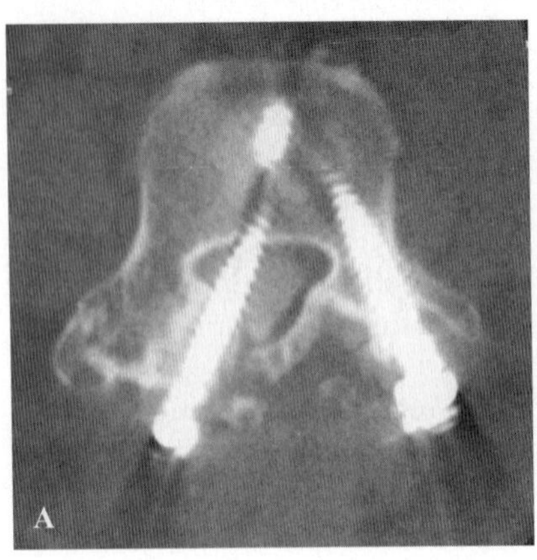
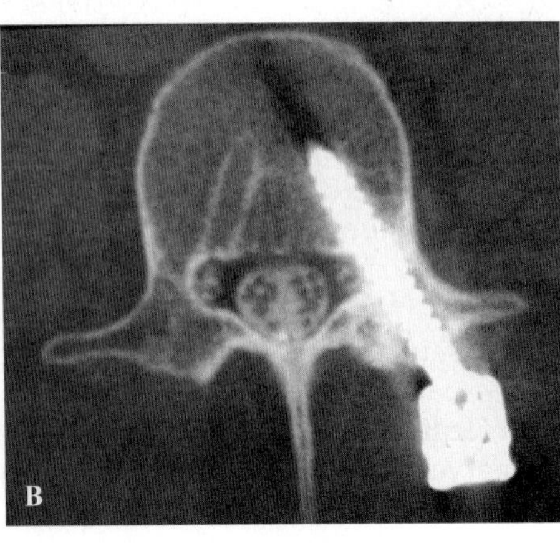

FIGURE 16–10. Poor pedicle screw placement. *A.* Axial CT demonstrating grossly inaccurate placement of pedicle screw on the right side. *B.* Another case. The left screw violates the medial cortex of the pedicle, but this is the asymptomatic side. The right screw of this construct already has been removed and its tract is still visible.

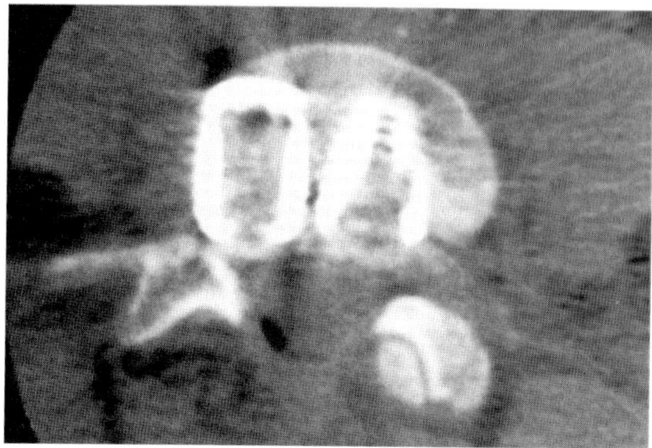

FIGURE 16–11. Violation of the right foramen by a titanium fusion cage. This patient underwent anterior lumbar interbody fusion procedure with titanium fusion cages and developed foot drop immediately thereafter. This postsurgical axial CT image demonstrates placement of the right cage extending to the intervertebral foramen. After the cage was "backed-out" a quarter turn, the neurological abnormality resolved.

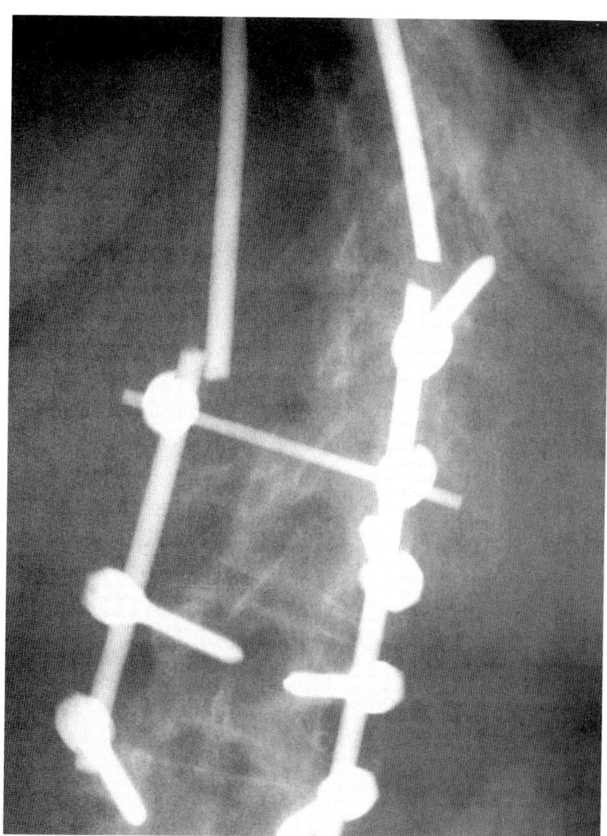

FIGURE 16–12. Broken rod. Frontal radiograph of the thoracolumbar junction in a patient with a degenerative scoliosis and a lower lumbar multilevel posterior fusion construct interconnected with rods into the thoracic spine. The rods broke singularly rather than simultaneously with different traumas.

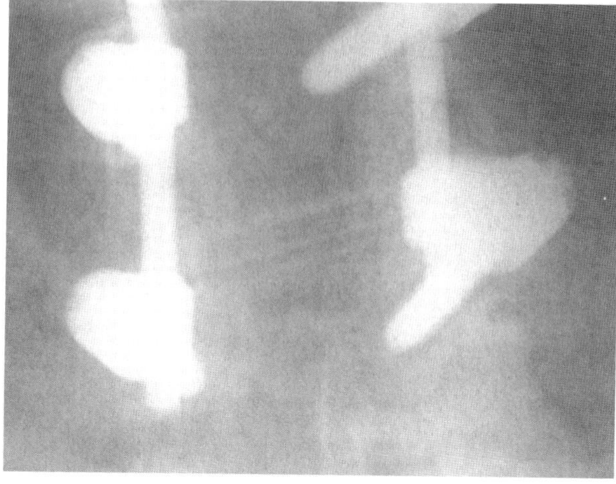

FIGURE 16–13. Loose pedicle screw. Chronic recurrent back pain in this patient prompted radiological reevaluation. Note the radiolucent halo around the lower left screw on the frontal view.

of the vertebra.[42] The common features in biomechanical descriptions of instability include increased mobility, abnormal spinal motion, and/or decreased stiffness of the functional spinal unit. The ability to demonstrate large movement is not always possible, which may be due to interpatient differences or the inability to move smoothly in maximum flexion.

Stress FE radiographs of the lumbar spine are in common use for the detection of gross instability patterns, despite existing controversy (Fig. 16–5). These dynamic techniques in the lumbar spine for

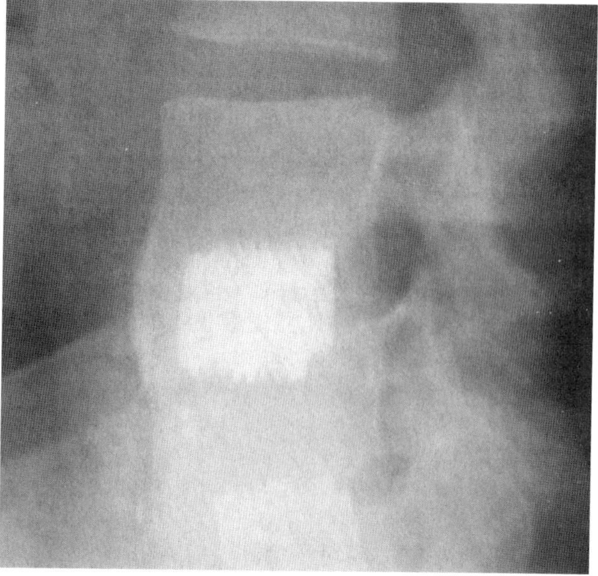

FIGURE 16–14. Successful fusion. A two-level anterior lumbar interbody fusion with titanium cages. Note the thick trabecular bone that bridges the interspace anterior to the cage.

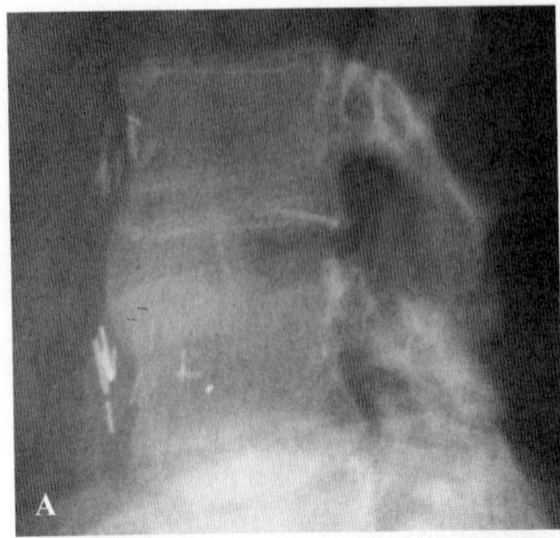

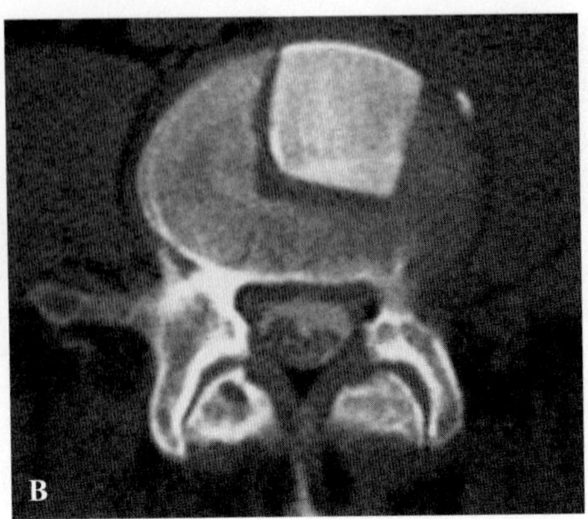

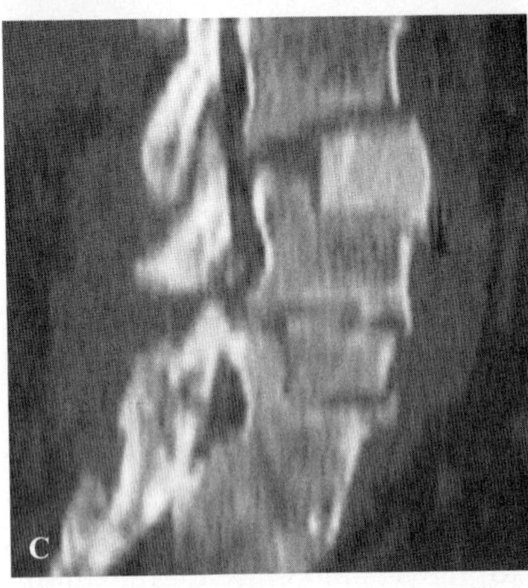

FIGURE 16–15. Pseudoarthrosis. *A.* This patient is status post two-level anterior lumbar interbody fusion procedure. The lateral view is suspicious for pseudoarthrosis. Note the apparent radiolucency surrounding the bone graft at L3–L4. *B.* Axial CT at L3–L4. There is a lack of incorporation of the graft. *C.* Sagittal reconstruction demonstrates complete absence of trabecular bone formation at the interfaces of the grafts at both L3–L4 and L4–L5 levels.

translatory and angular motion present technical and visual problems and have not been subjected to study for accuracy and reliability. They do, however, provide a semiquantitative means to evaluate end point anteroposterior motion characteristics.[43] When used to measure sagittal translatory movement in patients with spondylolisthesis, the overall performance of these methods have been good, notwithstanding the difficulty in determining the osseous landmarks used for the measurements.[44]

The question of position for FE studies has been addressed by Wood et al. [45] They studied intervertebral motion in spondylolisthesis with FE views in standing and decubitus position. In their study 31 of 50 patients displayed abnormal translation, but 18 had abnormal motion only when in lateral decubitus position, and only 4 of the 50 had more abnormal motion while standing.

The use of lumbar sidebending films for the determination of instability is less clear.[46] Pitkanen and Manninen showed that FE films more frequently revealed signs of instability than sidebending films (84 versus 50 patients). Intertechnique agreement was poor. The signs of instability on sidebending films were best correlated with the findings of angular motion and posterior sliding instability on FE films. Therefore, sidebending films may be complementary to FE films, but are probably unlikely to be helpful on a routine basis.[47]

Some declare that the FE radiographic evaluation is not useful. Using a computer-assisted program and passive radiographs in their study, Dvorak et al. concluded that these types of studies do not aid in differentiating the underlying pathological conditions.[48] In their study of asymptomatic individuals Hayes et al. concluded that FE radiography was a questionable study as a primary determinant of lumbar intersegmental instability. This was based on their finding of widely variable "norms" of angular and translatory movement. For instance, 20% of their cases had more than 4 mm of translational shift at L4–L5.[49]

Others have reported increase in anteroposterior translation in unstable segments.[50] For instance, Boden et al. attempted to define the utility or futility of FE examinations. They looked at dynamic motion rather than static positions and found that 42% of the normal subjects had at least one level with a static displacement greater than 3.0 mm in either flexion or extension, but only 5% had a dynamic AP translation greater than 3.0 mm. They continue to use less than 3.0 mm as a cutoff limit for normal anteroposterior translatory shift on dynamic studies.[51] Unfortunately, in actual practice lumbar spine movements are influenced by various factors besides the pathological

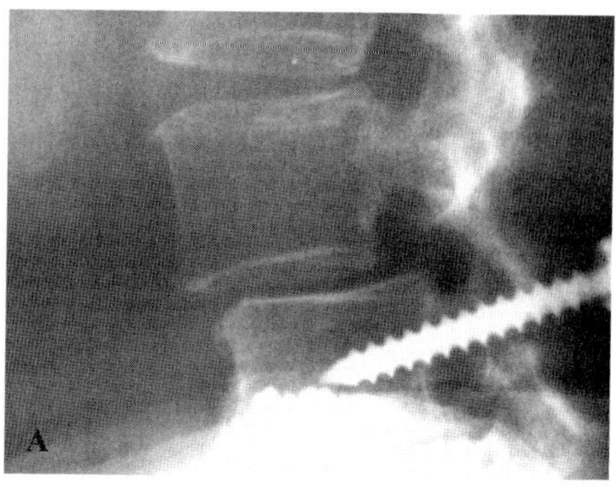

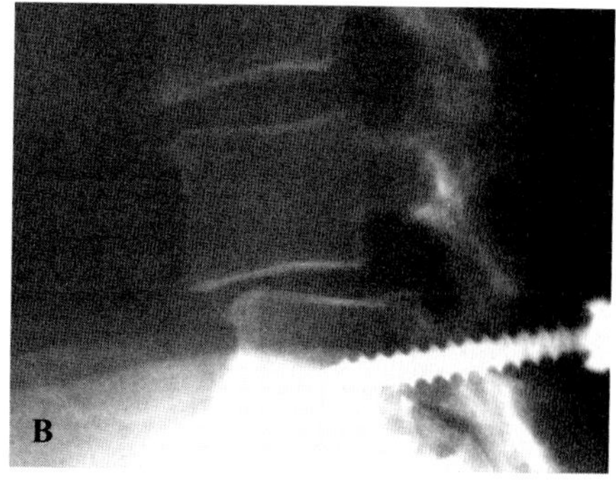

FIGURE 16–16. Degenerative spondylolisthesis above a fusion construct. *A.* The appearance on this lateral view seems straight forward with decreased disc spacing and anterolisthesis. The question of any degree of intersegmental motion is resolved by an FE study. *B.* Lumbar flexion demonstrates both translatory and angular shift of L3 on L4. In cases like these it is important to understand the nature of specific pain generator(s) that may represent active components of the patient's pain syndrome.

status of the motion segment. For instance, a patient who is in pain and has muscle spasm becomes problematical to study dynamically and FE does not always provide accurate information.[52]

When dealing with postsurgical cases, the concept of deterioration and destabilization of adjacent articulations is of critical importance (Fig. 16–16). Following lumbar fusion, both the sacroiliac joints and proximal articulations take on increased stress. Patients with persistent or recurrent pain need to be worked up for both internal disc disruption (discogenic pain) and instability. Figure 16–17 demonstrates such a case.

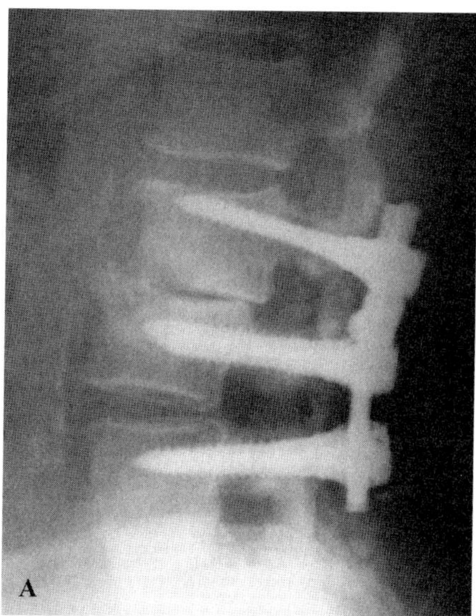

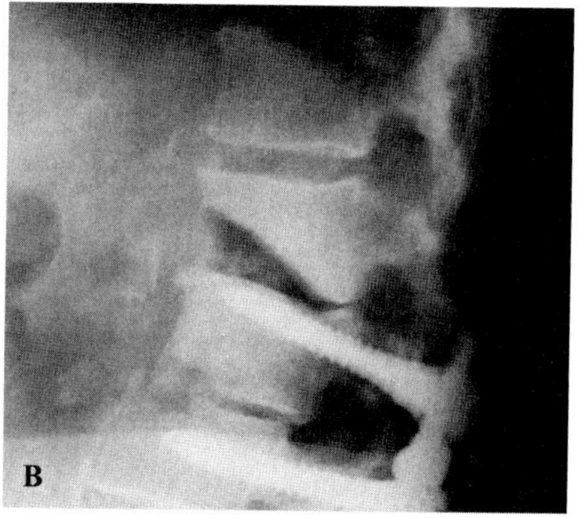

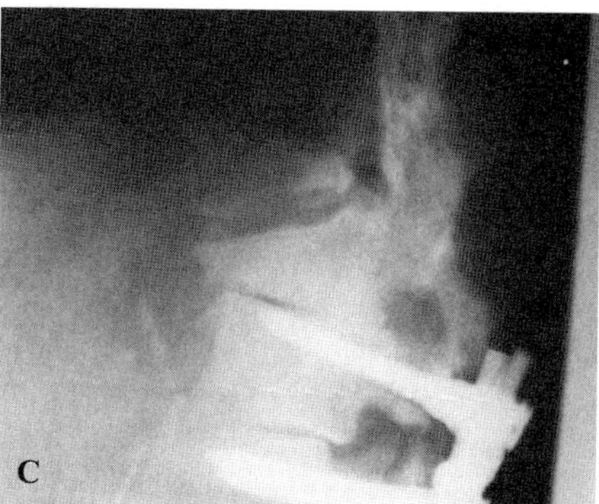

FIGURE 16–17. This patient has had "successive" ascending fusion procedures over several years, and the placement of a spinal cord stimulator for pain control. *A.* The lateral image demonstrates a somewhat thinned disc interspace above the existing construct between L2–L4. The patient had experienced ongoing pain after the latest procedure. *B.* Extension; *C.* flexion. Less than a year later after the most recent procedure the L1–L2 interspace has become destroyed, along with the anteroinferior aspect of the vertebral body. Note the angular movement between the flexion and extension excursions.

Clinical Pearl: Proximal (or distal) motion segment deterioration after a fusion procedure may be alarmingly rapid. It should NEVER be assumed that intersegmental stability is normal in these cases. FE studies are an important imaging tool.

There are important lessons to be learned in circumstances like these. In some cases the issue of instability is clear, but in others the presence or absence of movement is anything but clear. Flexion and extension studies may provide that clarification. Furthermore, there should be no hesitation to reimage if there is failure to achieve significant clinical improvement with the treatment plan, when there has been interim exacerbation or when pain suddenly arises without explanation. The patient's plan may need to be restrategized, perhaps with advanced imaging studies.

While plain radiographs reveal static end point relationships, they do not provide information on detailed motion throughout the flexion and extension excursion. Frymoyer et al. have called attention to the possibility of an instability catch, midpoint between end ranges on FE views, thereby missing the segmental abnormality.[53]

VIDEOFLUOROSCOPY

As an imaging tool, videofluoroscopy (VF) has been sporadically used for quite some time to evaluate the quality and quantity of spinal motion. This type of study goes beyond end point stress views, allowing quantification of motion between the end ranges. Previously, cineradiography produced motion images that were difficult to evaluate. Today the images are digitized. The Quebec task force studied VF in 1987 and did not support its use as a clinical tool in the lumbar spine on the basis of lack of standardization with training and protocols, and its reliability of findings when compared with the clinical correlation (Quebec task force, 1987).

There have been few studies utilizing this technique. Video characterization of lumbar movement was performed in a study by Kanayama et al., which revealed deformation behavior of normal lumbar discs while undergoing flexion and extension of the trunk.[54] This study demonstrated that during flexion, disc deformation increased rapidly after a certain delay from the start of trunk motion, and reached maximum value before the finish of trunk motion. Time lags in motion response occurred and each disc deformed, not simultaneously, but stepwise from the upper to the lower level. Kanayama's work reveals the phenomena of lumbar spinal kinematics that may provide understanding of intersegmental instability.[54]

Early techniques encountered high radiation exposure and difficulty in adjusting for out of plane images. Calibration of multiplanar motion, measurements of lumbar angular rotation, and instantaneous centers of rotation in the coronal plane have been carried out by Breen et al.[55] Images were digitized from an image intensifier. Observer error occurred in marking coordinates and scaling the image presented by the computer's monitor. Out-of-plane images caused some distortion. Also there was some loss of image quality as a result of scattered radiation from the soft tissues. Nevertheless, this technique may have some value in the light of its efficiency and low x-ray exposure to patients.[56]

More recently Zheng et al. reported encouraging findings of the kinematic analysis of the lumbar spine.[57] Digital VF was used to produce 2D image sequences of the spine in motion. Their images exhibited noise degradation enhanced by the very low radiation dosage. Under such circumstances, the determination of vertebral position within the image sequence may be challenging. Their technique used a combination of spine kinematic measurements with a solid model of the human lumbar spine for visualization of the spine in motion. Edge detection was improved. A dynamic visualization package was developed in order to view the moving lumbar spine from any angle and viewpoint.

Despite the remaining questions about sensitivity, specificity, and reliability of standard FE studies of the lumbar spine, they remain in regular use and often provide practical information. While they often fail to detect excessive motion or to augment the visibility of a halo, they often do allow the identification of unusual and abnormal degrees of movement indicating instability. Videofluoroscopic imaging of the lumbar spine has never gained any far-reaching enthusiasm for its use in general or specialty spine practices. Protocols and standardization are still lacking, and reliability and comparison to clinical findings have still not been adequately studied.

Clinical Pearl: FE examinations of the lumbar spine are important studies when there is suspicion of intersegmental instability based on clinical findings, subjective complaints, or conventional radiographic signs of degenerative disc thinning and traction spur formation. The understanding of excessive motion may not be otherwise understood and the use of FE projections should NOT be constrained categorically. On the other hand, lateral bending views offer little information not gleaned on standard and FE views, and their use should NOT be routine. At the present time there is no convincing evidence of the utility or reliability of VF in lieu of FE studies.

COMPUTED TOMOGRAPHY

During the 1980s, CT became the preferred imaging for spinal investigations beyond conventional radiography. This preference later decreased to a secondary role with the introduction of MRI in the mid-1980s. Recently, there have been technical advances in CT. Single breath-hold acquisitions of 25–30 seconds are possible with spiral CT, and multidetector scanners have scan times that are two to eight times faster. Image-processing techniques including multiplanar reconstruction (MPR) and volumetric 3D imaging provide capabilities that are critical in some spine imaging cases.

CT uses a thin collimated x-ray beam rotating through a 180-degree arc. The beam is equal to the defined slice thickness. Nowadays scanners use a slip ring technology that allows the acquisition of two axial slices per rotation of the x-ray tube (helical or spiral CT). Contiguous multiplanar reconstructed images are possible. While the obtained spatial resolution is less than that of conventional radiographs, the contrast resolution of CT is dramatically better than conventional radiography (approximately 100 times). The sharply collimated x-ray beam provides greater soft tissue detail than do plain films.

The CT image is produced based on mathematical measurements of the attenuation of a well-collimated x-ray beam passing through a section of anatomy. Contrast in the image derives from the differences in attenuation based on electron density and the effective anatomic number of the individual tissue components.

The CT image is not recorded in a conventional radiographic manner. A curvilinear array of radiation detectors is present as a fixed ring. The detectors measure the amount of radiation passing through the patient and form an image based on the differential absorption of the x-rays. Each array detector responds by downloading numeric data to the system's computer. The computer assigns a numeric value to the attenuation data from each radiation detector. The relative attenuation coefficient (μ) is expressed as a CT number or Hounsfield unit (HU). This number may vary from -1000 to $+1000$ HU. Pure water is equal to 0 HU, air is -1000 HU, and cortical bone and metal are $+1000$ HU. These data are portrayed on an image matrix made up of pixels (picture elements) each containing the attenuation value of the imaged anatomy in that sector. The CT image is a map of the linear attenuation values of the tissue. The matrix is usually 512×512 pixels.

The inability of a patient to remain motionless during the study remains a problem with the CT examination, as are some metallic objects (surgical hardware, shrapnel, etc). Beam-hardening artifacts may be created by the presence of some fusion cages, pedicle screws, rods, and plates. Nevertheless, in many instances the environs of the spinal canal is imaged well (Figs. 16–10 and 16–11). As might be expected obese patients often produce a suboptimal study.

Indications and Uses of Computed Tomogarphy

Overall, CT is a powerful and versatile tool in the adjunctive diagnosis of musculoskeletal pathology, especially in discerning complex spatial relationships. The high contrast between low-density fat and the higher density intervertebral disc and nerve roots allows for highly accurate delineation of nerve root impingement. Indeed, CT became increasingly important because of its high-resolution cross-sectional depiction of the soft tissues and bony components of the spine. Sagittal and coronal multiplanar reconstructed images also help in the diagnosis of alignment and rotational abnormalities. Reformatted data produce images of somewhat lesser resolution in other planes. Three-dimensional images often provide unique visual perspectives compared to traditional planes of imaging. These 3D techniques are adjunctive to other modalities. They have demonstrated greatest usefulness in complex spine fractures and fracture–dislocations, cases with marked degenerative change, and in complicated anomalous formations. They are less useful with soft tissue abnormalities. The indications for lumbar CT examinations are listed in Table 16–1.

Trauma

The widespread availability, speed, and versatility of CT have made it a mainstay in evaluating acute spine trauma. High-resolution CT allows for excellent noninvasive evaluation of osseous detail and adjacent soft tissues of the spine, particularly the complex anatomy

TABLE 16–1. Indications for CT

- Degenerative disease
  - Posterior facets: hypertrophic change, facet cysts
  - Stenosis and related stenotic features
  - Vacuum facet, vacuum SI, vacuum disc
- Disc herniation, particularly far lateral herniation
- Ligamentous ossification: OPLL, ligamentum flavum, anulus fibrosus
- Trauma: retropulsed fragment(s), avulsions, posterior rim fractures, arch and facet fractures
- Spondylolysis/spondylolisthesis: pars integrity and evidence for healing, hypertrophic callus at the pars or lamina
- Neoplasia
- Infection and inflammatory process: provides high spatial resolution and exceptional detail of cortical bone, detects small areas of erosion or lysis, gas, and foreign bodies
- Complex congenital bony anomalies, dysraphism, diastematomyelia, meningocele, lipomeningocele
- Postoperative: evaluation of fusion, grafts, placement, and integrity of hardware
- Postmyelography CT: spinal canal and neuroforaminal stenosis, conjoined nerve root

in areas that do not image well with conventional radiographs. A prime example is occult and complex fractures. Indeed, CT is the examination method of choice in evaluation of spinal trauma. While the routine use of CT for screening purposes is not advocated, it is appropriate for those patients who are otherwise not reliably examinable.

The thoracolumbar junction is very susceptible to injury. The orientation of the facet joints and gross differences in the thoracic versus lumbar ranges of motion help to account for this propensity.

In the trauma case, CT can usually discern bone, blood, disc, and foreign bodies, although in cases like these MRI would provide significant additional information about the contents of the spinal canal and foramina. It has the added benefit of accurately detecting concomitant thoracic cage and abdominal abnormalities including vascular injuries with minimal respiratory misregistration.

It is very useful for compression and burst injuries in providing additional information with respect to retropulsed fragments (Fig. 16–6*B*). It also provides improved detail of the crush pattern and vital information with respect to the integrity of the spinal canal and individual arch elements.

The posterior vertebral arches are seen in great detail with CT, which is in contrast to a more limited evaluation of the posterior elements with MRI. This is especially true of laminar fracture and articular facet fracture. Posterior disruption of the ligamentous complex gives rise to a naked facet appearance on CT. The actual visualization of the ligament disruption proper is better seen on MRI.

Posterior Arch and Facets

CT with MPR allows for excellent delineation of the lumbar facet joints, their orientation, alignment, and spacing as well as any degree of erosion, cystic change, or marginal proliferation. Laminar thickening, capsular calcification, and synovial facet cysts and synovitis may also be visualized. DISH and OPLL often exhibit hyperostosis adjacent to the facet articulations in addition to central canal involvement. CT with MPR is excellent for evaluation of the pars interarticularis (Fig. 16–4*D*).

Disorders of the Intervertebral Discs

There are several pitfalls in the CT diagnosis of disc disruption. Nonparallel scanning through the plane of the intervertebral disc may create the false appearance of a disc herniation. The steep lumbosacral angle sometimes exceeds the maximum gantry angle. This places the posterior margin of the L5 disc posterior to the L5 body. In these instances there should be no compression of the thecal sac. A similar situation may arise in cases of spondylolisthesis and scoliosis. Conjoined nerve roots may also simulate the mass effect of a herniated disc. They may cause a soft tissue density in the anterior epidural space along the course of the exiting root and may obliterate the local epidural fat. The mass effect of a confluence of the epidural veins also may be similarly confusing.

The CT findings of disc herniation are similar to that of MRI: focal or broad-based alteration of the margin of the disc with displacement or compression of the thecal sac or neural elements; obliteration of the epidural fat; and calcification or gas within the disc herniation. Sequestered disc fragments are often surrounded by fat. CT is, however, useful in showing disc calcifications.

While the calculation of CT attenuation values (HU) is helpful in the differentiation between certain tissues, it has not been helpful for the disc proper. CT images do not allow for the differentiation between anulus fibrosus and nucleus pulposus, or direct evidence for contained versus noncontained disc herniations. In this regard MRI is far superior to CT, and it has expanded our understanding of intervertebral disc pathology. Another example is the differentiation of a conjoined nerve root, which remains difficult with conventional CT because of the similarity in the density of a herniation and the nerve root.

The computed tomographic differentiation between postoperative scarring from recurrent herniation is difficult. CT is better than myelography alone. Previously, CT with contrast was used to differentiate enhancing scar from nonenhancing disc. MRI with contrast is now the procedure of choice because of the decreased incidence of contrast reactions.

Stenosis

CT is the best choice for evaluation of the bony spinal canal and intervertebral foramina. Congenital stenosis usually demonstrates uniform narrowing over several segments, decreased AP dimension of the canal, short and thick pedicles, and decreased interpedicular distances. On the other hand, degenerative stenosis exhibits nonuniform stenosis with hypertrophic changes from the articular facets, thickening of the ligamentum flavum, generalized bulging or frank herniation of the disc(s), posterior vertebral body osteophytes, and obliteration of the epidural fat.

Clinical Pearl: CT is superior for the evaluation of the vertebral canals in cases of stenosis.

Visualization of the lateral recesses and foramina is excellent with CT. The boundaries of the lateral recess are *anterior* (posterolateral margin of the vertebral body and disc), *posterior* (superior articular process), and *lateral* (pedicle). Normally the lateral recess measures $\geq$5 mm. The boundaries of the intervertebral foramen are *superior* (pedicle above), *inferior* (pedicle below), *anterior* (posterior aspect of vertebral bodies and intervertebral discs), and *posterior* (pars interarticularis and apex of the superior articular process of the inferior vertebra).

CT affords excellent visualization of Paget's disease and good correlation with conventional radiographs. Stenosis occurs in Paget's disease because of bony enlargement. Facet arthropathy often occurs when there is trabecular remodeling of the articular processes. DISH and ossification of the posterior longitudinal ligament (OPLL) are often associated with central stenotic effects and they are imaged ideally with CT.

Sacroiliac Joints

The overlying bowel pattern often obscures visualization of the sacrum and sacroiliac joints on conventional studies (Fig. 16–7*A* and 16–7*B*). Not only does CT provide superior anatomic detail for the detection of sacral fracture, stress fractures, sacroiliitis, infection, and tumor, but it is also sensitive to pelvic bleeding in cases of pelvic trauma or aneurysm.

Postsurgical Evaluation

With prominent and annoying metallic artifact in the postsurgical setting, CT or CT myelography with MPR allows the questions of fusion status and stability, graft incorporation, graft migration, hardware placement, and hardware integrity to be settled when unanswered by MRI (see Figs. 16–10, 16–11, 16–15*B*, and 16–15*C*).

Clinical Pearl: CT provides the best information concerning hardware placement, loosening, and osteosynthesis at a graft/bone or cage/bone interface.

Infection

Osteolysis and fragmentation of the vertebral end plates may be depicted earlier on CT than on conventional imaging (Fig. 16–9*C*). Sometimes there is extension into the posterior arches and paraspinal soft tissue. The paraspinal soft tissues are visualized well on CT and abscesses often contain gas.

Tumors

MRI has largely replaced CT for the study of spinal neoplasms, except for the visualization of cortical erosions and calcified tumor matrices. Osteochondromas uncommonly involve the spine, but they may appear as an extension of the vertebral arch in close association to the spinous and transverse process.

CT–MYELOGRAPHY

In the 1970s, Amipaque (metrizamide) was introduced and replaced Pantopaque (iophendylate) as the contrast agent for myelography. Pantopaque had to be removed following a myelographic procedure as the residual contrast could lead to arachnoiditis. Metrizamide gets absorbed into the bloodstream, does not cause arachnoiditis, and can be used in combination with a CT examination (CT-myelography; CTM).

After the introduction of the opaque contrast medium into the subarachnoid space the spinal cord and nerve roots may be outlined. The low viscosity of the water-soluble contrast permits filling of the nerve roots and better visualization. Abnormalities of the dura or arachnoid may thereby be appreciated. Myelography demonstrates the nerve root sheaths to their termination near the dorsal root ganglion.

Flexion and extension views may be helpful with myelography if dynamic stenosis is suspected, particularly with patients in the upright position.

Today, with water-soluble contrast, CT is almost always performed at the conclusion of standard myelography as a complimentary examination adding the advantages of the cross-sectional and MPR perspective (Fig. 16–18). Current nonionic contrast agents have a much lower incidence of side effects and

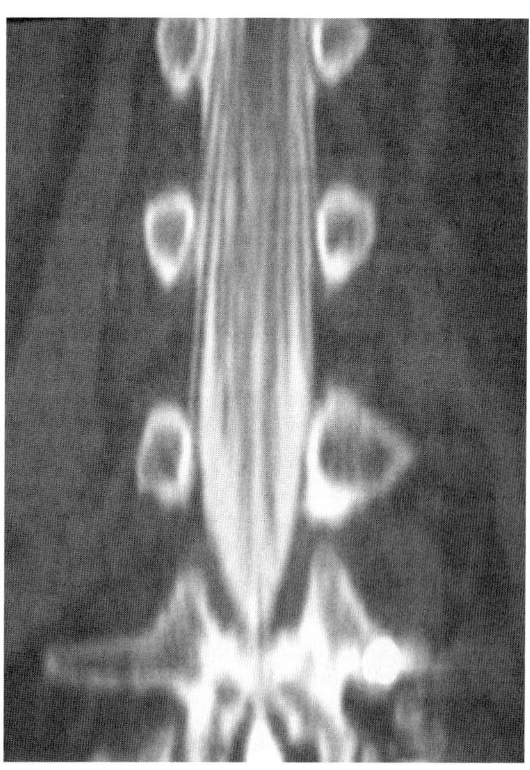

FIGURE 16–18. CTM. Coronal reformatted image showing the fine detail of the distribution of the individual terminal fibers of the cauda equina.

allergic reactions. With the introduction of small (26- or 27-gauge) needles with blunt tips, the occurrence of spinal headaches and other complications has been markedly reduced and patient tolerance to the procedure has increased significantly.

There is an ongoing controversy as to the utilization of CT alone or in conjunction with myelography (CTM) for the diagnosis of degenerative disease including stenosis. Nowadays in many spine-specialty centers CTM is extensively used to sort through the pathoanatomy and search for a better understanding of the pain generators in lumbar spine cases (Fig. 7–9B).

Despite the strong use of MRI, CTM is still considered by some to be the gold standard for demonstrating the soft tissue and bony changes that result in nerve root and spinal cord compression.[58]

Some studies have shown that conventional myelography is superior to plain CT in the assessment of root compression in the lateral recesses. Bartynski and Lin conclude in their study that MRI significantly underestimates root compression caused by degenerative changes in the lateral recess.[59] While MRI is excellent for characterization of the degenerative disc proper and for disc protrusion, conventional myelography and CT are important supplemental studies necessary to confirm degenerative nerve root impingement in the lateral recess as the cause of radiculopathy. These studies can be performed to confirm the findings at MRI or when looking for foraminal disc herniations that may have been missed at MRI.

CT is also used for guidance during interventional procedures such as facet injections or laser ablation techniques. However, in most centers fluoroscopic guidance is preferred. CT scanners dedicated for injection procedures are not available at most centers. C-arm fluroscopic techniques are quicker, more flexible, and better suited for most lumbar spine procedures.

Post-discography CT is discussed in Chapter 17 (see also Fig. 6–3B).

MAGNETIC RESONANCE IMAGING

After its introduction into clinical use in the early to mid-1980s, MRI rapidly replaced CT scanning as the modality of choice for most spine imaging, despite its far greater cost and greater susceptibility to motion artifacts. The initial lofty expectations that MRI would fully elucidate all facets of pathomorphology and obviate the need for other techniques has not occurred.

Few controlled studies have been done to compare and contrast it with other imaging modalities. Important advantages of MRI include the lack of ionizing radiation, multiplanar capability over a wide spine area, and a wide array of pulse sequences that permit much greater tissue contrast and characterization as compared to CT. Indeed, MRI is sensitive to an entire spectrum of phenomena to which radiography is totally insensitive.

MRI Physics

The detailed physics of MRI is complicated and can prove to be a quagmire for all but the most intrepid physics enthusiasts. The intent here is to provide the reader with enough understanding of the basic physics to understand image production, artifacts, and the pulse sequences in common use. Detailed discussion of MRI physics can be found in numerous books detailing MRI.

There is little similarity with the physics of ultrasonography or conventional radiography. Unlike CT, which depends upon multiple thin slices of radiation that are "backplotted" through Fourier transform, MRI requires no ionizing radiation to the patient in order to obtain images. Instead, MRI uses magnetic fields and radiofrequency (RF) waves. A powerful magnet (e.g., 0.1–1.5 T) is used to align tissue protons parallel to the magnetic field. Following this, an RF pulse is generated perpendicular to the magnetic field, causing the protons to be "knocked down" at an angle to the magnetic field (90 degrees for most standard spin echo sequences). Once the RF pulse is completed, the tissue protons "relax" back into their parallel state relative to the magnetic field. As they relax they emit back the energy they gained with the RF pulse. This energy, in the form of a *signal*, is detected by receiver coils in the MRI scanner, and through Fourier reconstruction based on step-wise changes in phase or frequency, and is localized in 3D space. Furthermore, each tissue in the body has differing signal characteristics, depending on the number and "freedom" of its protons. These same characteristics in turn determine how quickly or slowly the protons realign in the main magnetic field after the RF pulse. Some tissues, such as water, have very "loose" or mobile protons that return very quickly to alignment in the magnetic field. Thus, water will give a very different signal from bone, where the existing protons are largely immobile. This helps explain why calcium appears dark on any sequence, since it cannot emit much signal (unless the associated calcium/bone is filled with fat or water).

The specific techniques for obtaining the MRI are called *pulse sequences*. The distinctiveness of the RF pulse determines the nature of the pulse sequence, of which there are an ever-increasing number on the MRI market.

These pulse sequences result from the manipulation of the RF pulse factor variables before acquisition

TABLE 16–2. Differences in Signal Intensity on T1-Weighted (T1W) Versus T2-Weighted (T2W) Images

Tissue	T1W	T2W
Cortical bone	Low	Low
Tendons and ligaments	Low	Low
Fibrocartilage	Low	Low
Muscle	Intermediate	Intermediate
Non-neoplastic tumour	Low-intermediate	Low/intermediate/possible high
Neoplastic tumor	Low-intermediate	Intermediate–high/possible low
Water,CSF	Low	High
Inflammation	Low	High
Proteinaceous fluid, abscess	Intermediate	High
Fat	High	High (slightly lower than on T1W)
Hemorrhage,acute	High	High
Hemorrhage,chronic	Low	High

of the scan: TR, TE, and RF angle. The TR (time to repetition: the time between generation of the RF pulses) and TE (time to echo: the length of time before sampling the energy or *echo* of the RF signal from the tissue) may be lengthened or shortened, and the RF angle (*flip angle*) increased or decreased (how far the proton is knocked down from the original upright position in the main magnetic field).

Tissues have inherent MRI properties that are termed T1 or T2 relaxation characteristics. Accordingly, the two most basic and important MRI sequences are termed *T1-weighted* and *T2-weighted,* which means that the study brings out or emphasizes these respective characteristics. A third important sequence is termed *proton density-weighted* (PD or intermediate-weighted), which brings out a useful mix of both T1 and T2 tissue properties. These sequences are termed spin echo (SE) and have been the mainstay of lumbar spine imaging. Table 16–2 itemizes the differences in signal intensities on T1-weighted and T2-weighted MR images. Figure 16–19 illustrates the differences between the T1-weighted and T2-weighted image.

T1-weighted pulse sequences are obtained with short TR (about 400–600 ms) and short TE (5–30 ms). T1-weighted images (also called fat images) have high signal-to-noise ratio (SNR) and produce excellent anatomical representation. On the other hand, T2-weighted sequences require a long TR (1500–3000 ms) and a long TE (60–120 ms). T2-weighted sequences emphasize the T2 properties of a tissue, especially its state of hydration and particularly the free extracellular fluid. Those sequences with long TR and short TE reflect the number of mobile hydrogen nuclei or spin density (PD).

Clinical Pearl: T1 and T2 relaxation are physical properties intrinsic to a tissue. The image character on the MR image is dependent largely upon a tissues' T1 and T2 properties and the number of mobile hydrogen ions.

A host of additional sequences have been developed that are useful for specific applications. They have been subject to frequent change and modification, and the same techniques are designated by different acronyms from different manufacturers. (The reader should not expect to remember the names of all the sequences, but there are some general classes of sequences that should be recognized.)

One of these is *T2** (T2 star). Such sequences use smaller flip angles (less than 90 degrees) and accentuate certain tissue properties such as fluid. Images are acquired more rapidly and they also may be used to reduce motion artifacts. Examples include *GRASS, FLASH,* etc.

Fast spin echo (turbo spin echo) sequences are now almost universally used to reduce scan time and increase spatial or contrast resolution.[60] These techniques show tissue properties that are similar to spin echo (T1 and T2-weighted sequences), but with some important differences such as brighter fat signal and decreased susceptibility artifact.

Both chemical fat-suppression and specific sequences such as STIR (short tau inversion recovery) have been developed that turn the normally bright fat

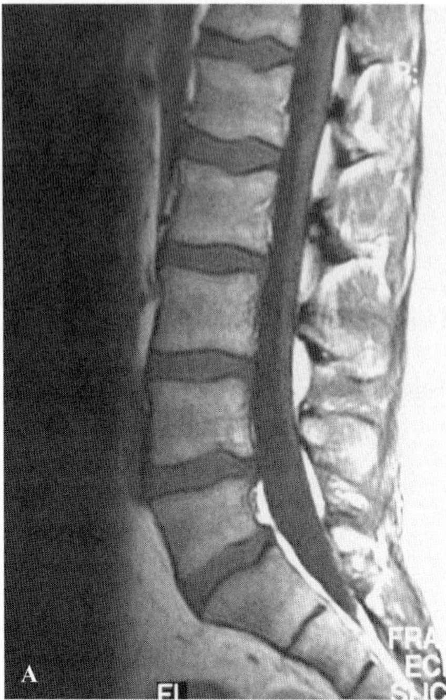

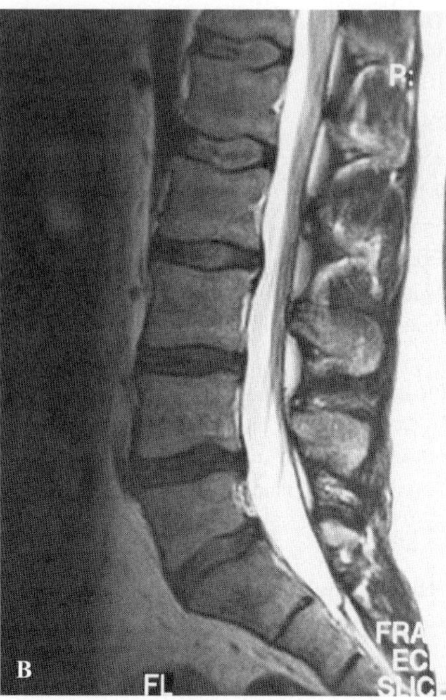

FIGURE 16–19. MRI appearance of the lumbar spine. *A.* Sagittal T1-weighted (T1W); *B.* sagittal T2-weighted (T2W). Subcutaneous fat is very high signal on both sequences. In the vertebra the normal proportion of red to yellow marrow is high so that vertebral bodies show medium to high signal with T1 and somewhat lower on T2W. The pattern of this signal may be homogeneous or inhomogeneous depending on the distribution of fibrous tissue and the marrow fat. End plates are low signal on both sequences. The appearance of the intervertebral disc reflects its water content. Normally the disc is low signal on T1W and high on T2W, unless water content has decreased. In this example the lower three discs have varying degrees of signal loss. The spinal cord and nerve tissues are intermediate in signal on T1W and somewhat lower on T2W. CSF is low on T1W and high on T2W. Note how conspicuous the posterior intervertebral disc is against the high signal of the CSF. On T1W images the signal of the anulus and longitudinal ligaments blend together imperceptibly with CSF.

signals to low signal (dark) so that fat can be differentiated from water (edema, infection, tumor, all bright on STIR).

Even more specialized sequences have been developed in the perpetual search for increased specificity or sensitivity in identifying tumor and metabolic/enzymatic abnormalities.

In addition to the various specific sequences, the technical parameters of how those sequences are obtained can be manipulated to shorten the time of the scan and improve tissue contrast or increase spatial resolution. One of these parameters is the NEX or number of excitations (acquisitions) that are obtained. With each acquisition (NEX), the same area is scanned identically and added to the collected data of the image. With each NEX, more signal is obtained and the image becomes less "noisy." However, doubling the NEX also doubles the time of the exam and increases the potential for motion artifact.

Slice thickness is also an important variable. Thinner slices exhibit greater spatial resolution (detail). However, the thinner slice also contains fewer signals and is therefore "noisier" and appears grainier. Increasing the NEX would help this problem. A compounding issue arises when using thinner slices, as it may take more time to get enough slices to cover the area of interest. Also, increasing the number of gradient phase or frequency steps can increase resolution, but may increase scan time or introduce artifacts.

Finally, field strength of the magnet is an important variable. Magnet strength is ranked from low field strength to high field strength: Ultralow (<0.1 T), low (0.1–0.3 T), midfield (0.3–0.6 T), and high field (>0.6 T). Signal strength increases in proportion to the strength of the magnetic field, so a larger magnet generates more signal than a smaller magnet, which improves image quality and decreases scan time. There are basic advantages of high-field systems including shorter imaging time, higher SNR, improved image resolution (both spatial and temporal), and thinner slice images.[61] However, small field strength magnets do have some strengths such as excellent ability to depict fat signal.

So, much like photography and conventional radiography, a variety of factors influence the appearance and usefulness of the final image. All of these variables must be taken into account in the quest to obtain an optimal scan. Scan time must be short enough to prevent motion, yet long enough to maximize SNR; slice thickness must be thin enough to get necessary detail but thick enough and with adequate spacing to provide enough signal and prevent bandwidth artifacts. Finally, the correct sequences and correct coils must be selected to optimize the scan and to obtain the necessary detail. Unfortunately, there is no one best pulse sequence or set of sequences that meets all clinical situations. Rather, an examination is best when specifically tailored to the patient and the diagnostic information desired. It behooves the practitioner to become acquainted with the various imaging techniques, advantages and disadvantages, and the availability at one's local MRI facility. Furthermore, the quality of the scan proper and quality of interpretation varies widely.[62,63]

Indications for MRI

MRI enjoys a number of advantages over CT for the evaluation of the spine. The lack of ionizing radiation, its multiplanar capability, and excellent contrast properties makes it the study of choice for most spinal pathology. In particular, MRI is indicated for disc pathology, suspected cord lesions, infection, bone marrow abnormalities, and spinal tumor (Table 16–3 lists the indications for MRI). However, in older patients with significant degenerative (osteophytic) disease, or in patients with suspected acute trauma (especially fracture), CT offers superior cortical detail.

Clinical Pearl: MRI is the procedure of choice for the study of most spinal pathology. However, some cases of osteodegenerative conditions and trauma may be better imaged with CT.

MRI with contrast is indicated (see Table 16–4) in cases of suspected infection (e.g., postoperative infection, suspected discitis, or epidural abscess), tumor (solid or intrathecal seeding, which may not be evident on nonenhanced sequences), suspected spinal AVM (for small-vessel enhancement), or in the postoperative setting when searching for recurrent herniation versus scar (Fig. 16–20). In cases of spinal surgery limited to the anterior approach (ALIF), contrast tends not to be helpful unless there is a suspicion of infection. Contrast may be helpful in cases of suspected adhesive arachnoiditis, as inflamed nerve roots show varying degrees of enhancement. Allergic reactions to MRI contrast tend to be less severe (nausea/vomiting, metallic taste, hives, shaking, chills) than those due to CT contrast (iodine). Life-threatening reactions are exceedingly rare with MRI contrast.

TABLE 16–3. Indications for Magnetic Resonance Imaging

- Simultaneous delineation of multiple soft-tissue and osseous abnormalities (multiplanar imaging over a wide area)
- Degenerative disease
- Disc lesions
- Stenosis and facet disease
- Dynamic lumbar studies
- Conjoined nerve roots
- Postoperative evaluation: DD of recurrent herniation and postoperative scar
- Infection: osteomyelitis, discitis, abscess formation
- Muscle injury, denervation
- Spondyloarthropathies
- Trauma: acute, pars stress reactions, and fracture
- Epidural hematoma
- Neoplastic disease: benign and malignant tumors of bone, METS, spinal cord tumors
- Marrow disorders
- Bony anomalies
- Tethered cord, syrinx, and related Arnold-Chiari malformation

Limitations/Drawbacks of MRI

Inherent tissue properties as well as certain technical factors of image acquisition make MRI subject to limitations and artifacts that are not found in conventional radiation-based imaging. The long and narrow tube of some high-field-strength MRI scanners present challenges for the claustrophobic patient. Indeed, claustrophobia remains a significant problem, occurring in 2%–5% of patients. Today there is a plethora of schemes to assist the space-challenged patient, which include mirrors, music, shorter bore magnets, and

TABLE 16–4. Indications for the Use of Contrast Enhanced MRI

- Suspected infection: post-operative infection, discitis or epidural abscess
- Tumor: solid or intrathecal seeding
- Suspected spinal arteriovenous malformation (AVM) for small-vessel enhancement
- Differentiation between recurrent herniation and postoperative scar
- Suspected adhesive arachnoiditis (inflamed nerve roots show varying degrees of enhancement)
- Inflammatory conditions

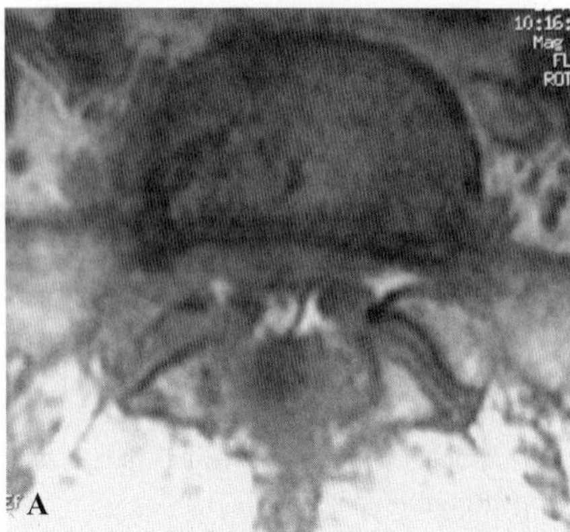

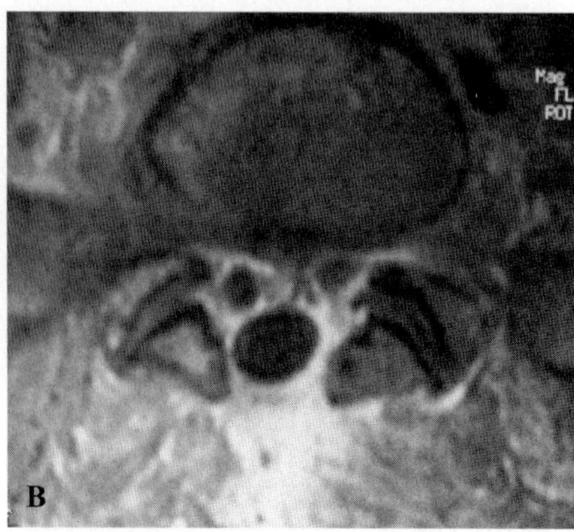

FIGURE 16–20. Laminectomy/discectomy. This patient underwent posterior decompression and experienced persistent symptoms. *A.* Noncontrast T1-weighted axial image at L5–S1. *B.* Postcontrast axial image through the same area showing enhancement around remnant disc tissue and the laminectomy defect area. Sometimes signal differences between the mass, the dural sac, and the disc margin may be sufficient so that scar tissue can be distinguished. More often they cannot be differentiated and contrast enhancement may be helpful. A nonenhancing anterior soft tissue mass that displaces the nerve root is suspicious for persistent or recurrent disc herniation. The anterior soft tissue mass may obliterate the epidural fat resulting in nonvisualization of the nerve roots.

scenic art painted on the magnet wall. In some cases a prone position may be helpful. A variety of anxiety reduction strategies have been developed to help patients cope with this problem; however, in actual practice almost all patients can tolerate closed MRI scanning following conscious oral sedation using agents such as Versed™, Valium™, or Benadryl™. For those few patients unable to tolerate closed scanning, either a wide (short) bore magnet or an actual open scanner will prove successful in almost all cases, but most open MRI systems have mid or low-field-strength magnets and therefore may produce poorer image quality compared to high-field-strength magnets.

CT is far less sensitive to motion artifact than is MRI. On CT scanning, motion will only degrade a single image out of perhaps 50–60 in an average scan. For the vast majority of MRI sequences a single movement, such as a cough or small shift in position will degrade not just one image, but every image in the sequence. For patients with persistent cough, Parkinsonian tremor, or involuntary tic or other motion, CT should be considered as an alternative.

MRI is substantially inferior to CT in the delineation of fine cortical structure including trabecular pattern, bony degenerative change, or subtle fracture line. MRI scanning is also inferior to CT in the assessment of neuroforaminal stenosis and particularly central stenosis, for which CTM remains the gold standard.

There are a number of well-known contraindications to MRI (see Table 16–5). These have been cataloged in a number of excellent references. A searchable database containing over 700 implants, devices, and objects that have been tested for MRI safety can be found at www.mrisafety.com. The more important contraindications include ferromagnetic aneurysm clips (more recent titanium clips may be safely scanned, but the exact clip model must be verified in writing before a scan is performed), cochlear

TABLE 16–5. Contraindications for MRI*

- Intracranial aneurysm clips
- Cardiac pacemakers
- Some prosthetic heart valves
- Implanted cardiac defibrillators
- Carotid artery vascular clamp
- Spinal cord stimulators (neurostimulators)
- Insulin infusion pump (implanted drug infusion device)
- Bone growth stimulator
- Metallic hardware,† devices‡, fragments
- Hearing aids and dentures (remove)
- Cochlear implants, ocular implants, penile implants
- Some shrapnel and bullets
- Intraoccular foreign bodies
- Tattooed eyeliner
- Some types of makeup

Note. These may be contraindicated unless tested and known safe at various magnetic strength levels. Surgical documentation of an implanted device is necessary, but not often known or available.

*May not apply to low-field imaging systems, i.e., Toshiba Access© 0.064T

†Post-operative MRI: In general, if the metallic object is a ëpassive implantí (no power in operation of the object) and made from non-ferromagnetic material (titanium, tantalum, elfiloy, MP35N, etc) the patient may undergo 1.5T examination immediately after surgery.

‡Weak ferromagnetic devices (intravascular coils, filters and stents become firmly fixed in 6–8 weeks following placement and are unlikely to be dislodged in a 1.5Tesla magnetic field.

implants, cardiac pacemakers, orbital metallic foreign bodies, active spinal stimulator devices and ferromagnetic metallic objects in close proximity to a critical structure such as the spinal cord or a major vessel. Ventriculoperitoneal (intracranial VP) shunts with metallic parts should not be scanned, as they may disconnect. Any active magnetic or electronic device will be deactivated by the magnetic field. Most surgical clips, caval filters, etc. are safe after the formation of granulation/scar tissue. In general, a reference frame of 6 weeks postoperatively is used to insure adequate immobilization of ferromagnetic surgical clips. In some cases, particularly large metallic objects such as those used in hip or shoulder replacements may cause local heating. Scanning should be terminated immediately in the rare event where a patient reports a "hot" sensation.

If there is a question as to whether a specific object is metallic, or is in close proximity to a critical structure (e.g., orbit or spinal cord), a two-view plain x-ray will usually resolve the issue.

MRI Artifacts

Because of the unique properties of magnetic imaging, MRI is subject to a number of artifacts. The most important of these are metallic artifacts, specifically those produced by ferromagnetic objects, which distort the alignment of protons in the scanner's main magnetic field.

In practice, even small magnetic objects may leave a large "black hole" or signal void in the image, with distortion of anatomy at the fringe of the artifact. Such spatial distortion may produce grossly erroneous measurements (e.g., canal and neuroforaminal diameters) and such images must be interpreted with caution.

Metallic artifacts from surgical hardware and micrometallic particles from surgical procedures often degrade the MR image. These can be mitigated by using sequences that minimize metallic artifacts (e.g., T1-weighted and fast spin echo) as opposed to those that maximize artifacts (e.g., T2-weighted images and particularly gradient-echo images). Sometimes, simply changing the imaging plane (e.g., adding coronal images) may be enough to remove the artifact from the area of interest.

Somewhat less common artifacts include banding artifacts, "wraparound" (an adjacent area wrapping into the area of interest, seen on very small fields of view) and chemical shift artifact (seen when tissues of markedly different chemical structure lie directly adjacent to one another, for instance, at the discovertebral interface).

Motion artifact is one of the most persistent and serious challenges to image quality. Swallowing, breathing, coughing, cardiac or vascular pulsations, subtle movement, and tremors all can degrade image quality. Technical reduction of motion may be achieved by the use of saturation bands placed over the heart or blood vessels, by reducing the scan time through the use of special sequences and by patient sedation or restraints.

Pathology

Degenerative Disorders For the average patient, MRI is the preferable examination of disorders of the lumbar spine because of its multiplanar capability, lack of ionizing radiation, better marrow evaluation, and superb tissue contrast. Occasionally unsuspected cystic lesions, like Tarlov cysts, and other soft tissue masses are often discovered fortuitously as a diagnostic bonus. MRI also is excellent for central canal evaluation including CSF, spinal cord proper, and descending nerves. The exception is central and neuroforaminal stenosis where MRI tends to overestimate the degree of stenosis due to "blooming" artifact, which is a form of magnetic susceptibility that artificially expands the adjacent cortical margins. CT myelography remains the preferred procedure for the evaluation of both and for evaluation of lateral recesses. Advanced degenerative change and DISH is often better evaluated by CT due to improved cortical detail.

Aging and degeneration produce classical MRI appearances in signal intensity and morphological character. MRI is excellent for the evaluation of all aspects of degenerative disc disease. The hallmark finding is decrease in signal intensity of the intrinsic aspect of the disc on T2-weighted images. Thinning of the disc interspace, disc bulging, and marginal hypertrophic change may be visualized on all sequences. The conspicuity of the intervertebral disc/CSF interface is much greater on T2-weighted and STIR images (Fig. 16–19). The usually darker disc can be seen especially well adjacent to the bright CSF on T2-weighted images (Fig. 6–4A). Early disc desiccation related to previous trauma, degenerative disease, or as a normal part of aging can be seen only on MRI.

The vertebral end plates may react to disc degeneration. Such change may take on several forms.[64] Type I change consists of vascular-reactive marrow and edema that appears as an area of low signal on T1-weighted and high on T2-weighted. Type II end plate change with progressive fatty marrow replacement demonstrates a zone of high signal on both T1-weighted and T2-weighted images. Type III change reflects bony accretion and sclerosis and appears as low signal on both T1-weighted and T2-weighted images. When sufficiently advanced, the Type III pattern is evident on conventional radiographs as end plate sclerosis.

Type I and II changes may enhance with contrast and must be differentiated from discitis and end plate infection. Some of these cases exhibit pain during discography. Type I Modic changes particularly are felt to relate to discogenic pain and perhaps instability.[65,66]

The terminology used to describe the various components of internal disc disruption (derangement) on MRI has been variable and confusing (see Chapter 6). Most disc herniations occur in discs that exhibit degenerative change. Focal abnormal anular contours measuring 3 mm assuredly have nuclear material beneath. An anular *bulge* is a concentric extension of the disc beyond the vertebral margin in a broad-based manner. It may also exhibit evidence for desiccation and decreased height. The term *protrusion* is used when there is focal- or broad-based extension of the anulus and either the outer anulus/posterior longitudinal ligament complex is intact or the base of the anular morphology is broader than the apex. Disc *extrusion*, on the other hand, represents a clear disruption of the anulus/posterior longitudinal ligament complex and/or the base of the abnormality is narrower than its apex in any imaging plane. Any degree of extension above or below the disc space represents migration of an extruded disc. For a disc to be *sequestered* it must be separated from the parent disc.

The mass effect of any degree of protrusion should also be correlated with the cross-sectional mensuration of the canal and the relationship to descending and exiting nerve roots. In some instances pre- or post-compressive swelling of the involved nerve root may be apparent. The imaged mass effect of disc protrusion is virtually always greater in appearance than the actual dimension. A cap of inflammatory reaction or granulation tissue contributes to the appearance of mass effect (Fig. 16–21).

Actual tear patterns include transverse tears at the discovertebral interface, concentric tears between lamellae of the outer anular bundles, and radial tears extending from the nucleus to the outer anulus.[67–69]

Anular tears with associated granulation tissue may be seen peripherally in any sector as a high-intensity zone on T2-weighted and STIR images (Fig. 6–4*A* and 16–4*B*). These same areas may enhance after administration of contrast on T1-weighted sequences. Granulation tissue has been reported in these same areas via biopsy.[70] Acute anular tears are seen only on MRI. These may appear as focal, linear, or circumferential abnormalities (See Figs. 6–3*A* and 6–3*B*). Anular tears are important to detect as a significant percentage are painful.

The various elements of stenosis are nicely portrayed with MRI. Bony hypertrophy and ligament (flaval) intrusion into the confines of the spinal canal and foramina is well depicted (see Figs. 7–7*A* and 7–7*B*). Synovial cysts are seen well on MRI (see Figs. 7–8*A* and 7–8*B*). Calcification within the disc or its periphery is not specifically evident on MRI however, and may be easier to identify on CT. Accurate measurements of canal dimensions can be made by computer.

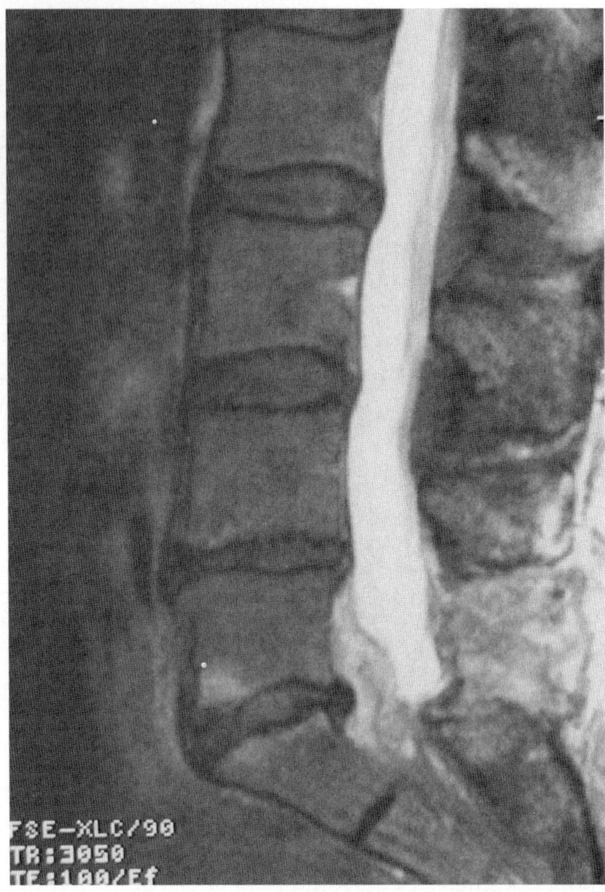

FIGURE 16–21. Laminectomy/discectomy. Sagittal T2-weighted image with fat saturation showing a large mass of granulation tissue/scar around the lumbosacral operative site, postdiscectomy, with a persistent disc protrusion.

MRI and CT myelography are both excellent for depiction of spinal cord compression. MR-myelography (MRM) is noninvasive. Coronal images are obtained using parameters to produce a "myelographic" appearance (TR 9000 ms, TE 272 ms, NEX 3, echo train length 32). However, this technique has been associated with a large number of false-positive and false-negative examinations when compared with conventional lumbar MRI.[71] Less than 64% of nerve root compression abnormalities and 72% of the disc protrusions noted on conventional MRI were seen with MRM.

Postoperatively, MRI with contrast (gadolinium) is the procedure of choice because of excellent enhancement of scar or granulation tissue as opposed to disc material, which remains dark following contrast

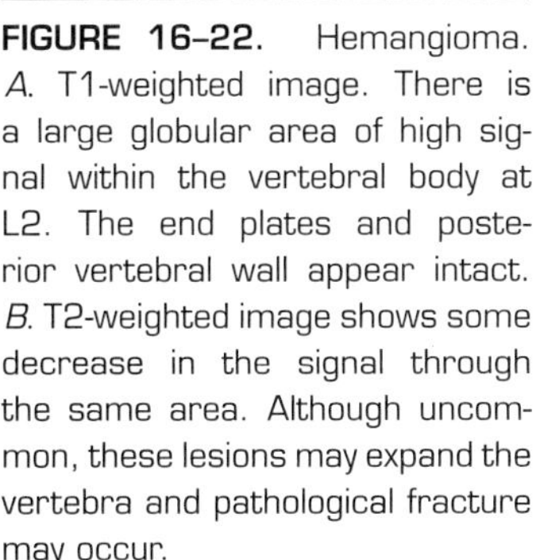

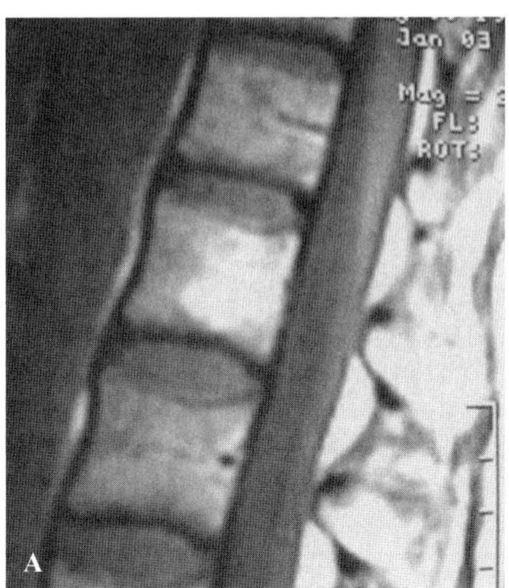

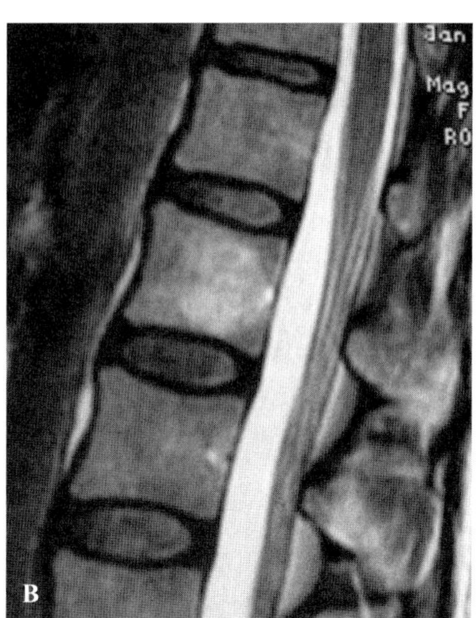

FIGURE 16–22. Hemangioma. *A.* T1-weighted image. There is a large globular area of high signal within the vertebral body at L2. The end plates and posterior vertebral wall appear intact. *B.* T2-weighted image shows some decrease in the signal through the same area. Although uncommon, these lesions may expand the vertebra and pathological fracture may occur.

(Fig. 16–20). Less consistent patterns of enhancement may be seen adjacent to a laminectomy defect. In addition, postoperative infection, subdural, or epidural hematoma are all better seen on MRI than on CT scan. Metallic artifact is usually minimal and quite focal because of the widespread use of titanium hardware. In some cases, CT myelography may be necessary as a supplement.

Bone Marrow Evaluation Early destructive changes in the spongiosa often go undetected with CT and conventional radiographs. These are also insensitive for the early detection of infiltrating neoplasms like metastatic adenocarcinoma, myeloma, leukemia and lymphoma, and other infiltrating processes affecting the bone marrow. MRI is more sensitive than bone scanning for detecting marrow tumor located in the axial skeleton.

Clinical Pearl: MRI is more sensitive than conventional radiographs and bone scanning for the detection of marrow tumor.

While MRI is the modality of choice for the evaluation of bone marrow lesions, especially metastatic disease, abnormal signal intensities are nonspecific, even in the face of known disease.

It is important to differentiate the exceedingly common and almost always incidental finding of a vertebral hemangioma from a pathological marrow lesion. Hemangiomas and fatty marrow islands may have a somewhat similar appearance. In most instances hemangiomas appears bright on both T1-wighted and T2-weighted sequences (Fig. 16–22). STIR or chemical fat-suppression may be helpful in turning these lesions dark, but occasionally they may contain water signal as well as fat, and may therefore remain at least partially bright on fat-suppressed sequences. The only other marrow lesion with a similar appearance is the exceedingly rare metastatic melanoma. Since melanin is paramagnetic, like gadolinium, it may appear bright on nonenhanced T1-weighted sequences. In clinical practice, unless the patient has a known or suspected history of melanoma, the bright T1-weighted marrow lesion may safely be assumed to be benign fatty lesions. Subacute hematoma, which can appear bright on T1-weighted images, would be exceedingly rare in the vertebral marrow proper.

Metastatic marrow lesions are usually, though not always, bright on T2-weighted and dark on T1-weighted sequences. This is due to their water content. Small round-cell tumors such as lymphoma or multiple myeloma may appear darker on T1-weighted and T2-weighted sequences because of the relative paucity of intercellular water in the tumor. Fibrotic and osseous lesions (e.g., bone islands, osteoid osteoma, and osteoblastoma) generally appear dark on all sequences because of the lack of any mobile protons.

The more typical metastatic marrow lesions consist of one or more rounded deposits that appear dark on T1-weighted and bright on T2-weighted and especially STIR sequences (Fig. 16–23). Some tumors such as lymphoma may be much more poorly defined, infiltrative, or may present as an inhomogeneous marrow pattern. Prior x-ray therapy causes the vertebral marrow included within the radiation port to appear bright on T1-weighted and T2-weighted sequences, particularly on FSE, due to diffuse fatty marrow replacement.

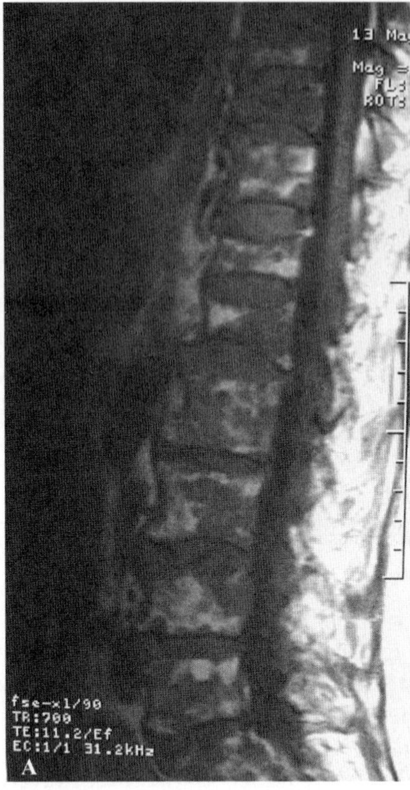

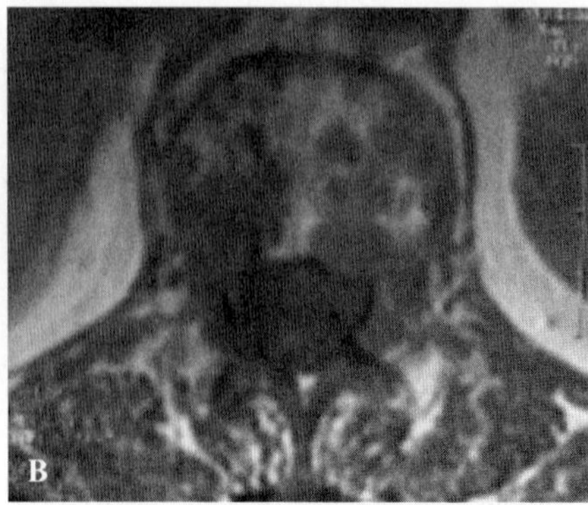

FIGURE 16–23. Metastatic disease. *A.* Sagittal T1-weighted image showing widespread diffuse involvement throughout the entire field of view. At the thoracolumbar region several segments exhibit end plate deformity and collapse. *B.* The axial view shows involvement of the pedicles and arch region and some cortical breakthrough into the spinal canal.

The signs of metastatic disease include multiple lesions, cortical expansion or "breakout" of the tumor, epidural extension, and known underlying malignancy. Enhancement is common with contrast but it usually does not aid in specificity. Gadolinium is helpful in ruling out CSF seeding from intracranial tumors, breast and some lung carcinomas, lymphomas, and other seeding tumors. It is also helpful in demonstrating epidural tumor spread.

Pathologic vertebral fracture is a common occurrence with malignancy, and must be differentiated from benign compression fracture. Clues indicating pathology include any adjacent soft tissue abnormality, marrow signal out of proportion to the fracture, extension of abnormal signal into the posterior elements, cortical expansion, and known history of malignancy. Benign fractures may have soft tissue abnormality if acute (because of hematoma) and extensive marrow signal change if there is acute marrow edema. Extensive fatty signal (bright on T1-weighted images) is characteristic of chronic benign fractures.[72,73] Multiple compression fractures in a patient with osteopenia or patients on chronic steroid medication are likely benign, especially with extensive fatty marrow replacement. A fracture in a patient with no or only minor trauma history must be considered malignant until proven otherwise. Abnormal marrow signal extending into the posterior elements is strongly suggestive of metastatic disease. Nuclear medicine bone scanning may be helpful to search for multiple lesions.

Metastases also must be differentiated from infection. The most important distinction is that metastatic disease usually spares the disc until very advanced stages. Even then it may not cross the disc space, whereas infection tends to be disc space centered. Also, infection tends to involve one or a few adjacent discs, whereas metastasis tends to be more widespread and scattered.

MRI is also useful for detecting marrow alteration indicating bony stress reaction at the posterior arch and particularly at the pars interarticularis. Hollenberg et al. have proposed an MRI classification system for bone stress reactions and spondylolysis.[74] These reactions are imaged best on fat-saturated T2-weighted images (Fig. 16–24).

Lesions of the Spinal Cord MRI is excellent for identifying lesions of the spinal cord. The intrinsic cord substance is not visualized with any other imaging modality. MS plaques appear bright on T2-weighted sequences, although they may be faint. MS plaques enhance with contrast only during the acute phase. Most spinal cord tumors enhance with contrast (Fig. 16–25). Spinal cord tumors may be extradural, intradural/extramedually (e.g., meningioma, schwannoma, neuroma), or intramedullary (e.g., astrocytoma, ependymona).

Clinical Pearl: MRI is the procedure of choice for identifying lesions of the spinal cord proper.

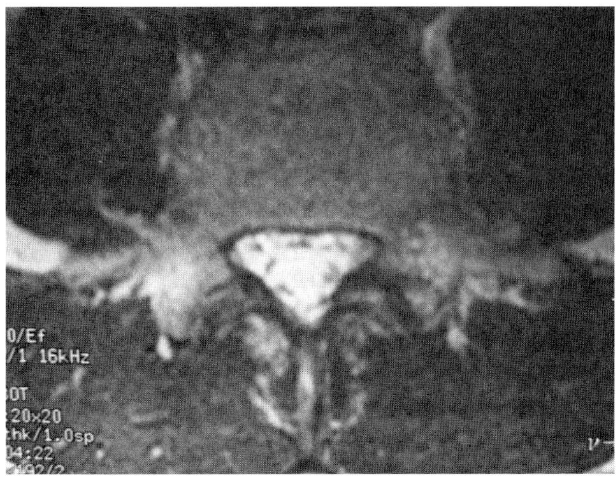

FIGURE 16–24. Lower lumbar axial T2-weighted MRI image with fat saturation showing heightened signal in the right posterior arch consistent with a pars stress reaction. There was no pars break defined on CT imaging.

On MRI a syrinx appears bright on T2-weighted and dark on T1-weighted sequences. These are well circumscribed and cystic, usually in the central cord, but may be more eccentrically positioned. These may cause spinal cord expansion. Except in those cases that are associated with Arnold-Chiari malformation, contrast should be added to aid in the differentiation of the other causes of cord syrinx (tumor, trauma, and infection).

Infection, Subdural Hematoma, and Epidural Hematoma MRI is the procedure of choice for suspected infection or suspected subdural or epidural hematoma. In the vertebral column, infection usually begins as a discovertebral focus. Contrast should always be used in cases of suspected infection. Early signs of infection include abnormal disc signal (often abnormally bright on T2-weighted images) or any disc enhancement. In the postoperative setting scattered or small areas of disc enhancement may be seen normally. Later signs include disc narrowing or poorly defined disc margins, epidural enhancement (epidural abscess), abnormal soft tissue signal enhancement surrounding the vertebrae, and abnormally decreased T1 and increased T2 signal with or without abnormal enhancement in the adjacent vertebrae (Fig. 16–8).

Tuberculosis tends to be somewhat atypical, as these infections may be more marrow centered and cause compression deformities with resultant kyphosis or "gibbus" deformities.

Epidural and subdural hematomas are readily demonstrated on MRI. They may develop spontaneously or be associated with anticoagulants therapy, trauma, or preexisting tumor or infection. Enhancement is variable but tends to be less than with epidural abscess. Infection and hematoma may coexist and often reflect neurosurgical emergencies, particularly if there is significant associated central spinal stenosis.

Acute Vertebral Trauma CT is the modality of choice for acute spine trauma in the nonpathological spine,

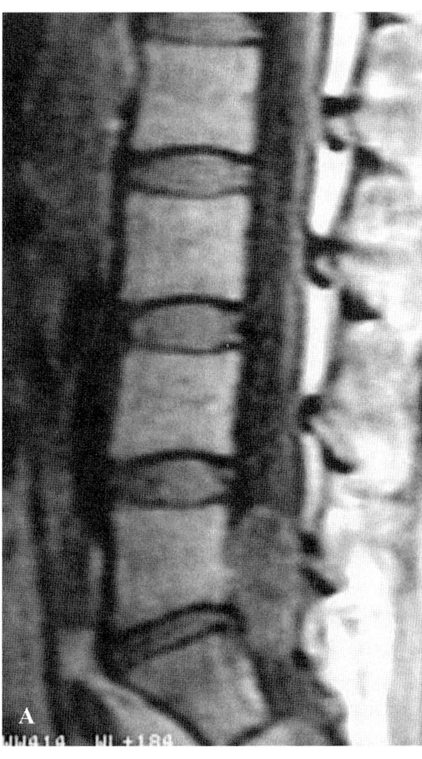

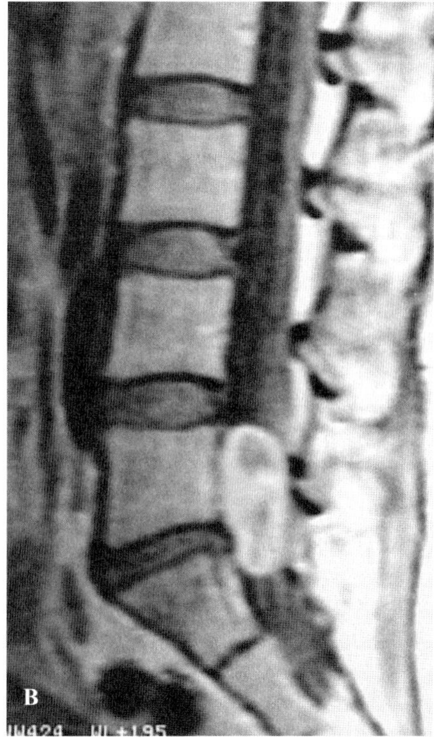

FIGURE 16–25. Neurofibroma. *A.* T1-weighted image without contrast. There is a large well-circumscribed, oval intradural extramedullary mass that fills the spinal canal at the level of L5–S1. The lesion is somewhat inhomogeneous with some areas isointense and others hypointense to the spinal cord. *B.* Contrast study. The lesion enhances peripherally and inhomogeneously suggesting cystic degeneration.

given the higher sensitivity for and delineation of associated fracture lines. Reformatted images may be used to evaluate alignment. CT is also far less susceptible to motion artifact, which is often a problem in the acute traumatic setting. CT is better for small avulsions and small posterior arch fractures. MRI can be helpful as an adjunct for evaluation of cord injury (bright areas of edema on T2-weighted images), cord compression, or cord or nerve root transection. MRI also is useful for excluding associated soft tissue or subdural hematoma. Fracture lines may or may not be seen as linear areas of decreased T1 and increased T2 signal, accompanied by marrow edema (broader areas of decreased T1 and increased T2 signal). Standard T1- and T2-weighted images should not be relied upon as the primary modality to exclude fracture; rather, STIR and fat-saturated T2-weighted images are much more sensitive.

DYNAMIC MRI

Although CT and MRI are presently the most frequently used noninvasive imaging methods for diagnosing stenosis, imaging of a supine patient may not demonstrate the degree of change in canal dimension that is possible by upright FE myelography. Marked variation in the severity of lumbar dural sac stenosis during flexion and extension has been shown in some patients.

The symptoms of lumbar spinal stenosis and intervertebral disc disease are often posture-dependent, and it is generally accepted that FE motions of the lumbar spine affect the capacity of the spinal canal and the mechanics of the intervertebral disc.

Currently, there is much interest in dynamic loading of the lumbar spine as well as weight-bearing and dynamic FE imaging. Axial loaded CT-myelography and MRI imaging has been accomplished with the patient recumbent and loaded in a portable device.[75] In 66 of 84 patients investigated in another study, there was a statistically significant reduction of the dural sac cross-sectional area in at least one site during axial compression in slight extension.[76] With change from flexion to extension and distraction to compression, up to 16% area reduction can be expected, along with a reduction in the mid-sagittal canal diameter of 2 mm.[77]

In the past, positional MRI had to be variously obtained with limited motion range and without weight-bearing effects. Weishaupt et al. have recently documented positionally related changes in the intervertebral canal measurements and nerve root compression not visible at conventional recumbent MRI. This study was performed on a mid-field strength scanner with the patients in seated position.[78]

An MRI system is available with capabilities to image in the upright, recumbent, and other nontraditional positions (Fonar©, 0.6 T). This opens investigation for patient scanning in positions of relevant clinical symptoms. Such studies may unmask and offer elucidation of dynamic kinetic-dependent anatomicopathological problems.

Conclusion

Except in those patients with advanced osteodegenerative diseases of the spine, suspected acute fracture or contraindication to scanning, MRI should be the modality of choice for evaluation of spine abnormalities. Even when an uncomplicated disc abnormality is suspected, an unexpected marrow, central canal, or cord lesion may be the cause of the patient's symptoms and may be entirely missed by conventional imaging. CT myelography remains the gold standard for precise delineation of central or neuroforaminal stenosis and root compression, but MRI is entirely adequate in most cases and is far superior to CT for most other applications.

NUCLEAR IMAGING

The development of bone-localizing diphosphonates occurred in 1972. Since then the techniques of nuclear bone imaging have become a common, safe, and indispensable diagnostic method that provides unique information about local and general bone metabolism. These studies often supply complimentary information for comparison with that derived from conventional radiography, CT, and MRI. While there is a negligible risk for reaction, it is contraindicated during pregnancy and while breast-feeding.

Bone scanning (*scintigraphy*) detects changes in bone physiology on the basis of high sensitivity to alteration in vascularity or osteogenesis. In other words, a lesion must exhibit metabolic activity in order to be detected. Purely destructive processes (without pathological fracture) such as myeloma usually result in a normal scan. While sensitivity to changes in bone metabolism is very high, the specificity is low and patterns of abnormal uptake may be produced by a number of different disorders. Therefore, as with other imaging modalities, bone scintigraphy may identify a focal abnormality, but provide only a differential diagnosis as to etiology. Interpretation of the images must be placed in the proper complimentary framework of clinical findings. Once a typical focus is located, conventional radiographs, CT, MRI, or biopsy can provide further clarification of the true pathology.

Clinical Pearl: Bone scanning techniques are very helpful in the search for occult destructive bone lesions, for example, METS. Their greatest

usefulness is in cases where conventional imaging is negative.

These techniques tend to be most valuable when the conventional radiograph is negative or questionable. Conversely, the nuclear medicine study is often unnecessary when other imaging is positive. Its application in oncology is well known and important since early detection may markedly influence patient management and outcome. In such cases multiple body areas are evaluated without additional exposure.

The principle of nuclear imaging depends on the selective uptake of the chosen radiopharmaceutical (compounds called tracers, labeled with a radioactive substance with sufficient energy level to be detected outside the body) by different body tissues. They are administered by means of an IV injection. The tracers produce gamma or x-radiation, and radiation dosage is about 0.7 rad to bone and 0.12 rad to whole body per mCi of tracer. Positron emission tomography (PET) on the other hand uses cyclotron-produced isotopes that emit positrons. It is based on new technological developments in nuclear medicine and digital imaging. PET is useful in evaluating physiological function of organs on a dynamic basis, including Parkinson's disease, seizure disorders, Alzheimer's disease, and others. It is also being used for the differentiation of benign and malignant tumors and for monitoring therapeutic response to tumor treatment.

Bone scintigraphy records the distribution of a radioactive tracer (usually Tc-99 methylene diphosphonate or MDP), in the skeletal system in planar (2D) or tomographic (3D) images. This may be performed in a whole body or limited mode. Anterior and posterior planar views are obtained with additional views as needed. Bone SPECT (single photon emission computed tomography) produces a tomographic image portrayal of tracer uptake.

Multiphasic bone scintigraphy consists of immediate blood flow images, intermediate soft tissue, and delayed bone images. The initial blood-pool phase is a dynamic sequence obtained as the tracer is injected. Intermediate static images usually follow within 15 minutes. Delayed images, planar or tomographic, are obtained in 2–5 hours. Occasionally even 24 hour delayed imaging is necessary. The *triple-phase scan* helps differentiate soft tissue abnormality from bone pathology and is useful, for instance, in assessing the approximate age of fractures from recent to remote.

The use of bone scintigraphy is very important in orthopedic practice. For example, consider the young patient with low back pain and lumbar extension pain provocation, but normal appearing conventional radiographs. Stress reactions and subtle stress fractures of the pars interarticularis are notoriously difficulty to define with conventional radiography. Active pars stress reactions and recent fracture or remodeling is usually clearly detected with bone scanning. Scintigraphy may also aid in estimating the age of a fracture. SPECT more accurately localizes a lesion in the transverse, coronal, or sagittal plane (Fig. 16–4C). MRI may demonstrate similar changes but often only with STIR sequences (Fig. 16–24). Common indications for bone scintigraphy are listed in Table 16–6.

TABLE 16–6. Common Indications for Bone Scintigraphy

- Unexplained (non-specific) bone pain
- Suspected (occult) fracture, including stress fracture, pars stress reactions and healing
- Osteomyelitis, discitis
- Arthritis
- Bone graft viability
- Neoplastic disease: primary tumors, METS, response to treatment
- Complex regional pain syndrome type I (reflex sympathetic dystrophy syndrome, RSDS)

Zoom magnification also improves resolution.[79–82] Rapid sequence pinhole collimation produces very high resolution of a specific area.

Other radiopharmaceuticals may be used in suspected infection and malignancy. The usefulness of Gallium-67 scanning includes the detection and follow-up of spinal infection and the detection and localization of tumors. Its greatest utility lies with lymphoma.[83] Indium-111 Tc-99m labeled leukocytes are most sensitive for acute infections of less than 4–6 weeks duration. Sensitivity declines with antibiotic therapy.[84] Tc-99m labeled colloid (albumin or sulfur) is used for regional bone marrow abnormalities.

BONE DENSITOMETRY

Osteoporosis is the most common cause of vertebral compression fractures. The differential diagnosis that must be considered with compression fracture includes various causes of osteomalacia, endocrinopathy, and malignancy as well.[85]

Spinal osteoporosis is a problem of epidemic proportions that carries significant morbidity. In the United States alone, about 1.5 million fractures are attributable to osteoporosis each year.[86] Osteoporotic vertebral compression fractures are now recognized as an increasingly common source of morbidity and mortality in the aging population. Previously, these fractures were assumed to be benign, and largely self-limited with few significant sequelae. Individual cohorts and population-wide analyses demonstrate high rates of chronic pain, functional decline, physiologic disorder, psychosocial dysfunction, and early mortality among patients with osteoporotic vertebral body compression fractures.[87]

Reduced bone mineral density (BMD) correlates well with osteoporotic compression fracture as well as increases risk for future fracture. The conventional radiographic evaluation is not sensitive for subtle fracture, and certainly not for risk for fracture in those patients without proven osteoporosis. It is well known that bone density loss of up to 50% often goes unrecognized (Fig. 16–1).

The understanding of the magnitude of the problem and awareness of preventative strategies has heightened, medical treatment and kyphoplasty has been developed, and technology for accurate BMD determination is now available.

Bone density determination has become an important aspect of patients at risk for osteoporosis. Several techniques have been used. These include single photon absorptiometry (SPA), dual photon absorptiometry (DPA), dual energy x-ray absorptiometry (DXA), quantitative computed tomography (QCT), and ultrasound transmission velocity and broadcast ultrasound attenuation. DXA is presently the technique most used in this determination. Advanced fan-beam DXA systems allow for practical, low-radiation dose scanning. Its precision allows for accurate follow up of patients. Serial examinations should be performed on the same equipment whenever possible.

Patients under 65 years of age and with multiple risk factors benefit from this determination, but those with previous fracture and no risk factors should also be scanned to determine a baseline status. Risk factors include early menopause (natural or surgical); no estrogen replacement; low calcium intake; family history of osteoporosis; small frame; Caucasian and Asian derivation; athletes with amenorrhea; and certain medications including diuretics, steroids, and anticonvulsants.[88]

The typical DXA examination consists of BMD measurements using anteroposterior lumbar spine and proximal femur sites. Patients with advanced degenerative disease may have overestimation of BMD. In such instances additional sites may be added, for example, a lateral lumbar spine. The latest generation equipment allows for fast scanning and improved image quality and the detection of vertebral osteophytes that may cause false BMD values.[89]

Clinical Pearl: DXA studies incorporating data from the lumbar spine and femoral neck are the standard determinations for measuring BMD. Measurements are readily attained and accurate. The *T* score correlates most closely with the diagnosis of osteoporosis, the estimation of risk of fracture, and the establishment of treatment strategies.

Measurements at the femoral neck and Ward's triangle are more sensitive than those at other peripheral areas.[90] Ward's triangle is the proximal femoral area enclosed by trabeculae from the principal compressive group, the secondary compressive group, and the tensile group. The lumbar spine is commonly scanned along with the hip. Sensitivity is greater in the lumbar spine with lateral imaging versus anteroposteriorly.[91]

It is important to relate the patient's BMD to the mean peak bone mass of healthy 25–30-year-old patients (termed *T* score), rather than age-matched reference ranges (*Z* scores) as the *Z* scores may underestimate the degree of loss and give a false sense of security.[92] The *T* score is the most relevant value clinically as it relates most closely with the diagnosis of osteoporosis, the estimation of risk of fracture, and the establishment of treatment strategies.

Osteoporosis is diagnosed when BMD is less than or equal to -2.5 standard deviations (SD) below peak bone mass (*T* score). *Established osteoporosis* is defined in patients with *T* scores less than −2.5 and have fractures. *Osteopenia* occurs when BMD falls between −1.0 SD and −2.5 SD below peak bone-mass (*T* score). Normal BMD is no more than 1 SD below the young adult mean value (*T* score).

The relationship between low bone mass and risk for fracture is strong. For every SD below peak bone mass in the spine, the fracture rate is increased 1.9-fold. In the hip, each SD loss increases the fracture risk rate 2.4-fold.

ULTRASOUND

Most recently there has been some interest in the feasibility of using diagnostic ultrasound for spine-related complaints. Moon et al. have addressed this issue relative to ligament injury at the thoracolumbar junction.[93] Their results show ultrasound to be less sensitive than MRI in predicting the status of the restraining ligaments. Furthermore, there have been no studies regarding the specificity and accuracy of these types of examinations. Ledsome et al. used ultrasound to directly measure distances between lumbar vertebrae.[94] McNally et al. was able to observe internal disc structure (between T11 and L3) in only 54% of individuals.[95] Naish et al. in their in vitro dog study showed correlation between obtained ultrasound images and the pathological condition of the intervertebral discs.[96] Exactly how accurately ultrasound is able to depict changes in the disc's structure is not currently known. Present studies only suggest a potential application for ultrasound imaging that to date has largely been unexplored.

For the time being, spinal diagnostic ultrasound is yet to be documented as a viable tool in the clinical setting.

SUMMARY

1. The diagnostic imaging tools available today are sophisticated and powerful. They offer much as one searches for the answers to clinical questions.
2. The patient history and clinical examination must never become secondary or considered inferior to the advances of technology. These data must be combined with, and understood in the light of, the imaging results.
3. The strategies for implementing an imaging plan should be based on the clinical question at hand and not on general statistics of information yield.
4. The results and importance of imaging findings are often only as good as the indications for the study.
5. The issue of cost containment must be considered and risk to the patient is also not to be ignored.

REFERENCES

1. Deyo RA, Diehl AK. Lumbar spine films in primary care: Current use and effects of selective ordering criteria. *J Gen Intern Med* 1986;1(1):20–25.
2. Leeds NE, Kieffer SA. Evolution of diagnostic neuroradiology from 1904 to 1999. *Radiology* 2000; 217(2):309–318.
3. Gray JE, Orton CG. Medical physics: Some recollections in diagnostic X-ray imaging and therapeutic radiology. *Radiology* 2000;217(3):619–625.
4. Brown PM, Zelt DT, Sobolev B. The risk of rupture in untreated aneurysms: The impact of size, gender, and expansion rate. *J Vasc Surg* 2003;37(2):280–284.
5. Meyerding WH. Spondylolisthesis. *Surg Gynecol Obstet* 1932;54:371–377.
6. Amato M, Totty WG, Gilula LA. Spondylolysis of the lumbar spine: Demonstration of defects and laminal fragmentation. *Radiology* 1984;153(3):627–629.
7. Libson E, Bloom RA. Anteroposterior angulated view. A new radiographic technique for the evaluation of spondylolysis. *Radiology* 1983;149(1):315–316.
8. Grogan JP, Hemminghytt S, Williams AL, et al. Spondylolysis studied with computed tomography. *Radiology* 1982;145(3):737–742.
9. Rothman SL, Glenn WV, Jr. CT multiplanar reconstruction in 253 cases of lumbar spondylolysis. *AJNR Am J Neuroradiol* 1984;5(1):81–90.
10. Saraste H, Brostrom LA, Aparisi T, et al. Radiographic measurement of the lumbar spine. A clinical and experimental study in man. *Spine* 1985;10(3):236–241.
11. Pitkanen MT, Manninen HI, Lindgren KA, et al. Segmental lumbar spine instability at flexion-extension radiography can be predicted by conventional radiography. *Clin Radiol* 2002;57(7):632–639.
12. Resnick D, Niwayama G. Radiographic and pathologic features of spinal involvement in diffuse idiopathic skeletal hyperostosis (DISH). *Radiology* 1976;119(3):559–568.
13. Denis F. The three column spine and its significance in the classification of acute thoracolumbar spinal injuries. *Spine* 1983;8(8):817–831.
14. Panjabi MM, Oxland TR, Kifune M, et al. Validity of the three-column theory of thoracolumbar fractures. A biomechanic investigation. *Spine* 1995;20(10):1122–1127.
15. Krueger MA, Green DA, Hoyt D, et al. Overlooked spine injuries associated with lumbar transverse process fractures. *Clin Orthop* 1996;327:191–195.
16. Miller CD, Blyth P, Civil ID. Lumbar transverse process fractures—A sentinel marker of abdominal organ injuries. *Injury* 2000;31(10):773–776.
17. Patten RM, Gunberg SR, Brandenburger DK. Frequency and importance of transverse process fractures in the lumbar vertebrae at helical abdominal CT in patients with trauma. *Radiology* 2000;215(3):831–834.
18. McFarland EG, Giangarra C. Sacral stress fractures in athletes. *Clin Orthop* 1996;329:240–243.
19. Leroux JL, Denat B, Thomas E, et al. Sacral insufficiency fractures presenting as acute low-back pain. Biomechanical aspects. *Spine* 1993;18(16):2502–2506.
20. Peh WC, Ooi GC. Vacuum phenomena in the sacroiliac joints and in association with sacral insufficiency fractures. Incidence and significance. *Spine* 1997;22(17):2005–2008.
21. Brahme SK, Cervilla V, Vint V, et al. Magnetic resonance appearance of sacral insufficiency fractures. *Skeletal Radiol* 1990;19(7):489–493.
22. Weber M, Hasler P, Gerber H. Insufficiency fractures of the sacrum. Twenty cases and review of the literature. *Spine* 1993;18(16):2507–2512.
23. Peh WC, Khong PL, Ho WY. Insufficiency fractures of the sacrum and os pubis. *Br J Hosp Med* 1995;54(1):15–19.
24. Major NM, Helms CA. Sacral stress fractures in long-distance runners. *AJR Am J Roentgenol* 2000; 174(3):727–729.
25. Rothschild BM, Poteat GB, Williams E, et al. Inflammatory sacroiliac joint pathology: Evaluation of radiologic assessment techniques. *Clin Exp Rheumatol* 1994;12(3):267–274.
26. Maigne JY, Guedj S, Straus C. Idiopathic coccygodynia. Lateral roentgenograms in the sitting position and coccygeal discography. *Spine* 1994;19(8):930–934.
27. Maigne JY, Doursounian L, Chatellier G. Causes and mechanisms of common coccydynia: Role of body mass index and coccygeal trauma. *Spine* 2000; 25(23):3072–3079.
28. Bernard TN, Jr. Lumbar discography followed by computed tomography. Refining the diagnosis of low-back pain. *Spine* 1990;15(7):690–707.
29. Osti OL, Fraser RD, Vernon-Roberts B. Discitis after discography. The role of prophylactic antibiotics. *J Bone Joint Surg Br* 1990;72(2):271–274.

30. Farber GL, Place HM, Mazur RA, et al. Accuracy of pedicle screw placement in lumbar fusions by plain radiographs and computed tomography. *Spine* 1995;20(13):1494–1499.
31. Sapkas GS, Papadakis SA, Stathakopoulos DP, et al. Evaluation of pedicle screw position in thoracic and lumbar spine fixation using plain radiographs and computed tomography. A prospective study of 35 patients. *Spine* 1999;24(18):1926–1929.
32. Shah RR, Mohammed S, Saifuddin A, et al. Comparison of plain radiographs with CT scan to evaluate interbody fusion following the use of titanium interbody cages and transpedicular instrumentation. *Eur Spine J* 2003.
33. Blumenthal SL, Gill K. Can lumbar spine radiographs accurately determine fusion in postoperative patients? Correlation of routine radiographs with a second surgical look at lumbar fusions. *Spine* 1993;18(9):1186–1189.
34. Siambanes D, Mather S. Comparison of plain radiographs and CT scans in instrumented posterior lumbar interbody fusion. *Orthopedics* 1998;21(2): 165–167.
35. Lin PM. Radiographic evidence of posterior lumbar interbody fusion with an emphasis on computed tomographic scanning. *Clin Orthop* 1989;242:158–163.
36. Burkus JK, Dorchak JD, Sanders DL. Radiographic assessment of interbody fusion using recombinant human bone morphogenetic protein type 2. *Spine* 2003;28(4):372–377.
37. Tullberg T, Brandt B, Rydberg J, et al. Fusion rate after posterior lumbar interbody fusion with carbon fiber implant: 1-year follow-up of 51 patients. *Eur Spine J* 1996;5(3):178–182.
38. Dvorak J, Froehlich D, Penning L, et al. Functional radiographic diagnosis of the cervical spine: Flexion/extension. *Spine* 1988;13(7):748–755.
39. Dvorak J, Panjabi MM, Novotny JE, et al. In vivo flexion/extension of the normal cervical spine. *J Orthop Res* 1991;9(6):828–834.
40. Dvorak J, Panjabi MM, Grob D, et al. Clinical validation of functional flexion/extension radiographs of the cervical spine. *Spine* 1993;18(1):120–127.
41. Knutsson F. The instability associated with disc degeneration in the lumbar spine. *Acta Radiol* 1944;25:259–609.
42. Frobin W, Brinckmann P, Leivseth G, et al. Precision measurement of segmental motion from flexion-extension radiographs of the lumbar spine. *Clin Biomech (Bristol, Avon)* 1996;11(8):457–465.
43. Matteri RE, Pope MH, Frymoyer JW. A biplane radiographic method of determining vertebral rotation in postmortem specimens. *Clin Orthop* 1976;116: 95–98.
44. Tallroth K, Ylikoski M, Landtman M, et al. Reliability of radiographical measurements of spondylolisthesis and extension-flexion radiographs of the lumbar spine. *Eur J Radiol* 1994;18(3):227–231.
45. Wood KB, Popp CA, Transfeldt EE, et al. Radiographic evaluation of instability in spondylolisthesis. *Spine* 1994;19(15):1697–1703.
46. Dupuis PR, Yong-Hing K, Cassidy JD, et al. Radiologic diagnosis of degenerative lumbar spinal instability. *Spine* 1985;10(3):262–276.
47. Pitkanen M, Manninen H. Sidebending versus flexion-extension radiographs in lumbar spinal instability. *Clin Radiol* 1994;49(2):109–114.
48. Dvorak J, Panjabi MM, Novotny JE, et al. Clinical validation of functional flexion-extension roentgenograms of the lumbar spine. *Spine* 1991;16(8):943–950.
49. Hayes MA, Howard TC, Gruel CR, et al. Roentgenographic evaluation of lumbar spine flexion-extension in asymptomatic individuals. *Spine* 1989;14(3):327–331.
50. Friberg O. Instability in spondylolisthesis. *Orthopedics* 1991;14(4):463–465.
51. Boden SD, Wiesel SW. Lumbosacral segmental motion in normal individuals. Have we been measuring instability properly? *Spine* 1990;15(6):571–576.
52. Sihvonen T, Partanen J, Hanninen O, et al. Electric behavior of low back muscles during lumbar pelvic rhythm in low back pain patients and healthy controls. *Arch Phys Med Rehabil* 1991;72(13):1080–1087.
53. Frymoyer J, Pope M, Wilder D. Segmental instability. In: Weinstein J, Weisel S, eds. *The lumbar spine.* Philadelphia: WB Saunders, 1990:612–636.
54. Kanayama M, Tadano S, Kaneda K, et al. A cineradiographic study on the lumbar disc deformation during flexion and extension of the trunk. *Clin Biomech (Bristol, Avon)* 1995;10(4):193–199.
55. Breen AC, Allen R, Morris A. Spine kinematics: A digital videofluoroscopic technique. *J Biomed Eng* 1989;11(3):224–228.
56. Breen A, Allen R, Morris A. A digital videofluoroscopic technique for spine kinematics. *J Med Eng Technol* 1989;13(1-2):109–113.
57. Zheng Y, Nixon MS, Allen R. Lumbar spine visualisation based on kinematic analysis from videofluoroscopic imaging. *Med Eng Phys* 2003;25(3):171–179.
58. Modic MT, Masaryk T, Boumphrey F, et al. Lumbar herniated disk disease and canal stenosis: Prospective evaluation by surface coil MR, CT, and myelography. *AJR Am J Roentgenol* 1986;147(4):757–765.
59. Bartynski WS, Lin L. Lumbar root compression in the lateral recess: MR imaging, conventional myelography, and CT myelography comparison with surgical confirmation. *AJNR Am J Neuroradiol* 2003;24(3):348–360.
60. Jones KM, Mulkern RV, Schwartz RB, et al. Fast spin-echo MR imaging of the brain and spine: Current concepts. *AJR Am J Roentgenol* 1992;158(6):1313–1320.
61. Bradley WG. Future cost-effective MRI will be at high field. *J Magn Reson Imaging* 1996;6(1):63–66.
62. Friedman DP, Rosetti GF, Flanders AE, et al. MR imaging: Quality assessment method and ratings at 33 centers. *Radiology* 1995;196(1):219–226.
63. Jarvik JG, Robertson WD, Wessbecher F, et al. Variation in the quality of lumbar spine MR images in Washington State. *Radiology* 2000;215(2):483–490.
64. Modic MT. Degenerative disorders of the spine. In: Masaryk TJ, Ross JS, eds. *Magnetic resonance imaging of the spine*. St. Louis: Mosby, 1994:80–150.

65. Braithwaite I, White J, Saifuddin A, et al. Vertebral end-plate (Modic) changes on lumbar spine MRI: Correlation with pain reproduction at lumbar discography. *Eur Spine J* 1998;7(5):363–368.
66. Weishaupt D, Zanetti M, Hodler J, et al. Painful lumbar disk derangement: Relevance of endplate abnormalities at MR imaging. *Radiology* 2001;218(2):420–427.
67. Yu SW, Haughton VM, Ho PS, et al. Progressive and regressive changes in the nucleus pulposus. Part II. The adult. *Radiology* 1988;169(1):93–97.
68. Yu SW, Haughton VM, Sether LA, et al. Anulus fibrosus in bulging intervertebral disks. *Radiology* 1988;169(3):761–763.
69. Yu SW, Sether LA, Ho PS, et al. Tears of the anulus fibrosus: Correlation between MR and pathologic findings in cadavers. *AJNR Am J Neuroradiol* 1988;9(2):367–370.
70. Pai RR, D'sa B, Raghuveer CV, et al. Neovascularization of nucleus pulposus. A diagnostic feature of intervertebral disc prolapse. *Spine* 1999;24(8):739–741.
71. Thornton MJ, Lee MJ, Pender S, et al. Evaluation of the role of magnetic resonance myelography in lumbar spine imaging. *Eur Radiol* 1999;9(5):924–929.
72. Yuh WT, Zachar CK, Barloon TJ, et al. Vertebral compression fractures: Distinction between benign and malignant causes with MR imaging. *Radiology* 1989;172(1):215–218.
73. Cuenod CA, Laredo JD, Chevret S, et al. Acute vertebral collapse due to osteoporosis or malignancy: Appearance on unenhanced and gadolinium-enhanced MR images. *Radiology* 1996;199(2):541–549.
74. Hollenberg GM, Beattie PF, Meyers SP, et al. Stress reactions of the lumbar pars interarticularis: The development of a new MRI classification system. *Spine* 2002;27(2):181–186.
75. Danielson BI, Willen J, Gaulitz A, et al. Axial loading of the spine during CT and MR in patients with suspected lumbar spinal stenosis. *Acta Radiol* 1998;39(6):604–611.
76. Willen J, Danielson B, Gaulitz A, et al. Dynamic effects on the lumbar spinal canal: Axially loaded CT-myelography and MRI in patients with sciatica and/or neurogenic claudication. *Spine* 1997;22(24):2968–2976.
77. Schonstrom N, Lindahl S, Willen J, et al. Dynamic changes in the dimensions of the lumbar spinal canal: An experimental study in vitro. *J Orthop Res* 1989;7(1):115–121.
78. Weishaupt D, Schmid MR, Zanetti M. Positional MR imaging of the lumbar spine: Does it demonstrate nerve root compromise not visible at conventional MR imaging. *Radiology* 2000;215:247–253.
79. Brown ML, Collier BD, Jr., Fogelman I. Bone scintigraphy. Part 1. Oncology and infection. *J Nucl Med* 1993;34(12):2236–2240.
80. Collier BD, Jr., Fogelman I, Brown ML. Bone scintigraphy. Part 2. Orthopedic bone scanning. *J Nucl Med* 1993;34(12):2241–2246.
81. Holder LE. Bone scintigraphy in skeletal trauma. *Radiol Clin North Am* 1993;31(4):739–781.
82. Brown ML, O'Connor MK, Hung JC, et al. Technical aspects of bone scintigraphy. *Radiol Clin North Am* 1993;31(4):721–730.
83. Front D, Bar-Shalom R, Israel O. The continuing clinical role of gallium 67 scintigraphy in the age of receptor imaging. *Semin Nucl Med* 1997;27(1):68–74.
84. Datz FL. Indium-111-labeled leukocytes for the detection of infection: Current status. *Semin Nucl Med* 1994;24(2):92–109.
85. Kim DH, Silber JS, Albert TJ. Osteoporotic vertebral compression fractures. *Instr Course Lect* 2003;52:541–550.
86. Riggs BL. Overview of osteoporosis. *West J Med* 1991; 154(1):63–77.
87. Truumees E. Medical consequences of osteoporotic vertebral compression fractures. *Instr Course Lect* 2003;52:551–558.
88. Cummings SR, Nevitt MC, Browner WS, et al. Risk factors for hip fracture in white women. Study of Osteoporotic Fractures Research Group. *N Engl J Med* 1995;332(12):767–773.
89. Felsenberg D, Gowin W, Diessel E, et al. Recent developments in DXA. Quality of new DXA/MXA-devices for densitometry and morphometry. *Eur J Radiol* 1995;20(3):179–184.
90. Blake GM, Fogelman I. Peripheral or central densitometry: Does it matter which technique we use? *J Clin Densitom* 2001;4(2):83–96.
91. Aoki TT, Grecu EO, Srinivas PR, et al. Prevalence of osteoporosis in women: Variation with skeletal site of measurement of bone mineral density. *Endocr Pract* 2000;6(2):127–131.
92. Kanis JA, Gluer CC. An update on the diagnosis and assessment of osteoporosis with densitometry. Committee of Scientific Advisors, International Osteoporosis Foundation. *Osteoporos Int* 2000;11(3):192–202.
93. Moon SH, Park MS, Suk KS, et al. Feasibility of ultrasound examination in posterior ligament complex injury of thoracolumbar spine fracture. *Spine* 2002;27(19):2154—2158.
94. Ledsome JR, Lessoway V, Susak LE, et al. Diurnal changes in lumbar intervertebral distance, measured using ultrasound. *Spine* 1996;21(14):1671–1675.
95. McNally DS, Naish C, Halliwell M. Intervertebral disc structure: Observation by a novel use of ultrasound imaging. *Ultrasound Med Biol* 2000;26(5):751–758.
96. Naish C, Mitchell R, Innes J, et al. Ultrasound imaging of the intervertebral disc. *Spine* 2003;28(2): 107–113.

CHAPTER

17

MINIMALLY INVASIVE APPROACHES TO THE EVALUATION OF LOW BACK SYNDROMES

Srdjan S. Nedeljković

OUTLINE

OBJECTIVES

1. Upon reading this chapter, the practitioner will gain an additional understanding of the relevant anatomy of the lumbar spine that can be responsible for the development of various pain syndromes.
2. The reader will learn the anatomical correlates of the clinical conditions that cause back pain.
3. The practitioner will gain knowledge of the techniques of discography, epidural steroid injections, epiduroscopy, facet injections, selective nerve root blocks, sacroiliac injections, and sympathetic blocks.

INTRODUCTION

Chronic pain represents a common complaint in industrialized countries, as reported by Bonica, who estimated that 30% of people in these countries report chronic pain.[1] In the United States, about 70 million people complain of chronic pain. Because up to 50 million are at least partially disabled by pain, this problem is a major cause of absence from work.[2] The greatest single cause of chronic pain is due to low back pain.

Fordyce stated that back pain is the second leading reason for physician office visits in the United States.[3]The annual incidence of low back pain in the United States is estimated at 5% of the adult population, with a lifetime incidence of 60%–85%.[4] When surveyed, 56% of persons reported some back pain during the preceding year, with 3% reporting low back pain of greater than 1-month duration.[5] Although 90% of patients will recover spontaneously within 2 weeks, the remaining patients constitute 40%–50% of referrals to pain clinics.[6]

Effective treatment of spinal pain is best accomplished once the source of the pain is known. Detailed knowledge of spine anatomy is a prerequisite for the

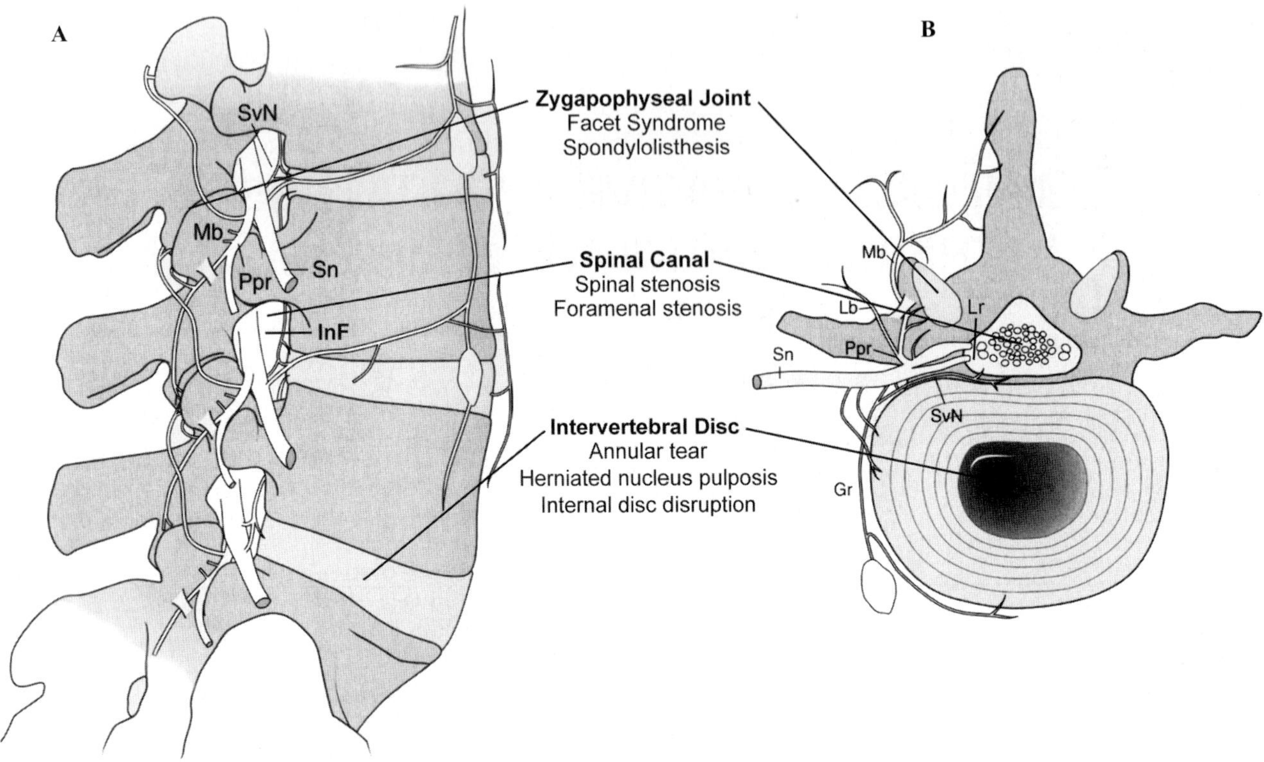

FIGURE 17–1. Lumbar spine innervation and pathology. Lateral (*A*) and transverse (*B*) views of the lumbar spine showing innervation of pain-generating structures. Sensory function to the intervertebral disc is provided via gray rami (Gr) from the sinuvertebral nerve (SvN). The zygapophyseal joint is innervated by the medial branch (Mb) off of the posterior primary ramus (Ppr) from the spinal nerve (Sn). The spinal nerve root can be compressed in the lateral recess (Lr) of the spinal canal or in the intervertebral foramen (InF). *Note*: Lb is lateral branch. *(From ref. 9.)*

rational diagnosis and treatment of spinal pain. The structures that may be the source of low back pain include the intervertebral discs, the posterior and anterior longitudinal ligaments, the nerve roots, the zygapophyseal joints, the sacroiliac joints, the regional musculoskeletal tissue, and the dural membrane.[7]

In spite of detailed knowledge of the anatomy of the spine, routine evaluations of back pain fail to reveal the diagnosis in up to 85% of cases,[8] as many of the pain-generating structures produce overlapping presentations. Because of the persistent and complex nature of low back syndromes, numerous procedures have evolved to more effectively address the problem for diagnosis, treatment, or a combination of both. These procedures play an integral part in the field of "pain medicine." This chapter will address the diagnostic aspects of low back syndromes, while Chapter 24 will cover a variety of treatment options.

CLINICAL CONDITIONS AND ANATOMICAL CORRELATES

Discogenic Pain

The disc is the largest avascular structure in the body. Its anatomical and physiological characteristics are addressed in detail in Chapters 2 and 6, while Chapter 6 also provides an overview of the pathological disc. Figure 17–1 provides an illustrative reference for this section, demonstrating lumbar spine anatomy, including innervation and pathology. Degeneration of the disc results from breakdown of proteoglycans in the nucleus pulposis and loss of cross-linkage of collagen proteins, resulting in a lower capacity to hold water.[10] This process leads to a weakened, desiccated disc. The repeated activities of everyday life, including axial, rotational, and shearing forces on the disc, lead to either microtrauma or macrotrauma to the annulus fibrosis. Development of small tears occurs in the outer annulus layer, with a gradual interruption of blood supply to the annular fibers. This condition may be the cause of nonspecific low back pain and usually resolves within a few weeks.

Acute annular tear may be the most common cause of low back pain.[11] The mechanism of injury is typically flexion, and patients may describe pain as beginning with a "pop" when bending over to lift. Pain is increased by bending forward, sitting, and is especially worse sitting in a car. Pain is usually nonradicular, as the disc is not compressing a nerve. Physical examination may reveal tight back muscles but

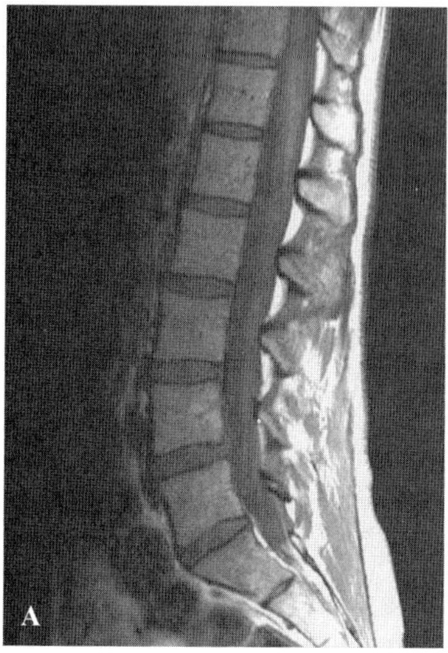

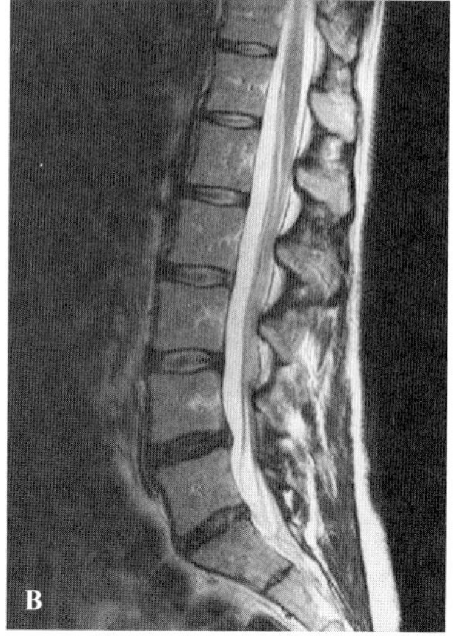

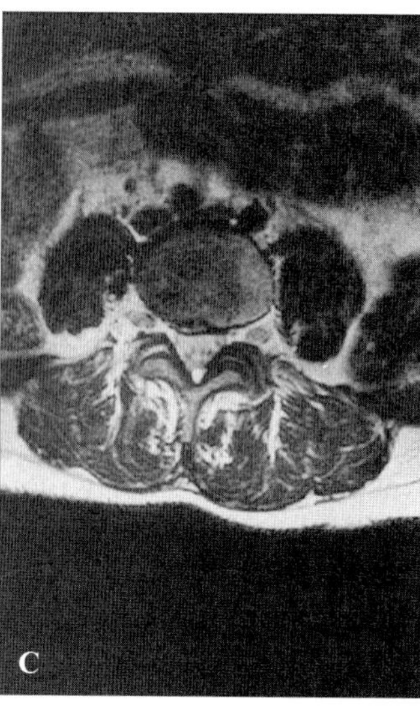

FIGURE 17–2. Herniated nucleus pulposis. *A.* Sagittal T1-weighted image of degenerative disc disease showing a protruding disc at the L4–L5 level, which is encroaching on the thecal sac. The T-1 image shows the vertebral bodies to be of higher intensity than the discs (brighter) and the spinal cord to be of higher intensity than the CSF. The CSF appears as black and the epidural fat appears as white. *B.* T2-weighted image of the same L4–L5 herniated disc. The vertebral bodies and the spinal cord appear to be of low intensity (darker) and normal discs appear lighter. The degenerated L4–L5 disc, however, appears to be darker, as it has lost some of its water content ("black disc phenomenon"). *C.* Axial T2-weighted view of this left-sided disc herniation, showing disc encroaching on the intervertebral foramen.

no neurological deficits. Patients often have difficulty flexing their backs but their straight-leg test is usually negative. Patients often respond to a short course of analgesics or anti-inflammatory drugs. Although injections can be done to the nerve supply of the ventral compartment—the sinuvertebral nerve, the communicating rami, and the sympathetic trunk—these injections are often unnecessary and have unproven benefit. Despite a paucity of research to date, an active rehabilitation program may prevent loss of functional ability and perhaps reduce the chances of reinjury.[12]

Internal disc disruption (IDD) is an ill-defined condition that has engendered a significant degree of interest over the past decade. It is characterized by low back pain with or without referred pain to the lower extremity. Pain results from axial or shearing forces loading the disc, which may cause tears in the annulus, inflammation, and abnormal movement of the spinal segment. Radiographically, patients may have a "black disc" on magnetic resonance imaging (MRI), representing loss of water content, and there may be evidence of an annular tear, which is visualized as a high-intensity zone. Discography can help confirm the diagnosis. Discography followed by computed tomography (CT) scanning is considered the "gold standard" for diagnosis because the discography reproduces the pain from IDD, and the injected radiocontrast dye then allows the best visualization of the disrupted disc using CT imaging.

Clinical Pearl: Effective treatment of spinal pain is best accomplished once the source of the pain is known. Detailed knowledge of spine anatomy is a prerequisite for the rational diagnosis and treatment of spinal pain.

Progressive annular disruption may result in a protrusion of nuclear material into the outer annulus and a bulging of the outer disc border. At first, the posterior longitudinal ligament can suppress the protrusion, commonly called a "contained" disc protrusion, but eventually the disc herniates into the spinal canal (noncontained disc herniation). Figure 17–2 demonstrates MRI views of a herniated nucleus pulposus. Herniation laterally may cause mechanical compression of the nerve root, but chemical and inflammatory mediators released from the disc can cause significant pain even without mechanical compression. In addition to direct nerve root irritation, nociception can arise from irritation of the outer annulus, posterior longitudinal ligament, anterior longitudinal ligament or dura. This may cause radicular or nonradicular pain.

The degenerating disc is not always painful. In a review of MRI studies in asymptomatic people, the prevalence of disc degeneration increased with age, and most patients with degenerative spine disease do not report pain.[13] The symptomatic early degenerative disc can be treated with a functional restoration program, examples of which are addressed in later chapters. A lumbopelvic stabilization program can balance loading of the disc and lessen shearing forces, leading to reduced back pain.

Herniation of the nucleus pulposis often results from a flexion-type injury that may be associated with lifting and twisting. Some patients may feel a "snap" at the time of injury. Pain can develop immediately or it may occur and worsen over the next several days. Pain results from stimulation of nociceptive tissues: nerve roots, the annulus, the anterior and posterior longitudinal ligaments, or the dura. If the disc herniates in the midline, patients will complain mainly of back pain. However, if the disc herniates posterolaterally, it may result in nerve entrapment and leg pain.

A very large disc herniation can cause spinal stenosis symptoms or lead to a cauda equina syndrome. Flexion, prolonged sitting, bending forward, or walking uphill generally increases pain from a herniated disc. On examination, there may be significant muscle spasm of the back musculature and range of motion is restricted, especially for flexion. The neurological exam findings are dependent on whether there is nerve root compression. Straight-leg raise (SLR) testing is often positive on the affected, ipsilateral leg. Radiological studies such as MRI or CT scan may confirm the presence of a neurocompressive disc lesion. Other conditions that can cause radicular symptoms and mimic pain from a herniated disc include myofascial pain, sclerotogenous pain from the zygapophyseal and sacroiliac joints, compartment syndromes, foraminal stenosis, epidural fibrosis, and peripheral neuropathies.

Patients with a herniated disc who require urgent surgical management are those who have cauda equina syndrome. If there is acute motor loss, the patient can be monitored and surgery may not be necessary if the patient's condition does not worsen.[14] Weber, in a landmark 10-year prospective study, compared patients with herniated discs who had operative treatment to those who had nonoperative management.[14] Although the surgical group had better results at 1 year, the difference at 4 years was not statistically significant, and the results in both groups were similar at 10 years. Because many patients improve rapidly, there is rarely a reason to operate if patients have less than 2–3 months of symptoms. Initial treatment options include analgesics, limitation of activities, and manual techniques and exercise to include a lumbar stabilization program. Injection therapies, such as epidural steroid injections and transforaminal nerve root injections, can decrease pain (refer to Chapter 24).

Spinal Stenosis

The etiology of spinal stenosis is multivariate and described in detail in Chapter 7 of this textbook. Degenerative changes in the discs and facet, or zygapophyseal, joints of the spine lead to instability and further mechanical disruption. The body responds to this condition by laying down new bone growth, which takes the form of osteophytes, in an attempt to stabilize the spinal motion segment. This results in narrowing of the neural foramen and the central canal. In the early stages of spinal stenosis, the intervertebral foramina will open with flexion and become narrow with extension, leading to pain with back extension. The intervertebral nerve root becomes irritated in this narrowed canal and suffers from compression, ischemia, and traction. In cases in which there is also a bulging or herniated disc, further narrowing of the canal may occur and an enhanced inflammatory response for the nerve root may result. Adhesions can form which lead to even more reduced mobility of the nerve root. Hypertrophy of the inferior articular zygapophyseal joint and thickening and bulging of the ligamentum flavum leads to central canal stenosis. Hypertrophy of the superior articular zygapophyseal joint narrows the lateral canal. Proliferation of bone that results from instability leads to stabilization at the expense of narrowing of neural canals and compression of neural elements.[11]

Spinal stenosis causes symptoms of neurogenic claudication, marked by either constant or intermittent low back pain that radiates to one or both legs, which is worsened by walking and relieved by rest. Although most cases of spinal stenosis are a result of degenerative changes that occur with aging, congenital spinal stenosis can also occur. Patients will often state that there is minimal or no pain with sitting or lying, but that pain occurs only with standing or walking. Walking worsens lower extremity symptoms, and the distribution of pain depends on the nerve roots involved. Central spinal canal stenosis is often marked by diffuse thigh numbness, pain, and heaviness.

On examination, it is found that stenotic patients often walk with a stooped-forward gait, using a cane or a walker for support. There is often a loss of lumbar lordosis, as extension of the back can exacerbate pain. Most patients with central canal spinal stenosis will have normal neurological exams. In patients with foraminal stenosis, motor, sensory, and reflex changes depend on the degree of nerve root involvement. Radiological examination confirms the diagnosis. CT scan shows bony and ligamentous changes best, but MRI scanning can also show the pathology behind the pain of spinal stenosis. In some patients, the disease is progressive and leads to substantial loss of function. In others, the stenosis stabilizes and patients learn to adapt.[15] Epidural steroid injections provide excellent relief in some patients, who may be helped by two to three injections per year. Diagnostic selective nerve root injections can help identify particular root compression and there may be a prolonged analgesic effect from the steroid. Surgery is an option for patients who do not respond to conservative measures, which is explained in Chapter 32.

Clinical Pearl: On examination, it is found that stenotic patients often walk with a stooped-forward gait, using a cane or a walker for support. There is often a loss of lumbar lordosis, as extension of the back can exacerbate pain.

Another condition that may cause spinal stenosis is spondylolisthesis (see Chapter 11). Pain may arise from the disc or posterior longitudinal ligament as a result of a shearing effect. Also, symptoms may arise from stenosis of the spinal canal or the exiting nerve roots, or from defects in the facet joints.[16] Unstable movement that may be associated with spondylolisthesis can worsen the clinical picture and result in increased pain. Instability of the spine can worsen stenosis with back flexion or extension, and the sheared disc may also cause pain. Conventional radiographic studies can confirm the diagnosis of spondylolisthesis, although lateral-view, flexion–extension studies are important to demonstrate actual instability.

Facet Arthropathy

The facet (zygapophyseal) joint is a true diarthroidal joint, with articular cartilage, subchondral cartilage, a capsule with a synovial lining, and a meniscus.[10] Despite its rather small size, the joint is richly innervated with nociceptors and capable of generating significant pain.[17] Degeneration of the joint typically first causes an inflammatory synovitis, which usually presents with nonspecific low back pain worsened with extension. This topic is reviewed in greater detail in Chapter 8. Often, symptoms improve with anti-inflammatory drugs. The initial stage of synovitis is usually followed by deterioration of the cartilage on the articular surface, which leads to abnormal motion of the joint and subluxation. Instability of the joint caused by progressive deterioration can result in degenerative spondylolisthesis. Facet disease can cause spinal stenosis by narrowing the lateral recess, leading to nerve root irritation or sciatica. Alternatively, tearing of the facet capsule, innervated by the medial branch of the dorsal ramus, can cause back pain with a referral pattern to the proximal leg. In order, perhaps, to diminish abnormal motion, calcium is deposited around the facet joints in the form of osteophytes, facet hypertrophy, and overgrowth of bone. This can result in narrowing of the intervertebral foramen and spinal stenosis.[10,11]

The clinical history in facet disease is that of nonspecific low back pain that may radiate to the buttocks and proximal legs to the knees. Pain is worsened by standing erect and can often be elicited by back extension or lying prone. The neurological exam is typically normal. There may be paravertebral tenderness on palpation over the joints. Radiological appearance alone has no direct correlation with painful joints.

The presence of painful facet joints can be confirmed by eliminating pain with injections of local anesthetic either directly into the joint or on the medial branch of the dorsal ramus that innervates the joint. In the lumbar region, either intra-articular or medial branch blocks (MBBs) can be done. Intra-articular injections may be a more specific block, as MBBs can anesthetize surrounding tissues that also may be causing pain. Treatment options include manual techniques and exercises to improve posture and conditioning and to relieve stress on the facet joints. If diagnostic MBBs provide relief of pain, radiofrequency lesioning (neurotomy) techniques can be used to provide a more long-term denervation of the painful area (see Chapter 24).

Clinical Pearl: The presence of painful facet joints can be confirmed by eliminating pain with injections of local anesthetic either directly into the joint or on the medial branch of the dorsal ramus that innervates the joint.

Back Pain After Spinal Surgery

Persistent pain after back surgery is a major concern and may be caused by multiple factors. Pain may result from the persistence or recurrence of any of the original causes of pain. Disc herniations can recur, spinal stenosis can redevelop, and the degenerative arthritic cascade may lead to new pain in adjacent or operated spinal levels. In addition, direct surgical trauma can lead to nerve injury and persistent pain in traumatized or instrumented bones.

Postsurgical scar tissue can develop in the spinal canal, and epidural adhesions can provoke continuous pain, independent of activity, which radiates either unilaterally or bilaterally. MRI with gadolinium, as noted in Figure 17–3, will confirm the presence of epidural scarring, which is commonly found after multiple "failed" back surgeries. Further surgical treatment typically becomes progressively more unsuccessful in this scenario. Epidural steroid injections are also poorly effective, as the injectate tends to flow along the "path of least resistance" and does not reach the intended area that is blocked by scar tissue. In some cases, paravertebral or transforaminal steroid injection techniques may prove to be more beneficial, as they allow clinicians a direct route to deliver treatment to the sensitized or inflamed nerve. Some have advocated the use of special directable catheters and epiduroscopy techniques, with injections of hypertonic saline and/or hyaluronidase, or the use of

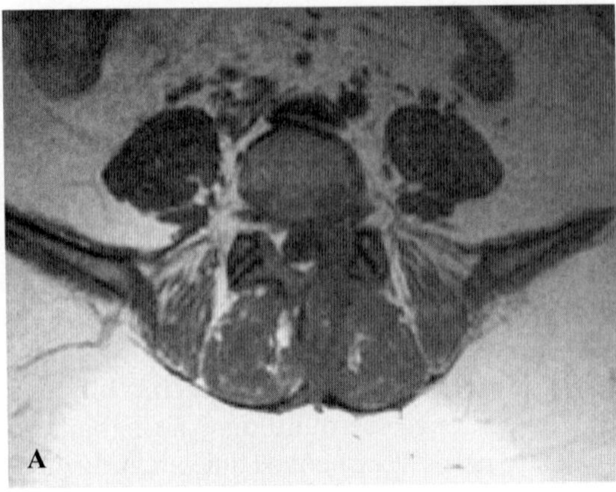

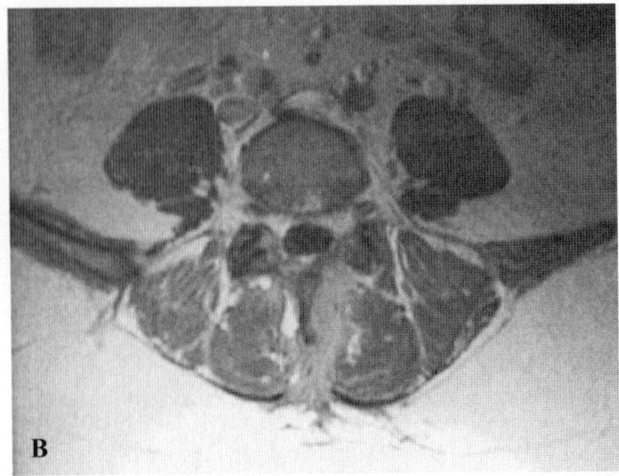

FIGURE 17–3. Epidural fibrosis after back surgery. Epidural scar tissue: After back surgery, epidural scarring and granulation tissue may form. This condition can often cause persistent pain and radiulopathy after lumbar surgery and is best seen on MRI with gadolinium. *A.* Axial T1-weighted view demonstrating the thecal sac (dark) surrounded by normal epidural fat on the right side (white) with a large mass in the anterior left region, which is abutting the thecal sac. It may be difficult to tell whether this mass is a recurrent disc or whether it is scar tissue. *B.* Enhancement with gadolinum shows that the disc does not enhance (remains dark) whereas the scar tissue is enhancing (appears brighter). There is also enhancement in the soft tissue scar posteriorly (appears brighter). *(Special thanks to Dr. Amir Zamani, Director of Neuroradiology at the Brigham and Women's Hospital in Boston, for contributing the images in Figures 17–2 and 17–3.)*

spinal cord stimulation for persistent radiating nerve pain (see Chapter 24).

Other Causes for Low Back Pain

Low back sprain/strain is an injury to the back muscles that can occur in patients after trauma. On examination, there is tenderness and spasm of the back muscles with diminished range of motion. There is increased pain with movement in any direction, and trigger points may be palpable. The neurological exam is typically normal in this common condition. Most patients recover in a few days to two weeks. Treatment includes resumption of normal activities, manual techniques such as manipulation, mobilization, and massage, exercises to recondition the back, and anti-inflammatory medications. Patients may also benefit from trigger point injections and a transcutaneous electro-nerve stimulator (TENS) unit. If pain continues, in many instances a structural basis will be its cause and await discovery.

Patients with low back pain who are inactive will develop consequences of muscle disuse and deconditioning. Muscles that support the trunk lose strength and endurance, including abdominal muscles, lumbar and thoracic paraspinal muscles, and quadriceps muscles, and many patients suffer from an overall loss of aerobic capacity.[11] Pain can result from inflammation and overuse of muscles that are weak and tight. Restoring muscle strength and endurance can improve stability and reduce stress on a painful torn annulus or inflamed facet joint, hopefully allowing it to heal. Overused muscles that are stressed beyond capacity become chronically shortened and have decreased blood flow, accumulating lactate and other algogesic substances within the tissue. Tight, weak muscles cannot optimally protect the spine, leaving it at risk for future pain and trauma.[11]

Other causes of low back pain include vertebral compression fractures, cancer, and infections. These diagnoses have been covered in detail in Chapter 10. The most common spinal cancers are those that metastasize from other organs, especially the lung, prostate, and breast. Pancreatic cancer is commonly associated with back pain. Visceral conditions, such as obstruction or inflammation of the bowel or ureters, as well as aortic dissection or angina pectoris, can present with back pain. Also to consider are rare rheumatological conditions, such as ankylosing spondylitis, psoriatic arthritis, sacroiliitis, and Reiter's and Behcet's syndromes.

DIAGNOSTIC PROCEDURES FOR LOW BACK PAIN: AN OVERVIEW

The primary method for diagnosis of low back pain and associated syndromes remains obtaining a comprehensive history and performing a physical examination. Certainly, the advent of CT scanning and MRI testing enhanced the ability of a clinician to better diagnose the cause of painful symptoms due to spinal degeneration and disease. However, the use of any diagnostic test in exclusion of a general clinical evaluation is prone to result in misdiagnosis. For example, there is a fairly high incidence of abnormal MRI in the absence of painful symptoms, especially in older patients.[13]

Pain management diagnostic procedures can be categorized by two contrasting strategies: those that increase and those that relieve the symptom generator(s). Provocative discography is an example of a procedure designed to localize a painful area (disc) by increasing the symptoms. Procedures that aim to decrease pain caused by the symptom generator include epidural injections, epiduroscopy, facet injections, selective nerve root blockade, and sympathetic blockade.

DISCOGRAPHY: USES AND CONTROVERSIES

Discography is a commonly used diagnostic method used to elucidate the source of pain in patients who suffer from low back pain or other spinal syndromes. It also provides information regarding the structural integrity of the intervertebral disc.

Schmorl first performed injections of intervertebral discs in a necroscopic study in 1929.[18] Lindblom later described discography in living patients in a European study published in 1948,[19] with the first US report published by Wise and Weiford in 1951.[20] At first, patients were given highly irritating, iodinated oil-based contrast that had low diagnostic sensitivity because of its highly irritating properties. Later, water-based contrast dye and improved imaging techniques led to increased diagnostic accuracy because of lower false-positive rates and sharper visual fields.

Technique

Discography is performed most often with the patient in the prone position. Typically, the L3–L4, L4–L5, and L5–S1 levels are identified fluoroscopically. A double needle technique, using a 22-gauge 7-in spinal needle through a short 18-gauge needle, or a single needle technique, using a 7-in 22-gauge needle, has been described. The needle is inserted 8–10 cm lateral to the midline from the side opposite to the pain directly into the L3–L4 and L4–L5 discs. At the L5–S1 level, the needle is inserted 1 cm lateral and proximal to the L4–L5 needle. The needle is advanced fluoroscopically to the nucleus pulposis, taking care not to leave the tip in the annulus fibrosis. An injection given into a normal annulus fibrosis will often cause pain, leading to a potential false-positive test result from discography.

An injection of normal saline is given, with a volume of 1–3 mL until resistance is encountered, and the pain response is graded on its location and radiation. Alternatively, nonionic contrast dye can be injected at a volume of 1–3 mL, and the volume of injection, quality of pain, and direction of abnormal tracking are documented. At least two levels of injection are required. Discography is positive if the injection recreates pain (described as "concordant pain") and the radiographic study (either concurrent x-ray or, better yet, postprocedure CT scan) reveals annular disruption. At least one of the other levels injected must have a negative response and a normal radiographic study, which is termed the "control level." Without a negative control level, a positive discogram is not considered to be a reliable test. Injecting local anesthetic into the disc should relieve pain, although this is not generally performed as part of a discography evaluation.

Clinical Pearl: The primary indication for discography is to diagnose patients with low back/leg pain whose CT/MRI studies failed to explain their pain.

Manometry

The issue of whether to perform manometry (a test to measure injection pressures) during a discography procedure is a controversial one. Although the International Spinal Injection Society (ISIS) has recommended manometry for all discography procedures, many practitioners believe that an experienced clinician can sense disc pressures based on feel alone. Others feel that intradiscal pressure readings have little bearing on whether a discography is positive or negative, and that these readings therefore have little predictive value in terms of diagnostics or therapeutic measures.

There are several commercially available manometry devices. On entering the disc, the clinician can use a manometer to assess the "opening" pressure of a disc, which is usually less than 15 pounds per square inch (PSI)[21]. As the disc is filled with contrast material, the pressure will increase. If pain occurs at low pressures, the test for that target disc is considered positive. Generally, injecting a disc to pressures higher than 100 PSI may damage the annulus,[21] and pain generation at these levels is not considered diagnostic. In a study by O'Neill and Kurgnasky,[22] pressure-sensitive discs had a mean pain threshold of 19.8 PSI with a standard deviation of 15 PSI. However, the false positive rate for discography was 100% at 50 PSI, 50% at 25 PSI, and 10% at 14 PSI. The false positive rate could not be calculated for discs with pain thresholds of less than 10 PSI.[22] In another study, pressures of 38.4 PSI and 69.7 PSI were needed to induce moderate or severe pain in patients with discogenic pain.[23] Because the standard deviations for these means were large, the pain thresholds overlapped between healthy controls and discs that caused moderate or severe pain.[24] Therefore, it is safe to conclude that there is currently no clear consensus relating specific figures for intradiscal pressures to the diagnosis of discogenic pain or to future responses to therapy. The best utility for manometry may be to compare abnormal discs to "control" discs in the same individual.

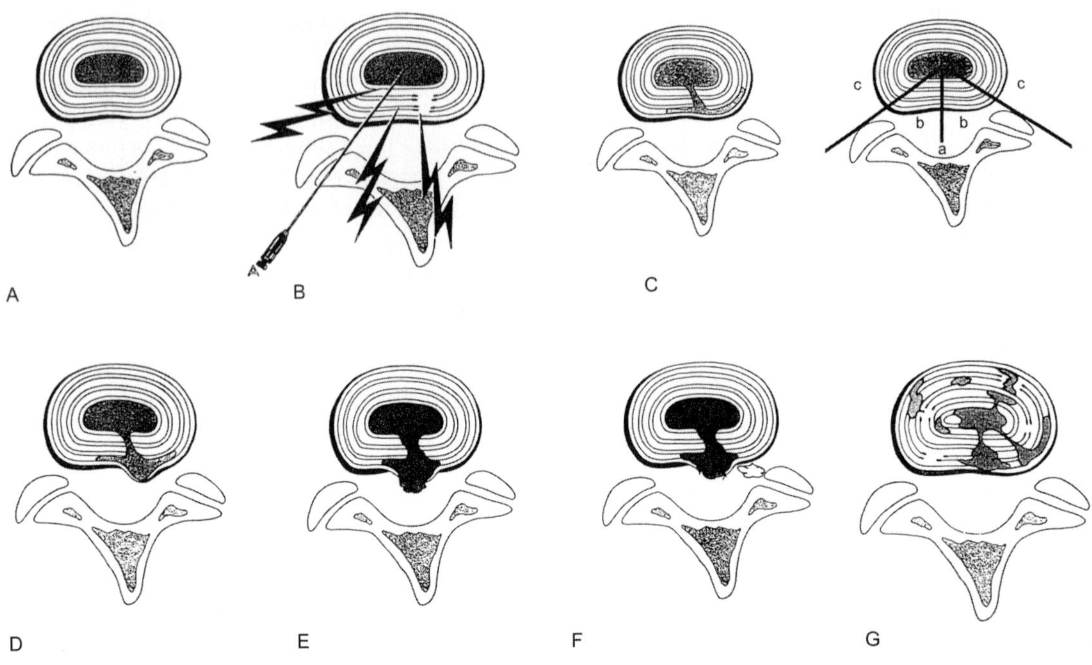

FIGURE 17–4. Morphologic changes in the intervertebral disc as seen with discography: *A.* normal CT discogram; *B.* minimal fissures in the annulus; *C.* radial fissuring (a, posteriorly; b, posterolaterally; c, laterally); *D.* protruding disc herniation (contained by the posterior longitudinal ligament [PLL]); *E.* extruded disc herniation (penetrating the PLL; *F.* sequestered disc herniation (note fragment in intervertebral foramen); *G.* internal disc disruption. *(Adapted from ref. 22.)*

Indications

Discography has been used as a diagnostic tool to diagnose disc herniation. Changes in discographic patterns can identify the morphologic changes of disc degeneration, and the location of pain that is provoked helps identify the level of pathology. Figure 17–4 demonstrates morphological changes that can be observed on discography. Discography may be used as a complement to myelography, providing better visualization of lateral disc herniations and discs at the L5–S1 level.[25] With the development of CT scanning, with its 92% diagnostic reliability rate, and MRI, which correlates with discography 89% of the time,[26] the indications for discography have become much more specific. For that reason, noninvasive testing with CT or MRI scanning is used as a first-line modality to diagnose patients with low back pain.

The primary indication for discography is to diagnose patients with low back/leg pain whose CT/MRI studies failed to explain their pain. In such patients, the CT/MRI either may be normal or it may show multilevel disc degeneration. Discography can identify the symptomatic level, confirming the source of discogenic pain among multiple degenerated discs. The internal morphology of stressed, pressurized discs can be studied and categorized. In a patient with a normal MRI, pain provocation by discography can identify subtle early signs of degeneration that are too early even for an MRI to identify.[27]

In addition, discography can help identify or exclude the disc as a source of pain in post-laminectomy patients. For patients after spinal fusion, discography can identify lateral and foraminal disc herniations. Discography clarifies which levels are appropriate for surgical fusion, establishes which are the normal discs, and more effectively assesses the lumbosacral junction. By revealing disc morphology, discography can be used to determine which type of surgery is advisable or whether the patient is a candidate for chemonucleolysis, intradiscal electrothermonucleoplasty (IDET), nucleoplasty, or spinal fusion.[28] Discography may have negative predictive value, in that patients who have pain with all levels injected are less likely to benefit from surgery. Finally, injecting cortisone intradiscally after discography may have a therapeutic effect, although one must carefully measure this benefit versus the increased risk of infection. When compared to other tests, discography is the only pain-provocative test that confirms whether a patient's symptoms are discogenic in origin.

Comparison of Discography and CT/MRI

Multiple studies have been conducted to assess the value of discography as a diagnostic tool. Collins compared discography to MRI in a prospective study of 29 patients and 73 lumbar levels.[29] There were 57 degenerative levels of the 73 levels tested. All of the patients who had symptom reproduction on discography also had degenerative changes on MRI (13 patients). Annular disruption was present (confirmed on discography) in 10 of the 13 symptomatic levels, compared to only 9 of 44 asymptomatic, degenerated levels. Although disc degeneration alone on MRI did not predict symptoms, the relationship was stronger when annular tears were visualized on MRI. Overall, there was a 90% correlation between MRI and discography, when looked at in terms of pain on discography and the presence of disc degeneration on MRI. Of the 16 nondegenerative levels on MRI, 4 patients had positive pain on discography, thus yielding a false-positive rate of 25%. However, some of these patients may have had early internal annular disruption without degenerative changes on MRI, as an interval of time must pass between disruption of the annulus and loss of water content to be reflected on MRI as decreased signal intensity.

Bernard concluded that discography was more sensitive than MRI, as 18 of 177 discs with normal T2-weighted images on MRI had abnormal discograms, with annular disruption confirmed by postdiscography CT scanning.[26] False-positive test results in discography can also occur from errant intra-annular injections. In this study of 250 patients ranging in age from 18 to 75 years who had discograms at 725 levels, 308 discs were normal and 417 were abnormal. Of the 417 abnormal discs, only 257 injections provoked the patients' typical pain complaints. The results of discography and characteristic disrupted annular pattern seen on CT scan were used to identify the level causing patients' symptoms. The results were also used to determine the type of disc disruption, whether herniation or epidural scarring was causing symptoms postoperatively, and whether the patient was a candidate for percutaneous or open discectomy. The conclusion of the Bernard study was that discography followed by CT influenced patient management in 93% of cases.

Jackson compared CT, myelography, discography, and discography followed by CT in 231 disc sites in an attempt to assess the accuracy of each technique, as confirmed by open surgical assessment.[30] Discography followed by CT provided the most accurate results (87%), compared to CT alone (74%), pain on discography (64%), and radiological findings on discography (58%). CT scanning alone was associated with a higher false-positive rate (24%) compared to discography (19%). For lumbar herniated nucleus pulposis, the radiological findings on discography are highly sensitive (81%) and pain reproduction on discography is highly specific (89%), thus making it a useful technique to evaluate patients with an equivocal diagnosis. A follow-up study compared MRI to CT scanning in determining the reliability of assessing early degenerative disc changes.[31] MRI was judged superior to CT in recognizing early degenerative process, with an accuracy of 76% versus 74% for CT scan. The false-positive rate of 15% for discography in this study is substantially lower than other published reports of up to 48%.

Vanharanta confirmed that the proportion of discs with deterioration increases with patient age, but that the percentage of patients who have pain associated with degeneration is higher in young patients.[32] Severely degenerated discs were painful in 82% of young patients but only in 57% of older patients, and there was a higher proportion of dissimilar pain on provocation in the older group. In an earlier study, exact or similar reproduction of pain on discography was more likely in patients with disc herniation and degeneration (82% and 80%) compared to other nonspecific low back pain (55%–60%).[33] Although MRI accurately reflects the degenerative changes that are confirmed with discography, patients with peripheral annular tears may be better identified by discography.

Clinical Pearl: Although MRI accurately reflects the degenerative changes that are confirmed with discography, patients with peripheral annular tears may be better identified by discography.

Moneta, in a study of 833 discs in 306 patients, confirmed a higher incidence of exact pain reproduction among patients with annulus rupture versus patients with only disc degeneration.[34] Since many patients with disc degeneration also have annular rupture, multivariate statistical techniques are required to rule out dependent variables and random effects. Disc degeneration alone is less likely to result in pain on discography than are annular ruptures; lumbar discs, which are more caudad, are more likely to elicit exact pain reproduction than more cephalad discs, while age has been demonstrated to have only a borderline association. Vanharanta (1987) also showed that with greater degeneration, discography was more likely to be painful, more likely to have exact reproduction of pain, and that disc disruption (i.e., annular tearing) was more likely to cause pain than disc degeneration (i.e., dehydration).[35] In this study, 20% of normal-appearing discs resulted in pain complaints when injected, which is a significant false-positive rate.

In a study assessing the role of discography in predicting surgical outcome, Colhoun studied 195 patients 2 years after surgery, 137 of whom had positive discography.[28] In patients with abnormal discs who had pain provocation on discography, 89% had a good surgical result compared to only 52% of patients with abnormal discs who did not have positive pain provocation on discography. This study analyzed the predictive value of symptom reproduction during discography, and most patients underwent subsequent fusion. Pain was most common with posterior annular tears (65%) with only 35% of patients with degenerated discs having pain. In patients who had morphologically abnormal but nonsymptomatic discs, 41 of 43 also benefited from surgery. This study found a high false-positive rate with provocation discography.

Some studies that report a high false-positive rate with discography have significant flaws. Holt reported a 37% false-positive rate in asymptomatic volunteers.[36] However, the "volunteers" for this study were prisoners at a state penitentiary, some of who may have had ulterior motives to claim pain. Also, irritating contrast material was used and there was a high failure rate of needle placement (failure to puncture disc in at least one level occurred in over 50% of patients).[37] Finally, Holt did not differentiate between symptom reproduction and simple pain on injection. As with all research, objective assessment of the methodology and results must be addressed to determine the value of each study.

Morphologic Changes

Several different classification systems have been devised to delineate morphologic changes associated with disc degeneration as seen on discography.[26,38,39] Various types of injections of contrast help to define the internal structure of the intervertebral disc and define whether there is internal disc disruption, contained herniation (within the posterior longitudinal ligament), foraminal herniation, lateral herniation, sequestered disc fragments, or recurrent disc herniation versus adhesive scar in postoperative patients.

Tournade described four stages of morphological damage as seen under x-ray after contrast injection into a disc.[38] In a normal disc, the nucleus pulposis is difficult to inject, forming a bilenticular image when imaged. Stage I describes a flattened nucleus with slight anterior–posterior fragmentation, resulting from a median protrusion between the layers of the interior and exterior posterior annulus. In Stage II, the nucleus is elongated anteriorly–posteriorly and fragmented with lateral annular fissures. Stage III demonstrates a fragmented, multilocular nucleus clustered in an anterior–posterior direction at the posterior fibers of the annulus. Stage IV includes a fissure of the posterior longitudinal ligament with herniation into the epidural space.

Bernard[26] also described a number of patterns on postdiscography CT scans (see Figure 17–4). Type I demonstrates a normal, asymptomatic nucleus pulposis. Type II is a normal nucleus pulposis with the existence of symptoms, suggesting the earliest stage of annular tearing. In Type III, annular tears cause radial fissures, mainly posteriorly and laterally. In Type IV, the nuclear material has protruded beyond the boundary of the annulus, and in Type V it has extruded (i.e., "noncontained" nucleus). Type VI represents a sequestered disc and Type VII exhibits total disc disruption.

A third classification system, the Dallas Discogram Description, presents a very different organizational approach than the previous measures. The Dallas system provides grades for annular degeneration, annular disruption, pain provocation, and the volume of contrast the disc accepts. It also a category for other comments about the procedure. Using this system, Sachs found a false-positive rate of 13%.[39]

Complications

The most feared complication for discography is discitis. The intervertebral disc is an avascular structure that receives its nutrition via passive diffusion and is ill equipped to defend itself against infection. Primary disc infections present as an increase in axial pain, fever, and elevated erythrocyte sedimentation rate (ESR). The infectious process devastates the disc, ultimately resulting in fusion of the vertebral bodies. Discitis has been reported to occur with an incidence of 0.1%–1.0%, and it can be complicated by epidural abscess, subdural empyema, and prevertebral abscess.[40–42] Some cases of discitis, on the other hand, are probably sterile.

The diagnosis of discitis is often delayed. Elevations in ESR occur on average 20 days postprocedurally, and bone scans become positive after about 33 days.[42] X-rays reveal narrowing of the disc space with endplate erosion, with about 50% of patients manifesting x-ray changes. Discitis causes destruction of the cartilaginous endplates, herniation of intervertebral discs to adjacent vertebral bodies, and replacement of the nucleus pulposis by granulation tissue.[43] The typical course of lumbar discitis is 8–11 weeks. Recommended treatment is with a 4-week course of intravenous antibiotics.

In addition to discitis, other complications reported from discography include retroperitoneal hemorrhage, subarachnoid injections, spinal cord injury, and vascular injury. Whether preprocedural prophylactic antibiotics are of benefit remains questionable. A study by Rhoten found that 2 g of cefoxitin administered intravenously had good penetration into the disc, with highest levels present 45–57 minutes after injection.[44] A second study confirms that cefoxitin can penetrate the intervertebral disc to destroy *Staphylococcus epidermidis*, but reiterates that antibiotics are quantifiable in the disc only 30–60 minutes after intravenous injection.[43] Thus, antibiotics are effective only if given prophylactically and they may not arrest the course of an already present infection. Some advocate the use of intradiscal cefoxitin 1 mg/mL given at the time of discography, although this is not universally accepted or routinely performed.

Clinical Pearl: In addition to discitis, other complications reported from discography include retroperitoneal hemorrhage, subarachnoid injections, spinal cord injury, and vascular injury.

Spinal cord compression is a rare complication from discography. The incidence of spinal cord compression from discography may be higher in patients with critical spinal stenosis or existing cord compression. Care should be taken when performing discography in patients with an element of spinal stenosis.

Discography is unlikely to induce herniation in normal discs. Damage to the disc would depend on the volume injected, the needle gauge, and the frequency of annular puncture. Nonetheless, this complication is only theoretical and has never been reported. Johnson looked at 80 levels of discography followed up 5–38 months later by a second discography.[41] There were no new abnormalities in previously normal discs.

After discography, patients may have a transient exacerbation of pain. This is usually of short duration, but may require treatment with analgesics or anti-inflammatory drugs. However, most patients can return to their usual activities by the next day. Rarely, irritation of nerve roots adjacent to the disc can cause a temporary radiculitis. These symptoms may be lessened with the typical treatments for neuropathic pain, including use of antidepressant- and anticonvulsant-type medications. Occasionally, simply applying ice to the area of the back near the site of needle puncture can relieve localized pain related to tissue and muscle trauma from the procedure.

There is no sound structural reason for sustained pain after discography. Carragee reported on this phenomenon in a study of asymptomatic patients who underwent a discography procedure.[42] None of the patients who had normal psychometric testing complained of prolonged pain after discography. However, patients with abnormal psychometric testing reported a 40% incidence of new low back pain after discography, and patients with somatization disorder reported a 66% incidence of new pain after discography. Patients with occupational disability were even more likely to report pain after discography, with an incidence of 80%.

PAIN-RELIEVING DIAGNOSTIC PROCEDURES FOR LOW BACK PAIN

Overview on the Utility of Diagnostic Blocks

A diagnostic neural blockade procedure consists of administering local anesthetic along or adjacent to a structure in the spine, which is thought to be causing pain. Figure 17–5 provides illustrations for three commonly utilized diagnostic blocks: epidural injections, selective nerve root blocks, and sympathetic blocks. Occasionally, steroids are used to enhance or prolong the effect of the block. The most common local anesthetics used are lidocaine, which has a duration of effect of about 45–90 minutes, or bupivacaine, which has a duration of effect of about 2–6 hours. In some patients, local anesthetic blockade can last much longer than the usual duration of effect. The mechanisms for this phenomenon are incompletely understood. The volume of injectate differs depending on the type of injection. Usually, nerve root and facet injections are done with 1.0–1.5 mL of local anesthetic, whereas epidural doses may be in the range of 3–5 mL, and lumbar sympathetic blockade is done with volumes of 5–10 mL. Generally, there is a lack of consensus regarding the optimal dose of local anesthetic to use for a diagnostic neural blockade procedure.

Using neural blockade procedures as a diagnostic modality can be problematic. Since pain is a subjective complaint, the reporting of pain and its relief can be influenced by nonanatomic factors as well as on organic pathology. Emotional, behavioral, social, financial, legal, and psychological factors may play a role. Therefore, whether a subject reports pain relief after a neural blockade procedure may be affected by such factors. Patient selection criteria may play a role, as some patients may have a desire to report a certain result, either consciously or subconsciously. Another issue is that of the placebo response, which may be influenced by patient expectations and a physician's convictions, along with possibly endogenous opioid mechanisms.[47,48]

There are neurophysiological issues that are problematic in the diagnosis of back pain with neural blockades. When a nerve block is done, three questionable assumptions are made.[45] First, it is assumed that the pathway of pain is in an exact location and impulses are carried along a fixed route. Second, it is assumed that the injection of local anesthetics abolishes the sensation of the intended nerves and no others. Third, the relief of pain is thought to be due only to blockade of the target pathway.[49] There is evidence that these assumptions are overly simplistic.

In addition, issues with local anesthetics and their delivery complicate neural blockade. Variable effects can be expected of local anesthetics, based on nerve fiber size, diffusion barriers, the length of the nerve exposed to the anesthetic, and the rate of firing of the axon.[49] Systemic effects of larger doses of local anesthetics can affect impulse generation from injured nerves, as shown in studies of systemic lidocaine infusion.[50,51]

Another issue is that of anatomical factors that may make the distribution and flow of a local anesthetic unpredictable and uncertain in terms of diagnostic reliability. For example, a "selective" nerve root block may not be selective if the volume of local

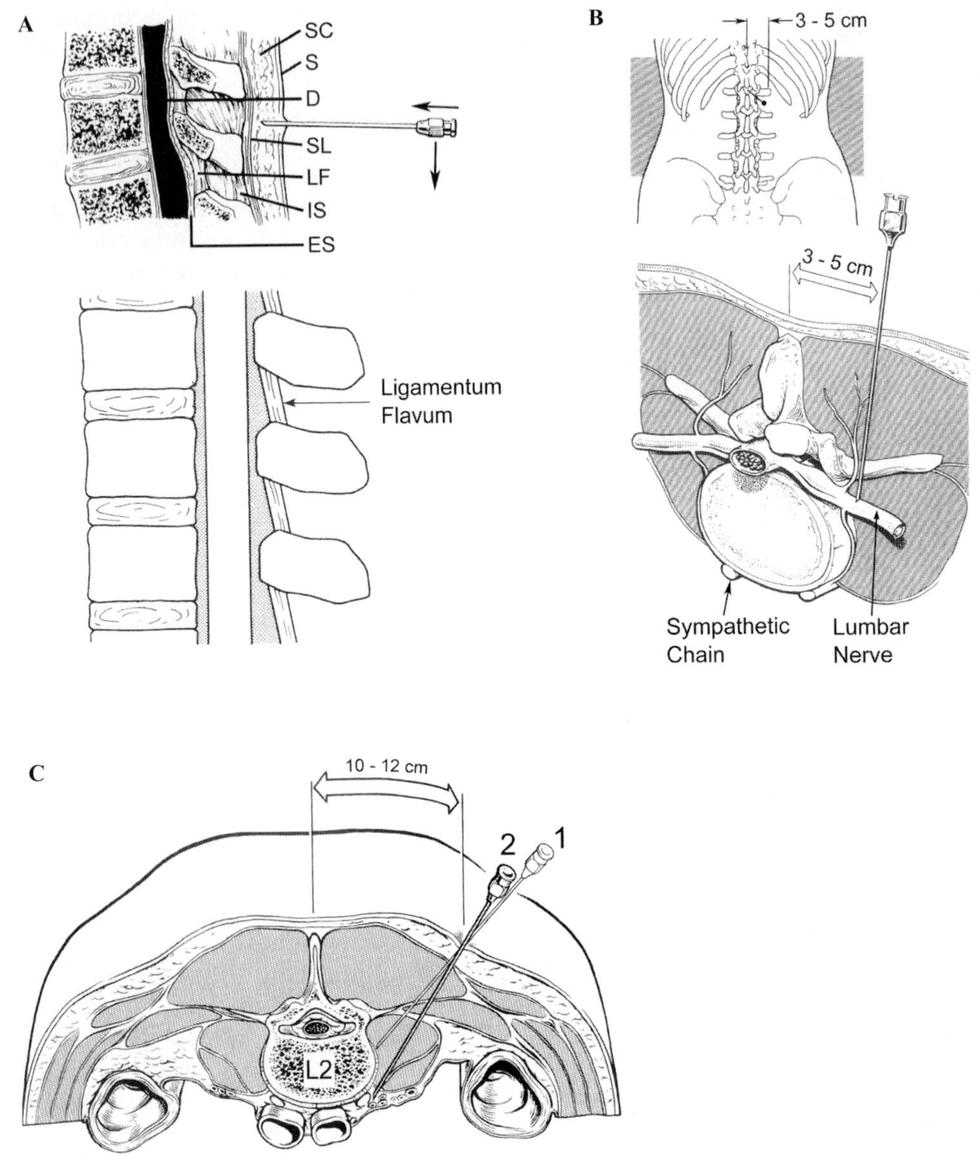

FIGURE 17–5. Overview of diagnostic nerve blocks. *A. Epidural steroid injection.* The needle passes through the skin (S), subcutaneous tissue (Sc), supraspinal ligament (SL), intraspinous ligaments (Is), ligamentum flavum (LF), and into the epidural space (ES), just superficial to the dura (D). *B. Selective nerve root block.* The needle is inserted 3–5 cm lateral to the midline and advanced cephalad, toward the pedicle and under the transverse process to lie in the exit of the intervertebral foramen. *C. Lumbar sympathetic block.* A needle is inserted 10–12 cm lateral to the midline, advanced to encounter the vertebral body (1), and then walked anteriorly to rest in the area of the sympathetic chain (2), anterolateral to the vertebral body. *(From: Cousins and Bridenbaugh, pp. 252 (A), 476 (B), and 433 (C).) (Adapted from ref. 9.)*

anesthetic injected spreads to the epidural space and affects adjacent nerve roots. On the other hand, if the local anesthetic does not really reach the nerve root and spreads instead along the vertebral body at the site of the sinuvertebral nerves or the sympathetic nervous system, then the implications of the block become completely different. If the patient is actually suffering from a primary muscular problem, injection of local anesthetic into the erector spinae or psoas muscles may lead to pain relief, making the injection of local anesthetic near the nerve root irrelevant. In other words, the risk of false-negatives and false-positives is quite high with any "diagnostic" nerve injection.

Clinical Pearl: Using neural blockade procedures as a diagnostic modality can be problematic. Since pain is a subjective complaint, the reporting of pain and its relief can be influenced by nonanatomic factors as well as on organic pathology. Emotional, behavioral, social, financial, legal, and psychological factors may play a role.

The net result is that clinicians should be aware of considerations that challenge the use of neural blockade as a diagnostic modality. Nonetheless, there is a wide clinical practice that advocates the use of nerve blocks as a way to help confirm or reject a diagnosis. The general recommendation is that neural blockade be used only as one method to answer the diagnostic dilemma of back pain. Great care should be taken in using the results of neural blockade procedures to decide on surgical interventions, for the reasons outlined above.

Epidural Steroid Injections

Some have advocated for the use of epidural steroid injections to determine whether a particular pain problem is caused by spine pathology. There are several reasons why the effects of epidural steroid injections are a poor predictor of actual pathology causing pain. First, epidural steroid injections can lead to pain relief from a number of diverse painful spine conditions, including annular tear, neurocompressive herniated nucleus pulposis, facet arthropathy, spinal stenosis, and foraminal stenosis. Since any of these conditions may respond to an injection, a beneficial response does not indicate which condition is the actual cause of pain.

Also, efficacy of an epidural steroid injection may depend on the flow of steroid to the affected area. In some cases, thin fibrous connective tissue bands may preclude the flow of steroid to the pain-generating area, such that an otherwise well-done injection can have variable effects on pain. The level of injection can be difficult to confirm precisely, especially in obese patients or in the elderly with scoliosis and significant degenerative changes. The injectate can flow to multiple levels, either cephalad or caudad from the needle, making it difficult to know where it is actually having its primary effect.

Finally, systemic effects of steroid can give patients a transient improvement in their condition, even if the medication is injected into a vein or into musculoligamentous tissue. For example, just because a patient with spinal stenosis seems to respond with improved pain and functional ability after an epidural steroid injection, it does not preclude the possibility that the response was due to systemic absorption of steroid. When the placebo response and sheer coincidence are taken into consideration, along with the aforementioned factors, the diagnostic efficacy of an epidural steroid injection is thrown into serious question.

Epiduroscopy

Spinal endoscopy has been advocated as a diagnostic and therapeutic tool to visualize the spinal cord and epidural space in patients with back pain. Endoscopy is done via a caudal approach by which a scope is inserted through the sacrococcygeal ligament and into the caudal canal. Usually, a catheter can be advanced cephalad to rest in the lumbar epidural space. This is the preferred approach to access the epidural space for patients who have had lumbar spine surgery and whose posterior anatomy may have been altered. A catheter is inserted with a fiberoptic scope, with an overall diameter of about 3 mm. Injured nerves are visualized, and medications are injected at the site of the presumed injury. Spinal endoscopy is a minimally invasive technique to treat back pain before further invasive surgical procedures are attempted. Inflammatory changes in injured nerves can be directly visualized, which may explain the location of the pain generator in patients with multiple levels of pathology on MRI scanning. In addition, medications can then be delivered directly to the inflamed tissue.

Several connective tissue bands have been identified in the epidural space using epiduroscopy.[52] These include a dorsomedian connective tissue band, called the plica mediana dorsalis. It has been postulated that these connective tissue bands may lead to erratic spread of epidural injectate, but this has not been substantiated.[53] The epidural space is known to change with age (see Chapter 8).

This technique may be helpful in the evaluation of patients who have persistent pain after back surgery. Epiduroscopy may confirm the presence of epidural fibrosis and be used as a guide for injection of steroids or hypertonic saline. Saitoh reports on two cases in which epiduroscopic adhesiolysis and irrigation led to pain relief in a patient with chronic low back pain and sciatica.[54] There have been no prospective studies to evaluate the efficacy or utility of epiduroscopy.

In pregnant women, epiduroscopy has been used to evaluate changes in epidural structure that may affect the spread of local anesthetic during epidural analgesia.[55] Pregnant women were found to have a narrower epidural space because of a greater density of epidural veins. The reasons for this finding include hormonal and mechanical changes induced by pregnancy, along with aortocaval compression and increased maternal blood volume.

Clinical Pearl: Epiduroscopy may confirm the presence of epidural fibrosis and be used as a guide for injection of steroids or hypertonic saline.

Another method to evaluate epidural anatomy is by injecting dye into the epidural space, either via the standard translaminar approach or via a caudal route. By directly visualizing dye spread radiographically, the clinician can potentially identify areas of obstruction, such as may be caused by fibrous adhesions after spinal surgery. As with endoscopic techniques, fluoroscopic imaging of the flow of contrast dye in the epidural space is dependent on a certain amount of subjective interpretation. There may be little relationship between the route of contrast dye spread and the cause of painful symptomatology. In many cases, the presence of epidural adhesions may be completely asymptomatic.

Potential complications of epiduroscopy include the occurrence of retinal hemorrhages due to increased CSF (cerebrospinal fluid) pressure from the injection of saline that is done during the procedure.[56] Decreasing the volume and rate of epidural injection can reduce this risk.

Facet Injections

In general, the literature supports the use of facet injections to delineate whether the source of spinal pain is from the facet joints. Mooney and Robertson showed that experimental back pain could be induced by stimulating the facet joints with an injection of saline,[17] and Marks showed that injecting into a facet joint can provoke local and referred pain.[57] However, although the facet joints can be a source of back pain, they are not the only source of pain, and anesthetizing the joint yields 8%–94% relief of pain, depending on the study.[58] As with other neural blockade procedures, the specificity of the block depends on limiting the spread of local anesthetic to block only the facet joint, which is compromised when local anesthetic spreads to the muscles, the epidural space, or to the nerve root. In addition to supplying the joint, the medial branch of the dorsal ramus supplies the local muscles, ligaments, and periosteum. Pain relief may occur from blockade of these structures, and not only the joint. Since the nerve supply to the spinal structures is multisegmental and because pain can result from any of these structures, diagnostic facet injections should be used only in the context of an overall evaluation and treatment plan.

Because uncontrolled single-facet injections have a poor specificity in the diagnosis of facet pain, various methods have been used to decrease their false-positive rate. Barnsley compared single diagnostic blocks to a double block technique in which local anesthetics of differing duration of effect were used.[55,56] Initial injections of either 2% lidocaine (short-acting) or 0.5% bupivacaine (long-acting) were given to 55 patients with neck pain of greater than 3 months duration after motor vehicle accident. Later, the block was repeated with the alternate local anesthetic. Only patients who had longer duration pain relief with bupivacaine (the longer acting drug) were considered to have a true positive response. Of the 60 joints injected, 16 had a false-positive response (27%). In the remainder, MBBs were deemed to be anatomically specific for the diagnosis of facet pain.

An issue arises on whether there are differences in results with intra-articular facet injections compared to MBBs. Intra-articular injections would be expected to be more specific for joint pathology, except in cases in which the injectate extrudes from the joint or it is injected pericapsularly. In terms of response, patients seem to have equivalent effect from either technique. Response to MBB facet injections has been found to predict results of radiofrequency denervation of the facet joints.[61,62] A more complete review of efficacy of facet injections and further facet joint procedures is given in the subsequent chapter on therapeutic efficacy of neural blockade (see Chapter 24).

Selective Nerve Root Blocks

Selective spinal nerve injections, commonly called paravertebral nerve root blocks, have been used for both the diagnosis and the treatment of spinal pain syndromes. Patients with radiating pain into a lower extremity can have abnormal radiographic results pointing out pathology at several spinal levels, and it may be difficult to determine the origin of a radiculopathy. Unfortunately, there are limitations in using spinal nerve injections to diagnose the source of pain.[49] First, pain can be caused by overlapping nerves. The injectate may spread nonselectively to other areas, such as the epidural space or other nerve branches. One cannot determine if the source of pain relieved by a nerve root block was within the nerve foramen or present more distally. The ability of a selective nerve root block to predict surgical outcome is questionable, as four studies showed a positive predictive value of 87%–100% but a negative predictive value of 27%–38%.[49] Other studies show that selective nerve blocks fail to predict the outcome of neuroablative procedures.

The general conclusion is that although selective nerve root blocks may be an excellent modality to deliver treatment to an area suspected of causing a painful spinal condition, this modality has limited diagnostic utility. This is outlined in North's 1996 study to evaluate the specificity of diagnostic nerve blocks in patients with sciatica due to lumbosacral spine disease.[63] North concluded that a positive response to a single nerve block lacks specificity, and that the role of diagnostic blockade should be to confirm management decisions supported by other clinical and diagnostic findings. More details on the use of selective spinal nerve blocks are given in Chapter 24.

Sacroiliac Joint Injections

The sacroiliac joint is the innervated articulation between the sacral bone and the iliac bone. It is a true diarthroidal joint that is supported by numerous ligaments and muscles that give it stability. Inflammation, trauma, degeneration, and mechanical disruption of this joint can result in pain. The prevalence of sacroiliac pain may approach 30% of patients who complain of low back pain.[64] Patients who have pain from the sacroiliac joint will usually complain of symptoms in the buttock, low back, and into the proximal lower extremity. Often, direct palpation over the joint will illicit pain. Radiographs, CT scanning, and bone scans may reveal signs of sacroiliac disease.

Sacroiliac injections are performed by inserting at least one needle into the joint and injecting local anesthetic and steroid. It is recommended that injections be done with guidance either fluoroscopically or by CT scanning to insure correct needle placement. Because of the numerous muscles and ligaments near the joint, postinjection pain relief does not reliably confirm that the sacroiliac joint alone is the pain generator. Since the sacroiliac joint covers a large area, some recommend the use of multiple needles to inject an adequate volume of local anesthetic to obtain pain relief.

Sympathetic Blocks

Lumbar sympathetic blockade has been used primarily as a modality to treat pain from lower extremity vascular insufficiency or from "reflex sympathetic dystrophy" of the lower extremity. Lately, there has been increasing question on the usefulness of sympathetic blockade as either a diagnostic or a therapeutic modality. There has been a recent consensus that many cases of reflex sympathetic dystrophy actually have no relationship with the sympathetic nervous system. This has led to the adoption of a new terminology for this syndrome, which is now called complex regional pain syndrome (CRPS).[65]

Clinical Pearl: Lumbar sympathetic blockade has been used primarily as a modality to treat pain from lower extremity vascular insufficiency or from "reflex sympathetic dystrophy" of the lower extremity. Lately, there has been increasing question on the usefulness of sympathetic blockade as either a diagnostic or therapeutic modality.

Because the contribution of the sympathetic nervous system is questionable in many cases of CRPS, the use of sympathetic blocks to determine a clinical diagnosis for these conditions is inappropriate. In terms of therapeutic efficacy, the role of these procedures has also been questioned. Also, similar to other diagnostic neural blockade procedures, sympathetic blocks lack specificity and are prone to anatomical factors that preclude their usefulness as diagnostic tools. For example, even a well-conducted sympathetic block may be incomplete because of poor spread of the injectate along the sympathetic chain. The block may not selectively block only the sympathetic chain, but may also block adjacent somatic structures and nerves. There may be a systemic local anesthetic effect throughout the body. For those reasons, as with the other diagnostic neural blockade procedures, the utility of sympathetic nerve blocks as a diagnostic tool is questionable at best.

CONCLUSION

The diagnosis of low back pain syndromes requires a sound knowledge of the presenting symptoms of various conditions causing spinal pain. Primarily, taking a careful history and performing a neurological and musculoskeletal examination provides a sound base for establishing the diagnosis. Imaging studies such as x-rays, CT scanning, and MRI can help distinguish one possible cause of back pain from another. However, many radiographic abnormalities are asymptomatic, thus reducing the specificity of these tests in determining the symptom generator.

Diagnostic dilemmas arise for cases in which multiple pathologies for causing pain are possible, and indeed multiple pathologies are found on radiographic imagery. In those cases, discography can help determine whether the pain symptoms are of a discogenic etiology and, if so, which disc is the primary cause of the symptoms. With regards to neural blockade procedures, their utility as a sole arbiter to determine the cause of a spinal pain condition is limited. However, as part of a comprehensive evaluation process, and by understanding their limitations, an astute clinician can utilize such techniques to help confirm or refute a particular diagnosis.

SUMMARY

1. Chapter 17 provided an overview of the clinically relevant anatomy as it pertains to spinal pain syndromes.
2. By describing the most common pain generators of the lumbo pelvic region, clinical rationale to utilize minimally invasive procedures was established.
3. A variety of minimally invasive diagnostic measures was described here.
4. The results of these tests can greatly assist the clinician in establishing a better understanding of the pain generator(s), which allows for a more cogent clinical strategy to be subsequently established.

REFERENCES

1. Bonica JJ. Importance of the problem. In: Andersson S, Bond M, Mehta M, Swerdlow M, eds. *Chronic noncancer pain.* Lancaster, UK: MTP Press Limited, 1987:13.
2. Fordyce WE. The problem. In: Fordyce WE, ed. *Back pain in the workplace: Management of disability in nonspecific conditions.* Seattle, WA: IASP Press, 1995:5–9, 19–23.

3. Lemrow N, Adams D, Coffey R, et al. The 50 most frequent diagnosis-related groups (DRGs), diagnoses, and procedures: Statistics by hospital size and location, DHHS Publication (PHS) 90–3465, Hospital Studies Program Research Note 13, Agency for Health Care Policy and Research, Public Health Service, Rockville, MD, September 1990.
4. Frymoyer J, Cats-Baril W. An overview of the incidence and costs of low back pain. *Ortho Clin North Am* 1991;22:263–271.
5. Sternbach RA. Survey of pain in the United States: The Nuprin pain report. *Clin J Pain* 1986;2:49–53.
6. Anonymous. Scientific approach to the assessment and management of activity-related spinal disorders. A monograph for clinicians. Report of the Quebec Task Force on Spinal Disorders. *Spine* 1987;12(Suppl 7):S1–59.
7. Derby R, Bogduk N, Anat D, Schwarzer A. Precision percutaneous blocking procedures for spinal pain. *Pain Digest* 1993;3:89–100.
8. Boden SD, Davis DO, Dina TS, Patronas NJ, Wiesel SW. Abnormal magnetic-resonance scans of the lumbar spine in asymptomatic subjects. A prospective investigation. *J Bone Joint Surg* 1990;72(3):403–408.
9. Manning DC, Rowlingson JC. Back pain and the role of neural blockade. In: Cousins MJ, Bridenbaugh PO, eds. *Neural blockade in clinical anesthesia and management of pain*, 3rd ed. Philadelphia: Lippincott-Raven, 1998;879–914.
10. Selby D. The structural degenerative cascade. In: White AH (ed), Schofferman J (assoc. ed). *Spine care*. St. Louis, MN: Mosby, 1995.
11. Schofferman J. Diagnostic decision making. In White AH (ed), Schofferman J (assoc. ed). *Spine care*. St. Louis, MN: Mosby, 1995:8–16, 41–51.
12. Fass A, Chavannes J, van Eijk TM, Gubbels JW. A randomized, placebo controlled trial of exercise therapy in patients with acute low back pain. Presented at the *20th Annual Meeting of the International Society for the Study of Lumbar Spine*, Marseilles, France, June 15–19, 1993.
13. Jensen MC, Brant-Zawadzki MN, Obuchowski N, et al. Magnetic resonance of the lumbar spine in people without back pain. N Engl J Med 1994;331:69–73.
14. Weber H. Lumbar disc herniation: A controlled, prospective study with ten years of observation. *Spine* 1983;8:131–140.
15. Onel D, Sari H, Donmez C. Lumbar spinal stenosis: Clinical, radiologic, therapeutic evaluation in 145 patients. *Spine* 1993;18:291–298.
16. Weinstein JN, Rydevik. The pain of spondylolisthesis. *Semin Spine Surg* 1989;1:100–105.
17. Mooney V, Robertson J. The facet syndrome. *Clin Orthop* 1976;15:149–155.
18. Schmorl G. Uber Knorpelknoten an der Hinterflache der Wirbelbandsheiben. *Fortsch Rontgenstr* 1929;40: 629–634.
19. Lindblom K. Diagnostic puncture of intervertebral disks in sciatica. *Acta Orthop Scand* 1948;17:231–239.
20. Wise RE, Weiford EC. X-ray visualization of the intervertebral disk. *Cleve Clin Q* 1951;18:127–130.
21. Cohen SP, Larkin TM, Barna SA, et al. Lumbar Discography: A Comprehensive Review of Outcome Studies, Diagnostic Accuracy, and Principles. *Regional Anesthesia and Pain Medicine* 2005;30:163–183.
22. O'Neill C, Kurgansky M. Subgroups of positive discs on discography. *Spine* 2004;29:2134–2139.
23. Giesecke T, Gracely RH, Grant MA, et al. Evidence of augmented central pain processing in idiopathic chronic low back pain. *Arthritis Rheum* 2004;50:613–623.
24. Shah RV, Everett CR, McKenzie-Brown A, et al. Discography as a diagnostic test for spinal pain: A systematic and narrative review. *Pain Physician* 2005;8:187–209.
25. Gresham JL, Miller R. Evaluation of the lumbar spine by diskography and its use in selection of proper treatment of the herniated disc syndrome. *Clin Orthop* 1969;67:29–41.
26. Bernard TN. Lumbar discography followed by computed tomography: Refining the diagnosis of low back pain. *Spine* 1990;15:690–707.
27. Zucherman J, Derby R, Hsu K, et al. Normal magnetic resonance imaging with abnormal discography. *Spine* 1988;13:1355–1359.
28. Colhoun E, McCall IW, Williams L, Pullicano VNC. Provocation discography as a guide to planning operations on the spine. *J Bone Joint Surg (BR)* 1988;70:267–271.
29. Collins CD, Stack JP, O'Connell DJ, et al. The role of discography in lumbar disc disease: A comparative study of magnetic resonance imaging and discography. *Clin Radiol* 1990;42:252–257.
30. Jackson RP, Cain JE, Jacobs RR, Cooper BR, McManus GE. The neuroradiographic diagnosis of lumbar herniated nucleus pulposus. I. -A comparison of computed tomography (CT), myelography, CT-myelography, discography, and CT-discography. *Spine* 1989;14:1356–1361.
31. Jackson RP, Cain JE, Jacobs RR, Cooper BR, McManus GE. The neuroradiographic diagnosis of lumbar herniated nucleus pulposus. II. A comparison of computed tomography (CT), myelography, CT-myelography, and MRI. *Spine* 1989;14:1362–1367.
32. Vanharanta H, Sachs BL, Ohnmeiss DD, et al. Pain provocation and disc deterioration by age: A CT/discography study in a low back pain population. *Spine* 1989;14:420–423.
33. Vanharanta H, Guyer RD, Ohnmeiss D, et al. Disc deterioration in low back syndromes: A prospective, multicenter CT/discography study. *Spine* 1998;13:1349–1351.
34. Moneta GB, Videman T, Kaivanta K, et al. Reported pain during lumbar discography as a function of anular ruptures and disc degeneration: A reanalysis of 833 discograms. *Spine* 1994;19:1968–1974.
35. Vanharanta H, Sachs BL, Spivey MA, et al. The relationship of pain provocation to lumbar disc deterioration as seen by CT/discography. *Spine* 1987;12:295–298.
36. Holt EP. The question of lumbar discography. *J Bone Joint Surg* 1968;50(A):720–726.
37. Simmons JW, Aprill CN, Dwyer AP, Brodsky AE. A reassessment of Holt's data on "The question of lumbar discography." *Clin Orthop Relat Res* 1988;237:120–124.

38. Tournade A, Patay Z, Tajahmady T, Braun JP, Million S, Schmutz, G. Contribution of discography to the diagnosis and treatment of lumbar disc hernation. *J Neuroradiol* 1991;18: 1–11.
39. Sachs BL, Vanharanta H, Spivey MA, et al. Dallas discogram description: A new classification of CT/discography in low back disorders. *Spine* 1987;12: 287–294.
40. Zeidman SM, Thompson K, Ducker TB. Complications of cervical discography: Analysis of 4400 diagnostic disc injections. *Neurosurgery* 1995;37:414–417.
41. Fraser RD, Osti OL, Vernon-Roberts B. Discitis after discography. *J Bone Joint Surg (Br)* 1987;69(B):26–35.
42. Guyer RD, Collier R, Stith WJ, et al. Disciitis after discography. *Spine* 1988;13:1352–1354.
43. Osti OL, Fraser RD, Vernon-Roberts B. Discitis after discography: The role of prophylactic antibiotics. *J Bone Joint Surg (Br)* 1990;72(B):271–274.
44. Rhoten RL, Murphy MA, Kalfas IH, Harn JF, Washington JA. Antibiotic penetration into cervical discs. *Neurosurgery* 1995;37:418–421.
45. Johnson RG. Does discography injure normal discs? An analysis of repeat discograms. *Spine* 1989;14:424–426.
46. Carragee EJ, Chen Y, Tanner CM, Hayward C, Rossi M, Hagle C. Can discography cause long-term back symptoms in previously asymptomatic subjects? *Spine* 2000;25:1803–1808.
47. Raja S. Nerve blocks in the evaluation of chronic pain: A plea for caution in their use and interpretation. *Anesthesiology* 1997;86:4–6.
48. Galer BS, Schwartz L, Turner JA. Do patient and physician expectations predict response to pain-relieving procedures? *Clin J Pain* 1997;13:348–351.
49. Hogan QH, Abram SA. Neural blockade for diagnosis and prognosis: A review. *Anesthesiology* 1997;86:216–241.
50. Kastrup J, Peterson P, Dejgard A, Angel HR, Hilsted J. Intravenous lidocaine infusion: A new treatment for chronic painful diabetic neuropathy? *Pain* 1987;28:69–75.
51. Tanelian DL, Maciver MB. Analgesic concentrations of lidocaine suppress tonic A-delta and C-fiber discharges produced by acute injury. *Anesthesiology* 1991;74:934–936.
52. Blomberg R. The dorsomedian connective tissue band in the lumbar epidural space of humans: An anatomical study using epiduroscopy. *Anesth Analg* 1986;65:747–752.
53. Hogan Q, Toth J. Anatomy of soft tissues of the spinal canal. *Reg Anesth Pain Med* 1999;24:303–310.
54. Saitoh K, Igarashi T, Hirabayashi Y, et al. Epiduroscopy in patients with chronic low back pain without remarkable findings on magnetic resonance imaging. *Masui—Jpn J Anesthesiol* 2001;50:1257–1259.
55. Igarashi T, Hirabayashi Y, Shimizu R, Saitoh K, Fukuda H, Suzuki H. The fiberscopic findings of the epidural space in pregnant women. *Anesthesiology* 2000;92:1631–1636.
56. Amirikia A, Scott I, Murray T, Halperin L. Acute bilateral visual loss associated with retinal hemorrhages following epiduroscopy. *Arch Ophthalmol* 2000;118:287–289.
57. Marks R. Distribution of pain provoked from lumbar facet joints and related structures during diagnostic spinal infiltration. *Pain* October 1989;39(1): 37–40.
58. Schwarzer AC, Aprill CN, Derby R. The false-positive rate of uncontrolled diagnostic blocks of the lumbar zygapophysial joints. *Pain* August 1994;58(2):195–200.
59. Barnsley L, Lord S, Wallis B, Bogduk N. False positive rates of cervical zygapophysial joint blocks. *Clin J Pain* 1993;9:124–130.
60. Barnsley L, Bogduk N. Medial branch blocks are specific for the diagnosis of cervical zygapophyseal joint pain. *Reg Anesth* 1993;18:343–350.
61. Lord SM, Barnsley L, Wallis BJ, McDonald GJ, Bogduk N. Percutaneous radio-frequency neurotomy for chronic cervical zygapophysial joint pain. *NEJM* December 5,1996;335(23):1721–1726.
62. McDonald GJ, Lord SM, Bogduk N. Long-term follow up of patients treated with cervical radiofrequency neurotomy for chronic neck pain. *Neurosurgery* 1999;45:61–68.
63. North RB, Kidd DH, Zahurak M, Piantadosi S. Specificity of diagnostic nerve blocks: A prospective, randomized study of sciatica due to lumbosacral spine disease. *Pain* 1996;65:77–85.
64. Schwarzer AC, Aprill LN, Bogduk N. The sacroiliac joint in chronic low back pain. *Spine* 1995;20:31–37.
65. Stanton-Hicks M, Janig W, Hassenbusch S, et al. Reflex sympathetic dystrophy: Changing concepts and taxonomy. *Pain* 1995;63:127–133.

CHAPTER

18

NEURODIAGNOSTIC APPROACHES TO THE EVALUATION OF LOW BACK SYNDROMES

Rand S. Swenson

OUTLINE

OBJECTIVES

1. To review the rational for neurodiagnostic testing in patients with low back syndromes.
2. To discuss the steps in validation of diagnostic tests for patients with low back syndromes.
3. To discuss the methodology, strengths, weakness and interpretation of neurodiagnostic tests for patients with low back syndromes.
4. To consider the proper role of neurodiagnostic testing in the evaluation of patients with low back syndromes.

INTRODUCTION

Back pain is among the most common disorders to afflict the human condition. Approximately 80% of humans will be significantly limited by back pain at some time in their life. This condition tends to be episodic and recurrent, although it can be chronic in a significant minority of patients. In this small percentage of individuals, back pain provides significant disability and is the most common cause of long-term disability in the United States.[1]

In most patients the precise cause of back pain cannot be identified with certainty. There are many potential pain-sensitive structures in the back, any of which may be the source of pain. Additionally, back pain may be caused by benign conditions or, in rare circumstances, may be due to a serious underlying disease. There is a complex interaction between disorders producing back pain and those resulting in symptoms of nerve root compression or irritation. Adding to the confusion is that some disorders affecting the nerve roots actually damage the axons or the myelin coverings (a process that will be referred to as radiculopathy) while others only result in inflammation or irritation (often referred to a radiculitis). Although these conditions may coexist, this is not a necessity and their presentations are quite different. For example, pure radiculopathy would be expected to result in weakness of innervated muscles or in decreased sensitivity of the innervated dermatome depending upon whether the ventral or dorsal root was affected, respectively. Furthermore, any myotatic reflex that is mediated through the ventral or dorsal root at that level would be expected to decrease. Radiculitis, on the other hand, is characterized by pain. This pain probably arises from a local inflammatory reaction and may be mediated by the nerves contained within the nerve roots and their coverings (the nervi nervorum). In this case there may be no actual loss of sensory or motor function and pain would be the dominant symptom. In this regard, radiculitis is similar to the irritation that can be present in any of the pain-sensitive tissues of the back except that the pain would be reproduced rather specifically by maneuvers that stress or traction the nerve roots. Because of the loss of function that is present in radiculopathy, this condition is commonly investigated with neurodiagnostic tests.

Several diagnostic procedures have been applied to low back pain (LBP) patients with varying goals. For example, blood tests such as erythrocyte sedimentation rate may be very helpful in the detection of rheumatologic, infectious, or neoplastic disease. Plain radiographs are useful in detecting osseous lesions (osteoporosis, fractures, dislocations, and metastatic disease). Imaging with magnetic resonance imaging (MRI), computed tomography (CT), discography, and/or myelography has become the "gold standard" for identification of radicular involvement by disc or foraminal encroachment. These procedures are discussed elsewhere.

Benign conditions (which have gone by several names including "nonspecific back pain" or "mechanical back pain") are far more common than other types of back pain.[2] Attempts to correlate anatomical imaging procedures with pain production have been disappointing, with the exception of the imaging of direct nerve root compression producing radiculopathy. The underlying cause of back pain is rarely identifiable with any degree of certainty and in many cases may be multifactorial. For example, back pain can result from local irritation of, or direct mechanical trauma to, pain-sensitive tissues (ligaments, muscles, joints, etc.). Pain may also arise from local chemical irritation of these sensitive tissues or from neurophysiological alterations in sensitivity of pain systems (as has been described in chronic experimental pain), such as spinal windup, central sensitization, and hyperalgesia. Additionally, it is possible that the initial injury may result in compensatory or adaptive mechanisms that may also result in pain such as muscle spasm. Because the underlying pathology or pathophysiology is not well understood, there are no diagnostic tests that have been consistently proven to directly confirm the presence of LBP. Diagnostic imaging, for example, has major limitations in this regard, with a high percentage of asymptomatic and otherwise healthy individuals showing what appear to be significant abnormalities such as degeneration of the disc or even frank herniation.

Another group of diagnostic procedures can be collectively grouped under the auspices of neurodiagnostic procedures. These procedures, used for assessing LBP and radiculopathies, are *not designed to determine the pain-sensitive tissue or underlying pathology.* Rather, these tests *have been designed to examine functional consequences of the condition.* It is with this in mind that the following discussion of neurodiagnostic approaches to low back syndromes takes place.

USES OF DIAGNOSTIC TESTS FOR BACK SYNDROMES

Many diagnostic tests have been applied to the evaluation of patients with low back disorders. There are eight common objectives for such testing (Table 18–1). First of all, tests may be used to rule out more serious problems contributing to back pain. These mostly include blood tests and images, as described above. A second goal is to determine whether there is injury to the nerves or nerve roots emanating from the spine. This type of testing has a long history, largely due to the possibility for surgical decompression of nerve roots or the spinal canal. A third goal is to try to identify the source of the back pain, that is, the pain-sensitive tissue. Most of these procedures have included diagnostic anesthetic blocks, under the theory that if the pain is blocked by a local anesthetic, the source of the pain has been determined. A fourth goal is to attempt to document the presence of back pain.

TABLE 18–1. Uses of Diagnostic Testing

1. Rule out more serious problems contributing to back pain.
2. Determine whether there is injury to the nerves and nerve roots.
3. Document the presence of back pain.
4. Identify spinal segmental abnormality.
5. Predict susceptibility to future or recurrent back pain.
6. Help design and monitor appropriate rehabilitation program.
7. Identify complicating factors.
8. Periodically monitor improvement or deterioration of a condition.

This goal is necessitated by the strong association between back pain and disability, leading to concerns about secondary gain in back pain.[1] The common involvement of psychosocial factors in back pain leads to frequent questions regarding the "organic" versus psychosocial nature of the pain. It also inspires a quest for "objective" measures of validation and quantification of pain. A fifth goal for diagnostic testing includes identification of spinal segmental abnormality. This motivation is particularly strong among practitioners who target therapies at local spinal disorders, such as practitioners of spinal manipulation. Some diagnostic procedures have been considered as methods to predict susceptibility for future or recurrent back pain. Other procedures have been proposed as a way to help design and monitor appropriate rehabilitation programs. Finally, some diagnostic tests have been devised to identify *intercurrent* problems, or complicating features, that may affect outcome. Some of these tests involve measurements of psychosocial factors potentially complicating the condition and will be addressed in Chapter 19. Others do fall into the realm of neurodiagnostic tests, such as the use of peripheral nerve conduction studies to detect peripheral nerve injury that may be mimicking radicular involvement.

It is clear that no single diagnostic procedure could hope to meet all eight of these diagnostic goals. Nonetheless, some neurodiagnostic procedures have been employed for more than a single purpose. It is important to consider these different objectives separately when discussing the value of particular diagnostic tests. A procedure that may be perfectly valid for one objective may be useless for others.

Diagnostic testing, in an attempt to validate the presence of back pain, is both the most interesting and the most controversial of topics. This mainly results from the frequency of medicolegal issues involving injury and disability. However, there is no current technology that is capable of taking such an image of pain. Therefore, all diagnostic approaches that attempt to document the presence of a painful condition involve the identification of various ramifications of the painful condition. Since most of those ramifications involve the nervous system, it is not surprising that many putative approaches are subsumed under the broad category of "neurodiagnostic approaches."

EVALUATION OF DIAGNOSTIC TESTS

From the above discussion, it should be apparent that in order to fully consider the diagnostic utility of a test, one must evaluate it in terms of the particular goal to which it is being applied. For example, needle electromyography may be considered to be a proven technique for the evaluation of radiculopathy, but this procedure is of no use in documenting whether a patient does or does not have pain. There are several steps involved in the evaluation and validation of diagnostic tests and it is critical to understand these steps if one is to appreciate the "state of the art" (Table 18–2).

TABLE 18–2. Variables That Need to be Known in the Validation of a Diagnostic Procedure

1. Comparison with gold standard*
2. Technical factors (independent of the condition to be examined) that affect the results of the test
3. Intraexaminer and interexaminer reliability
4. Stability over time in the absence of intervention or clinical change
5. Determination of sensitivity and specificity for the particular condition
6. Determination of positive and negative predictive values in the populations to which the test is being applied
7. Independence of some variables from voluntary control (if the test is being used as independent verification of the condition)

*If the gold standard is sufficiently established, this is the single most important step in validation of a diagnostic test.

A common method for evaluation of diagnostic procedures is by determination of the range of findings seen in "normal" individuals. This is a common method used for establishing normal values in blood testing. Anyone who is outside of 95% confidence levels is considered to be abnormal. It should be immediately apparent that there are significant problems applying this standard since it is critical to have a precise definition of "normal." This is particularly difficult when dealing with conditions such as LBP. Additionally, this method cannot provide any information about the significance of the abnormal findings, whether they are above or below these normal ranges.

The second common method of validation of a diagnostic test is by comparison of the test with a gold standard diagnostic test for the disorder. The principal limitation of this procedure is that it requires a well-documented gold standard for comparison. In the case of low back disorders, one might consider diagnostic imaging to be the gold standard for compressive radiculopathy. Therefore, a significant amount is known about the diagnostic utility of neurodiagnostic tests for this condition. However, there is no such gold standard test for "nonspecific" LBP much less for segmental abnormalities such as joint dysfunction, preventing such comparison. Clearly, this is a major limitation in the development of diagnostic tests for back pain.

When these methods of validating diagnostic procedures are not possible (as in most cases of back pain), the evaluation of a diagnostic test becomes much more difficult and requires a long series of steps. The first step requires determination of whether the diagnostic test observation is reliable. Can an examiner reproduce the finding on separate occasions (intraexaminer reliability)? Can others reproduce the same results (interexaminer reliability)? Are the findings stable over time in the absence of intervention or change in the condition?

The second step in this process involves comparing test performance of patients with the selected problem (back pain, in this case) with that of normal individuals. Sensitivity (the fraction of patients with the problem who test positive) and specificity (the fraction of individuals without the condition who test negative) of the test may be computed from these data. Of course, this requires the ability to define a population of individuals with and without the condition.

Once these values are known, several additional steps are required. The most important and often overlooked statistics in determining the clinical utility of a diagnostic test are the positive and negative predictive values. A positive predictive value computes how frequently a positive finding will actually indicate the presence of the clinical problem in the group of patients to which it is applied. For example, a test could have perfect sensitivity and only a 1% false-positive rate, but if this test is used to screen 1000 individuals, only 1 of who has the condition, the test will label 10 normal individuals as having the "abnormality" for every real abnormality that it identifies. The negative predictive value is also important and indicates how frequently a negative value truly indicates the absence of the clinical problem. In practice, it is often difficult to determine these values because additional data must be known regarding the frequency of the problem in the population to whom the test is being applied.

Once this information is known about a test, there is a final step in its validation that is often overlooked. This step is critical whenever the variable that is being measured is under voluntary control and particularly if the patient may have some motivation to be abnormal on the test. This is of particular concern in the case of back pain where tests may be needed to confirm the presence of a subjective complaint or to address the issue of secondary gain. Therefore, if the variable is under voluntary control, it must be demonstrated that there are detectible differences between individuals with the condition and those who attempt to mimic the condition.

With all of the steps involved in the validation of clinical tests, it is no wonder that there are few fully validated diagnostic tests for any back condition and none for "nonspecific" or "mechanical" back pain. This chapter will attempt to identify the strengths and weaknesses in the literature of the most commonly utilized neurodiagnostic procedures, as well as promising approaches and current gaps in the literature.

Before going on to discuss the various neurodiagnostic tests that have been applied to the low back, it is important to consider the meaning of the test. For example, does deconditioning or limited range of motion affect the test independent of the low back disorder? If so, this may greatly affect the interpretation of the test. This may also affect the positive and negative predictive values, since the appropriate comparison population would have similar states of conditioning and mobility.

The neurodiagnostic tests that have been proposed for back pain fall into several categories. Electromyography has generated the greatest number of articles by far, as well as the greatest number of different approaches. Somatosensory evoked potentials (SSEPs) have been used in several ways for the assessment of patients with back pain. Thermography, which examines certain aspects of neural control, represents a third basic approach. There have been some attempts at development of more objective and quantitative sensory tests as well. We will discuss each of these, in turn.

ELECTRODIAGNOSIS

Electromyography

Electromyography (EMG) refers to the electrical detection of signals arising from the depolarization of skeletal muscle. These signals may be detected from skin surface electrodes or from needles placed directly within the muscle. Typically, these two types of recordings are used for different purposes, with needle recording used to detect the behavior of individual muscle fibers and motor units, while surface recordings are used to detect overall muscle activity in particular positions or actions. For example, surface electrodes may record EMG activity at rest or in specific static postures or may evaluate the activity of muscles in particular motions or during fatiguing contractions. The surface EMG signal may be mathematically investigated. The most common forms of evaluation include integration or "root mean square" computation. These assess the overall amount of electrical signal. Other methods of signal processing include computing the frequency of waveforms, the power spectrum of the signal or "wavelets" within the signal. Furthermore, all of these methods can be applied while at rest or fatigued, in a static upright posture or during movement.

The high level of interest in EMG in the evaluation of back syndromes derives from clinical observation of alteration in paraspinal muscle tension in many such patients and theoretical constructs of back syndromes that incorporate abnormalities in the function or activity of these muscles. Given all of the possible EMG approaches to investigating back pain and the high clinical interest, it is no wonder that there are more studies of EMG than of any other neurodiagnostic approach to the evaluation of back pain and radicular syndromes.

Needle EMG Needle EMG is designed to investigate the amplitude and morphology of the electrical signal within skeletal muscle. There are specific findings that develop with recent denervation of muscles. In this situation, individual denervated muscle fibers become highly sensitive to mechanical stimuli as well as to chemical stimuli in the microenvironment surrounding the muscle fiber.

Clinical Pearl: There are changes in denervated muscle that can be detected by needle EMG.

A normal muscle is electrically silent when recording from a needle electrode. Movement of the needle normally elicits a brief burst of depolarization from muscle fibers (called *insertional activity*). This burst of activity ends immediately upon termination of the movement. At that point, electrical silence is restored. The only place within the muscle that is not electrically silent is the motor end plate. There are two types of electrical activity that can be seen in this region at rest, miniature end plate potentials and end plate spikes. These can be distinguished from abnormal resting discharges, but they require care in identification. This provides a particular challenge for beginning electromyographers, since end plate spikes can be misinterpreted as evidence of denervation or of increased insertional activity and membrane instability. This is the reason that it is recommended that electromyographers take care to avoid the end plate region if at all possible. This also contributes to difficulty in the needle evaluation of the paraspinal muscles where end plates can be found scattered throughout the muscles. The usual electromyographic test will examine more than 10 spots within the muscle before making a determination as to the normality of insertional and resting activities.

After resting electromyographic activity and insertional activity are assessed, the patient is asked to voluntarily contract the muscle. Contraction takes place by activating motor neurons to the muscle, each of which is connected to many muscle fibers scattered throughout the muscle (termed a *motor unit*). The electrical signal that is recorded as a "motor unit potential" (MUP) comes from the integration of the electrical signals arising from the discharge of the several muscle fibers within recording distance of the tip of the needle (typically 1–3 mm) that are attached to the same motor neuron (Fig. 18–1*A*). The amplitude of the MUP is dependent on the density of the muscle fibers attached to

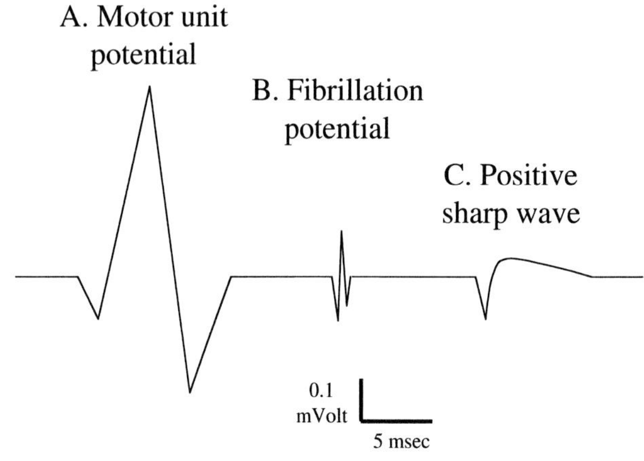

FIGURE 18–1. Morphology of normal motor unit potentials (*A*), fibrillation potentials (*B*), and positive sharp waves (*C*). The latter two are common findings in recent (1 week to 1 year) of denervation. Please note the calibration bar at the bottom, indicating the typical amplitude and duration of the potentials.

that one motor neuron, and is remarkably uniform for most clinically tested muscles, being between 0.3 and 3.0 mV. Additionally, MUPs usually have only one or two upward peaks. As the strength of contraction is slowly increased, motor units are recruited in a very orderly sequence. Each active motor unit increases its firing frequency to a defined level (usually around 10 discharges per second), at which point an additional motor unit is recruited. This process is quite orderly and can be quantified (recruitment pattern). Delayed recruitment (i.e., excessive firing rate of individual units prior to the recruitment of an additional unit) is a reflection of loss of motor units within the muscle. The final step in the EMG assessment of a muscle (a step which may not be necessary if everything else has been normal) involves maximal contraction. During such contraction, the electrical activity should fully obscure the baseline (termed a full interference pattern). Incomplete interference pattern is considered to be a reflection of loss of motor units in a muscle, though it can also be seen with diminished effort.

Needle EMG evaluates the integrity of the motor unit, that is, the motor neuron, motor axon, and the muscle to which it is attached. There are a series of changes that can be quantified after damage to the axon. It is noteworthy that these changes are triggered by actual disruption of the motor axon and develop in an orderly sequence that can help determine the timing of the injury. It is also noteworthy that these changes are not seen with damage to sensory axons, nor do they occur following damage to the myelin of the motor axon (assuming that the axon, itself, is undamaged). This is interesting because damage to myelin can result in complete block of motor conduction and even produce complete paralysis of the muscle without any of the changes that are associated with denervation. Additionally, damage to the central nervous system above the level of the motor neuron (such as by cervical spinal cord trauma or stroke) can result in complete paralysis without any abnormality on needle EMG except incomplete (or absent) interference pattern.

Following denervation, a series of events take place in the individual denervated muscle fibers that can be detected as abnormal electrical signals. First of all, over the period of a week or two, the denervated muscle fiber becomes progressively more mechanically irritable. Therefore, electrical discharges provoked by movement of the needle can outlast the actual movement by more than a second. This is termed *increased insertional activity.* Although this is not particularly specific, it does indicate that the muscle is excessively irritable. Muscle fibers also become chemically sensitive to their microenvironment and their membranes can also become unstable enough to produce spontaneous activity. This can be recorded as depolarization of individual muscle fibers. The spontaneous depolarizations of the individual fibers appear as fibrillation potentials (Fig. 18–1*B*) and positive sharp waves (Fig. 18–1*C*). These do not occur in normal muscles since the normal muscle fibers are only responsive to the activation of their motor unit. Typically, it takes more than a week for such potentials to develop, and they will disappear with complete degeneration of the denervated muscle fiber in 6 months to 1 year as the denervated muscle fiber completely degenerates. Needle EMG is very sensitive for the detection of these signals and they most often reflect denervation, although they may also occur in severe muscle disease or injury. An example of this can be seen in the area of a surgical scar, where fibrillations and positive sharp waves may simply be a reflection of the damage to muscles and the scarring process in muscles. Abnormal EMG findings in the area of prior surgical treatment (such as the back) must always be evaluated with some caution. Outside of the above caveats, the finding of fibrillations and positive sharp waves is the most reliable and objective test that there is for damage to motor axons to the muscle between 1 week and 6–12 months ago (or ongoing damage). Unfortunately, the finding of fibrillation and positive sharp waves is often termed *acute denervation*, although acute in this case refers to weeks and months.

Clinical Pearl: Needle electromyographic studies of paraspinal muscles are unreliable in a region of prior lumbar spine surgery.

Reinnervation of muscle is an ongoing process, occurring whenever a muscle is partially denervated. This process typically involves the development of sprouts from adjacent, unaffected motor nerve fibers that ultimately contact at least some of the denervated muscle fibers especially right in the area of other normally innervated muscle fibers. This process results in the development of clusters or clumps of reinnervated muscle fibers attached to individual motor neurons (remember that the normal motor unit has individual muscle fibers scattered throughout the muscle). Typically these motor units become significantly larger both in amplitude and in duration, since the needle is likely to be recording from more muscle fibers in this clump. Also, the MUPs often become more irregular (termed *polyphasic*) (Fig. 18–2). This process takes months and indicates the presence of chronic denervation. It should be noted that the needle study is much less sensitive to the process of reinnervation than it is to the findings of fibrillations and positive sharp waves seen with recent denervation.

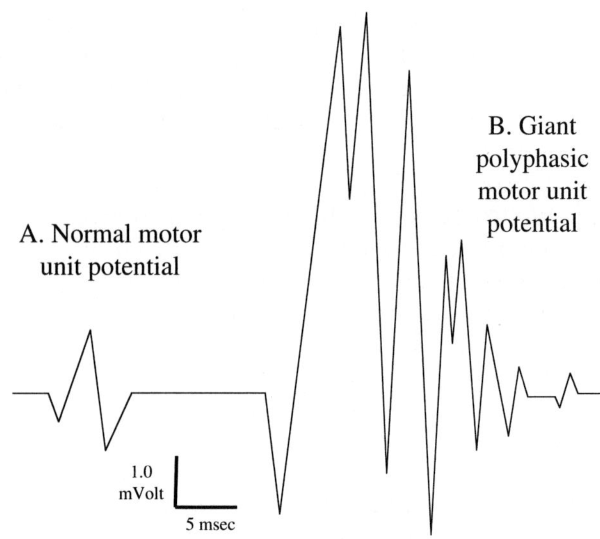

FIGURE 18–2. Morphology of giant, polyphasic motor unit potentials, often seen in denervating conditions of greater than a few months duration. Please note that the calibration bar is different in scale to that in Figure 18–1.

Clinical Pearl: There are changes in electrical signal seen in denervated muscle starting within the first 2 weeks, which can be present for 6–12 months (acute denervation). Other changes are seen beginning within several months and increasing with time (chronic denervation).

The typical needle EMG examination involves sampling a number of muscles. Its ability to localize a lesion depends on sampling muscles innervated by the same nerve but different nerve roots, muscles innervated by the same nerve root but different nerves, and muscles innervated at different locations along the course of the nerves. Paraspinal muscles can be very useful in this regard because nerve root damage will tend to produce abnormalities in these muscles as well as the muscles in the limbs (helping to distinguish a radiculopathy from a plexopathy or peripheral neuropathy, for example). However, needle studies in the paraspinal muscles can be difficult to interpret because of the frequency of prior surgery in the area, the overlap in innervation of the various nerve root levels (preventing precise localization), the distribution of motor end plates throughout the muscles, and the small amplitude of the motor unit potentials (making them closer in amplitude to fibrillation and positive sharp waves). Furthermore, it is very difficult to assess recruitment with voluntary contraction in these muscles because of the difficulty in activating them in a controlled manner. Considering all of these issues, it is clear that although paraspinal needle studies may be critical to the assessment of the level of involvement (i.e., nerve root or more peripheral), the results must be interpreted with care and hence requires interpretation by a skilled electrodiagnostician. Additionally, in the absence of denervation in more peripheral muscles the findings must be interpreted with caution.

Clinical Pearl: Denervation of paraspinal muscles is common in radiculopathy but should not be found in plexopathy or peripheral neuropathy.

The validation of needle EMG procedures for radiculopathy has largely been through comparison with gold standards for radiculopathy, such as imaging and/or surgical findings. There are definite limitations to the needle study in the investigation of patients with back and limb pain. First of all, EMG has never been shown to be helpful for evaluating any condition other than radiculopathy or damage to the dorsal primary ramus of the nerve. Furthermore, there must be actual axonal damage to motor nerve fibers in order to produce the findings of acute or chronic denervation. Therefore, it is no wonder that the needle electromyographic study is not abnormal in all patients with radiculopathy. The sensitivity for identification of radiculopathy ranges between about 70% and 90%.[3–5]

Clinical Pearl: Needle EMG is the most validated electrodiagnostic test for radiculopathy. However, it is only 70%–90% sensitive.

The issue of the specificity of needle EMG has been rather controversial. One recent study of 75 asymptomatic subjects without evidence of radiculopathy reported that there were no denervation potentials seen in any of the subjects.[6] Of course, this would suggest 100% specificity. However, this study was not done in a blinded fashion. There have been two very rigorous studies of the electromyographic activity in normal subjects that have reached somewhat different conclusions. Both of these studies showed that asymptomatic individuals could have signs of denervation, including fibrillation potentials and positive sharp waves in the paraspinal muscles. Haig and colleagues[7,8] performed a very systematic study in which 35 normal subjects each had EMG evaluation of 57 defined spots in the lumbar spine. These were intermixed with a series of patients with suspected radiculopathy. Electromyographers blinded to the patients' clinical status performed the evaluations. These investigators report that there is significantly more evidence of denervation in patients with radiculopathy than without. On the other hand, about half of their "normals" showed at least one site in the lumbar paraspinal muscles to have evidence of denervation. The fact that most of these sites clustered around the lowest part of the lumbar spine lead them to conclude that the small amount of denervation seen in these "normals" was probably due to clinically unrecognized nerve injury in this mechanically vulnerable area. Around the same time, a study published by Date and colleagues[9] reported that 14.5% of 65 asymptomatic subjects showed at least some spontaneous activity (i.e., fibrillations or positive sharp waves). They were not as systematic in their recordings, but they did make the interesting observation that the frequency of abnormality increases with the age of their "normal" subjects. They urged caution in the interpretation of the paraspinal EMG findings in middle-aged or older patients. Of course, since the prevalence of back disorders increases with age, an additional interpretation of their findings is that these older, asymptomatic individuals may have some minor and clinically unrecognized nerve injury. Nonetheless, minor abnormalities on the paraspinal needle study cannot be interpreted as unequivocal proof of radiculopathy, particularly in the absence of confirmatory clinical observations or other evidence such as confirmatory EMG findings in appropriate muscles of the limb (see below). The greater the abnormality (i.e., the number of locations that are abnormal as well as the number and persistence of the abnormal potentials) and the younger the patient, the more likely it is that abnormalities in paraspinal muscles represent actual nerve root damage. Therefore, paraspinal needle EMG findings require careful interpretation and correlation with the remainder of the exam (clinical, radiographic, and electrodiagnostic) and should not be considered in isolation. This is especially true given the technical problems that are known to complicate the test.

Clinical Pearl: As many as 14.5% of normal subjects might have signs of acute denervation in paraspinal muscles. Therefore, findings in the paraspinal

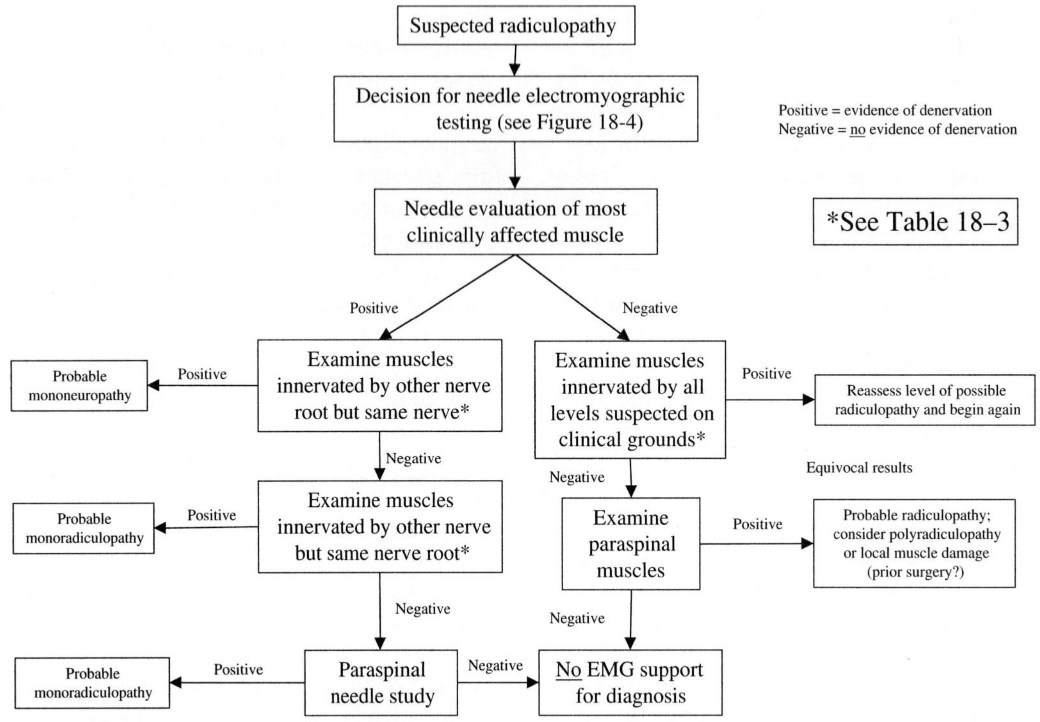

FIGURE 18–3. Algorithm for needle EMG of suspected radiculopathy.

muscles should be interpreted in context of the remainder of the electrodiagnostic examination as well as the clinical picture.

The paraspinal muscles, even the multifidi (which are the most segmental of the tested muscles), have an overlapping innervation. This makes it difficult to diagnose a particular level of nerve root injury based solely on the paraspinal findings. Most of the specificity of needle EMG for discriminating the level of the radiculopathy is afforded by examination of muscles of the lower limb (Fig. 18-3). Of course, this requires the electromyographer to have detailed knowledge of the innervation of these muscles (Table 18–3). The investigation of radiculopathy requires determination of the degree of denervation seen in the muscles and then the determination of the common shared nerve roots for the muscles shown to be abnormal. In the formulation of the list of muscles to be examined there are several considerations. Muscles supplied by the same nerve but different nerve roots should be examined, since a finding of abnormality in both of these muscles would suggest that the problem is more likely to be in the nerve rather than in the nerve root. Similarly, it is helpful to examine muscles supplied by the same nerve root but by different nerves since abnormalities in this muscle pair would direct attention to radiculopathy. A common example of this is the use of the tibialis anterior and tibialis posterior to help define L5 radiculopathy. Since both of these muscles are extensively innervated by L5, but since a different peripheral nerve supplies them, findings can help distinguish peroneal nerve injury from L5 radiculopathy (a common clinical conundrum). It is also useful to examine muscles that receive innervation at different levels along the same nerve because if the muscle that is innervated higher in the leg is normal while the lower one is abnormal, this would suggest a focal peripheral neuropathy between the levels of innervation of the two muscles. An example of this would be the tibialis anterior and the short head of the biceps femoris, which are both innervated by the peroneal nerve but one above the knee and the other below. Damage to the peroneal nerve at the level of the knee would affect the tibialis anterior but not this part of the biceps, for example. The presence of focal neuropathies may be confirmed with nerve conduction studies (see below).

Clinical Pearl: The needle electromyographic examination requires the testing of several muscles in order to determine a level of damage. Muscles supplied by the same nerve root but different peripheral nerves, and muscles supplied by different nerve roots but the same nerve should be tested.

Surface EMG Surface recordings of the electromyographic signal are of no use in the diagnosis of nerve root damage. However, there is an extensive literature on the electromyographic evaluation of LBP patients

TABLE 18-3. **Common Muscles Utilized in the Examination of Possible Lumbar Radiculopathy**

Muscle	Peripheral Nerve	Nerve Root (Minor)
Iliopsoas	Lumbar plexus	L2-3
Adductor longus	Obturator	(L2) L3-4
Quadriceps	Femoral	(L2) L3-4
Gluteus medius	Superior gluteal	L5 (S1)
Gluteus maximus	Inferior gluteal	L5-S1 (S2)
Semime mbranosus	Tibial part of sciatic	L5 (S1)
Biceps femoris short head	Peroneal part of sciatic	(L5) S1
Tibialis anterior	Deep peroneal	L4-L5
Extensor hallucic longus	Deep peroneal	L5 (S1)
Extensor digitorum brevis	Deep peroneal	L5 (S1)
Peroneus longus and brevis	Peroneal	L5 (S1)
Tibialis posterior	Tibial	L5 (S1)
Flexor digitorum longus	Tibial	L5-S1
Lateral gastrocnemius	Tibial	(L5) S1 (S2)
Medial gastrocnemius	Tibial	S1-2
Soleus	Tibial	S1-2
Abductor digiti minimi	Lateral plantar	S1-2
Abductor hallucis	Medial plantar	S1-2

Muscles in bold type are the more commonly used. Nerve root segments in parentheses represent minor contributions.

without radicular symptoms. This interest has largely resulted from clinical observation of alteration in paraspinal muscle tension in many patients with back pain and from theoretical constructs of back pain that predict abnormality in the function or activity of these muscles. The two most common models of muscular involvement in LBP are the "muscle spasm" model, which would predict excessive amounts of muscular activity, and the "muscle insufficiency model," which would predict decreased activity (or perhaps high levels of fatigue). To a large extent these two models are mutually exclusive and it is unclear whether there may be subpopulations of LBP patients fitting into each model. It is possible that some of the variability in outcomes between and within studies of surface EMG may arise from the enrollment of subjects with fundamentally different response properties of back muscles. Given the interest in the behavior of muscle tissue in back pain patients and the variability of responses, it is perhaps no surprise that there are more studies of surface EMG than of any other neurodiagnostic approach to the evaluation of back pain.

Clinical Pearl: Surface EMG cannot detect the changes of denervation in muscle.

It is relatively easy to record electrical signals from muscle in the lumbar paraspinal region through electrodes applied to the skin surface. There are several technical hurdles to be overcome in standardizing the recording and in determining the most appropriate methods for evaluation of the resultant signals. Additionally, it is difficult to determine what muscles are being recorded from, and even whether signals are being detected from the muscles that are most important. For example, various movements that have been shown to activate deep paraspinal muscles may not be detected on surface recording. Additionally, it is difficult to determine the degree of contribution of remote muscles to the signal that is being detected. All of these factors lead to serious theoretical concerns that must be addressed when considering the utility of surface EMG to evaluate segmental dysfunction.

It should be noted that surface EMG is a commonly utilized tool in research. While it is routinely used in measuring biomechanical and kinesiological activity in that setting, discussion regarding neuroelectrical testing in research exceeds the parameters of this clinical chapter. However, surface EMG presents an excellent example of how a tool may be broadly utilized in one field (research, for example) without being accepted in another seemingly similar venue (clinical utilization, for example).

With these factors in mind, the major proposed uses of surface EMG will be considered. These include static EMG recordings, dynamic EMG recordings, ambulatory EMG, spectral pattern analysis, and wavelet analysis.

Static Surface EMG The earliest method of surface EMG evaluation of back muscles examined signals in static positions. These studies are considered under the heading of "static EMG" (sEMG) despite the fact that these procedures really incorporate two distinct entities. The first procedure is of EMG recording while the back muscles are "at rest" (such as lying prone) and the other is performed in posturally active, static positions (such as sitting or standing). Of course, it could be argued that even quiet standing is a dynamic situation, but that designation will instead be reserved for those procedures that are designed for specific activation of paraspinal muscles.

There have been three main motives behind the attempts in correlating surface EMG and back pain. First of all, there is the strong motivation to develop objective findings to correlate with back pain. This goal requires a high level of proof, as well as the additional step of determining the degree to which the finding can be mimicked by voluntary activity. After all, these

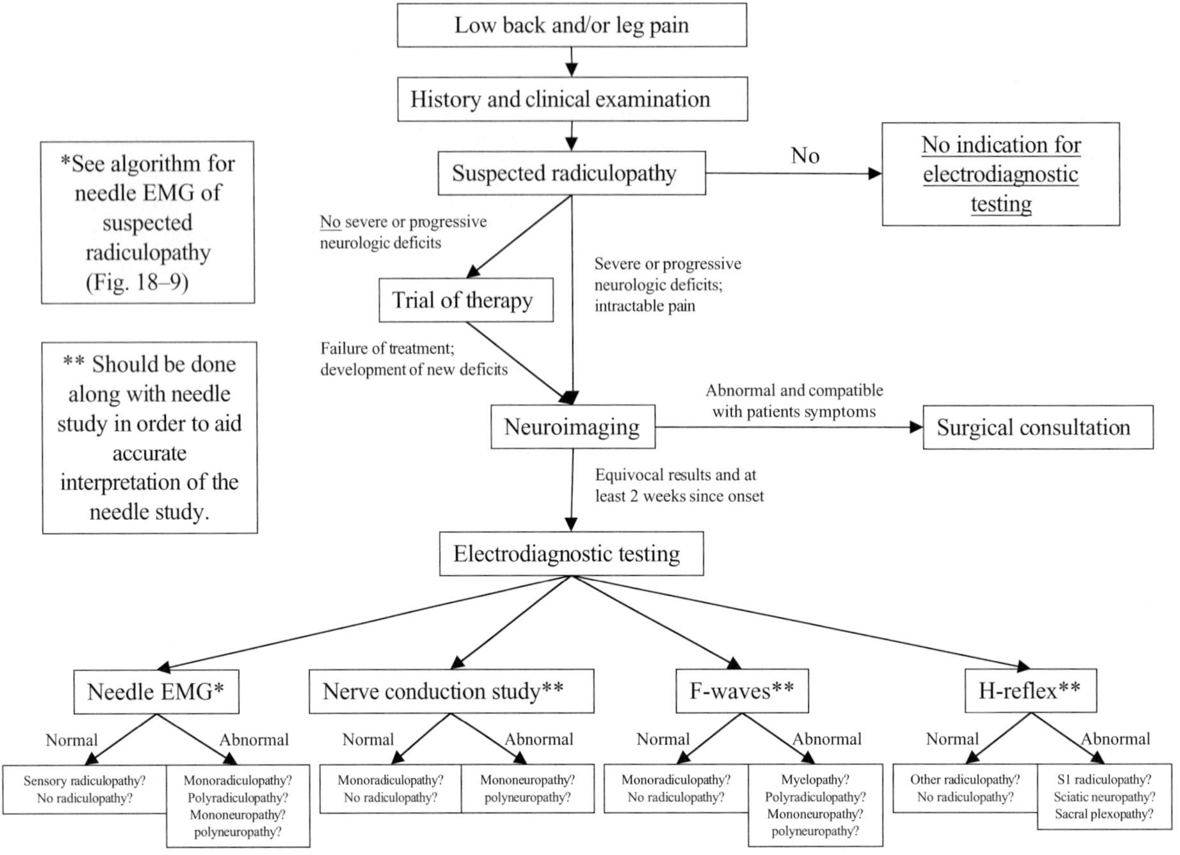

FIGURE 18–4. Algorithm for electrodiagnostic evaluation of patients with low back syndrome.

tests are likely to be applied to individuals who have potential motivations to voluntarily influence the outcome. Unfortunately, most of these procedures have not been subjected to such scrutiny. Secondly, therapeutic approaches might be designed to alter this variable, thereby improving back pain. Finally, sEMG has been proposed as a method of identifying sites of lesions requiring treatment.

The majority of interest in static surface EMG recordings has focused on the first goal, which is the potential to objectively validate the LBP complaint. This has been quite controversial and studies have produced varied results. For example, there are literature reports saying that patients with back pain have significantly increased sEMG signal.[10,11] However, there are other reports that lumbar sEMG is not different[12–14] or diminished [15,16] in patients with LBP when compared with normal individuals or with the same LBP patients at times of diminished pain. While it is likely that some of this difference is technical or due to patient selection, the disparate findings are truly difficult to reconcile and have led to skepticism relative to the value of the procedure. For example, the Therapeutics and Technology Assessment Subcommittee of the American Academy of Neurology did an assessment of the clinical utility of surface EMG in 2000.[17] They concluded that sEMG is unacceptable as a diagnostic tool for the evaluation of LBP. Other reviewers have reached the same conclusion.[18]

Cram and colleagues are the leading proponents of the use of scanning, static sEMG in the evaluation of back pain. They have reported that sEMG signals could be acceptably reproduced over three trials, each separated by an hour, with surface contact electrodes in both sitting and standing postures.[19] They found that upper back EMG signals correlate directly with the level of pain and that lower back EMG signals are inversely correlated with pain (more pain, lower signal) in patients with between 2 and 6 months of pain.[16] However, in light of difficulty reconciling the large number of studies done on the topic, significantly more work will be needed to overcome the general skepticism about the value of this application of surface EMG.

There have been reports of the use of static, postural EMG for identification of segmental spinal lesions.[20] This research, which the authors suggest may correlate with underlying manipulatable lesions, is hampered by the lack of a gold standard for the identification of such lesions as well as by the theoretical concerns of spatial specificity of the surface recordings, since the electrical signal can be detected many centimeters from the site of generation of the signal. These authors report that left–right asymmetry in EMG signal in static postures correlated with the presence of back pain and confirmed the observations of others relative to problems with normal "flexion-relaxation" in patients with LBP (see below). However, in the absence of a gold standard for comparison, many factors remain to be determined before this procedure can be accepted. These steps include determination of specificity and sensitivity; the stability of the finding without intervention; the predictive value of the finding; the level of voluntary control; and, given the technical limitations of surface recording from deep muscles, the spatial distribution of the surface electromyographic signals from these muscle groups. The fact that other investigators have not found consistent and reliable sEMG correlates of back pain means that extensive clinical studies are still necessary in order to validate any clinically useful measures for static paraspinal EMG procedures.

Dynamic Surface EMG Because of the inconsistent results of studies correlating sEMG with lower back pain, investigators began a search for other correlates of back muscle pain and "spasm." This subsequently spawned the investigation of muscular response to dynamic positions as a predictor of pain. Studies have suggested that averaged EMG has at least an acceptable level of reproducibility, and that this reproducibility is better at higher load levels,[21] suggesting that dynamic EMG may be better than static EMG.

The most consistent and common finding is that patients with LBP frequently do not show the normal relaxation of paraspinal muscles during the latter phases of trunk flexion (so-called *flexion-relaxation*). Several investigators have shown this to be a reasonably consistent finding [12,22–25] and that the degree of this loss correlates with the amount of LBP and/or disability.[26] However, there are several potential explanations for this observation. It is certainly possible that pain results in a "withdrawal-type" reflex reaction in back muscles, preventing full flexion. Such reflexes in paraspinal muscles to deep, painful stimuli have been demonstrated in animal models.[27] In this regard, the lack of reflex relaxation would be considered to be a type of involuntary "guarding" and, as such, could represent an independent measure and potentially valuable confirmation of the presence of back pain. However, it is equally possible that patients were simply prevented from reaching a position of rest at the end of the range of motion or that they voluntarily limited their motion. In this case, the finding of lack of flexion-relaxation could simply represent a behavioral epiphenomenon of back pain. Ahern and colleagues [13] emphasized this point, identifying several abnormalities on dynamic EMG testing between normals and LBP patients. These abnormalities included the lack of flexion-relaxation as well as abnormal responses during rotation. They emphasized the need for further investigation in order to determine the precise causes of the findings.

A study by Watson and colleagues[28] did not find any correlation between flexion-relaxation and the level of back pain, but rather found a correlation with fear of movement. On this basis, they suggested that flexion-relaxation might be heavily influenced by conscious or unconscious psychological factors rather then being a purely physiological measure. However, this was a small study and further work is clearly necessary before accepting this view.

Some studies have evaluated tasks other than flexion. Soderberg and Barr[29] found no difference during lifting tasks between patients with chronic back pain and normal patients during motion. However, they did find that paraspinal muscle contraction was maintained for a longer time after the task in the LBP patients. Triano and Luttges[30] reported that 80% of subjects with a recent history of LBP had asymmetrical EMG signals during nonpainful postural tasks, a finding rarely seen in their control subjects. Other researchers have also documented this asymmetrical neuromuscular function in similar cases.[31]

Ahern et al.[13] reported that there was increased paraspinal EMG signal between controls and LBP patients during several movements. However, Nouwen and colleagues[22] reported more divergent results than Ahern et al., finding that flexion was the only movement during which normal and LBP patients differed, with the normal patients demonstrating flexion-relaxation.

Comparing EMG signal and trunk muscle strength has been proposed as a method of evaluating LBP patients. However, van Dieen and Heijblom[32] reported that the high degree of variability in these measures limits clinical utility. Robinson et al.[33] adopted a somewhat different approach and looked at changes in EMG signal with fatiguing exercise, finding that there were differences in patterns of fatigue between chronic LBP patients and controls. They proposed that the specific pattern might be useful in identifying patients with insincere efforts rather than patients with true LBP. However, most of the work on fatigue patterns of muscles in LBP patients has been done with spectral analysis (see below), requiring somewhat more sophisticated signal analysis equipment.

Two groups of investigators[34,35] have independently reported abnormal patterns of activation of synergistic muscles such as the multifidi and oblique muscles during trunk rotation in LBP patients. However, their data do not show this to be a consistent enough finding to be of clinical diagnostic utility.

Interestingly, these abnormal patterns were not found to improve following intensive rehabilitation.[35] However, it must be noted that other investigators have reported that intensive rehabilitation can improve complementary trunk rotator muscle patterns of abnormal EMG signal[36,37] suggesting potential differences in the rehabilitation program on the part of these groups.

Another approach to the dynamic evaluation of the function of trunk muscles in LBP has examined the response reaction time of muscles to sudden shifts in position (e.g., by jerky movement of a seat). It has been reported that the muscle response is significantly delayed in LBP patients compared to controls[38] and that the LBP patients also demonstrated greater variability in muscular response times. On the basis of these findings, it is not clear whether this delay in reaction is a result of pain or is itself a contributory cause of the development of the symptom constellation, which is an intriguing possibility.

The reliability of the surface recording procedures and the appropriateness of various EMG measures has been questioned. Koumantakis et al.[39] examined fatiguing contractions of the lumbar paraspinal muscles from LBP patients and controls. They reported that the integrated signals (which are a common mathematical method of quantifying the surface EMG) were not particularly reliable, while the frequency spectral analyses were significantly better in terms of reliability. These kinds of observation lead to a large number of studies using the frequency spectra of the EMG under dynamic and often fatiguing conditions (see below).

At the present time, it would appear that loss of flexion-relaxation is a common finding in patients with LBP. However, this can be significantly affected by behavioral factors, potentially limiting its utility as a completely objective evaluative tool. Additionally, although most studies have seen at least some correlation of this phenomenon with the severity of back pain, this has not been a universal observation, hampering its use as a quantitative tool. Therefore, it would appear that significantly more investigation would be needed before accepting dynamic surface EMG as part of a routine investigation of patients with back pain.

Clinical Pearl: Absence of normal flexion-relaxation is the most studied sEMG finding in patients with "nonspecific" LBP.

Ambulatory EMG Ambulatory EMG monitoring has been attempted in patients with LBP.[40,41] While the limited amount of data ensure that the results of these studies is extremely preliminary, patients with LBP appear to have higher levels of integrated EMG signal than do normal subjects. However, given the difficulties in drawing clear conclusions about the integrated EMG signal in LBP patients under rigorously controlled situations (see the prior section), it is not surprising that few investigators have expended the effort to report data in the uncontrolled ambulatory setting. It would appear that ambulatory EMG monitoring is at a very early investigational stage at this time.

Spectral Analysis Spectral analysis is a tool that quantifies the specific frequencies of surface EMG waveforms. These waveforms, in turn, reflect the character of the muscle fiber types making up the muscle and that are active under any particular set of circumstances.[42] Spectral analysis is typically done under a degree of sustained and usually fatiguing contraction, making it a variant of the dynamic studies described above.[43,44] During such fatiguing contractions, the EMG signal undergoes a frequency compression that can be recorded and plotted in healthy individuals and in patients with various disorders of the spine. Spectral analysis is attractive since it is a measure outside of voluntary control and can be examined in an objective manner.

There does appear to be a fairly broad range of normal[45] and significant variability over time in normal individuals.[46] This would limit sensitivity of the test in detecting patients with subtle abnormalities and may also limit the utility of the procedure in evaluating therapeutic outcome. Nonetheless, many studies have shown differences between LBP patients and normals.

For example, Greenough and colleagues[47] report that spectral analysis of the lumbar spine muscles discriminates LBP patients from normals with a sensitivity of 76% and a specificity of 81%. Klein et al.[48] reported that spectral analysis of signals during maximal voluntary contraction of extensor muscles was able to correctly categorize rowers with and without back pain with 66% sensitivity and 71% specificity, although these values could even be improved upon if the measures were retaken during a short recovery period following the contraction. De Luca reported that spectral analysis testing during fatiguing contraction distinguishes 84% of patients with LBP from normals,[49] results that have basically been confirmed by others.[50–53]

Although the results from these reports are promising, several issues remain before applying spectral analysis to the clinical evaluation of patients. First of all, studies to date have employed a limited number of subjects leading to concern about the generalizability of the findings. Additionally, deconditioning (which is common in patients with back pain) can be a confounding variable. Although there are some data to suggest that patients with LBP can be distinguished from simple deconditioning of back muscles, it is clear that deconditioning must be considered in examination protocols, especially when they involve fatiguing contractions. Furthermore, it is possible that the altered spectral pattern may be a reflection of patients at risk for LBP rather than a result of the painful condition, again, having implications on the interpretation of findings.

It is not known whether rehabilitation protocols can normalize the EMG spectral pattern in patients with LBP. This is an important consideration if the test is to be used in monitoring progress or results of treatment. Spectral analysis has generally been applied with controlled, relatively simple contraction of back extensor muscles, since it is substantially more difficult to control sustained contractions during more complicated, coupled movements, such as rotation. Finally, the utility of this procedure in screening asymptomatic individuals (such as in industrial population) to determine risk of LBP is not known.

Given the increase in recent literature regarding this procedure, one would expect that the answer to some of these questions will soon become available. This is likely to increase interest in the potential clinical and research applications of EMG signal analysis. The main limiting factor is likely to be the range of normal along with the effects of deconditioning that may affect the sensitivity for detecting clinically relevant changes.

Clinical Pearl: Signal-processing technology holds some promise for the identification of clinically meaningful phenomena in LBP patients.

Wavelet Analysis Spectral analysis of EMG signal is useful for evaluating the EMG signal during static positions. Quite recently, two groups of investigators have been engaged in examining the potential for using wavelet analysis of electromyographic signals following transient trunk movements.[54–56] This has the advantage of being able to evaluate patients during motion and also shows changes with fatigue that are different in patients with and without back pain. The application of wavelet analysis to the evaluation of LBP and rehabilitation is much earlier in development than either standard dynamic EMG or spectral analysis, and will require substantially more validation.

Summary of Surface EMG in Back Pain Despite great interest in surface EMG in the evaluation of LBP, there are many technical and theoretical barriers that must be overcome before these procedures will be of accepted clinical use. The Therapeutic and Technology Assessment Subcommittee of the American Academy of Neurology investigated the utility of surface EMG in 2000.[17] On the basis of the available literature at the time, they discounted the value of surface EMG in being able to identify individuals with back pain or of being able to predict risk of future back pain. Significant advances have been made even over the brief interval since then, particularly in terms of the use of advanced methods of signal processing. However, the application of surface EMG procedures to clinical practice, in this author's opinion, remains to be realized. As such, surface EMG must at this time be considered "investigational" and that its value is likely to depend on advanced signal-processing technology, probably under controlled load conditions. It is expected that several categories of responses will be identified, some of which will likely correlate with risk for development of LBP, while others are more likely to reflect current problems. The procedure holds promise for identifying patients who will benefit from particular forms of rehabilitative protocols and may, at some point, be a useful adjunctive tool for stratifying treatments and monitoring progress.

Clinical Pearl: Surface EMG is a common research tool but it has not been validated as a method for objective verification of underlying spinal pathology.

Nerve Conduction Velocity Studies

Nerve conduction velocity (NCV) studies are frequently performed as part of the electrodiagnostic consultation in patients with radiculopathy. However, these studies should be normal if radiculopathy is the only problem affecting the patient. Nerve conduction studies can test sensory or motor nerve fibers and can determine both the speed of conduction as well as the amplitude of the electrical signal evoked following stimulation of a nerve.

Clinical Pearl: Nerve conduction studies in the limb should be normal in cases of uncomplicated radiculopathy. These are useful for distinguishing coexistent problems that may be complicating diagnosis.

Motor Conduction Studies Motor conduction studies are performed by stimulating a motor nerve while recording the response from one or more of its target muscles (Fig. 18–5). It is important to note that the electrical signal that is being recorded following motor nerve stimulation (called the compound muscle action potential [CMAP]) is actually generated by the muscle, and therefore is quite large. When motor nerve fibers are stimulated close to the muscle, the amount of time before the muscle starts depolarizing is called the *terminal latency*. (The term "LATENCY" refers to the duration of the interval between the stimulus and the responses). This value includes both the amount of time that it takes the nerve to conduct from the point of stimulation to the motor end plates in the muscle

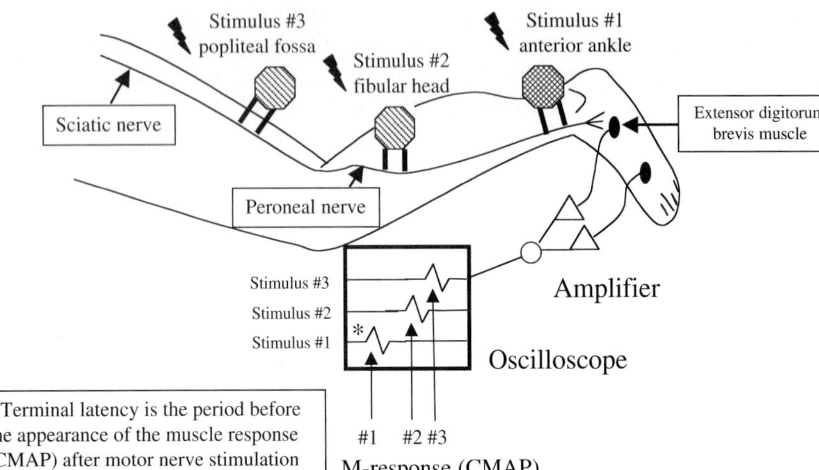

FIGURE 18–5. Method of motor nerve conduction studies. Surface recordings are made between a pair of electrodes applied over a muscle innervated by the stimulated nerve (in this case the extensor digitorum brevis muscle with stimulation of the deep peroneal nerve). Stimulus #1 at the ankle produces a compound muscle action potential with terminal latency seen in the lowest tracing (shown by the*). Stimulation at progressively higher levels of the nerve produces CMAP after progressively longer delays. Conduction velocity in the peroneal nerve can be calculated by dividing the distance between the stimulation points by the difference in time between the onset of the CMAP.

as well as the amount of time for the neuromuscular junction to activate the muscle. Strictly speaking, the terminal latency does not directly measure nerve conduction (because it also includes the neuromuscular junction activation phase) but it is a reasonable reflection of nerve conduction over this segment of the nerve in the absence of uncommon neuromuscular diseases. There are tables of normal for the terminal latencies of defined lengths for each of the major motor nerves of the limb. Abnormal prolongation of this value is often of benefit in the detection of distal entrapment neuropathies. Once a terminal latency has been recorded, the motor conduction velocity can be determined by stimulation of another, more proximal site along the motor nerve. The computation of motor nerve conduction velocity requires knowing the distance between the two simulation sites and the difference in the terminal latencies recorded from the more distal and more proximal sites. Dividing the distance by the time gives the NCV over the segment in between the stimuli.

Sensory Conduction Studies Sensory conduction velocity is an easier measure to compute, but is more technically difficult to record (Fig. 18–6). This test can be done in either an orthdromic (i.e., distal stimulation and proximal recording) or an antidromic (i.e., proximal stimulation and distal recording) direction. In order to be sure that sensory nerve conduction is being recorded, either the stimulation point or the recording electrode (or both) must be over a part of the nerve that does not contain motor nerve fibers. Examples include the lateral femoral cutaneous nerve, the sural nerve, or the superficial peroneal nerve. The recording is made directly from the sensory nerve (the evoked response is called the sensory nerve action potential [SNAP]) and therefore is quite small (about a thousand times smaller than the CMAP). The distance between the site of stimulation and recording is divided by the latency (i.e., the amount of time between the electrical stimulus and the SNAP) to determine the sensory nerve conduction velocity over the segment. Of course, the SNAP is quite small in amplitude, and recordings must be done in a rather meticulous fashion to avoid artifact.

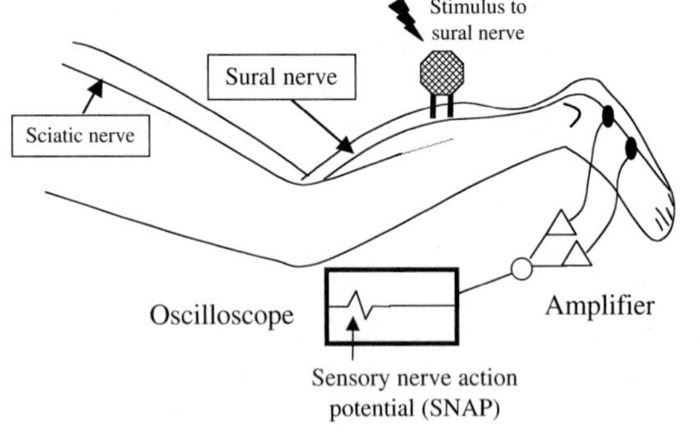

FIGURE 18–6. Method of sensory nerve conduction studies. Recordings are made through a pair of surface electrodes applied over the course of the nerve that is to be stimulated. In this case, recordings are from the sural nerve on the lateral side of the foot with stimulation of that nerve in the posterior calf. Conduction velocity can be calculated by dividing the distance between the stimulus and recording points by the difference in time between the onset of the SNAP.

NCV Limitations The sites from which nerves can be directly stimulated and from which the nerve or appropriate muscles can be recorded limit sensory and motor nerve conduction studies. For example, this makes the technique poorly suited to the investigation of nerve root problems since it is both difficult to directly electrically stimulate and record from a nerve root because of its deep location and multiple surrounding structures. Other common technical problems in nerve conduction studies include difficulties locating the nerves and measuring the course of a nerve (particularly for those nerves that follow a winding or bending course).

Measuring NCV Results

The results of nerve conduction studies are compared to tables of normal and also to the values in an unaffected limb of the same individual. There are normal values for both sensory and motor conduction (as well as for terminal latency). For example, a good rule of thumb is that motor nerve conduction should be at least 40 m/s in the lower limb, while sensory nerve conduction should be at least 35 m/s. Normal aging can slow the conduction velocity as can low temperature of a limb. In the elderly it may be impossible to record some sensory nerve conduction, such as from the sural nerve. There are tables that may be used to adjust normal values with extremes of age and limb temperature.

The two values that are most important in a nerve conduction study are the speed of conduction and the amplitude. The speed is a reflection of the diameter of the axons and, most importantly, the thickness of the myelin sheath. Most of the conditions that damage nerves result in at least some injury to the myelin covering the axons. During recovery from focal neuropathy a thinner and less well-developed myelin sheath is produced, slowing conduction. Of course, this slowing would be the greatest in the area of the damage. Additionally, many conditions such as compressive neuropathy, preferentially damage the largest, fastest conducting fibers. This also contributes to slowing (as manifest by decreased conduction velocity). Actual blockage of conduction or damage to significant numbers of axons can result in a decrease in size, or distortion of the recorded signal. The decrease in amplitude of signal is not as sensitive to injury as is the decrease in NCV, since a substantially higher percentage of nerve fibers would have to be blocked or killed in order to produce a noticeable loss of amplitude.

Conventional sensory and motor nerve conduction studies should be normal in patients with an uncomplicated radiculopathy (i.e., a monoradiculopathy without complicating conditions such as polyneuropathy or peripheral entrapment neuropathies). There are several reasons for this. The motor conduction studies are usually normal because the mixed nerves that are stimulated in the limb are composed of several nerve roots. Even a large amount of damage to one of these nerve roots does not affect the conduction in motor axons from other roots. In the case of sensory conduction studies, the damage due to radiculopathy is typically proximal to the dorsal root ganglion, leaving the sensory axon that extends into the limb unimpaired. Finally, the greatest abnormality in nerve conduction is found at the level of the injury. In the case of radiculopathy, the damage is quite proximal. Since it takes highly specialized procedures to stimulate the nerve roots proximal to the area of nerve root damage, the segment of greatest damage is not tested by conventional nerve conduction studies.

The preceding discussion would suggest that sensory and motor nerve conduction studies have no place in the investigation of radiculopathy. However, many patients with suspected radiculopathy have additional problems such as a polyneuropathy or focal entrapment neuropathy that complicate their assessment. In fact, one of the more common electrodiagnostic consultation is for the patient with weakness in foot and toe dorsiflexion (such as in foot-drop), with a consideration as to whether this is due to L5 radiculopathy or to peroneal neuropathy (such as often occurs at the level of the knee). The focal entrapment neuropathy is usually detected quite easily by nerve conduction studies across the knee, providing a major contribution to the overall assessment. Other examples of the utility of nerve conduction studies in the investigation of the patient with suspected radiculopathy include helping to distinguish upper lumbar radiculopathy from meralgia paresthetica and the investigation of the patient with numbness of the feet (since this may result from radiculopathy, polyneuropathy, or focal sensory nerve damage).

Nerve conduction studies may be of great help in the patient with more than one problem complicating their evaluation (e.g., a radiculopathy plus a focal entrapment neuropathy). These studies may alter the interpretation of needle electromyographic studies (e.g., by demonstrating that denervation of the abductor hallucis is due to a tarsal tunnel syndrome, rather than being a reflection of an S1 radiculopathy). Finally, nerve conduction studies may provide data that are critical for the proper interpretation of evoked potential data and the data from "late potentials," including F-waves and H-reflexes that are described below.

Clinical Pearl: Nerve conduction studies should be done as part of the evaluation for potential radiculopathy since sensory and motor symptoms in lower extremity may be caused by conditions such as polyneuropathy (such as occurs with diabetes

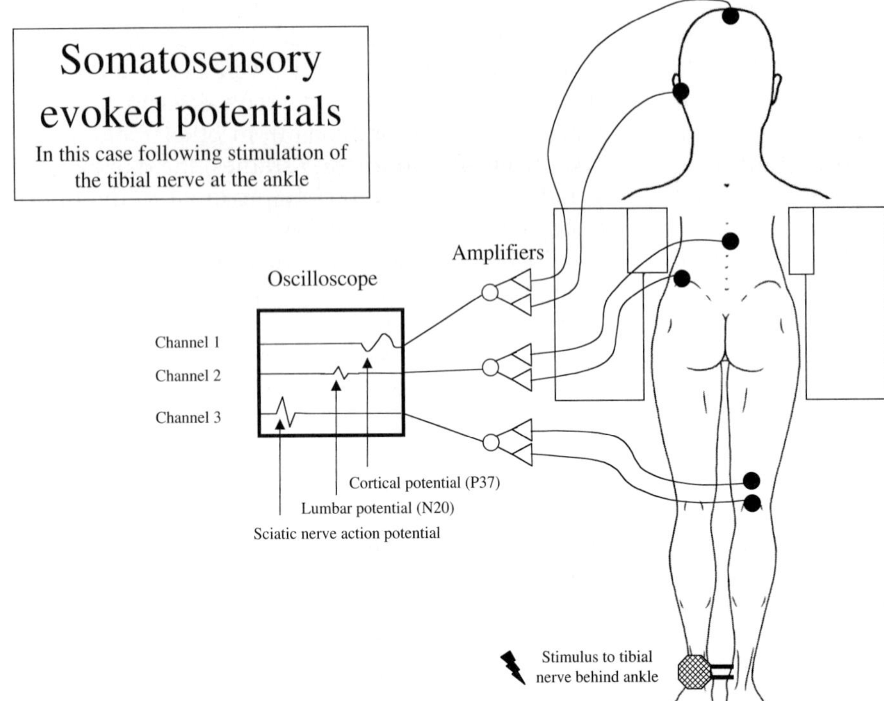

FIGURE 18–7. Method of somatosensory evoked potentials (SSEPs) testing. The stimulus can be delivered to a mixed nerve (as in this case, with tibial nerve stimulation) or to a dermatome (dermatomal somatosensory evoked potentials). The recordings are made through pairs of electrodes (one an active electrode and the other a reference electrode) applied to sites along the sensory system. These typically include electrodes along more proximal portions of the nerve in question, over the lower spinal cord and over the motor area of the 2 cerebral cortex. The signals are fed through amplifiers into different channels of the recording device for display. The timing of the waveforms and the time in between the various waves are recorded and compared to a table of normal values and to the unaffected side.

mellitus or other systemic conditions) or focal neuropathy (such as with entrapment neuropathies). Data from the nerve conduction studies may be critical for interpretation of needle EMG findings, for example.

Evoked Potentials Evoked potentials are responses in the nervous system to stimulation of a sensory pathway. Clinically, this includes stimulation of a sensory nerve in the limb (somatosensory evoked potentials—SSEPs), the visual system (visual evoked potentials), or the auditory system (brain stem auditory evoked potentials). These techniques have the potential for investigating the integrity of the pathways of sensory transmission all the way from the point of peripheral activation through the cerebral cortical representation.

The procedure for recording evoked potentials requires placement of a low-impedance surface electrode over several portions of the nervous system, followed by repeated activation of the sensory system. The minute electrical responses that are evoked by stimulation (for SSEPs, this usually consists of electrical stimulation of sensory or mixed nerves in the limbs) are recorded and averaged over many trials. This averaging eliminates background "noise" and the normal ongoing electrical nervous system activity that is often much larger than the signal evoked by the stimulus. In the case of SSEPs, usually over 500 stimuli are needed in order to obtain reliable, reproducible responses. Damage to the sensory pathway decreases the speed of conduction (much as was described in the section on nerve conduction studies), although diminished amplitude (which normally has a higher degree of inherent variability) may also be seen.

Somatosensory Evoked Potentials Of the three types of clinically useful evoked potentials, SSEPs have been investigated in terms of potential to detect damage to nerve roots, although there have also been some intriguing recent studies of responses evoked directly from paraspinal muscle stimulation.

SSEPs are produced by activation of the large-diameter peripheral nerve sensory fibers (Fig. 18–7). These nerve fibers include many that are conveying sensation from muscles as well as those from touch and pressure receptors in the skin and deeper tissues. Pain fibers contribute little (if anything) to the normal, clinical evoked potential. This limits the utility of the procedure for investigation pain physiology or damage to pain pathways.

Clinical Pearl: SSEPs evaluate only the largest sensory nerve fibers and the dorsal column medial lemniscal pathways through the central nervous system.

Compressive neuropathies tend to affect the larger diameter sensory fibers first. This is due to the higher metabolic demand of the large axons, the greater demands for maintaining membrane stability, and the size and fragility of the myelin layers surrounding these fibers. The effects of nerve root injury can result from mechanical damage to the axon, from the generation of inflammatory chemicals in the area, or from the impaired blood flow or tissue oxygenation. These may damage the axon directly or by injuring the myelin (the sheath that is responsible for the high conduction velocity of these axons). As described previously, repair of damaged myelin results in an axon that conducts more slowly than before the damage. Just as with nerve conduction studies, decreased amplitude of evoked signals may also reflect damage; however, since amplitude is a significantly more variable measure, only large differences in amplitude can be interpreted as reflecting pathology.

Most clinical SSEPs are done by stimulation of large-diameter mixed nerves of the periphery (such as the median, ulnar, peroneal, or tibial nerves). These nerves are composed of sensory nerve fibers from many nerve roots, limiting the ability to identify damage to a single nerve root.[57] While there has been some discussion of the value of mixed nerve SSEPs in the identification of radiculopathy (such as by using the peroneal nerve SSEP for the L5 nerve root),[58] most investigators have not found this to be of particular value. However, there are some conditions in which multiple nerve roots are compressed (such as by lumbar spinal stenosis) where evoked potentials might be of greater utility.[59] However, in this setting, neuroimaging studies such as MRI are probably of greater use and the electrophysiological studies are probably only helpful as an adjunctive procedure if there is a question regarding the clinical significance of the imaging findings.

Clinical Pearl: Mixed nerve SSEPs (e.g., from tibial nerve or peroneal nerve stimulation) are of limited help in investigation of monoradiculopathy. They are better at detecting polyradiculopathy (such as with lumbar spinal stenosis) or damage to spinal cord sensory pathways (myelopathy).

Dermatomal Somatosensory Evoked Potentials Dermatomal somatosensory evoked potentials (DSSEPs) are a type of SSEP that involves the recording of potentials evoked following the stimulation of particular skin regions that are innervated by individual nerve roots (autonomous zones). Occasionally, sensory nerves that supply these autonomous zones may be stimulated directly (such as the sural nerve for the S1 nerve root or the superficial peroneal nerve for the L5 root). This procedure is often called *segmental somatosensory evoked potentials* although the principle is similar to DSSEPs.

DSSEPs are a highly controversial topic. There have been many studies examining DSSEPs in lumbar radiculopathy.[60] However, differences in technique and disagreements about the acceptable definitions of abnormality have significantly colored the interpretation of the literature. For example, Scharff et al. reported that a great majority of patients with documented radiculopathy have abnormal lower limb DSSEPs.[61] However, it has been pointed out that using their liberal criteria for abnormality, the procedure loses specificity.[62] A position paper presented by the American Academy of Neurology in 1997 has acknowledged this controversy and was unable to reach definitive conclusions regarding the utility of DSSEPs in the investigation of radiculopathy.[63] This is particularly true because of highly variable reports relative to the specificity of the test. The conclusion of the committee that DSSEPs were "investigational" is probably warranted based on the literature available in 1997. Unfortunately, there has not been sufficient subsequent investigation to clarify ambiguities identified by the committee. Therefore, a more favorable assessment of the procedure cannot be supported at the present time.

Clinical Pearl: Because of issues regarding specificity and standardization of technical details, DSSEPs should be considered "investigational."

Paraspinal Muscle Evoked Potentials Zhu and colleagues[64] have made the intriguing observation that there are abnormal somatosensory potentials evoked by magnetic stimulation of paraspinal muscles in areas that show palpable hypertonicity. Interestingly, these abnormal potentials have been shown to normalize by effective treatment. This observation provides interesting insights into the physiology of muscle hypertonicity in the back. However, whether it will ever prove to be a useful evaluative tool in clinical practice remains to be seen.

Late Potentials Late potentials are electrodiagnostically elicited responses in muscle that appear following stimulation of motor nerves. They have been termed *late-potentials* because they take substantially longer to appear than the responses that are recorded during the motor nerve conduction study (described in the section on nerve conduction studies as the CMAP). There are two distinct types of late responses, the H-reflex (Fig. 18–8) and the F-response (Fig. 18–9).

Clinical Pearl: Late potentials should be done in concert with motor nerve conduction studies since

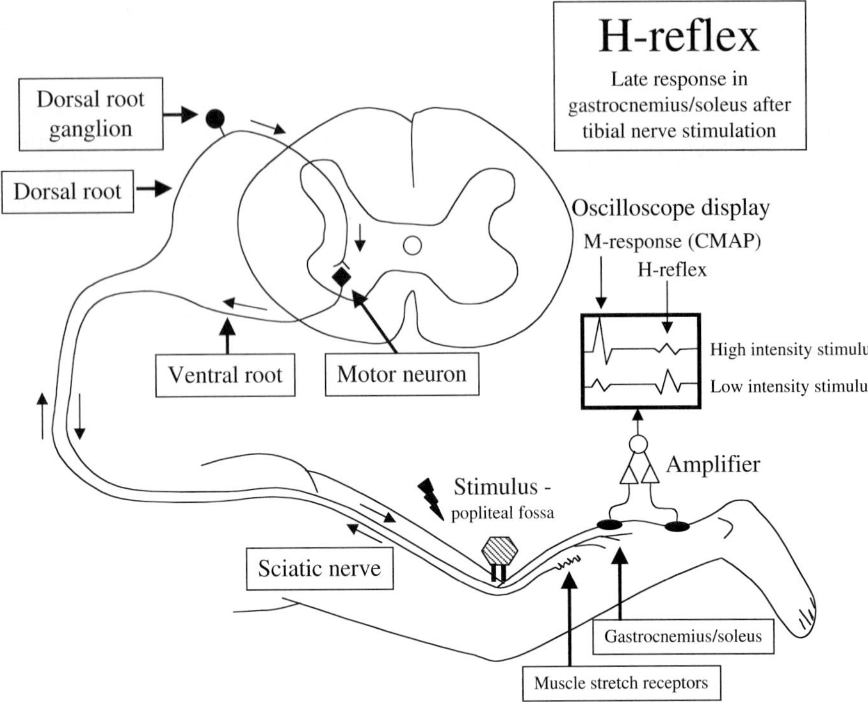

FIGURE 18–8. Method of H-reflex testing. The stimulus is delivered to the tibial nerve in the popliteal fossa, with recordings from the calf muscles. With low intensities of stimulation, the axons from muscle stretch receptors are preferentially stimulated, resulting in a reflex response in the calf muscles. This reflex follows the same course as the Achilles reflex. Wih higher intensity stimulation, the H-reflex becomes smaller, and the primary response that is seen is due to direct activation of motor axons to the calf muscles (which, of course, appears much sooner than the reflex). Results are compared to a table of normal values and to the unaffected side.

interpretation of an abnormally delayed F-wave or H-reflex requires knowledge of motor conduction in the distal limb.

Clinical Pearl: Late potentials (F-responses and H-reflexes) should be done bilaterally since side-to-side difference is a more sensitive indicator of abnormality than slowing of the absolute latency.

H-Reflex The first type of "late response" is called the H-reflex, named in honor of Hoffmann, who first described this response in 1918. The pathway for this

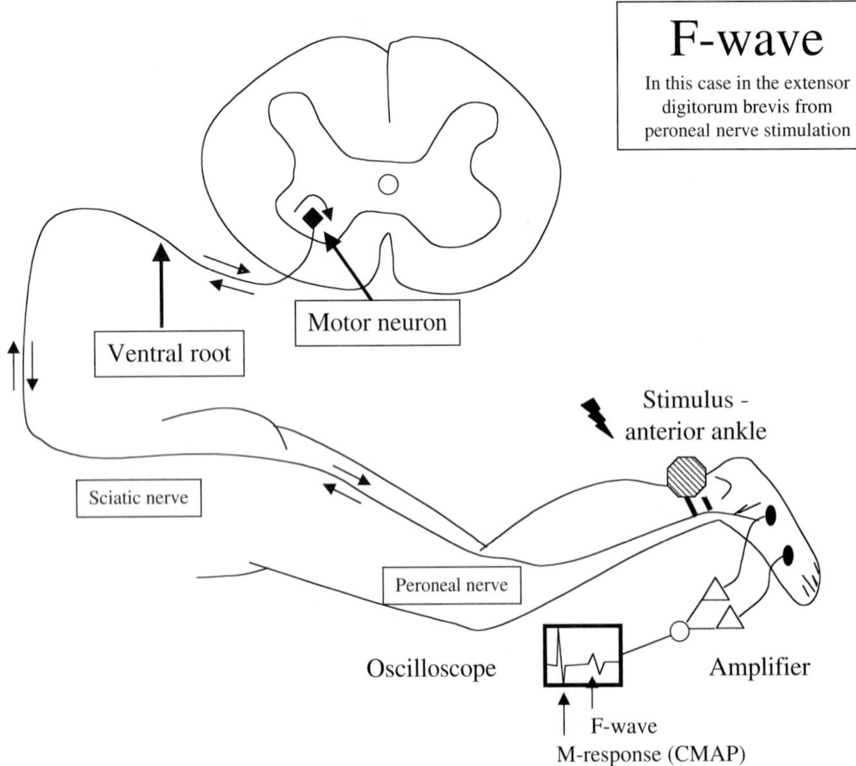

FIGURE 18–9. Method of F-wave testing. The stimulus is delivered to a motor nerve (in this case the peroneal at the level of the ankle) with recordings from one of the muscles to which it is attached. High-intensity stimulation results in the generation of an action potential that propagates in both directions, i.e., directly to the muscle (producing a rapid response—a CMAP) and back toward the motor neuron cell body. A percentage of these motor neurons will result in a second action potential that will then course all the way back down the axon to the muscle, resulting in a small, delayed response. Results are compared to a table of normal values (corrected for height) and to the unaffected side.

reflex and the significance of abnormalities are easiest to understand by recognizing that it is basically an electrical test of the muscle stretch reflex. It is most commonly tested by electrical stimulation of the tibial nerve, with recordings from the gastrocnemius/soleus muscle complex (i.e., the triceps surae) (Fig. 18–8). Therefore, this response utilizes the same neural pathway as the ankle jerk reflex.

In discussing the H-reflex it is helpful to know some of the technical details of the procedure. Electrical stimulation will depolarize the largest, most heavily myelinated nerve fibers at lower stimulus intensities than those required to activate small nerve fibers. Since the largest nerve fibers in a peripheral nerve are those arising from muscle stretch receptors, there should be an intensity of the stimulus that is capable of activating muscle stretch afferent nerve fibers without directly activating many motor nerve axons (which are slightly smaller in diameter). When muscle stretch sensory fibers are stimulated (whether it be by electrical activation of axons or by tapping the tendon of the muscle), a monosynaptic reflex contraction will be elicited in the muscle. Because this response must traverse the sensory axon all the way back to the spinal cord before synapsing on the motor neuron, and since the motor response must then traverse the length of the motor axon to the triceps surae muscle, this reflex takes a long time (at least in electrodiagnostic terms). That is where the designation of "late potential" comes from. Theoretically, this reflex can be elicited from virtually any muscle that has a motor nerve that can be stimulated. However, in practical terms, only the triceps surae muscle produces H-reflexes that are reliable enough to be clinically useful. Therefore, when a clinical electrodiagnostic procedure reports an H-reflex, the test has evaluated the integrity of the reflex arc from the tibial nerve through the spinal cord and back to the triceps surae. Damage to any portion of the reflex arc, including the sciatic nerve or the sensory or motor nerve root, can result in loss or slowing of the reflex response. Additionally, the amplitude of response (expressed as a ratio of the reflex response to the maximal response that can be elicited in the muscle by direct electrical stimulation of motor axons—the so-called H/M_{max}) is also reliable enough to be of diagnostic value. Since the H-reflex is mediated primarily over the S1 nerve root (just like the ankle jerk reflex), it is a sensitive test for S1 radiculopathy. However, once the reflex arc has been damaged, it often does not return to normal (making the test less useful in investigation of the question of recurrent radiculopathy). While this may be viewed as an electrical test of the ankle jerk, or Achilles' tendon reflex, there are some differences that should be noted. For example, as opposed to the clinical ankle jerk, the H-reflex can be precisely quantified (both in terms of latency and amplitude) and, therefore, may be a more useful index to follow with time or treatment.

H-reflexes can be elicited from almost any limb muscle. However, from a practical perspective, with the notable exception of the triceps surae muscle, the responses are not reliable enough to be of general clinical use. This limits the H-reflex to being a fairly sensitive and quantitative test of sciatic nerve and S1 nerve root function. Certainly, this can be of great, albeit restricted utility in investigating patients with suspected S1 radiculopathy.[65]

Clinical Pearl: The H-reflex is a sensitive indicator of S1 nerve root function, though it can also be affected by damage to the proximal sciatic nerve or sacral plexus.

F-Response The second type of late potential is the F-response. This is a response that can be seen to occur in muscles during a motor nerve conduction study long after the initial contraction of the muscle, the CMAP (described in the section on nerve conduction studies). While the CMAP usually appears within several milliseconds (depending on how close the stimulus point is to the muscle), depending on the stimulus site, another response can be recorded in the muscle up to around 50 milliseconds later (Fig. 18–9). Since this response was first recorded in *foot muscles*, it came to be known as the *F-response*. Over time it was found that this late response was not actually a reflex in conventional terms. The electrical impulse runs proximally along the motor axon from the site of initiation of the action potential. When the depolarization being conducted in an antidromic direction along the motor axons reaches the motor neurons in the spinal cord, a percentage of these motor neurons are activated a second time. This results in an efferent discharge that is conducted down the axon to the muscles themselves. This second, later activation produces a small muscle contraction that is termed the F-response. Because the number of motor neurons that are reactivated is somewhat unpredictable, the amplitude of this signal is variable and, therefore, amplitude measurements are of little use. However, delay in the F-response indicates some slowing of conduction of the motor axon. Since the F-response traverses more proximal portions of the motor axons (twice, in fact), it may be useful in the investigation of radiculopathy.[66–69] However, since most muscles are innervated by more than one nerve root, and since the integrity of a relatively few motor axons is all that is required to elicit an F-response, this is not particularly sensitive for damage to single nerve roots. Furthermore, since sensory nerve roots do not participate in this response, a radiculopathy that only affects sensory nerve fibers would not affect this response. Studies have suggested that F-responses may be of greater use in investigating cases of suspected lumbar spinal stenosis, where they may provide some physiological measure of nerve function to accompany the imaging findings.[70] This is because spinal stenosis, by its very nature, involves several nerve roots.

Clinical Pearl: F-responses are mediated over several nerve roots. Therefore, they are rarely abnormal in monoradiculopathy.

THERMOGRAPHY

Thermography, either through direct skin contact or through infrared detection, has been touted as a method for evaluation of back pain and for detection of radiculopathy.[71] This method has had a particular interest for chiropractors since certain chiropractic techniques have historically used a thermocouple for identification of segmental dysfunction.

Several groups have investigated thermography in patients with radiculopathy.[72,73] For example, Harper and colleagues[72] have reported that infrared thermography was quite sensitive in detecting patients with radiculopathy. This is similar to the findings by other investigators.[74,75] However, the procedure was highly nonspecific and they concluded that thermography is of little or no utility in the diagnosis of lumbosacral radiculopathy,[74] a sentiment echoed by other investigators.[76]

Thermography has also been touted as an independent and objective correlate of pain. There are reports that patients with back pain have regions of increased warmth of the skin,[77] while chronically painful limbs associated with back pain are cool.[80] Although studies have indicated correlation between symptoms and thermographic findings, most of the criteria outlined as "evidence" in Table 18–1 have not been met. For example, when dealing with symptoms such as LBP (as opposed to radiculopathy, for example), there is no gold standard against which to compare findings. The various elements necessary to determine positive and negative predictive values are also not known and the various factors that can influence the thermographic pattern are poorly understood. It is no wonder then that the Therapeutic and Technology Assessment Subcommittee of the American Academy of Neurology did not find sufficient evidence to indicate the value of this procedure in the evaluation of back pain.[79] This position was echoed by a systematic review of studies up through 1991[80] and in a more recent study comparing the diagnostic accuracy of thermograms in patients with and without low back symptoms.[81]

Clinical Pearl: Because of issues of specificity, thermography should be considered "investigational" with regard to application to the study of patients with back pain or radiculopathy.

The issue of whether there are thermographic findings indicating segmental dysfunction has been a thorny, albeit important one for practitioners who utilize manual techniques such as manipulation and mobilization. Hindering this assessment is the lack of a universally accepted gold standard for the identification of the underlying segmental abnormalities and the relative unreliability of clinical methods for the identification of such abnormalities. Keating and colleagues[82] found some concordance between examiners for the identification of large temperature differentials, although this level of agreement was not all that impressive. Plaugher and colleagues reported slightly better levels, but still with unimpressive agreement levels.[83] More recently, attempts are underway to develop automated, reliable methods of temperature pattern detection.[84,85] Should such methods prove to have high internal consistency, the long process of attempting validation as a diagnostic protocol will need to be completed before general acceptance as a useful clinical tool.

There has been discussion of the utility of thermography for the investigation of type I complex regional pain syndrome (CRPS type I—formerly known as reflex sympathetic dystrophy). This is a condition that can complicate the clinical course of several painful problems, including back pain. Part of the criteria for assessment of this condition includes abnormalities in neurovascular function, often reflected as changes in temperature. Therefore, it should not be surprising that thermography is quite sensitive for detecting the problem. Gulevich and colleagues[86] evaluated 185 patients with chronic pain, comparing results with a consensus clinical evaluation. They used a thermal stress protocol for thermographic evaluation, finding that this had 93% sensitivity and 89% specificity (for a 90% positive predictive value and 94% negative predictive value in their patients with chronic pain). Their findings were quite supportive of those by Bruehl and colleagues,[87] who also considered the effects of various cutoff points for determining normality. As with any test, changing cutoffs to improve sensitivity (and negative predictive value) will decrease specificity (and positive predictive value). At the current state of knowledge, conventional thermography is not sufficiently specific to be diagnostic of CRPS type I.[80] While it does appear that ancillary maneuvers, such as thermal stress responses, may improve the utility of the test, and despite inherent limitations in the clinical criteria for CRPS,[88] thermography still must be considered as an adjunct to the clinical evaluation of the condition.

Despite a long history, thermography at this point can only be considered investigational in terms of use in evaluation of back pain or segmental dysfunction. Although it appears to be sensitive in the detection of radiculopathy, its lack of specificity impairs usefulness for the assessment of this condition. It may be a useful adjunct to the clinical examination in the assessment of CRPS type I.

QUANTITATIVE SENSORY TESTING

Purely sensory complaints are common in clinical practice. Many of these take the form of pain, but symptoms of diminished sensation or "numbness" are also frequent. Although SSEPs evaluate sensory pathways, there are limitations of this procedure, which are outlined above. At the present time, SSEPs and sensory nerve conduction studies are the only truly objective tests of sensory function. However, there has been an increase in quasi-objective measures of sensory function over the past 15 years. These range from very low-tech (such as the sensitivity for detection of vonFrey hairs) to more high-tech methods, including threshold studies for detection of vibration and for the determination of electrical current perceptual threshold (CPT).[89–91] The term *quasi-objective* is used to describe these procedures because they still rely on the patient's report of a subjective sensory phenomenon. Therefore, although these tests may be quantitative and while they may have some built-in control procedures, they cannot be considered as completely objective validation of an otherwise purely subjective complaint. They often function as useful screening methods for patients prior to performing more objective (and presumably more expensive or invasive) procedures. However, if consistent results are obtained over several trials, the results can approach a degree of objectivity as long as the limitations inherent in the procedures are not ignored. The particular strength and utility of this type of testing resides in the ability to follow the progress of a known condition (such as carpal tunnel syndrome or diabetic neuropathy) where deterioration may be an important determinant in therapeutic intervention. This device was evaluated by the Technology Assessment Committee of the American Academy of Electrodiagnostic Medicine,[92] which pointed out several important technical issues that remain with this method of sensory evaluation. Their conclusion in this 1999 review was that there was insufficient information to draw conclusions about the usefulness of this form of sensory testing. Unfortunately, most of these limitations have not been conclusively addressed by subsequent studies.

SUMMARY

1. Several neurodiagnostic procedures have been investigated relative to their ability to provide useful data in patients with LBP.
2. The main goals of diagnostic testing in LBP patients have included those listed in Table 18–1.
3. Diagnostic tests require validation. The steps involved in validation of diagnostic tests are listed in Table 18–2.
4. Diagnostic tests for radiculopathy have typically been validated by comparison with gold standards, including diagnostic imaging and findings at surgery.
5. The validation of diagnostic testing for segmental abnormality or for the objectification of lower back symptoms has been hampered by lack of gold standards.
6. Needle EMG, evoked potential testing, and thermography have been applied to the evaluation of radiculopathy by comparison with gold standard tests.
    (a) Needle EMG is the most established and reliable of the electrodiagnostic procedures for the diagnosis of radiculopathy, although its sensitivity is only approaching 80%, with specificity above 85%. Although there are normal individuals who have signs indicating denervation in paraspinal muscles, this test can be diagnostic of radiculopathy when the findings in paraspinal muscles are accompanied by supportive findings in limb muscles. It may be of particular use when imaging and clinical findings are equivocal, although results must be interpreted with great caution in patients who have had prior spine surgery.
    (b) Mixed nerve SSEPs have limited use in the investigation of radiculopathy, though they may be of some clinical use in the assessment of neurogenic claudication (with spinal stenosis). Dermatomal potentials must be considered investigational at this time because of concerns about lack of specificity and debate about the appropriate limits to ranges of normal (affecting sensitivity).
    (c) Thermography is sensitive for radiculopathy, but also highly nonspecific, negating its utility for this condition.
7. Surface EMG procedures have been extensively discussed in relation to the investigation of LBP.
    (a) Static surface recordings have yielded variable results. It is not clear whether these variable results are simply a reflection of different patient populations or technical factors, or whether these results are reflections of important underlying clinical phenomena. Therefore, they

cannot be recommended for clinical diagnostic use at this time.

(b) Dynamic EMG testing (at least in terms of the flexion-relaxation response) appears to be a common and physiologically important correlate with LBP. However, significant questions remain about the diagnostic specificity of this observation and about the potential utility of EMG evaluation in other ranges of motion. Therefore, any findings on such studies can oy be considered to be confirmatory of assessments made by other clinical means.

(c) Abnormalities in the spectral EMG pattern are common in LBP patients during fatiguing contractions, although the diagnostic significance of these findings requires more investigation prior to the realization of any clinical application.

(d) Procedures such as ambulatory EMG and wavelet analysis are in early developmental stages. Therefore, they are not recommended for clinical diagnostic use at this time.

8. NCV studies are commonly used in patients with suspected radiculopathy. Radiculopathy will not alter peripheral nerve conduction studies. The primary use of nerve conduction studies is in evaluating potential peripheral entrapment neuropathy that can mimic radiculopathy or that can complicate its assessment. Nerve conduction studies are also helpful in the evaluation of findings of evoked potential studies and of the so-called *late potentials*.
9. Late potentials can be of use in the detection of lumbosacral radiculopathy. The H-reflex is an objective and reliable test of the Achilles reflex arc and, therefore, is a good indicator of S1 nerve root function. F-wave is a test of the complete length of motor axons in any peripheral motor nerve (such as the tibial or peroneal). However, since these nerves contain contributions from more than one nerve root, monoradiculopathy rarely produces a definable abnormality. The F-wave may be a better test of conditions that involve more than one nerve root (such as lumbar spinal stenosis).
10. SSEPs investigate the course of large-fiber sensory pathways from the periphery to the cerebral cortex. Potentials evoked by stimulation of large mixed nerves (such as the tibial or peroneal) are rarely abnormal in monoradiculopathies because each of these nerves is composed of several sensory nerve roots. Dermatomal evoked potentials may be more useful, but there are too many gaps in the literature to recommend them as more than "investigational" in nature.
11. Thermography has not been proven to be helpful in the evaluation of nonspecific back pain, segmental dysfunction, or radiculopathy despite extensive literature and a long history of use. Therefore, it is not recommended for clinical diagnosis of these conditions. It is also not specific for, and therefore not diagnostic of, CRPS type I (previously, reflex sympathetic dystrophy). However, it may contribute to the overall clinical assessment of these patients.
12. Quantitative sensory testing is a quasi-objective test that adds little to the clinical diagnosis of radiculopathy, much less to objectifying back pain. It may be useful to follow changes over time of sensory abnormalities that have been diagnosed and documented by other means.

REFERENCES

1. Andersson GB. Epidemiological features of chronic low-back pain. *Lancet* 1999;354:581–585.
2. Swenson RS. Lower back pain: Differential diagnosis, a reasonable clinical approach. *Neurol Clin N Am* 1999;17:43–63.
3. Weber F, Albert U. Electrodiagnostic examination of lumbosacral radiculopathies. *Electromyogr Clin Neurophysiol* 2000;40:231–236.
4. Braune HJ, Wunderlich MT. Diagnostic value of different neurophysiological methods in the assessment of lumbar nerve root lesions. *Arch Phys Med Rehabil* 1997;78:518–520.
5. Knuttson B. Comparative value of electromyographic, myelographic and clinical–neurological examinations in diagnosis of lumbar root compression syndrome. *Acta Orthop Scand* 1961;49(Suppl):1–135.
6. Tomasella M, Crielaard JM, Wang FC. Dorsal and lumbar paraspinal electromyographic study. Multi-MUP analysis and drawing up normal values in a reference population. *Neurophysiol Clin* 2002;32:109–117.
7. Haig AJ, LeBreck DB, Powley SG. Paraspinal mapping. Quantified needle electromyography of the paraspinal muscles in persons without low back pain. *Spine* 1995;20:715–721.
8. Haig AJ, Talley C, Grobler LJ, et al. Paraspinal mapping: Quantified needle electromyography in lumbar radiculopathy. *Muscle Nerve* 1993;16:477–484.
9. Date ES, Mar EY, Bugola MR, et al. The prevalence of lumbar paraspinal spontaneous activity in asymptomatic subjects. *Muscle Nerve* 1996;19:350–354.
10. Grabel JA. Electromyographic study of low back muscle tension in subjects with and without chronic low back pain. *Dissert Abstr Int Ch* 1973;3:60–62.
11. Ambroz C, Scott A, Ambroz A, et al. Chronic low back pain assessment using surface electromyography. *J Occup Environ Med* 2000;42:660–669.
12. Arena JG, Sherman RA, Bruno GM, et al. Electromyographic recordings of low back pain subjects and nonpain controls in six different positions: Effect of pain levels. *Pain* 1991;45:23–28.
13. Ahern DK, Follick MJ, Council JR, et al. Comparison of lumbar paravertebral EMG patterns in chronic

low back pain patients and non-patient controls. *Pain* 1988;34:153–160.
14. Miller DJ. Comparison of electromyographic activity in the lumbar paraspinal muscles of subjects with and without chronic low back pain. *Phys Ther* 1985;65:1347–1354.
15. Linsinski P. Surface EMG in chronic low back pain. *Eur Spine J* 2000;9:559–562.
16. Traue HC, Kessler M, Cram JR. Surface EMG topography and pain distribution in pre-chronic back pain patients. *Int J Psychosom* 1992;39:18–27.
17. Pullman SL, Goodin DS, Marquinez AI, et al. Clinical utility of surface EMG: Report of the therapeutics and technology assessment subcommittee of the American Academy of Neurology. *Neurology* 2000;55:171–177.
18. Nouwen A, Bush C. The relationship between paraspinal EMG and chronic low back pain. *Pain* 1984; 20:109–123.
19. Cram JR, Lloyd J, Cahn TS. The reliability of EMG muscle scanning. *Int J Psychosom* 1994;41:41–45.
20. Leach RA, Owens EF Jr, Giesen JM. Correlates of myoelectric asymmetry detected in low back pain patients using hand-held post-style surface electromyography. *J Manipulative Physiol Ther* 1993;16:140–149.
21. Danneels LA, Cagnie BJ, Cools AM, et al. Intra-operator and inter-operator reliability of surface electromyography in the clinical evaluation of back muscles. *Manual Ther* 2001;6:145–153.
22. Nouwen A, Van Akkerveeken PF, Versloot JM. Patterns of muscular activity during movement in patients with chronic low-back pain. *Spine* 1987;12:777–782.
23. Sihvonen T, Partanen J, Hanninen O, et al. Electric behavior of low back muscles during lumbar pelvic rhythm in low back pain patients and healthy controls. *Arch Phys Med Rehabil* 1991;72:1080–1087.
24. Kaigle AM, Wessberg P, Hansson TH. Muscular and kinematic behavior of the lumbar spine during flexion-extension. *J Spinal Disord* 1998;11:163–174.
25. Shirado O, Ito T, Kaneda K, et al. Flexion-relaxation phenomenon in the back muscles. A comparative study between healthy subjects and patients with chronic low back pain. *Am J Phys Med Rehabil* 1995;74:139–144.
26. Triano JJ, Schultz AB. Correlation of objective measure of trunk motion and muscle function with low-back disability ratings. *Spine* 1987;12:561–565.
27. Stubbs M, Harris M, Solomonow M, et al. Ligamento-muscular protective reflex in the lumbar spine of the feline. *J Electromyogr Kinesiol* 1998;8:197–204.
28. Watson PJ, Booker CK, Main CJ. Evidence for the role of psychological factors in abnormal paraspinal activity in patients with chronic low back pain. *J Musculoskeletal Pain* 1997;5:41–56.
29. Soderberg GL, Barr JO. Muscular function in chronic low-back dysfunction. *Spine* 1983;8:79–85.
30. Triano JJ, Luttges M. Myoelectric paraspinal response to spinal loads: Potential for monitoring low back pain. *J Manipulative Physiol Ther* 1985;8:137–145.
31. Lariviere C, Gagnon D, Loisel P. The comparison of trunk muscles EMG activation between subjects with and without chronic low back pain during flexion-extension and lateral bending tasks. *J Electromyogr Kinesiol* 2000;10:79–91.
32. van Dieen JH, Heijblom P. Reproducibility of isometric trunk extension torque, trunk extensor endurance, and related electromyographic parameters in the context of their clinical applicability. *J Orthop Res* 1996;14:139–143.
33. Robinson ME, Cassisi JE, O'Connor PD, et al. Lumbar iEMG during isotonic exercise: Chronic low back pain patients versus controls. *J Spinal Disord* 1992;5:8-15.
34. Ng JK, Richardson CA, Parnianpour M, et al. EMG activity of trunk muscles and torque output during isometric axial rotation exertion: A comparison between back pain patients and matched controls. *J Orthop Res* 2002;20:112–121.
35. Lu WW, Luk KD, Cheung KM, et al. Back muscle contraction patterns of patients with low back pain before and after rehabilitation treatment: An electromyographic evaluation. *J Spinal Disord* 2001;14:277–282.
36. Mooney V, Gulick J, Perlman M, et al. Relationships between myoelectric activity, strength, and MRI of lumbar extensor muscles in back pain patients and normal subjects. *J Spinal Disord* 1997;10:348–356.
37. Lindgren KA, Sihvonen T, Leino E, et al. Exercise therapy effects on functional radiographic findings and segmental electromyographic activity in lumbar spine instability. *Arch Phys Med Rehabil* 1993;74:933–939.
38. Radebold A, Cholewicki J, Polzhofer GK, et al. Impaired postural control of the lumbar spine is associated with delayed muscle response times in patients with chronic idiopathic low back pain. *Spine* 2001;26: 724–730.
39. Koumantakis GA, Oldham JA, Winstanley J. Intermittent isometric fatigue study of the lumbar multifidus muscle in four-point kneeling: An intra-rater reliability investigation. *Manual Ther* 2001;6:97–105.
40. Jalovaara P, Niinimaki T, Vanharanta H. Pocket-size, portable surface EMG device in the differentiation of low back pain patients. *Eur Spine J* 1995;4:210–212.
41. Sherman RA, Arena JG, Searle JR, et al. Development of an ambulatory recorder for evaluation of muscle tension-related low back pain and fatigue in soldiers' normal environments. *Mil Med* 1991;156:245–248.
42. Jurell KC. Surface EMG and fatigue. *Phys Med Rehabil Clin N Am* 1998;9:viii–ix, 933–947.
43. Ng JK, Richardson CA. Reliability of electromyographic power spectral analysis of back muscle endurance in healthy subjects. *Arch Phys Med Rehabil* 1996;77:259–264.
44. Thompson DA, Biedermann HJ. Electromyographic power spectrum analysis of the paraspinal muscles. Long-term reliability. *Spine* 1993;18:2310–2313.
45. Peach JP, Gunning J, McGill SM. Reliability of spectral EMG parameters of healthy back extensors during submaximum isometric fatiguing contractions and recovery. *J Electromyogr Kinesiol* 1998;8:403–410.
46. Elfving B, Nemeth G, Arvidsson I, et al. Reliability of EMG spectral parameters in repeated measurements of back muscle fatigue. *J Electromyogr Kinesiol* 1999;9:235–243.

47. Greenough CG, Oliver CW, Jones AP. Assessment of spinal musculature using surface electromyographic spectral color mapping. *Spine* 1998;23:1768–1774.
48. Klein AB, Snyder-Mackler L, Roy SH, et al. Comparison of spinal mobility and isometric trunk extensor forces with electromyographic spectral analysis in identifying low back pain. *Phys Ther* 1991;71:445–454.
49. De Luca CJ. Use of the surface EMG signal for performance evaluation of back muscles. *Muscle Nerve* 1993; 16:210–216.
50. Peach JP, McGill SM. Classification of low back pain with the use of spectral electromyogram parameters. *Spine* 1998;23:1117–1123.
51. Mannion AF, Connolly B, Wood K, et al. The use of surface EMG power spectral analysis in the evaluation of back muscle function. *J Rehabil Res Dev* 1997;34: 427–439.
52. Oddsson LI, Giphart JE, Buijs RJ, et al. Development of new protocols and analysis procedures for the assessment of LBP by surface EMG techniques. *J Rehabil Res Dev* 1997;34:415–426.
53. Roy SH, De Luca CJ, Emley M, et al. Classification of back muscle impairment based on the surface electromyographic signal. *J Rehabil Res Dev* 1997;34: 405–414.
54. Pope MH, Aleksiev A, Panagiotacopulos ND, et al. Evaluation of low back muscle surface EMG signals using wavelets. *Clin Biomech* 2000;15:567–573.
55. Sparto PJ, Parnianpour M, Barria EA, et al. Wavelet analysis of electromyography for back muscle fatigue detection during isokinetic constant-torque exertions. *Spine* 1999;24:1791–1798.
56. Sparto PJ, Jagadeesh JM, Parnianpour M. Wavelet analysis of electromyography for back muscle fatigue detection during dynamic constant-torque exertions. *Biomed Sci Instrum* 1997;33:82–87.
57. Wilbourn AJ, Aminoff MJ. AAEE minimonograph#32: The electrophysiologic examination in patients with radiculopathies. *Muscle Nerve* 1988;11:1099–1114.
58. Walk D, Fisher MA, Doundoulakis SH, et al. Somatosensory evoked potentials in the evaluation of lumbosacral radiculopathy. *Neurology* 1992;42:1197–1202.
59. Kondo M, Matsuda H, Kureya S, et al. Electrophysiological studies of intermittent claudication in lumbar stenosis. *Spine* 1989;14:862–866.
60. Swenson RS. Dermatomal somatosensory evoked potentials: A review of the literature. *J Neuromusculoskeletal Syst* 1994;2:45–51.
61. Scharff TB, Dallman DE, Toleikis JR, et al. Dermatomal somatosensory evoked potentials in the diagnosis of lumbar root entrapment. *Surg Forum* 1981;32:489–491.
62. Aminoff MJ, Goodin DS, Barbaro NM, et al. Dermatomal somatosensory evoked potentials in unilateral lumbosacral radiculopathy. *Ann Neurol* 1985;17: 171–176.
63. Anonymous. Assessment: Dermatomal somatosensory evoked potentials. The American Academy of Neurology, Therapeutics and Technology Assessment Subcommittee. *Neurology.* 1997;49:1127–1130.
64. Zhu Y, Haldeman S, Hsieh CY, et al. Do cerebral potentials to magnetic stimulation of paraspinal muscles reflect changes in palpable muscle spasm, low back pain, and activity scores? *J Manipulative Physiol Ther* 2000;23:458–464.
65. Dhand UK, Das SK, Chopra JS. Patterns of H-reflex abnormality in patients with low back pain. *Electromyogr Clin Neurophysiol* 1991;31:209–213.
66. Tang LM, Schwartz MS, Swash M. Postural effects on F wave parameters in lumbosacral root compression and canal stenosis. *Brain* 1988;111(Pt 1):207–213.
67. Linden D, Berlit P. Comparison of late responses, EMG studies, and motor evoked potentials (MEPs) in acute lumbosacral radiculopathies. *Muscle Nerve* 1995;18:1205–1207.
68. Toyokura M, Murakami K. F-wave study in patients with lumbosacral radiculopathies. *Electromyogr Clin Neurophysiol* 1997;37:19–26.
69. Braune H, Wunderlich MT. Diagnostic value of different neurophysiological methods in the assessment of lumbar nerve root lesions. *Arch Phys Med Rehabil* 1997;78:518–520.
70. Kondo M, Matsuda H, Kureya S, et al. Electrophysiological studies of intermittent claudication in lumbar stenosis. *Spine* 1989;14:862–866.
71. Pawl RP. Thermography in the diagnosis of low back pain. *Neurosurg Clin N Am* 1991;2:839–850.
72. Harper CM Jr, Low PA, Fealey RD, et al. Utility of thermography in the diagnosis of lumbosacral radiculopathy. *Neurology* 1991;41:1010–1014.
73. Thomas D, Cullum D, Siahamis G, et al. Infrared thermographic imaging, magnetic resonance imaging, CT scan and myelography in low back pain. *Br J Rheumatol* 1990;29:268–273.
74. Chafetz N, Wexler CE, Kaiser JA. Neuromuscular thermography of the lumbar spine with CT correlation. *Spine* 1988;13:922–925.
75. Gillstrom P. Thermography in low back pain and sciatica. *Arch Orthop Trauma Surg* 1985;104:31–36.
76. So YT, Aminoff MJ, Olney RK. The role of thermography in the evaluation of lumbosacral radiculopathy. *Neurology* 1989;39:1154–1158.
77. Rubal BJ, Traycoff RB, Ewing KL. Liquid crystal thermography: A new tool for evaluating low back pain. *Phys Ther* 1982;62:1593–1596.
78. Uematsu S, Jankel WR, Edwin DH, et al. Quantification of thermal asymmetry. Part 2. Application in low-back pain and sciatica. *J Neurosurg* 1988;69:556–561.
79. Anonymous. Assessment: Thermography in neurologic practice. The American Academy of Neurology, Therapeutics and Technology Assessment Subcommittee. *Neurology* 1990;40(3, Pt 1):523–525.
80. Hoffman RM, Kent DL, Deyo RA. Diagnostic accuracy and clinical utility of thermography for lumbar radiculopathy. A meta-analysis. *Spine* 1991;16:623–628.
81. Leclaire R, Esdaile JM, Jequier JC, et al. Diagnostic accuracy of technologies used in low back pain assessment. Thermography, triaxial dynamometry, spinoscopy, and clinical examination. *Spine* 1996;21(11):1325–1330.
82. Keating JC Jr, Bergmann TF, Jacobs GE, et al. Interexaminer reliability of eight evaluative dimensions of lumbar segmental abnormality. *J Manipulative Physiol Ther* 1990;13:463–470.

83. Plaugher G, Lopes MA, Melch PE, et al. The inter- and intraexaminer reliability of a paraspinal skin temperature differential instrument. *J Manipulative Physiol Ther* 1991;14:361–367.
84. Owens EF Jr, Stein T. Computer-aided analysis of paraspinal thermographic patterns: A technical report. *Chiro Res J* 2000;7:65–69.
85. Hart J, Boone WR. Pattern analysis of paraspinal temperatures: A descriptive report. *J Vertebral Subluxation Res* 2000;3:1–8.
86. Gulevich SJ, Conwell TD, Lane J, et al. Stress infrared telethermography is useful in the diagnosis of complex regional pain syndrome, type I (formerly reflex sympathetic dystrophy). *Clin J Pain* 1997;13:50–59.
87. Bruehl S, Lubenow TR, Nath H, et al. Validation of thermography in the diagnosis of reflex sympathetic dystrophy. *Clin J Pain* 1996;12:316–325.
88. Harden RN, Bruehl S, Galer BS, et al. Complex regional pain syndrome: Are the IASP diagnostic criteria valid and sufficiently comprehensive? *Pain* 1999;83:211–219.
89. Dotson RM. Clinical neurophysiology laboratory tests to assess the nociceptive system in humans. *J Clin Neurophysiol* 1997;14:32–45.
90. Pitei DL, Watkins PJ, Stevens MJ, et al. The value of the neurometer in assessing diabetic neuropathy by measurement of the current perception threshold. *Diabetic Med* 1994;11:872–876.
91. Franzblau A, Werner RA, Johnston E, et al. Evaluation of current perception threshold testing as a screening procedure for carpal tunnel syndrome among industrial workers. *J Occup Med* 1994;36:1015–1021.
92. Anonymous. Technology review: The Neurometer Current Perception Threshold (CPT). AAEM Equipment and Computer Committee. *Muscle Nerve* 1999;22:523–531.

CHAPTER

19

BIOPSYCHOSOCIAL FACTORS IN LOW BACK SYNDROMES

Jake Epker and Andrew R. Block

OUTLINE

OBJECTIVES

1. To provide clinicians with a foundation for considering these issues from an evaluation and treatment perspective. Specifically, the goals are as follows:
2. Review some of the basic psychosocial issues frequently observed in patients with chronic pain that can serve as barriers to optimal treatment response.
3. Provide clinicians a template for briefly screening for selected psychosocial risk factors.
4. Provide suggestions about how to preliminarily reduce the influence of some risk factors.
5. Provide a template for when to refer patients for a behavioral medicine evaluation and what to expect from the psychologist when this occurs.
6. Provide examples of how behavioral medicine treatment is coordinated with conservative medical care to achieve optimal treatment outcome.

INTRODUCTION

Perhaps one of the greatest challenges facing healthcare professionals involved in treating patients with chronic pain is the issue of psychosocial barriers to recovery. While previous chapters have discussed the etiology and assessment of low back syndromes, the psychosocial component cannot be ignored. It has been well established that a variety of psychosocial factors play a significant role in the lives of patients with chronic pain, with many of these factors maintaining or exacerbating pain.

PAIN AND THE BIOPSYCHOSOCIAL MODEL

Pain is arguably one of the most pervasive forms of stress in the industrialized countries. Pain accounts for 80% of all visits to physicians in the United States, with the treatment of chronic pain costing approximately \$125 billion annually.[1] Close to 50 million Americans experience some degree of disability, whether it is temporarily or permanently. Similarly, the cost of back pain in the United Kingdom has been estimated at approximately \$9 billion, when treatment, lost production, and disability benefits are factored.[2] Cross-cultural comparisons of patients from the United States, Mexico, Japan, Italy, and New Zealand who were treated at specialized pain treatment centers demonstrate a high degree of disruption in many areas of functioning across industrialized countries.[3] Lengthier episodes of pain (e.g., chronic pain) impact individuals in a variety of ways.

Pain is generally considered acute if it lasts for less than 6 weeks. Acute pain serves as a physiological signal that something is wrong.[4] One of the keys to acute pain is that it typically enables the clinician to identify the underlying cause of pain, based on the location, pattern, and description of the pain symptoms. *Alternatively, chronic pain lacks the same degree of diagnostic utility and instead tells only that something is wrong somewhere in the patient's life.* The source of this pain may lie with biological, psychological, or social difficulties. More often, there is typically a combination of such factors contributing to the chronic pain condition. These observations led to the development of the biopsychosocial model.

Clinical Pearl: Psychosocial variables are more likely to have a greater influence on chronic back pain disability than on the back pain itself.

Many studies investigating factors that place individuals with acute low back pain at risk for becoming chronic and disabled have identified psychosocial variables as playing a strong contributory role.[5,6] In addition, Volinn[7] emphasized that psychosocial variables are more likely to have a greater influence on chronic back pain disability than on the back pain itself. Such studies highlight the important role that psychosocial variables play in chronic pain. As the duration of the pain increases, a combination of biopsychosocial factors may serve to maintain the pain condition.

Clinical Pearl: When pain perception, suffering, and pain behavior expand beyond the initial stimulation of pain receptors, patients may experience high levels of pain and display greater pain behavior than can be explained by the tissue damage alone.

The biopsychosocial model[8,9] considers nociception as the foundation of the various aspects of the pain experience (see Fig. 19–1). When pain perception, suffering, and pain behavior expand beyond the initial stimulation of pain receptors, patients may experience high levels of pain and display greater pain behavior than can be explained by the tissue damage alone. As chronicity lengthens, a patient's life may become consumed by pain and its psychosocial consequences. Emotional distress in the form of depression, anxiety, anger, or frustration may come to dominate a person's mood. Friends and loved ones may respond to the individual with either disbelief since they cannot directly observe the cause of the pain or else in a solicitous manner that may tend to reinforce pain

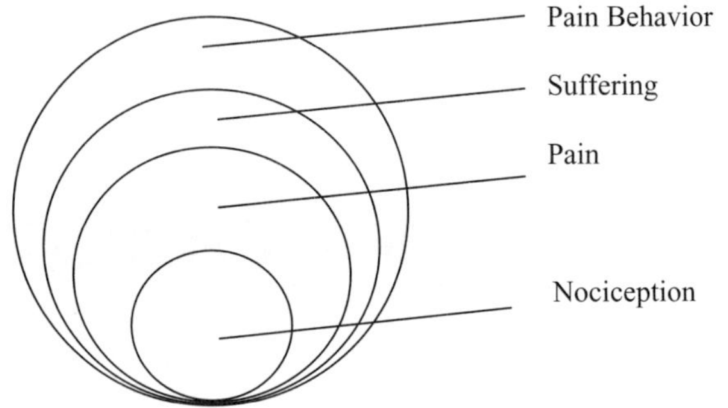

FIGURE 19–1. The biopsychosocial model of pain. *(Adapted from Loeser.[9])*

behavior. Fordyce et al.[10] noted that pain behavior initially elicited by nociception could persist beyond normal healing time because behavioral responses can lead to positive consequences, such as solicitous attention from a spouse, financial compensation, and/or avoidance of unwanted responsibilities. In either case, maintenance of the "sick-role" can be fraught with a number of psychological and social considerations.

Thus, the biopsychosocial model has important implications for the evaluation and treatment of pain. First, it points to the importance of examining and treating the psychosocial factors associated with excessive pain behavior, emotional distress, and poor treatment response. Second, the model suggests that effective treatment of chronic pain conditions require the inclusion of diagnostic and treatment components to address these psychosocial sequelae of chronic pain.

Pain can be identified and produced from any anatomical site that is innervated. However, spine-related pain, in particular low back pain, is considered one of the archetypal chronic pain syndromes and is the most prevalent condition with which people present for conservative care. Much research has been conducted regarding psychosocial aspects of chronic low back pain. While the biopsychosocial model clearly implies an ongoing interaction of various factors, several will be discussed independently here. As noted previously, these are several of the most commonly observed barriers to optimal treatment outcome.

Clinical Pearl: Depression, anger, anxiety, and somatization (i.e., high pain sensitivity) are four broad emotional categories that have frequently been cited in the literature as being prevalent in the lives of patients with chronic pain.

Emotional Aspects

All chronic pain conditions can be associated with a wide range of affective experiences.[11] Depression, anger, anxiety, and somatization (i.e., high pain sensitivity) are four broad emotional categories that have frequently been cited in the literature as being prevalent in the lives of patients with chronic pain. While there remains debate regarding the etiology of such emotional states (i.e., which comes first, chronic pain or emotional distress in the forms discussed below), it is clear that consideration of such conditions is essential for understanding and effectively treating many chronic pain patients.

Depression Depression, or dysthymia, is perhaps the most frequently cited classification of emotional distress observed in patients with chronic pain.[12,13] In the United States, the mental health field uses the *Diagnostic and Statistical Manual for Mental Disorders*, Fourth Edition,[14] to determine whether individuals meet criteria for diagnoses of depressive disorders. From a psychiatric perspective, the criteria for a major depressive disorder can be found in Table 19–1.

Lindsay and Wyckoff[15] found that up to 85% of patients with chronic pain fit the diagnostic criteria for clinical depression. Interestingly, it has also been found that 39% of patients with chronic pain have a history of depression that precedes the onset of pain.[16] This suggests that with many depressed chronic pain patients, what clinicians are observing may be an exacerbation of a preexisting emotional disturbance. In addition, the fact that many of the symptoms or consequences of chronic pain are also found in depressed patients (e.g., sleep and appetite disturbance, concentration problems, and social withdrawal) is further evidence of the overlap between conditions. Following the biopsychosocial model, which posits an interaction between variables, it seems that depression and pain interact in such a way that a vulnerable patient enters a vicious cycle of ongoing pain, emotional difficulty, and decreased physical functioning, with each factor exacerbating the overall level of emotional distress and physical dysfunction. For instance, a person with a history of depression may develop a discopathy that causes persistent, daily pain. The individual could become limited with regard to daily activities, isolate himself or herself more frequently, and engage in a more sedentary lifestyle. This combination exacerbates the depressed mood and contributes to deconditioning, each of which exacerbates pain.

TABLE 19–1. Criteria for a Major Depressive Disorder According to the Diagnostic and Statistical Manual of Mental Disorders

A. Five or more of the following symptoms have been present during the same 2-week period and represent a change from previous functioning; at least one of the symptoms is either (1) depressed mood or (2) loss of interest or pleasure.*
   1. depressed mood most of the day, nearly every day, as indicated by either subjective report (e.g., feels sad or empty) or observation made by others (e.g., appears tearful)
   2. markedly diminished interest or pleasure in all, or almost all, activities most of the day, nearly every day (as indicated by either subjective account or observation by others)
   3. significant weight loss when not dieting or weight gain, or increase or decrease in appetite nearly every day
   4. insomnia or hypersomnia nearly every day
   5. psychomotor agitation or retardation nearly every day (observable by others, not merely subjective feelings of restlessness or being slowed down)
   6. fatigue or loss of energy nearly every day
   7. feelings of worthlessness or excessive or inappropriate guilt nearly every day
   8. diminished ability to think or concentrate, or indecisiveness, nearly every day
   9. recurrent thoughts of death (not just fear of dying), recurrent suicidal ideation without a specific plan, or a suicide attempt or a specific plan for committing suicide

B. The symptoms do not meet criteria for a mixed episode.

C. The symptoms cause clinically significant distress or impairment in social occupational or other important areas of functioning.

D. The symptoms are not due to the direct physiological effects of a substance (e.g., a drug of abuse, a medication) or a general medical condition (e.g., hypothyroidism).

E. The symptoms are not better accounted for by bereavement (i.e., after the loss of a loved one, the symptoms persist for longer than 2 months).

* Do not include symptoms that are clearly due to a general medical condition.

Clinical Pearl: Employees who placed blame for an injury on the employer had poorer pain treatment outcomes.

Anger Anger is another common emotional consequence of chronic pain with which individuals must cope. Fernandez et al.[17] report that 86% of patients with chronic pain seen in an outpatient setting experience anger that is of greater intensity than that reported by age-matched pain-free individuals. Often this anger is directed at insurance companies and the health-care system. In addition, among individuals who report work-related injuries and are treated through a workers' compensations insurance company, the incidence and expression of frustration and anger may be even greater, with patients frequently blaming the insurance carrier for their status. The target of the patient's anger is significant in that it may influence treatment outcome. DeGood and Kiernan[18] found that employees who placed blame for an injury on the employer had poorer pain treatment outcomes. These researchers also found that patients who made these attributions also had higher levels of mood disturbance than those who did not make such attributions. Turk and Fernandez[19] have suggested that patients who are angry, blame others for their difficulties, and are rebellious toward authority figures may respond more poorly to treatment because they fail to form a therapeutic alliance with the treatment team.

Anxiety Anxiety is another common emotional state observed and studied in patients with chronic pain.[20,21] In acute pain, many activities, including those that are pleasurable or neutral (i.e., neither desirable nor undesirable), may induce or exacerbate pain. Such activities are viewed as aversive and tend to be avoided; that is, fear of inducing or increasing pain level leads to avoidance of activities. This fear and avoidance can be generalized to an increasing number of activities, including simple motor behaviors (e.g., walking, sitting, standing), leisure activities, and sexual behavior, significantly contributing to self-limiting behavior in a number of areas (i.e., the person chooses to limit or restrict the behavior). In addition, anxiety is typically accompanied by activation of the sympathetic nervous system, with the resultant increased muscle tension and sympathetic activation serving to exacerbate existing pain conditions.[22] This can lead to increased avoidance of situations and activities in which the patient experiences anxiety and/or muscle tension, as the patient makes every effort to avert the increases in pain that invariably accompany them. As more activities are avoided, a person's motivation and stimulation can dwindle, with a sense of depression and worthlessness being exacerbated as well.

Somatization Somatization, or pain sensitivity, is arguably the most problematic emotional factor associated with chronic pain. Early psychological theories were presented regarding the role that psychological difficulties play in physical complaints when associated with minimal identifiable pathophysiology. Freud and others[23,24] argued that protracted physical complaints in the absence of identifiable physiological damage are the result of unconscious psychological or emotional conflicts being converted into physical complaints. This is the origin of the term *conversion disorder*. Although there is little direct evidence to support this,[25] there nevertheless exists a converging body of evidence demonstrating that a large proportion of patients with chronic pain may be excessively sensitive to pain.

First, studies using the Minnesota Multiphasic Personality Inventory (MMPI) indicate that the most common personality profile seen in patients with chronic pain involves elevations on the Hypochondriasis and Hysteria scales.[26] These scales typically indicate sensitivity to physical symptoms, disease conviction (i.e., strong, rigid belief that only medical factors modulate pain), a tendency for exacerbation of physical symptoms in times of stress, and denial of psychological problems.[27] Patients with such elevations on the MMPI typically respond poorly to both conservative treatment for chronic pain[28] and surgical intervention (see Chapter 35).[29,30]

Second, controlled research has documented the presence of excessive pain sensitivity in patients with chronic pain. For example, Schmidt[31] used a cold-pressor test (immersion of the forearm in an ice water bath) and found that patients with chronic pain reported higher levels of pain and tolerated the water for shorter periods of time than did a control group. Block et al. [32] found that MMPI elevations on the Hypochondriasis and Hysteria scales were associated with false-positive test reports of pain for patients undergoing provocative discography, a presurgical diagnostic test for disc herniation (see Chapter 17). Therefore, somatization is a characteristic that seems to contribute to the protracted nature of pain for many chronic pain patients.

Clinical Pearl: The ways in which spouses, family, friends, coworkers, and strangers respond to a person with chronic pain will have a tremendous impact on that individual through processes such as reinforcement and punishment.

Relationships

The primary relationships of a patient with chronic pain may be some of the most frequently overlooked aspects of his or her condition by primary care clinicians. In part, the occurrence and severity of depression that occurs in physical disorders such as chronic pain are associated with a lack of social support.[33] In addition, marital distress and conflict can contribute to poor adaptation to living with chronic pain.[34] The ways in which spouses, family, friends, coworkers, and strangers respond to a person with chronic pain will have a tremendous impact on that individual through processes such as reinforcement and punishment.

Seminal work recognizing and conceptualizing this phenomenon among patients with chronic pain is generally attributed to Fordyce.[35] According to this behavioral perspective, chronic pain sensation arises from nociception, but pain behavior may be maintained by reinforcement. Various factors can contribute to such reinforcement. For example, receiving increased attention from a spouse when pain is communicated through groaning or limping would tend to reinforce, or increase the likelihood, that such behavior continues. Similarly, disability or workers' compensation payments may serve to reinforce "sick-role" behavior, thus extending the length of disability and decreasing the likelihood that one will return to improved functional status as quickly as possible.

Besides the role that reinforcement plays in influencing pain behavior, patients with chronic pain also have to contend with lay people's ignorance of their condition and the ways in which pain can have a pervasive influence in different areas of life. Essentially, many people are not knowledgeable about chronic pain or the biopsychosocial model and therefore may not understand the ways in which pain, emotional distress, and other factors can interact with one another. Chronic pain is typically not observable by others. Many individuals with chronic pain have friends and family members who cannot comprehend the degree of pain with which the patient must cope on a daily basis. This, in turn, can lead to a greater sense of isolation and a perception by the patient that he or she is alone and without support. Add to this the fact that many people do not understand the ways in which pain, emotional distress, and other nonmedical factors can interact and exacerbate one another, and there exists the potential for even greater despondency, frustration, and social isolation for the individual with pain. Often patients perceive that others, including many of the health-care providers they have seen, believe them to be "faking it," embellishing their complaints, or that the pain is "all in their head." Such attributions, whether real or imagined, can negatively impact a person's mood, sense of social support, and trust in the health-care system.

Spousal ("Significant Other") Reinforcement Among the different relationships that people maintain, perhaps one of the most influential is that with one's spouse or "significant other." One's spouse has the opportunity to provide reinforcement and or punishment in response to pain-related behavior. Block et al.[36] demonstrated that spousal reinforcement might strongly impact pain behavior. Patients whose spouses were highly solicitous (i.e., provided frequent attention by offering to take over responsibilities or duties for the patient) reported higher pain levels in the presence of their spouse than in the presence of a ward clerk, whereas patients with minimally solicitous spouses did not demonstrate this. More recent research has shown that solicitous spouses may influence actual pain behavior.[37] In the presence of solicitous spouses, patients with chronic pain exhibit decreased walking time on a treadmill and have greater pain report than do patients with nonsolicitous spouses.

Conversely, an aggressive spouse and a more contentious spousal relationship can provoke chronic illness behavior. This may occur when one spouse feels the disabled spouse is no longer able to shoulder their share of the household duties, often feeling resentful for the added burden of work. Sociological and cultural stereotypical views may come into play, interfering with alternative household duties. For example, the disabled husband who always financially supported the family may resent the new role of "homemaker" while the wife goes to work, despite the fact that he is physically capable of performing these domestic duties. He may react to this perceived "demasculinization" in his status with aggressive behavior or by noting intolerable pain with such activity, further reinforcing his pain behavior.

Clinical Pearl: Patients who are injured on the job are often faced with at least some disincentive for improvement, for they typically receive worker's compensation benefits, including medical coverage and financial benefits in the form of supplementary income, while avoiding the rigors of actually working for such benefits.

Vocational Factors

Aspects of a person's employment status can negatively influence pain behavior by either reinforcing it or by serving as a disincentive for recovery. Factors such as job attitude, assignment of blame, and worker's compensation can all play a role in a patient's behavior. One often-cited study prospectively evaluated 3000 aircraft workers and found that workers with a high level of job dissatisfaction were 2.5 times more likely to incur a job-related back injury than workers who were satisfied with their jobs.[38] Once an injury has occurred, individuals who blame the employer for the injury tend to have greater mood disturbance and poorer pain treatment outcome than do patients who either refrain from assigning blame or else blame someone other than the employer.[18]

Patients who are injured on the job are often faced with at least some disincentive for improvement, for they typically receive worker's compensation benefits, including medical coverage and financial benefits in the form of supplementary income, while avoiding the rigors of actually working for such benefits. Patients receiving such benefits have been shown to have poorer treatment outcome for pain than patients who do not receive such benefits.[39,40] This has led to the conclusion that "compensability" is one of the strongest predictors of excessive disability among patients with chronic pain.[41] In a meta-analysis of studies of compensated patients, Rohling et al.[42] identified 32 studies that contained quantifiable data for treatment and control groups. The researchers concluded that compensation is related to increased reports of pain and reduced treatment efficacy. The results of this meta-analysis suggest that this relationship is likely causal and Rohling et al. statistically demonstrated that if compensation were eliminated as a variable, the experience of chronic pain would decrease by an average of 24%.

Once an individual is injured and/or physically limited such that he cannot perform the type of work to which he is accustomed, added suffering can occur.

For instance, many patients in this situation report feelings of worthlessness and low self-esteem, as they view their role as a worker and a provider, especially if they are the primary financial support of the family, as lost. The same can be said for the patient's role as a husband, wife, or parent. This can be a significant contributor to depression, fear about the future, and hopelessness. In addition, the financial implications for lost wages and, if disability status persists, lost benefits can be staggering to an individual and his or her family.

Impact on Children

Since many people with chronic pain are in their "employment years" and may have dependent children, it is important to briefly address some of the ways that a person's chronic pain and disability can impact both the patient and his/her children. In one scenario, the patient is spending more time at home, but is no longer able to play or interact with the children in a typical manner. It might be difficult, if not impossible, to lift, carry, or hold young children. Similarly, it can be difficult to engage in physically oriented activities, such as throwing a ball, athletics, camping, rough-and-tumble play, etc., with children of any age. Even a parent's ability to walk or stand for extended periods, as is required to go to the fair, zoo, or shop at the mall, is limited. These types of activities are then often avoided. When a patient experiences these types of hindrances in typical parent–child interactions, it can contribute to feelings of worthlessness, inadequacy as a parent, and depression, similar to the vicious cycle previously described. In addition, the parent may become more irritable and demonstrate significantly less frustration tolerance. When this occurs, there is a greater likelihood of the parent responding in a punishing manner to the children, or else avoiding interactions all together to prevent such a response.

Children can also observe and learn from the interaction among parents.[43] The typical stresses that occur in a relationship with chronic disability of one of the partners were already discussed. The parent who avoids unpleasant tasks or situations by retreating into the safe enclave of increased pain in the end teaches their child a strategy for avoiding disagreeable scenarios. In the same light, the parent who embellishes their pain with inappropriate body movement or moaning to underscore their suffering teaches their child how to demonstrate future illness for optimal effect. On a more generic level, it is important to understand that the parents and other influential persons in the maturing child's life serve as role models in a positive or negative way. Therefore, any of the above noted issues that briefly cover the psychosocial barriers to recovery can serve as veritable training sessions in the child's psyche for future chronicity when the opportunity arises in adulthood.

All of these factors can negatively impact a child's emotional development. In particular, childhood development suggests that young children (e.g., 5–10 years) are likely to internalize such interactions as evidence of their own inadequacy or unlovability. Thus, both the parent and the children can suffer as a result of chronic pain conditions. For clinicians, understanding the myriad ways that chronic pain can have a devastating impact in all areas of a person's life provides an opportunity to take a more holistic perspective in order to identify and address biopsychosocial components of chronic back pain.

Clinical Pearl: The way that a person thinks, his attitudes, and beliefs can all impact the overall presentation and treatment outcome.

Cognitive Factors

Thus far the focus has been on emotional and behavioral factors that influence pain. However, another major psychological phenomenon that needs to be addressed is cognitions. The way that a person thinks, his attitudes, and beliefs can all impact the overall presentation and treatment outcome. Two major areas of cognitions that have been researched are irrational beliefs and coping strategies.

Some patients hold irrational beliefs about pain (see Table 19–2). Such individuals may believe that a minor setback indicates the occurrence of a major injury (i.e., catastrophizing) or may erroneously attribute blame for an injury and its sequelae to themselves (i.e., personalizing). Similarly, some individuals have "emotional reasoning." This means that they believe that their feelings about the pain must be true simply because they believe them to be true. Such irrational beliefs about pain have been shown to be predictive of high pain levels, high levels of depression, and poor treatment outcome.[44,45]

Coping strategies refer to the specific thoughts or behaviors in which a person engages to manage pain or emotional reactions to pain.[46] One way to organize coping strategies is to divide them along three dimensions: conscious cognitive coping, self-efficacy, and pain avoidance. Conscious cognitive coping includes techniques such as ignoring the pain and using positive self-statements, such as "I can overcome the pain." Self-efficacy refers to an individual's perceived ability to control or decrease the pain. Pain avoidance includes hoping/praying that the pain will decrease without a plan for accomplishing such a reduction and praying. Research has shown that higher self-efficacy is frequently associated with lower pain intensity and enhanced physical functioning.[47] Pain avoidance has

TABLE 19–2. Several Types of Irrational Beliefs with Examples from Patients with Chronic Pain

1. *All-or-nothing thinking* (also referred to as black-and-white thinking): You view a situation in only two categories instead of on a continuum.
   Example: "If I cannot have complete pain relief, then treatment is a failure."
2. *Catastrophizing:* You predict the future negatively without considering other, more realistic outcomes.
   Example: "If my pain persists, I won't be able to do anything at all."
3. *Emotional reasoning:* You think something must be true simply because you "feel" (actually believe) it so strongly, while ignoring or discounting evidence to the contrary.
   Example: "I feel (believe) this treatment is going to cure my pain, so it must/will."
4. *Mind reading:* You believe you know what others are thinking, failing to consider other, more likely possibilities.
   Example: "My doctor referred me to a psychologist, he must think this pain is all in my head."
5. *Overgeneralization:* You make a sweeping negative conclusion that goes far beyond the current situation.
   Example: "Because I can't physically perform my previous job, I'm not able to perform any job."
6. *Personalization:* You believe you are the cause of some negative event over which you had no influence, without considering more plausible explanations for the event.
   Example: "My doctor spent only 15 minutes with me because he doesn't care about me."

been shown to be maladaptive and can lead to poorer treatment outcome.[48] Given the role that different cognitive coping styles can have on pain and response to treatment, it can be argued that this is yet another psychosocial factor that needs to be evaluated and addressed as part of a comprehensive evaluation of individuals with chronic pain.

The aforementioned studies highlight the important role that psychosocial factors play in transition from acute to chronic pain and in the maintenance and exacerbation of chronic pain conditions. Several reviews have summarized the results of many of the studies that address this topic. The National Advisory Committee on Health and Disability of New Zealand performed one such review. Kendall et al.[49] reviewed the literature related to acute low back pain patients developing a chronic and disabling condition and identified several psychosocial variables that place patients at risk for developing chronic problems (see Table 19–3). These variables have been collectively coined as "yellow flags" to emphasize their importance, just as "red flags" emphasize the serious disorders, including cancer, fractures, and systemic diseases (see Chapter 10).

TABLE 19–3. Categories of Psychosocial "Yellow Flags" with Examples of Each Category

1. Attitudes and beliefs about pain
   (a) fear avoidance—belief that activity will cause pain or injury
   (b) catastrophizing
   (c) belief that pain is uncontrollable
   (d) belief that pain must be eliminated before normal activity can be attempted
2. Behaviors
   (a) substance abuse history or excessive medication use
   (b) reduced participation in or withdrawal from activities of daily life
   (c) avoidance
   (d) use of extended rest
   (e) sleep quality reduced since onset of pain
   (f) history of noncompliance or "doctor shopping"
3. Compensation
   (a) lack of financial incentive to return to work
   (b) history of ineffective case management
   (c) disputes regarding compensation
4. Diagnosis and treatment
   (a) sanctioning of disability by health professionals
   (b) conflicting diagnoses
   (c) diagnoses leading to catastrophizing and fear
   (d) lack of satisfaction with previous treatment
   (e) advice to withdraw from daily activities or work
5. Emotion
   (a) depression
   (b) fear of pain or disability
   (c) anxiety of heightened awareness of body sensations
   (d) stress
6. Family
   (a) overprotecting partner
   (b) solicitous behavior by partner
   (c) socially punitive responses
   (d) history of abuse
   (e) history of model for chronic pain behavior
7. Work
   (a) belief that work is harmful
   (b) unsupportive or unhappy work environment
   (c) negative experience of management or absence of interest from employer

While the aforementioned variables may be common material for the mental health professional, consideration of evaluating patients in terms of the multitude of psychosocial factors that may play a role in their presentation to the primary care clinic may seem a daunting task to the nonmental health specialists. However, it is not necessary for such health-care professionals to assess for all of these factors. Rather, a basic understanding of the types of variables that may be present and a plan of assessment supply the clinician with the tools necessary to address such potential problems.

CLINICIAN'S GUIDE TO ASSESSING PSYCHOSOCIAL RISK FACTORS

Once familiar with many of the psychosocial risk factors that can contribute to chronicity and poor treatment outcome, the clinician's first step is to inquire about the most common risk factors that are considered "yellow flags." Following identification of risk factors, they need to be addressed clinically. While aspects of this can and should be initially accomplished by the primary health-care provider,[2] there will be times a referral to a mental health professional, with training and experience in behavioral medicine, will be indicated. However, it can be argued that the responsibility for attending to these risk factors and for monitoring for their presence over time falls on the patient's clinician, who usually has the greatest access to the patient and serves as the "gatekeeper" for pain-related treatment. Assessments of the types of risk factors that are both clinically relevant and lend themselves to relatively easy identification are discussed next. While the other factors identified in this text are important as well, the domains discussed here lend themselves to relatively straightforward assessment.

Clinical Pearl: The responsibility for attending to these risk factors and for monitoring for their presence over time falls on the patient's clinician, who usually has the greatest access to the patient and serves as the "gatekeeper" for pain-related treatment.

Assessment

One option for assessing for many of these risk factors is to incorporate questions into either the initial intake paperwork or else into the initial patient interview. For example, inquiring about depression, anger, anxiety, attribution of blame (especially in work-related injuries or accidents), and the quality of spousal relationships would be valuable information to obtain. Having the patient rate each emotion on a scale from 0 to 10 could assess depression, anger, and anxiety. Attribution of blame and work-related attitudes could be determined by either an open-ended question (e.g., "I blame my pain on __________" or "Please describe the good and bad parts of your work") or else a forced choice response (e.g., "I blame my pain on [choose one or more]: (a) my boss; (b) workplace conditions; (c) myself; (d) God; (e) there's no one to blame, it just happened."). The current nature of the marital relationship could be addressed with a single question (e.g., "I consider my relationship with my spouse/significant other to be: (a) excellent; (b) good; (c) adequate; (d) poor").

TABLE 19–4. Waddell's Tests for Nonorganic Signs of Low Back Pain

1. Tenderness
   (a) Superficial—pain in response to light pinch of the skin
   (b) Nonanatomical—deep tenderness distributed over an area too wide to be localized to one source
2. Stimulation
   (a) Axial loading—low back pain when pressing on patient's head
   (b) Rotation—low back pain when rotating shoulders and pelvis
3. Distraction
   (a) Straight-leg raise—pain experienced when tested formally, but not when tested with distraction
4. Regional disturbances
   (a) Weakness—"giving away" of muscles that cannot be explained on localized, neurological basis
   (b) Sensory—diminished sensation to pinprick or light touch in a nonneurological pattern
5. Overreaction
   (a) The observation of excessive verbalization, facial expression, or other overly dramatic behaviors

Somatization tendencies refer to high pain sensitivity. Paying close attention and evaluating for symptom magnification during the physical evaluation could be helpful here. Waddell et al.[50] identified a set of five "nonorganic signs" (the so-called Waddell signs) that can indicate a patient is being strongly influenced by factors other than the nociception generated by damaged tissue (see Table 19–4). While it can be argued that one or more of these signs could serve as a false-positive indicator, the presence of three or more is generally considered clinically significant and suggests there are nonmedical psychosocial issues that need to be addressed. Similarly, paying close attention to the presence of exaggerated pain behaviors and looking for potential inconsistencies from one environment to another (e.g., pain behavior is different in the waiting room than during the examination) would be helpful as well.

Histories of substance abuse and/or evidence that a patient is using medications excessively (i.e., beyond the recommended dosage or frequency) are important risk factors to identify. At times, a warning sign that this may be occurring can be seen by a history of "doctor shopping." A history of noncompliance or frequent changes in treating physicians should be considered a yellow flag regardless of whether or not a patient has a history of substance abuse. Finally, whenever the patient is involved in pending litigation related to the injury/pain or the patient is receiving worker's compensation benefits, these should also be considered risk factors for poor outcome.

For clinicians who are interested in taking a slightly more detailed approach to the assessment of emotional distress so that the data gathered are more precise and measurable, consideration of assessment self-report questionnaires is recommended. For example, the Symptom Checklist 90-Revised (SCL-90-R)[51] is a brief self-report questionnaire that covers an array of symptoms clusters, including depression, anxiety, hostility, and somatization. It takes less than 15 minutes for most individuals to complete it and can be scored on a computer, with a profile generated upon completion of scoring. The profile contains standardized scores in the aforementioned domains and includes normative data from a sample of patients seeking outpatient treatment. This allows for assessment with less chance of "overpathologizing" patients' complaints. For instance, it is normal for a person with a medical problem to report some degree of somatic and emotional symptoms. Comparing a chronic pain patient's results to other outpatients enables the clinician to be more confident that any emotional distress identified is not the result of typical symptoms, but rather a result of symptoms in excess of what other individuals with medical health problems report. In addition, the SCL-90-R has been shown to be sensitive to change in clinical status[52,53] and patients generally do not object to completing the questionnaire.[54] Therefore, it can potentially be used as an outcome measure for assessing change in emotional status over the course of treatment. If a patient scores above a T-score of 65 on any of the aforementioned scales, this suggests significant distress in that area and thus consideration of a referral to a behavioral medicine specialist would be warranted. In addition, repeated administration and comparison of scores (i.e., before and after procedures or other aspects of treatment) can provide information as to whether identified domains of emotional distress are changing in a desired direction. When scores remain elevated, or else when scores become elevated, during the course of medical treatment, a referral to a mental health specialist should be strongly considered.

Another brief self-report questionnaire that can be used as a screening instrument is the Pain Patient Profile (P-3).[55] The P-3 is a 44-item self-report, multiple-choice measure designed to help identify patients who are experiencing emotional distress associated with a primary complaint of pain. This measure takes less than 15 minutes to complete and is designed for use with patients experiencing pain as a result of physical trauma (e.g., motor vehicle accident or work-related injury), disease, or illness. The P-3 has a validity indicator and three clinical scales: Depression, Anxiety, and Somatization. Thus, it is similar to the SCL-90-R in that it focuses on several of the primary emotional domains discussed in this text. The P-3 was "normed" on a sample of patients with pain. Therefore, elevations on one or more of the scales suggest emotional distress in excess of what is typically seen in patients with pain and indicate there may be a need to address that atypical area of functioning. When a patient elevates two or more scales, a referral to a behavioral medicine specialist is recommended. The benefits of this measure include a presentation of results in a one-page summary sheet that is easy to understand, with graphic comparisons of the patient's scores to the normative sample and to a nonpain community sample. Once the measure is used to establish a clinical baseline, the measure can subsequently be used to monitor a patient's progression over time.

Clinical Pearl: Being familiar with the basic types of psychosocial issues that may be present in a patient allows the primary health-care provider to express an understanding to the patient that such phenomena exist, are real, and are important.

Addressing the Psychosocial Factors

Even before identifying potential psychosocial risk factors for poor outcome, clinicians can do much to address the impact that these variables can have on pain developing into a chronic state. Being familiar with the basic types of psychosocial issues that may be present in a patient allows the primary health-care provider to express an understanding to the patient that such phenomena exist, are real, and are important. *As opposed to avoiding or minimizing such variables, they should be normalized.* This can be accomplished through either printed materials or direct conversation that address the "normalcy" of experiencing any of the aforementioned psychosocial sequelae to pain, including the emotional distress and the impact on relationships that often occurs when living with pain. Some clinicians may even opt to provide each new patient with a brief letter of introduction to these topics (see Table 19–5). This helps patients feel more "normal" in their experiences, reduces the anxiety that the awareness of these factors produces, and assists in rapport building between physician and patient, as the patient then recognizes that the clinician has a fuller understanding of the various ways that chronic pain impacts a person's overall quality of life. In addition, in the event that referral to a behavioral medicine specialist is made, the patient will be less likely to interpret this as a sign that the referring physician believes the patient's pain is "all in his head" or that the patient "is crazy."

Primary health-care providers can also potentially improve patient outcomes by addressing specific aspects of the patients' functioning prior to them becoming chronic. Education and information can help to address some of the emotional aspects of pain,

TABLE 19–5. Sample Letter of Introduction for Behavioral Medicine Evaluation

Behavioral Medicine Evaluation

Pain is more than just an unpleasant sensation. It is a condition that can affect much of a person's existence. Patients may become depressed, angry, or tense. Dependency on others may increase, and interpersonal and marital difficulties may arise. As pain continues, the combination of emotional, physical, and financial problems can lead to increased difficulties in coping, thus making recovery from pain more difficult.

It is widely recognized that physical injuries can have devastating effects. Therefore, physicians routinely refer patients to a psychologist with expertise in addressing problems related to chronic pain.

What a behavioral medicine evaluation means—and what it does not mean:
A visit with a psychologist does not mean that the pain is imaginary or "all in your head". It is not a sign of weakness. Rather, most patients welcome the opportunity to talk about the case with a professional in order to help:

- Discover that many other individuals experience similar frustrations
- Find ways of overcoming depression or other emotional conditions associated with pain.
- Find ways of reducing pain and stress without excessive medication.
- Maximize your opportunities for recovery from surgery or rehabilitation.

What is the evaluation like?
The evaluation normally consists of an interview and the administration of brief questionnaires. In the interview you will be asked about your feelings and emotions; problems you may have had coping with the injury or pain; family problems that may have developed; your strengths and weaknesses; your personal, educational, and work goals; stressors in your life; and questions you may have regarding your condition.

You may have some concerns about confidentiality. You can feel certain that any issues you discuss with a psychologist will be treated with the utmost respect for your privacy. If you are covered by workers' compensation insurance, your insurance carrier is entitled to copies of any written reports. Therefore, please let us know if you wish to keep certain topics out of any written report. No other outside agency or physician may receive copies of your report unless you provide written approval to do so.

There will be a charge for the evaluation, which includes interpretation of the findings and preparation of a written report.

What about insurance coverage?
Insurance companies generally understand and appreciate the role of psychology, yet vary in terms of reimbursement for these services. If you have any questions about your insurance coverage for a behavioral medicine evaluation, please contact your carrier or our office.

If you have further questions regarding this service, please do not hesitate to contact our office at (800) 555-XXXX.

especially anxiety, fear, and beliefs about an injury. For example, in addition to performing thorough examinations, providing considerable information regarding the course of illness, treatment, and functional goals can help to reduce fear and debunk false beliefs about injury. Several studies demonstrating the effectiveness of early prevention included a strong educational/informational component to the intervention.[56,57] In addition, recommending maintenance of daily activities can be quite beneficial. In a review of the literature, Waddell et al.[58] found that advice to continue typical activities and stay active, despite the presence of pain, consistently results in a faster return to work, less disability, and fewer recurrent problems than "treatment as usual" without such emphasis.

The algorithm in Figure 19–2 was created to assist with conceptualization of the process of identification and treatment of psychosocial risk factors. Since many patients will present with acute problems that can be remedied within a short time frame, it is not necessary to extensively evaluate each patient's psychological functioning upon the initial visit. However, including certain "yellow flag" questions in the intake forms as described above and looking for dramatic adjectives when describing pain can help clinicians identify those patients who could then be administered a psychological screening measure on the next visit. As can be seen, the authors recommend that the comprehensive evaluation include assessment and regular reassessment of medical and psychosocial risk factors for poor outcome. The risk factors that can be readily identified through interview and observations by the primary health-care provider have been discussed previously and are identified under the title *Medical/Physical Examination*. In addition, tools to assess major domains of emotional distress are covered under the title *Assessment of Emotional Risk Factors*. In all cases, it is recommended that emphasis be placed on education and information, normalizing the patient's

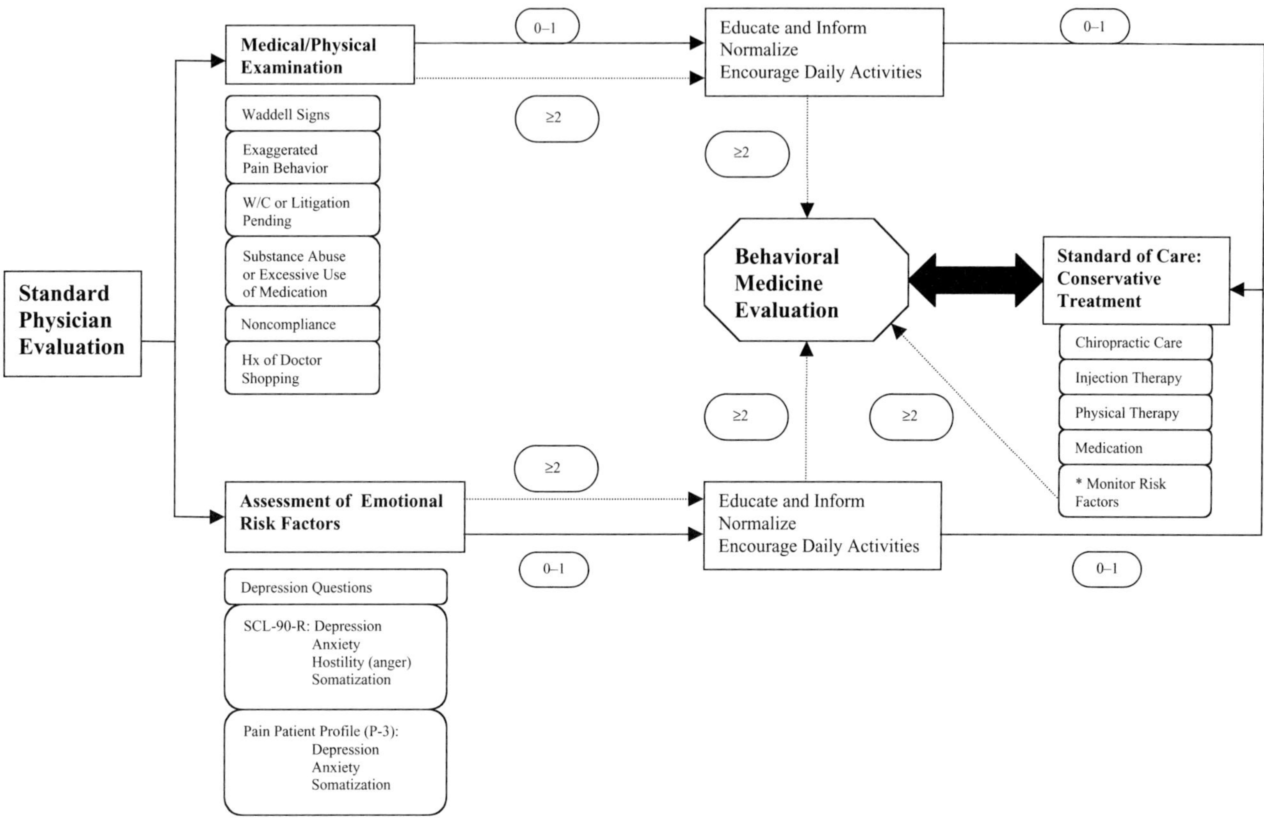

FIGURE 19–2. Algorithm for assessment of psychological risk factors and referral.

experience, and encouraging maintenance of typical daily activities, as such emphasis is likely to improve treatment outcome and reduce the risk of emotional distress.

Once a patient is identified as possessing one or more psychosocial risk factors for poor outcome, the next question the clinician must answer is: "What do I do now?" For those patients who present with minimal (i.e., 0–1) psychosocial risk factors, the standard conservative treatment is likely sufficient, with continued normalization and monitoring of these risk factors. If the patient's psychosocial status changes such that additional risk factors are identified over time, then referral for a behavioral medicine evaluation is warranted. Likewise, if the severity of the risk factors identified appears to be a major obstacle to positive treatment response, then referral would again be appropriate.

Clinical Pearl: Any major psychosocial risk factors that are identified should be addressed with a treatment plan whose intention is to minimize those factors so that the optimal *global* treatment response can be achieved.

If a patient has two or more such risk factors, the authors suggest that consideration of a referral to a mental health professional is warranted. Ideally, this referral should go to a professional with training in behavioral medicine and who has experience working with patients with chronic pain. The mental health professional should be licensed and be able to demonstrate a working knowledge of the basic medical aspects of chronic pain conditions. Before making a referral to mental health clinicians, it might be helpful to ask them to share their experience in working with patients with low back pain.

Once the referral has been made, it can be expected that the behavioral medicine specialist will evaluate the patient, often using both personal interview and psychometric testing, to more fully examine the presence and severity of the aforementioned psychosocial risk factors for poor outcome, and then communicate the results of this evaluation to the referring clinician. Any major psychosocial risk factors that are identified should be addressed with a treatment plan whose intention is to minimize those factors so that the optimal *global* treatment response can be achieved. In this manner, the referral to a mental health professional should not be viewed as "bouncing" the patient, but rather as an opportunity to acquire adjunctive expertise so that the functional restoration goals can be achieved as efficiently as possible. Most patients will typically also be participating in traditional conservative treatment, as indicated in the algorithm by the heavily shaded arrow between the behavioral medicine consultation and standard of care. In this way, patients are participating in both modalities, utilizing the behavioral medicine treatment to help optimize conservative treatment outcome. While the specific psychological treatment techniques used in these cases are beyond the scope of this text, in general the referring clinician should expect that the majority of behavioral medicine interventions will be relatively time-limited (e.g., 4–12 sessions versus years of psychological therapy), with a focus on cognitive-behavioral treatments.

In all cases, the intensity and duration of intervention by the behavioral medicine specialist will vary depending on the type and severity of psychological disturbances and psychosocial risk factors identified. In some cases, this intervention might be minimal, requiring only 1–2 sessions to address a problem, such as fears about a procedure based on misconceptions and irrational beliefs (i.e., thinking errors). In other cases, where there is a moderate degree of psychosocial disturbance, the mental health provider could work with the patient once a week for several weeks while the patient is involved in conservative care treatment. In extreme cases, in which the degree of psychopathology is severe and there are a large number of psychosocial risk factors, it is conceivable that the majority of intervention offered to the patient could be more psychologically oriented.

Besides involvement by the behavioral medicine specialist, there will likely be times when it is also necessary to refer to a specialist who can manage psychotropic medications. Obviously, this referral can be made by the primary health-care provider, but it can also be initiated by the psychologist. This referral is most likely to occur when a patient presents with significant psychological distress across several domains, such as a person with a long history of depression, who is experiencing panic attacks and appears to have become addicted to one or more substances.

Clinical Pearl: Ideally, in treatment settings where a team of specialists provides care, regular staffing meetings, in which treatment plans and pertinent issues of patient care are discussed, can be quite helpful in achieving outcome goals.

While it may be obvious, it is important to note that patient outcome is going to be impacted by communication among clinicians. Even when there are only two health-care providers involved in patient care, communication is important. As the complexity of a patient's care increases, this communication becomes imperative for successful outcome. This typically can occur through either telephone updates, if time permits, or else through regular provision of progress notes to update one another on the treatment goals and response to treatment. Ideally, in treatment settings where a team of specialists provides care, regular staffing meetings, in which treatment plans and pertinent issues of patient care are discussed, can be quite helpful in achieving outcome goals.

Patients present with varying levels of psychosocial risk factors that serve as potential barriers to functional improvement and response to medical treatment. This text attempts to provide a relatively straightforward paradigm for conceptualizing the primary health-care professionals' role in assessing and addressing such risk. The conservative care clinician's primary responsibility is to make the initial assessment, educate, inform, normalize, monitor for changes over time, and then refer to a behavioral medicine specialist, as indicated. Subsequently, the recommendations made by the behavioral medicine specialist will be dependent upon the results of a more thorough biopsychosocial evaluation.

Clinical Pearl: The conservative care clinician's primary responsibility is to make the initial assessment, educate, inform, normalize, monitor for changes over time, and then refer to a behavioral medicine specialist, as indicated.

Practical Utilization: Scenarios and Case Studies

What follows are descriptions of several typical scenarios, based on the type and severity of psychosocial risk factors, that are likely to occur. These scenarios can be thought of as lying on a continuum from least to greatest involvement of psychosocial risk factors. A case study for each scenario is included to elucidate the potential role of the psychologist and the interplay of medical and psychologically oriented treatments.

Scenario 1: In the simplest of cases, the patient presents to the clinic and is assessed in a typical fashion. As with many patients who have been living in pain for many months, a patient may present with two or more risk factors for poor outcome and therefore be referred for a behavioral medicine consultation, as indicated in Figure 19–2. If the results of the behavioral medicine evaluation indicate that the psychosocial risk factors are limited to those identified, then it may be that no additional psychological treatment is recommended, but rather the patient is maintained solely in clinician recommended conservative care that is appropriate for his or her particular condition.

Case Study 1: The patient is a 59-year-old male who had fractured his left ankle in a work-related injury. He had undergone surgery to repair the fracture. A steel plate was inserted with hardware. Postsurgical evaluation by the referring physician indicated that the left ankle showed remarkable loss of range of motion with rather significant swelling and tenderness circumferentially. The left knee was modestly tender as would be noticed with early chondromalacia or patellofemoral syndrome. Examination of the spine was normal, except for the lumbar facets, which were somewhat irritable as noted on extension, lateral bending, and rotation. The right sacroiliac joint was deranged as noted on Gillette's, Gaenslen's, sacral thrust, Thomas', Patricks', and march tests. The physician noted that this was not surprising given the avoidance of weight bearing on the left lower extremity. Diagnoses by his physician included complex regional pain syndrome, type I (CRPS type I) of the left ankle, lumbar spondylosis, and right sacroiliac joint dysfunction. The presence of depression was noted by subjective rating, as were concerns (i.e., anxiety) about his future employability and finances. In addition, since this was a work-related injury, it was a worker's compensation case. The patient was referred for behavioral medicine evaluation to more fully examine the psychosocial sequelae of his injury.

Two weeks prior to the behavioral medicine evaluation, the patient received a selective nerve root block with transforaminal epidural steroid injection under C-arm fluoroscopy. He stated that this significantly helped reduce the pain in his left lower extremity, although now he was experiencing constant numbness in that area. He had also been using a muscle stimulator to treat the lumbar pain. The patient denied other significant medical complaints. Current medications included Bextra (for inflammation and pain), Topamax, Zanaflex, and Effexor. The patient had no history of substance abuse nor did he smoke cigarettes.

Work history indicated that the patient had worked for 20 years for a local city agency. He indicated that he enjoyed his work and that it was "a good job." At the time of this evaluation, he was receiving worker's compensation benefits in the form of medical treatment. He had returned to work in a light duty capacity full-time. Family history indicated that the patient had been divorced for approximately 7 years, following a 6-year marriage. He stated that he had three daughters, aged 12, 11, and 8 years. His daughters lived with their mother, but he had full visitation on the weekends. He also had two siblings that were supportive.

The claimant reported that his mood was generally "normal," but that he had been worried about his finances. His affect (i.e., outward expression of emotion) was bright and consistent with an euthymic (i.e., normal, nondepressed) mood. He indicated that he was sleeping well and that the current medications had improved his sleep. He denied significant problems with short-term memory or concentration. He also noted that his appetite had been good and his energy was adequate during the day. He denied suicidal ideation and did not appear to meet criteria for a mood disturbance. Along these lines, he had no history of psychiatric treatment. Psychometric testing confirmed that the patient was free of significant psychopathology, as measured by the SCL-90-R. In addition, testing demonstrated that he perceived himself to have a moderate degree of control over his pain and that he used a number of adaptive coping strategies, including ignoring the pain and changing his thoughts when in pain. Testing revealed that he did not tend to catastrophize when in pain.

As can be seen in the above report, the patient presented with relatively few of the psychosocial risk factors for poor treatment outcome. Therefore, the recommendations following this evaluation were limited to continuation of conservative treatment, with regular monitoring of his psychosocial status. No psychological follow-up was scheduled, but the patient was encouraged to contact either his physician or the psychologist who performed the evaluation should he notice a significant deterioration in his mood or coping abilities. Likewise, the patient's physician was informed of the same and encouraged to refer the patient back for additional evaluation if his status should decline significantly.

Scenario 2: A second scenario would be one in which the results of the behavioral medicine evaluation indicate that there are a moderate number and severity of psychosocial risk factors that require attention. In such cases, the psychologist might recommend several sessions of behavioral medicine intervention in order to address these risk factors. Oftentimes, cognitive-behavioral treatment, which focuses on short-term, time-limited solution or problem-solving approaches, would be introduced in order to help the patient learn more effective means of coping with both their chronic pain and any emotional distress that is present. At the same time, the patient would continue to participate in standard medical treatment, receiving whatever medications, injections, and other treatment or combinations of treatments that are deemed most appropriate by his or her primary care clinician. The goal in such a scenario would be to help minimize the impact of psychosocial risk factors on the patient's presentation, thus removing barriers to optimal response to medical treatment.

Case Study 2: The patient is a 34-year-old female who presented at a pain management physician's office with complaints of cervical pain, migraines, and lumbar pain that had lasted for approximately 6–7 months. Medical records indicated a history of three motor vehicle accidents 6 years previous. Several physicians, who found no definable diagnosis, had evaluated her within the past 6 months. She had not responded to previous treatment with short-acting narcotic medication. The referring physician's evaluation of her cervical region indicated extreme tenderness along the greater occipital nerve root, positive spring test at C3, C5, and C7, and paraspinal muscle spasticity with scattered myofascial trigger points. There was positive spring at T12, L3, L4, and L5, with tenderness along the L2–L3 and L3–L4 lumbar facet joints bilaterally. At the time of behavioral medicine evaluation, pain-related medical diagnoses included cervicogenic headache, cervical spondylosis without myelopathy, bilateral greater occipital neuralgia, and cervical intervertebral disk disruption.

The physician observed her to be quite tearful. She expressed hopelessness and anxiety about her physical status and lack of response to previous treatment. The clinician also observed a moderate degree of dramatic responses in regards to pain. Therefore, she was referred for a behavioral medicine evaluation for more thorough evaluation of the role that depression, anxiety, and potential somatization were playing in her overall presentation, with appropriate treatment recommendations.

The patient indicated that approximately 6 months previous she began to experience pain in her cervical and lumbar regions, along with tingling and numbness in her right hand. Apparently, following evaluation by several different physicians, it was determined that she had been bitten just prior to the onset of these symptoms by what was determined to be a black widow spider. Following multiple bites, she spent 3 days in the hospital and she reported that she experienced numerous neurological difficulties, including problems with memory, tremors, as well as sleep disturbance. She also noted that she had been experiencing migraine headaches for the past 5–6 months, with each one lasting approximately 3–4 days. At one point during the previous multiple medical evaluations, prior to the determination that a black widow spider bit her, she had been diagnosed with fibromyalgia.

Prior to the behavioral medicine evaluation, she had been involved in physical therapy and had been undergoing passive rehabilitative physiotherapeutic modalities, including the use of a muscle stimulator. On the day of her psychological evaluation, she rated her pain level as a 7 on a scale of 0–10. Although she exhibited continuous bracing and guarding behavior (i.e., movement patterns and posture), this pain rating was somewhat higher than would have been expected given her overall presentation. Current medications included Topamax, Zanaflex, Darvocet, and Effexor. She had no history of substance abuse or any significant psychiatric history. She noted that prior to her current medication regimen, she would go for several days without sleeping. With the current medications, she was sleeping approximately 6 hours per night.

Brief family history indicated that the patient was a homemaker and was involved in homeschooling her children. She reported that she had four children, aged 14, 11, 6, and 4 years of age. She stated that she had been married for the past 6 years and that her husband had been supportive during this episode of chronic pain. However, she noted that he had been worried about her and agitated with the misdiagnoses and the slow pace at which she received treatment. As noted previously, it had been 6 months from the time of pain onset until the behavioral medicine evaluation. Similarly, she began treatment with her current physician 5 months post-pain onset. In addition to her chronic pain, she identified additional major stressors that included raising her four children and taking care of an uncle with Alzheimer's disease and Parkinson's disease.

The patient described her mood as depressed and irritable. Her affect was tearful and consistent with dysthymic/depressed mood. As noted previously, she experienced significant sleep disturbance for the past 6 months, although her current medications seemed to be helping with sleep. She endorsed significant problems with both short-term memory and attention/concentration for the past 6 months. She described her energy as "sluggish, but functional." She indicated no major changes with her appetite and she denied suicidal ideation. In addition, she noted that she was experiencing a significant sense of worthlessness and uselessness since this episode of pain and migraine headaches had begun.

Behavioral medicine treatment recommendations for this patient included primarily cognitive-behavioral therapy, with a focus on enhancing her ability to cope with pain and depression. In particular, it was recommended that the patient undergo relaxation training and behavioral modification techniques in order to enhance her ability to complete daily activities without exacerbating pain (i.e., pacing). In addition, special attention was focused on enhancing her sense of control and self-efficacy. This information was communicated to the treating physician and it was recommended that conservative treatment continue as planned. Along these lines, the fact that the patient's sleep had improved significantly with current medications was communicated to the physician as well.

The patient returned approximately 3 weeks after the initial evaluation to begin treatment. At the onset of this follow-up session, she rated her pain level as a 6 and her stress level as a 4, each on a scale of 0–10. She was provided a brief educational component to explain how relaxation training works and the ways in which a stress/pain response affects a person's physiological functioning. Subsequently, she was taught several relaxation techniques, including diaphragmatic breathing, autogenic training, and visual imagery. At the conclusion of this treatment, the claimant shed several tears and reported that she had experienced significant relief. She also noted that this was the first time she had felt such relief from pain since this episode began several months previous. She rated her pain level as a 3 and the stress level as a 0; thus she had achieved elimination of the stress level and a 50% reduction in pain. Interestingly, the patient noted that although she felt relieved, she was experiencing a fair degree of guilt secondary to her perception that in some way, she did not deserve to "take a break" and treat herself to the relaxation. Brief cognitive techniques were used to help reframe the use of relaxation as a means of taking care of herself in order to enhance her efficacy with taking care of others, such as her children and husband. Subsequently, within the context of the same session, additional relaxation and imagery/self-hypnotic work was done to assist with reducing the pain. At the conclusion, she reported that she experienced equitable levels of stress relief compared to the first exercise, the pain was lowered and quite tolerable, and she was free of guilt as well. She was encouraged to use these techniques over the course of the next 2 weeks and then return for follow-up.

She was unable to return for the second session until 4 weeks later. At that session, she noted that she had been able to use these techniques effectively on her own. She also reported that she perceived she was coping more effectively with pain and that her mood had improved significantly (i.e., less depression, hopelessness, and anxiety). In addition, she noted improved interactions with family members and increased participation in daily activities. At the second session, the relaxation/self-hypnosis work was repeated to reinforce and enhance her abilities with self-regulation (e.g., self-efficacy). She was able to gain a favorable response similar to the first session. She was scheduled for a third session, but had to cancel it because of a family vacation. Her care is still ongoing, and she was encouraged to return on an "as needed" basis. In the meantime, we anticipate that she will be able to receive optimal benefit from the conservative care she currently receives (i.e., injections and supervised physical therapy) and, ultimately, require significantly less use of medications in order to manage her pain.

Scenario 3: A third scenario would be one in which, following the behavioral medicine evaluation, it is determined that there are numerous psychosocial barriers for recovery, such that the patient is not likely to be able to benefit from typical conservative medical treatment without substantial reduction in the psychosocial barriers. In such instances, the recommendation would be that the primary focus of treatment initially shifts to psychosocial domains, with specific recommendations determined by the particular risk factors with which the patient presents. In such cases, the goal would be to treat these symptoms so that these obstacles or barriers could be minimized or even removed. In addition, the patient would be consistently monitored and reevaluated to determine the point at which these factors had been minimized such that the patient is more able to benefit from standard care. Often, with such patients, it is recommended that nonpsychosocial treatment be limited to the most conservative means available, with more invasive procedures being postponed until the patient has been stabilized from the standpoint of minimizing psychosocial risk factors for poor treatment outcome.

Case Study 3: The patient is a 61-year-old female who had been wheelchair-bound for approximately 3 years secondary to chronic ischemic problems in her lower extremities. The patient's medical history was positive for chronic obstructive pulmonary disease, reflux, Hepatitis B, diverticulitis, hypertension, severe peripheral vascular disease, and atherosclerotic coronary artery disease. Physician evaluation of the spine identified bilateral greater occipital nerve tenderness, bilateral paraspinal muscle tightness and scattered myofascial trigger points in the cervical and lumber regions, as well as bilateral sacroiliac joint dysfunction that was more severe on the left than on the right. Pain-related diagnoses included CRPS type I of the left lower extremity, status post acute ischemic injury, bilateral sacral iliac dysfunction, and spondylosis of the cervical and lumber spine without myelopathy. She had a long history of depression for which she had been under the care of a psychiatrist and counselor for approximately 10 years. In addition to depression, the clinician noted inconsistencies that suggested exaggerated pain behavior. The patient was initially referred for behavioral medicine evaluation as a part of a comprehensive evaluation for her candidacy for a spinal cord stimulator trial to treat cervical and upper left extremity pain. Given the presence of several risk factors for poor outcome, the referring physician requested assistance with determination of her psychosocial readiness for surgery.

Two days prior to the behavioral medicine evaluation, the patient apparently had engaged in unusual and strange behavior that was potentially dangerous to her. Her daughter, who accompanied her to the appointment, reported that she discovered the patient repeatedly attempting to drive her automatic wheelchair through a doorway in her house that was not wide enough to accommodate it. It was discovered later that another physician had prescribed a new medication recently and she was experiencing what was determined to be delirium. Fortunately, a home health nurse had identified the onset of the delirium-based behavior as occurring subsequent to the addition of new medication and she recommended discontinuation of it. This appeared to be assisting with clearing of the symptoms.

On the day of the behavioral medicine evaluation, the patient's thinking was still clouded and she was experiencing significant difficulties with attention and short-term memory. She also noted that she had no memory of events from the past several days, including the events 2 days prior. She indicated that she was coping with several recent stressors related to family situations. In addition, she identified a long history of emotional and physical abuse, as well as the death of her son 1 year prior. She presented with exaggerated pain behaviors, and the issue of potential excessive medication use had been introduced as well. At the psychological evaluation, her affect was especially tearful and labile. She endorsed depressed mood, but indicated that her depressed mood had been under control until approximately 3 months prior to the past week. Along with depressed mood, the claimant endorsed severe sleep disturbance, decreased energy, poor appetite, problems with attention and concentration, and problems with short-term memory. She denied suicidal ideation. While psychometric testing was not performed on the day of this evaluation because of the patient's cognitive status, the psychologist's opinion was that she presented with a high degree of pain sensitivity (i.e., somatization).

As noted above, the patient presented with a substantial medical history and it was discovered that four different physicians were prescribing her medications for the various conditions. While this was not a case of "doctor shopping" and the patient was not receiving pain medications from more than one physician, nevertheless it was determined that there had been little communication amongst these physicians and this was seen as a contributing factor to the recent delirium. In addition, the patient expressed concerns about the number of medications she was taking and indicated that she desired to decrease them as much as possible.

Given the patient's mental status at the time of evaluation and the numerous psychosocial barriers to optimal treatment response that had been identified during the evaluation, it was recommended that a decision to pursue a trial of spinal cord stimulation therapy be placed on hold pending the outcome of behavioral medicine intervention and medical stabilization of the patient. Along these lines, the recommendation was made that the referring physician, in this case the pain management physician, take the lead role in coordinating the prescription efforts of the various physicians involved in the patient's care. In addition, the patient's concerns regarding the number of medications she was taking was communicated to the physician, so that every effort could be made to adhere to her wishes to minimize these.

As noted previously, the claimant had a 10-year history of depression. However, since she was receiving treatment from a psychiatrist and counselor and the depression had been well controlled until the past week, no effort was made to provide additional services for the depression. However, feedback was given to both the psychiatrist and the counselor and, after consulting with each of them, brief behavioral medicine treatment was pursued. The goal was to utilize self-hypnosis with a focus on pain management to help enhance the patient's sense of control over aspects of the pain.

The patient was unable to return for approximately 1 month, but was then seen for behavioral medicine follow-up. She presented with more euthymic mood and was fully oriented. Initially, the focus of treatment was on the relaxation response with imagery for deepening. While she was able to become more relaxed, no significant alterations in sensations, which would be consistent with having entered a deeper hypnotic state, were noted. As before, it was recommended that the patient continue treatment with her psychiatrist and counselor for her mood and return in several weeks for additional hypnotic work. She returned in approximately 3 weeks, at which time her mood remained euthymic and stable. She was reporting significant pain in her left lower extremity with shooting pain and alterations in temperature. Hypnosis was used again, with a focus on altering the sensations toward increased warmth. While this was moderately successful, it was determined that the patient's mood and psychosocial status were substantially improved to the point that she would be an adequate candidate for spinal cord stimulation therapy. This was communicated to the treating physician, who then began to make necessary arrangements on the basis of his assessment of her medical condition. The patient was scheduled to return several weeks following the trial in order to reassess her status and determine what additional, if any, behavioral medicine evaluations might be of benefit to help enhance treatment outcome. We anticipate that she will achieve a moderate response from implantation therapy, with ongoing conservative and psychiatric care.

Scenario 4: In yet another scenario, shifting along a continuum of the severity of psychosocial risk factors, the results of a behavioral medicine evaluation could reveal that an individual presents with a number and severity of psychosocial risk factors such that he or she is extremely unlikely to benefit from any of the treatments offered. In such instances, a recommendation for discharging the patient could be made. Obviously, this decision would not be made lightly and would be a result of collaboration between the behavioral medicine specialist, treating physician, and other health-care providers involved in the multidisciplinary treatment of the patient. However, it is the case that there are patients who are so invested in the "sick-role" and present with such a high number and severity of medical and psychosocial risk factors that there is little chance of them benefiting from conservative treatment. Such patients could be referred to an inpatient functional rehabilitation setting if one is available in their area.

Case Study 4: The patient is a 47-year-old male who reported that he was injured approximately 21 months previously in a work-related injury. He reported that he was carrying a heavy pipe with two other workers, but that his back was injured when each of them stepped into a low spot and the majority of the load was left on him. The patient had been previously evaluated by several clinicians (i.e., more than 10) and had received a number of injections and physical therapy, with no significant reduction in pain. Several clinicians had determined that the patient was dependent on opioid medication. In addition, the patient reported a history of "seizures," but radiological and diagnostic studies had been normal.

Physical examination identified bilateral greater occipital nerve tenderness and positive anterior cervical thrust shear (ACTS) at C6–C7, with a positive spring at C5 and C7. He had remarkable spasmodic paraspinal musculature bilaterally more so on the right than on the left with scattered myofascial trigger points. His cervical facets on the right at C4–C5, C5–C6, and C6–C7 were hypomobile on palpation. He had a positive spring at T5 and T6 with remarkably hypertonic paraspinal musculature in the upper to mid thoracic level with scattered myofascial trigger points and tenderness over the facets. He had a positive spring at L3 and L4, bilateral paraspinal muscle hypertonicity, scattered myofascial trigger points, and tenderness about the lumbar facets, which was exacerbated by flexion and rotation. The right sacroiliac joint showed tenderness and was anteriorly rotated in an up-slipped position as noted by Gillette's, Gaenslen's, sacral thrust, Thomas', and Patrick's tests. The diagnoses included the following: cervical, thoracic, and lumbar intervertebral disk disruption; myofascial pain syndrome; cervicogenic headache; cervical spondylosis without myelopathy; and bilateral greater occipital neuralgia. In addition, the clinician noted the presence of depression, anxiety, and opioid dependence, as evidenced in the medical records.

Among other treatment modalities, the patient's current pain management physician was considering implantation of an interthecal medication pump to assist with pain management. However, as noted previously, the patient had received numerous injections, physical therapy, and other conservative modalities, with none producing a substantial reduction in pain. In addition, the physical therapist involved in his care reported that, in her professional opinion, his effort was suboptimal and that he came to therapy in order to avoid discharge and potential elimination of medication prescriptions.

The patient was referred for behavioral medicine evaluation because of concerns about the number of risk factors for poor treatment outcome that had been identified. At the time of this evaluation, the claimant was receiving worker's compensation benefits, which was in the form of medical treatment, and he was involved in litigation in order to reach a settlement with the insurance company. He presented with pain "from my neck down to my low back." He rated his pain level as a 5, but he exhibited minimal pain behaviors. Clearly his pain rating was significantly higher than would be expected given his pain behavior. The patient noted that pain was increased by "any type of movement," as well as sneezing, coughing, driving, turning his head, and standing or sitting for more than 20 minutes. He also stated that the only thing that decreased his pain level was medication. As noted previously, the medical records indicated that several physicians were concerned about substance dependence. Along these lines, the patient stated, "I feel better than I have in months" as a result of taking an extra six narcotic analgesic pain pills per day. Current medications were reported to include MSContin, Bextra, Zanaflex, Topamax, Effexor, and Xanax.

He stated that the benzodiazepine (e.g., Xanax) had initially been prescribed a number of years prior to the injury by a psychiatrist for "nerves." However, a psychiatrist had not treated the patient since then; instead he relied on his primary care physician to supply the Xanax. The patient noted that he was prescribed 2 mg t.i.d., but that he was about to run out before his refill was due because he took up to 10 mg at a time over the course of a day. The patient had a history of alcohol abuse predating the injury as well, but stated that he had not consumed any alcohol in one and a half years. When discussing his current situation, the patient consistently referred back to the pain as being his primary problem. He noted that previous efforts to "cut back on Xanax" resulted in significant exacerbation in pain, as well as symptoms that he referred to as "seizures and blacking out."

The claimant indicated that his mood was depressed and irritable. He exhibited affect consistent with a depressed and anxious mood. He reported significant problems with sleep, appetite, short-term memory, and low energy. The results of psychometric testing, including his MMPI-2 profile, indicated that there was a strong psychological component to his physical complaints, with these tending to increase in times of stress. Testing data also indicated that his somatic concerns bordered on being delusional in nature.

As a result of this evaluation, it was recommended that more invasive pain management procedures, such as implantation of a medication pump, be removed as a treatment option for this patient. In addition, the recommendation for a referral to a psychiatrist for pharmacological management of his preexisting and current psychiatric symptoms was made. Finally, given the patient's history of benzodiazepine and narcotic dependence, it was recommended that strict limits be set with the patient, with clear communication that any violations would result in his immediate discharge. Behavioral medicine intervention was not recommended in this case because it was determined that the patient's lack of insight and investment in identifying his problem as being primarily medical in nature would prohibit him from benefiting from such treatment. Finally, given the above noted factors, the recommendation was made to the patient's case manager at the worker's compensation insurance company that efforts be made to settle his case so that the patient could begin to "get on with his life." The suggestion was made that he would likely not benefit substantially from any of the medical treatments offered until he had received appropriate psychiatric treatment and his worker's compensation case had reached closure. At the request of the insurance company, one follow-up session was scheduled to provide the patient with feedback regarding this evaluation and to provide encouragement to pursue psychiatric treatment. Although he expressed an understanding and agreed to make these arrangements, several months later he had not done so.

SAMPLE REPORT

For demonstration purposes, a copy of the report generated from this initial evaluation is presented below

Behavioral Medicine Evaluation

Patient: XXX
SSN:
Date of Evaluation:
Referral Source: Dr. YYY

History of Illness:

XXX is a 47 year-old male who was presented with reports of pain "from my neck down to my low back." He stated that the pain began in 12/00 when he was injured while carrying a heavy pipe with two co-workers. To date, the patient has received conservative treatment in the form of injection therapy, physical therapy, and medication management. Apparently, none of these have provided substantial reduction in the patient's report of pain. However, he noted that on the day of this evaluation, "I feel better than I have in months." He reported that this was achieved by taking an "extra 6 pain pills per day." Medical records indicate that several physicians have noted problems with substance dependence for this patient in the past two years. In addition, he has a history of alcohol abuse and benzodiazepine dependence pre-dating this injury.

Current medication include: Xanax 2 mg TID; Prilosec; MS Contin 15 mg BID; Bextra 10 mg QHS; and Topamax 25 mg QPM. The patient reported that he quit taking Effexor 150 mg QAM because "it can cause seizures" and is no longer taking Zanaflex because his prescription expired. Medical records note a history of medication non-compliance within the past two years, with the patient regularly choosing which medications to take and which not to take, despite recommendations by his treating physicians to the contrary.

The patient reported that he has not consumed alcohol in 1.5 years, that he smokes 1–1.5 packs of cigarettes per day, and that he does not use illicit street drugs. However, as noted above, he has a history of alcohol abuse and dependence on Xanax. Currently, he reported that he takes up to 10 mg of Xanax at a time. He reported a recent history of "seizures" and "blacking out" when he has attempted to "cut back on Xanax." Medical records indicate that any such episodes have likely been the result of withdrawal from benzodiazepine addiction.

Mr. XXX reported that he saw a psychiatrist a number of years ago for problems with his "nerves" and several doctors have recommended that he be treated by a psychiatrist for pre-existing emotional difficulties. However, the patient has not followed up with these recommendations on a regular basis.

On the day of this evaluation, the patient rated his pain level as a 5, stating that this is as low as his pain ever goes. However, his pain behavior was inconsistent with this pain rating, as he exhibited much less pain behavior than would be expected given this rating. For example, he displayed minimal shifting and no guarding, bracing, or grimacing. He rated his worse pain as a 10, with pain made worse by "any type of movement," sneezing, coughing, turning his head while driving, standing for more than 20 minutes, sitting for more than 20 minutes, and walking for more than 10 minutes. He stated that medication is the only thing that helps reduce pain.

Past medical history is also positive for a broken back, pelvic bone, and hip when the patient was 18 years old. It reportedly took 8 months before he could walk although he required no surgery.

Brief Social History:

Mr. XXX reported that he has been married for 6 years to his third wife. He indicated that she has been supportive, although medical records indicate significant marital distress. His children are adults and live independently. He reported that in addition to his wife, he has many friends who are a good source of support for him.

Mr. XXX reported that he completed high school and that he had no major academic difficulties.

He stated that he worked in industrial construction "all my life," but had been employed for approximately one year by his current employer at the time of the injury. He currently receives medical benefits from the Worker's Compensation insurance company, but has not received any supplemental income payments since 4/02. He has retained an attorney to assist with these matters. He also retained another attorney to help him acquire Social Security Disability Benefits, which he currently receives. He has not worked since the injury in 12/00.

Mental Status:

Mr. XXX presented in casual attire and appeared older than his stated age. Although he appeared somewhat anxious and irritable, with mild psychomotor agitation, he maintained good eye contact and was cooperative throughout the evaluation.

Speech was normal in pace and volume and consistent with educational and cultural background. He was alert and fully oriented. Thoughts appeared to be logical and goal-directed. There were no loose associations or confusion apparent. He denied current hallucination, delusions, obsession, and compulsions. There was no evidence of a formal thought disorder.

The patient reported that his mood was irritable and depressed. He exhibited affect consistent with dysthymic and anxious mood. He reported significant problems with sleep disturbance, poor energy, appetite, and short-term memory. However, he also indicated that his energy had improved in the past few days prior to this evaluation. He stated that he has to "force myself to eat." He denied suicidal ideation.

Tests Administered:

Minnesota Multiphasic Personality Inventory–2 (MMPI-2); Coping Strategies Questionnaire-Revised (CSQ-R); Multidimensional Pain Inventory (MPI)

Tests Results:

On the MMPI-2, Mr. XXX responded in an honest and forthright manner, producing a valid and interpretable profile. His profile suggests that he is experiencing acute emotional distress, but that much of his psychological distress is chronic in nature.

His scores suggest that he is experiencing significant emotional distress, primarily in the form of depression and anxiety. However, his profile is also suggestive of excessive bodily concerns that could border on being delusional in nature. He is likely to present with multiple physical complaints, including epigastric symptoms. Such patients tend to have a strong psychological component to their illnesses, but see themselves as medically ill and seek medical treatment. Patients with such profiles tend to lack insight into the role that emotional or psychological factors play in their presentation of physical ailments. For this patient, much of his emotional distress is expressed through magnification of and a focus on his physical complaints.

On the MPI the patient's response indicates that he is reporting a high level of pain severity and pain related interference that exceeds that of most chronic pain patients. At the same time, he perceives himself to have minimal control over his physical functioning, pain, or other areas in his life. These factors contribute to him having a Dysfunctional coping style. In addition, his wife likely reinforces pain behavior, which further exacerbates his "sick role" behavior and serves as an obstacle to him engaging in adaptive behaviors.

On the CSQ-R, the patient's primary response to pain is catastrophizing. This means that when he perceives his is in pain, he tends to view his circumstances in a worse case scenario and he may "give up" when in pain. Such an approach tends to exacerbate a sense of worthlessness about the self and hopelessness about the future, thus exacerbating depression.

Overall, the testing results suggest that the patient has a long-standing tendency to utilize physical malfunctioning as a means of expressing psychological or emotional distress. He has little insight into this phenomenon and such patients tend to receive minimal benefit from psychological treatment, as their primary focus in on perceived physical malfunctioning. Nevertheless, the patient also engages in coping responses that are dysfunctional and thus he may benefit from cognitive behavioral therapy aimed at helping him to develop more adaptive coping responses.

Diagnostic Impression:

Axis I: Anxiolytic Dependence With Physiological Dependence
Undifferentiated Somatoform Disorder
Depressive Disorder NOS
Anxiety Disorder NOS

Axis II: Personality Disorder NOS

Axis III: chronic pain

Axis IV: unemployment; limited finances

Axis V: Current GAF = 60; Highest GAF past year = 60

Summary and Recommendations:

XXX is 47 year-old male who reported that he was injured in 12/00 in a work-related accident. Since that time, he has been treated by numerous physicians of various specialties and has undergone a Functional Capacity Evaluation. The results of many of the diagnostic tests performed have generally been reported as being within normal limits. In addition, the results of the FCE clearly indicate less than optimal effort and inconsistencies between subjective report and objective findings.

The results of this evaluation suggest that the patient experiences long-standing psychological distress that tends to be displayed through manifestation and magnification of physical symptoms. He has poor insight into the role that this emotional distress plays in his physical presentations. In addition, he has a long history of dependence on benzodiazepines and is abusing his current narcotic pain medication. These factors suggest a poor prognosis for this patient.

Mr. XXX could likely benefit from treatment for his depression and anxiety from a psychiatrist. This has been recommended to him on several occasions, but he is not currently pursing such treatment. A psychiatrist could provide treatment for his emotional distress while addressing potential medical concerns as he is taken off benzodiazepines and narcotics. Such treatment might best be provided in the context of an inpatient facility. However, as noted previously, these appear to be long-standing issues that pre-date the patient's reported injury. In addition, given his tendency to focus on physical symptoms, he may show minimal motivation to pursue such treatment. Along these lines, he is not likely to benefit from traditional behavioral medicine intervention, as he is likely to participate minimally due to a focus on physical versus psychological symptoms.

I appreciate the opportunity to evaluate this interesting patient. If there are any questions or if I can be of further assistance with Mr. XXX's care, please feel free to contact me at your convenience.
Jake Epker, Ph.D.
Licensed Psychologist

SUMMARY

1. This chapter reviews many of the psychosocial risk factors that have been shown to be associated with chronicity and poor response to treatment among patients with low back pain.
2. A model is provided to assist primary health-care providers and spine specialists in their efforts to conceptualize assessment of these risk factors and make use of behavioral medicine consultations. When a number of such risk factors are identified, it is appropriate and recommended that such a referral be made.
3. In presenting this treatment paradigm, practical aspects of integrating behavioral medicine with conservative medical treatment are also addressed so that clinicians can have a better understanding of what to expect when such a referral is initiated.
4. The integration of specialties such as these, with regular communication between health-care providers, increases the likelihood that psychosocial risk factors will be identified and effectively addressed so that patients with chronic low back pain can be helped to achieve optimal treatment outcome.

REFERENCES

1. Frymoyer JW, Durett CL. The economics of spinal disorders. In: Frymoyer JW, ed. *The adult spine*, 2nd ed. Philadelphia: Lippincott-Raven, 1997:143–150.
2. Higginson G. Clinical Standards Advisory Group. *Qual Health Care* 1994;3(Suppl):12–15.
3. Sanders SH, Brena SF, Spier CJ, Beltrutti D, McConnell H, Quintero O. Chronic low back pain patients around the world: Cross-cultural similarities and differences. *Clin J Pain* 1992;8(4):317–323.
4. Grzesiak RC. Psychologic considerations in temporomandibular dysfunction: A biopsychosocial view of symptom formation. *Temporomandibular Disord Orofacial Pain* 1991;35(1):209–226.
5. Fenerstein M, Berkowitz SM, Peck CA. Musculoskeletal-related disability in U.S. Army personnel: Prevalence, gender, and military occupational specialties. *J Occup Environ Med* 1997;39:68–78.
6. Sanders SH. Risk factors for the occurrence of low back pain and chronic disability. *Am Pain Soc Bull* 1995;5:1–5.
7. Volinn E. Back pain and associated disability in the United States. *Am Pain Soc Bull* 1996;6(6):8.
8. Melzack R, Wall PD. Pain mechanisms: A new theory. *Science* 1965;150:971–979.
9. Loeser JD. Concepts of pain. In: Stanton-Hicks M, Boas R, eds. *Chronic low back pain*. New York: Raven Press.
10. Fordyce WE, Lansky D, Calsyn DA, Shelton JL, Stolov WC, Rocket DC. Pain measurement and pain behavior. *Pain* 1984;18:53–65.
11. Gaskin ME, Greene AF, Robinson ME, Geisser ME. Negative affect and the experience of chronic pain. *J Psychosom Res* 1992;36:707–713.
12. Banks SM, Kerns RD. Explaining high rates of depression in chronic pain: A diathesis-stress framework. *Psychol Bull* 1996;119:95–110.
13. Romano JM, Turner JA. Chronic pain and depression: Does the evidence support a relationship? *Psychol Bull* 1985;97:18–34.
14. American Psychiatric Association. *Diagnostic and statistical manual of mental disorders*, 3rd ed. Washington, DC: Author.
15. Lindsay P, Wyckoff M. The depression-pain and its response to antidepressants. *Psychosomatics* 1981;22:571–577.

16. Polatin PB, Kinney RK, Gatchel RJ, Lillo E, Mayer TG. Psychiatric illness and chronic low-back pain. The mind and the spine—Which goes first? *Spine* 1993;18:66–71.
17. Fernandez E, Clark TS, Ruddick-Davis D. A framework for conceptualization and assessment of affective disturbance in pain. In: Block AR, Kremer EF, Fernandez E, eds. *Handbook of pain syndromes: Biopsychosocial perspectives*. Mahwah, NJ: Lawrence Erlbaum Associates, 1998.
18. DeGood DE, Kiernan B. Perception of fault in patients with chronic pain. *Pain* 1996;64:153–159.
19. Turk DC, Fernandez E. Personality assessment and the Minnesota Multiphasic Personality Inventory in chronic pain: Underdeveloped and overexposed. *Pain Forum* 1995;4(2):104–107.
20. McCracken LM, Gross RT, Aikens J, Carnrike CLM. The assessment of anxiety and fear in persons with chronic pain: A comparison of instruments. *Behav Res Ther* 1996;34:927–933.
21. Brown FF, Robinson ME, Riley JL, Gremillion HA. Pain severity, negative affect, and microstressors as predictors of life interference in TMD patients. *CRANIO* 1996;14:63–70.
22. Flor H, Birbaumer N, Turk DC. The psychobiology of chronic pain. *Adv Behav Res Ther* 1990;12:47–84.
23. Breuer J, Freud S. *Studies in hysteria*. New York: Basic Books, 1895.
24. Engle GL. "Psychogenic" pain and the pain-prone patient. *Am J Med* 1959;26:899–918.
25. Gamsa A. The role of psychological factors in chronic pain. 2. A critical appraisal. *Pain* 1994;57:17–29.
26. Keller LS, Butcher JN. Assessment of chronic pain patients with the MMPI-2. *MMPI-2 Monographs*, Vol. 2. Minneapolis: University of Minnesota Press, 1991.
27. Graham JR. *The MMPI-2: Assessing personality and psychopathology*. New York: Oxford University Press, 1990.
28. Kleinke CL, Spangle AS. Predicting treatment outcome of chronic back pain patients in multidisciplinary pain clinic. Methodological issues and treatment implications. *Pain* 1988;33:41–48.
29. Block AR. *Presurgical psychological screening in chronic pain syndromes: A guide for the behavioral health practitioner*. Mahwah, NJ: Lawrence Erlbaum Associates, 1996.
30. Riley JL, Robinson ME, Geisser ME, Wittmer VT, Smith AG. Relationship between MMPI-2 cluster profiles and surgical outcome in low-back pain patients. *J Spinal Disord* 1995;8:213–219.
31. Schmidt AJM. The behavioral management of pain: A criticism of a response. *Pain* 1987;30:285–291.
32. Block AR, Vanharanta H, Ohnmeiss D, Guyer RD. Discographic pain report: Influence of psychological factors. *Spine* 1996;21:334–338.
33. Rodin G, Craven J, Littlefield C. *Depression in the medically ill: An integrated approach*. New York: Brunner/Mazel, 1991.
34. Faucett JA. Depression in painful chronic disorders: The role of pain and conflict about pain. *J Pain Symptom Manage* 1994;9:520–526.
35. Fordyce WE. *Behavioral methods in chronic pain and illness*. St. Louis: C.V. Mosby, 1976.
36. Block AR, Kremer EF, Gaylor M. Behavioral treatment of chronic pain: The spouse as a discriminative cue for pain behavior. *Pain* 1980;9:243–252.
37. Lousberg R, Schmidt AJ, Groenman NH. The relationship between spouse solicitousness and pain behavior: Searching for more evidence. *Pain* 1992;51:75–79.
38. Bigos SJ, Battie MC, Spengler DM, et al. A prospective study of work perceptions and psychosocial factors affecting the report of back injury. *Spine* 1991;16:1–6.
39. Davis RA. A long-term outcome analysis of 984 surgically treated herniated lumbar discs. *J Neurosurg* 1994;80:415–421
40. Hudgins WR. Laminectomy for treatment of lumbar disc disease. *Tex Med* 1976;72:65–69.
41. Frymoyer JW, Cats-Baril WL. An overview of the incidences and cost of low back pain. *Orthop Clin Am* 1987;22:263–271.
42. Rohling ML, Binder LM, Langhinrichsen-Rohling J. Money matters: A meta-analytic review of the association between financial compensation and the experience and treatment of chronic pain. *Health Psychol* 1995;14:537–547.
43. Hasvold T, Johnsen R. Headache and neck pain: Family learnt illnesses behavior? The Bardu Musculoskeletal Study, 1989—1990. *Fam Prac* 1996;13(3):242–246.
44. Keefe FJ, Brown GK, Wallston KA, Caldwell DS. Coping with rheumatoid arthritis pain: Catastrophizing as a maladaptive strategy. *Pain* 1989;37:51–56.
45. Gil KM, Abrams MR, Phillips G, Keefe FJ. Sickle cell disease pain: Relation of coping strategies to adjustment. *J Consult Clin Psychol* 1990;57:725–737.
46. Brown GK, Nicassio PM. Development of a questionnaire for the assessment of active and passive coping strategies in chronic pain patients. *Pain* 1987;31:53–64.
47. Jensen MP, Turner JA, Romano JM, Karoly P. Coping with chronic pain: A critical review of the literature. *Pain* 1991;47:249–283.
48. Rosensteil AK, Keefe FJ. The use of coping strategies in chronic low back pain patients: Relationship to patient characteristics and current adjustment. *Pain* 1983;17:33–44.
49. Kendall NA, Linton SJ, Main CJ. *Guide to assessing psychosocial yellow flags in acute low back pain: Risk factors for long-term disability and work loss*. Wellington, New Zealand: Accident Rehabilitation and Compensation Insurance Corporation of New Zealand and the National Health Committee, 1997.
50. Waddell G, McCulloch JA, Kummel E, Venner RM. Non-organic physical signs in low back pain. *Spine* 1980;5:117–125.
51. Derogatis LR. *SCL-90-R: Administration, scoring and procedures manual-II for the revised version*. Towson, MD: Clinical Psychometric Research, 1983.
52. Spinhoven P, Linssen ACG. Behavioral treatment of chronic low back pain. I. Relation of coping strategy use to outcome. *Pain* 1991;45:29–34.
53. Wallis BJ, Lord SM, Bogduk N. Resolution of psychological distress of whiplash patients following treatment by radiofrequency neurotomy: A randomized, double-blind, placebo-controlled trial. *Pain* 1997;73:15–22.

54. Bernstein IH, Jaremko ME, Hinkley BS. On the utility of the SCL-90-R with low-back pain patients. *Spine* 1994;19:42–48.
55. Tollison CD, Langley JC. *Pain patient profile*. Pearson Assessments.
56. Indahl A, Velund L, Reikeraas O. Good prognosis for low back pain when left untampered: A randomized clinical trial. *Spine* 1995;20:473–477.
57. Linton SJ, Hellsing AL, Bergstrom G. Exercise for workers with musculoskeletal pain: Does enhancing compliance decrease pain? *J Occup Rehabil* 1996;6: 177–190.
58. Waddell G, Feder G, Lewis M. Systematic reviews of bed rest and advice to stay active for acute low back pain. *Br J Gen Pract* 1997;47(423): 647–652.

PART

IV

CONSERVATIVE TECHNIQUES FOR LOW BACK SYNDROMES

CHAPTER

20

MANIPULATION TECHNIQUES FOR LOW BACK SYNDROMES

Paul D. Hooper and Craig E. Morris

OUTLINE

OBJECTIVES

1. To define and describe spinal manipulation.
2. To understand the clinical rational for spinal manipulative procedures for low back syndromes.
3. To understand different approaches to spinal manipulation.
4. To understand manipulation under anesthesia for low back syndromes.
5. To understand indications, precautions and contraindications for spinal manipulation.
6. To understand important evidence-based literature regarding spinal manipulation.

INTRODUCTION

The use of manipulation of various parts of the body is not new. In fact, manipulation of the spine, or spinal manipulative therapy (SMT), has been used in some manner by almost every civilization for centuries.[1–2] For more than a century, doctors of chiropractic, medicine, and osteopathy, in addition to physical therapists, have popularized SMT. Recently, triggered largely by the growth in popularity among the population, and a growing research database supporting its efficacy, the use of SMT has increased significantly in a number of countries around the world.

Low back pain is one of the most, if not the most, common condition for which SMT is utilized. For example, utilization studies demonstrate that most patients presenting to a chiropractor to be treated with SMT have a primary complaint of low back pain.[3] These studies are helpful in understanding the type and variety of conditions treated with this modality. This chapter will explore the use of SMT in the treatment of the various low back syndromes that are presented throughout this text.

MANIPULATION

Definition and Description of Manipulation

Manipulation has been defined as the application of manual forces to the body and includes a wide variety of methods and/or techniques. It may be done manually or mechanically, actively or passively. The manipulation procedure may incorporate the use of long body levers, as seen in the "lumbar roll," which produces rotation of the lumbar spine using the legs and upper trunk as levers (see Fig. 20–1). These techniques are sometimes referred to as "indirect" techniques since they do not use a contact directly on the target joints being manipulated. The manipulation may also be applied using short levers. In this case, a direct contact is made on the spinous and/or transverse processes of adjacent spinal segments. Consequently, these short lever procedures are sometimes referred to as "direct" techniques.

In addition to variations in the contacts utilized, manipulation techniques also vary depending on the type of thrust that is delivered. The manipulation may be performed using a rapid (high-velocity), short (low-amplitude) thrust. Variations of this high-velocity, low-amplitude (HVLA) thrust include a rapid application of force combined with an equally rapid withdrawal. Other clinicians may incorporate the use of mechanical aids or devices in an attempt to deliver a more controlled or reproducible thrust, or to generate additional force during the delivery of the manual thrust. Several examples of these mechanical aids can be seen: (1) the Activator Adjusting Instrument (AAI), (2) flexion–distraction manipulation, and (3) "drop" tables. Each of these methods is described in detail in other sources and the reader is referred to reference 6 for more information. Finally, in some select circumstances, manipulation may be performed while the patient is under sedation. This method, referred to as manipulation under anesthesia or MUA, is described in detail later in this chapter.

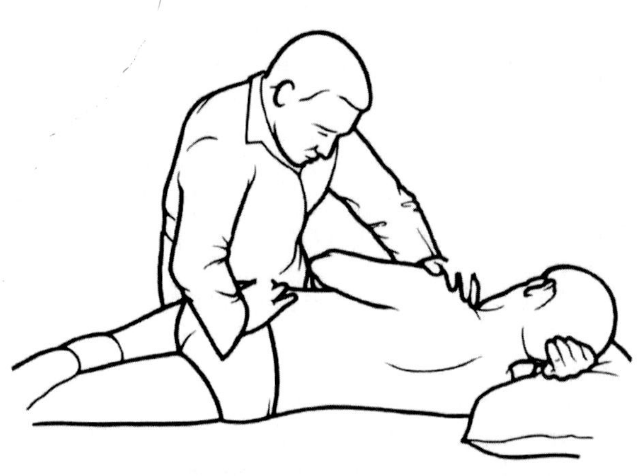

FIGURE 20–1. Long-lever side-lying manipulation. *(Adapted from Kenna and Murtaugh.[5])*

Objectives of Manipulation

While a large variety of styles and techniques of manipulation exist, there are also a number of different objectives stated for their use. Some authors claim that manipulation primarily addresses joint dysfunction and is, therefore, best utilized in the presence of joint hypomobility.[4,5] Others claim that the objectives are to realign the joints of the spine and to "normalize" the spatial relationship of the disc.[6] Still others claim that manipulation should be used with the purpose of "restoring normal articular relationship and function as well as reestablishing neurological integrity, thereby influencing physiological processes".[7]

In general, the objectives of spinal manipulation are to

1. relieve pain and discomfort,
2. improve posture and locomotion,
3. improve local function,
4. improve function elsewhere in the body, and
5. enhance the sense of well-being.

With regard to patients with low back pain, spinal manipulation is probably most often used in an attempt to reduce pain and to restore spinal function. Evans states that the effects of HVLA include[8]

1. a release of entrapped synovial folds or plica,
2. relaxation of hypertonic muscles by sudden stretching,
3. disruption of articular or periarticular adhesions, and
4. unbuckling of motion segments that have undergone disproportionate displacements.

With this in mind, the literature supporting the effect of SMT on patients with low back pain will be addressed later in this chapter.

Types of Manipulation Techniques

High-Velocity, Low-Amplitude Manipulation (Thrust Techniques) The high-velocity, low-amplitude (HVLA) thrust involves the application of a force that uses a rapid (high-velocity) manual force that is delivered with a controlled and relatively shallow (low-amplitude) thrust. While the forces used can be relatively high, care is taken to properly position the patient and to deliver a thrust in a manner that (a) attempts to isolate the force to the target region or joint, and (b) utilizes the most advantageous direction. For this particular type of SMT to be performed successfully, the patient must be as relaxed as possible at the time the thrust is delivered. By definition, the HVLA utilizes the combination of positioning, relaxation, and speed of thrust to successfully accomplish the SMT.

Oftentimes, the HVLA technique is accompanied by an audible "click" or "pop." This audible release, called joint "cavitation," is one of the factors that distinguish these techniques from other manual therapy interventions.[9] Brodeur reviewed the literature on the audible release associated with HVLA manipulation. He stated that it is caused by a sudden decrease in intracapsular pressure, which in turn, causes dissolved gasses within the synovial fluid to be released into the joint cavity. This may be explained by the fact that during the "crack" associated with a joint manipulation, there is a sudden joint distraction. This distraction occurs in less time than that required to complete the stretch reflexes of the periarticular muscles, and it is proposed that the cavitation process is generated by an elastic recoil of the synovial capsule as it "snaps back" from the capsule/synovial fluid interface. In addition, the sudden joint distraction is likely to be a high impulse acting on the ligaments and muscles associated with the joint. Brodeur, therefore, suggests that the cavitation process provides a simple means for initiating the reflex actions and that without the cavitation it would be difficult to generate the forces in the appropriate tissue without causing muscular damage.[10] Meal and Scott state that the crack is a consistent double-peak wave accompanied by a drop in tension that occurs immediately after the first sound wave. This sound indicates separation of the articular surfaces.[11]

Protopapas and Cymet state that the articular release is a physiologic event that may or may not be audible. However, after an articular release, there is a difference in joint spacing with an increase in the distance between articular surfaces. They also note that not all noise that emanates from a joint signifies an articular release.[12] Evans states that there appears to be two separate modes of action from joint manipulation: (1) intra-articular mechanical effects and (2) neurophysiological effects. He continues that the cavitation should not be an absolute requirement for the mechanical effects to occur but may be a reliable indicator for successful joint gapping.[10]

Several authors have attempted to identify from where (i.e., from which joint) the audible noise originates. Reggars and Pollard looked at the relationship between the side of head rotation and the side of joint cavitation for the cervical spine. Their research suggests that there is a higher occurrence of joint cavitation on the ipsilateral side to head rotation, which may have implications for the lumbar spine.[13] Beffa and Mathews state that there is no statistically significant correlation between the anatomical location of cavitation sounds and the particular SMT technique selected.[14]

Whether or not the audible cavitation is clinically significant is not clear. There is some evidence that the audible sound adds some value to the manipulation. For example, Colloca et al. state that thrust SMT in human subjects was found to stimulate spinal nerve root responses.[15] However, other investigators disagree. Flynn et al. looked at the relationship between joint cavitation and symptomatic improvement with spinal manipulation in patients with low back pain. They suggested that the occurrence of a cavitation would not improve the odds of achieving a dramatic reduction in symptoms, and that there is no relationship between this noise during sacroiliac region manipulation and improvement in range of motion (ROM), pain, or disability in individuals with nonradicular low back pain. Additionally, they state that the occurrence of a cavitation did not improve the odds of a dramatic improvement with manipulation treatment.[16]

Herzog et al. investigated whether the audible release associated with SMT or the velocity of the thrust provokes an activation of spinal muscles. Electromyographical (EMG) activity was observed consistently 50–100 milliseconds after the onset of each of the rapidly delivered manipulations, whether or not the treatment resulted in an audible release. In contrast, for slower manipulation procedures, there was never any visible EMG activity of the target muscles, whether or not the treatment resulted in an audible release or not. The authors suggest that high-velocity thrusts elicit muscle activation, whereas slow force application does not. They also state that the audible release does not (by itself) evoke muscle activation or a joint proprioceptive reflex response as has been previously speculated in the literature.[17]

In a study looking at neurophysiological responses to SMT, the authors state that thrust SMTs in human subjects were found to stimulate spinal nerve root responses that were temporally related to the onset of vertebral motion.[18] There may also be some potential for a psychological, or even placebo, effect, stemming from the audible release, as evidenced by Evans' statement that this may be a reliable indicator of successful joint gapping.[10]

Recent research provides further insights into the neurophysiological effects of SMT. Pickar noted that a theoretical framework exists from which hypotheses regarding these effects can now be developed.[21] Dishman and Bulbubian demonstrated a profound but brief reduction of alpha motoneuronal excitability.[22] These inhibitory effects have been found to be regional,[23] whereas the central response is that of motor facilitation.[24] Finally, a new preliminary report by Sung et al. measured abrupt changes in the lumbar paraspinal muscle mechanoreceptors of six cats following biomechanical loading simulating SMT, suggesting that these afferents may play a role in the neurophysiological responses and paving the way for further studies.[25]

Non-Thrust Techniques While many individuals utilize the thrust or HVLA techniques described in the previous section, some practitioners remain cautious about the magnitude of the forces involved, while still incorporating manipulation as one of their treatment tools. Rather than relying solely on the thrust techniques, a variety of nonthrust techniques have been developed and used over the years. These methods have been popular with varying groups of clinicians and are referred to as "oscillation," "articulation," or "mobilization" techniques. They include the use of repetitive, rhythmic movements that are performed within the available range of joint motion. Unlike the HVLA thrust techniques, these procedures are performed within the patient's ability to resist. They are not typically accompanied by the audible release that is common to the HVLA thrust techniques; however, joint cavitation may sometimes occur. These techniques are described in greater detail in Chapter 23 of this textbook.

Mechanically Assisted Manipulation Techniques There are a number of relatively common manipulation techniques that incorporate the use of various forms of mechanical devices. These devices include handheld adjusting instruments (e.g., AAI), adjusting tables with "drop" pieces (e.g., Thompson table), and motorized adjusting tables (e.g., Leander table).

Handheld adjusting devices. Recent surveys show that approximately two thirds of all chiropractors use these or similar devices at some point in their practice.[26] The rationale for using these mechanical aids varies both with the device being used and with the understanding and preference of the practitioner. As an example, many clinicians utilize the AAI in an attempt to deliver a precise and repeatable manipulative thrust (see Fig. 20–2). To this end, a fair amount of research has been performed to determine the exact amount of force that is delivered.[27,28] Some practitioners use these devices in an attempt to enhance the thrust, while others use them out of concern for the amount of force that may be delivered manually.[29] Some practitioners feel that the long cylindrical shape allows for more specific lines of drive, although Ross has questioned this.[30] Still others incorporate these devices on occasion in areas where manual contact may be difficult. These techniques are often referred to as "low force" techniques. However, this term may actually be a misnomer, as the forces can vary significantly depending on the device, its setting, and application.

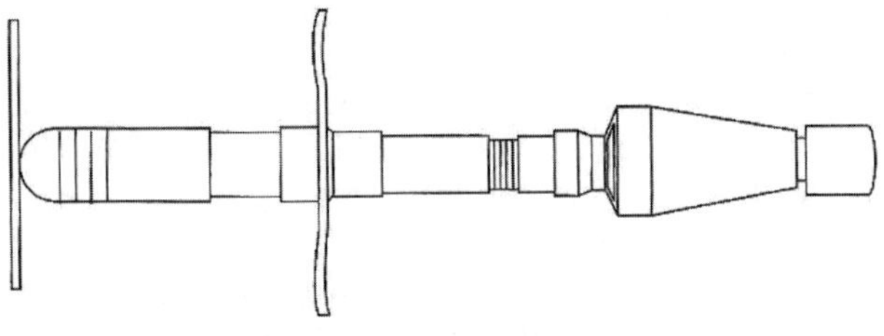

FIGURE 20–2. Handheld adjusting instrument: the AAI. *(Adapted from Fuhr et al.[31])*

Adjusting tables with "drop" pieces were popularized by Clay Thompson.[32] His "drop tables" remain popular among a number of clinicians in order to enhance the delivery of force used in their manipulative techniques. Many of these tables incorporate separate pieces or segments that are designed to "drop away" when force is applied. This sudden dropping away of the table segment has the additional advantage of adding speed and decreasing the resistance to the manual forces that are being applied and may, therefore, reduce the amount of force necessary.

Motorized tables. One of the innovative adjusting devices is the motorized adjusting table. These tables provide a constant up and down movement that is used by the clinician to facilitate the manipulative thrust. Typically, the thrust is applied at a particular point during the travel of the table, at a point where muscular inhibition is apparently increased causing a decrease in muscle tone. Using the movement from the table, the amount of force required to deliver the manipulative thrust is reduced during this relaxation phase. These techniques represent a motorized form of the traction-assisted manipulation techniques described in the next section.

Traction-Assisted Manipulation Techniques One form of manipulation that is particularly popular within the chiropractic profession includes the addition of gentle traction forces that are applied during the procedure in an attempt to assist the manipulation. These techniques, which date back to Hippocrates (see Chapter 1), were brought to modern times by McManis, and more recently by Cox.[33] These procedures were previously referred to as "flexion–distraction," but have recently been renamed as "traction-assisted" manipulation. The procedures are designed for use with patients with either low back pain and/or neck pain. Typically, the patient is placed prone on a table that consists of several separate pieces. The patient is positioned with their ankles strapped to the lower portion of the table and a gentle traction force is applied in a caudad direction. A roll is often placed under the patient's abdomen in order to increase the lever

TABLE 20–1. Special Considerations for Lumbar Spine and Pelvic MUA

Indications	Contraindications	Preoperative Evaluation	Operative Procedure and Physician Qualification
Acute and chronic lumbar, pelvic, or lower extremity musculoskeletal syndromes nonresponsive to conservative management	Absolute; Hypermobility/instability Unstable spondylolisthesis	X-ray films of lumbar spine and pelvis including AP, lateral, and both oblique projections, supplemented by flexion/extension lateral and side-bending AP motion studies	Articulatory and high-velocity thrust techniques that do not pull unnecessary rotary torque through segments of the lumbar spine
Somatic dysfunction considered to be a significant component of such syndromes	Relative; Herniated nucleus pulposus with extruded free fragment Advanced spondylosis and spondylarthrosis	Supplemental imaging studies (CT, MRI, myelography, or discography) as indicated by history and physical examination	Physician competence for techniques just described
Lumbar disc syndrome without evidence of acute neurological deficit, nonresponsive to conservative care	Progressive neurological deficit of lower extremity	Complete neurological and physical examination Electrodiagnostic studies (EMG and NCV) as indicated by history and physical examination	

Source: From Greenman.[40]

effect, optimizing the mechanical advantage. However, as Cox states, "The roll is not necessary if the patient already has one naturally provided."[34] A specific contact, utilizing the clinician's cephalad hand, is made at the target spinal segment to stabilize the superior aspect of the motor unit. At the same time the caudal portion of the table is moved in a rhythmic upward and downward motion (i.e., floor to ceiling). This procedure repetitively places the lumbar spine in both a flexed and distracted position. During the application, the clinician applies various manual forces to specific lumbar segments in an attempt to alleviate pain and dysfunction.

Manipulation Under Anesthesia Manipulation of the anesthetized patient is neither a new concept nor a new procedure. In fact, as early as 1846, Bigelow suggested this approach as an example of new clinical possibilities for the reduction of dislocations.[35] In addition, JB Mennell, a pioneer in modern manual and physical medicine, discussed the use of anesthesia with joint manipulation in his 1920 textbook.[36] MUA continued to enjoy some degree of acceptance and utilization in the ensuing decades, at least in North America. As an example, Siehl and Bradford reported on 87 patients with low back pain who underwent MUA procedures from 1950 to 1952. They reported that greater than 60% of these cases responded with good or excellent results.[37] Gradually, MUA gained acceptance, only to decrease in popularity among orthodox medical practitioners, perhaps because of the general negativity regarding manipulation, greater focus on invasive procedures, or the likely combination of both.

Spinal MUA remained a focus of interest among various osteopathic physicians in the 1960s and 1970s, with papers by Beckett and Francis,[38] who reported on 723 spinal MUA cases, and Morey,[39] who discussed MUA for both spinal and extremity conditions. Of particular importance is a case study by Greenman who provided clinical criteria for the use of spinal MUA. He presented indications, relative contraindications, and absolute contraindications for lumbar and pelvic MUA[40] (see Table 20–1).

With its introduction into the chiropractic profession in the late 1980s, MUA gained renewed interest. This came at a time when chiropractors were first allowed privileges in either a hospital or outpatient surgical center. Several authors have reported case studies illustrating successful treatment of patients with MUA. Francis presented one of the first chiropractic papers on spinal MUA, describing the successful resolution of a case of chronic back pain and leg pain.[41] Similarly, Alexander reported on a case study in which the patient, a golf professional with a lumbar postlaminectomy syndrome, evidence of epidural fibrosis, and recurrent disc herniation, underwent spinal MUA. The patient returned to play 2 weeks post-treatment without further complications.[42] Davis et al. reported successful results in two cases of failed back surgery syndrome.[43] In a unique report, Ben-David and Raboy discussed three successful cases of a single spinal MUA procedure, each immediately followed by an epidural steroid injection (ESI). The authors theorized that the spinal MUA works by lysing adhesions and loosening fibrotic tissue, and that the ESI would reduce inflammation created by the MUA trauma and inhibit reformation of such fibrotic and adhesive tissues. They did not advocate this combination of MUA/ESI as a standard treatment, "but rather suggesting an alternative path out of the therapeutic dead ends we all at times reach."[44]

West et al. presented the largest published case study involving chiropractic spinal MUA to date.[45] The authors discussed 177 cases of patients (17–65 years old) who underwent MUA. The procedure was routinely performed three times serially, and 168 of the 177 patients completed the program. With regard to the low back pain, a 60.1% decrease in pain was reported by 11-point visual analog scale (from a pre-MUA average of 7.27/10 to a post-MUA average of 4.91/10 to 2.96/10 six months following MUA). They reported a decrease in medication usage, a measurable increase in motion, and a significant increase in the percentage of those who returned to work. It should be noted that the treatment strategy for these cases was one that also included medication, rehabilitation, and counseling.[45] Unfortunately, there are no known randomized MUA trial studies currently available.

Serial Applications of Spinal MUA

One of the criticisms for the use of spinal MUA is that it is routinely performed serially, with some protocols recommending three or more procedures. Several authors have attempted to explain the rationale for such multiple treatments. Mennell stated that each manipulation procedure would likely affect different adhesive structures. He also suggested that too aggressive treatment might actually harm the patient by creating an inflammatory response, thereby creating the formation of new adhesions.[36] Using a similar argument, Beckett and Francis recommended this procedure be performed serially to prevent severe reaction and shock by attempting too much with one procedure.[38]

In the discussion of an MUA case involving the cervical spine of an acute patient, Hughes stated that serial applications, which he dubs the Texas Chiropractic College (TCC) protocol, are now considered the industry standard.

Complications

Lewin, in his 1955 textbook, discussed complications from spinal MUA that included dislocation of the hip, paralysis of the external popliteal or peroneal nerves, and avulsion of the Achilles tendon from the triceps surae muscle.[46] Haldeman and Rubinstein reported on 16 cases of cauda equina syndrome associated with spinal MUA.[47] However, these may be misleading because there is evidence that more recent MUA protocols appear to significantly reduce morbidity rates.[48] Indeed, Kohlbeck notes, "There are no recent reports of complications following MUA as currently administered, using lighter anesthetics and less manipulative force."[49]

Spinal MUA Procedure

As previously noted, the spinal MUA procedure is performed in a hospital or outpatient surgical center. The patient is placed under general anesthesia, and two clinicians perform the procedure, a primary and an assistant surgeon. The term *surgeon* is used because of the operating room setting, the use of anesthesia, and the fact that these types of procedures have been historically been called *closed surgical procedures*. However, this descriptor may be inappropriate if a clinician without a surgical license uses it. The assistant may be involved in performing manipulation or may simply assist in safely transferring the patient's positions and holding them in place in order for the primary surgeon to perform the manipulations. Prior to the performance of the manipulations, the patients are passively stretched to lengthen the thoracolumbopelvic and lower extremity myofascial tissues.

The patients are typically placed in a side-lying position and a manipulation is performed on each side of the lumbar spine and sacroiliac joints. If the thoracic spine is included, the manipulation is generally performed in a supine position. The typical procedure requires approximately 15 minutes from the time the patient is placed under general anesthesia till the time he or she is taken away from the operating room.

Postoperative Management

The patients are typically released the same day of the procedure, often provided with medication for pain and instructions to use ice applications for pain. The patients were generally instructed to perform specific stretches and to remain as physically active as tolerable. Follow-up treatment consisting of additional in-office manipulation and a graded exercise rehabilitation program is instituted. West et al. describe a post-MUA protocol that essentially covers these topics.[45]

Summary

Spinal MUA remains an enigmatic approach to acute and chronic spinal conditions. It has not been universally accepted as a procedure for regular utilization in the health-care world, as questions of use, efficacy, and relative safety remain. A variety of approaches have been devised for the procedure, such as single and serial procedures. Clearly, it should not be considered a stand-alone procedure, but as one part of a more complex strategy that includes myofascial lengthening and mobilization during the procedure, and also follow-up counseling and rehabilitation.

Spinal MUA presents an interesting and contrasting procedure, i.e., an abundance of case studies stating impressive results contrasted by a dearth of quality research, utilizing today's standards. Until quality trials that meet today's standards are performed, spinal MUA must remain a promising, experimental option rather than an accepted clinical procedure. Clinicians who perform spinal MUA should ethically inform the patients of its investigational status so that appropriate informed consent is provided.

MANIPULATION AND LOW BACK PAIN

The Role of Manipulation in Low Back Pain

Although it is a widely used tool, the question remains: what is the role of manipulation in the management of patients with low back pain? Should it be a primary treatment tool or should it be used sparingly and under clearly defined purposes? To those familiar with its application, manipulation is a primary tool that has far-reaching benefits and little risk. To others, however, manipulation involves a broad range of procedures that have, at best, a placebo response. Based largely on available evidence, manipulation has received positive recommendations as a treatment modality by a number of government-sponsored committees that have developed treatment guidelines for acute low back pain (United States, AHCPR[50]; Canada, QTF[51]; United Kingdom, CSAG[52]; New Zealand, ACC[53]; and most recently the European Guidelines for Acute Back Pain[54]) In fact, one government commission (Canada) recommended practitioners of spinal manipulation over other health-care professionals as the first contact physician for patients with back pain.[55]

Indications for Manipulation

It is reasonable to conclude that manipulation has its most direct effect on the synovial joints of the spine, although this remains theoretical. If so, then it should be most effective on patients presenting with dysfunction of these joints, i.e., facet or sacroiliac syndrome. However, numerous studies have demonstrated the efficacy of spinal manipulation on a wide range of conditions. Perhaps, since manipulation is a mechanical treatment, it might be considered that it is most likely to have a positive impact on low back pain that stems from some form of mechanical deficit. However, recent papers have emphasized the neurophysiological response, so reflexive actions from mechanical stimuli appear to influence the response.[56,57]

Contraindications, Precautions, and Treatment Modifiers

As with any form of treatment, there are clinical scenarios and conditions that create an increased measure of risk. In some instances, these conditions may simply make the clinician more cautious. An example would be a patient who is concerned or tentative about receiving SMT. Other times, the presence of such concerns may actually contraindicate the use of the procedure entirely. For instance, the presence of a local spinal tumor, fracture, or osseous infection would preclude the use of spinal manipulation. The following table provides a list of conditions, or "red flags" that add concern, although the reader is directed to Chapter 10 for a detailed explanation of red flags.

Fortunately, the majority of adverse effects arising from SMT is of a short duration, is not particularly serious, and commonly improves with time and without therapeutic intervention. Although these may result in some temporary pain or inconvenience, they often go unreported. More serious complications, however, have deservedly gained considerable attention, but appear to be exceedingly rare. In spite of the large numbers of manipulation procedures performed, there are relatively few reports of serious complications.[58,59]

Injuries from lumbar spine manipulation are relatively rare, with the most frequently reported complication being the prolapse of a herniated intervertebral disc resulting in a cauda equina syndrome.[60–62] Because of the paucity of research documenting per- and post-manipulation morphological disc changes, it remains speculative whether the manipulation cause herniation/prolapse or merely provokes a preexisting condition. The other painful complication of lumbar or thoracic manipulation is spraining of the costovertebral or costochondral joints during rotation of the trunk. Table 20–2 lists the total numbers of reported complications of lumbar manipulation over an 80-year period. The generally accepted contraindications for manipulation of the lumbar spine are provided in Table 20–3 and, for the most part, are based on common clinical sense. They include the following:

- compromised bone structure (i.e. fractured or significantly weakened)
- severe or progressive neurological deficit
- acute or inflammatory joint disease
- bleeding disorders
- inadequate examination procedures
- inadequate manipulative training and skills

TABLE 20-2. **Complications from Low Back SMT Reported Causes (1911–1991)**

Age/Sex	Initial Complaint	Therapy Involved	Outcome
39/M	Right sciatica with mild left leg symptoms	Forced lumbar lordosis	Decompressive laminectomy with slight relief
32/F	Recurrent lumbosciatica	Chiropractic manipulation	Relief with discectomy
	Sciatica	Standard manipulation	
52/M	S1 sciatica	Five treatments by chiropractor	Death from infection following surgery
45/M	Lumbalgia	Medical manipulation	Surgery with residual lumbalgia
41/F	Back pain and leg weakness	Chiropractic manipulation	Incomplete relief from surgery 12 days later
55/M	Lumbalgia	Chiropractic manipulation	Surgery-discectomy; residual defects
46/M	Sciatica	Medical manipulation	Surgery; residual mild bilateral paresis
39/M	L5 sciatica	Chiropractic manipulation	Surgery; residual sphincter loss
31/M	Achondroplasia, low back pain	Chiropractic manipulation	Surgery; leg weakness, neurogenic bladder
62/M	Back and leg pain	Chiropractic manipulation	Surgery; leg braces, self-catheterization
36/F	Back and leg pain	Chiropractic manipulation	Surgery; perineal hypalgesia, self-catheterization

Source: Adapted from Haldeman and Rubinstein.[47]

In addition to the more serious consequences, there are several minor or temporary adverse effects. These have been divided into the following categories,[64] in increasing order of severity:

1. *Exacerbating reaction*: Subjective discomfort of the patient, not influencing his or her working ability, which is quickly reversible.
2. *Aggravating reaction*: Objective worsening of the preexisting state, with decreased work capacity. This may take longer or require other treatment to return to baseline.
3. *Reversible complication*: The precipitation of a new injury that requires special diagnostic and/or therapeutic interventions, and which is reversed by appropriate treatment.
4. *Irreversible complication*: The precipitation of tissue damage that leads to some form of permanent impairment.

Manipulation of the Low Back

Manipulation of the lower back has been used by a variety of clinicians throughout recorded history. This section will attempt to describe some of the more commonly used manipulation procedures.

Long-lever, side-lying manipulation. This commonly used manipulation procedure is performed with the patient in a side-lying position. The lower arm is tucked under the patient with the patient lying on the back of the shoulder, as shown in Figure 20–1. The upper leg is flexed, with the foot being hooked behind the lower knee. The contact hand is placed on the appropriate part of the lumbar spine (e.g., spinous

TABLE 20-3. **Contraindications for High-Velocity Manipulation Techniques on the Lumbar Spine**

Local fractures
Severe osteoporosis
Multiple myeloma
Osteomyelitis
Local primary bone tumors
Local metastatic bone tumors
Paget's disease
Progressive neurological deficit
Local spinal cord tumors
Cauda equina syndrome
Structural instability (ex/unstable spondylolisthesis)
Inflammatory phase of rheumatoid arthritis (spinal)
Inflammatory phase of ankylosing spondylitis
Inflammatory phase of psoriatic arthritis (spinal)
Reiter's syndrome
Congenital bleeding disorders
Acquired bleeding disorders
Inadequate physical and spinal examination
Inadequate manipulative training and skills
*Under certain circumstances, soft tissue or joint mobilization procedures may still be appropriate.

Source: Adapted from Haldeman et al.[63]

process of lumbar vertebra), with the stabilizing hand placed on the shoulder. The patient's torso is rotated slightly in order to produce tension under the contact hand. Once the patient is sufficiently relaxed, the clinician delivers a thrust through the contact hand. Variations of this manipulation may also be used to produce movement in the sacroiliac joint. The long leverage provides a mechanical advantage to the clinician to facilitate the delivery of the manipulative force.

b) *Short-lever, side-lying manipulation (push–pull).* This manipulation procedure is performed with the patient positioned similarly to that described above. In this technique, however, the clinician makes a more direct contact on the joints to be manipulated, with both hands making contact with the segments to be manipulated. The fingers of one hand make a contact superior to (i.e., cephalad) the spinous process of the lower vertebra of the involved segment (e.g., L5). The other hand makes a contact below (i.e., caudal) the spinous process of the upper vertebra (e.g., L4). The patient is positioned by pushing away with the lower forearm, while pulling toward with the upper forearm (see Fig. 20–3). As before, when the patient is relaxed, the thrust is delivered through the contacting fingers. The direct contact provides an additional measure of control over the longer lever described earlier.

Traction-assisted manipulation. In this procedure, the patient is positioned prone on the treatment table. The ankles are strapped to the caudal portion of the table and the patient holds onto the handrails. The center portion of the table is released and the clinician takes hold of the lever. The clinician places a contact hand on the vertebral segment involved and the table is gently moved up and down and from side to side. As the table is moved, there is a gentle traction force applied via the ankle straps.

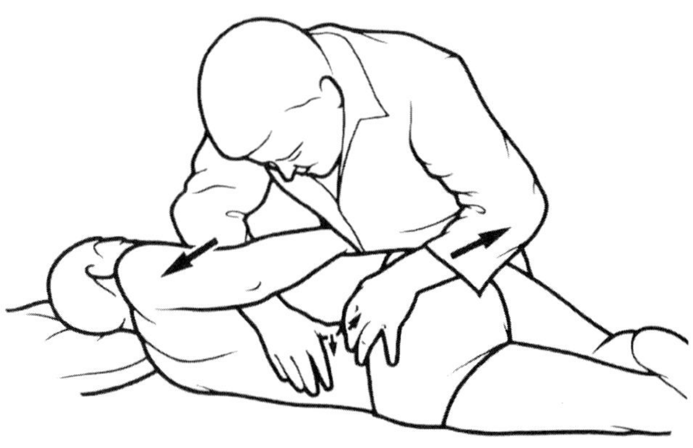

FIGURE 20–3. Short-lever side-lying manipulation. *(Adapted from Kenna and Murtaugh.[5])*

LITERATURE REVIEW

Is There an Ideal Candidate for Manipulation?

Because of the dramatic increase in the biomechanical aspects of low back syndromes (see Chapters 5 and 11), it would appear that the use of manipulation might be beneficial on a wide variety of problems. One question, however, that remains to be answered is: Is there an ideal candidate for manipulation? Several investigators have looked at this question. Stig et al.[65] looked at the recovery patterns of patients who were treated with chiropractic spinal manipulative therapy for long-lasting or recurrent back pain. They included patients with episodes that had lasted at least 2 weeks, and who had pain of at least 4 weeks duration in the prior 12 months. Fifty percent of the patients were found to be significantly better within 4 visits or 2 weeks of starting chiropractic care, and 75% were much better by 12 visits. In a study with similar findings, Axen et al.[66] stated that the chance of being recovered by the fourth visit was only 30% if all of the following criteria were present:

- no improvement immediately after one visit,
- no decrease in pain at visit 2,
- no decrease in disability reported at visit 2, and
- an uncommon reaction to the first treatment (local pain or fatigue lasting more than 24 hours, new radiating pain, or other reactions).

Flynn et al.[67] noted common features in patients with low back pain who were most likely to respond to SMT:

- segmental dysfunction/pain upon springing over lumbar facets,
- acute onset of pain <16 days,
- no pain distal to the knee,
- limited hip internal rotation, and
- low fear-avoidance beliefs score

The authors state that the presence of four out of five of these variables increased the probability of success with manipulation from 45% to 95%. Thus, patients with three or less of these variables present had less than a 50% chance of satisfactory recovery.[68]

In a study[69] designed to identify factors associated with reduced likelihood of benefit from manipulation, 75 subjects received a spinal manipulation intervention for a maximum of two sessions. Of these, only 20 subjects (28%) did not improve. Six variables were identified with an inability to improve with manipulation:

- longer symptom duration,
- having symptoms in the buttock or leg,
- absence of lumbar hypomobility,

- less hip range of motion,
- less discrepancy in left-to-right hip medial rotation range of motion, and
- a negative Gaenslen's sign (a sign of sacroiliac inflammation).

Manipulation and Low Back Syndromes

Acute and Subacute Low Back Pain Since the most common reason for the use of spinal manipulations administered each year (30% to 50%) is for the treatment of low back pain,[70,71] much of the investigations into the effectiveness of SMT has focused on this area.[72–74] As an example, more than 40 randomized controlled trials (RCTs) involving SMT have been published with approximately two thirds of the studies analyzing the effect of SMT on low back pain. These randomized trials involving SMT have been the subject of several extensive reviews and meta-analyses, which will be discussed later.[75–80]

In addition to RCTs, uncontrolled prospective and retrospective case studies have also been published. Unfortunately, since there is a wide variation in manipulation techniques, and skill levels among those techniques, that have been used, compounded by poor descriptions of procedures used, these studies have been difficult to interpret. Because it is a clinical art, there is also a wide variety of manipulative skills among clinicians. In addition, there is wide variation in the percentage of patients with low back pain who respond favorably to spinal manipulation: from 51% of inpatients hospitalized for low back pain[81] to over 90% in patients seen in a private practitioner's office.[82]

Manipulation has been compared to a variety of other treatment modalities. When compared to bed rest and analgesia,[83] analgesia alone,[84] short-wave therapy, heat, exercise and massage,[85] or mobilization,[86] manipulation appears to be a significantly more effective method of treating acute low back pain. A study by Coxhead[87] suggests that combining treatments was more effective than using a single treatment protocol. When manipulation, traction, exercise, and corsets were offered at the same time, the improvement rate increased from 69% for a single treatment protocol to 88%. Patients were also less likely to return for further treatment if they had received multiple treatment modalities.

Some of the controlled clinical trials have compared the results of manipulation to different forms of placebo treatments as well as many of the recognized conservative forms of treatments for low back pain. In many cases, positive results were not seen on reexamination of patients after different periods of treatment.[88,89] In other cases, positive results were seen to varying degrees.[86,90]

Glover et al.[91] found a relatively crude long-lever manipulation to be significantly more effective than the placebo only in those patients who had pain for less than 7 days. On the other hand, Berquist-Ullman and Larsson[72] showed significant improvement of more specific articulating and mobilizing techniques over the placebo. The patients undergoing manipulation showed less pain after 6 weeks, less sick leave following treatment, and a decreased tendency to change their occupation.

Studies at the University of California at Irvine have helped to rule out the psychological effect of laying on of hands.[89,92–94] By selecting patients who were unable to tell the difference between a manipulative thrust and a simple massage, it was possible to demonstrate that something intrinsic to the manipulation appeared to cause improvement of symptoms in patients with low back pain.

It would appear that the positive effects of manipulation occur either immediately after the manipulation is given or within the first 4–6 weeks of treatment. Attempts at evaluating the long-term effects of manipulation using a brief, 2- to 4-week, treatment period have not demonstrated any significant differences over control subjects at 3 or 12 months.[72,94,95] And, although certain practitioners of manipulation commonly use intermittent or regular manipulation, no investigations have as yet been undertaken to determine the long-term effect of these protocols.

Ottenbacher and DiFabio[96] in their review of 57 studies on manipulation/mobilization noted that those studies that did not employ random assignment were more likely to support manipulation/mobilization. Furthermore, the use of manual therapy in conjunction with other therapies was more effective, especially when treatment effects were measured immediately after therapy. These observations again stress the need for properly controlled and defined research protocols before conclusions can be reached.

In a recently published study, McMorland and Suter[97] examined the outcome of patients receiving chiropractic treatment for uncomplicated mechanical neck and/or low back pain. A total of 119 patients were included in the study, with the treatment consisting of spinal manipulation, soft tissue treatments, home care, ergonomic, return-to-work instructions, and rehabilitative exercises. Patients were stratified based on duration and severity and statistically significant reductions in disability and pain scores were seen in all groups. Also, Bronfort et al.[98] reviewed 39 RCTs of SMT and mobilization. They state that minimal clinically important differences in patient-oriented outcomes were identified when SMT was compared with other therapies. Recent European Guidelines suggest considering referral for spinal manipulation for patients who are failing to return to normal activities.[99]

Chronic Low Back Pain There is growing evidence that SMT may be useful for the treatment of acute, uncomplicated lower back pain. The case for manipulation in the treatment of more chronic conditions, however, is less convincing. In 1985, Cassidy and Kirkaldy-Willis[100] reported on 283 patients who were unresponsive to other conservative measures, and were treated in a hospital-based setting with SMT. The authors found that some patients with low back pain and/or sciatica responded to manipulation. As might be expected, those without radiation of symptoms below the knee responded significantly better than those with distal radiation of pain. Patients with nerve compression syndromes, nerve root entrapment, and central spinal stenosis also had a lower improvement rate, but significant improvement was reported in 50% of patients with lateral entrapment and 36% with central stenosis. As a side note, the authors also suggested that clinicians who perform manipulation should do it often in order to develop and maintain optimal skills.

Two prospective studies have looked at the use of SMT in patients with chronic low back pain. The first was an RCT that was published in the *British Medical Journal*.[101] This study compared the application of clinic-based chiropractic manipulation (HVLA thrust techniques) to a hospital-based treatment. In the second follow-up study, Waagen et al.[90] reported that chiropractic manipulation was both subjectively and objectively more effective at relieving low back pain when measured against a manual placebo treatment and an outpatient family practice approach. The beneficial effect of SMT appeared to be more evident with time and, according to the authors, produced a long-term benefit in comparison to hospital outpatient programs.

Andersson et al. reported on the effect of osteopathic SMT plus standard medical treatment (83 patients) compared to more standard medical therapies (72 patients). All patients experienced back pain for at least 3 weeks but less than 6 months. Patients in both groups improved during the 12-week treatment period, with no statistically significant differences between the groups. However, the SMT group required significantly less medication and used less physical therapy.[102] In a similar study, outcomes data for 93 chiropractic patients and 45 medical patients with chronic recurrent low back pain were compared. Patients treated by chiropractors showed greater improvement and satisfaction at 1 month compared to those treated by family physicians; however, it was suggested that nonclinical factors may have played an important role.[103] Bronfort et al.[104] compared the use of trunk exercise combined with either SMT or NSAID therapy and found equal short- and long-term improvements in pain and disability. Recently, the UK BEAM Trial Team stated that manipulation followed by exercise achieved a moderate benefit at 3 months and a small benefit at 12 months.[105] In addition, the team also looked at the cost effectiveness of adding spinal manipulation, exercise classes, or manipulation followed by exercise to "best care" in general practice. They state that spinal manipulation is a cost-effective addition to "best care," and that manipulation alone probably gives better value for money than manipulation followed by exercise.[106]

Low Back Pain with Radiculopathy While the use of SMT in patients with nonradicular low back pain is becoming increasingly more accepted, the use of SMT in patients with neurological signs and/or symptoms, especially those with lumbar intervertebral disc syndromes, remains controversial. Several studies have demonstrated successful outcomes for patients with nerve root compression and intervertebral disc herniation. Mathews and Yates[107] reported a reduction of disc herniation in each of five patients treated with SMT. Other early studies using myelography have failed to demonstrate any change in discal structures, although evidence of symptom relief has been shown.[108]

The use of less invasive imaging (e.g., CTs and MRIs) has made pre- and posttreatment evaluation of disc herniation feasible. Cassidy et al.[109] reported on 14 patients undergoing side posture manipulation for lumbar disc herniation. All patients received CT scans before and 3 months after treatment. After a daily course of side posture manipulation (2–3 weeks), 13 of the patients achieved significant clinical improvement and relief. There was a small decrease in size in 5 patients, with 1 patient showing a significant decrease in the size of the disc herniation.

After reviewing the literature on the treatment of lumbar intervertebral disc herniation by side posture manipulation, Cassidy et al. suggested that manipulation is worth trying in these patients.[109] In their review, the authors state that the uncontrolled studies show a 50%–80% improvement rate in symptom relief in disc herniations treated with SMT.[110,111] Nwuga[112] in a weakly controlled study felt that lumbar side posture rotational manipulation was superior to conventional physiotherapy, adding support to this position.

In a case report, Morris[113] describes the nonsurgical treatment of an acute S1 radiculopathy resulting from a large L5–S1 disk herniation. The patient presented with an array of symptoms that included severe lower back pain. In addition, the patient had pain, paresthesia, and plantar flexion weakness of the left leg, an absent left Achilles reflex, left S1 dermatome hypesthesia, and left gastrocnemius/soleus weakness. A variety of conservative manual treatments were used, including McKenzie end-range maneuvers, flexion distraction, and side posture manipulation. Chapter 22 discusses McKenzie treatment protocols and emphasizes that trial courses of combined manual methods, such as McKenzie techniques and manipulation, can be quite effective. The patient returned to modified work 27 days after the onset of symptoms, and was discharged as asymptomatic after 50 days and 20 visits, although the left S1 reflex remained absent. Despite this improvement, a follow-up MRI demonstrated no change in the size or contour of the herniation. In a similar case of sciatica associated with discogenic lower back pain, Bergmann and Jongeward[114] discuss the use of manipulative therapy in a patient who suffered from lower back and left leg pain, decreased sensation in the dorsum of the left foot and toes, and a disc herniation demonstrated by CT. The patient was initially treated with ice followed by flexion–distraction therapy. Side posture manipulation was added after the first three treatments, and the patient was released from care after nine treatments. The authors suggest that lumbar disc herniation with neurological deficit and radicular pain does not contraindicate the judicious use of manipulation, and there is ample evidence to suggest that a course of conservative care, including spinal manipulation, should be completed before surgical consultation is considered.

Although current studies suggest that SMT may offer some promise in the treatment of lumbar radiculopathy, several authors have questioned the methodological quality of many of the studies.[98,115,116] Clearly, more quality studies are needed to clarify the appropriate utilization of SMT for radicular syndromes.

Meta-Analyses

Despite the shortcomings of some of the published research, there are now sufficient studies to be able to perform meta-analyses.[115–117] The authors of a meta-analysis of 23 randomized controlled clinical trials by Andersson[118] concluded that SMT is consistently more effective in the treatment of low back

TABLE 20–4. Clinical Characteristics of Patients Most Likely to Benefit From SMT

Author	Study	Findings
Stig et al.[65]	Patients with episodes that lasted at least 2 weeks, and pain of at least 4 weeks in the prior 12 months	50% of patients were found to be significantly better within 4 visits or 2 weeks of starting chiropractic care 75% were much better by 12 visits
Axen et al.[66]	The chance of being recovered by the fourth visit was only 30% if all of the following criteria were present	No improvement immediately after 1 visit No decrease in pain at visit 2 No decrease in disability reported at visit 2 An uncommon reaction to the first treatment
Flynn et al.[67]	Patients with low back pain most likely to respond to SMT	Segnmental dysfunction/pain upon springing over lumbar facets Acute onset of pain <16 days No pain distal to the knee Limited hip internal rotation Low fear-avoidance beliefs score
Fritz et al.[69]	Study designed to identify factors associated with an inability to benefit from manipulation	Longer symptom duration Having symptoms in the buttock or leg Absence of lumbar hypomobility Less hip range of motion Less discrepancy in left-to-right medial hip ROM A negative Gaenslen's sign

Source: From Haldeman et al.[63]

pain than are any of the comparison treatments. The authors state that the average patient receiving spinal manipulation is better off than from 54% to 85% of the patients who received the comparison treatment.

In a blinded review of randomized clinical trials, Assendelft et al.[119] noted that chiropractic seems to be an effective treatment of back pain. After extensive review of the literature, the RAND Corporation convened two panels of physicians and chiropractors and subjected the topic to a consensus process they had developed for other treatment modalities. A relatively high level of consensus was obtained.[120] Table 20–4 is a summary of the characteristics of patients determined likely to benefit from spinal manipulation by this process.

In a systematic review of the literature to assess the efficacy of SMT for patients with low back pain, Koes et al.[115] identified 36 randomized clinical trials comparing manipulation with some other treatment. Scores were assigned on a scale of 0–100 for quality of methods, the conclusion of authors regarding spinal manipulation, and the results based on the main outcome measure. Although most of the studies were of poor quality (highest score was 60), 19 (53%) showed favorable results for manipulation. Five of the studies (14%) reported positive results in one or more subgroups only. Among the five studies with highest scores (50–60 points), three were positive and two were positive only for a subgroup of the study population. Twelve trials included patients with acute low back pain only. Of these, five reported positive results, four reported negative results, and three reported positive results in a subgroup of the study population only. There were eight trials that focused on patients with subacute or chronic low back pain. Of these, five reported positive results, two were negative, and no conclusion was presented in one study. Sixteen of the studies included an effect measurement of at least 3 months, and in six of these the authors reported positive effects of manipulation. The authors conclude that while the efficacy of SMT for patients with acute or chronic low back pain has yet to be demonstrated with sound RCTs, there are indications that manipulation might be effective in some subgroups of patients.

SUMMARY

1. Spinal manipulation remains a popular modality of treatment for low back syndromes.
2. As evidence-based medicine increasingly gains popularity around the world, the scientific support for SMT appears to have grown. This has been most recently bolstered by the European Guidelines for acute and chronic low back pain, the first truly international evidence-based guidelines.
3. Further research is needed to clarify how to best utilize SMT, what types of patients would be best suited to receive a SMT, and for which conditions it would be most efficacious.

REFERENCES

1. Lomax E. Manipulative therapy: A historical perspective from ancient times to the modern era. In: Goldstein M, ed.*The research status of spinal manipulative therapy*. NINCDS Monograph No. 15. DHEW Publication No. (NIH) 76–998, Bethesda, MD, 1975.
2. Lomax E. Manipulative therapy: A historical perspective. In: Beurger AA, Tobis JS, eds. *Approaches to the validation of manipulative therapy*. Springfield, IL: CC Thomas, 1976:205–216.
3. Schiotz EH. Manipulation treatment of the spinal column from the medical–historical viewpoint (NIH Library translation). *Tidschrift For Laegeform* 1958;78:359–372.
4. Breen AC. Chiropractors and the treatment of back pain. *Rheumatol Rehabil* 1977;16:46–53.
5. Kenna C, Murtagh J. *Back pain and spinal manipulation: A practical guide*. Sydney: Butterworths, 1989.
6. Haldeman S. *Principles and practice of chiropractic*, 3rd ed. New York: McGraw-Hill, 2004.
7. Willis KW. *Managing low back pain*, 2nd ed. Baltimore: Williams & Wilkins, 1988.
8. Schafer RC, Faye LJ. *Motion palpation and chiropractic technique: Principles of dynamic chiropractic*. Huntington Beach, CA: The Motion Palpation Institute, 1989.
9. Plaugher G. *Textbook of clinical chiropractic: A specific biomechanical approach*. Baltimore: Williams & Wilkins, 1993
10. Bergmann TF. Various forms of chiropractic technique. *Chiro Tech* 1993;5(2):53–55.
11. Evans DW. Mechanisms and effects of spinal high-velocity, low-amplitude thrust manipulation: Previous theories. *J Manipulative Physiol Ther* May 2002; 25(4):251–262.
12. Gibbons P, Tehan P. Patient positioning and spinal locking for lumbar spine rotation manipulation. *Man Ther* August 2001;6(3):130–138.
13. Brodeur R. The audible release associated with joint manipulation. *J Manipulative Physiol Ther* March/April 1995;18(3):155–164.
14. Meal GM, Scott RA. Analysis of the joint crack by simultaneous recording of sound and tension. *J Manipulative Physiol Ther* September 1986;9(3):189–195.
15. Protopapas MG, Cymet TC. Joint cracking and popping: Understanding noises that accompany articular release. *J Am Osteopath Assoc* May 2002;102(5): 283–287.
16. Reggars JW, Pollard HP. Analysis of zygapophyseal joint cracking during chiropractic manipulation. *J Manipulative Physiol Ther* February 1995;18(2):65–71.
17. Beffa R, Mathews R. Does the adjustment cavitate the targeted joint? An investigation into the location of

cavitation sounds. *J Manipulative Physiol Ther* February 2004;27(2):e2.
18. Colloca CJ, Keller TS, Gunzburg R. Biomechanical and neurophysiological responses to spinal manipulation in patients with lumbar radiculopathy. *J Manipulative Physiol Ther* January 2004;27(1):1–15.
19. Flynn TW, Fritz JM, Wainner RS, Whitman JM. The audible pop is not necessary for successful spinal high-velocity thrust manipulation in individuals with low back pain. *Arch Phys Med Rehabil* July 2003;84(7):1057–1060.
20. Herzog W, Conway PJ, Zhang YT, Gal J, Guimaraes AC. Reflex responses associated with manipulative treatments on the thoracic spine: A pilot study. *J Manipulative Physiol Ther* May 1995;18(4):233–236.
21. Pickar J. Neurophysiological effects of spinal manipulation. *Spine* September/October 2002;2(5):37–71.
22. Dishman J, Bulbubian R. Spinal reflex attenuation associated with spinal manipulation. *Spine* October 1, 2000;25(19):2519–2524.
23. Dishman J, Cunningham B, Burke J. Comparison of tibial nerve H-reflex excitability after cervical and lumbar spine manipulation. *J Manipulative Physiol Ther* June 2002;25(5):318–325.
24. Dishman J, Ball K, Burke J. Central motor excitability changes after spinal manipulation: A transcranial magnetic stimulation study. *J Manipulative Physiol Ther* January 2002;25(1):1–9.
25. Sung P, Kang Y, Pickar J. Effect of spinal manipulation duration on low threshold mechanoreceptors in the lumbar paraspinal muscles: A preliminary report. *Spine* January 1, 2005;30(1):115–122.
26. Christensen MG, Kerkoff D, Kollasch MW, Cohn L. *Job analysis of chiropractic: A project report, survey analysis and summary of the practice of chiropractic within the United States*. Greeley, CO: National Board of Chiropractic Examiners, 2000.
27. Keller TS. Engineering—In vivo transient vibration analysis of the normal human spine. In: Fuhr AW, Green JR, Collaca CJ, Keller TS, eds. *Activator methods chiropractic technique*. St. Louis: C.V. Mosby, 1997:Chapt. 22.
28. Keller TS, Colloca CJ, Fuhr AW. Validation of the force and frequency characteristics of the Activator™ adjusting instrument: Effectiveness as a mechanical impedance measurement tool. *J Manipulative Physiol Ther* 1999;22(2):75–86.
29. Herzog W, Kats M, Symons B. The effective forces transmitted by high-speed, low-amplitude thoracic manipulation. *Spine* 2001;26(19):2105–2111.
30. Ross JK, Bereznick DE, McGill SM. Determining cavitation location during lumbar and thoracic spinal manipulation: Is spinal manipulation accurate and specific? *Spine* July 1, 2004;29(13):1452–1457.
31. Fuhr AW, Colloca CJ, Green JR, Keller TS. *Activator methods chiropractic technique*. St. Louis: C.V. Mosby, 1997.
32. Bergmann TF, Peterson DH, Lawrence DJ. *Chiropractic technique: Principles and procedures*. New York: Churchill Livingstone, 1993:748–749.
33. Cox JM. *Low back pain: Mechanism, diagnosis and treatment*, 5th ed. Baltimore: Williams & Wilkins, 1990.
34. Cox J. *Cox Flexion Distraction Seminar*. Whittier, CA: Los Angeles College of Chiropractic, 1998.
35. Bigelow HJ. Insensibility during surgical operations produced by inhalation. *Boston Med Surg J* 1846;35:309–317.
36. Mennell JB. *Massage, its principles and practice*. by London: J & A Churchill, 1920;213–215.
37. Siehl D, Bradford, W. Manipulation of the low back under general anesthesia. *J Am Osteopathic Assoc. (Orthoped Suppl)* December 1952;8(1):239–241.
38. Beckett RH, Francis R. Spinal manipulation under anesthesia. In: Lawrence DJ, ed. *Advance in Chiropractic*. Vol. 1. St. Louis: Mosby-Year Book, 1994;325–340.
39. Morey LW Jr. Osteopathic manipulation under general anesthesia. *J Am Osteopathic Assoc* March 1978; 73:127–135.
40. Greenman P, Manipulation with the patient under anesthesia. *J Am Osteopathic Assoc* September 1992; 1159–1170.
41. Francis R. Spinal manipulation under general anesthesia: "A chiropractic approach in a hospital setting." *ACA J Chiropractic* December 1989;12:39–41.
42. Alexander GK. Manipulation under anesthesia of lumbar post-laminectomy syndrome patients with epidural fibrosis and recurrent HNP. *ACA J Chiropractic* June 1993;6:79–82.
43. Davis CG, Fernando CA, da Motta MA. Manipulation of the low back under general anesthesia: Case studies and discussion. *JNMS* Fall 1993;1(3):126–134.
44. Ben-David B, Raboy M. Manipulation under anesthesia combined with epidural steroid injection. *JMPT* November/December 1994;17(9):605–609.
45. West DT, Matthews RS, Miller MR, Kent GM. Effective management of spinal pain in one hundred seventy-seven patients evaluated for manipulation under anesthesia. *J Manipulative Physiol Ther* June 1999;22(5):299–307.
46. Lewin P. *The disc and its syndromes*. Philadelphia: Lea & Febiger, 1955:19.
47. Haldeman S, Rubinstein SM. Cauda equina syndrome in patients undergoing manipulation of the lumbar spine. *Spine* December 17,1992;17(12):1469–1473.
48. Haldeman S, Kohlbeck FJ. Medication-assisted spinal manipulation. *Spine J* July/August 2002;2(4):288–302.
49. Kohlbeck F. Medication-assisted spinal manipulation. In: Haldeman S, ed. *Principles and practice of chiropractic*, 3rd ed. New York: McGraw-Hill, 2005;850–859.
50. AHCPR. Management guidelines for acute low back pain. Rockville MD: Agency for Health Care Policy and Research, US Department of Health and Human Services, 1994.
51. Spitzer WO. Scientific approach to the assessment and management of activity-related spinal disorders. A monograph for clinicians. Report of the Quebec Task Force. *Spine* 1987;12:51.
52. Clinical Standards Advisory Group report on back pain. London: HMSO Publication Center, December 1994.

53. ACC. *New Zealand acute low back pain guide*. Wellington, NZ: Accident Rehabilitation & Compensation Insurance Corporation of New Zealand and the National Health Committee, 1997.
54. Airaksinen O, Hildebrandt J, Mannion AF, et al. European guidelines for the management of chronic nonspecific low back pain. Management Committee of COST B13, Palma de Mallorca, 2004.
55. Manga P, Angus D. Report on chiropractic. *CMAJ* October 15, 1994;151(8):1107–1108; author reply 1108, 1110.
56. Dishman JD, Burke J. Spinal reflex excitability changes after cervical and lumbar spinal manipulation: A comparative study. *Spine* May/June 2003;3(3):204–212.
57. Pickar JG. An in vivo preparation for investigating neural responses to controlled loading of a lumbar vertebra in the anesthetized cat. *J Neurosci Methods* July 15, 1999;89(2):87–96.
58. Ladermann JP. Accidents of spinal manipulation. *Ann Swiss Chiro Assoc* 1981;7:161–208.
59. Shekelle PG, Adams AH, Chassin MR, Hurwitz EL, Brook RH. Spinal manipulation for low-back pain. *Ann Intern Med* October 1, 1992;117(7):590–598.
60. Richard J. Disk rupture with cauda equina syndrome after chiropractic adjustment. *NY State J Med* September 15, 1967;67(18):2496–2498.
61. Gallinaro P, Cartesegna M. Three cases of lumbar disc rupture and one of cauda equina associated with spinal manipulation (chiropraxis) *Lancet* February 19, 1983;1(8321):411.
62. Markowitz HD, Dolce DT. Cauda equina syndrome due to sequestrated recurrent disk herniation after chiropractic manipulation. *Orthopedics* July 1997;20(7):652–653.
63. Haldeman S, Hooper PD, Phillips RB, Scaringe JG, Traina AD. Spinal manipulative therapy. In: *The adult spine: Principles and practice*, 2nd ed. Frymoyer JW, ed. Philadelphia: Lippincott-Raven, 1997:1837–1861.
64. Dvorak J, Kranzlin P, Muhlemann D, Walchli B. Musculoskeletal complications. In: Haldeman S, ed. *Principles and practice of chiropractic*, 2nd ed. Norwalk, CT: Appleton and Lange, 1992;549–577.
65. Stig LC, Nilsson O, Leboeuf-Yde C. Recovery pattern of patients treated with chiropractic spinal manipulative therapy for long-lasting or recurrent low back pain. *J Manipulative Physiol Ther* May 2001;24(4):288–291.
66. Axen I, Rosenbaum A, Robech R, Wren T, Leboeuf-Yde C. Can patient reactions to the first chiropractic treatment predict early favorable treatment outcome in persistent low back pain? *J Manipulative Physiol Ther* September 2002;25(7):450–454.
67. Flynn T, Fritz J, Whitman J, et al. A clinical prediction rule for classifying patients with low back pain who demonstrate short-term improvement with spinal manipulation. *Spine* December 15, 2002;27(24):2835–2843.
68. Flynn T, Fritz J, Whitman J, Wainner R, Magel J, Rendeiro D, Butler B, Garber M, Allison S. A clinical prediction rule for classifying patients with low back pain who demonstrate short-term improvement with spinal manipulation. *Spine* December 15, 2002;27(24): 2835–2843.
69. Fritz JM, Whitman JM, Flynn TW, Wainner RS, Childs JD. Factors related to the inability of individuals with low back pain to improve with a spinal manipulation. *Phys Ther* February 2004;84(2):173–190.
70. Breen AC. Chiropractors and the treatment of back pain. *Rheumatol Rehabil* 1977;16:46–53.
71. Nyiendo J, Phillips RB, Meeker W, Kunsler G, Jansen R, Menon M. A comparison of patients and patient complaints at six chiropractic college teaching clinics. *J Manipulative Physiol Ther* 1989;12:79–85.
72. Berquist-Ullman M, Larsson U. Acute low back pain in industry. *Acta Orthop Scand* 1977;170(Suppl): 1–117.
73. Tobis JS, Hoehler FK. Musculoskeletal manipulation in the treatment of low back pain. *Bull NY Acad Med* September 1983;59(7):660–668.
74. Korr IM. *Neurobiologic mechanisms in manipulative therapy*. New York: Plenum Press, 1978.
75. Anderson R, Meeker WC, Wirick BE, Mootz RD, Kirk DH, Adams A. A meta-analysis of clinical trials of spinal manipulation. *J Manipulative Physiol Ther* March/April 1992;15(3):181–194.
76. Assendelft WJ, Koes BW, Knipschild PG, Bouter LM. The relationship between methodological quality and conclusions in reviews of spinal manipulation. *JAMA* December 27, 1995;274(24):1942–1948.
77. Koes BW, Assendelft WJ, van der Jeijden GJ, Bouter LM, Knipschild PG. Spinal manipulation and mobilisation for back and neck pain: A blinded review. *BMJ* November 23, 1991;303(6813):1298–1303.
78. Bronfort G, Haas M, Evans RL, Bouter LM. Efficacy of spinal manipulation and mobilization for low back pain and neck pain: A systematic review and best evidence synthesis. *Spine J* May/June 2004;4(3):335–356.
79. Ernst E. Chiropractic spinal manipulation for neck pain: A systematic review. *J Pain* October 2003;4(8): 417–421.
80. Koes BW, Bouter LM, van der Heijden GJ. Methodological quality of randomized clinical trials on treatment efficacy in low back pain. *Spine* January 15, 1995;20(2):228–235.
81. Chrisman OD, Mittnacht A, Snook GA A study of the results following rotatory manipulation in the lumbar intervertebral disc syndrome. *J Bone Joint Surg* 1964;46A:517–524.
82. Fisk JW. Manipulation in general practice. *NZ Med J* September 1971;74(471):172–175.
83. Coyer AB, Curwen IHM. Low back pain treated by manipulation: A controlled series. *BMJ* March 19, 1955;19:705–707.
84. Evans DP, Burke MS, Lloyd KN, Roberts EE, Roberts GM. Lumbar spinal manipulation on trial. Part 1. Clinical assessment. *Rheumatol Rehabil* 1978;17:46–53.
85. Edwards BC. Low back pain resulting from lumbar spine conditions. A comparison of treatment results. *Aust J Physiother* 1969;15:104–110.

86. Hadler NM. A benefit of spinal manipulation as adjunctive therapy for acute low-back pain: A stratified controlled trial. *Spine* September 1987;12(7):702–706.
87. Coxhead CE. Physiotherapy in low back pain. *Nurs Mirror Midwives J* January 13, 1977;144(2):57–59.
88. Doran DML, Newell DJ. Manipulation in treatment of low back pain: A multicentre study. *BMJ* 1975;2:161–164.
89. Buerger AA. A clinical trial of rotational manipulation. In: *Pain Abstracts*, Second World Congress on Pain, Montreal, Canada. International Association for the Study of Pain, *Seattle* 1978;1:248.
90. Waagen GN, Haldeman S, Cook G, Lopez D, DeBoer KF. Short term trial of chiropractic adjustments for the relief of chronic low back pain. *Manual Med* 1986;2:63–67.
91. Glover JR, Morris JG, Khosla T. Back pain: A randomized clinical trial of rotational manipulation of the trunk. *Br J Ind Med* 1974;31:59–64.
92. Brunarski DJ. Clinical trials of spinal manipulation: A critical appraisal and review of the literature. *J Manipulative Physiol Ther* 1984;7:243–249.
93. Buerger AA. A clinical trial of spinal manipulation. *Fed Proc* 1979;38:1250.
94. Hoehler FK, Tobis JS, Buerger AA. Spinal manipulation for low back pain. *JAMA* 1981;245:1835–1838.
95. Sims-Williams H, Jayson MIDC, Young SMS, Baddeley H, Collins E. Controlled trial of mobilization and manipulation for patients with low back pain in general practice. *BMJ* 1978;2:1338–1340.
96. Ottenbacher K, DiFabio RP. Efficiency of spinal manipulation/mobilization therapy. A meta-analysis. *Spine* 1985;10:833–837.
97. McMorland G, Suter E. Chiropractic management of mechanical neck and low-back pain: A retrospective, outcome-based analysis. *J Manipulative Physiol Ther* June 2000;23(5):307–311.
98. Bronfort G, Haas M, Bouter LM, et al. Efficacy of spinal manipulation and mobilization for low back and neck pain: A systematic review and best evidence synthesis. In Bronfort G, ed. *Efficacy of manual therapies of the spine* [Thesis]. EMGO Institute: Amsterdam, the Netherlands, 1997.
99. van Tulder MT, Becker A, Bekkering T, et al. European guidelines for the management of acute nonspecific low back pain in primary care. Management Committee of COST B13, the Netherlands, 2004.
100. Cassidy JD, Kirkaldy-Willis WH. Spinal manipulation for the treatment of chronic low back and leg pain: An observational study. In: Buerger AA, Greenman PE, eds. Empirical approaches to the validation of spinal manipulation. Springfield, IL: CC Thomas, 1985:119–148.
101. Meade TW, Dyer S, Browne W, Townsend J, Frank AO. Low back pain of mechanical origin: Randomized comparison of chiropractic and hospital outpatient treatment. *BMJ* 1990;300:1431–1437.
102. Andersson GB, Lucente T, Davis AM, Kappler RE, Lipton JA, Leurgans S. A comparison of osteopathic spinal manipulation with standard care for patients with low back pain. *N Engl J Med* November 4, 1999;341(19):1426–1431.
103. Nyiendo J, Haas M, Goodwin P. Patient characteristics, practice activities, and one-month outcomes for chronic, recurrent low-back pain treated by chiropractors and family medicine physicians: A practice-based feasibility study. *J Manipulativc Physiol Ther* May 2000;23(4):239–245.
104. Bronfort G, Goldsmith CH, Nelson CF, et al. Trunk exercise combined with spinal manipulative or NSAID therapy for chronic low back pain: A randomized, observe-blinded clinical trial. *J Manipulative Physiol Ther* 1996;19:570–582.
105. UK BEAM Trial Team. United Kingdom back pain exercise and manipulation randomized trial: Effectiveness of physical treatments for back pain in primary care. *BMJ* December 11, 2004;329(7479):1377–1385.
106. UK BEAM Trial Team. United Kingdom back pain exercise and manipulation randomized trial: Cost effectiveness of physical treatments for back pain in primary care. *BMJ* December 11, 2004;329(7479): 1381–1385.
107. Mathews JA, Yates DAH. Reduction of lumbar disc prolapse by manipulation. *J Bone Joint Surg* 1964; 46-A:517–524.
108. Chrisman OD, Mittnacht A, Snook GA. A study of the results following rotatory manipulation in the lumbar intervertebral disc syndrome. *Journal of Bone and Joint Surgery* 1964;46A:517–524.
109. Cassidy JD, Thiel HW, Kirkaldy-Willis WH. Side posture manipulation for lumbar intervertebral disk herniation. *J Manipulative Physiol Ther* February 1993; 16(2):96–103.
110. Chrisman OD, Mittnacht A, Snook GA. A study of the results following rotatory manipulation in the lumbar intervertebral disc syndrome. *J Bone Joint Surg* 1964;46A:517–524.
111. Kuo PP, Loh Z. Treatment of lumbar intervertebral disc protrusions by manipulation. *Clin Orthop* 1987;215:47–55.
112. Nwuga VCB. Relative therapeutic efficacy of vertebral manipulation and conventional treatment in back pain management. *Am J Phys Med Rehabil* 1982;61:273–278.
113. Morris CE. Chiropractic rehabilitation of a patient with S1 radiculopathy associated with a large lumbar disk herniation. *J Manipulative Physiol Ther* January 1999;22(1):38–44.
114. Bergmann TF, Jongeward BV. Manipulative therapy in lower back pain with leg pain and neurological deficit. *J Manipulative Physiol Ther* May 1998;21(4):288–294.
115. Koes BW, Assendelft WJ, van der Heijden GJ, Bouter LM. Spinal manipulation for low back pain: An updated systematic review of randomized clinical trials. *Spine* 1996;21:2860–2871.
116. van Tulder MW, Koes BW, Bouter LM. Conservative treatment of acute and chronic nonspecific low back pain: A systematic review of randomized controlled trials of the most common interventions. *Spine* 1997;22(18):2128–2156.

117. Shekelle PG, Adams AH, Chassin MR, Hurwitz EL, Brook RH. Spinal manipulation for low-back pain. *Ann Intern Med* October 1, 1992;117(7):590–598.
118. Andersson GB. Factors important in the genesis and prevention of occupational back pain and disability. *J Manipulative Physiol Ther* January 1992;15(1): 43–46.
119. Assendelft WJ, Koes BW, van der Heijden GJ, Bouter LM. The effectiveness of chiropractic for treatment of low back pain: An update and attempt at statistical pooling. *J Manipulative Physiol Ther* October 1996;19(8):499–507.
120. Shekelle PG, Adams AH, Chassin MR, Hurwitz EL, Brook RH. Spinal manipulation for low-back pain. *Ann Intern Med* October 1, 1992;117(7):590–598.

CHAPTER

21

THE BIOMECHANICS OF SPINAL MANIPULATION

Walter Herzog

OUTLINE

OBJECTIVES

1. To critically review the scientific information on the biomechanics of spinal manipulation with focus on (a) the external forces exerted by clinicians on patients, (b) the vertebral movements caused by these forces, and (c) the internal forces transmitted by structures such as intervertebral discs and vertebral arteries during spinal manipulation
2. To critically review the physiological and neuromuscular effects caused by spinal manipulation with focus on (a) reflex activation, (b) reflex inhibition, and (c) the Hoffmann (H-) reflex response associated with spinal manipulation

INTRODUCTION

Background

Spinal manipulation has been a subject of great historic interest for the treatment of a number of maladies, including various spinal syndromes. A quick glance at the existing scientific evidence regarding spinal manipulation in the early 1980s, whether from the chiropractic, osteopathic, or medical literature, showed that it was largely based on anecdotal evidence and hearsay. Therefore, scientific research was initiated in 1985 at the University of Calgary in this fascinating field. With a background in biomechanics, researchers at the University of Calgary initially focused on establishing the forces exerted during spinal manipulation, the corresponding spinal (vertebral) movements, and determining the loading of internal structures through spinal manipulation.

However, soon following the initial "mechanical" experiments, it became obvious that spinal manipulations gave "physiological" results that might produce beneficial treatment effects. Therefore, goals were set to quantify some of the "neurophysiological" effects that were produced during spinal manipulation. A precise understanding of the location of the origins of the audible releases associated with spinal manipulation that motivated these studies was also sought. The interpolated-twitch-technique-measured cavitation sounds and electromyographic (EMG) activities triggered by spinal manipulation were all introduced at this time. These techniques then served students, post-doctoral trainees, and clinicians to perform a series of critical experiments that helped elucidate the neurophysiological effects associated with spinal manipulation. These studies form the nucleus of this chapter.

Definition of Biomechanics

Biomechanics is the science that deals with the external and internal forces acting on (or in) a biological system, and the effects produced by these forces. Typically, "effects" are understood to be mechanical in nature (displacements, velocities, accelerations, etc.); however, in the context of this chapter, "biological" or "physiological" effects will be included that are produced by spinal manipulation. But the line will be drawn at psychological and social effects that might be associated with spinal manipulation. Such effects will not be treated here, with the exception of studies in which placebo or sham treatments were considered.

Spinal Manipulation

The art of spinal manipulation has many facets, origins, and interpretations. In the context of this chapter, spinal manipulations are treatments of high-speed (or high-velocity) and low-amplitude produced by the thrusting of a hand (contact) on specific parts of the spine. All spinal manipulations in our studies were given by full-time practicing chiropractors. Short consideration will also be given to Activator™ and Integrator™ manipulations that mimic, to a certain degree, the high-speed, low-amplitude thrust provided by the manually applied spinal treatments.

Purpose

The purpose of this chapter is to briefly review the existing data on the mechanics of spinal manipulation and to relate the mechanical events to the accompanying neurophysiological effects, such as reflex responses, muscle inhibition, and EMG occurrences. The review will be based on our own experiences, and therefore should not be considered a total treatment of the biomechanics and neurophysiology of spinal manipulation. Rather, it should be seen as a review with focus on specific topics.

THE BIOMECHANICS OF SPINAL MANIPULATION

The External Forces Applied during High-Speed, Low-Amplitude Spinal Manipulative Treatment

When performing a high-speed, low-amplitude spinal manipulative treatment, three phases can be identified on the corresponding force–time plot (Fig. 21–1): the preload phase, the thrust phase, and the resolution phase.

Clinical Peral: When performing a high-speed, low-amplitude spinal manipulative treatment, three phases can be identified on the corresponding force–time plot (Fig. 21–1): the preload phase, the thrust phase, and the resolution phase.

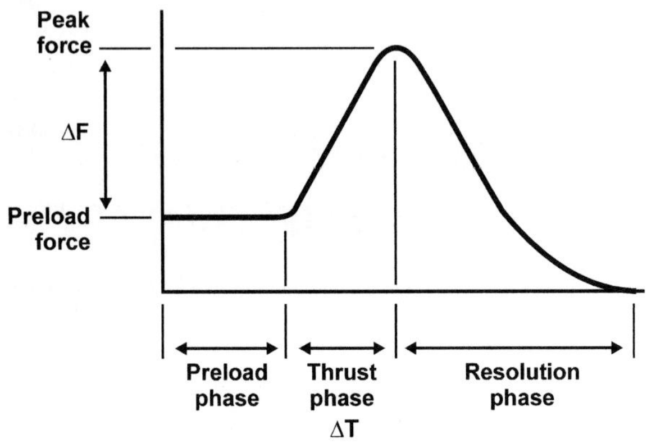

FIGURE 21–1. Schematic representation of the force–time history of a spinal manipulative treatment and selected definitions of force parameters.

The *preload phase* allows the clinician to make a good contact with the thrusting hand(s) on the target point on the spine. In this phase, the target joint is typically moved to the endpoint of the physiologic range of motion. Therefore, any additional force (that occurs during the thrust phase) is believed to move the target joint beyond the normal range of motion, into the so-called paraphysiological zone. The preload phase typically lasts for 5–10 seconds. Oftentimes, the clinician will synchronize the end of the preload phase with an "external" event, for example a specific point in the patient's breathing cycle. The end of the preload phase is typically associated with a small unloading, a pumping-like action, to initiate the following thrust phase (Fig. 21–2).

The *thrust phase* follows the preload phase without delay. The thrust phase is considered the actual spinal manipulative treatment. In this phase, the clinician attempts to apply a precisely defined force magnitude in a defined direction to the target point. The thrust is given at a high speed, and the rate of force increase is substantial. Thrusts to the cervical spine typically last less than 100 ms; thrusts to the thoracic and lumbar spine, as well as to the sacroiliac joint, typically last less than 200 ms (Table 21–1). In this short time frame, forces of up to 1200 N may be given to the patients (unpublished observations); 1200 N is a force equivalent to 1.5 times the weight of an 80-kg (176-lb) individual.

Average peak forces given during the thrust phase of spinal manipulations depend strongly on the site of treatment. Average peak forces for treatments on the cervical spine are in the order of 100–150 N (Table 21–1, Fig. 21–3), often with little or no preload force preceding the thrust. Average peak forces across a number of chiropractors and subjects are approximately 300–500 N in our laboratory (Table 21–1), although we have

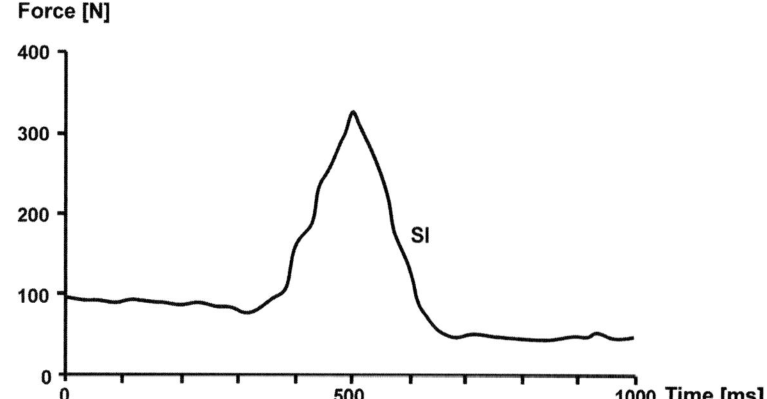

FIGURE 21–2. Mean ($n = 6$), representative force–time curve for high-speed, low-amplitude manipulative treatments to the sacroiliac joint (SI) using the Thompson technique. The treatments were performed by the same chiropractor on six different patients.

measured forces in excess of 1000 N from individual chiropractors, as mentioned above (unpublished observations).

Based on results from a variety of studies in which the forces applied by chiropractors on patients were directly measured (and not calculated or derived based on an inverse dynamics approach[7]), the following general statements can be made:

- The peak thrust forces vary greatly across clinicians.[2,8]
- The peak thrust forces vary for a given clinician depending on the patient.[8,9]
- The peak thrust forces vary greatly depending on the treatment site; cervical treatments typically give smaller peak thrust forces than treatments at any other location of the spine.[5,8–11]
- The peak thrust forces were statistically significantly related to the preload forces for a given practitioner. In practice that means that if a clinician produced a greater preload force in one patient compared to another, then the peak thrust force and the change in force from preload to peak force (Fig. 21–1) tended to be greater as well.[12]
- The time of thrust application (Δt, Fig. 21–1) was approximately 50–150 ms for cervical manipulations, and 100–200 ms for manipulations at all other segments of the spine. As such, the time of thrust application was the only variable in the force–time curves that appeared to be similar across clinicians and patients.

From the above findings, one might conclude that the peak thrust force magnitude (and the associated rate of change in thrust force) is not a determinant of a successful treatment, as different (successful) clinicians reach greatly different peak force magnitudes in their treatments. However, the time period within which the thrust force is completed seems "invariant," and therefore might possibly be the trademark of successful clinical treatments. We will come back to the idea of a successful treatment later in this chapter.

Clinical Peral: From the above findings, one might conclude that the peak thrust force magnitude (and the associated rate of change in thrust force) is not a determinant of a successful treatment, as different (successful) clinicians reach greatly different peak force magnitudes in their treatments.

The *resolution phase* follows the treatment thrust, and is associated with the release of the thrusting hand(s) from the patient. It is highly variable among clinicians, and is typically not considered relevant for the clinical success of the treatment. For lack of any evidence (and scientific study on the resolution phase), I will not attempt to provide any further details on this final phase of the force–time curve of spinal manipulations.

Vertebral Movements Associated with the Treatment Thrust of Spinal Manipulations

About 10 years ago, one of the primary questions of the biomechanics of spinal manipulation was: Is there relative movement of adjacent vertebrae during the treatment thrust? Obviously, a clinician always feels movement of the spine in the thrust phase (Fig. 21–1); however, until recently it was not clear whether this movement was caused exclusively by relative movements of nontarget spinal segments that moved within the normal range of motion, or if some of this movement was caused by the target vertebrae moving in the paraphysiological zone.

There are a series of studies in which relative vertebral movements were assessed for treatments using the Activator™ instrument[13–15] or using low-speed, low-force manipulations.[16,17] In these studies, substantial relative movements between adjacent vertebral bodies were measured, but the peak forces were of magnitudes similar or smaller than the preload forces measured during high-speed, low-amplitude spinal manipulation. Therefore, these movements likely occurred within the normal range of motion and are of little relevance here.

TABLE 21–1. **Summary of Selected Force–Time Characteristics of Spinal Manipulative Therapy**

Source	Site	Treatment Technique	Measurement Technique	Preload Force (N)*	Preload Force (N)	Peak Force (N)*	Peak Force (N)	Treatment Time (ms)*	Treatment Time (ms)*	Time to Peak (ms)*	Time to Peak (ms)*
Wood/Adams[1]	SI	Thompson technique	Simulator			257 ± 76R 254 ± 82L			175–547		
Hessel et al.[2]	SI	Thompson technique	EMED		20–180		250–450 220–550	271 (1) 280 (2)	200–420		
Herzog et al.[3]	SI	Thompson technique	EMED	88 ± 78		328 ± 78					
Herzog et al.[3]	T4	Posterior-to-anterior, hy-pothenar	EMED	139 ± 46		399 ± 119				150 ± 77	
Triano/Schultz[4]	C	R, L rotate	Force-plate inverse dynamics			123 R 111 L			200–300		
Kawchuk et al.[5]	C 1, 2	Toggle technique	EMED	2 ± 2	0–11	118 ± 16	99–140	102 ± 15	90–120	48 ± 15	30–65
Kawchuk et al.[6]	C 1, 2	Lateral break	EMED	40 ± 5		102 ± 7				87 ± 3	
Kawchuk et al.[6]	C 1, 2	Gonstead technique	EMED	25 ± 7		110 ± 6				92 ± 5	
Kawchuk et al.[6]	C 1, 2	Rotation technique	EMED	29 ± 4		41 ± 5				79 ± 4	

Note: SI, sacroiliac.

*Values represent mean ± SD.

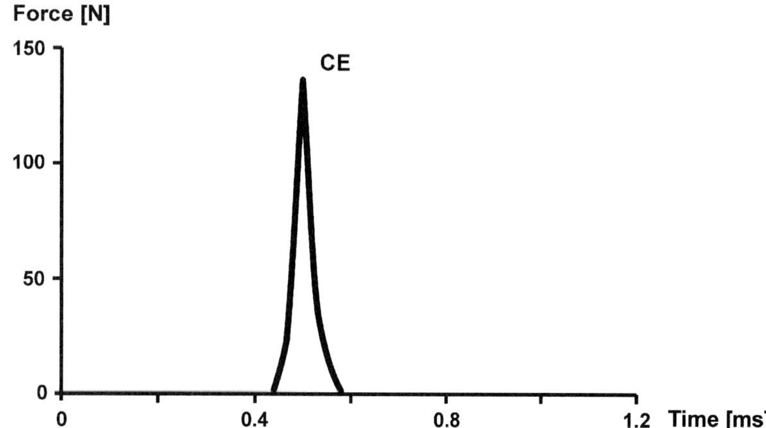

FIGURE 21–3. Representative force–time history of a spinal manipulation on the cervical spine.

In order to test whether there was relative movement of vertebral bodies in the paraphysiological zone of the treatment thrust, Gál and collaborators[18] performed a study in which the three-dimensional movements of vertebrae T10–T12 were quantified following the application of preload forces during the treatment thrust. In order to do this, two bone pins were embedded in each of the three target vertebrae in two human cadaveric specimens.[18,19] The spinal manipulations consisted of straight posterior-to-anterior thrusts using a reinforced hypothenar contact on the transverse process of the target vertebra. Each bone pin contained a series of markers that were digitized from high-speed film (100 frames/s). The thrust forces were recorded using a thin, flexible pressure pad (EMED Inc., Munich).

The mean preload and peak forces were 82 and 532 N, respectively ($n = 30$).[18,20] Absolute posterior-to-anterior and lateral displacements of the vertebrae were 6–12 and 3–6 mm, respectively (Fig. 21–4*A*). Relative axial and sagittal rotations during the treatment thrust were 0.4–1.2 and 0.1–1.8 degrees, respectively (Fig. 21–4*B*). Only the relative axial and sagittal rotations were statistically significant; none of the relative linear displacements showed consistent trends.

Why should straight posterior-to-anterior thrusts to the transverse process cause rotations of adjacent vertebral segments? Imagine that the force applied by the clinician is as shown schematically in Figure 21–5. If we further assume that the axis of rotation is somewhere along the anterior–posterior axis of symmetry of the vertebra, the force applied to the transverse process will tend to displace the vertebra anteriorly and will produce an axial rotation, as shown in the figure. However, one cannot just consider a vertebral body in isolation. One must visualize that the target vertebra is also bracketed by a vertebra above and below the target segment (Fig. 21–5). As the target vertebra is displaced anteriorly, the adjacent vertebrae will be "dragged" along because of their attachment to the target vertebra. This will cause sagittal rotation of the adjacent vertebrae relative to the target vertebra, as shown in Figure 21–5. The relative axial and sagittal rotations of T10, T11, and T12 measured in the studies by Gál et al.[18–21] were in exact agreement with the theoretically expected relative movements made using Figure 21–5.

Therefore, based on the results by Gál et al.[18–21] (and these still appear to be the only studies of relative, three-dimensional movements of human vertebrae

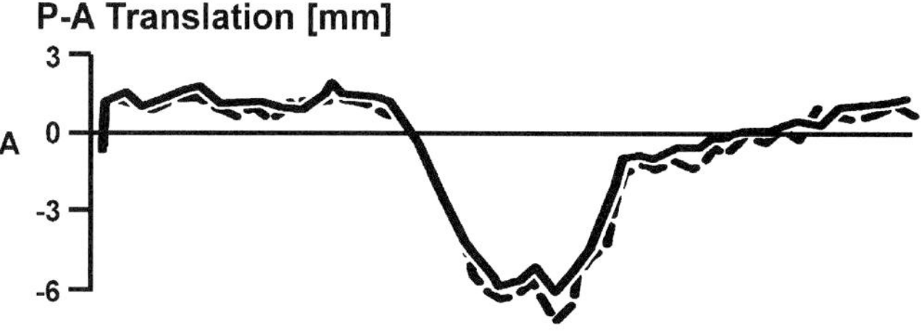

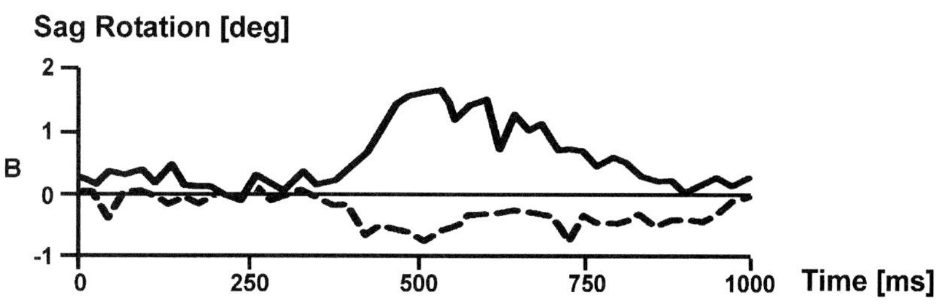

FIGURE 21–4. Posterior-to-anterior translations (*A*) and sagittal rotations (*B*) of T10 and T12 during a posterior-to-anterior thrust to the transverse process of T11 in a fresh, unembalmed, post rigor, human cadaver. Displacements were recorded after the application of the preload force; therefore, the linear and angular displacements shown are likely in the paraphysiological zone.

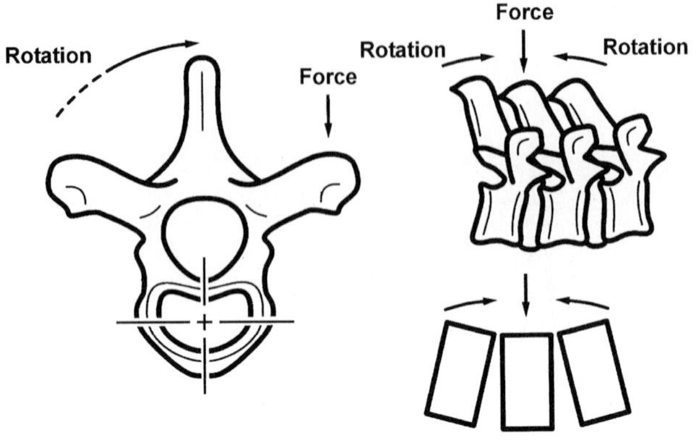

FIGURE 21–5. Schematic illustration of a spinal manipulative force on a vertebral body and its effect on the target and neighboring vertebrae. A straight posterior-to-anterior force to the transverse process of a vertebrate (as shown) will likely cause an anterior displacement and an axial rotation (clockwise, in the example shown) of the target vertebrae. Because of the anterior displacement of the target vertebrae, the adjacent vertebrae will likely undergo a sagittal rotation (in opposite directions, as indicated by the arrows).

during high-speed, low-amplitude spinal manipulations), it appears that vertebral bodies adjacent to the target vertebra will undergo relative movements in the so-called paraphysiological zone during spinal manipulation.

Internal Forces Associated with Spinal Manipulations

In a book published in 2000, Herzog stated "there are no measurements of internal forces during spinal manipulative treatments." Internal forces were defined as the forces carried by body internal structures, such as the transverse or spinous processes, ligaments, muscles, intervertebral discs, blood vessels, nerves, etc. Obviously, some of these structures are of particular interest in the analysis of spinal manipulation as they are thought to carry substantial loads (e.g., discs) or because they are implicated in injuries following spinal manipulation (e.g., blood vessels).

There are currently two reports on internal forces during spinal manipulation. The first deals with changes in intradiscal pressure during lumbar spinal manipulation,[22] and the second deals with the forces and elongations of the vertebral artery during high-speed, low-amplitude treatments of the neck.[23] Maigne and Guillon[22] inserted a pressure sensor into lumbar intervertebral discs and measured the intradiscal pressure in two cadaveric specimens exposed to two spinal manipulative treatments. They found an increase in intradiscal pressure (0.65 bars ± 0.2 bars) in the initial phase of the thrust. They interpreted the increase in pressure as being caused by the relative rotation of the adjacent vertebral bodies that is produced by the manipulative thrust. They then found a decrease in pressure in the second part of the thrust that was partly associated with recoil from the thrust and a traction of the lumbar spine. The authors speculated that there might be two beneficial effects of the *pressure decrease in the second part of the manipulative thrust*: (1) a decreased pressure may help a protrusion to be sucked back into the center of the disc, and (2) the pressure decrease was thought to provide a more uniform pressure distribution on the end plates of the discs, and so reduce stress on the end plates and possibly reduce pain. However, because of the small number of specimens ($n = 2$) and individual tests ($n = 5$), no generalizations of these data can, and should, be made about the effects of spinal manipulative treatments on disc pressure. Also, the measurements were made at a single location within the disc, whereas one must expect that intradiscal pressures vary as a function of location. Since it is not known what pressures are required to cause damage to a disc, we cannot relate the pressure increase during the treatment thrust to a failure load. Finally, it must be remembered that all measurements were made in cadavers; therefore any changes in material properties from a live patient to the specimens used here would not be accounted for. Muscular reflex responses observed in patients would likely not influence the first part of the pressure measurements (i.e., the increased pressures) because it typically takes 50–200 ms from the onset of the treatment thrust until the appearance of muscle reflex responses. And, accounting for the electromechanical delay, muscle forces would likely only occur approximately 150–300 ms after the onset of the thrust, that is, just about at the end of the intradiscal pressure increase. However, disc pressure decreases 200–300 ms after the onset of the treatment thrust, which coincides precisely with the expected reflex increase in muscle force observed in live subjects.[24] Therefore, the observed decrease in intradiscal pressure observed in the cadaveric specimens may be offset, or reversed, in real subjects by increases in muscle force. Thus, we should be careful when interpreting Maigne and Guillon's beneficial effects of the intradiscal pressure decreases in cadavers, as they may not occur in real subjects because of the reflex increase in muscle force.[22]

Clinical Peral: We should be careful when interpreting Maigne and Guillon's beneficial effects of the intradiscal pressure decreases in cadavers, as they may not occur in real subjects because of the reflex increase in muscle force.[22]

Symons et al.[23] quantified the forces and strains in the vertebral artery in situ during spinal manipulation. The study was motivated by the increasing concern of the safety of neck manipulations and the risk of stroke in the vertebrobasilar system.

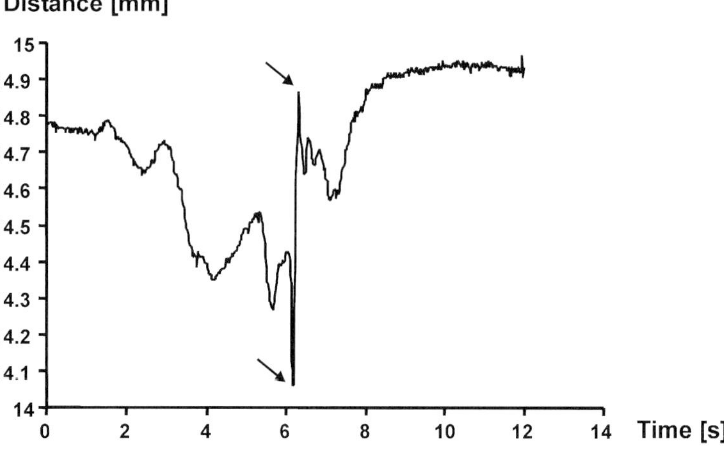

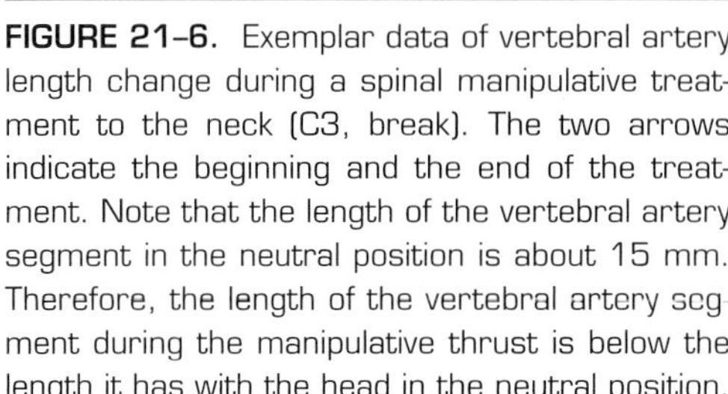
FIGURE 21-6. Exemplar data of vertebral artery length change during a spinal manipulative treatment to the neck (C3, break). The two arrows indicate the beginning and the end of the treatment. Note that the length of the vertebral artery segment in the neutral position is about 15 mm. Therefore, the length of the vertebral artery segment during the manipulative thrust is below the length it has with the head in the neutral position.

Strain measurements were obtained in six vertebral arteries at the C0–C1 and the C6-subclavian artery level using sonomicrometry. Strains were determined for a series of clinically relevant range of motion tests, diagnostic procedures, and spinal manipulations. Following the in situ testing, the vertebral arteries were dissected free and force–strain relationships up to mechanical failure were obtained using an Instron (1122) materials testing machine.

Spinal manipulative treatments on the contralateral side of the cervical spine resulted in an average strain of 6.2 ∀ 1.3% to the distal segment (C0–C1) of the vertebral artery, and 2.1 ∀ 0.4% strain to the proximal (C6-subclavian artery) segment (Fig. 21–6). These strain values were similar or lower than the strains recorded during diagnostic and range of motion testing. Failure strains of the vertebral arteries were 39%–62%. Therefore, the strains sustained by the vertebral arteries during spinal manipulation were found to range from about one sixth to one thirtieth of the failure strain.

Symons et al.[23] concluded that the strains of the vertebral arteries during spinal manipulations were an order of magnitude smaller than the failure strain. Therefore, they concluded that under normal circumstances, a single, typical spinal manipulation is unlikely to mechanically disrupt the vertebral artery. Needless to say that these two isolated studies on internal forces associated with spinal manipulation do not allow us to gain insight into the internal mechanics of these treatment procedures. There is much research to be done, and much opportunity, in this area of scientific investigation.

Clinical Peral: Symons et al.[23] concluded that the strains of the vertebral arteries during spinal manipulations were an order of magnitude smaller than the failure strain. Therefore, they concluded that under normal circumstances, a single, typical spinal manipulation is unlikely to mechanically disrupt the vertebral artery.

THE NEUROPHYSIOLOGICAL EFFECTS ASSOCIATED WITH SPINAL MANIPULATION

Reflex Activation of Muscles during Spinal Manipulative Treatments

It has been hypothesized that the thrust-like forces produced during high-speed, low-amplitude treatments elicit reflex responses, which in turn may influence spinal health in a variety of ways—reflex inhibition of hypertonic muscles,[25–28] reduction of pain,[26,27,29] and short-term reflex activation of skeletal muscles of the back[24,30] and upper limbs,[24] to name but a few of the possibilities. Theoretically, the reflex responses (or inhibitions) may be elicited from a variety of receptors, including the various mechanoreceptors in the capsule of spinal facet joints, pain receptors, cutaneous receptors, and the proprioceptors of skeletal muscles: the muscle spindles and Golgi tendon organs.

During and following spinal manipulation, a variety of observations have been made which may be related to reflex pathways that were evoked during the treatment. These anecdotal observations frequently revolve around the musculature, for example, the relaxation of hypertonic muscles following a treatment. And, as suggested by the anecdotal observations in clinical practice, many of the reflex activities can be, and have been, measured using EMG recordings from the skeletal musculature. Wyke[29] measured an increase in activation of selected forelimb muscles in the cat when distracting cervical facet joints. Herzog et al.,[24] Suter et al.,[30] and Herzog[31] recorded reflex activation of originally silent musculature that was local and distant to the site of manipulation during and immediately following spinal manipulative treatments. Herzog[32] also observed a complete deactivation of

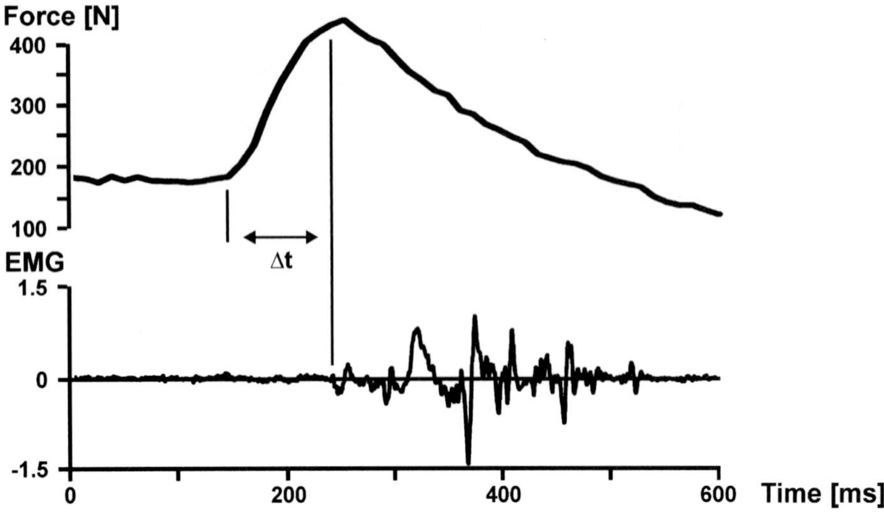

FIGURE 21–7. Representative force–time and EMG–time history of a spinal manipulative treatment on the thoracic spine. The EMG reflex response follows the onset of the treatment thrust by about 50–200 ms (Δt).

hypertonic spinal musculature following spinal manipulation in a single patient. Finally, Fuhr and Smith[14] recorded reflex responses following Activator treatments in humans and dogs.

EMG reflex responses always occur during or immediately following high-speed, low-amplitude spinal manipulative treatments. For treatments on the thoracic spine, the reflex responses occur within about 50–200 ms following the onset of the treatment thrust[24,30](Fig. 21–7). The EMG response signals last for approximately 100–400 ms and then disappear completely.

In a study aimed at determining the frequency and extent of reflex responses elicited by spinal manipulation, Herzog et al.[24] recorded the EMG responses of 16 neck, back, arm, and leg muscles for high-speed, low-amplitude spinal manipulations from the neck to the lower back and sacroiliac joint (Fig. 21–8). Ten young asymptomatic subjects were used. It was found that each treatment produced distinct and consistent reflex responses in a target-specific area. The reflex responses occurred within 50–200 ms following the onset of the treatment thrust and lasted for approximately 100–400 ms. The responses resembled normal voluntarily elicited EMG signals, suggesting that the reflex responses were of multireceptor origin and were elicited asynchronously.

Reflex responses were measured over a large area of the back, and for some treatments consistently occurred in the arm and leg musculature (Fig. 21–9). It was concluded from the results of this study that high-speed, low-amplitude spinal manipulation produces consistent reflex responses in the back, arm, and leg musculature. Since reflex responses were measured far away from the treatment area, it was further concluded that spinal manipulation might have beneficial effects at locations far removed from the specific treatment site.[24]

In a similar study to that of Herzog et al.[24], Symons et al.[33] determined the EMG reflex responses of the same 16 muscles as shown in Figure 21–8 using Activator treatments. Spinal manipulative treatments in this study were delivered with an Activator II instrument to nine asymptomatic volunteers at six sites bilaterally (C3/4, T2/3, T6–8, T11/12, L2–4, and the sacroiliac joint). The reflex responses were measured using bipolar surface EMG electrodes. Data were collected at 2000 Hz.

During spinal manipulation treatments using high-speed, low-amplitude thrusts, reflex responses occurred in 100% of all cases, they were of multireceptor origin, and they occurred over a large area.[24,34] In contrast, treatments with the Activator instrument resulted in observable reflex responses in 68% of all treatments.[33] Furthermore, the responses always

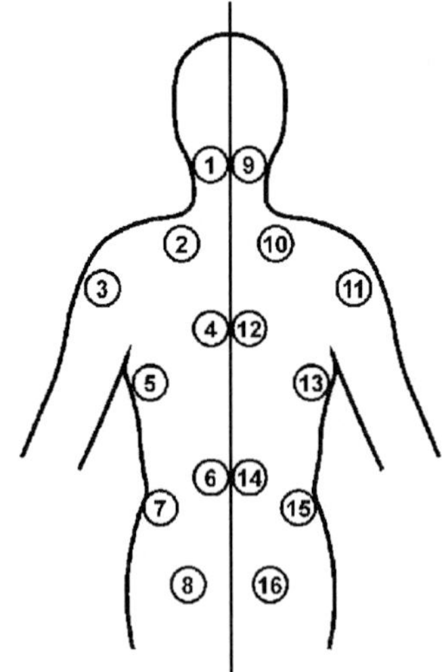

FIGURE 21–8. Schematic representation of the 16 EMG measurement sites chosen for evaluating the reflex responses associated with spinal manipulative treatment.

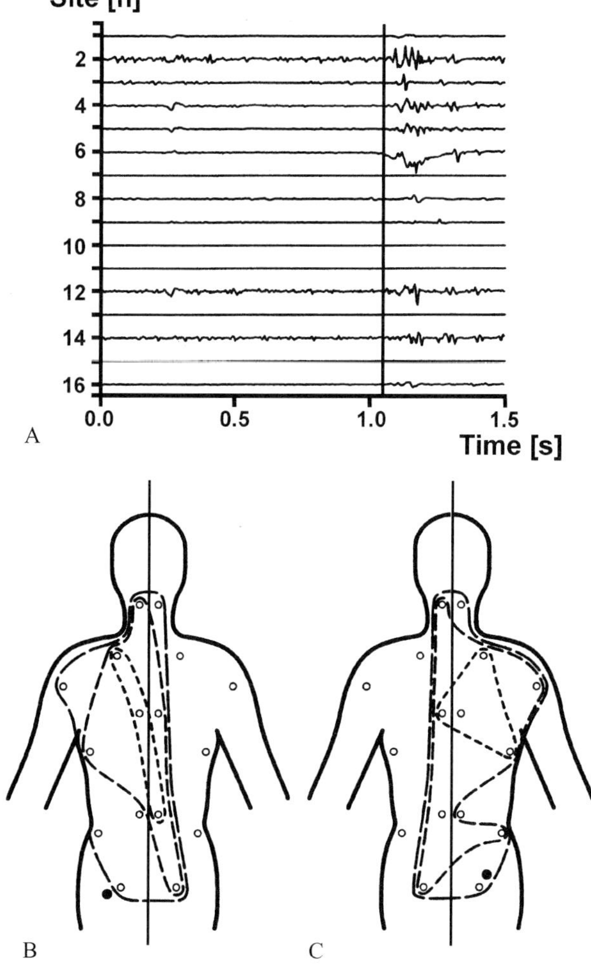

FIGURE 21–9. *A.* Exemplar data of reflex responses following spinal manipulative treatment. The vertical line just after time = 1.0 s indicates the onset of the treatment thrust. Parts *B* and *C* show the site of treatment application (filled dot), and the short-dashed, medium-dashed, and large-dashed lines indicate a 100%, 80%, and 50% occurrence of reflex response measured by the electrodes enclosed within the various lines.

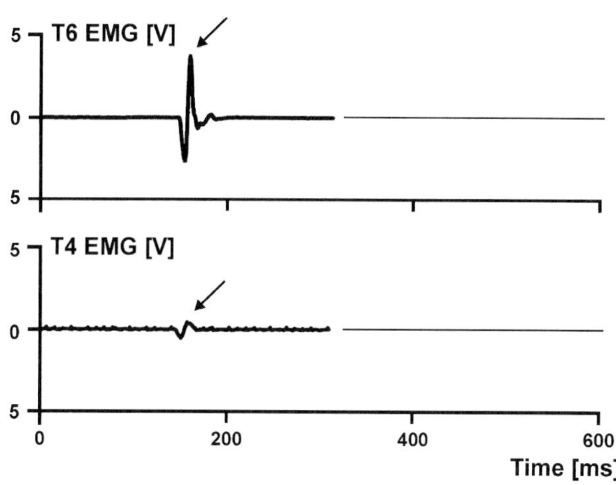

FIGURE 21–10. Representative EMG–time histories of the spinalis muscle at the level of T6 and T4 for an Activator treatment on the level of T6. Note the clear, single-compound motor unit action potential-like response at T6 and the almost imperceptible response at T4. There were no further responses at any of the other EMG electrode recording sites.

occurred close to the treatment site ipsilaterally (Fig. 21–10), and they were detected in muscles that had an attachment site on the vertebral body that was adjusted. Finally, the responses always had a characteristic shape reminiscent of that of a compound motor unit action potential (Fig. 21–10). Therefore, it was concluded, that, in contrast to the manual treatments,[24,34] activator treatments resulted in a local response directly at the target site, and the reflex responses were associated with a single proprioceptor group, likely the muscle spindles.[33]

Reflex Inhibition and Spinal Manipulation

Joint pain and swelling are known to cause muscle inhibition through reflex pathways. Muscle inhibition is defined here as the inability to maximally activate muscles during a full effort voluntary contraction. Often, a small level of muscle inhibition is observed in normal, asymptomatic populations.[35] However, injury, pain, swelling, surgery, and other joint problems have been associated with levels of muscle inhibition that clearly exceed the levels observed in asymptomatic populations.[36–38] The magnitude of muscle inhibition has also been shown to depend on the muscle group tested,[35] and the joint angle at which testing is performed.[39]

Recently, reflex inhibition in hypertonic musculature as well as changes in muscle inhibition for patient populations have been studied in conjunction with spinal manipulation for the first time. Herzog et al.[24] showed that in some patients presenting with muscle hypertonicity, muscle stiffness and activation were reduced to normal levels following a single episode of treatment (Fig. 21–11). However, it must be emphasized that this observation was not consistent across all subjects tested. Therefore, Figure 21–11 has the character of a single case study. Also, it is not known why hypertonicity and hyperactivation were reduced successfully by spinal manipulation in some patients but not in others. But the above observation (Fig. 21–11) should remind us that under some circumstances, painful hypertonicity could be treated successfully with a single manipulative treatment. Although the mechanisms underlying the decrease in activation of hypertonic musculature is not understood, one possible pathway might involve a decrease in alpha-motoneuron excitability caused by spinal manipulation. In accordance with this idea, decreases in the soleus H-reflex have been observed following sacroiliac joint manipulation[40] and changes

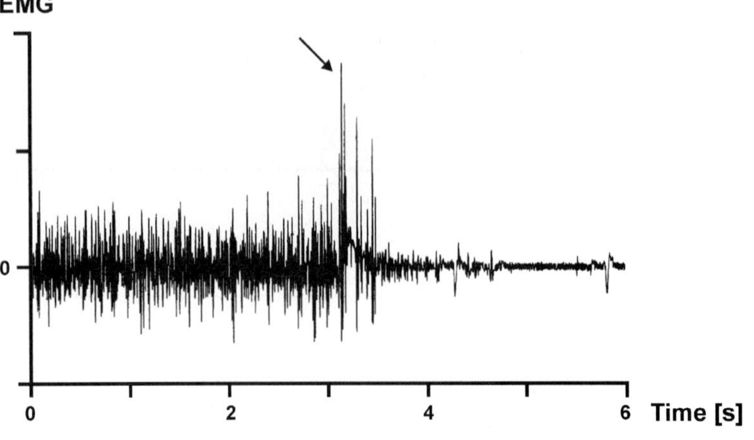

FIGURE 21–11. EMG–time history of a hypertonic muscle before, during, and after spinal manipulation. Before the treatment, the muscle showed a high EMG activity and was said to be stiff (motion palpation). During the treatment, the EMG activity increased (arrow), presumably because of reflex activation produced by the treatment. Following the treatment, the EMG was silent (except for occasional heartbeats) and the muscle was found to be relaxed and soft (motion palpation).

in the H-reflex have also been found following spinal manipulation in patients with unilateral disc herniation.[41]

Clinical Pearl: Herzog et al.[24] showed that in some patients presenting with muscle hypertonicity, muscle stiffness and activation were reduced to normal levels following a single episode of treatment.

Recently, we investigated the effect of spinal manipulation of the sacroiliac joint on knee extensor inhibition for patients with anterior knee pain. A first study was designed as a clinical outcome study with 18 patients with anterior knee pain and an associated sacroiliac joint dysfunction. Patients received a high-velocity, low-amplitude thrust to the sacroiliac joint in a side-lying position. Knee extensor inhibition was evaluated using the twitch interpolation technique[35,42,43] before and after treatment. Muscle inhibition decreased from about 25% to 20% for the patient population. For the knee extensors, an inhibition of 10% is typically found for a normal reference population. Therefore, although there was a decrease in muscle inhibition observed following treatment, the inhibition values remained significantly larger than those for normal, asymptomatic people.

The above study was designed as a clinical outcome study. This design has the advantage that it represents best what happens in the real clinical setting. However, from a scientific point of view, it is hard to elucidate why the treatment effect was observed, since training effects, or placebo effects, could have produced the decrease in muscle inhibition observed above. Therefore, the above study was repeated using a randomized controlled, double-blind study with 28 patients with anterior knee pain.[44] Patients were randomly assigned to the treatment or the control group. The treatment group received a sacroiliac joint manipulation, as in the previous study. The control group underwent the same diagnostic procedures as the treatment group but received only a sham manipulation. Knee extensor inhibition was assessed before and after the (sham) treatments. It was found that the only significant change in knee extensor inhibition occurred in the experimental leg of the treatment group (the leg with the anterior knee pain; Fig. 21–12). No such effects were found in the contralateral leg (no pain) or in the experimental or contralateral leg of the control group. These results indicate that it was the spinal manipulation, rather than a training or placebo effect, which caused the decrease in muscle inhibition. However, as in the clinical outcome study, muscle inhibition values after spinal manipulation in the patient group remained significantly higher, on average, than those observed in an asymptomatic reference population.[44] The precise mechanisms underlying the decrease in knee extensor inhibition following sacroiliac joint manipulation are not known at present.

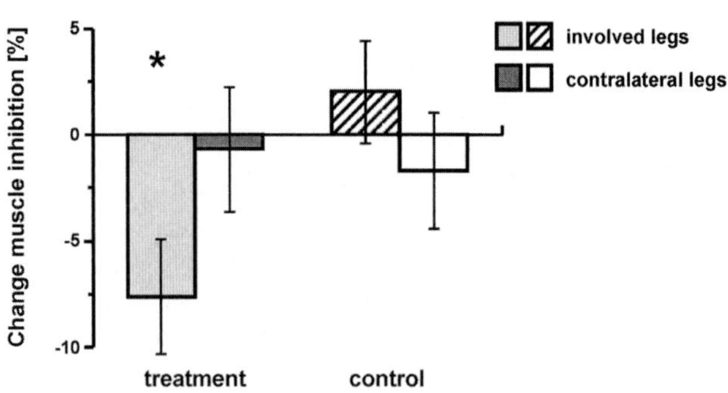

FIGURE 21–12. Change in muscle inhibition for the involved and the corresponding contralateral legs from before to after spinal manipulative treatment of the sacroiliac joint. Note that the only significant decrease in muscle inhibition occurred in the involved legs that were treated.

The H-reflex Response Associated with Spinal Manipulation

The tibial nerve Hoffmann (H-) reflex provides a neurophysiological index of alpha-motoneuron pool excitability. H-reflex responses under well-controlled experimental conditions have been carried out prior and following spinal manipulation, in order to determine if alpha-motoneuron pool excitability changes as a function of spinal manipulation.[40,41,45–47]

Knee extensor inhibition in patients with sacroiliac joint problems has been shown to decrease following spinal manipulation,[44] suggesting that alpha-motoneuron pool excitability is increased. In contrast, hypertonic muscle activity prior to spinal manipulation has been shown to disappear in some (but not all) patients following treatment, suggesting that alpha-motoneuron pool excitability may be decreased (at least temporarily) following treatment.[24] Although appearing contradictory at first glance, the findings from these studies are similar in that they both suggest manipulation may normalize muscle activity. Direct measurement of the H-reflex pre- and postspinal manipulation may provide insight into how alpha-motoneuron pool excitability changes as a function of spinal manipulation.

Cramer et al.[45] found no change in the H-reflex response of patients with acute low back pain following five treatments over a 10-day period. However, short-term effects might have been missed, as the patients were not evaluated immediately following spinal manipulation, as was done in other studies. Also, patients with abnormal H-reflex latencies were excluded from the analysis.

Murphy et al.[40] found a small (12.9%) but statistically significant decrease of the H-reflex following prone sacroiliac joint manipulation in asymptomatic subjects ($n = 34$) using a pelvic drop of about 10 mm. Likely, although it was not described explicitly, H-reflex responses were measured immediately following the spinal manipulation, while the subjects remained in the prone position.

Floman et al.[41] assessed changes in the H-reflex response in patients ($n = 24$) with unilateral disc herniation at L5–S1 with mass effect on the involved S1 root and without other lumbar spine pathology as viewed on CT (computed tomography) imaging or MRI (magnetic resonance imaging). Patients were between 20 and 50 years and presented with sciatica along the distribution of the S1 nerve root. All patients had a positive straight-leg raising test, most of them at less than 40 degree and the rest at less than 60 degree. In 16 of the 24 patients, the Achilles tendon reflex was diminished or absent. None of the patients displayed a motor deficit. Thirteen of these patients showed an abnormally decreased H-reflex amplitude and/or latency. In these patients, H-reflex amplitude was significantly increased following spinal manipulation in the side-lying position. Patients who did not show an abnormal reflex response did not show changes in the H-reflex amplitude or latency following manipulation.

Dishman and Bulbulian[47] reported a significant decrease in the H-reflex amplitude following lumbar spine manipulation and mobilization in the side-lying position in 17 asymptomatic subjects. H-reflex assessments were made immediately following manipulation or mobilization by turning the subjects from the side-lying into the prone position. The H-reflex amplitude was found to be transient (about 30 seconds). Of course, reorientation of subjects from the side-lying to the prone position could have influenced the H-reflex measurements. In order to test this hypothesis, we performed a study similar to that by Dishman and Bulbulian,[47] except that the H-reflex responses were determined in the side-lying position, and so patients were not reoriented following treatment. No changes in H-reflex response were found when treatments and H-reflex determination were performed in the side-lying position. However, when subjects were turned from a side-lying into a prone position, either after spinal manipulation or no manipulation, the transient decrease of the H-reflex response observed by Dishman and Bulbulian[47] was reproduced. Therefore, we concluded that the decrease in H-reflex amplitude observed by Dishman and Bulbulian[47] was not associated with the spinal manipulation, but was an artifact of the repositioning of the subjects.

In summary, studies on changes in the H-reflex responses following spinal manipulation are inconsistent. Therefore, no firm conclusions about the effects of spinal manipulation on alpha-motoneuron excitability may be drawn, at present.

CONCLUSION

Based on our research over the past 16 years on the mechanics and neurophysiology of spinal manipulation, the following conclusions may be drawn:

- The forces applied by chiropractors to patients during high-speed, low-amplitude spinal manipulations are substantial and may exceed the body weight of the clinician.
- These forces cause relative movements of adjacent vertebral bodies in the paraphysiological zone.
- These forces do not appear to load internal structures (e.g., the vertebral artery) to a significant degree.
- Spinal manipulations apparently produce multi-segmental reflex responses that are associated with a variety of afferent pathways.

- Activator treatments produce reflex responses segmentally that are likely caused by muscle spindles exclusively.
- Spinal manipulation has been found to alleviate muscle inhibition in patient populations.
- Spinal manipulation has been found to decrease hypertonicity in some (but not all) patients.
- Spinal manipulation alone does not appear to influence the alpha-motoneuron pool excitability as evaluated by the H-reflex response in asymptomatic subjects or patients with no prior abnormalities in the H-reflex response. However, in patients with decreased H-reflex amplitudes or increased latency times, alpha-motoneuron excitability appears to increase following spinal manipulation.

Because of the widespread and costly nature of the problem to all industrialized countries, there is a real need to identify a paradigm for the beneficial effects of spinal manipulation in patients with back pain. At present, such a paradigm cannot be formulated, as the number of scientific studies in this area is small, and not systematic enough to allow the derivation of firm conclusions.

It will be a challenge in the future to systematically tackle the most pertinent research questions associated with spinal manipulation. In order to do that successfully, much more basic science study in the area of spinal manipulation is required. Outcome studies, epidemiological research, and cost–benefit analyses may provide the reasons for doing manipulation-related research, but such studies cannot provide the answers that will help establish spinal manipulation on firm scientific grounds.

SUMMARY

1. The forces applied by clinicians to patients during high-speed, low-amplitude spinal manipulations are substantial and may exceed the body weight of the clinician.
2. These forces cause relative movements of adjacent vertebral bodies in the paraphysiological zone.
3. These forces do not appear to load internal structures (e.g., the vertebral artery) to a significant degree.
4. Spinal manipulations apparently produce multisegmental reflex responses that are associated with a variety of afferent pathways.
5. Activator treatments produce reflex responses segmentally that are likely caused by muscle spindles exclusively.
6. Spinal manipulation has been found to alleviate muscle inhibition in patient populations.
7. Spinal manipulation has been found to decrease hypertonicity in some (but not all) patients.
8. Spinal manipulation alone does not appear to influence the alpha-motoneuron pool excitability as evaluated by the H-reflex response in asymptomatic subjects or patients with no prior abnormalities in the H-reflex response. However, in patients with decreased H-reflex amplitudes or increased latency times, alpha-motoneuron excitability appears to increase following spinal manipulation.

REFERENCES

1. Wood J, Adams A. Forces used in selected chiropractic adjustments of the low back: A preliminary study. *The Research Forum, Palmer College of Chiropractic* 1984;1:16–23.
2. Hessel B, Herzog W, Conway P, et al. Experimental measurement of the force exerted during spinal manipulation using the Thompson technique. *J Manipulative Physiol Ther* 1990;13:448–453.
3. Herzog W, Zhang Y, Conway P, et al. Cavitation sounds during spinal manipulative treatments. *J Manipulative Physiol Ther* 1993;16:523–526.
4. Triano J, Schultz A. Motions of the head and thorax during neck manipulations. *J Manipulative Physiol Ther* 1994;17:573–583.
5. Kawchuk G, Herzog W, Hasler E. Forces generated during spinal manipulative therapy of the cervical spine: A pilot study. *J Manipulative Physiol Ther* 1992;15:275–278.
6. Kawchuk G, Herzog W. Biomechanical characterization (fingerprinting) of five novel methods of cervical spinal manipulation. *J Manipulative Physiol Ther* 1993; 16(9):573–577.
7. Andrews J. Biomechanical analysis of human motion. *Kinesiology* 1947;4:32–42.
8. Herzog W, Conway P, Kawchuk G, et al. Forces exerted during spinal manipulative therapy. *Spine* 1993; 18:1206–1212.
9. Herzog W. *Clinical biomechanics of spinal manipulation*. Philadelphia: Churchill Livingstone, 2000:1–228.
10. Conway P, Herzog W, Zhang Y, et al. Forces required to cause cavitation during spinal manipulation of the thoracic spine. *Clin Biomech* 1993;8:210–214.
11. Herzog W. Biomechanical studies of spinal manipulative therapy. *JCCA* 1991;35:156–164.
12. Herzog W. Mechanical and physiological responses to spinal manipulative treatments [invited review]. *J Neuromusculoskeletal Syst* 1995;3:1–9.
13. Keller T, Nathan M, Kaigle A. Measurement and analysis of interspinous kinematics. In: *Proc Intl Conf Spinal Manipualtion*, 1993:51.
14. Fuhr A, Smith D. Accuracy of piezoelectric accelerometers measuring displacement of a spinal adjusting instrument. *J Manipulative Physiol Ther* 1986;9:15–21.
15. Smith D, Fuhr A, Davis B. Skin accelerometer displacement and relative bone movement of adjacent

vertebrae in response to chiropractic percussion thrusts. *J Manipulative Physiol Ther* 1989;12:26–37.
16. Lee R, Evans J. Load–displacement–time characteristics of the spine under posteroanterior mobilization. *Aust J Physiother* 1992;38:115–123.
17. Lee M, Svensson N. Effect of loading frequency on response of the spine to lumbar posteroanterior forces. *J Manipulative Physiol Ther* 1993;16:439–446.
18. Gál J, Herzog W, Kawchuk G, et al. Biomechanical studies of spinal manipulative therapy (SMT): Quantifying the movements of vertebral bodies during SMT. *JCCA* 1994;38:11–24.
19. Gál J, Herzog W, Kawchuk G, et al. Measurements of vertebral translations using bone pins, surface markers and accelerometers. *Clin Biomech* 1997;12(5):337–340.
20. Gál J, Herzog W, Kawchuk G, et al. Forces and relative movements during SMT to an unembalmed post-rigor human cadaver: Peculiarities associated with joint cavitation. *J Manipulative Physiol Ther* 1995;18: 4–9.
21. Gál J, Herzog W, Kawchuk G, et al. Movements of vertebrae during manipulative thrusts to unembalmed human cadavers. *J Manipulative Physiol Ther* 1997;20: 30–40.
22. Maigne J, Guillon F. Highlighting of intervertebral movements and variations of intradiskal pressure during lumbar spinal manipulation: A feasibility study. *J Manipulative Physiol Ther* 2000;23:531–535.
23. Symons B, Leonard T, Herzog W. Internal forces sustained by the vertebral artery during spinal manipulative therapy. *J Manipulative Physiol Ther* 2002;25: 504–510.
24. Herzog W, Scheele D, Conway P. Electromyographic responses of back and limb muscles associated with spinal manipulative therapy. *Spine* 1999;24(2):146–152.
25. Gillette R. A speculative argument for the coactivation of diverse somatic receptor populations by forceful chiropractic adjustments. *Manual Med* 1987;3: 1–14.
26. Haldeman S. Spinal manipulative therapy in sports medicine. *Clin Sports Med* 1986;5:277–293.
27. Raftis K, Warfield C. Spinal manipulation for back pain. *Hosp Pract (Off Ed)* 1989;15:89–90,95–108.
28. Zusman M. Spinal manipulative therapy: Review of some proposed mechanisms, and a new hypothesis. *Aviat Space Environ Med* 1996;32:89–99.
29. Wyke B. *Aspects of manipulative therapy.* Glasgow E. F., Twomey L, Scull E, and Kleynhans A, ed. Publisher: Churchil Livingstone, 1985:72–77.
30. Suter E, Herzog W, Conway P, et al. Reflex response associated with manipulative treatment of the thoracic spine. *J Neuromusculoskeletal Syst* 1994;2:124–130.
31. Herzog W. On sounds and reflexes. *J Manipulative Physiol Ther* 1996;19:216–218.
32. Herzog W. *Mechanical, physiologic, and neuromuscular considerations of chiropractic treatments.* Advances in Chiropractic, Volume 3. New York: Lawrence, 1996: 269–285.
33. Symons B, Herzog W, Leonard T, et al. Reflex responses associated with activator treatment. *J Manipulative Physiol Ther* 2000;23(3):155–159.
34. Herzog W, Kats M, Symons B. The effective forces transmitted by high-speed, low-amplitude thoracic manipulation. *Spine* 2001;26(19):2105–2110.
35. Belanger A, McComas A. Extent of motor unit activation during effort. *J Appl Physiol* 1981;51(5):1131–1135.
36. Hurley M, Jones D, Wilson D, et al. Rehabilitation of quadriceps inhibited due to isolated rupture of the anterior cruciate ligament. *J Ortho Rheum* 1992;5: 145–154.
37. Suter E, Herzog W, Bray R. Quadriceps inhibition following arthroscopy in patients with anterior knee pain. *Clin Biomech* 1998;13:314–319.
38. Suter E, Herzog W, De Souza K, et al. Inhibition of the quadriceps muscles in patients with anterior knee pain. *J Appl Biomech* 1998;14:360–373.
39. Suter E, Herzog W. Extent of muscle inhibition as a function of knee angle. *J Electromyogr Kinesiol* 1997;7: 123–130.
40. Murphy BA, Dawson N, Slack JR. Sacroiliac joint manipulation decreases the H-reflex. *Electromyogr Clin Neurophysiol* 1995;35:87–94.
41. Floman Y, Liram N, Gilai A. Spinal manipulation results in immediate H-reflex changes in patients with unilateral disc herniation. *Eur Spine J* 1997;6:398–401.
42. Merton P. Voluntary strength and fatigue. *J Physiol* 1954;123:553–564.
43. Hales J, Gandevia S. Assessment of maximal voluntary contraction with twitch interpolation: An instrument to measure twitch response. *J Neurosci Methods* 1988;25:97–102.
44. Suter E, McMorland G, Herzog W, et al. Conservative lower back treatment reduces inhibition in knee-extensor muscles: A randomized controlled trial. *J Manipulative Physiol Ther* 2000;23(2):76–80.
45. Cramer G, Humphreys C, Hondras M, et al. The H_{max}/M_{max} ratio as an outcome measure for acute low back pain. *J Manipulative Physiol Ther* 1993;16(1):7–12.
46. Humphreys C, Triano J, Brandl M. Sensitivity study of H-reflex alterations in idiopathic low back pain patients vs. a healthy population. *J Manipulative Physiol Ther* 1989;12(2):71–78.
47. Dishman J, Bulbulian R. Spinal reflex attenuation associated with spinal manipulation. *Spine* 2000;25(19): 2519–2525.

CHAPTER

22

McKENZIE PROTOCOLS FOR MECHANICAL TREATMENT OF THE LOW BACK

Steven L. Heffner, Robin McKenzie, and Gary Jacob

OUTLINE

OBJECTIVES

1. Assimilate the information from the subjective history and clinical evaluation forms into a proper treatment protocol for the patient.
2. Treat the postural syndrome.
3. Treat the dysfunction syndrome.
4. Recognize and treat the seven derangement syndrome categories.
5. Recognize an irreducible derangement.
6. Discuss proper treatment of a relevant lateral shift.
7. Discuss proper treatment of a deformity.

INTRODUCTION

Assessment principles and protocols for McKenzie low back methods were discussed in detail in

Chapter 15. A thorough understanding of such assessment is a necessary precursor for the clinician to then integrate the strategies and skills of the low back McKenzie treatment approaches that are covered in this chapter.

Clinical Pearl: Once the subjective history and mechanical evaluation has been performed on the initial office visit, the McKenzie practitioner should have an idea as to which mechanical category the patient may belong.

Depending upon the syndrome, a specific self-treatment program is prescribed for home use.

The treatment programs for each of the three mechanical syndromes, postural, dysfunction and derangement are discussed. Included are illustrations, *clinical pearls,* and a case study of each syndrome to assist the reader in better appreciating the clinical concepts, decision making, and treatment of each particular syndrome.

Acute patients who receive proper mechanical treatment typically experience a rapid decrease and/or abolition of symptoms. Chronic conditions, however, can be quite different, with an initial temporary, exercise-related aggravation of symptoms being quite common. This should be explained to patients prior to the onset of the treatment phase as part of an ethical and informed patient communication. Conversely, the clinician should not place too much emphasis on the risk and severity of symptom exacerbation as this may deter the patient from complying with the treatment program and performing the necessary movements and/or positions.

Finally, the three most important things to do with the patient is to *Educate, Educate, and Educate!*

GENERAL COMPARISON OF PROCEDURAL EFFECTS OF THE THREE SYNDROMES

The postural syndrome is generally not affected by mechanical maneuvers performed by the clinician or by him/herself. The goal is therefore to isolate and subsequently instruct the patient to avoid the offending position(s).

Restoration of function or movement of the adaptively shortened tissue is the goal of the dysfunction syndrome. Therefore, frequent repetition of restricted end-range exercises is the necessary mechanical strategy.

Reduction of the derangement by alteration of the position/shape of the semiviscous nucleus/annulus is the goal of the derangement syndrome. Therefore, restricted end-range loading for a prolonged period of time is the necessary mechanical strategy for this syndrome.

McKENZIE TREATMENT PROTOCOLS WITH CASE STUDIES

To demonstrate the practical integration of McKenzie assessment and treatment protocols, case studies and subsequent treatment summaries are presented for each of the three syndromes.

Case Study 1

Jana is a 23-year-old female office worker whose postures and stresses during work involve mainly sitting at a computer console area and transmitting data. She is active in aerobics and weight training, in addition to performing typical household cleaning chores.

Her anatomical pain diagram reveals a midline, symmetrical, low back pain that has gradually moved up into the lower thoracic area. These symptoms have been present for several months and appeared to be worsening. There was no single precipitating event that suddenly provoked her symptoms.

Jana's pain is intermittent and the only movement or position that produces her symptoms is sitting. Bending, standing, walking, and lying have no effect. She feels worse as the day progresses but feels fine during the morning and late evening. She has no complaints while she is moving about.

Her sleep is not disturbed, while bladder function and gait are normal. She has had no previous history of back pain.

Further investigation reveals that a couple of hours of sitting were initially required to produce Jana's pain. However, this has progressed over the past two weeks to the point that 15 minutes of sitting produces her symptoms.

Previous treatment consisted of anti-inflammatory medication prescribed by her family physician, which was of no benefit.

There is no history of major or pertinent surgery, recent accidents, and/or unexplained weight loss. She did not have night pain that awakened her nor had she taken steroid medication for a prolonged period.

Differential Diagnosis: Postural syndrome vs. derangement vs. another unknown condition.

Following the initial history, Jana was asked if she had any symptoms while sitting through the questioning without back support. She indicated that about halfway through the history her symptoms began and continued.

She was then instructed to sit erect, producing a lordosis in her low back. When asked if there was any change in her symptoms, she remarked that her symptoms abolished shortly after sitting up straight.

This strengthens the postural syndrome diagnosis but does not rule out derangement syndrome since postural correction can abolish their symptoms also.

Mechanical Assessment (see Figs. 15–1 and 15–2 for McKenzie Assessment Sheets) Range of motion testing (see movement loss section of figure) revealed no loss of mobility in all arcs.

Jana had no pretest pain, and repetitive movements in the sagittal and coronal planes did not produce any symptoms.

At this point it is probably a postural syndrome due to the fact that *a derangement must have a movement loss*, and repetitive movements in at least one direction produce pain.

Strategically speaking, when utilizing McKenzie protocols, one should rule out a derangement first before treating anything else. Therefore, the patient was instructed to perform repetitive forward flexion exercises 15 repetitions every 2 waking hours for the next 24 hours. If the condition is a derangement then flexion of the lumbar spine will produce and worsen the symptoms. If it is a postural syndrome there will be no effect.

Jana returned the next day with no change in her symptoms from flexion. This effectively ruled out derangement syndrome.

Clinical Pearl: Strategically speaking, when utilizing McKenzie protocols, one should rule out a derangement first before treating anything else.

Diagnosis Postural syndrome

Treatment of Postural Syndrome Although it was discussed in detail in Chapter 15, the key characteristics of the postural syndrome are as follows:

- intermittent pain
- time factor
- pain produced by maintenance of posture/position
- symptoms provoked by position, but not by movement
- no deformity (relevant to pain)
- no loss of movement
- no provocative signs/no pathology
- aged 30 years and under (usually)
- sedentary workers (underexercised)
- often have cervical and thoracic pain also
- often have days at a time without pain
- no pain while active and moving
- pain is local to the spine (not referred)

Postures involved: Figure 22–1*A* demonstrates an example of a typical patient with the postural syndrome.

Treatment: Instructing the patient to maintain a sustained, poor posture and subsequently recreating their pain confirms the presence of the postural syndrome. The ability to recreate these symptoms helps to convince the skeptical patient that their posture is indeed the causative factor. Once the postural syndrome is the accepted diagnosis of patient and clinician, the focus then turns to the abolition of the pain by correcting the posture.

To obtain the correct sitting posture, one must be acquainted with the extreme of the good and the bad postures. The "slouch/overcorrect" maneuver is performed to learn this motor skill. The patient should sit on the edge of the chair and allow the lumbar spine to slouch into a fully flexed position and allow the head and chin to protrude. He/she must smoothly move or transition into a fully erect sitting position, with a maximal lumbar lordosis and head held directly over the spine with a retracted chin. This postural motion should be repeatedly performed in a smooth and flowing manner from the extreme of the good to the extreme of the bad (see Fig. 22–1*A* to 22–1*C*).

To maintain the correct sitting posture when sitting for prolonged periods of time it is essential to maintain a lordotic posture at all times. The lumbar spine may be held in lordosis in two ways:

(a) *Actively* by conscious control of the lordosis while sitting without a backrest.
(b) *Passively* by the use of a lumbar support while sitting with a backrest.

Case Study 2

Cameron is a 35-year-old construction worker who has not been working for the past 8 weeks. Prior to that, he had been working at modified duties (i.e., no forward bending) following lumbar spine laminectomy/discectomy.

His anatomical pain diagram reveals central low back pain at the beltline.

The pain has been present for approximately 8 weeks, beginning shortly after returning to forward bending movements postoperatively.

Cameron's pain is intermittent. It is worsened while bending forward, but is relieved when he straightens his back up. Sitting, rising from sitting, walking, and lying have no effect on his symptoms. There is no change or effect from the diurnal cycle. Whether he remains still or is moving about makes no difference.

Cameron's sleep is not affected. His gait is normal, as is his bowel and bladder function. He had low back pain with right sciatica previously that seemed to resolve with the required above-mentioned surgery.

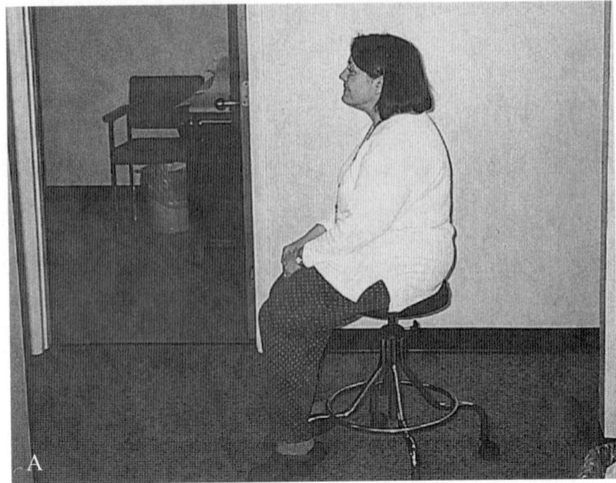

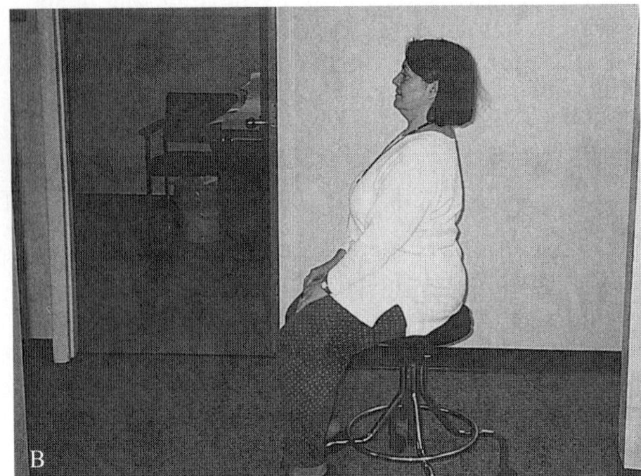

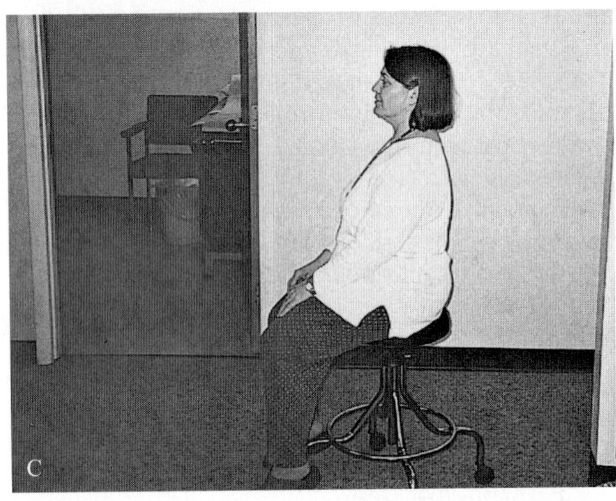

FIGURE 22–1. (*A*) The typical slouched posture of the postural syndrome. This position is used as part of the recurrent postural correction movements as the patient transitions to an extremely erect posture as shown in (*B*). The patient then starts to return to the initial slouched posture, with the neutral erect posture shown in (*C*) being found at around the halfway point of the postural transition. The patient should then be instructed that this neutral position represents the desired posture.

Postsurgical treatment involves anti-inflammatory and analgesic medication prescribed by the surgeon. Home exercises consist of straight-leg raise 10 repetitions, three to four sets per day, and walking up to 2 miles daily.

Cameron denies any recent accidents or unexplained weight loss.

He presents with poor seated posture during the history and denies increased symptoms in this position. He was instructed to sit erect, which had no subsequent effect on his symptoms.

Differential Diagnosis: Derangement syndrome vs. dysfunction syndrome vs. unknown third diagnosis

Mechanical Assessment Cameron had moderate loss of movement in flexion, which was painful. He has no pretest pain present.

Flexion in standing (FIS) provokes end-range pain (ERP). Repetitive FIS has continued ERP with each movement but this pain does not last once the flexion maneuvers are discontinued. All other sagittal and coronal movements have no effect on his symptoms.

Neurological testing was unremarkable for the lower extremities bilaterally.

This clinical picture is consistent with a dysfunction. In contrast, a derangement will have improved symptoms with repetitive movements in one direction and will worsen in another, generally the opposite, direction.

To remain conservative, one should assume that it is a derangement and send him home to perform extension in standing (EIS) exercises, performing 15 repetitions every 2 hours over the next waking 24–48 hours. Cameron must also sit with a lumbar roll to maintain a lumbar lordosis. The rationale for this protocol is that if it is a derangement, then the EIS and postural correction may very well decrease the symptoms and improve the flexion movement loss.

If there is no change in symptomatology following this protocol, then one should further rule out the derangement by having Cameron perform repetitive flexion movements (standing or sitting or lying) over the next 24–48 hours. If it is a posterior derangement the condition will worsen and mobility in flexion will decrease even more. Of course a moderate to severe increase in pain before the 24 hours has elapsed would require the patient to discontinue the repetitive flexions, as the findings are confirmed and one must avoid a severe exacerbation of symptoms. However, if there is no overall increase in symptoms with repetitive flexion maneuvers, it is not a derangement.

Diagnosis Dysfunction syndrome

Treatment of the Dysfunction Syndrome The key characteristics of the dysfunction syndrome include

- intermittent pain
- no time factor
- pain produced at end position or movement of shortened structures.
- pain relief with relief of stress/unloading shortened tissue
- always a loss of function/movement
- no deformity (not rapidly reversible)
- test movements reproduce pain but does not worsen as a result
- over 30 years of age except where trauma or derangement is the causative factor
- poor posture often underexercised

Treatment: The symptoms of dysfunction are more related to movement and become evident in the difficulty or inability of the patient to accomplish end range of movement, most frequent in the extremes of flexion and extension. These will remain present until the length of the shortened tissues is increased and the end range of movement is improved. This will be achieved in 4–6 weeks, provided the treatment procedures are used in a precise manner.

Clinical Pearl: The very nature of adaptive shortening of soft tissues adjacent to articular structures prohibits the rapid recovery of function in a few days.

Stretching must be performed in a way that it allows elongation of ligamentous structures and scar tissue without causing microtrauma. Pain produced by stretching should stop shortly after the stress is released.

To achieve the lengthening of adaptively shortened soft tissues it is not sufficient to perform stretching once a week, neither is it sufficient to do this once a day. *The stretches must be performed every 2–3 hours on a daily basis. This usually needs to be continued for a 4- to 6-week period or until the patient can fully stretch without any ERP.*

If no strain pain is produced during the performance of the exercises for the recovery of the lost movement, the contracted soft tissues are not being sufficiently stretched to enhance elongation of the shortened structures.

The following instructions must be given to the patient:

- stretch in the direction of movement loss and ERP
- allow elongation without microtrauma
- pain produced by stretching must stop shortly after release of stress
- persisting pain afterwards indicates overstretching
- peripheralization should never occur
- stretching must be strong enough to reproduce discomfort or some pain
- must be performed regularly during the day (15/2 hours)

Case Study 3

Andrei is a 40-year-old truck driver who drives long distances and then unloads and reloads his trailer. This involves frequent bending, lifting, and twisting. He enjoys doing yard work and minor repair projects at home.

His anatomical pain diagram reveals pain on the right side of the low back, buttock, posterior thigh, lateral calf, and foot. He relates that his symptoms began 2 weeks prior to his initial office visit.

Andrei states that he was lifting boxes at work and felt a sudden pain in his low back. He continued to work through the day with no increase in pain. Upon waking the next morning, he found that he could not get out of bed because of severe low back and right leg pain. This persisted despite 2 days of bed rest. He consulted his family doctor, who subsequently sent him for an MRI and prescribed pain and anti-inflammatory medication.

The medication allowed him to tolerably ambulate but the leg pain did not abate.

Andrei's pain in the back and leg was constant but it did vary in intensity. He also had loss of movement because of the pain.

Bending, sitting, rising from sitting, walking, and lying prone or on his right side worsens his symptoms. He wakes up with the symptoms, which last through the day and remain painful through the evening.

Lying on his back with his knees bent temporarily decreases his pain. The pain wakes him up three to four times every night and he changes positions frequently through the night.

A previous history of low back pain indicated localized low back pain numerous times over the past several years which would resolve within a few days with over-the-counter anti-inflammatory medication and rest.

Previous treatment for this episode of pain included a referral for physical therapy, which included moist heat, electrical stimulation, and ultrasound modalities for 1 week, which only provided temporary pain relief.

MRI testing revealed a mild–moderate L4–L5 right posterolateral HNP with evidence of L5 nerve root encroachment.

Andrei denied previous surgeries, accidents, and unexplained weight loss.

The patient could not sit for more than a few seconds, so he was instructed to lie in his most comfortable position, which was left-sided.

Mechanical Assessment Andrei could not sit in an erect manner, and even a poor posture was briefly tolerated. He presents with a left forward antalgic lean while standing.

Movement loss testing revealed a major loss of flexion, extension, and right-side gliding. He could cross midline from left- to right-side gliding although it was extremely painful.

Repeated standing test movements were not initially performed because of marked pain with all movements. Therefore, he was placed in a prone position. This position was also very painful; therefore his hips were shifted away from the leg pain (i.e., to the left). This increased his low back pain but moved the leg pain up (centralized) to his mid calf, abolishing his lateral foot symptoms.

Keeping his hips to the left he was instructed to repetitively perform extension in lying (EIL) to as far as tolerated. He began with 1/3 of his normal end-range extension and increased the range to 2/3 end-range EIL with repetition. With the increased mobility his leg symptoms disappeared and moved up to the mid thigh. The thigh, buttock, and low back pain amplified. The lower leg pain remained better indicating that *centralization* was taking place.

After 20 EIL with left-side gliding were performed, the symptoms remained centralized but did not recede further up the leg.

Andrei was then instructed to get off the table while maintaining a lumbar lordosis. Upon standing, the pain radiated back to the knee but not below. His antalgia was also abolished.

He was instructed how to maintain a posturally correct seated posture, sitting with his buttock and back against the chair (a roll caused peripheralization). Once the pain in his leg started to return, he was instructed to stand up.

Diagnosis Derangement 5 with a relevant lateral component vs. a second unknown diagnosis.

The real question is whether the derangement is reducible or not. If reducible, this patient will improve with movements/positions in a certain direction.

Treatment Sit with buttocks/back against a firm chair as long as tolerated. Every hour lie prone with hips shifted away from the side of pain as long as tolerated. Before getting up perform EIL with hips shifted to left with the goal of locking the elbows at end-range elbow extension. One would discontinue this maneuver if this peripheralizes his symptoms.

The patient is then instructed to return to the office in 24 hours for follow-up.

Day 2: The patient returned with increased low back and buttock pain but abolished foot/leg/thigh pain. This was considered to be an improvement because Andrei's symptoms had centralized.

Movement loss assessment revealed increased flexion and side gliding to the right.

The treatment procedure was performed and he could "lock out" his elbows without provoking any leg pain. EIL without hips away peripheralized the symptoms.

Side gliding in standing (SGIS) right was performed without any peripheralization. Status post SGIS right centralized the pain to the right-sided low back.

Andrei was sent home with the same postural correction and to perform SGIS right 10–15 repetitions every 1–2 hours. He was instructed to discontinue these maneuvers if the pain peripheralized and return to Day 1 movements. He was instructed to return in 24 hours for follow-up.

Day 3: Andrei has had no leg pain in 2 days, but his back pain persists at a slightly increased level. SGIS right movements have become pain-free. Sitting is now tolerated for 15 minutes.

Movement loss assessment shows flexion described as moderated loss and extension as improved.

EIS was attempted and it produced only central increase in symptoms that did not remain worse. A lumbar roll was attempted and was well tolerated.

Andrei was instructed to perform EIL 10–15 repetitions every 1–2 hours. If the symptoms worsened, he was to return to frontal movements as before. He was instructed to return in 24 hours for follow-up.

The patient has now reduced the derangement from a 5 to a 1. An explanation of derangement syndrome treatment protocols is as follows.

DERANGEMENT TREATMENT STRATEGY

Mechanical treatment is dependent upon the mechanical diagnosis for derangements. Derangements that are considered to be *anterior* require strategies containing a flexion component, and those that are considered to be *posterior* contain strategies containing an extension component. In most cases, these may be conducted within the sagittal plane, but flexion and extension strategies may, in other cases, be combined with coronal or transverse motions for the best mechanical and symptomatic responses. In cases where movements outside the sagittal plane may be considered beneficial, disc derangement in nonsagittal directions may be considered. Derangements then can be considered to have anterior, posterior, or lateral components.

McKenzie classifies derangements into seven categories on the basis of the location of symptoms and the presentation of fixed antalgias responsive to end-range loading in directions other than that within which complaints are caused.[1]

A limerick to remember this, known as "Jacob's Deranged Poem,"[2] is a practical way to remember the seven derangement categories, which are explained in Table 22–1.

Derangements 1 through 4 do not have symptoms below the knee.

Derangements 1 through 6 concern derangements determined to have a posterior component after examination.

Derangement 7 would include all anterior derangements (those derangements) responsive to flexion and/or worsened by extension.

For the lumbar spine, derangement 7 typically presents with a fixed lordosis, for the cervical spine this is rarely the case. Regarding derangements 1 through 6, a pattern can be seen. These derangements represent "couplets" (1 and 2, 3 and 4, 5 and 6), with the odd numbered derangement of the couplet representing a symptom pattern (1 = central or symmetrical, not beyond the knee/elbow; 3 = unilateral, not beyond the knee/elbow; 5 = unilateral, beyond the knee/elbow). The odd number derangements of the couplets indicate the same symptom pattern as the lesser odd number with the *addition* of an antalgia (2 = kyphosis; 4 = acute scoliosis, called torticollis in the cervical spine; 6 = acute kyphosis or scoliosis).

Some differences should be noted between the lumbar and cervical spine regarding this classification system.

Frequently, with the lumbar spine, derangement 7 is accompanied with a fixed lordotic deformity, while this is rarely encountered in the cervical spine.

Treatment of the Derangement Syndrome

The theoretical model for the derangement syndrome involves the concept of displacement of the semiviscous nucleus annulus. Figure 22–2 presents an excellent visual description of the derangement syndrome,

TABLE 22–1. Derangement Categories with *Jacob's Deranged Poem*

Derangement 1	*One is central*
Central or symmetrical symptoms	
Rarely buttock symptoms	
No postural deformity	
Derangement 2	*Two is kyphotic*
Central or symmetrical symptoms	
With or without buttock or thigh symptoms	
Deformity of kyphosis	
Derangement 3	*Three is unilateral*
Unilateral or asymmetrical symptoms	
With or without buttock or thigh symptoms	
No deformity	
Derangement 4	*Four is scoliotic*
Unilateral or asymmetrical symptoms	
With or without buttock or thigh symptoms	
With scoliotic deformity	
Derangement 5	*Five is in the leg*
Unilateral or asymmetrical symptoms	
With leg symptoms distal to the knee	
No deformity	
Derangement 6	*Six is all the worse*
Unilateral or asymmetrical symptoms	
With leg symptoms distal to the knee	
With scoliotic deformity	
(Anterior Derangement)	
Derangement 7	*Seven is the reverse of the first*
Central or symmetrical symptoms	
Rarely buttock symptoms	
Accentuated lumbar lordosis	

Source: From Jacob.[2]

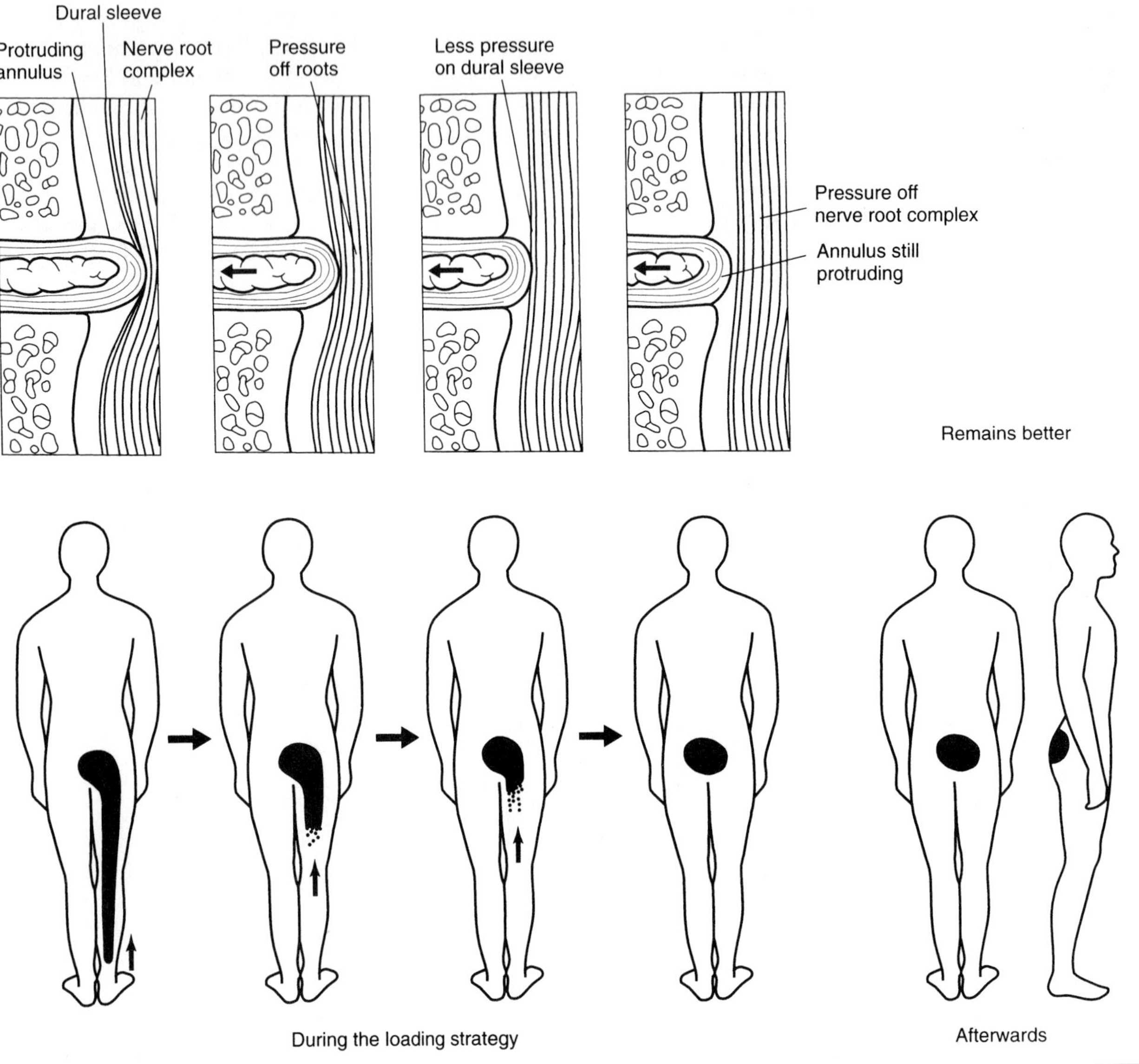

FIGURE 22–2. The theoretical model of the centralization phenomena in which pain recedes to the torso (i.e., center of the body) from the periphery on the leg as the protruding annulus fibrosis recedes from the neural canal with end-range loading strategies. *(Reprinted with permission from Murphy[3]).*

in which the reduction of the protruding annulus coincides with the centralization phenomena that was discussed in Chapter 15. There are scores of references that provide evidence for the basis of this theory; however the present state of knowledge, the actual events that occur with the development and reduction in the derangement syndrome are not fully known.

History:

- men more than women
- age 20–55 years
- worse with prolonged sitting or rising from sitting
- worse stooping or bending
- better walking
- better lying

Characteristics:

- often constant pain
- time factors (diurnal cycle)
- pain brought on or increased by certain movements/positions (repetition/sustaining usually worsens pain)
- pain decreased or abolished by othermovements/positions (repetition/sustaining usually improves the condition)
- always a loss of movement/function

- deformity of kyphosis/scoliosis is common
- deformity of accentuated lordosis uncommon

Acute Kyphosis Posterocentral derangement (indicating D2)

Acute Scoliosis Posterolateral derangement (indicating D4,6)

Acute Accentuated Lordosis Anterior or anterolateral derangement (indicating D7)

Test movements:

- peripheralization of symptoms occurs during development of the derangement
- centralization of symptoms occurs during reduction of the derangement
- rapid and lasting changes following test movements indicate derangement
- if test movements or positions cannot reduce symptoms, annular wall may be breached (noncontained nucleus)

Treatment steps:

1. Reduction of derangement
2. Maintenance of reduction
3. Recovery of function
4. Prevention of recurrence/prophylaxis

McKENZIE DERANGEMENT PROGRESSIONS

A meticulous history and range of motion examination is much more important when patients present without any apparent antalgia as opposed to the presentation with antalgia.

Derangement 2 represents a kyphotic deformity, derangement 4 represents a scoliotic deformity, and derangement 7 represents a lordotic deformity. In these cases, the treatment protocols can be predicted for the majority of individuals so classified.

Clinical Pearl: Derangement 2 (fixed kyphosis) can typically be treated with the "extension principle."

Derangement 7 (fixed lordotic deformity) can typically be treated with the "flexion principle."

Only on rare occasions do these derangements require the addition of a loading vector outside the sagittal plane.

For a derangement 4 (scoliotic) deformity, protocols typically involve reducing the deformity in the coronal plane (with side gliding in the lumbar spine and lateral flexion; see Fig. 22–3*A* and 22–3*B*) after which the extension principle is employed, i.e., the spine is treated as a derangement 2. These treatment strategies could therefore be considered as sagittal/extension protocols, merely preceded by coronal/lateral maneuvers.

Considering these protocols individually, the purported predictability of when the various derangements would require which protocols would be as follows.

Extension protocols: Derangement 2 would almost always require this maneuver. Expectations would then result in the expected order of appropriateness of these treatment strategies (derangement 1 greater than derangement 3; greater than derangement 5; greater than derangement 6, with a kyphotic component). Coronal and lordotic deformities are not considered amenable to this treatment strategy.

Coronal then extension protocols: Derangement 4 would be most amenable to this combination. Next to this, the decreasing frequency of expectations would be derangement 6, with a coronal component,

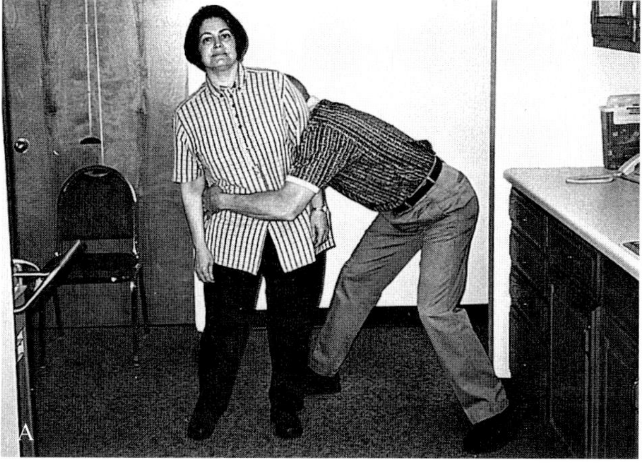
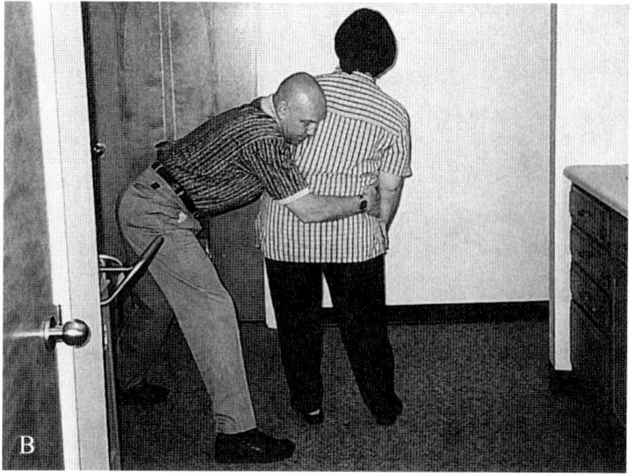

FIGURE 22–3. The side gliding maneuver from the anterior (*A*) and posterior (*B*) view, which is designed to remove the coronal/lateral component from the derangement syndrome.

derangement 3, derangement 5, and derangement 1. Derangement 7 would not be expected to be amenable to "coronal then extension" end-range loading strategies.

Flexion loading protocols: By definition, only derangement 7 would respond to flexion end-range loading strategies.

RELEVANT LATERAL COMPONENT

As previously noted, loading outside the sagittal plane may at times be appropriate. It is then assumed that the individual has a "relevant lateral component," i.e., response to loading outside the sagittal plane (see Fig. 22–3*A* and 22–3*B*). This can be true even when presenting complaints are central, as in the occasional response of a derangement 1 to unilateral loading technique.

TREATMENT OF DERANGEMENTS 1–7

Treatment of Derangement 1

This is central or symmetrical pain across L4–L5, with rarely any buttock or thigh pain and no deformity.

This indicates a minor posterior disc disturbance. Derangement 1 patients can self-treat. It is undesirable to use manual techniques in the first 24 hours.

Treatment

1. Reduction by application of extension principle
2. Maintenance of reduction by
   - maintenance of lordosis
   - sitting with lumbar support
   - frequent performance of extension exercises
3. Recovery of function by
   - flexion procedures (lying first)
   - followed by extension procedures
4. Prophylaxis
   - continuation of exercises as directed
   - follow advice (especially regarding the avoidance of, or proper mechanics associated with, prolonged bending and sitting)

Clinical Pearl: The treatment aim in derangement syndrome is to reverse derangements 2–6 by shift correction or extension principle to resemble derangement 1 (centralization).

Treatment of Derangement 2

This is central or symmetric pain across L4–L5, with or without buttock and or thigh pain, with deformity of lumbar kyphosis.

This indicates a major posterocentral disc disturbance. It is a progression of derangement 1 and can easily worsen to a derangement 4 or 6 unless one is careful.

Treatment

1. Reduction of deformity until the prone position can be obtained easily
2. Further treatment as for derangement 1

Clinical Pearl: Self-treatment procedures for posterior derangements can typically commence when the patient is able to lie prone.

Treatment of Derangement 3

This involves unilateral or asymmetrical pain across L4–L5 with or without buttock or thigh pain and no deformity.

This is a minor posterolateral disc disturbance and is a progression of derangement 1.

Treatment

1. Reduction as for derangement 1
2. If no centralization or reduction of pain occurs, the application of unilateral procedures is indicated
3. Once centralization or reduction of pain is achieved, further treatment is as for derangement 1

Treatment of Derangement 4

This is a unilateral or asymmetrical pain across L4–L5 with or without buttock or thigh pain and with deformity of lumbar scoliosis.

This is typically a major posterolateral disc disturbance and can be considered a progression of derangement 2 or 3.

Treatment

1. Reduction of derangement
   - lateral shift correction for lateral component of derangement
   - extension procedures for reduction of posterior component
   - maintenance of lordosis for stabilization of reduction
2. If following reduction of deformity no centralization occurs the application of unilateral technique is necessary
3. Once centralization is achieved, further treatment is as for derangement 1

Treatment of Derangement 5

This is a unilateral or asymmetrical pain across L4–L5 with or without buttock or thigh pain. There is leg pain extending below the knee.

The pathogenesis is a posterolateral disc disturbance with impingement on nerve root and dural sleeve.[3] Sciatica is usually intermittent, rarely constant. It is a progression of derangement 3 or 4.

Intermittent Sciatica This may be caused by a disc bulge. Flexion in both standing and lying enhance pain; repetition worsens symptoms. It may be caused by an adhesive or tethered nerve root. This is labeled as an adherent nerve root, and flexion in standing enhances pain but repetition does not necessarily worsen the symptoms.

Treatment of an Adherent Nerve Root

1. Stretching by flexion procedures
2. Followed by extension procedures to prevent recurrence of derangement

Treatment of Disc Bulge Reduction of derangement as treatment of derangements 1 or 3.

Treatment of Derangement 6

This is a unilateral or asymmetrical pain across L4–L5 with or without buttock or thigh pain. There is leg pain extending below the knee and a deformity of sciatic scoliosis.

The most frequent cause is a major posterolateral disc disturbance with impingement on the nerve root and dural sleeve.[3] Sciatica is usually constant. It is a progression of derangements 4 and 5.

Treatment If movement or postures/positions *do not* reduce sciatica: no treatment utilizing movement or positions is possible at this stage.

If sciatica is reduced by movement or positions then proceed with a reduction of deformity as with derangement 2 or further reduction as for derangements 3 and 1.

Treatment of Derangement 7

This is a symmetrical or asymmetrical pain across L4–L5 with or without buttock and/or thigh pain and a deformity of accentuated lordosis.

This involves an anterior or anterolateral disc disturbance.

Treatment Reduction of derangement utilizing flexion procedures.

CONCLUSION

This chapter is written to broaden health-care professionals' approaches for sound and effective management of their patients' low back syndromes. The instructions provided are aimed at allowing the patient the opportunity to take greater responsibility for his or her own recovery. It is hoped that in departing from the usual "hands-on" pathway so dear to the hearts of many clinicians, the emphasis will shift from patient dependence on treatment to patient independence. A vast number of treatments delivered by health-care providers for the abolition of musculoskeletal conditions are usually unnecessary, and their effectiveness is often unproven.[4] Eventually, all health-care practitioners involved in the field of musculoskeletal syndromes must provide the education that will enable the patient to practice "autotherapy."[5]

Research clearly indicates that the only intervention that consistently appears beneficial across a wide range of spinal and nonspinal musculoskeletal problems is exercise. The following are several quotes from recent studies on treatment of musculoskeletal disorders:

> One can draw a number of conclusions, however. First, and importantly, exercise appears to be the best modality. Strengthening muscles protects the joint. Secondly, most of the machines that plug into the wall are acting as flashy placebos.[6]
>
> In common with other areas of musculoskeletal rehabilitation, the evidence strongly supports exercise (except possibly in the rare case of true radicular back pain) and a cognitive behavioral approach to pain management.[7]

1. It has been the authors' intention in this chapter to describe the treatment of the mechanical syndromes utilizing the McKenzie approach as related to musculoskeletal pain.
2. This discussion included how to gather data about patient problems, assess changes, manage different mechanical conditions, and to rapidly conclude whether a condition will respond to mechanical therapy.
3. It is the hope of the authors that this text will assist those clinicians who are perplexed by the failure of many interventions to "cure" their patients' problems, and who seek endorsement for an approach that demands patient involvement as a logical way forward for the health-care profession.

SUMMARY

1. The hope is from reading this chapter the clinician understands that exercise is the most beneficial evidence based treatment for spinal and non-spinal musculo-skeletal problems.
2. When finished the clinician should be able to distinguish between the three mechanical syndromes: postural, dysfunction and derangement, and their respective treatment per McKenzie protocol.

3. The primary goal of this chapter is for the clinician to understand that McKenzie therapy's primary objective is for patient self-treatment and the "empowerment" of the patient concerning their spinal condition(s).

REFERENCES

1. McKenzie RA. *The lumbar spine: Mechanical diagnosis and therapy*. Lower Hutt, New Zealand: Spinal Publications, 1981.
2. Jacob G. Teaching syllabus: Mechanical diagnosis and therapy of the lumbar spine. Teaching Syllabus: Los Angeles College of Chiropractic Post graduate Rehabilitation Diplomate Course, Whittier, California, October, 1996.
3. Murphy D. *Conservative management of cervical spine syndromes*. New York: McGraw-Hill Medical Publishers, 2000.
4. Maigne JY. Classification des lesions discales lombaires. *Rev Med Orthop* 1992;30:5–8.
5. van der Windt DAWM, van der Heijden GJMG, van der Berg SGM, ter Riet G, de Winter AF, Bouter LM. Ultrasound therapy for musculoskeletal disorders: A systematic review. *Pain* 1999;81:257–271.
6. McKenzie RA, May S. *The human extremities: Mechanical diagnosis and therapy*. Lower Hutt, New Zealand: Spinal Publications, 2000.
7. Clark AK. Effectiveness of rehabilitation in arthritis. *Clin Rehab* 1999;13 S1:51–62.
8. Pruett DW, Griffin MR. Published trials of non-medical and noninvasive therapies for hip and knee arthritis. *Ann Intern Med* 1994;121:133–140.

CHAPTER

23

MOBILIZATION METHODS FOR LOW BACK SYNDROMES

Craig E. Morris, Muffit Jensen, and Vladimir Janda

OUTLINE

OBJECTIVES

1. Provide a summary of commonly utilized mobilization strategies for low back syndromes.
2. Describe a new organizational structure for relaxation, release and stretch methods.
3. Describe mobilization techniques for low back syndromes.
4. Explain mobilization method management strategies.
5. Emphasize the importance of teaching patients independent self mobilization methods.

INTRODUCTION

The locomotor system describes an individual's capacity to move within his or her environs via neuromusculoskeletal activity. Morphology and physiology are interdependent aspects of this complex system. Structural changes therefore result in functional alterations and vice versa.

Morphological alterations can occur within soft tissues (i.e., skin, muscle, fascia, etc.) and joints, leading to postural compromise, motor control difficulties (i.e., incoordination), and associated pain syndromes.[1–3]

A shortened soft tissue, such as myofascial tissue, is a common morphological alteration. Shortened myofascial tissues lead to compromised function of antagonists, a scenario described in Chapter 13 as *muscle imbalance*. For example, structural shortening of hip flexors in ice hockey players correlates with reduced hip extension.[4] Local muscle imbalances can progress to more regional or global alterations, such as Janda's stereotypical postural syndromes. The nature and degree of locomotor system alterations manifest in many ways, requiring a variety of approaches to assess and correct these changes.

Chapter 5 discussed functional aspects of lumbopelvic stability and also touched upon the etiological aspects of motor control dysfunction to this region that is so strategically relevant to human locomotion. Chapter 9 addressed the dynamic and nondynamic nature of physiological and pathological muscle function, emphasizing the myofascial trigger point (TrP) phenomena. Chapters 12 and 13 covered various approaches to the physical examination, designed to isolate the symptom generator(s), and described additional assessment skills for chronic pain syndromes commonly used for clinicians who integrate manual therapeutic methods in their practice. The reader is directed to those chapters in order to establish a broader clinical foundation from which to build competence in manual techniques.

This chapter will continue with this line of clinical reasoning, discussing manual maneuvers to restore soft tissue and joint mobility to improve locomotor function. These methods will be organized into two basic topics: mobilization techniques for the soft tissues and also for the joints.

Soft tissue mobilization techniques comprise a variety of approaches designed to normalize soft tissue tone. The complex interrelationships of the various target tissues, including skin, fascia, muscle, ligament, tendon, and nerves, and their unique mechanical and neurophysiological properties require explanation to allow the clinician to appreciate a plethora of available treatment methods.

For the purpose of this chapter, joint mobilization will be defined as manual joint techniques *without thrust* (i.e., high-velocity, low-amplitude [HVLA] force). Joint mobilization methods will be addressed later in the chapter, following the discussion on soft tissue techniques. Thrust manipulation, utilizing HVLA methods, was covered in Chapter 20.

Finally, it is important to understand that the integrative action of the nervous system prohibits any manual method to solely affect the target soft tissue or the joint because of various global reflexive responses of stimulated exteroceptors or proprioceptors.[5] In addition, techniques described here as soft tissue methods for the sake of organization, such as muscle energy techniques, were designed to target joints also. Therefore, soft tissue techniques can affect joint mobility and vice versa.

Reasonable Expectations

It stands to reason that the manual skills described in this chapter cannot be *taught* here. Obviously, the art of mobilization and myofascial lengthening techniques require a practical, hands-on teaching environment. An in-depth explanation of manual techniques is also beyond the parameters of this chapter. Indeed, entire books are dedicated to individual methods described in the ensuing pages. Several excellent textbooks devoted to mobilization techniques serve as references for this chapter and the reader in search of deeper understanding is directed to those texts. This chapter can nevertheless provide an outline for the learning process of, an appreciation of the rationale for, and potential benefits derived from the appropriate utilization of soft tissue and joint mobilization methods.

TERMINOLOGY AND BACKGROUND INFORMATION

Manual techniques are described and taught in a variety of ways. Because of the lack of standardization, confusion with terminology and contradictory approaches to methods using the same name ensue. In order to overcome such *terminological chaos*[6] the following section are designed to provide clarification of various methods that will be described later.

Relaxation, Release, and Stretch

Practitioners commonly hear of manual techniques designed to normalize soft tissue tone described as relaxation, release, or stretch techniques. There are no universally accepted definitions of these three terms, and they at times appear to be interchangeable. However, the lead author considers all three to be unique, and within their differences lie important subtleties for the clinician who aims toward mastery of mobilization techniques. In addition to categorizing these terms in a manner that can assist in a more organized learning process, clarifying these terms can assist clinicians in more effective communication.

For the purpose of this chapter, the lead author will describe the three muscle lengthening techniques.

Briefly defining each term can help to provide an initial insight into their individuality.

1. Relaxation (Definition: An intrinsic reduction of tension; to loosen). A minimal load directed at the dynamic, contractile component of the muscle to increase tissue length and reduce tone. This method utilizes the understanding of the muscle spindle and gamma system, as discussed in Chapter 9, in order to alter the muscle tone via the neurologically mediated process of inhibition. Because muscle contractibility can be altered reflexively, this is a relatively brief technique. It is quite pleasant because it requires little muscle contraction, perhaps 1 or 2 on a scale of 10, on the part of the patient. In fact, the chances for failure increase with increased loading due in part to nociceptive stimulation, which is facilitory. It must also be performed gently, without any sudden movement or loading, in order to avoid the stretch reflex. The reduction in tone, or inhibition, comes from within the patients themselves, defining the *relaxing* nature of this strategy. Therefore it must, by design, be painless, and yet the clinician must adaptively and gently maintain the same minimal load to lengthen the patient's muscle as the dynamic component relaxes. Finally, the clinician should be careful to avoid increasing the loading during the relaxation, focusing on maintaining a consistent, light pressure throughout.

2. Release (Definition: To set free or to let go). A mild to moderate load is used for this method, which is directed more toward the nondynamic connective tissue component of muscle and fascia. Because this tissue is slow to shorten, it generally requires a longer period compared to the other two techniques to make an effect. This is also a technique that can load the tissues along the line of a muscle, or in any other direction. A prolonged load can also lengthen the dynamic contractile muscle tissue. Like the relaxation technique, the degree of clinician loading, or hand pressure, should remain constant throughout the procedure. Release methods are quite practical for regions where a broad, flat region with a multiplex of tissue layers of varying vectors, such as the posterior lumbar region, is present. However, the other two techniques (i.e., relaxation and stretch) are typically quicker, and therefore more practical if it is determined that the fascia requires little, if any, lengthening.

3. Stretch (Definition: To forcefully extend one's body, or limbs; to strain). This method requires a relatively greater load to the tissue than the previous two. It is meant to target the noncontractile portion of the muscle, the ground substance, although it affects the contractile tissues also by forcefully overcoming any resistance such as stretch reflex. In contrast to a relaxation or release, increases in loading can occur during the procedure and may in fact improve the results. Stretch procedures have the benefit of being relatively quick, but there are additional issues to consider when increasing the loading to a patient, such as increased risk of pain and injury. As such, the clinician must screen the patient who is a candidate for stretch to ensure that he or she can safely tolerate the procedure.

TABLE 23–1. Techniques Based On Specific Lesion Palpated

Condition	Treatment
Skin/fascial restriction	Skin rolling, skin release
Fascial/muscle restriction	Myofascial release, self-stretches
Muscle hypertonicity due to postural shortening	Specific MET, static stretching, PFS, PIR
Myofascial pain syndrome	TrP release, PIR, spray and release
Muscle adhesion	Muscle stripping, Graston©IART, myofascial release, fascial slider
Tendon/ligament scarring due to sprain/strain	Cross-friction massage, Graston®IART
Joint restriction	Joint mobilization, S/cS, self-mobilization, joint manipulation,† MET
Nerve/dural adhesion	Neuromobilization

†See Chapter 20.

The clinician must therefore decide which one or combination of these techniques is most appropriate for the patient: relaxation techniques which are safe but have less effect on the noncontractile tissues, stretch techniques which effect the noncontractile tissues but carry the risk of additional force, or the release maneuver which uses a relatively moderate degree of force (i.e., less than relaxation but more than stretch) that can be multivectored but requires additional time.

Table 23–1 indicates what techniques to employ once palpation has led to the determination of the specific lesion.

Active, Passive, and Semiactive Procedures

Techniques can be divided into *active* and *passive* procedures, in addition to a combination of each that the lead author describes as *semiactive* procedures.

Active procedures require the patient's *participation in the activation* (i.e., muscular contraction) of *the target tissues* and/or region. For example, an active technique to lengthen the iliopsoas would entail contraction of that target muscle.

Passive approaches only require the patient's presence as the clinician performs all of the work. The patient simply relaxes during the procedures.

Semiactive procedures are those that require the patient's participation, but do not activate the target tissues and/or region being treated. For example, procedures that utilize visual or respiratory *synkinesis* (to be discussed later) to normalize low back tissues would fall under the category of a semiactive procedure.

An active method will entail having the patient contract the target muscle or group of muscles to move a body part or resist against some load. Active and semiactive techniques utilize today's understanding of neurophysiological aspects of inhibition and facilitation, which is discussed below in *Neurophysiological Strategies*.

Direct versus Indirect Methods

Manual techniques can also be divided into *direct* and *indirect* methods. Direct methods describe manual techniques directed *at* the target tissue. For example, a direct skin technique utilizes a skin contact on the target skin region and a direct fascial technique directly loads the sub-dermal target fascia. A direct muscle technique may use a skin contact over the belly of the target muscle.

Indirect methods lengthen target tissues using manual techniques or contacts directed at nontarget tissues. This is especially beneficial for those tissues and body regions where a mechanical advantage can be utilized by using a joint as a fulcrum, or where a direct mechanical advantage is difficult to obtain. For example, an indirect method often requires a contact of a distal joint whose motion affects the target tissue. Relaxation of the rectus femoris muscle, in the modified Thomas position (see Chapter 13), requires a contact of the ipsilateral tibia, extending the hip and flexing the knee, as a lever. Therefore, the target muscle (i.e., rectus femoris) can be lengthened once the hip and knee motions bring the target muscle to its barrier despite no *direct* manual loading.

Oscillatory Methods

Oscillatory mobilization provides another set of options that can be quite effective. Oscillations can be divided into proactive, reactive, and passive oscillations.

Proactive oscillatory techniques are those that have the patient perform the movements while the clinician resists the motion. The clinician resistance can stop all motion (isometric), and can even provide resistance through the arc of motion (isotonic) in either concentric (i.e., shortening muscle contraction), eccentric (i.e., lengthening muscle contraction), or both motions. In addition, the clinician can control the speed of the oscillations of the motion, from rapid (three to four times per second) to slow (perhaps once every 2 or 3 seconds. In providing the resistance, the clinician controls the arc of motion.

Reactive oscillatory techniques are those that have the clinician perform the movement while the patient resists the motion. As with the proactive method, motions can be in a variety of speeds, isotonically, isometrically, and also concentrically, eccentrically, or both. The clinician must provide concise explanation to the resistive patient, who must exercise greater control than in the proactive method.

Passive oscillatory techniques are those that have the clinician perform all of the force while the patient remains relaxed. The speed of the oscillations is considered to be of critical importance for passive oscillations. The clinician is advised to speed up and slow down the frequency, sensing for greater relaxation and release. The optimal oscillation frequency varies between patients, target body regions, or tissues, and often even during the same oscillatory mobilization as the patient adapts to treatment.

The ability to quickly attempt variations in oscillatory methods and alter the technique *as the patient responds* provides another example of increasing expertise involved in manual mobilization techniques.

Neurophysiological Strategies

An understanding of neurophysiology allows the clinician to employ procedures to alter dynamic muscle function to assist in normalizing joints and soft tissues. These measures are designed to reduce or increase muscle contractability. A neurologically mediated reduction in function, for example muscle function, is termed *inhibition* (Latin *inhibitus* = to hold back or hinder), whereas neurologically mediated increased function is called *facilitation* (Latin *facilis* = easy). This chapter will use two types of inhibition: *reciprocal inhibition*[5,6] and *autogenic inhibition*[7,8]. Reciprocal inhibition reflexively reduces target muscle activity as its antagonist contracts. For example, reciprocal inhibition of the target biceps brachii will occur while the ipsilateral triceps brachii contracts. In contrast, autogenic, or postcontraction, inhibition reflexively reduces target muscle function following the completion of a contraction and a brief latency period. For example, autogenic inhibition of the target biceps brachii occurs following its own contraction and the brief latency period.

A subcategory of inhibition and facilitation is known as *synkinesis*. The Greek translation for this is "with motion." Synkinesis methods *reflexively* affect the target muscle function by either increasing inhibition or facilitation. The two methods of synkinesis mentioned in this chapter will be *visual* and *respiratory* synkinesis. In most cases, inspiration or shifting the eyes toward the side ("ipsiversive") of muscle activity is facilitory, while expiration or shifting the eyes away

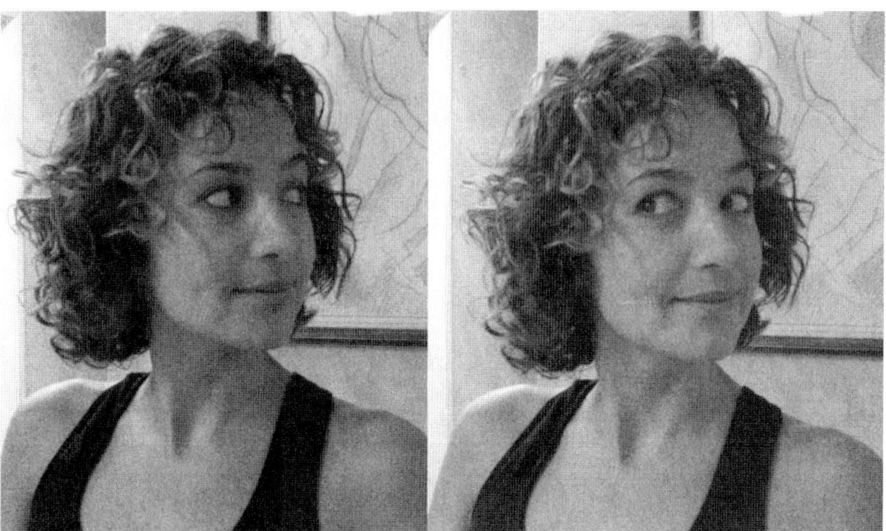

FIGURE 23–1. The "Morris maneuver" teaches the clinician and student to appreciate the impact of synkinesis methods, while differentiating weakness from inhibition. On the left, the eyes shift in the direction of the rotating head (ipsiversive gaze). On the right, the eyes shift away from the rotating head (contraversive gaze), which requires greater muscular effort to achieve the same degree of rotation.

from the side ("contraversive") of muscle activity is inhibitory.[8] The lead author has observed that visual synkinesis techniques seem to have a greater effect on the upper body and upper extremities than on the lower half. Respiratory synkinesis techniques tend to be more effective than visual synkinesis for the lower half, although the former can be effective for the upper half also. Expertise in the utilization of both allows the practitioner to be able to judge the efficacy of either or both techniques for the specific needs of each patient.

Despite the above explanation, clinicians tend to incorrectly consider inhibition and weakness to be synonymous terms. In the same manner, facilitation and strengthening are improperly considered equal expressions. Understanding the differences between these terms, as explained above, is considered crucial to the clinician who desires mastery of manual mobilization techniques. Janda named the so-called "Morris maneuver," proposed by the lead author, to quickly teach clinicians and students the difference between these terms and the immediate impact of synkinesis methods. To perform the maneuver, a clinician is instructed to shift the eyes to one side and rotate the head in the *same* direction (example: eyes shift to the right and head shifts to the right). After returning the head and eyes forward, the person is then instructed to shift the eyes to the opposite side while rotating the head to the original side (example: eyes left and head right). The person will invariably notice that he or she must work much harder to achieve the very same head rotation compared to the previous action, simply by changing from an ipsiversive to a contraversive gaze! Figure 23–1 demonstrates the Morris maneuver.

The final introductory neurophysiological topic of interest for this chapter concerns reduction of muscle resistance in order to normalize myofascial tissue. Stretch reflex (also known as myotatic reflex or the Liddell–Sherrington reflex) is an autogenic excitation, or facilitation, that must be addressed to reduce risks of patient injury from overload. Therefore, inhibitory strategies described above will be integrated into various methods later in the chapter in order to neutralize the stretch reflex.

Technique Guide: *Look for the symbol* 📖 **HOW TO** *for easy step-by-step instructions on various techniques, and the symbol* ⌛ **HOW OFTEN** *for guidelines on treatment frequency.*

SOFT TISSUE TECHNIQUES

Skin Restriction

If skin drag or resistance was perceived during the palpatory examination, its nature and etiology must be investigated. One will find a restricted skin barrier to springing assessment, in addition to increased moisture via locally increased sympathetic activity. As previously noted, increased local sensitivity is often present, which helps to define the term *hyperalgesic zone* (HAZ). Local joint dysfunction, trigger points (TrPs), scleratogenous pain, and autonomic dysfunction can cause this event. If it is decided that direct treatment may be of benefit, it can be dealt with using skin release or skin rolling methods. Depending on the size of the area being treated, the fingertips or hands placed flat on the skin can be used.[8,9]

As with all manual methods, skin release and skin rolling are designed to be simultaneously diagnostic and therapeutic. Recurrence of the HAZ will suggest that an underlying problem exists and that the clinician should search elsewhere for the culprit. Skin techniques are quite subtle, so the practitioner should remember to compare the HAZ with surrounding skin or the patient's contralateral skin region, which will hopefully provide a "control" (i.e. a normal comparison) to determine normotonic springing and skin drag.

Skin Release

Procedure: Passive
Method: Direct
Facilitation/inhibition: No

HOW TO

1. Lightly contact the skin between finger pads almost touching one another.
2. Lightly separate the fingers with minimal force to the barrier and wait for the release.
3. Hold up to 10 seconds or more. An "ease" will be felt as the tissue releases.
4. Recheck to see if normal springing is restored and skin drag is normalized.
5. Compare in several different directions.

HOW OFTEN

Results are generally achieved quickly, but multiple areas may be affected. Scan areas for involvement and treat as needed.

Skin Rolling

Procedure:	**Passive**
Method:	**Direct**
Facilitation/inhibition:	**No**

Skin rolling can also be performed if there is a skin, subdermal, or perhaps a fascial restriction present. It can generally be thought as a type of release, although it can at times require a rather forceful approach, more along the line of stretch. Some areas respond favorably to skin rolling such as the region over the iliac crest in addition to the thoracolumbar fascia, but some areas where the skin is tighter or more adhered, this technique may be impractical as well as quite painful to the patient.

HOW TO

1. A fold of skin is lifted and rolled between the fingers in a linear or "U" shape, as seen in Figure 23–2.
2. For deeper fascia, a pulling type of maneuver, in which one envisions a separation of the tissue layers, can be effective.

HOW OFTEN

Results are generally achieved quickly, but multiple areas may be affected. Scan areas for involvement and treat as needed.

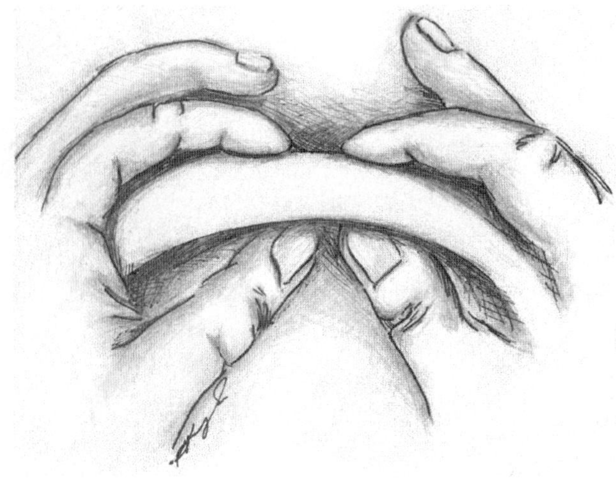

FIGURE 23–2. The skin rolling technique is effective for superficial and deeper tissues. A "U-shaped" skin rolling method adds another dimension to separate and mobilize various tissue layers.

Fascial/Muscle Restriction

Fascia is a tough fibroelastic tissue that spreads throughout the body in a three-dimensional web from head to foot functionally without interruption. The contiguous nature of the so-called fascial system was discussed in Chapter 2, with an emphasis placed on its proprioceptive role in addition to its stabilizing role in the locomotor system. Fascia envelops every muscle, organ, blood vessel, and bone. Therefore, local tissue tensions (due to factors such as trauma, poor posture, tissue creep, scar tissue, adhesions, inflammation, etc.) can effect the tissue tone and function of distant body regions via this contiguous fascial network (Fig. 23–3). Shortened fascia can even have an effect on the movement of bones and joints, leading to painful syndromes.

Brief stretching alone will not release fascia because of its tenacious collagenous makeup. Repeated and prolonged loading, as defined earlier by release maneuvers, has proven to be more effective. Of course, prolonged, painless, moderate loading also tends to inhibit muscle contraction, allowing one to then focus on the fascial restriction.

Myofascial Release[10,11] (Fig. 23–4)

Procedure:	**Passive or semiactive**
Method:	**Direct**
Facilitation/inhibition:	**Optional**

HOW TO

1. Apply gentle pressure to the restricted tissue and then wait. The load should be applied along the fascial plane, or as close to it as possible. Patience

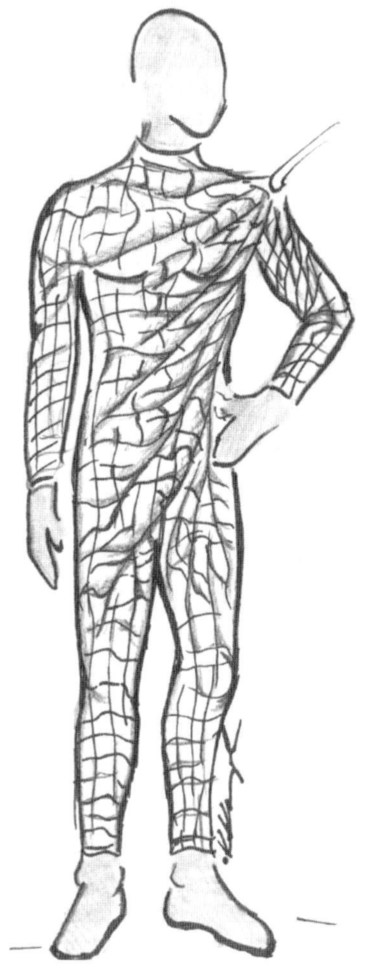

FIGURE 23–3. The fascial system forms a contiguous elastic meshwork of tensile tissue, analogous to a subdermal sweater.

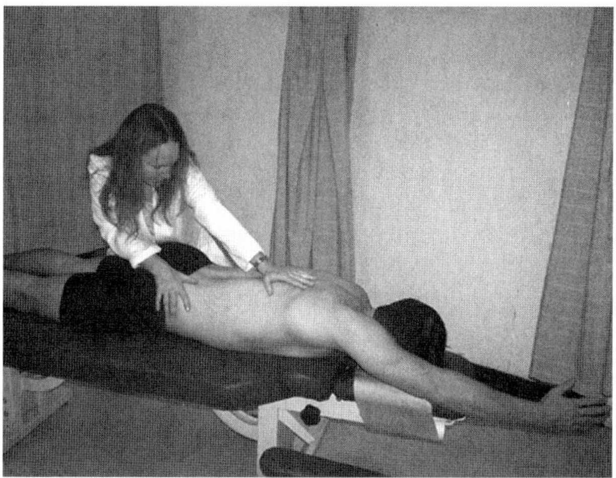

FIGURE 23–4. Myofascial release utilizes strategies that load the target tissue along the plane of the fascial sheaths.

is often required until the tissue releases. The initial releases are often from hypertonic muscle tissue. Some clinicians integrate a patient muscle contraction and then postcontraction release during this phase to speed muscle inhibition and more efficiently localize the fascia.

2. Continue loading along the same vector until a firmer collagenous barrier is reached.
3. Hold contact without additional pressure for at least 60–120 seconds, or until the release is completed.
4. The release is generally gradual and slow.
5. Follow tissue until movement ceases.
6. Because of the multidirectional and continuous nature of fascia, palpate for restricted fascia in other vectors and adjacent body regions. If restrictions are found, repeat the above protocols.

HOW OFTEN

Because of the gentleness of this technique, it can be done daily if needed. However, patient self-stretches, performed multiple times daily, can be quite helpful once the directions of release are understood.

Fascial "sliders." Once the clinician obtains the necessary understanding and skills for assessment and implementation of manual methods, the combinations of methods can be customized to the specific needs of each patient. Many of the techniques presented here are offshoots of prior methods, as a part of the evolutionary process in this field of treatment.

Fascial sliders (FS) are the lead author's variation of myofascial release, of the active and passive oscillations of muscle energy techniques, and of neural mobilization techniques discussed later in the chapter. To appreciate the rationale behind FS requires some explanation. Fascial sliders take into account the sliding layers of the contiguous fascial system in the thoracolumbosacral region.

A key component among these layers include the *erector spinae aponeurosis* (ESA), an *independent* sheet of connective tissue arising from caudal thoracic erector spinae fibers. The ESA traverses the lumbar region, essentially sliding *independently*, along the longitudinal axis, *superior to* the lumbar erector spinae. The ESA is responsible for up to 50% of force in lumbar extension.[12] Figure 23–5 demonstrates the independent, longitudinal ESA. Conversely, the lumbar erector spinae lie deep to the ESA and therefore appear to act independently of the more cephalad thoracic erector spinae.[12]

Fascial sliders also incorporate the work of Vleeming et al.[13,14] who found that the thoracolumbar fascia (TLF) and sacroiliac ligaments provide a functionally continuous bridge between the low back, pelvis, and lower extremities to facilitate load transference during bipedal activities such as gait. Finally, the FS technique

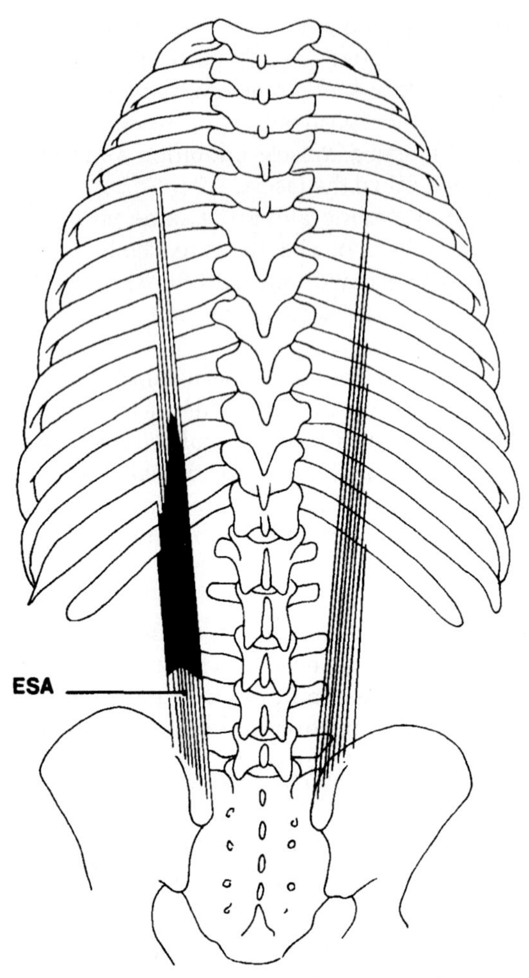

FIGURE 23–5. The erector spinae aponeurosis (ESA) is a broad sheet of tendinous fibers arising from the caudal tendons of the thoracic erector spinae (longissimus thoracic [LT] and caudal thoracic fibers of the iliocostalis lumborum [IL]). As illustrated, the ESA extends inferiorly in a longitudinal axis, which is superior to and independent of the lumbar erector spinae. The ESA inserts into the ilia and sacrum. *(Reprinted with permission from Bogduk.[12])*

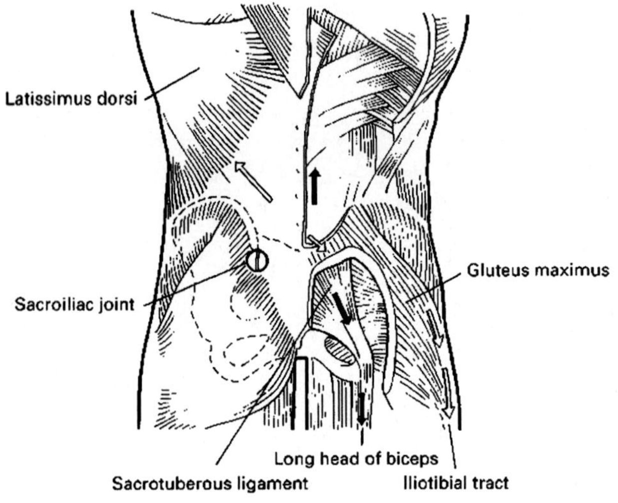

FIGURE 23–6. Schematic of the posterior myofascial functional loop that allows for multidimensional force transference from the torso to the pelvis and lower extremity. *(Reproduced with permission from Vleeming et al.[13])*

also utilizes the recent understanding of the importance of the latissimus dorsi and its ipsilateral and contralateral (i.e., crossing the midline barrier thought to exist by the spinous processes) contribution to force transference, along with the transverses abdominis, to the posterior layer of the TLF and along the kinetic chain.[15] Figure 23–6 demonstrates the functionally chained contralateral latissimus dorsi, bilateral TLF, ipsilateral long dorsal ligament, and ipsilateral biceps femoris. It should be emphasized that these findings were not original, but merely confirmatory of the so-called loops and slings that were described in prior decades to explain diagonal myofascial functional chains.

Fascial sliders are designed to address myofascial adhesions, such as occurring in posttraumatic and postsurgical back cases, although the same event may occur with less trauma and prolonged inactivity.

Fascial sliders incorporate the sliding nature of the myofascial system by utilizing oscillating superior and inferior myofascial migrating movements. Superior thoracolumbar myofascial motion occurs with the "hip hike" maneuver described in Chapter 13. It was inspired by the heel-walking test to assess L5 motor function. The hip hike is a motion that is essentially a unilateral pelvic elevation, designed to draw the ipsilateral iliac crest cephalward using key muscles such as the ipsilateral quadratus lumborum and external oblique musculature. Sacroiliac motion is believed to occur in the form of ipsilateral counter nutation and contralateral rotatory lumbar motion, although the kinesiological aspects of this coupled motion are beyond the parameters of this chapter.

A second strategy for superior myofascial migration occurs actively by instructing the patient to raise his or her arm overhead, raising the limb as far as possible. This scapular elevation affects the latissimus dorsi and its contiguous posterior TLF connection previously mentioned. A passive superior myofascial migration strategy can occur by having either the clinician or an assistant traction the arm superiorly.

Caudal myofascial sliding occurs passively when the clinician inferiorly tractions the target leg. An active inferior sliding strategy can be used as the patient attempts to lower the target hip in a motion opposite of the hip hike.

The active coupled motion of the hip hike is believed to provide autogenic inhibition along the key transitional region of the torso, pelvis, and lower extremities, *providing an excellent opportunity for long axis soft tissue and joint mobilization methods*. The vector of loading can extend superiorly in an ipsilateral or a contralateral direction, or a combination of both via the latissimus dorsi depending on whether one or both arms are elevated.

HOW TO

1. The patient is placed prone on the table with the feet off the end of the table. The arms rest on the table, one or both placed overhead in relation to the patient.
2. The clinician, stationed at the end of the table, firmly grasps the ankle of the patient's target leg.
3. The clinician distracts the leg caudally. As the leg and ipsilateral pelvis are lowered, an inferior fascial sliding of the TLF will occur.
4. The patient is then instructed to elevate the contralateral shoulder and arm (e.g., "reach your arm high overhead"). As this occurs, the clinician reduces the caudal distraction of the target leg, allowing it to migrate superiorly because of fascial system tensioning and thoracolumbar sliding (see Fig. 23–7).
5. The patient is then instructed to gradually lower the shoulder as the target leg is again distracted inferiorly as before.
6. This is repeated for 5–10 times.
7. The same procedure is then performed on the contralateral leg.
8. The same method is used involving the ipsilateral arm.
9. The same method is then used involving both upper extremities simultaneously.

The clinician may be able to facilitate the FS by instructing the patient to actively elevate the hip on the same side as the contact leg. This "hip hike," in conjunction with the overhead arm elevation, increases the cephalward myofascial migration.

Many variations of this technique can be utilized, such as instructing the patient contract the latissimus dorsi by grasping an overhead bar and pulling up to utilizing respiratory synkinesis methods.

HOW OFTEN

Because of the gentleness of this technique, it can be done daily if needed. However, postsurgical patients can experience increased pain and edema because of lysing of fascial adhesions, especially in the perisacral region. In those instances, local applications of cryotherapy is recommended, with FS performed no more than three times weekly.

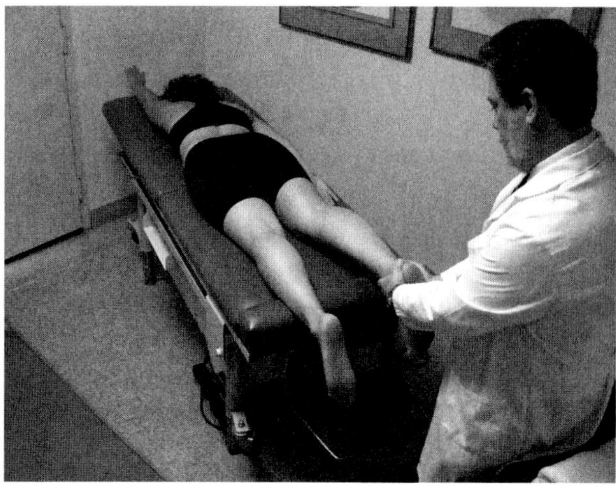

FIGURE 23–7. Fascial slider (FS) technique with cephalad fascial shift.

MUSCLE HYPERTONICITY

Muscle Energy Techniques

Muscle energy technique (MET), a method developed by Mitchell Sr.,[16] is designed to restore mobility by utilizing the understanding of neuromusculoskeletal function following pathological changes in locomotion by restoring the muscle to its optimal resting length and normalize joint mobility.

Originally designed to increase joint motion and decrease muscle tone by inhibiting the facilitated segment, a concept first proposed by Korr[17], these techniques have become an increasingly popular method to create optimal muscle length through specific muscular facilitation and inhibition. This can be accomplished by strategic muscle contractions of varying intensities (depending on which MET is utilized) with specific body positions. A plethora of variations in MET methods are possible, which far exceeds the parameters of this summary chapter. The physiological basis of how these techniques work was presented in Chapter 9. This chapter will discuss the following METs:

1. Postfacilitation stretch (PFS)
2. Postisometric relaxation (PIR)

Specific patient positions for individual muscles are detailed under the heading *Specific Muscle Positioning for METs or Stretching* later in this chapter. These positions can be utilized for any of the METs, as well as when using spray and release.

Postfacilitation Stretch (PFS)[11,18] This is designed to lengthen the noncontractile tissue once the dynamic tissue has been inhibited, especially when the contractile tissue is shortened. With this technique, the clinician does not have to overcome the contractile tissue, which would require greater force to overcome and thus increase the chance of patient injury. The energy expenditures of the clinician during manual techniques must also taken into consideration, from both a safety standpoint and also because the clinician typically sees multiple patients per day and must save his or her energy to assist others. Because of the resilient nature of the target shortened, nondynamic collagenous component of muscle, significant force must be utilized to successfully lengthen these tissues during the post-facilitation (autogenic) inhibition period.

Procedure: **Active**
Method: **Indirect**
Facilitation/inhibition: **Yes**

HOW TO

1. Position the patient so the target muscle(s) is shortened to approximately 50% capacity in order to activate the greatest number of motor units (V. Janda, personal communication, 2002). The patient and clinician should be placed in positions that provide stability for the patient and the optimal mechanical advantage for the clinician.
2. The patient is instructed to aggressively contract against the examiner's resistance for 7–10 seconds using maximum strength. The clinician must resist all motion as the patient contracts.
3. The patient is instructed to suddenly and completely relax. The clinician then waits for a second or two to allow for a brief latent period of muscular inhibition, before quickly and aggressively stretching the muscle. While there may be minimal discomfort during the stretch, stretching should continue if there is pain. It is important that the patient completely relax. The patient may first have taught how to relax immediately by mimicking the timing of a moderate contraction followed by a moderate stretch until such time that the patient becomes comfortable with the timing of the procedure.
4. The inhibitory period follows for about 10–15 (use 12) seconds, which is the period of stretching. Stretch must be performed with an even speed.
5. Following the stretch, the muscle is returned to its earlier, prestretched position, which again recruits the most motor units. This position is held for 10–20 seconds before repeating the same facilitation procedure and subsequent stretch.
6. Depending on the effect of the previous stretch (i.e., as the range of motion [ROM] increases), begin the next stretch at the midpoint of the motion where the greatest number of motor units would again be recruited. If there is no improvement, begin again at the same midpoint as before.
7. Stretch three to five times; more than five times may cause the muscle to become sore and hypertonic, reversing any benefits gained by the stretch.

HOW OFTEN

The practitioner should obtain good results within 6–10 visits. Frequency should be no more often than every other day. Waiting more than a few days, however, may allow the muscle to fully return to its pre-PFS length. The patient should perform home stretching exercises to complement the in-office stretches, but should not be allowed to perform endurance or strengthening exercise to muscles that are being stretched during the treatment period.

Postisometric Relaxation (PIR) Mitchell Sr. developed this method under the auspices of an MET, although Lewit later altered and renamed the modified approach.[19,20] PIR differs from PFS in that the forces generated by patient and clinician are not maximal, but rather minimal. PIR is designed to inhibit the target tissues, the contractile aspects of the striated muscle, via autogenic inhibition. Lewit also modified this gentle and subtle technique, integrating synkinesis techniques designed to facilitate or inhibit the respiratory or visual synkinesis measures. Antagonistic, or reciprocal, inhibition strategies, based upon Sherrington's second law by contraction of the antagonist(s) to the target muscle, may also be utilized to speed the muscle balancing process.

Procedure: **Active**
Method: **Indirect**
Facilitation/inhibition: **Yes**

HOW TO

1. Isolate the target muscle and lightly lengthen it to the barrier (the point where it meets first resistance).
2. Instruct the patient to contract the target muscles with minimal force (approximately 10% of the patient's force) for 8–10 seconds as the clinician resists any patient motion.
3. Instruct the patient to relax completely. As the muscle relaxes, the clinician maintains the same light pressure, feeling the muscle lengthen as it relaxes after a brief latency period (i.e., 1–3 seconds). This autogenic inhibition can slowly continue for more than 10 seconds, and the clinician should wait for the lengthening relaxation phase to finish before repeating the procedure.

4. The clinician must be certain to avoid returning any of the increased motion gained following PIR, as this new position becomes the starting point for the next PIR cycle.
5. Repeat three to five times or until no further gain is achieved.

There are six additional strategies that may improve the results:

1. Increasing the time for which the contraction is held.
2. Increasing the contraction, which is not to exceed 30% capacity.
3. Visual synkinesis (eye movements toward the target muscle are usually facilitory and away are inhibitory).
4. Respiratory synkinesis (inspiration is usually facilitory, while expiration is usually inhibitory).
5. Antagonist contraction (contraction of the antagonist to the target muscle causes reflex inhibition of the target muscle).
6. A combination of two or more of the above.

HOW OFTEN

See comments under *Post-Facilitation Stretch* (PFS)

Contraindications of METs[8,21,22]

1. These techniques should not be used during the acute phase of a condition.
2. Differentiate between limited joint movements (i.e., capsular adhesion versus joint blockage), since the technique will not reduce the capsular adhesion.
3. Do not use the technique if the patient is unable to relax. The patient must be able to relax immediately.
4. Do not use the technique in the presence of primary muscle disease or rheumatoid arthritis.

Self-Static Stretching The practitioner must appreciate his or her practical limitations during an office visit. To supplement and assist in restoring proper function, "home work" is often given to the patient in the form of one or more self-stretches performed multiple times daily. These stretches are directed at the hypertonic muscles to restore optimal muscular length, although they will also increase the motion of joints affected by the target muscle(s). Several self-stretches are demonstrated later in the chapter under the heading of *Self-Mobilization*. There are many books available in which pictures can be copied and given to the patient as a reminder and guide to proper positioning.

HOW OFTEN

It is important to stretch a minimum of two times per day, holding each static stretch given for 30–60 seconds.

Myofascial Pain Syndrome

As described in Chapter 9, myofascial pain syndrome is described as a characteristic referred pain pattern from a specific skeletal muscle[6,7] *in which only a small portion of fibers within a muscle become taut and hypertonic*. A diagnosis of myofascial pain syndrome in this specific sense requires the clinical identification of TrPs that reproduce the pain pattern described by the patient.

TrP Release (aka Ischemic Compression) Nimmo was a leader in integrating TrP work into clinical practice. He termed the procedure the receptor tonus technique.[23] Nimmo used deep pressure applied directly over the irritable lesion to produce what he believed was an ischemic compression effect. This can be used on both active and latent TrPs. The term "ischemic compression" was made popular by Travell and Simon.[24,25] However, this term appears to be contradictory, since a TrP is already an ischemic event. Thus, the recommended term used today is "trigger point release."

Procedure: **Passive**
Method: **Direct**
Facilitation/inhibition: No

HOW TO

1. Apply sustained digital pressure to the TrP within the target muscle for 20–60 seconds.
2. Increase pressure as the sensitivity decreases and the tension of the TrP wanes.
3. Release pressure when the TrP subsides, or it is no longer tender to pressure.
4. Follow with passive lengthening of the target muscle or muscle group.

Because of the gentleness of this technique, it can be performed daily if needed. However, self-stretches of target muscles and a functional stabilization program to improve motor control can reduce the necessity for numerous repetitions of this method.

HOW OFTEN

1. Repeat daily for 1–2 weeks
2. Suspend treatments for 2–3 days if soreness develops.

3. As noted above, self-stretches of target muscles and a functional stabilization program to improve motor control can reduce the necessity for numerous repetitions of this method.

Spray and Release (aka Spray and Stretch) Travell and Simons developed this method[24,25] to eliminate TrPs. Cold fluorimethane spray was thought to inhibit pain and motor neuron activity, while the subsequent, specific loading was thought to biomechanically lengthen the target tissue and disrupt the TrP nodule. The authors believe that the technique should be called *spray and release* based on the gentleness of techniques as described earlier in this chapter. A vapocoolant spray such as Flouri-Methane can be used, although this method has become controversial because of the negative effects of fluorocarbons on the ozone layer.

Procedure: Passive
Method: Direct (spray) and indirect (release)
Facilitation/inhibition: No (i.e., while no active inhibition or facilitation techniques are used, the cold spray is thought to produce a reflexive inhibition allowing for a more effective release afterward)

HOW TO

1. Patient positioned comfortably.
2. Flouri-Methane sprayed over involved muscle. Direct spray at 3060 degrees angle to the skin surface. Spray two to three times, each covering 10 cm/s.
   (a) Sweep spray parallel to muscle fibers
   (b) Sweep spray toward TrP
3. Muscle involving TrP is then gently loaded until release.
4. After release
   (a) Apply moist heat to involved muscle for 10–20 minutes
   (b) Instruct patient to move (i.e. actively) through an entire range of motion that fully contracts and lengthens the involved muscle.

HOW OFTEN

1. Repeat daily for 1–2 weeks.
2. Suspend treatments for 2–3 days if soreness develops.
3. As noted above, self-stretches of target muscles and a functional stabilization program to improve motor control can reduce the necessity for numerous repetitions of this method.

Postisometric Relaxation (PIR) See *Muscle Hypertonicity* section above. This technique is quite effective for the treatment of myofascial TrPs.

Specific Muscle Positioning for METS or Myofascial Lengthening

These position guidelines are used for any MET (Ex/PFS, PIR, etc.) of choice. The specific patient position is dependent on patient comfort together with the effectiveness of treatment being performed. If one MET is not successful, try another. If one position is not favorable, try another.

The modified Thomas position is an extremely practical position for applying MET techniques to various muscles of the hip. This positioning and the specific assessment methods for each of these muscles, in addition to several other key lumbopelvic muscles and joints, were addressed in detail in Chapter 13. As previously noted, the assessment skills described in Chapter 13 are considered vital in order to better utilize the techniques in this chapter. Table 23–2 outlines practical MET position maneuvers. The reader is referred to the descriptions and illustrations in Chapter 13 to better understand the descriptions provided in Table 23–2.

Tendon/Ligament/Fascial Adhesions/Scarring[26]

Recurrent microtrauma to tendons or ligaments cause a proliferation of fibroblasts and initiation of an inflammatory cascade, resulting in the laying down of new collagen along the normal lines of stress. Whether using an instrument or one's hands, the final goals are the same: to increase motion, improve function and with this, hopefully decrease pain. Four popular techniques for tendon/ligament scarring include instrument-assisted release techniques (IART), cross friction, Active Release Technique (ART®), and muscle stripping.

IART (Instrument-Assisted Release Technique)

Procedure: Passive
Method: Direct
Facilitation/inhibition: No

Instrument-assisted manual techniques are not new to the field of manual therapy. These are tools designed to enable clinicians to effectively mobilize scar tissue, fascial restrictions adhesions, and reduce hypertonicity. There are several such tools available for clinicians. These include the Graston® instruments and the newer Sound-Assisted Soft Tissue Mobilization (SASTM®) tools. Both designed by the same inventor, the Graston instruments use specially designed handheld, stainless steel instruments to accomplish this task while the SASTM instruments are made of a polymer (Fig. 23–8). Both types of IARTs offer the clinician several benefits, including reduced stress to

TABLE 23–2. Positioning for Myofascial Lengthening Techniques

Muscle	Patient Position	Doctor Position	Lengthen By
Iliopsoas	Supine in a modified Thomas position	Bracing patient to maintain proper position	Apply downward load to the extended target thigh
	Prone with target hip extended and knee flexed. The non-target leg off the table with foot stabilized on the floor	The leg remaining on the table is flexed by clinician at the knee and lifted off the table	Trying to induce increase hip extension Caution not to extend from the lumbar spine
Rectus femoris	Supine in a modified Thomas position	Bracing patient to maintain proper position	Maintain target hip extension while flexing the knee beyond 90 degrees
	Prone	Contact target leg, flexing at knee	Draw the target heel to ipsilateral buttock
Tensor fascia latae	Supine in a modified Thomas position	Bracing patient to maintain proper position	Draw target leg medially while maintaining hip extension
	Side-lying (target side up) backed up against stabilizing clinician	Stabilize patient from behind the low back	Load target leg down toward floor while stabilizing the pelvis (i.e., target hip is moved posteriorly and medially)
Hamstrings	Supine	Elevate the target leg SLR style	Without posterior pelvic rotation bring one leg up in flexion until the barrier is reached
Piriformis	Supine with the target hip slightly flexed	Grasp target leg, drawing thigh to clinician's chest	Load thigh, compressing hip and internally rotate hip
Single-joint hip adductors	Supine in a modified Thomas position	Bracing patient to maintain proper position	Load the target leg off the table outward
Erector spinae	Seated	On either side of the patient	Bend the patient between their spread legs. Watch for thoracic kyphosis
Quadratus lumborum	Prone	Grasp target side ankle	Traction leg in the caudal direction making sure movement occurs at the pelvis
Quadratus lumborum	Side-lying effected side down with the top leg bent and braced in front of the other leg	Lift target leg up	Continue leg elevation (i.e., hip flexion) to barrier
Gastrocnemius	Supine	Passive dorsiflexion of ankle with extended knee	Try for increased dorsiflexion
Soleus	Supine	Passive dorsiflexion of ankle with the knee flexed	Try for increased dorsiflexion
Latissimus dorsi	Prone	Grasp both the wrists of the patient Elevate arms overhead	Distract arms superiorly
Latissimus dorsi	Side-lying	Grasp target wrist Elevate arm overhead	Distract target arm superiorly
Diaphragm	Seated, slightly slumped forward	Standing behind patient with arms around patient's thorax and grasping anterior, inferior costal margins	Distract inferior costal soft tissue caudalward as patient exhales

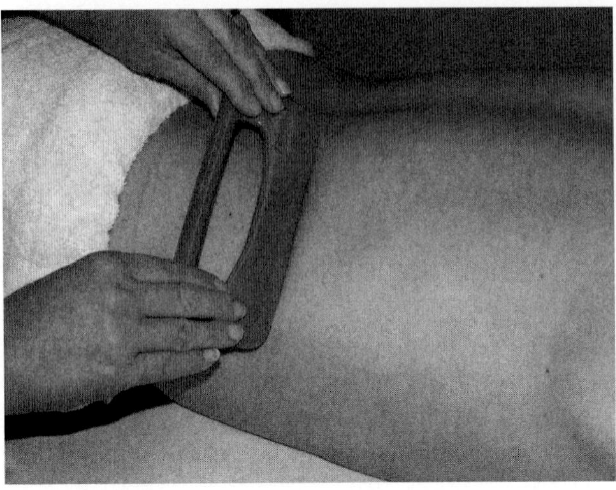

FIGURE 23–8. Sound assisted soft tissue mobilization (SASTM®) instruments are a popular and effective type of instrument-assisted release technique (IART).

the clinician's hands and increased sensitivity of deep fibrotic tissues.

Graston and SASTM are not the only IARTs, although the lead authors of this chapter have found them to be extremely effective for tendon/ligament scarring, muscle adhesion, fascial restriction, as well as acute and chronic bursitis. Another type of IART is the Intracell® devise. The specific methods and frequency of IARTs vary by method.

Cross-Friction Massage

Procedure: **Passive**
Method: **Direct**
Facilitation/inhibition: No

Cross-friction massage is generally used for tendon and ligament scarring. This technique can be employed over the iliolumbar ligament, sacrotuberous ligament, as well as over the supraspinous ligament and the many tendons that connect to the pelvis and greater trochanter. Cross friction is based on the premise that pressure and movement across the normal direction of the tendon or ligament (right angles) is used to synthesize, remodel, and repair the collagen fibers in the favored direction. This is advantageous because scar tissue should heal along the normal lines of stress, but adhesions can lead to fibrosis and immobilization of not only the soft tissues surrounding the injury, but also the local joints.

HOW TO

1. Use a reinforced finger (i.e., one finger over another) to contact the ligament or tendon at a right angle without the use of creams.
2. Make sure that the clinician's finger and underlying skin move as one contiguous tissue repeatedly traverses across the target tissue with as much pressure as the patient can tolerate.
3. Increase friction as a new level of anesthesia is reached.
4. A minimum of 10 minutes is required, but may be done to a maximum of 20 minutes.

Ultrasound used before cross friction may be useful in softening the tissue.

HOW OFTEN

1. Depends on the condition being treated, however two to three times weekly is typical unless the patient becomes too sore with this frequency.
2. Usual response time for an overuse syndrome is 2 weeks to 2 months.
3. Perform every other day.
4. Stop if friction aggravates the condition.

Other contraindications include inflammation, hematoma, and calcification.

Neural Mobilization[27]

The final target soft tissue to mobilize for this chapter is nervous tissue and its supporting structures. The nervous system is a continuous tract and like any other tissue is susceptible to compression or adhesions, leading to adverse neural tension. Because it is the most sensitive of all tissues, the importance of the consequences of adverse neural tension cannot be overstated.

Restricted neural mobility can occur anywhere along the neuraxis, nervous tissue, and supporting structures housed within the axial skeleton, and also continuing into the periphery. Butler likened the mobility of the nervous system to a brake cable traversing through a tube, able to slide along independent of its protective cover. Such adaptability to mechanical changes is vital. For example, Breig found that the length of the spinal column increased by 5–9 cm in flexion compared to extension.[28] In addition, Smith et al. found in a cadaveric study of 10 specimens that the L4, L5, and S1 nerve roots moved between .5 and 5 mm caudally during the supine straight-leg raise (SLR) maneuver.[29]

Mobilization of the nervous system, or neuromobilization, describes manual techniques designed to assess and restore the mobility in the spinal canal, of the exiting nerve roots, and also along the periphery. An understanding of neural anatomy and kinesiology can then allow one to utilize manual strategies for the diagnosis and treatment of restricted neural mobility. It must be emphasized that, unlike previous target

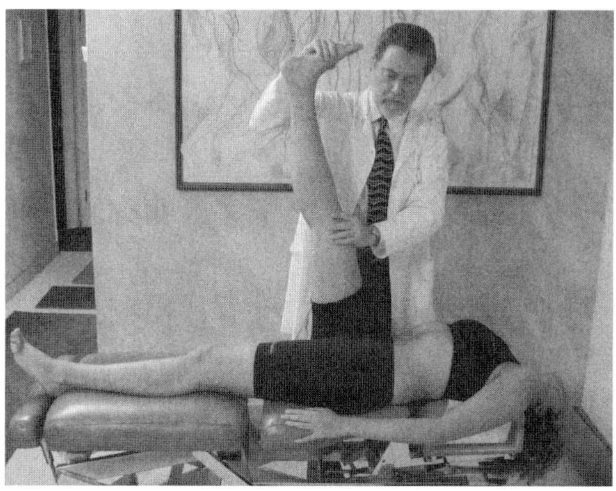

FIGURE 23–9. Neural mobilization ("nerve flossing") technique utilizing cervical extension and SLR with foot dorsiflexion to perform caudal glide along the neuraxis and the lower limb.

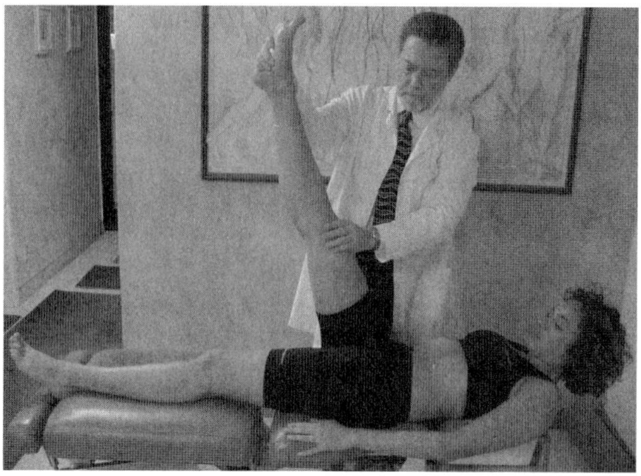

FIGURE 23–10. Neural mobilization ("nerve flossing") technique utilizing cervical flexion and reduced SLR with foot plantar flexion to perform cephalad glide of the neuraxis.

soft tissues, *neuromobilization is not designed to stretch or lengthen the nerve, but rather to free it from restrictive perineural structures*. These techniques have gained the nickname of "sliders" because they promote sliding of the neuraxis during mobilization. This method has also been called "neural flossing" because the repetitive and oscillating motion of nerves through tight spaces is analogous to the common dental practice.

With regard to low back syndromes, the most important mobilization techniques involve variations of the supine SLR maneuver. Briefly explaining, flexing, internally rotating, and/or adducting the hip, extending the knee, dorsiflexing, and/or inverting the foot/ankle all cause a caudalward, or inferior, translation of the neuraxis and peripheral nerves. Superiorly, cervical extension reduces the length of the neural canal, allowing for greater caudal neuraxial glide when combined with an SLR maneuver (Fig. 23–9). Combinations of these maneuvers therefore effectively increase the neural mobilization inferiorly, while the order of which joint is moved *isolates* the regional neural tensioning. Therefore, an SLR with internal hip rotation and hip adduction will traction the neuraxis inferiorly, with increased isolation of tension at the exiting lumbar nerve roots and hip region. If one were to then flex the knee, this would reduce the nerve root and hip region tension, while ankle dorsiflexion and internal rotation would then increase neural tension to the lower leg, allowing the clinician to isolate various target neural branches as desired.

Reducing the caudal neuraxial glide can be accomplished by reversing the above maneuvers. However, if a superior neuraxial glide is desired, then combinations such as plantar flexion, reduced SLR, and cervical flexion will accomplish this quite nicely (Fig. 23–10).

Once the target neural tissues have been isolated and tensioned, a repetitive, oscillating sequence of caudalward and cephalward maneuvers creates the desired neural mobilization.

In addition to a supine maneuver, this can also be performed with the patient in a seated position, the most common of which involves a forward-flexed head and torso, known as the "slump" posture.

Neural mobilization techniques utilize oscillating methods of increased and reduced tensioning in order to gradually release the nervous tissue from its restrictive environs. Greater overall translation occurs if one also utilizes superior neuraxis translation strategies, as occurs with cervical spine flexion. In contrast, cervical extension reverses superior neuraxis progression.

This chapter presents a cursory overview of this topic. Butler describes the principles and practice of neural tension tests and mobilization maneuvers in detail and the reader is referred to this source for further information.[27]

JOINT MOBILIZATION

Restricted joint motion has been variously described by different names from multiple perspectives, but all share a common principle in that the joint motion is reduced.

Joint Restriction

Mobilization

Procedure: **Passive**
Method: **Direct**
Facilitation/inhibition: **No**

The biomechanics of spinal manipulation of an HVLA delivery system was discussed at length in

TABLE 23–3. Manipulation vs. Mobilization

Manipulation	Mobilization
Generally associated with an audible sound	Usually no audible sound
High velocity, low amplitude	Low velocity, gradual graded movements
Limited palpatory feedback during thrust	Ongoing palpatory feedback during mobilization
Sudden force	Gradual force
Often performed through pain	Rarely performed through pain

Chapter 20. HVLA manipulation is the most supported method of manual treatment for acute and chronic low back pain. One of its practical strengths is its relative quickness in clinical use. However, a drawback is that the clinician loses full control of the dynamic changes occurring in the joint for a split second during the thrust. Another drawback is that the force exerted requires a stable joint complex to withstand the sudden load and this entails a degree of risk. There are times though when the clinician may prefer another approach to restore joint function. If this is indeed the case, then joint mobilization may be instituted in lieu of a manipulative procedure.

Joint mobilization is a safe, gentle, and effective alternative to manipulation, although they can at times be effective allies in reaching the goal of improved function. The main differences between these techniques are contrasted in Table 23–3.

Mobilization involves varying degrees of force to the joint, although gentle movements should be first utilized, especially in cases of severe pain. One of the most important requirements for mobilization is that the patient must be as relaxed as possible. Activation of the patient's muscles that stabilize the joint will compromise the effectiveness of the procedure. Indications for mobilization are listed in Table 23–4.

TABLE 23–4. Indications for Joint Mobilization

To restore joint mobility when motion is restricted because of adhesion, hypertonicity, fascial restriction, or joint blockage
Can be performed prior to or following manipulation to ensure proper joint mobility
HVLA thrusting manipulation is not tolerated well by the patient
Joint hypomobility
When pain is to be avoided
Acute conditions

Graded Mobilization Strategies. In order to better appreciate various mobilization techniques and the appropriate utilization of each, Maitland describes grades of oscillatory mobilization as well as sustained mobilizations.[30] Some important guides used to determine the optimal mobilization strategy are pain production, hypertonicity, patient apprehension, and severity of joint limit restriction.

Grades of Oscillatory Mobilization:

Grade I: Small amplitude movement at beginning of range
Grade II: Large amplitude movement within active range (but not at end of range)
(Grades I and II are considered slow stretches and are used primarily for pain relief.)
Grade III: Small amplitude movement up to limit of range
Grade IV: Large amplitude movement at limit of range
(Grades III and IV do affect the barrier and have a mechanical effect on the joint)
Grade V: High velocity thrust at limit of range (See chapter)

Grades of Sustained Mobilizations:

Tx. I: Small amplitude movement with no appreciable movement
Tx. II: Sustained movement within ROM to the restriction (i.e., the first barrier of resistance)
Tx. III: Sustained movement at end of range through the restriction

HOW TO

Three to four mobilizations of a joint lasting approximately 30 seconds each. If the joint is painful, decrease the time and number of repetitions.

Mobilization Techniques The following procedures comprise a collection of methods described by various referenced authors. In many cases, the lead author has modified them.

The following icons will be used to organize the procedures:

Ⓟ Patient position
Clinician position
ⓘ Clinician contacts
Key to unlocking this joint

Sacroiliac Mobilization

Procedure: **Passive**
Method: **Direct**
Facilitation/inhibition: **No**

The sacroiliac (SI) joint, because of its size, morphology, and unique function (see Chapters 2, 5, and 8) can be effectively mobilized by separating the mobilizations into an upper and lower joint technique. These approaches are adapted from Lewit.

HOW TO

A. Upper SI mobilization[8]

Ⓟ Patient position

The patient is placed in a side-lying, hook-lying position, ensuring that he or she is well balanced (i.e., neither swaying forward or backward) in order to avoid activation of pelvic stabilizing muscles. For patients with a broad pelvis and narrow legs, a pillow placed between the knees will reduce unwanted regional tension caused by hip adduction.

Clinician position

The clinician sits on the table in the space provided by the patient's side-lying, crook-lying (hip-flexed at 45 degrees and knee-flexed at 90 degrees) legs. The clinician is facing toward the patient's head.

Clinician hand contacts

One of the clinician's hands contacts the patient's lateral and *superior* aspect of sacral base, just medial to the posterior superior iliac spine (PSIS) and the SI joint. There are two recommended contacts here. Lewit recommends the dorsum of the second and third proximal phalanges, while the pad of the thumb traverses the target SI to contact the PSIS. This allows for improved differentiation of SI motion during mobilization. A second option is to make the sacral contact with the hypothenar pad (see Fig. 23–11).

The other hand contacts the patient's ipsilateral anterior superior iliac spine (ASIS). This should be a soft palmar contact, as a hard contact on the bony ASIS is uncomfortable and will cause the patient to become protective and tense.

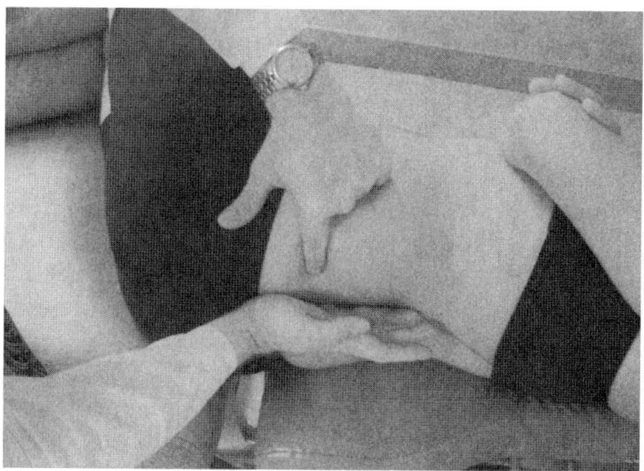

FIGURE 23–11. The contact for the side-lying superior SI joint mobilization is critical. Note that the hypothenar contact is medial to the SI joint. The thumb contacts PSIS to aid the reader in clarifying anatomical landmarks, spanning the joint to more effectively determine joint motion.

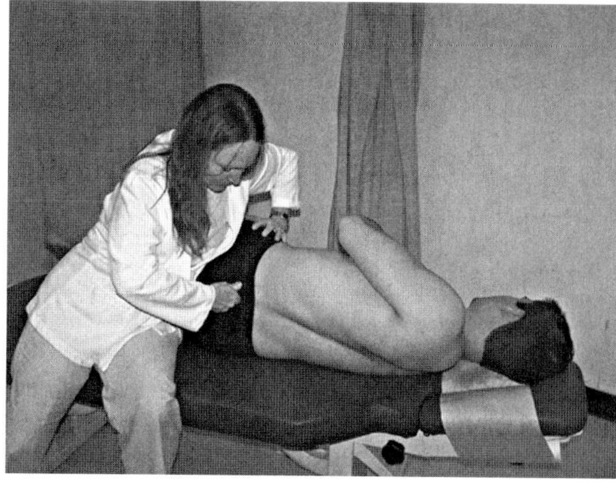

FIGURE 23–12. The side-lying upper SI joint mobilization maneuver.

The clinician then lowers his or her arms so that the forearms are horizontally opposing each other.

Key to unlocking this joint

The clinician then lightly compresses the hands together in a scissor-like motion, which loads the superior SI joint. Graded mobilization strategies can then be used. As mobility increases, the clinician can then add a "rocking"-type of motion, with added compression of the most superior aspect of the joint during scissoring oscillations. This is designed to mimic nutation and counternutation motion of the superior SI joint (see Fig. 23–12).

B. Lower SI mobilization[8]

Ⓟ Patient position

The patient is placed in a side-lying, hook-lying position, ensuring that he or she is well balanced (i.e., neither swaying forward or backward) in order to avoid activation of pelvic stabilizing muscles. For patients with a broad pelvis and narrow legs, a pillow placed between the knees will reduce unwanted regional tension caused by hip adduction.

Clinician position

The clinician sits on the table in the space provided by the patient's side-lying, crook-lying (hip-flexed at 45 degrees and knee-flexed at 90 degrees) legs. The clinician is facing toward the patient's head.

Clinician hand contacts

One of the clinician's hands contacts the patient's lateral sacrum, just medial to the *inferior* aspect of SI joint. There are two recommended contacts here. The first is to make the contact with the thenar pad. A second option is to make the inferior sacral contact with the hypothenar pad.

The other hand contacts the patient's ipsilateral ASIS. This should be a soft palmar contact, as a hard contact on the bony ASIS is uncomfortable and will cause the patient to become tense.

The clinician then lowers his or her arms so that the forearms are horizontally opposing each other.

Key to unlocking this joint

The clinician then lightly compresses the hands together in a scissor-like motion, which loads the inferior SI joint. Graded mobilization strategies can then be used. As mobility increases, the clinician can then add a "rocking"-type of motion, with added compression of the most inferior aspect of the joint during scissoring oscillations. This is designed to mimic nutation and counter-nutation motion of the inferior SI joint (see Fig. 23–13).

Coccyx. The coccyx presents a unique challenge because of its regional morphology. It is a segmented, osseous peninsula surrounded by soft tissue, embedded within the gluteal crease and in proximity to the anus. Appropriate, efficacious and safe coccygeal mobilization techniques can be of great benefit to suffering patients. It is important to remember that the peri-coccygeal tissue encompasses the posterior pelvic floor myofascial tissues. Assessment of the coccyx was covered in Chapter 13. Janda demonstrated the following technique (F.A.I. course Redendo Beach, California 2001):

Ⓟ Patient position

Prone on the table with a roll placed underneath the pelvis to flex the hips and elevate the coccygeal region.

Clinician position

Standing alongside the table at the level of the patient's mid-thighs, and the clinician's torso faces toward the head of the table.

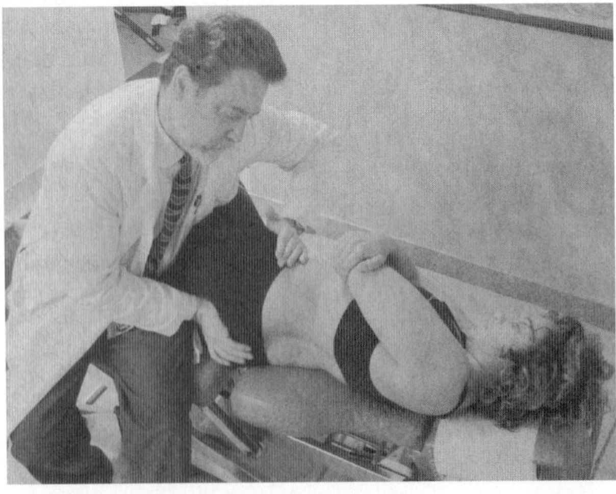

FIGURE 23–13. The lower SI joint mobilization maneuver.

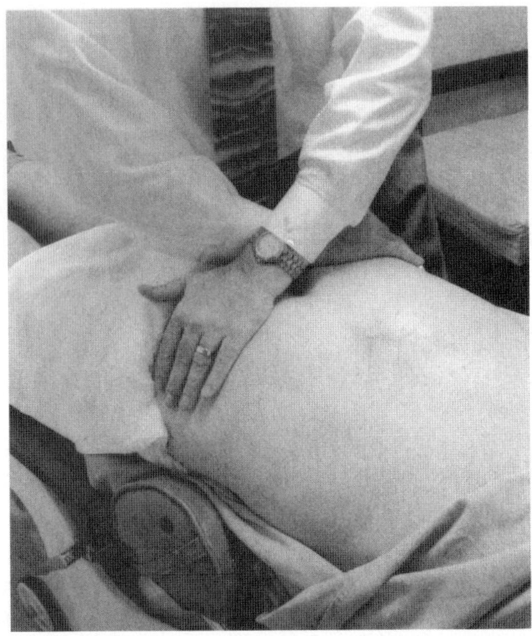

FIGURE 23–14. Coccygeal mobilization technique. The clinician's bilateral palmar contacts immediately lateral to the coccyx, scissored arm position, and lateral versus anterior loading are vital for successful mobilization—so is the patient's ability to activate the pelvic floor musculature.

Ⓘ Clinician contacts

The palms are placed on the buttocks, with the proximal hand positioned along each side of the coccyx. The fingers of each hand are parallel with and in opposition with the other, and the arms are placed in a scissor-like position. Although a broad palmar contact is established, the greatest load is placed on the "heels" of the palms (proximal thenar and hypothenar eminences), just lateral to the coccyx (see Fig. 23–14).

Key to unlocking this joint(s)

The clinician tensions the pericoccygeal tissues by drawing the tissues on each side of the coccyx laterally. The clinician must focus on lowering his or her elbows to provide a greater lateral loading instead of a posterior to anterior load. Increasing the posterior to anterior load tends to stabilize the coccyx, reducing the effectiveness of the mobilization maneuver. Once the peri-coccygeal tissue is taken to the barrier of resistance, this contact is maintained.

Meanwhile, the patient is instructed to draw the pelvic floor *inward* and *upward*. This is often a confusing instruction, so further clarification is necessary. For males, they are instructed to attempt to draw the scrotum up (i.e., inward or superiorly), a maneuver that they can easily understand and usually perform. For females, they can be instructed to perform a Kegel maneuver, a common exercise to improve pelvic floor function. If they are unfamiliar with this maneuver, then they can be instructed to draw the muscles of the pelvic floor up in the same manner that they would suddenly interrupt the urine flow during urination. Female patients typically understand and comply with this explanation. It is important that the patient does not simply contract the buttocks, as the gluteus maximus tends to have less effect on the coccyx than the pelvic floor musculature.

The coccygeal mobilization occurs as the patient contracts and relaxes the pelvic floor while the clinician maintains the bilateral peri-coccygeal contact. Several oscillations are generally required to achieve the mobilization.

Lumbar Spine Rotational Mobilization[8] As described in Chapter 4, lumbar rotation is actually a coupled motion due to anatomical restrictions from the zygapophyseal joints. Nevertheless, the low back practically rotates bilaterally on its axis and segmental restrictions can be improved using a simple rotational strategy.

HOW TO ?

Ⓟ Patient position

The patient is placed in a prone position on the table.

Clinician position

The clinician stands at the side of the table at the level of the patient's waist.

ⓘ Clinician contacts

The clinician reaches across the patient's body and places the caudal hand along the lateral and anterior aspect of the contralateral iliac crest. This is performed in a manner that allows for posterior rotation of the pelvis and lumbar spine as the clinician retracts his or her contact arm and the grasped ilium. The clinician's cephalad hand then makes a thumb pad contact along the lateral aspect of the ipsilateral spinous process of the lowest mobile lumbar segment, typically L5 (Fig. 23–15).

Key to unlocking this joint

The mobilization is performed as the clinician rotates the contralateral pelvis posteriorly while holding a firm contact of the spinous process (i.e., interfering with its rotation along with the pelvis).

Once the joint is mobilized, the clinician can then move to the adjoining superior segment and repeat the procedure if a joint restriction is observed. Of course, with each succeeding level, there will be additional joint play due to the additional joints between the target spinous process and ASIS contact.

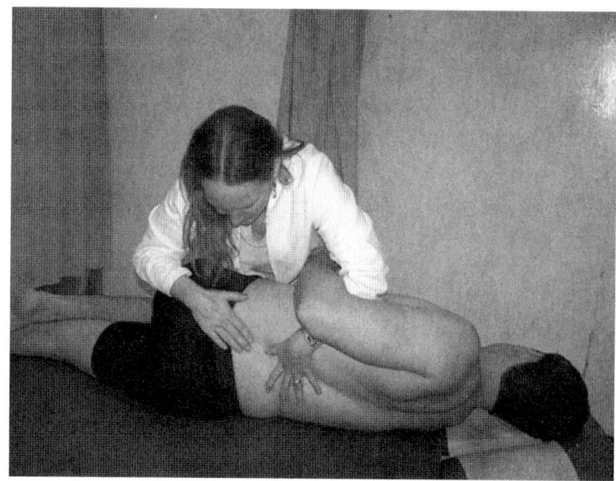

FIGURE 23–15. Lumbar rotational mobilization technique. This technique also targets segmental or short multisegmental spinal muscles such as the multifidi.

Once the lumbar joints are corrected on one side, the clinician then switches sides and repeats the procedures for contralateral joint rotational mobilization.

Lumbar Spine A–P Mobilization[8]

Ⓟ Patient position

The patient is placed in a side-lying, hook-lying position on the table. Both knees are just off the side of the table, while the lower legs remain on the table. The patient's lumbar spine should be in a relaxed neutral or slightly lordotic (i.e., as opposed to a rounded, or kyphotic) position. A high table, preferably one that approximates the clinician's waist level, is preferable.

Clinician position

The clinician stands, facing the table and next to the patient's flexed knees.

ⓘ Clinician contacts

The clinician places the patient's knees into his or her lower abdomen. The clinician then reaches across the table and contacts the patient's lowest mobile lumbar spinous process with the finger pad of the third digit. The other finger pads are placed alongside the third digit, but with a less firm contact. The finger pads of the other hand are placed on top of the fingers of the contact hand for increased digital stability (Fig. 23–16).

Key to unlocking this joint

The clinician then simultaneously moves his or her abdomen forward (i.e., driving the patient's knees, thigh, and pelvis posteriorly) while drawing the

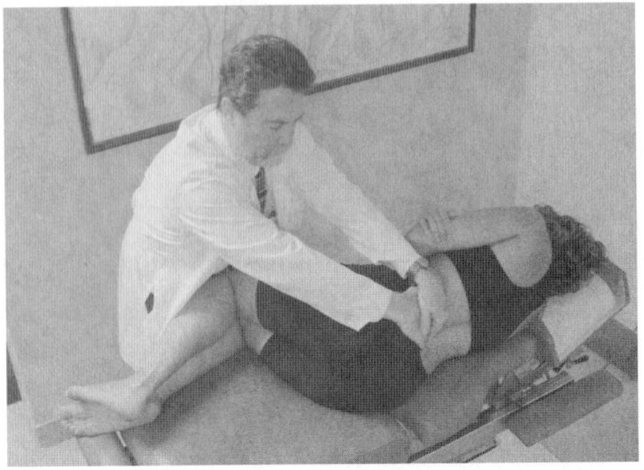

FIGURE 23–16. Lumbar A-P mobilization.

target spinous process closer (i.e., anteriorly) with the contact hands. Mobilization occurs in the anterior–posterior (A–P) plane using graded oscillations.

This maneuver is then repeated at each successive, superior joint.

Lumbar Distraction Mobilization[8] Lumbar distraction, or long axis, mobilization is a very gentle technique that can be extremely effective in reducing low back tightness. It is not a specific technique, but rather a generic maneuver. Another great benefit is that it requires a minimal amount of clinician strength, utilizing instead strategic mechanical advantages to traction the patient's torso inferiorly.

HOW TO

Ⓟ Patient position

The patient is placed in a supine, hook-lying position on the table.

Clinician position

The clinician stands along the side of the table, approximating the level of the patient's pelvis. The clinician then elevates the patient's legs, a partial bilateral SLR maneuver. Then the clinician elevates his or her caudal leg, placing that foot on the table under the patient's thighs. The clinician's thigh should then be horizontal as the foot rests on the table.

ⓘ Clinician contacts

The clinician then lowers the patient's legs, placing them so that the patient's popliteal creases are resting on the clinician's horizontal thigh. The patient's lower legs are then lowered until the legs come to rest on the clinician's horizontal thigh. Some clinicians prefer to cross the patient's lower legs, which is merely a matter of preference. The clinician places one or both hands on the patient's lower leg, at approximately the ankle.

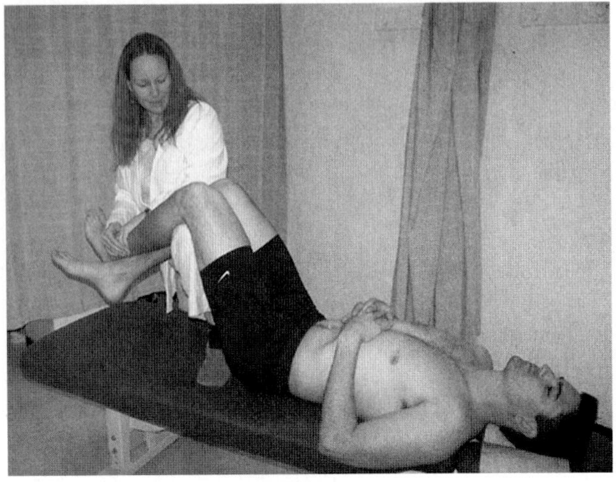

FIGURE 23–17. Lumbar distraction mobilization.

Key to unlocking these joints

With the patient in position, the clinician slightly moves the horizontal thigh caudalward on the table to provide a slight distraction. The clinician then lowers the patient's ankle while maintaining a firm position with the horizontal leg. The downward motion of the lower leg causes an inferior traction of the lumbopelvic region. As the clinician releases the lower leg, the lumbopelvic distraction is reduced. Repetitive oscillations of this maneuver can then be performed (Fig. 23–17).

Pubic Symphysis Mobilization[31] The symphesis is not easily mobilized in a direct manner because of

1. Difficulty in gaining the mechanical advantage for a strong joint,
2. A small and sensitive contact area,
3. Complication of the proximity of the genitalia.

Therefore, an indirect mobilization method can be quite practical. The recommended technique is a type of muscle energy procedure adapted from Greenman, who considers this a "shotgun technique" because of its nonspecific corrective strategy. This approach is divided into two parts, an abduction strategy (A) and an adduction strategy (B).

HOW TO

A. Pubic Symphysis Hip Abduction Technique

Ⓟ Patient position

The patient is placed on the table, next to the edge, in a supine, hook-lying position (i.e., with the hips flexed at 45 degrees° and knees at 90 degrees). The knees and feet should be together, with the feet resting on the table.

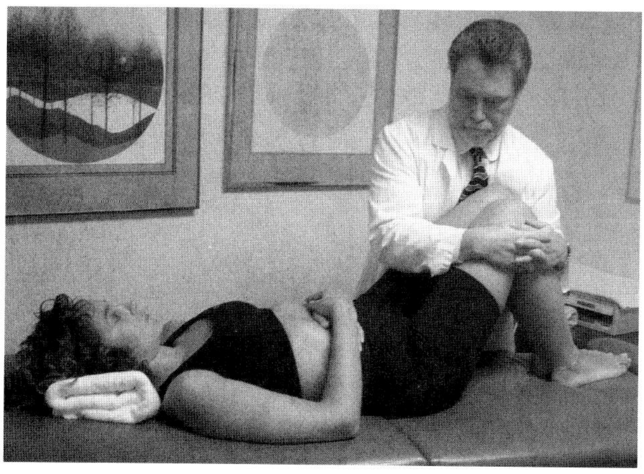

FIGURE 23–18. Pubic symphysis hip abduction technique.

Clinician position

The clinician stands along this side of the table (on either side of the patient), facing the table, at the level of the patient's knees.

Clinician contacts

The clinician firmly grasps the patient's flexed knees, drawing them against his or her torso (Fig. 23–18).

Key to unlocking this joint

The patient is instructed to externally rotate the thighs, attempting to draw the knees apart for 3–5 seconds. The clinician should have a clear mechanical advantage, so no patient leg motion should occur. This isometric activity should be repeated three times.

B. Pubic Symphysis Hip Adduction Technique

Patient position

The patient is placed on the table, next to the edge, in a supine, hook-lying position (i.e., with the hips flexed at 45 degrees and knees at 90 degrees). The knees are fully abducted while the feet remain together.

Clinician position

The clinician stands along this side of the table (on either side of the patient), facing the table, at the level of the patient's knees.

Clinician contacts

The clinician reaches across the table to grasp the patient's contralateral knee. The elbow of the same contact arm is then placed medial to the patient's ipsilateral knee. In this manner, the clinician's arm forms a type of wedge to stop hip adduction. The clinician's other hand is placed on the patient's ipsilateral knee for added stability (Fig. 23–19).

Key to unlocking this joint

The patient is instructed to draw the knees together for 3–5 seconds. The clinician should again have a clear mechanical advantage, so no patient leg motion should occur. This isometric activity should be repeated three times.

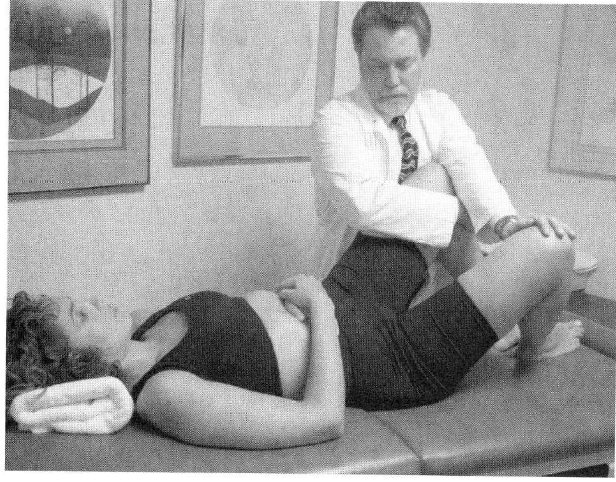

FIGURE 23–19. Pubic symphysis hip adduction technique.

Hip Mobilization[8,31] The hip joint is a clinically deceiving joint because referred pain coming from this joint can extend to the low back, SI joint, groin, thigh, and knee. Mobilization techniques must be carefully planned because of the size of the joint and challenges involved in gaining a mechanical advantage because of the torso and involved limb. The clinician must therefore strategize to use his or her body in a manner that can neutralize these mechanical disadvantages, while utilizing a contact that allows for fine palpation to monitor subtle changes in the hip joint during mobilization.

HOW TO

Patient position

The patient is supine for this procedure, lying close to the same side of the table as the target hip (i.e., left edge of table for left hip joint). The target hip is positioned in the hook-lying position.

Clinician position

The clinician typically kneels alongside the table, next to the target hip and facing toward the head of the table.

Clinician contacts

The clinician then elevates the target leg and places it to rest on his or her shoulder. The clinician then places both hands around the proximal thigh, firmly interlacing the fingers along the anterior aspect to form one functional unit.

Key to unlocking this joint

The clinician then elevates his or her torso slightly, bringing the foot of the target leg off the table and then

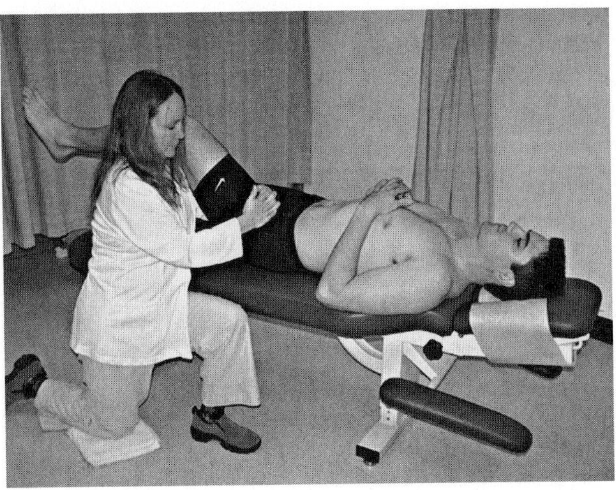

FIGURE 23–20. Hip mobilization technique.

maneuvering the target hip to approximately 90 degrees of flexion. The mobilization strategy entails the coupled movements of the bent leg on the clinician's shoulder and the interlaced hands at the anteromedial thigh. The clinician should then lightly distract the hip joint by moving his or her body away from the target hip (Fig. 23–20).

With the hip in this relaxed, distracted position, the clinician can then mobilize the joint in an A–P direction, a medial to lateral motion, in circumduction, in varying degrees of hip abduction or adduction, or any combination of these.

HOW OFTEN

1. Can be performed daily if there is no joint soreness. If there is soreness, wait until it has passed.
2. Success should be seen in 4–5 days.
3. Increased symptoms are common, but if pain persists, stop treatment and reevaluate patient.

Contraindications to Mobilization A list of absolute contraindications is provided:

Metastatic or neoplastic disease in the target joint(s)
Cauda equina syndrome
Tri-level lumbar root signs (i.e., motor compromise from L4 to S1)
Inflammatory arthritis in the target joint(s)
Infection of target region
Bone disease in the target joint(s)
Fracture in the region of the target joints
Severe neurological signs such as long tract signs

Self-Mobilization

Procedure: **Semiactive**
Method: **Direct**
Facilitation/inhibition: No

Once a mobilization has been performed, joint self-mobilizations can be performed to help maintain restored motion. Also, a series of self-stretches, using any one or combination of strategies described in this chapter, can be quite helpful. As previously mentioned, self-mobilization and self-stretches frequently involve the same maneuver, with the only difference being the sited target tissue. For example, a hip-flexor stretch is also a hip mobilization technique.

A great deal of empowerment can be achieved when the patient assists in his or her own care, as the locus of control is transferred to the patient. In order to speed recovery, daily repetitions of self-mobilization can be an effective adjunct to in-office treatment. Self-mobilization is gentle and slow, and should be as specific as possible.

HOW TO

Procedure: **Active**
Method: **Direct**
Facilitation/inhibition: No

The patient lies on his or her side with the affected SI joint up. The lower leg is extended. The patient then stabilizes the pelvis by bending the upper leg and placing the knee against the table. The upper hand is then placed at the PSIS and the patient tries to gap the SI joint by springing pressure in an anterior and inferior direction. Once in position with the correct contact, the patient is instructed to contract his or her biceps in an oscillating manner, which provides a load to the SI in the prior vector (Fig. 23–21).

Lumbopelvic Spine[8]

A. Flexion and Extension

The patient can perform this by getting onto their hands and knees, called the quadruped position, with their spine in a neutral position. They are then trained to sway (i.e., extend their lumbar region as they draw the abdomen closer to the floor) and arch (i.e., flex their lumbar region as they pull their abdomen away from the floor.) their back within their tolerable range. This motion has many names, with the "cat-cow" being quite popular.

Knee-chest stretches are a more aggressive form of flexion self-mobilization. The patient lies supine and grasps the knees with both hands, interlacing the fingers for additional stability. The patient then can attempt to extend the thighs and low back as the hands isometrically held maintain the flexed position for 5–10 seconds. The patient then relaxes the legs and back and subsequently draws the knees closer to the chest. This self-stretch/mobilization is typically repeated two to four times (Fig. 23–22).

Low back self-mobilization in extension can be more aggressively performed with the press-up

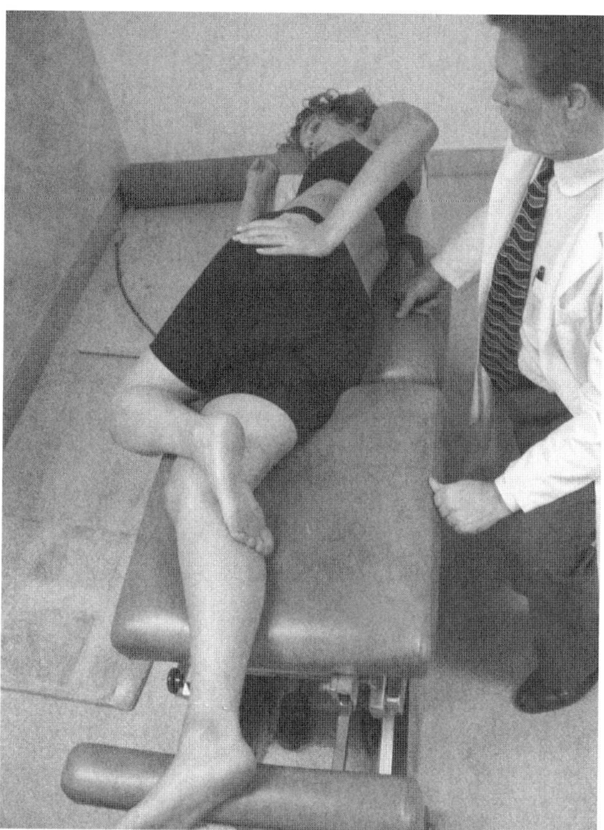

FIGURE 23–21. Self-mobilization for SI joint.

maneuver. The patient is placed in a prone position and performs a modified push-up by elevating the shoulders while the pelvis remains on the floor or table. The musculature of the abdomen and lumbopelvic region must remain relaxed for this procedure to allow for end-range low back extension (Fig. 23–23).

If carried out in a standing position, the patient can place their hands on the segment(s) that need

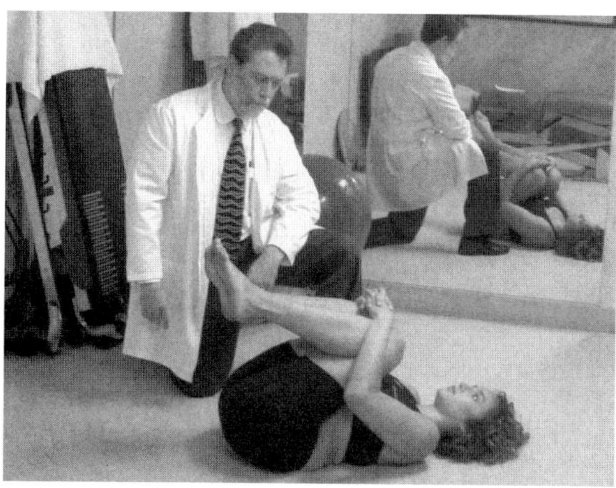

FIGURE 23–22. Self-mobilization technique for the lumbar flexion and lengthening of the erector spinae.

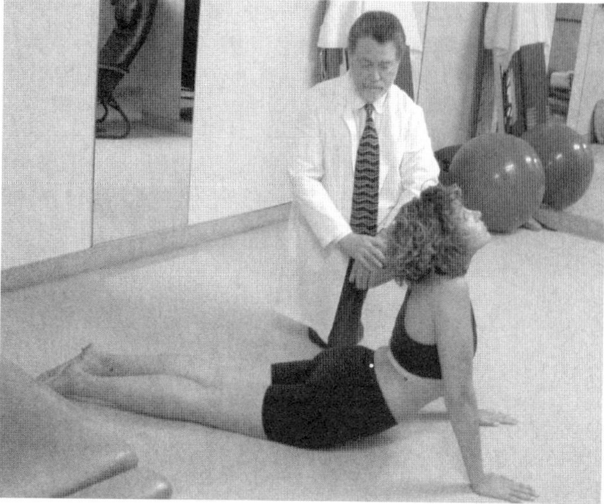

FIGURE 23–23. Self-mobilization techniques for lumbar extension and lengthening of the rectus abdominis.

motion, and bend forward or backward from that fulcrum. Because of additional spinal loading associated with this maneuver, standing end-range extension and flexion self-mobilization should be reserved for end-stage activities once increased lumbopelvic mobility is demonstrated.

B. Rotation

The patient lies on a table on his or her side (e.g., left) with the target side (right) up. The bottom leg (left) is extended at the hip and knee. Depending on the lumbar level to be mobilized, the upper (right) leg, flexed at the knee, is brought into hip flexion (i.e., less hip flexion for lower lumbar segments, and more for higher segments). In this position, the patient's flexed right hip and knee are several inches above the table. The patient uses the bottom (left) arm to grasp and pull the bent (right) knee, gently rolling the leg and hip over (down toward the table) and rotating the pelvis and low back.

C. Lateral Flexion

This self-mobilization can be performed in the standing position. The thumbs are used to wedge against the spinous process and the patient then attempts to bend over that point.

D. Hip Extension

This can be performed in a kneeling position, with the target musculature being the iliopsoas. The patient kneels on the target knee, with the opposite leg placed in front, with the foot flat on the floor for added stability. The lumbopelvic region is placed in a neutral position and the abdominal muscles isometrically contracted. The patient then shifts forward by contracting the ipsilateral gluteus maximus, causing extension of the ipsilateral iliopsoas. It is important for the patient to remain upright, as a forward lean will reduce the degree of hip extension and compromise the effectiveness of the stretch. In some cases, a taut ipsilateral rectus femoris may become taught before the iliopsoas due to the flexed knee, necessitating that the rectus be lengthened first. If the patient experiences knee pain from this kneeling position, a pillow may be placed under the knee or the lengthening can be performed on a bed to dampen the load.

E. Hip Abduction

Another strategy for self-mobilization utilizes the lever effect of the lower extremity and the gravity. This strategy is termed *gravity-induced postisometric relaxation* by Lewit.[8] The patient is placed in a side-lying position near the bottom of the table with the target hip up and the target leg extended and hanging off the bottom of the table. The patient is stabilized by holding on to both sides of the table and also by bearing weight on the hip- and knee-flexed lower (i.e., nontarget) extremity. The weight of the extended target leg will cause it to be lowered until the abductors of the hip come to tension. The patient can then slightly contract the abductor for several seconds before again relaxing it and allowing the load from gravity to lengthen the target abductor and, ergo, lower the leg.

F. Hip Adduction

Hip adductor stretches should be divided into those that span one or two joints.

Single-joint hip adductors: These can be performed in an upright position with the knee of the target leg flexed in order to isolate the single-joint hip adductors. The patient can kneel on both knees with the legs apart. The patient then laterally shafts the pelvis to the contralateral side of the target leg in order to lengthen the target hip adductors.

If the patient has difficulty kneeling because of knee pain, he or she may try performing this maneuver on a soft surface such as a bed to see if that is tolerable.

Two-joint hip adductors: These can be performed upright in a standing position with the legs extended to ensure that the two-joint hip adductors are lengthened. The patient stands with the feet wide apart and shifts the pelvis to the contralateral side, opposite of the target.

G. Hip External Rotation

This can be performed while lying supine. The patient flexes the target leg at the hip and knee and rotates the lower leg medially to rest the ankle region on the contralateral thigh. With this "figure 4" position established, the patient then flexes the contralateral hip, pulling that limb and the flexed, rotated target limb closer to the chest. The hands can be placed, with fingers interlaced, around the thigh of the contralateral thigh to more effectively draw the limbs closer to the torso (Fig. 23–24).

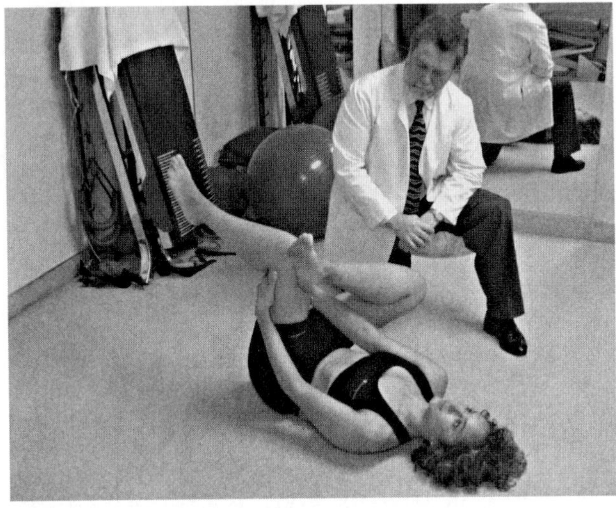

FIGURE 23–24. Self-mobilization technique for external hip rotators.

HOW OFTEN

The patient can self-mobilize multiple times daily if it does not increase the pain.

Strain/Counterstrain (S/CS)

Strain/counterstrain is a system developed by Jones to correct joint dysfunction of acute or chronic traumatic origin.[32,33]

Its goal is to reestablish proper joint proprioception by utilizing the technique strain/counterstrain, which utilizes "EASE" of a tender point within a muscle as a guide to the success of the treatment.

HOW TO

1. Contact the tenderest point with as much pressure as one would place on a closed eye.
2. Move the body part into the position that decreases the tenderness under the contact finger by 70% (EASE). The position is usually the position in which the injury happened.
3. Hold for at least 90 seconds.
4. Initial 5–10 seconds: A reset of the CNS theoretically occurs.
5. Next 30–45 seconds: The theoretical vascular phase occurs. One might feel a pulse, a change in tissue texture, or a warming sensation. These are all believed to be associated with vascular/fascial release mechanisms.
6. Last 30–45 seconds: The theoretical lymphatic phase occurs. Tissue palpation changes from boggy and swollen to nearly normal.
7. Perform the same procedure on the other side (tender points are generally bilateral).

⌛ HOW OFTEN

1. No more than five tender points should be treated at a single session.
2. Treatment can be every other day unless the patient is too sore from the prior treatment.

Confounding Factors

One must also remember that other health factors can create a resistance to stretch, which can alter soft tissue tensions/tones. Briefly, confounding issues can include endocrine, immune, gastrointestinal, genitourinary, neurological, and psychological disorders, as well as nutritional deficiency, use of medication, and chemical abuse.

Management Strategies

A word of caution is necessary with regard to mobilization strategies. It is important to remember that increased mobility places greater demands on the locomotor system to maintain functional stability. In cases of suddenly increasing mobility by, for example, 50% prior to mobilization, it is wise to consider whether the patient is sufficiently functionally and symptomatically stable to accommodate the additional burden and sustain sufficient motor control. For example, a patient presenting with acute mechanical lumbosacral region pain, demonstrating an anterior pelvic tilt and tight hamstrings, may be a poor choice for hamstring lengthening techniques. This is because the hamstrings may be acting to stabilize the lumbopelvic region, preventing a greater anterior pelvic tilt. Ergo, lengthening them may increase the anterior tilt, destabilizing the region and provoking the condition. Therefore, the clinician who utilizes mobilization methods must either

1. Proceed slowly, gradually increasing motion to ensure that the patient is sufficiently functionally stable to accommodate the increased mobility, or
2. Be prepared to make a trade-off by replacing the restrictive tissue with improved functional stability. For example, a sensorimotor training program, designed to effectively improve joint stability via improved co-contraction, could be instituted directly after mobilizing techniques. Sensorimotor training techniques are described in Chapters 26 and 27.

The importance of the understanding of this concept cannot be overstated, for it differentiates the clinician from the technician. The clinician understands, incorporates, and integrates the multifaceted physiological aspects of the condition and ensuing treatment. The technician merely observes a problem and tries to resolve it without the understanding of the causation or potential sequelae associated with this strategy. The clinician who repeatedly lengthens the same shortened tissue or restricted joint without investigating the etiology of the recurrences is, after all, acting as a technician.

Monitoring Progress

After the initial few visits utilizing mobilization and myofascial balancing methods, a number of questions should be answered to determine the degree of benefit for this therapeutic approach.

1. Did those involved (i.e., the patient and the clinician) note a difference during or following treatment?
2. Is this the only therapy required for the patient's condition, or should other in-office or home activities be included?
3. Did the methods performed set up a chain reaction of improved function, such as better posture or gait, or increased motion or exercise capacity?
4. Did the therapy restore joint or soft tissue function to allow other rehabilitation strategies to then be effectively performed?
5. Did the benefits from therapy last until the next visit?
   (a) If not, the clinician should probably look elsewhere for a dysfunctional chain or other cause of recurrence. Or, the patient's activities (i.e., poor postural, sleeping, or working habits) may be undermining case progress.
   (b) If so, these methods can be discontinued in order to focus on other techniques and exercises designed to restore global functional restoration and promote patient independence.
6. Finally, are the mobilization methods and other treatment strategies, such as patient education, creating an environment for the patient to overcome barriers to recovery and become increasingly independent for self-care?

Once these questions have been answered, one can proceed accordingly, always remembering that the soft tissue or joint lesion may be only one piece in a very complex puzzle.

SUMMARY

1. This chapter provided a brief overview of mobilization and myofascial balancing techniques for low back syndromes. These techniques can be utilized individually, together with other manual techniques, and in combination with exercise,

psychotherapy counseling, and host of other therapeutic measures.

2. The techniques described in this chapter vary between authors, and indeed between patients treated by those authors, depending on the response of the patients. For example, if the target tissue or joint responds quickly to a given technique, the clinician can then proceed without completing the prescribed time or repetitions.
3. With time and experience, the delineated distinction between techniques, which is considered necessary for the learning process, becomes less distinct as the clinician integrates various combinations to dynamically respond to each specific situation.
4. Excellence in the field of mobilization allows the clinician not only to determine appropriate methods, locations, and tissues to be targeted, but also to ascertain the nature and degree of change that occur during and following treatment.
5. Proficiency in these methods does not advance rapidly, although the authors recommend that clinicians and students interested in this field aspire to master each of the skills outlined here.
6. It should be noted that a great deal of emphasis was placed upon self-mobilization techniques, those performed by the patient without clinician assistance. This is by design, as every opportunity to teach the patient self-reliance instead of clinician reliance must be taken. Once the merit of the mobilization or myofascial lengthening technique is established, and it is determined that repetitions of these methods are necessary, the patient can and must be taught to perform them well and independently, away from the clinic.
7. It must be assumed that training to perform these techniques optimally will require more than one visit, so the clinician must review and correct the techniques at subsequent visits until they are either perfected or no longer necessary because of patient improvement. In this way, mobilization and myofascial lengthening techniques are not a clinical endpoint, but rather a stepping-stone on the way to independent patient functional restoration.
8. Once the target tissues have been mobilized, a functional stabilization strategy may become necessary for chronic conditions. These topics will be discussed in Chapters 26 and 27 of this textbook.

REFERENCES

1. Janda V. Muscles as a pathogenic factor in back pain. In: *Proceedings of the International Federation of Orthopedic Manual Therapists*, New Zealand, 1980.
2. Bullock-Saxton JE, Janda V, Bullock MI. The influence of ankle sprain injury on muscle activation during hip extension. *Int J Sports Med* August 1994;15(6):330–334.
3. Garsden LR, Bullock-Saxton JE. Joint reposition sense in subjects with unilateral osteoarthritis of the knee. *Clin Rehabil* April 1999;13(2):148–155.
4. Tyler T, Zook L, Brittis D, Gleim G. A new pelvic tilt detection device: Roentgenographic validation and application to assessment of hip motion in professional ice hockey players. *J Orthop Sports Phys Ther* November 1996;24(5):303–308.
5. Sherrington CS. *The integrative action of the nervous system*. London: Archibald Constable & Co., Ltd., 1906.
6. Janda V. Differential diagnosis of muscle tone in respect of inhibitory techniques. In: Paterson JK, Burn L, eds. *Back pain, an international review*. Dordrecht, The Netherlands: Kluwer Academic Press, 1990:196–199.
7. Moore JC. The Golgi tendon organ: A review and update. *Am J Occup Ther* April 1984;38(4):227–236.
8. Lewit K. *Manipulative therapy in rehabilitation of the motor system*, 3rd ed. Oxford, England: Butterworth-Heinemann, 1999.
9. Chaitow L. *Palpation and assessment skills*. Edinburgh: Churchill Livingstone, 2003.
10. Barnes JF. Myofascial release: The search for excellence, a comprehensive evaluatory and treatment approach.Paoli, PA: Rehab Services, Inc. and Myofascial Release Seminar, 1990.
11. Hammer W. *Functional soft tissue examination and treatment by manual methods*. Gaithersburg, MD: Aspen Publication, 1999:535–540.
12. Bogduk N. *Clinical anatomy of the lumbar spine and sacrum*. Edinburgh: Churchill Livingstone, 1997:114–120.
13. Vleeming A, Pool-Goudzwaard AL, Stoeckart R, van Wingerden JP, Snijders CJ. The posterior layer of the thoracolumbar fascia. Its function in load transfer from spine to legs. *Spine* April 1, 1995;20(7):753–758.
14. Vleeming A, Pool-Goudzwaard AL, Hammoduglhlu D, Stoekart R, Snijders CJ, Mens JM. The function of the long sacroiliac ligament: Its implication for understanding low back pain. *Spine* March 1, 1996;21(5):556–562.
15. Barker P, Briggs C, Bogeski G. Tensile transmission across the lumbar fasciae in unembalmed cadavers: Effects of tension to various muscular attachments. *Spine* January 15, 2004;29(2):129–138.
16. Mitchell F. Motion discordance. In: *Yearbook of the Academy of Applied Osteopathy*, Carmel, CA, 1967:1–5.
17. Korr I. Spinal cord as organizer of the disease process. J Amer Osteo Assoc 1976;76:35–45.
18. Janda V. *FAI Manual Medicine Workshop*, Redondo Beach, CA, 2002.
19. Lewit K. Postisometeric relaxation. *Cas Lek Cesk* 1980; 119(15/16):450–455.
20. Lewit K, Simons DG. Myofascial pain: Relief by post-isometric relaxation. *Arch Phys Med Rehabil* August 1984;65(8):452–456.
21. Dutton M. *Manual therapy of the spine: An integrated approach*. New York: McGraw Hill, 2002 p. 254.

22. Chaitow L. *Soft tissue manipulation: A practitioner's guide to the diagnosis and treatment of soft tissue dysfunction and reflex activity*. Thorsens: Rochester, Vermont, 1987: 209.
23. Schneider M, Cohen J, Laws S. *The collected writings of Nimmo and Vannerson: Pioneers of chiropractic trigger point therapy*. Pittsburgh, PA: Schneider, 2001.
24. Simons D, Travell J, Simons L. *Myofascial pain and dysfunction: The trigger point manual*, Vol. 1, 2nd ed. Baltimore: Williams & Wilkins, 1999.
25. Travell J, Simons D. *Myofascial pain and dysfunction: The lower extremities*, Vol. 2. Baltimore: Williams & Wilkins, 1992.
26. Oschman JL. *Energy medicine, the scientific basis*. New York: Churchill Livingstone/Harcourt Publishers, 2000:52–55.
27. Butler DS. *Mobilisation of the nervous system*. Melbourne: Churchill Livingstone, 1991.
28. Breig A. *Adverse mechanical tension in the central nervous system*. Stockholm: Amquist & Wiskell, 1978.
29. Smith S, Massie J, Chesnut R, Garfin S. Straight leg raising. Anatomical effects on the spinal nerve root with and without fusion. *Spine* June 15, 1993;18(8):992–999.
30. Maitland GD. *Vertebral manipulation*, 5th ed. Oxford: Butterworth-Heinemann, 1998.
31. Greenman P. *Principles of manual medicine*. Baltimore: Williams & Wilkins, 1996.
32. Jones LH. *Strain and counterstrain*. Colorado Springs, CO: Academy of Applied Osteopathy, 1981.
33. Chaitow L, Bradley D, Gilbert C. *Multidisciplinary approaches to breathing pattern disorders*. Edinburgh: Churchill Livingstone, 2002.

CHAPTER

24

MINIMALLY INVASIVE PROCEDURES FOR THE TREATMENT OF LOW BACK SYNDROMES

Srdjan S. Nedeljković

OUTLINE

OBJECTIVES

1. To gain an understanding of the common minimally invasive procedures used for the treatment of low back pain.
2. To learn about the indications and outcomes for these procedures.
3. To gain knowledge on the confounding factors that make it difficult to study the efficacy and outcomes of neural blockade procedures.

INTRODUCTION

Earlier chapters of this textbook have addressed the etiology and assessment of low back syndromes. More recent chapters have discussed some therapeutic approaches to this challenging and broad set of conditions. Chapter 17 provides a brief overview of the minimally invasive diagnostic approaches important in evaluating low back syndromes. This chapter will now integrate the minimally invasive, therapeutic aspects of nonsurgical management for these conditions.

In order to have success in the management of spinal pain syndromes, a reliable differential diagnosis is a first requirement. However, it is important to realize that because of the multisegmental innervation of the spine, making a specific diagnosis for what is causing pain is often a very difficult task. Using neural blockade procedures to treat back pain may not be successful for a number of reasons: (1) The incorrect nerve is blocked, (2) the neural input to the painful structure is incompletely blocked, or (3) the nerve block procedure itself is inadequate to correct the cause of pain.

There are numerous complicating factors that can influence the success or failure of a neural blockade procedure for pain management. There is evidence that the sympathetic nervous system may play a role in pain symptoms, such that blockade of a peripheral nerve alone fails to reduce pain. Indeed, anatomical and histopathological studies confirm that the sympathetic nervous system plays a role in spinal pain, as studies have shown that sprouting of sympathetic fibers in the dorsal root ganglion occurs after peripheral nerve lesions. Also, blocking any type of nerve pathway may be nonspecific. For example, sympathetic blocks themselves are nonspecific since they also block sensory pathways, and dorsal compartment blocks are nonspecific since there is spill over to the sympathetic pathways. Ventral compartment blocks, such as blockade of the sinuvertebral nerve, also overflow to the communicating rami as well as the spinal nerves. Finally, there are few good studies that validate the usefulness of nerve blocks in the treatment of low back pain. The only possible exception is for epidural steroid injections, which mainly have a short-term benefit, and facet injections, for which good evidence exists of their efficacy for neck pain, but there are no good studies looking at results for low back pain.

Despite the lack of scientific evidence to support their use, there are a variety of management options for patients who suffer from one or more of the common conditions causing low back pain. For some painful conditions, evidence exists to support the use of a particular procedure, whereas for other conditions the data is incomplete, although it is often a clinician's judgement that patients will benefit. Finally, there are certain patients who as a group can be predicted to have a poor outcome from any interventional procedures used for pain control. This chapter will provide an overview of the various neural blockade procedures that are commonly used for the treatment of low back pain, with attention given to outcomes and results of these procedures.

Many types of minimally invasive interventions have been used for chronic or acute low back pain.

TABLE 24–1. The Efficacy of Various Procedures to Typical Low Back Syndromes

Painful Condition	ESI	Facet	SCS	MPT
Discogenic disease	++			+++
Herniated nucleus pulposus	+++			++
Spinal stenosis	+++	+	+	++
Foramenal stenosis	+	++	+	+
Facet arthropathy	++	+++		+++
Myofascial pain				+++
"Failed back" pain			++	+

Note: ESI = epidural steroid injection; Facet = facet injection; SCS = spinal cord stimulation; MPT = manual and physiological therapeutics. Each (+) represents efficacy of treatment.

These include epidurolysis of epdirual adhesions (either with hypertonic saline or hyaluronidase), epidural phenol injections, long-term catheterization with infusions of epidural local anesthetics, sympathetic blocks or radiofrequency of sympathetic nerves, intradiscal injections, etc. However, among the most common neural blockade procedures are steroid injections into the epidural space (which can be done either translaminar or transforamenally), facet injections, and spinal cord stimulation. As shown in Table 24–1, manual and physiological therapeutics, with or without transcutaneous nerve stimulation, are useful for most patients with low back syndromes, and an aerobic muscle-strengthening program should be instituted promptly in almost all patients.

COMMON PROCEDURES FOR THE TREATMENT OF LOW BACK PAIN

Spinal Injection Therapies

Epidural Steroid Injections Lumbar epidural steroid injection (ESI) is the most widely used invasive, nonoperative treatment for low back pain and sciatica. The use of ESI was first reported in 1952,[1] with the first English language report in 1961.[2] ESI are used on the presumption that lumbosacral radiculopathy involves a significant inflammatory component of the nerve root, which may be evoked by chemical or mechanical irritation.[3] By delivering a full dose of steroid directly to the site of neural or perineural inflammation, nerve root irritation can be lessened. Steroids decrease inflammation by inducing the biosynthesis of phospholipase A_2 inhibitor.[4–6] Phospholipase A_2 liberates fatty acid substrates required for prostaglandin synthesis, and various prostaglandins (PGE_2 for instance) are thought to cause hyperalgesia. Steroids have also been shown to suppress ectopic discharges from neuromas[7] and suppress ectopic neural discharges from injured nerve fibers.[8]

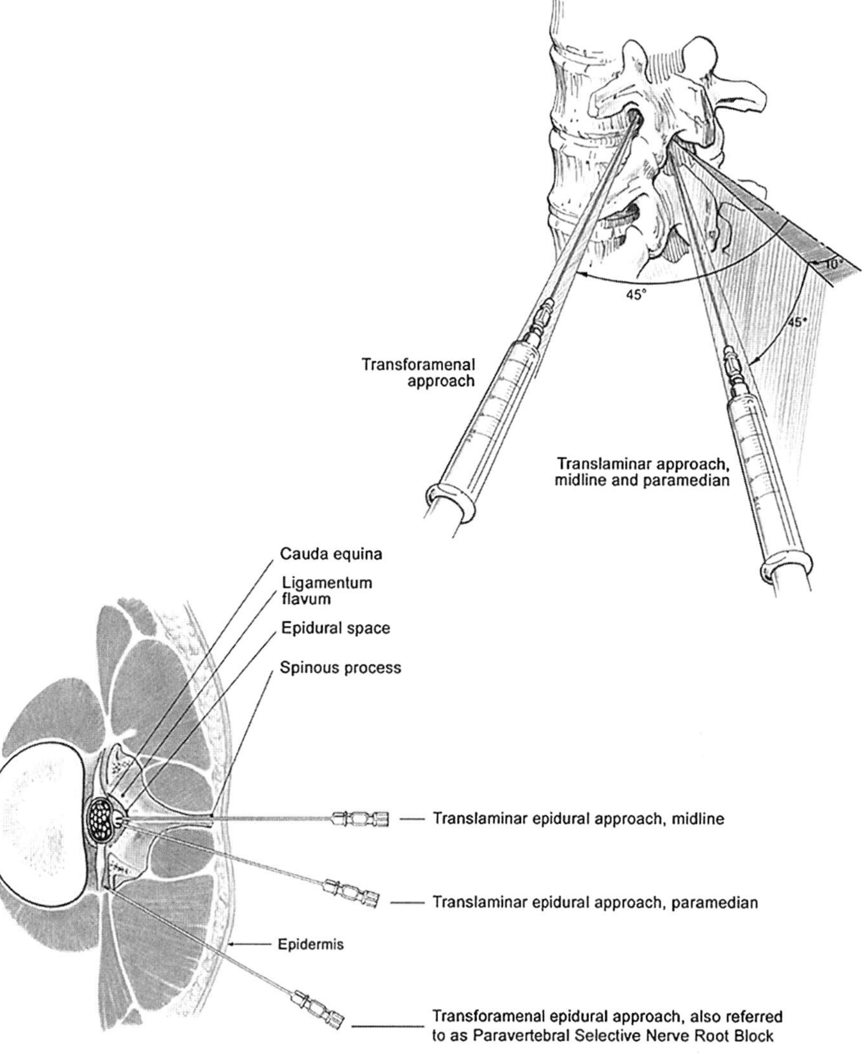

FIGURE 24–1. Methods of epidural steroid injection. Three common approaches to the epidural space are shown. The needle may be inserted either via a midline or paramedian translaminar approach, traversing the area between the spinous processes. In cases where there are significant calcifications of the interspinous ligaments, the needle may be inserted via a transforamenal approach. This technique is also known as a "paravertebral nerve root injection." *(Modified from Katz*[10]*.)*

They may have an anesthetic effect on unmyelinated C fibers.[9]

Clinical Pearl: Lumbar epidural steroid injection (ESI) is the most widely used invasive, nonoperative treatment for low back pain and sciatica.

In most instances, lumbar ESIs can be performed with the patient in the sitting position. This makes it easier to identify the midline in obese patients and the effects of gravity may increase the likelihood of the epidural injectate bathing the sacral segments. An alternative position to sitting is prone position, which is preferred by a number of clinicians. The following surface anatomy is identified: midline spinous processes, iliac crests (line drawn between highest point passes through L4 spinous process), and posterior superior iliac spine (PSIS) (line drawn through PSIS crosses S2 level). After local infiltration, an 17-gauge Tuohy needle is introduced in the desired interspace. Using loss of resistance to saline or air, the epidural space is located. A glass syringe and extension tubing filled with saline are connected to the epidural needle. The extension tubing is held vertically and acts as a manometer, with the column of saline falling into the epidural space and fluctuating with heart beat and breathing, thus providing verification of accurate needle placement. Figures 24–1 and 24–2 demonstrate typical minimally invasive approaches to the epidural space.

Medication is placed into the barrel of the syringe and allowed to infuse by gravity. Preservative-free normal saline is used to flush the tubing at the end of the injection to lessen the chance of fistula formation. Typical medications would include a mix of methylprednisolone (120 mg) with 0.5% lidocaine (3 mL), injected as close as possible to the level of pathology. Although larger volumes of local anesthetic have been used, there is no evidence that large volumes of anesthetic improve efficacy. Usually, three injections are given, 1 month apart, based on patient's response. It is advised to give injections at least 2–3 weeks apart, as it may require that long for the steroid to exert its beneficial effect. Also, more frequent injections can result in accumulation of steroid and increase the likelihood of undesirable steroid side effects. For these reasons, in our practice, we usually ask patients to return after 1 month for their second or third steroid injections. After a series of three injections, it is my clinical experience that there is no further benefit in giving more than three sequential epidural injections, and there is no scientific evidence to support giving a greater number of injections in sequence. However, should a patient respond to a series of epidural injections and then develop pain in the future, this treatment option may again be offered.

Multiple studies have been published over the past 35 years regarding the efficacy of ESI. In most cases, the cause for the patients' symptoms, the criteria used for patient selection, and the follow-up has varied. The general conclusion is that although short-term pain relief due to ESI occurs in many patients, there is a reduction in benefit over time[12]: from 90% to 70% by 6 months[13] and from 68% to 42% by 2 years.[14] Some have questioned whether the efficacy of ESI is an improvement over the natural history of the disease,[15] as patients with acute symptoms are most likely to improve with any modality of treatment (68%–82% of the control group in this study improved without ESI).[16–19] Overall, the efficacy of ESIs has been difficult to establish,[20] although many practitioners believe in their effectiveness. Beliveau showed that giving epidural injections with steroids was more efficacious than giving them without[21] (*see Outcomes of Neural Blockade for Pain Relief* section for further discussion on outcomes of ESIs). Patients with prolonged duration of pain, nonradicular diagnosis, lack of employment, and a history of smoking are less likely to benefit from this treatment.[22]

The best results of treatment with ESIs are seen in patients with a subacute history of back and leg pain. It is recommended to avoid ESI for patients with less than 1 week of pain, as many will start to improve without injection. Better results have been confirmed in patients who have not had back surgery. Patients who have pain as their only symptom of sciatica have a greater chance of improvement when compared to patients who have motor, reflex, or other sensory disturbance. Patients with bony abnormalities usually respond poorly compared to patients with bulging discs and acute radiculopathy, although there is often significant improvement due to ESI in patients with spinal stenosis.[23] As with most treatments for chronic pain, better results are found in patients without psychological overlay and workmen's compensation issues.

Complications from ESI can be divided into two groups: technical and those relating to steroid effects. Although extensive clinical experience confirms the safety of ESI, the loss of resistance technique has been associated with a 2.5%–5% incidence of dural puncture,[24] with the risk being greater laterally where there is a thinner epidural space. The incidence of postdural puncture headache for patients undergoing ESIs (who have inadvertent dural punctures) does not differ from that of the patients who have dural punctures for other reasons.[25] There is a remote possibility of anterior spinal artery ischemia with lateral needle placement in the intervertebral foramen.[26] This may occur from injury of the artery of Adamkiewicz, which enters via the intervertebral foramen most commonly at T11–T12 on the left and which supplies the thoracolumbar anterior spinal artery. Placement of the needle in the intervertebral foramen near the dural cuff may cause paresthesia or radicular pain (1.3%).[12] If the needle is off midline, epidural veins are more likely to be encountered and bleed. A needle inserted into a facet joint, richly innervated with nociceptors, may cause severe pain with paravertebral muscle spasm. Transient exacerbations of pain with injection are thought to be secondary to injecting large volumes of solution quickly into a noncompliant epidural space. Plummer, in a retrospective study of 313 patients, showed that 12% had pain on injection. The pain response varied from dull, ill-localized discomfort, to excruciating unilateral or bilateral radicular pain.[27] This is thought to be due to altered compliance of the epidural space and may be more frequent in patients with spinal stenosis, epidural metastasis, or vertebral collapse. Rare complications resulting from ESI include spinal anesthesia and intraocular hemorrhage, which is thought to be due to increased CSF pressure caused by injections of large volumes.[28,29]

In spite of overwhelming clinical experience that ESIs have no deleterious effect on neural or perineural tissues, this remains an area of controversy, and some groups have cautioned about the use of ESI.[30,31] Methylprednisolone contains 30 mg/mL of polyethylene glycol, which is an alcohol and a nonionic detergent. It was first used intrathecally in 1960[32] as treatment for lumbar radiculopathy for the "failed back" surgery syndrome in 3000 patients, with good results. Boines showed 80%–90% improvement in patients with multiple sclerosis.[33] However, later studies have purported that intrathecal steroids can cause significant neuronal and meningeal damage, leading to an 80%–100% incidence of adhesive arachnoiditis, aseptic meningitis, transient inability to micturate, conus medullaris syndrome (similar to cauda equina syndrome, but with upper motor neuron signs), and other problems.[31,34,35] Polyethylene glycol, in much higher quantities, is a known toxin, resulting in necrosis of connective tissues and muscles, and causing demyelinating lesions in nerves.[36] Although steroids are given epidurally under the assumption that there is no connection between the epidural and subarachnoid spaces, this has been found to be untrue, since arachnoid villi subtend the subarachnoid, subdural, and epidural spaces.[37]

When the literature is reviewed carefully, it becomes evident that a proven causal effect is lacking between ESI and arachnoiditis. Experimental data in animals fails to confirm a relationship between subarachnoid steroid injection and arachnoiditis, and in Abram's review of 64 series of ESI in nearly 7000 patients, there were no reports of arachnoiditis.[38] The few cases of aseptic meningitis were not associated with any permanent morbidity.

Regarding side effects from systemic steroids, plasma cortisol levels can be depressed for at least 2 weeks after ESI.[39] Also, the effects of *depot steroid* may not be fully apparent for about 2 weeks. Because of these two reasons, the author does not usually offer patients more than one epidural steroid injection per month. Other steroid side effects that have been reported include development of Cushing's syndrome, sodium retention, changes in serum glucose levels, and cases of steroid "psychosis."[40,41] These are more likely with higher doses of steroid that are injected in rapid succession. The author completes a trial of ESI after three injections, as there is no proof that more than three injections confer any added benefit. Contraindications for ESI include abnormal coagulation studies and infection.

Selective Spinal Nerve Injections and Caudal Steroid Injections Two variations on the technique of performing an ESI are "selective spinal nerve injections" and "caudal steroid injections." Selective spinal nerve injections, also known as paravertebral root injections or transforamenal ESIs, are given by positioning a needle at the exit of the spinal nerve root in an intervertebral foramen. Positioning a needle within the intervertebral foramen allows for an injection of steroid directly along an inflammed or irritated nerve root. By directly depositing steroid along the nerve root, a more pronounced pain relieving effect may be possible. Fluoroscopic guidance is necessary to achieve a successful selective nerve injection, and contrast dye is usually used to ensure that the injectate flows along the intended nerve. A typical dose of steroid given for a selective spinal nerve injection ranges from 40 to 80 mg of methylprednisolone. This technique is useful for patients who have had spinal surgery and who have scarring, fusion material, or disruptions of their epidural space that make a translaminar ESI unfeasible.

Clinical Pearl: Positioning a needle within the intervertebral foramen allows for an injection of steroid directly along an inflammed or irritated nerve root. By directly depositing steroid along the nerve root, a more pronounced pain relieving effect may be possible.

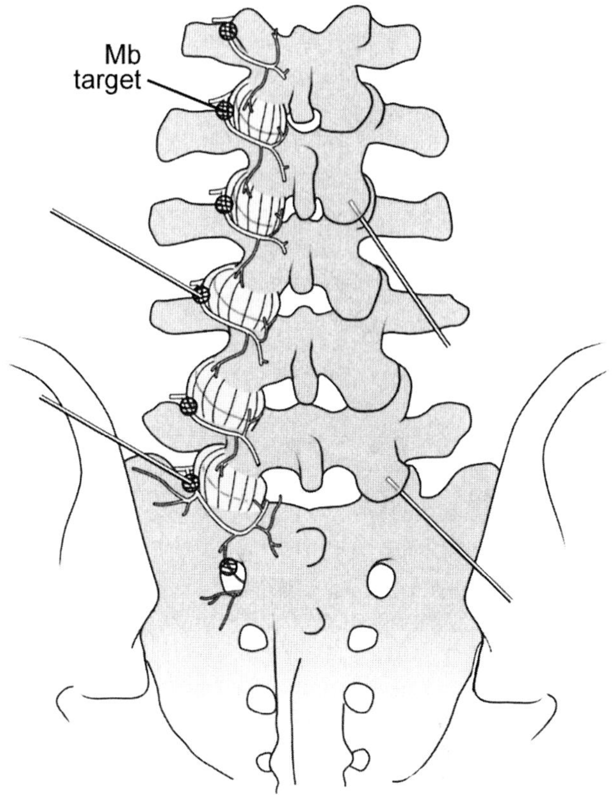

FIGURE 24–2. Lumbar zygapophyseal joint blocks: medial branch and intra-articular (facet injections and radiofrequency lesioning). The needle placements for medial branch (left) and intra-articular (right) injections of the lumbar spine are shown. The joint capsule has been removed on the right to show an intra-articular injection. The targets for medial branch block are indicated on the left (hatched circles). *(Adapted from Manning and Rowlingson.*[42]*)*

A caudal steroid injection involves inserting a needle through the sacrococcygeal ligament and into the caudal space. Often, an epidural needle is used, such that an epidural catheter can be advanced within the caudal canal until it reaches the lumbar epidural space. Thereby, an injectate of steroid can be given in the caudal space or wherever the epidural catheter tip is located. The caudal approach is often used for patients who have an inaccessible epidural space via the lumbar approach due to spinal surgery or scarring. Also, an epidural catheter advanced via a caudal approach can be positioned directly along the nerve root presumed to be causing pain. In order to position a catheter inserted via a caudal approach to the site of spinal pathology, fluoroscopic guidance is recommended. The dose of steroid given via a caudal steroid

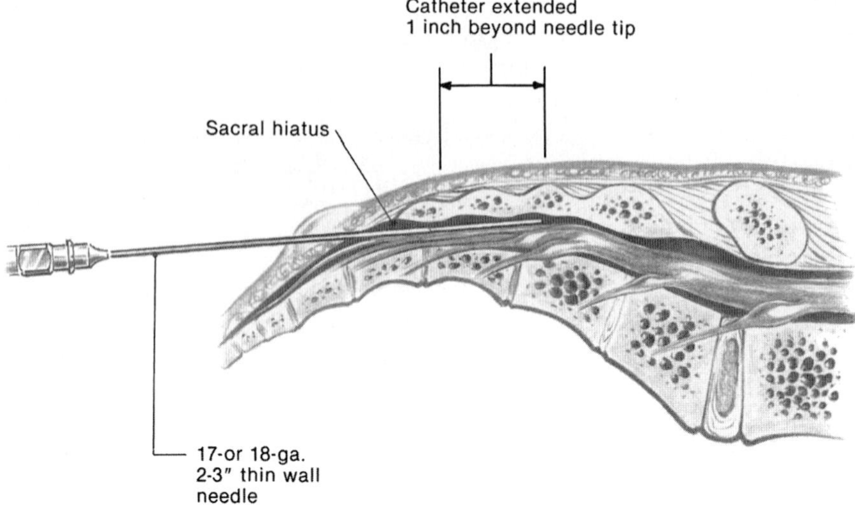

FIGURE 24–3. Caudal steroid injection. Sagittal view of the caudal epidural space showing a needle inserted through the sacrococcygeal ligament. Often, a catheter can be threaded up into the caudal space, directly accessing the lumbar epidural space. This technique may be useful for patients who have had lumbar laminectomy and have had posterior spinal fusion procedures. *(From Katz[11].)*

injection is about the same as that used for a typical ESI, or about 120 mg of methylprednisolone.

Facet Injections and Radiofrequency Lesioning Procedures

As described in greater detail in Chapter 17, the facet (zygapophyseal) joint is richly innervated and can be an important source of low back pain. Whether back pain is caused by facet joint pathology can be confirmed by injecting anesthetic either directly into the joint or to the medial branch of the dorsal ramus that innervates the joint. Figure 24–3 provides an illustration of common approached to the target zygapophyseal joint or medial branch. If a local anesthetic blockade of the facet joint reliably reduces or eliminates pain, then treatment can be accomplished by either steroid injections or by performing radiofrequency lesioning (RFL) procedures. Often, steroids are given as part of the diagnostic facet procedure. As such, steroid injections of the facet joints may provide pain relief for a prolonged time. However, if facet steroid injections fail to provide long-term relief of back pain, the patient may be a candidate for RFL of the facet joints.

Radiofrequency current acts by heating tissues as a result of electrical resistance. This differs from electrocautery, in which the tip of the cautery device is the heated element. Thereby, RFL is more similar to microwave technology. In pain management practice, RFL uses low levels of continuous sinusoidal radiofrequency current, causing a coagulative necrosis of both myelinated nerve fibers and unmyelinated fibers.[43] Particular attention needs to be given to correct application of the dispersive pad, as faulty contact or uneven pressure on the skin can cause severe burns.

The lesion size depends on the strength and duration of electrical current, the electrode tip size, temperature, and the water content of the tissue. To create an adequate lesion, it is necessary to reach temperature equilibrium, which occurs when heat loss and lesion temperature is constant. This depends on current density at the tip of the needle, the fluid loss that results from lesioning, the electrode tip size, and the vascularity of the tissues.[44]

Percutaneous RFL has been used for many conditions in a variety of anatomic locations. The most extensive literature and success rates are for lumbar or cervical zygapophyseal (facet) denervation; therefore, RFL is most commonly utilized for these procedures. Results for low back pain are best for patients who suffer from axial or mechanical back pain and who present without true radiculopathy below the knee. Patients who have symptoms of back pain on extension, tenderness over the zygapophyseal joint, and radiological confirmation of zygapophyseal disruption are good candidates[45,46] (see *Outcomes of Neural Blockade for Pain Relief* section later in this chapter). Patients with previous back surgery, psychological issues, or who are involved in litigation due to work injuries are less likely to respond favorably to this type of therapy.[46] The medial branch of the dorsal ramus innervates the zygapophyseal joint, and this becomes the neural target for RFL. Before proceeding with RFL, it is important to perform a diagnostic medial branch block with local anesthetic, as discussed in Chapter 17. A positive block is one that gives relief with 1–2 mL of local anesthetic, which lasts as long as the duration of effect for that anesthetic.

Several terms have been occasionally used to describe RFL of the facet joints. An appropriate analogous term is radiofrequency neurotomy. The other commonly used description, radiofrequency rhizotomy, is a misnomer. By definition, rhizotomy specifically means disruption of a nerve root, which is not done during RFL of the facet joints. Instead, an RFL facet procedure targets only a branch of the dorsal ramus, which itself arises from the nerve root.

In order to perform an RFL procedure, it requires C-arm fluoroscopy and sterile conditions. Although some advocate the use of sedation, almost all patients can tolerate an RFL procedure well with just local anesthesia. Also, unsedated patients are able to better report their areas of stimulation, making the procedure easier and less risky in terms of potential nerve injury.

First, the dispersive pad is placed on the patient, who is in the prone position and draped in a sterile fashion. The radiofrequency target sites are visualized, being at the union of the transverse apophysis and the superior articular process. A 100 mm or 150 mm, 22-gauge needle is used, and it is important to check that the RFL electrode fits through this needle and the tip is located just at the end of the bare metal tip of the cannula. The needle is Teflon coated, except for its 5-mm active tip.

Next, the integrity of the system is confirmed by checking the impedance, which should be between 400 and 700 Ω, once the needle has been placed. Next, sensory stimulation is performed to replicate the patient's pain and confirm proper placement. Stimulation may be described as a tingling in the local area or a pressure sensation. Stimulation is performed at 50 Hz at currents up to 1 V.

Clinical Pearl: Percutaneous RFL has been done for many conditions in a variety of anatomic locations. The most extensive literature and success rates are for lumbar or cervical zygapophyseal (facet) denervation; therefore, RFL is most commonly utilized for these procedures.

Finally, motor testing is done at 2 Hz with currents up to 4 V.[47] If this causes movement in the lower extremity, the electrode may be too near the anterior motor root and the needle must be repositioned prior to lesioning. Twitching locally in the back is common and acceptable. Lateral fluoroscopy is used to confirm that placement of the needle is not too far anteriorly placed. Once proper needle placement is confirmed, 1 mL of 2% lidocaine is injected to anesthetize the area prior to lesioning. Lesioning is performed at a temperature of 80° C for 90 seconds. This procedure is then repeated on each targeted zygapophyseal joint.

The expected result of RFL is temporary denervation and anesthesia of the target zygapophyseal joint. The success of denervation varies upon the degree of neurotomy achieved and the speed with which the medial branch regenerates. The typical length of time it takes for these nerves to regenerate is from 4 to 6 months. Theoretically, this period would provide a window of opportunity, once the pain generator(s) are neutralized, for a lumbopelvic stabilization program, a return to regular activities, and a disruption of the chronic pain cycle.

Epidural Neuroplasty (Lysis of Adhesions) Hemorrhaging and subsequent scarring can cause epidural adhesions, which occur in the epidural space after laminectomy. Also, leakage of disc material, as found with a herniated nucleus pulposus, can result in fibrocyte deposition and an inflammatory response in the epidural space. A leaking disc releases lactic acid, cytokines, histamine, and other foreign proteins that cause chemical irritation and trigger an autoimmune reaction that can lead to adhesions.[48] Although epidural adhesions themselves are not painful, they can produce radicular symptoms by causing compression and/or tethering of the nerve root, sensitizing it, and leading to swelling and ischemia of the nerve.[49] Direct mechanical pressure from scar tissue can impair blood supply and result in decreased nutrient transport to the nerve roots. Changes in permeability of the endoneural capillaries results in intraneural edema, which leads to intraneural fibrosis.[48] Ultimately, central sensitization and hyperalgia may occur as the chronic radicular syndrome evolves, with adhesions making the nerve root even more sensitive to mechanical stimuli.

The rationale behind epidural neuroplasty, also called epidurolysis of adhesions, is to deliver anti-inflammatory medications (such as steroids and hypertonic saline) to shrink nerve root swelling, and to use hypertonic saline and hyaluronidase to mechanically and chemically break up adhesions. Injecting steroid alone near the area of epidural scarring may be effective in some patients. However, in other cases it can be ineffective since the adhesions themselves prevent the steroid from reaching its intended site, the edematous, constricted nerve root. Epidural neuroplasty is a potential alternative to surgical re-exploration and excision of scar tissue, since more surgery can lead to yet more adhesions and neural compromise.

The diagnosis of epidural adhesions is made best by gadolinium-enhanced MRI, which will allow visualization and highlight scar tissue surrounding the affected nerve root. In some cases, it is difficult to distinguish scar tissue from other pathologies, such as a recurrent herniated disc, but a gadolinium-enhanced MRI test remains the "gold standard" for diagnosing epidural adhesions. In some patients, scar tissue may be asymptomatic, which underlies the importance of correlating MRI findings with the clinical picture. Epidural adhesions can also be seen with *epidurography*. Epidurography is a technique in which the epidural space adjacent to the adhesions is accessed and contrast medium is injected. The contrast takes the path of least resistance, bypassing the adhesions and thereby delineating their location, as seen under fluoroscopy.

Any such injections into the epidural space can cause further spinal compression and should be done incrementally. Patients should be alert to report any new neurological symptoms during the procedure.

Indications for performing epidural neuroplasty include any conditions that lead to epidural adhesion formation. These would include "failed" spinal surgery, disc disruption, vertebral compression fractures, scar formation after meningitis or infection, and may include failure to respond to a trial of spinal cord stimulation or spinal opioids.[50] Most often, patients are deemed not to be surgical candidates. Patients must be advised of the potential side effects. Inadvertent injection of local anesthetics intravascularly or into the intrathecal space can cause hypotension, temporary paralysis, or seizures. Injections of hypertonic saline intrathecally can cause permanent bowel and bladder dysfunction, paralysis, and sexual dysfunction.[48] As with other spinal procedures, there are risks of infection and catheter shearing.

The technique for epidural lysis of adhesions has been developed and improved by Dr. Gabor Racz, from Texas Tech Institute. In his report of experience with over 2500 patients, there have been no serious neurological complications, with only one case of difficulty voiding, which lasted 1–2 weeks, and one case of perineal numbness that lasted 1–2 months.[50] The procedure is done in an operating room environment, with the patients lightly sedated and with IV access. Patients must be able to report weakness or other neurological changes during the procedure. Monitors are placed, including EKG, automated blood pressure cuff, and pulse oximetry. C-arm fluoroscopy and water-soluble contrast are used.

For lower lumbar epidurolysis, the patient is placed prone on the fluoroscopy table with a pillow under the abdomen and the legs abducted to ease access to the caudal canal. The caudal space is entered with a 16-gauge epidural needle, usually 1–2 cm from the opposite side of the midline to allow advancement of the needle toward the affected side. The needle is advanced to the S2 or S3 vertebral body such that the intrathecal space is not entered. Needle placement is confirmed by lateral and AP fluoroscopic images and by negative aspiration for CSF and blood. Then, 10 mL of water soluble contrast is injected to further confirm that the needle is not in the intrathecal or intravascular space. Intrathecal spread will cause dye to spread centrally and cephalad, whereas intravascular spread will be marked by immediate runoff of the contrast. An additional injection of 14 mL of bupivacaine 0.25% with steroid 40 mg can be given incrementally to prove that the injectate is not intrathecal.[50] A rapid development of motor/sensory loss indicates an unintended spinal placement, in which case the procedure is aborted.

If proper needle placement outside of the thecal sac is confirmed, a directable, flexible-tipped catheter is advanced into the adhesions. After negative aspiration, additional contrast is given through the catheter to prove its placement within or nearby to epidural adhesions. Then, hyaluronidase is injected, followed by 0.25% bupivacaine with 40 mg steroid.[51] The catheter is then affixed to the patient's back and the patient is observed for neurological deficits. If there are none, the patient is injected with 10 mL of 10% hypertonic saline, while in the recovery room. On the first postprocedure day, the patient is brought back for a second injection, which also consists of 10 mL 10% hypertonic saline. The series is concluded after the third dose of hypertonic saline, which is given on the second postprocedure day, and then the catheter is removed. These injections are painful, but usually only for about 5 minutes, and therefore, local anesthetic is injected each day prior to the hypertonic saline. The administration of steroid and hypertonic saline is thought to break up epidural adhesions and shrink nerve swelling. Hyaluronidase is thought to dissolve epidural adhesions via its ability to disrupt proteoglycans.[52]

Intravenous antibiotics are given during hospitalization, and oral antibiotics are given for 5 days after discharge. Rehabilitation is aggressively pursued to improve strength and tone, and there is often an improvement in pain and motor function. The technique is modified slightly for cervical, thoracic, and lumbar injections, such that the volume of hypertonic saline given is 4 mL for cervical, 6 mL for thoracic, and 8 mL for lumbar injections.[50]

Clinical Pearl: The rationale behind epidural neuroplasty, also called epidurolysis of adhesions, is to deliver anti-inflammatory medications (such as steroids and hypertonic saline) to shrink nerve root swelling, and to use hypertonic saline and hyaluronidase to mechanically and chemically break up adhesions.

The complications from epidural neuroplasty are primarily related to unintended subarachnoid injection of either the local anesthetic or hypertonic saline. Paralysis and bowel and bladder dysfunction are of greatest concern, as are infection and the general risks of steroid use. Some recommend performing urodynamic studies to document the existence of preexisting subclinical neurogenic bladder, which may be due to an underlying pathological process such as constrictive arachnoiditis.[48] Rapid injections into the epidural space may cause unintended increases in CSF pressure, which can lead to cerebral hemorrhage, visual disturbances, headache, and decreased spinal blood flow.[48] Patients should be advised to be aware of signs and symptoms of infection, such as fever, nausea and vomiting, neck stiffness, increased pain, and neurological changes.

Outcome data for the effectiveness of epidural neuroplasty are sparse. Arthur reported on 100 patients, half who received hyaluronidase in addition to hypertonic saline, in which 81% of the hyaluronidase group compared to 68% of the non-hyaluronidase group had significant pain relief.[53] In about 86%–88% of patients, the relief dissipated by 6 months. There are no studies that apply stringent outcome criteria, such as improvement in physical function or return to work. To the author's knowledge, there are no studies that look at outcomes of epidural neuroplasty in a double-blind, prospective manner, or that compare this technique to either placebo or other techniques.

Subarachnoid and Epidural Neurolysis Neurolytic types of injections are used primarily for cancer pain management, and their use is not advocated for the treatment of nonmalignant painful conditions. Subarachnoid and epidural neurolysis carries the risk of unpredictable spread of injectate, which may cause unwanted motor or sensory neurological deficit. For patients with cancer, the resultant chemical rhizotomy can control refractory localized pain syndromes, especially in the chest wall, limbs, and perineum. In performing subarachnoid blockade, the patient is positioned so that the dorsal columns of the spinal cord are isolated. Hyperbaric phenol sinks to the downward-facing dorsal columns, whereas hypobaric alcohol will rise to upward-facing dorsal columns. Inadvertant spread of injectate may affect anterior motor nerve segments, with resultant motor loss (occurs in 5%–20% of cases) and a loss of bladder and rectal function (occurs in 5%–60% of cases).[54] Motor function usually does improve, at least partially, over time. These procedures are limited to patients with tumor invasion and destruction of nerves or plexii, and for those who already have irreversible neurological deficits, including bowel and bladder dysfunction.

Neurosurgical techniques have been used for pain management, but these are mainly of historical interest. Results are highly variable and mixed, and patients can develop significant complications from such procedures, including exacerbation of pain or creation of a new pain syndrome. These techniques include surgical rhizotomy, cordotomy, hypophysectomy for pituitary ablation, and cingulotomy. Cordotomy involves lesioning the anterolateral spinothalamic tract, resulting in contralateral loss of pain and temperature sensation. This procedure is most often done percutaneously. Up to 90% of patients have immediate results, with 50% pain-free after 1 year,[54] but neurological complications can be devastating. Neurosurgical techniques for pain management are not recommended for nonmalignant pain states.

Spinal Neuromodulation

Spinal Cord Stimulation Spinal cord stimulation (SCS) is a technique of implanting a permanent device for long-term stimulation of the spinal cord in order to treat intractable pain. Since its inception in the late 1960s, this technique has had increasing efficacy as the technology has improved and patient selection criteria have become better known[55] (see *Outcomes of Neural Blockade for Pain Relief* section). SCS is used primarily for the treatment of neuropathic pain. Neuropathic pain is such that might arise from diabetes, peripheral nerve injuries, lumbosacral radiculopathy, postherpetic neuralgia, phantom limb, multiple sclerosis, central poststroke pain, CRPS (complex regional pain syndrome, previously called reflex sympathetic dystrophy), and other such conditions. Most of these conditions can be treated with medications, nerve blocks, and other therapies that may be prescribed in a multidisciplinary pain center, but a portion of patients may continue to experience pain in spite of aggressive medical management. This group of patients may be candidates for SCS.

The mechanism for efficacy of SCS is not known. The original *gate control theory*, as postulated by Melzack and Wall in 1965,[56] purports that electrical stimulation of large afferent nerve fibers inhibits pain transmission in the dorsal horn of the spinal cord. Evaluation of the parameters of SCS and anatomical and electrical properties of the dorsal columns of the spinal cord seems to substantiate this as a primary mechanism of action.[57] Another theory proposes that electrical stimulation cancels neuropathic pain messages in the spinothalamic tract via noradrenergic and seritonergic pathways.[58] Most hypothesis point to a segmental inhibitory process at the dorsal horn, but supraspinal mechanisms are also likely involved.[59]

The possible indications for SCS are many, and there are many studies that attempt to define outcomes of this therapy for various pain states. With regards to low back pain, SCS is effective for neuropathic pain in the limbs and works best when there is minimal axial pain.[60] A common indication in the USA is for a patient with failed back surgery syndrome, who may have pain related to scarring of nerve roots. In Europe, where the incidence of both spinal surgery and the failed surgical back are far less, the most common indication is for end-stage peripheral vascular disease. In such cases, SCS has been shown to improve pain, improve microcirculation, decrease amputation rates, and improve healing of ulcers.[61] Some studies have identified predictors of poor outcome for SCS (such as psychiatric comorbidity, work injuries related to litigation issues, active drug addiction, the lack of a clear-cut diagnosis, and nonstatic pain states, e.g., such as cancer), but the results have varied.[62,63]

Proper protocols for SCS initially require placement of a trial electrode for several days. Patients are placed prone on a fluoroscopy table and kept awake to monitor response. Under local anesthesia, an epidural needle is placed in the spine, similar to the technique for epidural analgesia but at a more acute angle to the skin and slightly paramedian to enable electrode manipulation. A stimulating electrode is then advanced into the epidural space under fluoroscopic guidance. The usual entry level for patients with low back pain or lower extremity pain is T12–L1, with the tip advanced in the posterior epidural space to the T10 level, although this may vary depending on elicitation of stimulation paresthesias. After the electrode (there may be one or two) reaches its radiological target, it is connected to a stimulating device, and the patient is stimulated in multiple configurations. The electrode and stimulation are manipulated until the patient reports paresthesias covering the entire pain area. Once the trial implantation is complete, the patient is discharged with a temporary externalized electrode coupled to a small belt-hung stimulating device for a trial period.

Clinical Pearl: A common indication in the USA is for a patient with failed back surgery syndrome, who may have pain related to scarring of nerve roots. In Europe, where the incidence of both spinal surgery and the failed surgical back are far less, the most common indication is for end-stage peripheral vascular disease.

Several criteria have been proposed to evaluate whether a trial of SCS is deemed successful prior to implantation. Most would agree that pain relief must be at least 50% and must be accompanied by patient satisfaction. If that is the case, a permanent electrode can be implanted. The temporary electrode is removed and a period of 2–3 weeks is allowed to pass so as to lower the risk of infection from multiple catheter insertions. When the permanent electrode is placed, it is positioned in the area where the maximal stimulation had been achieved during the trial. Figure 24–4 demonstrates a variety of spinal cord stimulator leads. Next, an incision is made in the skin at the site of needle insertion, the needle is removed, and the electrode is sutured to the supraspinous ligament. The electrode with its lead extension is then tunneled under the skin and around the flank to the abdomen or to the gluteal region. A subcutaneous pocket is fashioned in either region, into which the stimulator generator is placed. The power generator is a thin disk, 1–2 in in diameter, similar to a pacemaker. Prior to closure, system integrity is checked with the console programmer. The device can be turned on and off and otherwise programmed as necessary by the patient using a handheld device.

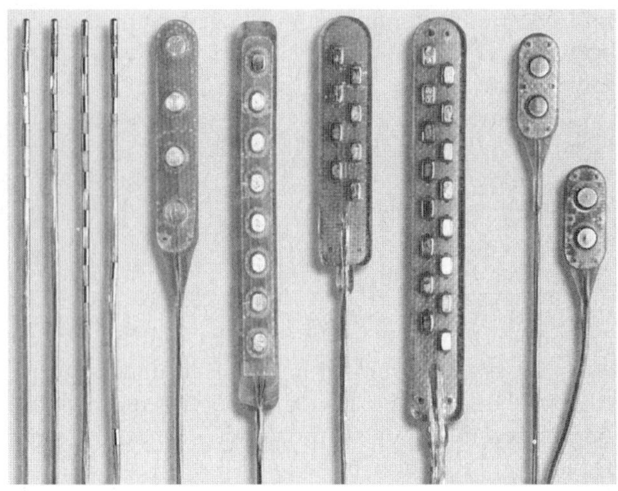

FIGURE 24–4. Types of spinal cord stimulator leads. These leads deliver electrical impulses to the spinal cord from an electrical generator device. The four cylindrical leads (left) can be place percutaneously. The plate-type leads (right) are placed surgically. *(Leads from Advanced Neuromodulation Systems, Inc.)*

Occasionally, patients who have had complex back surgery or who have otherwise abnormal spinal anatomy require an open surgical SCS implantation. This occurs in cases in which the SCS electrode cannot be advance into the epidural space because of posterior epidural scar tissue. In this case, a spine surgeon, often working alongside a pain management specialist, can perform a partial laminectomy at the T10–T11 level to allow direct placement of the electrode(s). Such procedures are relatively rare, but may be the only way to successfully utilize SCS in these patients.

Complications from SCS include infection, electrode migration, and loss of analgesia.[64,65] Infection is the most feared complication, with the incidence being at about 5%. Most infections are eradicated only by explanting the entire system. Epidural space infections are rare, and most infections are superficial.[60,62] Electrode migration, fracturing, or fibrosis at the tip can occur in up to 25% of patients, and this may require surgical repositioning or replacement of the electrode.[66] Often, catheter reprogramming performed noninvasively can restore stimulation in the desired area. Loss of analgesia despite persistent paresthesia from the electrode can occur, but its causes and treatment are unknown. The batteries for SCS devices typically last about 5–7 years and require surgical replacement when they are no longer functioning.

Intrathecal Pumps and Their Agents The use of intrathecal opioids provides another modality to treat both chronic nonmalignant pain and pain related to cancer. The challenge is in picking the appropriate patients for use of this type of drug delivery system. It is inappropriate to implant a spinal delivery system for a patient who has a very limited life expectancy, in whom pain relief can be accomplished by oral or single injection therapies, and in whom the complications of intrathecal therapy outweigh the potential benefits. Implantation of devices for delivery of intrathecal or epidural opioids, local anesthetic solutions, and clonidine is for the 5%–10% of patients who respond poorly to pharmacological treatments, injections, other conservative measures, and surgical treatments. A large number of these patients may suffer needlessly because alternative pain management techniques are either not known or not practiced in the community.

The treatment of back pain with spinally (meaning by the epidural or the subarachnoid route) administered opioids, either alone or in combination with local anesthetics or clonidine, has become more utilized. The effectiveness of therapy is contingent on the nature and source of the pain syndrome. Nociceptive pain usually responds well to systemic opioid therapy, and this includes many patients with mechanical back pain. Most failures of systemic opioid therapy, when excluding factors such as undertreatment with too low a dosage, knowledge deficiency, and patient compliance issues, are in patients who suffer from neuropathic pain.[67] Systemic opioid therapy may also fail in a number of patients who have basically adequate analgesic control, but occasional severe movement-related pain.

The indication for implantation of spinal delivery systems is primarily for patients in whom the oral route of analgesic medication either provides inadequate pain relief or causes unacceptable side effects. Also, patients who continue to have pain in spite of surgical treatments for back pain may also be appropriate candidates for intrathecal infusion therapies. Many of these patients will suffer from intractable axial back pain, or other diffuse axial pain syndromes. Prior to implantation, the patient must first undergo a preimplantation trial with a temporary catheter. The trial must confirm that the patient is responding well to this type of therapy with minimal side effects. In addition, implantation should occur only in situations where the patient is educated about the system and adequate facilities are present for its maintenance. Finally, the patient's psychological status must be stable and favorable. Patients who suffer from drug dependence and use pain for secondary gain or to obtain more narcotic medications are not good candidates for implantation. Intrathecal opioid therapy for nonmalignant pain is still controversial. Some types of patients who may be good candidates are those with "failed" spinal surgery syndrome, intractable neuropathic pain, or pain due to vascular ischemia.

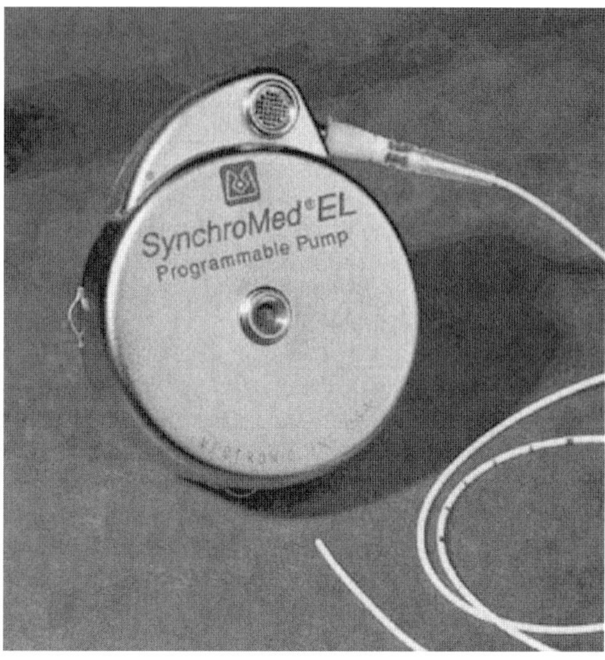

FIGURE 24–5. Intrathecal pump delivery system with intrathecal catheter. *(Pump photo courtesy of Medtronic, Inc.)*

Totally implanted infusion pumps have the advantage of delivering higher cerebrospinal fluid levels of morphine with lower plasma levels and fewer supraspinal side effects. In a typical delivery system, medication is placed in a reservoir of 18 mL. Figure 24–5 demonstrates an intrathecal pump delivery system, while Figure 24–6 demonstrates the intrathecal placement of the catheter amongst the surrounding anatomy. Once implanted, programmable pumps can be accessed readily without penetrating the patient. It is recommended that the medication reservoir be accessed at least every 3 months. Complications from spinal opioids include nausea and vomiting, urinary retention, and respiratory depression, but these are unlikely in patients who are already tolerant to the effects of systemic opioids. There is also a small risk of CSF leak, spinal headache when first implanted, and meningitis. Spinal opioid therapy can be continued for years, and medications other than morphine can be given to improve the quality of analgesia (i.e., bupivacaine, clonidine, baclofen).

Choosing Between Intrathecal or Epidural Systems An important issue is the choice between intrathecal versus epidural infusion.[69] One advantage of subarachnoid infusions is that catheter-tip fibrosis is less of an issue than with the epidural route. Therefore, infusions may be continued for longer than 6 months with subarachnoid catheters, whereas epidural catheters

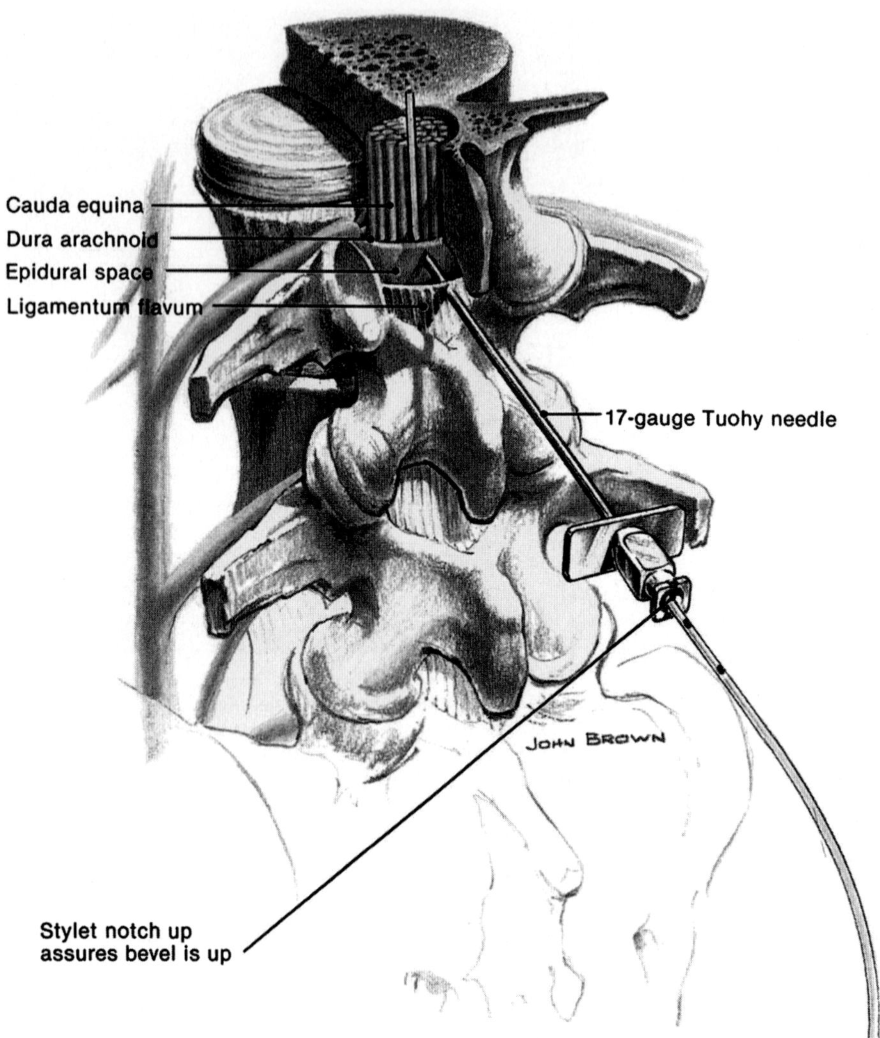

FIGURE 24–6. Intrathecal catheter placement. Lumbar spine anatomy showing needle placement and catheter in intrathecal space. Epidural space is indicated as well. *(From Katz.*[68])

may stop being effective by that time. Recently, several cases of intrathecal catheter granuloma formation have been reported, occasionally causing neurological deficits and increased pain,[70–72] but this phenomenon appears to be rare. The potential for development of catheter tip fibrosis with epidural catheters is the major reason why most patients with persistent back pain syndromes are candidates only for intrathecal therapy. Epidural therapy tends to be utilized for periods of time that are shorter than 2 weeks.

With subarachnoid infusions, lower doses of opioids are used, and therefore, lower rates of systemic side effects from the opioids can be expected versus epidural infusion. If the need arises, other intrathecal medications can be administered, such as local anesthetics, clonidine, and baclofen. Disadvantages of intrathecal catheters include risk of meningitis, persistent headaches, subcutaneous spinal fluid hygromas, and CSF leaks leading to subdural hematoma.[69] It may also be more difficult to titrate local anesthetics or opioids to achieve segmental analgesia.

The major advantage of epidural catheters is the ease and convenience of making changes in doses and types of medications delivered, which can be done by family members or home health agencies with a simple telephone order. Therefore, local anesthetic can be added to infusions when the patient's pain becomes resistant to opioid infusions alone, as in cases where a prolonged trial of infusion therapy is given prior to proceeding with an implant. In addition, there is less risk of a spinal leak, most infections are confined to the skin entry site, lower CSF levels of drug are present after bolus dosing, and additional dosing of medication on an as needed basis is more feasible and can be done at home. The main disadvantage of the epidural approach is the development of catheter tip fibrosis in 3–6 months, which makes the infusion lose efficacy.[73] Other potential disadvantages are irritation of the skin entry site and wound breakdown. When infections occur, most are superficial or in the catheter subcutaneous track and not epidural. Most infections can be managed conservatively without surgery by applying topical care and systemic antibiotics, and by explanting catheters for deep track and epidural infections.[74,75] If an epidural abscess develops and neurological deficits begin, neurosurgical debridement may be necessary.

Clinical Pearl: With subarachnoid infusions, lower doses of opioids are used, and therefore, lower rates of systemic side effects from the opioids can be expected versus epidural infusion. The major advantage of epidural catheters is the ease and convenience of making changes in doses and types of medications delivered, which can be done by family members or home health agencies with a simple telephone order.

Extraspinal Injection Therapies

Trigger Point Injections Although many cases of low back pain are due to mechanical spine disorders, in some patients the primary source of pain is myofascial dysfunction. Abnormalities in the muscles and connective tissues can cause hyperirritable bundles of tissue called trigger points (TrPs).[76] The key component of myofascial pain syndrome, chapter nine of this text explains the etiological and diagnostic aspects of TrPs in detail. Patients with TrPs will have muscle tenderness, loss of range of motion, and often a taut band of tissue apparent on palpation which can offer refer pain to distant anatomical sites. To reduce the TrP, injections of saline, steroid, or dry needling have been used as treatments.

Studies by Garvey and Hong show that injections of either lidocaine or lidocaine with steroid are equally effective for treating TrPs as is the technique of dry needling.[77,78] However, Travell and Simon clearly state that steroids are contraindicated for TrPs and instead recommend procaine or a derivative thereof.[76] To date, there are no controlled studies evaluating the clinical response to trigger point injections, although there have been many case reports and case series showing efficacy of this type of treatment for low back pain, lumbar radicular symptoms, chest pain, abdominal and pelvic pain, tendinitis, and focal dystonias. Most clinicians believe that TrP injections should be limited to a series of three or four injections, accompanied by a myofascial stretching/release and/or rehabilitation program.

Botulinum Toxin Botulinum toxin is one of a series of "muscle relaxant" medications that are used in patients with chronic pain. Muscle relaxants include medications in the mephenesin class as well as quinine, baclofen, tizanidine, dantrolene, benzodiazepines, and now botulinum toxin. Drugs in the mephenesin class are the most widely prescribed muscle relaxants used in pain management.[79] Unfortunately, there are no studies to compare the safety and efficacy of these drugs to others, and the mechanism of action is not understood. Most likely, they work by depressing polysynaptic reflexes over monosynaptic reflexes, but they provide significant muscle relaxation only at the expense of sedation.[79]

Botulinum toxin A is a neurotoxin that has several potential uses that can benefit a patient with chronic muscular pain. Produced by the bacterium, *Clostridium botulinum*, which can be found in food poisoning and as a biological weapon, it is one of the most deadly poisons known, causing death by muscle paralysis. Botulinum toxin exists in at least seven different serotypes, with the primary structure that of a light and a heavy polypeptide chain connected by a disulfide bond.[80] It was first injected clinically into overactive muscles in 1980 as a treatment for strabismus.[81] Since 1989, it has been approved in the United States by the Federal Drug Administration for the treatment of strabismus, blepharospasm, and cervical dystonia, and recently (2002) for the treatment of wrinkles.[82] Botulinum toxin has been used to treat excessive muscle contraction from various causes, including cervical dystonia (torticollis), spasticity of the calves and legs in cerebral palsy, spasmodic dysphonia, and the focal dystonia of the limbs that causes writer's cramp and musician's cramp.[83]

The site of action of botulinum toxin is the neuromuscular junction, where the toxin binds and prevents the release of acetylcholine. For some reason, the toxin seems to prefer to bind to the more active neuromuscular junction rather than the less active, thus producing muscle weakness without necessarily blocking voluntary control.[84] It is also theorized that the toxin may have some central nervous system effects, reversing inhibitory mechanisms in dystonia. There may be decreased input along sensory fibers in patients who receive botulinum toxin, or there may be changes in spinal cord neurons.[85,86] Botulinum toxin A is one of the serotypes now marketed, along with botulinum toxin B, which has been studied as a treatment for cervical dystonia. Since antibodies have been found to develop in 2% of patients receiving the A serotype and in 10% of patients after 1 year of repeated use of the B serotype, some patients can become resistant to the effects of botulinum toxin.[80,87,88] In such cases, it is possible that a new serotype will more be effective when antibodies have developed to one serotype.

The effective dose of botulinum toxin will vary, depending on the size of the muscle, the degree of weakness desired, and the commercial preparation of the formulation.[89] The effects of a single injection rarely last more than 3 months. Local side effects are primarily those of muscle weakness, but this lasts usually only 1–2 weeks. Systemic side effects are rare in doses up to several hundred units, but are a result of neuromuscular junctions being affected in various parts of the body, causing a sluggish pupillary response, reduced variability in heart rate, and impaired emptying of the gallbladder.[87,90,91]

Botulinum toxin has been found to have many uses outside of pain management.[92] It is injected into the internal urethral sphincter to improve detrusor sphincter dyssynergia. Injections into the lower esophageal sphincter improve dysphagia in patients with achalasia. Injection into the papilla of Vater improves symptomatic biliary disease and can predict whether endoscopic sphincterotomy will succeed. When injected into the external anal sphincter, it allows healing to occur from chronic anal fissure. Dermatologists use botulinum toxin to treat wrinkles from muscle contraction in the glabellar furrows and lateral canthal rhytids. Cholinergic sweat glands can be blocked, providing a treatment for unpleasant axillary hyperhidrosis. Injection of botulinum toxin into the pericranial muscles can reduce tension headache and migraine. By decreasing spasticity from stoke, multiple sclerosis, Parkinson's disease, and spinal cord injury, botulinum toxin can improve range of motion and enhance body hygiene.[93] When compared to surgical options, which are available for some of these conditions, botulinum toxin is often a better-tolerated and more cost-effective method of treatment.

Clinical Pearl: The site of action of botulinum toxin is the neuromuscular junction, where the toxin binds and prevents the release of acetylcholine. For some reason, the toxin seems to prefer to bind to the more active neuromuscular junction rather than the less active, thus producing muscle weakness without necessarily blocking voluntary control.

Botulinum toxin is useful for the treatment of various painful conditions, such as torticollis and some site-specific myofascial pain that is marked by palpable dystonia and well-localized TrPs.[94,95] By relaxing painful muscle spasm, botulinum toxin can enable the patient to proceed with beneficial rehabilitation and increase range of motion. With the help of rehabilitation, it is hoped that the inciting cause for the muscle spasm will subside such that the condition does not recur when the effects of botulinum toxin abate. In a randomized, double blind study of 31 patients with low back pain of more than 6-months duration, botulinum toxin injection was compared to placebo.[96] At 3 weeks after injection, 73% of subjects who received botulinum toxin had at least 50% pain reduction compared to 25% of those who received saline. At 8 weeks, 60% of those who received the drug had more than 50% pain relief, compared to 12.5% of those who received saline. Regarding functional ability, based on the results of the Oswestry Low Back Pain Questionnaire, after 8 weeks, 67% of patients who received botulinum toxin had improvement compared to 19% of those who received saline. In most cases, the effects of the drug diminished after 3–4 months.

Minimally Invasive Procedures for Discogenic and Vertebral Pain

Intradiscal Electrothermonucleoplasty Therapy Chronic pain from a discogenic origin is a significant cause of low back pain, possibly affecting 40% of all patients with low back pain.[97] Although in many persons the pain will subside within 1–3 months, some cases will progress to become more frequent and chronic. A number of these patients may respond to ESIs, manual techniques, modalities, exercise, and pharmaceutical agents, but in some individuals the pain may persist in spite of reasonable nonoperative measures. Intradiscal electrothermal therapy (IDET) is a possible treatment for some of these patients. Other options include managing pain and its functional limitations with medications and additional chronic pain management techniques, or to have the patient undergo surgical management, which primarily consists of interbody fusion with or without instrumentation.

The intervertebral disc is known to be a potential generator of pain. Nociceptors are present in the outer third of the annulus fibrosis as well as in the anterior and posterior longitudinal ligaments. Nerve fibers have been shown to grow into degenerated and disrupted discs.[98,99] Buckling of the disrupted annulus can lead to increasing mobility of the adjacent spinal segments, which can cause further fissuring of the annulus, sensitizing both mechanoreceptors and nociceptors and leading to chronic pain.[100] Also, an inflammatory chemical neuronitis can occur from release of nuclear materials. Inflammatory mediators and enzymes released as part of the degenerative process may stimulate nociceptors and result in pain. Both intradiscal mechanical and neural irritation can result from internal disc derangement. Therefore, even discs that do not directly compress or affect a nerve root can cause back pain and leg and buttock pain without true radiculopathy.

IDET involves inserting a 17-gauge, 6-in needle into a symptomatic disc and then threading a heat conducting 18-gauge catheter (30 cm long with a 6 cm active tip) to rest along the interior wall of the annulus[101] (see Fig. 24–7). The position of the introducer needle and the catheter in the nucleus of the disc should be confirmed fluoroscopically. The catheter should rest along the posterior border of the interior part of the annulus, and it should coil past the midline. Occasionally, bilateral catheters may be necessary to cover the entire area of the annulus. The catheter is heated to a temperature of 90°C, which corresponds to a tissue temperature of 75°C.[102] The entire heated portion

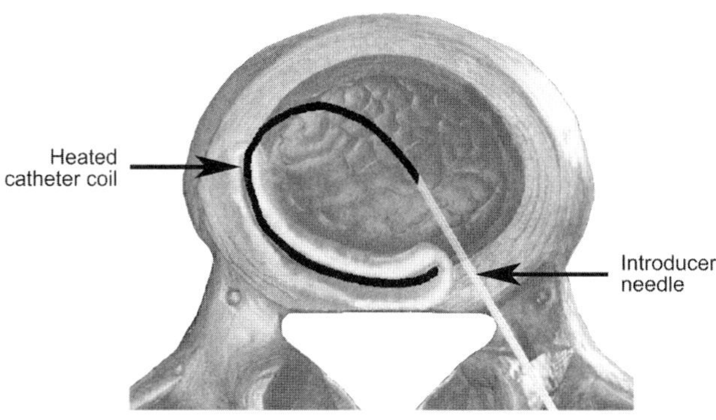

FIGURE 24–7. Intradiscal electrothermonucleoplasty. A 17-gauge 6-in needle is inserted into a lumbar disc. A heat conducting 18-gauge catheter (30-cm long with a 6 cm active tip) is positioned to rest along the inner wall of the annulus. *(From Oratec Interventions, Inc.)*

of the catheter must lie within the disc. If radicular symptoms develop during heating, the catheter should be repositioned to avoid nerve root injury. The catheter temperature is heated to 65°C and gradually increased to 90°C over 13 minutes (2 degrees per minute) and then kept at that temperature for a total duration of treatment of about 16 minutes.[101] There is usually a reproduction of the patient's usual pain during this time. Prior to removing the catheter, intradiscal antibiotics may be given. Typically, there is at first an increase in pain (1–2 weeks), followed by pain improvement 6–12 weeks after the procedure. Patients are advised to avoid any bending or twisting motions for at least 6 weeks after the procedure and driving or sitting should be limited to 30 minutes during that time. A lumbar corset is prescribed to be worn for the first 6–8 weeks after the treatment.[102] Athletic activities can be resumed after 5 or 6 months.

Intradiscal thermal lesioning is thought to work by two primary mechanisms. The intervertebral disc, being relatively avascular, tends to hold heat and maintain temperature during lesioning.[103] By heating the disrupted annulus, the resulting collagen shrinkage can lead to a stabilization of annular fissures. Collagen contraction, thickening, and remodeling can occur, leading to changes in the biomechanics of the disc and resulting in stabilization of the disrupted disc. The remodeling that occurs can lead to a reduction of disc volume and intrdiscal pressure, which may also reduce pain.[102] Heat-induced changes in annular collagen may lead to healing of an annular fissure.[104] In addition, thermocoagulation of nociceptors occurs at a temperature of 55°C–65°C, and this thermal injury of nerves is thought to lead to pain reduction. With IDET, heat is transferred to the tissues from the catheter, with feedback to the power generator to maintain the target temperature.[102] Cadaveric studies confirm that intradiscal temperatures of up to 76°C are reached with IDET, but that the maximum temperature measured outside the wall of the disc is 42.9°C, which is a safe temperature range for the surrounding structures. Similar temperatures were recorded in living subjects.[102] Direct lesioning of nociceptors may be an important mechanism of action for IDET.

Intradiscal thermal lesioning differs from radiofrequency lesioning (RFL) of the disc. With radiofrequency, heat is generated as a result of high alternating current density in the tissue.[105] A discrete tissue lesion occurs, but it is confined to the nucleus, with insufficient heating of the outer annulus.[106] Therefore, inserting a radiofrequency probe into the nucleus has not been found to yield good results for discogenic pain,[107] whereas better results can be expected if the annulus itself is heated.[108] Another difference between IDET and RFL is that a navigable catheter, which transfers heat directly to the annulus, is used in IDET.

IDET (intradiscal electrothermal coagulation therapy, or intradiscal electrothermal treatment) is recommended for patients with[102,103,109]

- function limiting low back disc pain for at least 6 months.
- lack of satisfactory improvement with progressive exercise, at least one ESI, a trial of rehabilitation, oral anti-inflammatory drugs, and activity modification.
- normal findings on neurological examination.
- negative straight leg raise test for radicular symptoms.
- MRI that does not show nerve compression.
- positive discogram, one which reproduces concordant pain at low pressurization (less than 1.25 mL dye volume) at one or more levels with adjacent control not demonstrating pain.

Exclusion criteria includes the following:

- Narrow disc height (less than 50%).
- Severe disc bulge through the annular ring or segmental instability.
- Very advanced signs of disc failure.
- Inflammatory arthritides, nonspinal condition mimicking back pain, medical disorders that preclude follow-up care, and prior surgery at the symptomatic level.

This procedure is not recommended for patients who may have psychosocial barriers, which would decrease the chance of improvement in pain. Such factors can be determined by utilizing measures outlined in Chapters 14 and 19. Patients should be made aware of and accept realistic expectations of outcome.[102] Such expectations would include a partial but not total reduction of back pain. Patients with spinal stenosis or significant disc herniations with nerve root compression are not good candidates for IDET. As indicated in the above criteria, patients who are candidates for IDET require a diagnostic evaluation that includes MRI and provocative discography that reproduces typical pain complaints. Younger patients, who are nonsmokers and who are motivated to improve, tend to fare better than other groups.[103]

Clinical Pearl: Both intradiscal mechanical and neural irritation can result from internal disc derangement. Therefore, even discs that do not directly compress or affect a nerve root can cause back pain and leg and buttock pain without true radiculopathy.

Several studies have examined outcomes following IDET. In a study of 25 patients with chronic low back pain due to discogenic disease and a mean duration of symptoms of 58.5 months, IDET was compared to spinal fusion or a chronic pain management program.[110] Patients were found to have an improvement in VAS scores (7.32 pretreatment mean improved to 3.58 posttreatment mean) as well as an improvement in physical function and narcotic consumption. In a study of 62 patients who were followed for at least 12 months after IDET,[109] pain (based on an 11-point Visual Analogue scale, VAS) and function (SF-36 scores) were found to improve in about 70% of patients, with 19% of patients showing no improvement in any scale. The mean change in VAS score was 3.0, and more than 90% of patients returned to work. Unfortunately, there was no comparative treatment group in this study. However, these improvements were comparable to the results of interbody fusion.[111] Traditionally, overall failure rates for lumbar fusion surgery approach 40%.[112]

When compared to patients undergoing a physical rehabilitation program, patients after IDET were found to have improved pain scores, improved disability, and less drug use. Karasek and Bogduk compared 35 patients treated with IDET to 17 patients who underwent standard physical therapy.[113] After 3 months, 4 of 17 patients obtained relief in the control group compared to 32 of 36 patients in the IDET group. Patients in the IDET group maintained these results at 6 and 12 months. Derby et al. reported on 32 patients with discogenic pain who underwent IDET. Patients were followed for 12 months, and the results were that 62.5% had a favorable outcome, 25% had no change in pain and function, and 12.5% had an unfavorable outcome after IDET.[101] The mean decrease in VAS was 1.84 and the mean decrease in Roland Morris Disability Questionnaire score was 4.03.

Wetzel et al. presented data on 2-year outcomes from IDET in abstract form at the 2001 annual meeting of the North American Spine Society.[114] Of the 74 patients enrolled in the study who underwent IDET, 18% (14 total) underwent additional back surgery. Overall, the mean reduction in VAS was 2.6 and there was an improvement in disability scores. In addition, there was a statistically significant reduction in leg pain in patients after IDET. An IDET registry created by the manufacturer was founded to study the results of this procedure. Thompson and Eckel's report on the first 100 patients enrolled in the registry found that there was an improvement in VAS of 3.1, and that patients tended to improve in terms of physical functioning.[115] There are yet to be any studies of IDET using strict, well-defined inclusion criteria and that are prospective and randomized with a control group. Because this is a relatively new procedure, no long-term results are yet available.

Few adverse outcomes have been reported from IDET procedures, with the number of IDET catheters used thus far being over 35,000.[116] Theoretically, because IDET is similar to discography, one would expect a risk of disciitis. Nerve root injury or cauda equina syndrome cannot be excluded as risks of this procedure. Contraindications to performing IDET include anticoagulation therapy and concurrent infection. In a cadaveric motion study of spinal segments after IDET, no destabilization of the spine was found.[117] Thus far, six cases of disc herniation have been reported in the level where IDET had been performed.[116] The most common mechanical complication is catheter breakage, with most catheters subsequently left in the disc, without causing further morbidity.

Nucleoplasty Nucleoplasty is the newest treatment for discogenic pain, and is available in the United States since October 2000. The procedure is intended to relieve pain from painful bulging discs that have not herniated through the annular ligament. In contrast to the IDET procedure, nucleoplasty is indicated for patients who have radicular leg pain along with their low back pain symptoms. Prior to performing the procedure, discography is necessary to confirm that the disc is indeed the pain generator. The nucleoplasty procedure is done under local anesthesia and fluoroscopic guidance, most often with the patient in a prone position.

The technical aspects and risk of performing nucleoplasty are similar to those of discography and the IDET procedure. Under fluoroscopic guidance, a specially designed needle (17-gauge, 6-in length) is inserted into the offending disc. During nucleoplasty, unlike the IDET procedure, it is recommended that the needle be inserted on the same side of the painful symptoms.[118] The needle is positioned in the outer layers of the disc. A nucleoplasty probe (called a "channelling wand") is inserted through the needle, and it is positioned within the disc. The tip of the probe utilizes bipolar radiofrequency current (100 Hz) in a non-heat-driven process, resulting in an ionization channel (vapor layer or plasma field) that disintegrates disc tissue.[119,120] On withdrawal of the probe, heat is given (40°C–70°C), with the idea being to coagulate and ablate adjacent tissue and shrink the newly created channel. A number of channels are then created within the disc (usually 6–12) by advancing and retracting the probe in a clockwise fashion. The disintegration and heating of disc material results in reduced pressure within the disc and therefore less compression on the adjacent nerve roots and pain-generating annular ligament.[121] Pain relief is thought to occur from reduced pressure of the remaining disc and a reduction in the size of the disc bulge.

Peer-reviewed efficacy data is lacking on this new modality. Most reports are from the Web site of the product's manufacturer.[119] Initial anecdotal experience suggests that this form of treatment may benefit patients with bulging discs, back pain, and radicular pain.[118] Pain relief occurs almost immediately after the procedure. Nucleoplasty, in comparison to IDET, produces lower temperatures within the disc, and some have postulated that it may have a lower chance of producing thermal injury to vertebral end plates.[122] However, if the probe is place closely to a nerve root, it may cause a sudden onset of radicular pain and lead to nerve injury. Therefore, patients should remain awake during the procedure, so they can report worrisome symptoms.

Chemonucleolysis Patients with a clear history of pain due to a herniated nucleus pulposis may be candidates for chymopapain chemonucleolysis. This procedure is one of a number of invasive techniques to alleviate back pain, which also includes surgical discectomy and microdiscectomy, percutaneous discectomy, and percutaneous laser discectomy. Studies have shown that chemonucleolysis has a success rate comparable to open discectomy and microdiscectomy.[123] Patients with a herniated disc may be considered for one of these treatments after a trial of conservative management. Chemonucleolysis was first done in 1963, and chymopapain injections into discs have been done for about 40 years.[124] However, this procedure is rarely done presently because of the fear of potentially fatal allergic reactions to chymopapain.

Candidates for chemonucleolysis should have only a single level disc herniation, as confirmed by MRI, and their pain should be primarily affecting the leg and not the back.[125] Chymopapain causes an enzymatic degradation of the nucleus pulposis, and it is approved only for the treatment of lumbar discs.[125] Contraindications to chymopapain injection include allergy to the drug, cauda equina syndrome, a sequestered disc, multiple back surgeries, progressive neurological deficits, spinal tumors, spinal stenosis, and spinal instability.[125] Patients who are obese, hypertensive, or who have a family history of stroke may be poor candidates for this procedure.

Clinical Pearl: Patients with a clear history of pain due to a herniated nucleus pulposis may be candidates for chymopapain chemonucleolysis. This procedure is one of a number of invasive techniques to alleviate back pain, which also includes surgical discectomy and microdiscectomy, percutaneous discectomy, and percutaneous laser discectomy.

The procedure entails inserting a needle into the affected disc and injecting chymopapain. Chymopapain, which is a derivative of papaya, dissolves nuclear material. Allergic anaphylactic reactions have been reported in 0.3% of patients and so premedication with benadryl and cimetidine is advocated by some.[125] In a review of 85 patients who received a second injection of chymopapain because of recurrent disc herniation, no allergic sensitivity reactions were seen.[126] The FAST (fluoroallergosorbent) test can be used to test for sensitivity to chymopapain.[125] Extra care should be taken for those who take β-blockers, as these drugs may blunt the effects of epinephrine, should anaphylaxis occur.

After the chymopapain injection, most patients experience immediate relief from pain. However, about 30% of patients may need up to 6 weeks to have relief of symptoms. some patients will have a transient flare of back pain.[125] Administering steroids periprocedure, using local anesthetic after injection, and giving anti-inflammatory drugs for some time after injection may lessen such flare ups.[125] Patients should limit physical activities for at least 3 months after the procedure. Chymopapain disc injections lead to a loss of disc height (average 15.8%), which does not reverse afterward on long-term follow-up.[127] Overall, between 1982 and 1991, 121 adverse events in 135,000 patients were reported to the Food and Drug Administration.[128] These included 7 cases of fatal anaphylaxis, 24 infections, 32 bleeding problems, 32 neurologic events, and 15 miscellaneous occurrences. Excess loss of disc height can lead to spinal instability. The risk of adverse events was less than that associated with laminectomy, and the long-term outcome reported was better than with laminectomy. Because of lower hospital stays, a cost savings is associated with chemonucleolysis over standard surgical treatments.[129]

The overall success rate after chymopapain chemonucleolysis ranges from 71% to 93%.[130] In a double-blind study of 30 patients treated with chymopapain injection compared to 30 patients who received only saline disc injection, after 10 years, 80% of the chymopapain group thought the injection was successful compared to only 34% of those who had received saline.[131] Long-term follow-up (7–20 years) of 3130 patients from 13 centers has shown a success rate of 77%.[130] Lecuire reported on 110 patients followed for 8–12 years after chymopapain injection and found excellent or good results in 63%, with 17% of patients having no pain relief after the procedure.[132] In a study of 200 patients with herniated discs, half of whom had surgical discectomy and half of whom had chymopapain injections, at 1 year, there was an 82% success rate for discectomy compared to an 87% success rate for the chymopapain group. Most other studies showed a somewhat better improvement in patients who had surgery (88% success rate) compared to those who received chymopapain (76% success rate).[133] In another study of patients with discogenic disease at either L4–L5 or L5–S1, good to excellent results were observed in 72% 5 years after receiving chymopapain injection, with a drop in the VAS from 8.5 to 0.7.[134]

Looking at functional results after chymopapain disc injections, Poynton reviewed 105 patients who were followed for a mean 12.2 years and assessed by the Oswestry Disability Questionnaire. An excellent or good response was seen in 67% of patients, with disciitis occurring in 5.7%.[135] Results from chymopapain injections have been poorer for patients receiving workers' compensation benefits.[136] Patients with new onset back pain with radicular symptoms have been found to have a more successful outcome with chymopapain injection compared to patients with a preexisting low back pain condition (85% success rate compared to 52% success rate).[137] In a review of 26 randomized controlled trials on the treatment of lumbar disc prolapse, 5 trials showed that chymopapain led to greater treatment success at 3–12 months than did placebo.[138] In this review, there was a 69% success rate with chymopapain injections compared to a 48% success rate in the placebo group at 3–12 months.

Vertebroplasty Vertebral compression fractures are an important cause of back pain, especially in elderly persons with osteoporosis. It is estimated that there are 700,000 compression fractures per year in the United States, resulting in 150,000 hospitalizations for pain control and medical management.[139] Also, patients with metastatic cancer, metabolic diseases, or those who use steroids chronically can develop fractures of the vertebral body. In addition to pain, vertebral compression fractures can cause decreased pulmonary function and gastrointestinal complications, ultimately leading to a higher morbidity and mortality. Compression fractures lead to a reduced forced vital capacity and forced expiratory volume (FEV_1).[140] Patients with thoracic compression fractures are more likely to have such problems, but these problems can occur even with lumbar fractures. Patients can develop sleep disorders, eat poorly, and become depressed and anxious.[141] There is a 25% increased risk of mortality for patients with compression fractures when compared to age-matched controls.[142]

Vertebroplasty is a procedure that involves the injection of a cement-like structure polymethylmethacrylate (PMMA) in a collapsed vertebral body, thereby reinforcing the fractured bone. By stabilizing the fractured vertebrae, pain can be diminished, patients can return to being ambulatory, and analgesic use can be curtailed. Overall, quality of life is improved. Vertebroplasty was first performed in France in the 1980s as a treatment for a patient with a vertebral angioma,[143] and is becoming increasingly popular throughout the United States. In addition to osteoporosis-related compression fractures, common indications for vertebroplasty include vertebral collapse from osteolytic metastasis, myeloma, hemangioma, and long-term corticosteroid therapy.[144] The surgical alternative to vertebroplasty is usually reserved for patients with neurological complications and most often involves anterior decompression with posterior fusion, usually with instrumentation.

After menopause, women become susceptible to developing osteoporosis, and therefore are prone to developing fractures of the hip and spine. Genetic factors, nutrition, and metabolic factors all play a role in the development of compression fractures.[145] Osteoporosis can lead to reduced mineral content in bone and decreased vertebral body strength, putting 30 million people in the US at risk for fractures.[145] The lifetime risk for developing a vertebral fracture is 16% for women and 5% for men. Of the 700, 000 vertebral fractures that occur in the United States each year, 18% occur in women over the age of 50 and 27% in women over the age of 65.[146] Treatments that are given to prevent the occurrence of compression fractures include hormone replacement (raloxifene, brand name Evista), bisphosphanates (alendronate, brand name Fosamax), and calcitonin (brand name, Micalcin). Patients may be given supplemental calcium and vitamin D. Most pharmacological agents require at least 1 year to reduce the level of osteoporosis.[147] Because bed rest leads to bone mineral loss and diminished muscle mass, a program of rehabitation and exercise should be implemented as soon as possible.

The usual presentation of a compression fracture is one of severe mid-line back pain. After vertebroplasty, pain relief and increased mobility are usually seen within 2–3 days.[148] Over a period of a few weeks, patients can decrease their pain medications and many will become pain free. Vertebroplasty offers an alternative to bed rest, pain medications, back bracing, and spinal stabilization surgery with hardware for spinal compression fracture cases. The procedure is performed for patients who identify pain in the same location that a compression fracture is seen on X-ray or MRI. A recent study found that 93% of patients had a mean pain improvement of 7.4 points on an 11-point VAS scale, with bone scan imaging being highly predictive of positive clinical response.[149] Although fractures with greater than 70% reduction of the original vertebral body height may be more difficult to treat, successful pain reduction can be obtained even in such cases.[150]

As noted, vertebroplasty is performed percutaneously by inserting an 11-gauge biopsy needle into a collapsed vertebra and injecting cement-like material (PMMA). A volume of cement of 3.5 mL, which is about 15% of the fill volume fraction, restores stiffness of the bone to prefracture levels,[151] and even volumes as low as 2 mL may restore strength.[152] Injections are usually done bilaterally (about 1.5–2 mL injected into each side), although unilateral cement injection may be adequate.[153,154] Other studies have shown that a medial-lateral bending motion ("toggle") occurs toward the untreated side with unilateral injections.[151] Also, increased pressure associated with a larger volume unilateral injection may increase the risk of cement extrusion. This substance hardens over a period of 10–20 minutes. Usually, the cement is mixed with an antibiotic and with barium to make it radiopaque. In the thoracic spine, the needle is inserted lateral to the pedicle and medial to the rib head. In the lumbar spine, the approach is posterolaterally.[145] A CT scan is then done to confirm spread and distribution of cement.

To avoid neurological complications, the technique is best done under local anesthesia, with the patient awake. Possible complications include bleeding, infection, pulmonary embolus, or leakage of cement into a blood vessel or into adjacent tissues. Most cases of cement leakage have no clinical significance.[155] Damage may theoretically occur from the heat of the cement. In a study to assess heat generated from polymerization of PMMA during vertebroplasty, it was found that temperatures did not rise above 41°C in the spinal canal, even though temperature in the center of the vertebral body rose as high as 60°C–70°C.[156] It is unknown whether this treatment may lead to increased bone resorption at the cement–bone interface or increased risk of fracture in treated or adjacent vertebrae due to changes in mechanical forces.[157] In 25 patients who had vertebroplasty and were followed for 12–84 months, it was found that there was a slightly higher risk of vertebral fracture in the vicinity of a cemented vertebra compared to an uncemented vertebra.[158]

Fluoroscopic guidance is certainly required, and in cases where visualization is poor, CT imaging may be necessary. Standard barium impregnated PMMA is often not sufficiently radiopaque to visualize and addition of other substances, such as tantalum or tungsten, may be necessary.[159] The images must clearly demonstrate that the needle tips are within the vertebral body. A thorough neurological evaluation should be performed after the procedure, and some clinicians advocate urgent decompressive surgery if postprocedure CT scans show cement in the spinal canal.[160]

Pain reduction of at least 50% and improved quality of life occurs in about 70%–90% of patients who undergo vertebroplasty.[159,161] Increased mobility has been found in 70%–80% of patients, with improvement after 1–2 days following the injection.[162] Martin evaluated 40 patients with vertebral tumors who were treated at 68 vertebral segment levels and reported a success rate of 80%.[148] The incidence of treatment failure was related mostly to poor patient selection or leakage of cement due to excess PMMA volume. In patients who had osteoporosis, one study reports that 95% had pain relief after vertebroplasty, compared to only 50% of patients with spinal tumors reporting pain relief.[163] Bone scanning can predict positive response to vertebroplasty.[149] As mentioned above, although cement leakage is seen in many patients, in most cases it does not cause clinical complications.[164] In a study of 159 patients who had undergone vertebroplasty, cement leakage into the epidural space occurred in 40.3% of patients.[165] A higher incidence of leakage was seen in patients who received injections above the T7 level and in those who received a larger volume of cement. Patients who had cement leakage had decreased pain relief immediately after the procedure. In addition, there have been reports of neurologic compromise and development of new radicular pain from cement extrusion causing constriction of the dural sac and nerve roots.[160,166] Cement uptake into the venous circulation can be complicated by pulmonary embolus of PMMA into the pulmonary arteries.[167] There is a suggestion that complications are more common in patients who have metastatic lesions rather than osteoporosis as a cause of their compression fracture.

Clinical Pearl: Vertebroplasty offers an alternative to bed rest, pain medications, back bracing, and spinal stabilization surgery with hardware for spinal compression fracture cases.

There is a lower risk of complications in patients who have vertebroplasty performed 3–4 weeks after their fracture.[145] In more acute fractures, there is a greater risk of bleeding and cement leak, perhaps because the venous plexus has not clotted and the fractured bone has not had a chance to partially consolidate. Contrast dye should be injected prior to cement injection to confirm that there is not extravascation into the spinal canal or epidural veins. Clinical outcomes of vertebroplasty may not depend on the age of fracture or duration of pain.[168] Successful clinical outcomes have been reported in patients with fractures as old as 2 years.[145] Pain relief can occur regardless of whether vertebral height is fully restored. In patients who had good to excellent pain relief from vertebroplasty, 100% of cases continued to show beneficial results after 1 month, 89% had benefit after 3 months, and 75% continued to do well after 6 months.[169]

OUTCOMES OF NEURAL BLOCKADE FOR PAIN RELIEF

Outcomes assessment for chronic pain is difficult to quantify. Since pain is a subjective complaint ("an unpleasant sensory and emotional experience"), it can be influenced by anatomic factors as well as nonorganic conditions. Emotional, behavioral, social, financial, legal, and psychological factors play a role, and it becomes difficult to compare the efficacy of an intervention when there are many potential outcomes measures. Some clinicians will look at relief of pain as measured by VAS, whereas others are more interested in improved mood and quality of life. Insurance companies and employers are more interested in return to work as a final outcome of therapy, and want proof that an intervention decreases health-care costs.

Discrepancies in outcomes occur not only because different outcome measures are employed, but outcomes results also differ because of the variety of patients seen, patient selection criteria, the types of procedures offered, whether or not a procedure was performed correctly, whether the presumed diagnosis is reliable, and based on the overall methodology of data collection. Patients may report improved outcomes simply because they want to satisfy their physician. Also, a placebo response cannot be ignored, and there may be both behavioral and physiological reasons for improvement with a placebo.[170,171]

In assessing outcomes, over the past several decades, the gold standard in scientific research has been the "double-blinded placebo-controlled prospective clinical trial." [172] To the contrary, many therapies in medicine are instituted based on clinician assessment and judgment, followed by a formal or informal case series. The empiric "gut feeling" of the physician becomes the basis of continuing the therapy, as it was for Bonica when he observed that analgesic blocks resulted in prolonged pain relief for some patients. In some cases, physicians are convinced that a certain therapy is effective, which may require years of "science" to prove or disprove. This may be the case for many of the neural blockade procedures done for pain.

In Chapter 17, the diagnostic utility of various types of neural blockade procedures was addressed. Several factors were also presented outlining limits in the usefulness of neural blockade for pain management. These included the assumption that clinicians understand the exact pathway that is causing pain, that local anesthetic given in a nerve block will abolish only the intended pain pathway, and that pain relief is only due to the neural blockade procedure.[173] In fact, each of these assumptions may be incorrect, thereby reducing their utility not only as a diagnostic tool, but also as a treatment tool.

In spite of these considerations in the use of neural blockade for pain management, there has been a long-standing clinical practice of their use. There are numerous studies that explore the usefulness of neural blockade as a therapeutic modality. The next part of this chapter will review outcomes data on several common pain management procedures, including facet injections, ESIs, selective spinal nerve injections, sympathetic blocks, intrathecal infusion therapy, and SCS.

Facet Injections and Radiofrequency Lesioning of Facet Joints

In 1911, Goldthwait while reporting on sciatica from lumbosacral sources first proposed the notion that the zygapophyseal joint may be a source of pain.[174] In 1927, Putti postulated, "Sciatica is a neuralgia caused by the pathological condition of the intervertebral foramen and intervertebral articulations."[175] Ghormley first used the term "facet syndrome" in 1933, and surgical fusion of the spine was performed to treat this condition.[176] In 1971, Rees developed a technique to surgically denervate the facet joint.177 Shealy modified this technique in 1975 to be done via a percutaneous RFL approach,[45,178] and in 1980, Bogduk proposed further modifications.[179] Since then, facet injection and neurolysis has been a popular therapy for the treatment of low back and neck pain. Figure 24–8 demonstrates fluoroscopic illustrations of zygapophyseal injections. The injectate solution includes radiopaque dye, which provides visual confirmation of correct anatomical placement.

Several studies look at whether there are clinical features that characterize patients with facet syndrome, and that could therefore predict response to facet injections, neurolysis, or back surgery. Jackson studied 127 variables in 454 patients who had low back pain with a normal neurological examination and no root signs.[180] Although they were unable to predict which patients would respond best to facet

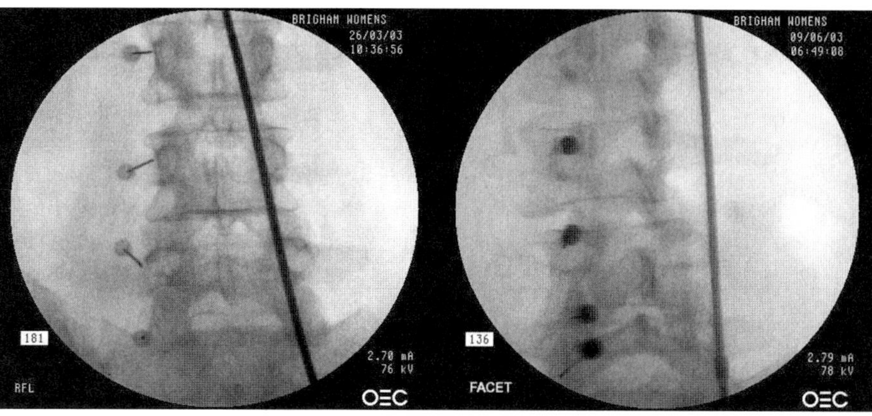

FIGURE 24-8. Facet (zygapophyseal joint) injections. Posteroanterior (left) and oblique (right) radiographs of the lumbar spine showing needles in position for medial branch blocks. With radiofrequency lesioning, the needles are advanced several millimeters off of the superior and medial aspect of the transverse process, at the junction of the transverse process with the superior articulating process of each facet joint.

injections, postinjection pain relief was seen more commonly in patients of older age, prior history of low back pain, normal gait, maximum pain on extension following forward flexion, and the absence of leg pain, muscle spasm, and aggravation of pain on Valsalva.

Revel randomized patients to receive either lidocaine or saline in the facet joint to assess the efficacy of single facet anesthesia versus placebo, and to determine the clinical criteria predictive of significant relief of low back pain after injection.[181] A positive result was one in which there was >75% pain relief after injection. Seven clinical criteria were examined, which were thought to be more highly prevalent in facet disease: age >65 years, pain not exacerbated by coughing, not worsened by hyperextension, not worsened by forward flexion, not worse when rising from flexion, not worsened by extension-rotation, and well relieved by recumbency. Lidocaine provided greater pain relief than did saline, and the presence of more than five of the seven clinical variables distinguished 92% of patients responding to lidocaine and 80% of those not responding to lidocaine. Thus, the presence of more than five of these seven clinical criteria can be used to select patients with low back pain who will respond to facet injections.

Revel's seven clinical variables were determined by a preceding study identifying predictors of a good response to facet injection.[182] A total of 90 maneuvers and symptoms were compared in a group of responders to facet injection to a group of nonresponders. Of the 40 patients, 22 were deemed responders to 1–4 facet injections, with 17 having a >90% response. The above seven variables were identified, and when four were present, facet injections had a sensitivity of 81.8% and a specificity of 77.8%.

Schwartzer questioned the ability of a single facet injection series to confirm the presence of clinical facet syndrome.[183] He conducted a prospective study to assess the prevalence and clinical features of patients with suspected pain from the lumbar facet joints. Of the 176 patients with low back pain, 47% of patients had response from lidocaine injections but only 15% had a >50% response to a confirmatory block with bupivacaine. Thus, the false positive rate of a single block was 38%. Response to both the lidocaine and confirmatory bupivacaine block was not predicted by the presence of any clinical features, such as site of pain, referral pattern of pain, and whether physical movements exacerbate pain.

The problem in determining which anatomical structure is causing back pain is that many structures can cause nonspecific neck and back pain, including the anterior longitudinal ligament, the posterior longitudinal ligament, the intervertebral discs, the dura, and the costovertebral ligaments, causing overlapping pain patterns. Although the facet joints are a source of pain, they are not often the only source of pain. Determining whether a patient has a clinical condition based only on response to a nerve block may be an errant form of circular reasoning. The specificity of the blockade depends on limiting the spread of the local anesthetic to block only the zygapophysis, which would be compromised when local anesthetic spreads to the surrounding structures. Pain relief may occur from blockade of these structures and not only the joint. As mentioned earlier, there may be technical issues in the performance of the block that cloud its outcome, and the placebo response must always be considered.

Because it is often difficult to definitively diagnose facet syndrome, radiological tests have been done to try to correlate radiographic abnormalities with symptoms. There is no correlation with symptoms, CT scans, and response to blocks.[184] In 63 patients with low back pain of more than 3 months and who underwent CT scan and local anesthetic block, there was no correlation between response to block and CT results. In addition, there was poor interobserver agreement between the radiologists interpreting the CT scans. Many patients with severe degenerative changes in the facet joints do not have pain, whereas the CT scan fails to reveal joint pathology in patients who are thought to have the syndrome.

Dolan looked at the value of SPECT (single photon emission computerized tomography) scans in identifying back pain likely to benefit from facet joint injection.[185] Of 58 patients with low back pain, 22 had facetal uptake of isotope on SPECT. Injections of lidocaine and methylprednisolone were then given to patients, i.e., the 22 who had positive scans and the 36 who had negative scans. Pain was assessed by the McGill Pain Questionnaire, Present Pain Intensity Score, and the VAS. At 1 month, all scores were reduced in the scan-positive patients, and at 3 months, the McGill scores were still lower in these patients. The scan-negative patients were no better. The frequency of improvement in scan-positive patients was 95% at 1 month, 79% at 3 months, with no significant difference to scan-negative patients seen at 6 months. Tenderness over the joint and osteoarthritis did not correlate with SPECT findings.

Clinical Pearl: The specificity of the blockade depends on limiting the spread of the local anesthetic to block only the zygapophysis, which would be compromised when local anesthetic spreads to the surrounding structures. Pain relief may occur from blockade of these structures and not only the joint.

Kaplan questioned the ability of lumbar medial branch blocks (MBB) to anesthetize the facet joint.[186] In a study of 18 asymptomatic individuals, contrast was injected into the lumbar facet joints to elicit pain. One week later, 15 subjects returned to undergo either saline or lidocaine MBB to correlate with the joints previously injected to elicit pain. The joints were once again provoked with contrast and the pain response was measured. All subjects who received saline MBB exhibited pain on injection, but eight of nine subjects who received lidocaine felt no pain. Thus, MBB successfully inhibited pain with capsular distension with a rate of 89%.

Facet injections given with local anesthetic, with or without steroid, are usually of short-term duration. The period of relative analgesia can be used to institute a rehabilitative program for the patient, which may lead to long-term improvement. If the patient's symptoms return, they may be under consideration for either facet neurolysis or surgical management. The question arises whether response to facet injection can predict surgical outcome or long-term benefit from radiofrequency neurolysis.

Several published studies that have attempted to correlate facet block with successful relief of pain after surgical fusion have shown unfavorable results. All of these studies are retrospective and most do not consider facet injection as the sole criterion in choosing which patient will have surgery. Lovely performed the first prospective study using MBB as the definitive criteria to chose patients for fusion.[187] A group of 91 patients with chronic low back pain and responsive to bracing underwent 197 facet injections. Of these, 28 patients had greater than 70% pain relief for more than 6 hours on three occasions, and this subgroup proceeded to have surgical fusion. Two other patients who had negative results from MBB also had fusion performed. Postoperatively, Prolo scores and self-assessment were used as outcome measures. Successful fusion was achieved in 23 of 30 patients. Of those with successful results, 19 of 23 had 90% pain relief with MBB, 3 of 23 had 50%–90% partial relief with MBB, and 1 patient had poor pain relief with MBB. Prolo scores improved from 3.9 to 7.7. Although there was no control group of patients who had negative results of facet blocks but underwent surgery anyway, the conclusion was that facet blocks can be used to successfully predict outcome in patients undergoing arthodesis for low back pain.

Percutaneous radiofrequency denervation of the spinal facets was reported by Shealy in 1975.[45] A 12-gauge needle with an electrode was inserted to the facet. Current was applied to test that the spinal nerve root was unaffected, and to stimulate an ache similar to the patient's original pain. A lesion was then done at 80°C. for 150 seconds. Patients were followed for more than 6 months. Of the 207 patients, group 1 consisted unoperated patients (57), group 2 included surgical patients without fusion (60), and group 3 included patients with multiple surgeries, an average of 4, (90 patients). Excellent results were seen as follows: group 1 = 36 of 57, group 2 = 15 of 60, and group 3 = 13 of 90. There was a higher rate of failure in patients who had undergone multiple operations and fusion. In addition to facet neurolysis, Shealy recommended an operant conditioning program with exercise, TENS, and rehabilitation.

Since then, numerous studies have shown the relative efficacy of radiofrequency procedures of the facet joints, although most of these studies have dealt with neck pain and the cervical spine. Lord evaluated percutaneous radiofrequency neurotomy (RFN) for chronic cervical zygapophyseal joint pain.[188] This was a double-blind randomized trial comparing patients who had RFL with multiple lesions at 80°C to a control group in whom a probe was inserted in the neck, but the temperature of the probe was not increased. The study group consisted of 24 patients (9 men and 15 women) with a mean age 43, who had pain of average duration 34 months after a motor vehicle accident. The source of pain was identified with double-blind placebo controlled local anesthetic confirmatory blocks. There were 12 patients in each group, and they were followed until they reported a return of pain to >50% of baseline. The median time elapsed to return of pain was 263 days in the radiofrequency group compared to 8 days in the control. At 27 weeks, 7 patients were free of pain in the radiofrequency group versus 1 patient in the control group. Thus, percutaneous RFN was shown to provide long-term relief in patients after whiplash injury.

McDonald also looked at the success of RFN for control of chronic neck pain in a group of 28 patients.[189] These patients also had controlled local anesthetic blocks, underwent RFN, and RFN was repeated if necessary. Complete relief of pain was initially achieved in 71% of patients. No patient who failed to respond to the first radiofrequency procedure had a good response to a second radiofrequency, but patients who initially responded well to radio frequency had relief reinstituted by a second radio frequency. The median duration of relief after the first procedure was 422 days and more than 219 days after the second procedure, with some patients still having relief when the study was closed. Outcome was not correlated with which operator performed the procedure, the type of electrode used, the litigation status of the patient, or the type of diagnostic block used to establish the diagnosis.

Radiofrequency cervical zygapophyseal joint neurotomy has also been used for the treatment of cervicogenic headache.[190] In this prospective study of 15 patients, outcome was assessed by evaluating the patients 1 week prior to the procedure and afterward for a short term (8 weeks), intermediate term (8.8 months), and long term (16.8 months). Outcome was measured by 100-mm VAS, a seven-point verbal rating scale, the number of headache days per week, and analgesic intake per week. RFN was found to reduce headache severity in 12 of 15 patients (80%) both at short-term and long-term follow-up. Mean VAS decreased 31.4 mm (short term) and 53.5 mm (long term). The average number of headache days decreased from 5.8 to 2.8 days. The average analgesic intake decreased from 17.5 pills to 3.4 pills per week. Although not a randomized trial, these results suggest a positive efficacy of RFN in the treatment of cervicogenic headache.

Radiofrequency denervation has also been studied for lumbar spine pain. Reports show favorable efficacy rates of radiofrequency to placebo, with success rates of 17%–83%.[191] North performed an analysis of prognostic factors in 82 patients who underwent MBB, 42 of whom had percutaneous radiofrequency denervation.[191] Patients were followed for 3.2 +/−2.0 years and 68% had experienced back surgery. Patients were selected for MBB if they had "mechanical" low back pain: pain exacerbated by exertion and prolonged sitting or standing, tenderness over the joints, absence of neurological deficits, absence of nonphysiologic signs, absence of obvious surgical lesions, and absence of posterolateral fusion. Patients had radiofrequency denervation if MBB resulted in more than 50% pain relief and were then assessed by measures including VAS, quality of life, and functional capacity. Of the 42 patients who had radiofrequency denervation, 45% had more than 50% pain relief 2 years later. Of the 40 patients who did not have RFL, 13% had more than 50% spontaneous improvement of pain in 2 years. Patients had improved capacity to perform acitivities of daily living and required fewer medications. Regarding prognostic factors for RFL, there were no factors that could predict long-term results. In particular, there was no association between prior lumbar surgery and success or failure of RFL. North cautioned that reversible blocks are poor predictors of further ablative procedures since MBB blocks are nonspecific and may numb sources of pain other than the joints. North also points out that regeneration of nerves may occur after RFL, deafferentation may exacerbate pain, and the small lesion of radiofrequency may be inadequate compared to the spread of local anesthetic given during the diagnostic block.

There are some negative reports also on outcomes of facet blocks, especially of diagnostic-type procedures with local anesthetic with or without steroid. Raymond pointed out that only 4 of 25 patients with low back pain had improvement with intra-articular facet injections, thereby doubting their usefulness.[192] The study methodology of this report can be questioned in that patient selection was very broad. Nonsurgical, postdiscectomy, fusion, and spondylolisthesis patients were all considered. Also, a very low volume of local anesthetic was used in the joint (<1 mL of 1% lidocaine), questioning whether the joint was adequately anesthetized. Carette's study was similarly flawed in that selection criteria for subjects were broad: all patients with chronic low back pain were included.[193] Intra-articular injections were compared to placebo, but only 20 mg of methylprednisolone was used. Patients were followed for 6 months, a point at which one would not expect to see long-term efficacy from steroid injections for a chronic problem. Both of these studies do not provide any confirmation that the intra-articular injections were actually given into the joint.

The major problem with the use of facet injections and RFL as diagnostic and therapeutic procedures is the likelihood that both neck and back pain are due to multiple causes. Facet syndrome may be accompanied by spondylosis, with narrowed intervertebral foramina, osteophytes, and degenerated intervertebral discs. The nerve supply to all of these structures is multisegmental, no radiological features are specific to chronic pain, and persistent pain can result from all of these. Bogduk performed a study of 318 patients with neck pain that was of a discogenic cause, due to facet syndrome, or a result of the combination of the two.[194] Of the group, 56 patients underwent both diagnostic discography and MBB. The results showed 11 patients had a positive response to discography, 13 had a positive response to MBB, and 23 had positive response to both MBB and discography. Thus, the most frequent outcome was that patients had pain from both sources, with most patients having pain from degeneration of both the discs and the facet joints. Bogduk subsequently concluded that both procedures can have false positive rates (although results of MBB are more specific if controlled double blocks are performed). Discography alone can be falsely positive if the disc is abnormal but not necessarily the only source of the pain, and MBB alone can be falsely positive if the joints are not the only source of pain. The point is made that the decision to proceed with surgery should be a careful one and not only based on the results of such diagnostic tests, since the specificity of these tests can be low.[194]

Epidural Steroid Injections

Epidural steroid injections remain the most commonly utilized pain management procedure. Although there is debate over the long-term pain relief that these injections provide, the evidence supports that these injections give temporary relief from low back pain on the order of several months.[20,195,196] Temporary relief of low back pain allows the original condition causing the pain to subside (i.e., if a herniated disc), creating an opportunity to maximize rehabilitative efforts while the symptoms are minimized and to return the patient to more normal function. McQuay's systematic review of over 15,000 studies evaluating outpatient services for chronic pain control as an outcome confirm that the evidence supports a beneficial short-term effect from ESIs.[197]

Epidural steroid injections have been used for a variety of pain syndromes, including ventral and dorsal compartment pain, segmental pain, epidural adhesions, and spinal stenosis. Although facet injections are the injection of choice for dorsal compartment pain, epidural steroids are often given first and have inconsistent results. Ventral compartment pain syndromes include annular tear and instability of the motion segment. These structures can be numbed by blockade of the sinu-vertebral nerve, the communicating rami, and the sympathetic trunk, but ESIs are a standard initial treatment for these conditions. Annular tears lead to leakage of the nucleus pulposis into the annulus, with symptoms of back pain, possible radiation to the leg with a positive straight leg raise test, and result in a positive discography.

An annular tear can be diagnosed with MRI, CT scanning, or discography. Discography is a powerful tool, being the only test to determine the pain generating level when multiple levels of the spine are diseased. Although false positive results can occur, discography followed by CT scanning is more accurate than CT scanning alone or MRI, which may not be accurate enough to reveal small tears.[198,199] Discography and MRI are equal in diagnosing annular tear, with a concordance rate of over 90%.[200] MRI shows degenerative changes in the disc better than discography, but may not denote an acute annular tear, and cannot determine which disc is the cause of pain if multiple discs are involved. Discography clarifies the relationship between imaging data and pain.

Clinical Pearl: ESIs have been used for a variety of pain syndromes, including ventral and dorsal compartment pain, segmental pain, epidural adhesions, and spinal stenosis. Although facet injections are the injection of choice for dorsal compartment pain, epidural steroids are often given first and have inconsistent results.

Epidural steroid injections have been used for the treatment of segmental nerve irritation, as caused by herniated nucleus pulposis or lateral recess stenosis. Patients will often have a radiating pain to a dermatome, positive straight leg raise, neurological deficit on exam, and radiological confirmation of nerve compression. Radiculopathy can be caused by segmental nerve irritation without compression. Although ESIs have been found to result in good short-term outcomes, studies have had conflicting results.[20,195,197] This may be due to differences in patient selection, different sites of administration, variable volumes of injectate, and the possibility of incorrect needle placement (which may occur in up to 30% of cases).[201] In addition, some studies report results 1 or 2 days after injection, whereas the full effect of the injected steroid may not be apparent for 6–10 days postinjection.

If the relief of the segmental pain syndrome is only temporary following ESIs, some advocate the use of radiofrequency percutaneous partial rhizotomy of the dorsal root ganglion. Although the rate of success is 22%–85%, test blocks have a high false positive rate (and do not predict outcome of neuroablation), and the procedure can be complicated by the development of permanent sensory loss and deafferentation pain.[52] In a study of percutaneous thermal lesioning of the dorsal root ganglion in patients with cervical pain and radiculopathy, there was initial pain relief in 75% of patients, but pain recurred in 33% of subjects.[202] Pain scores on a 0 to 10 point VAS scale decreased from 7.2 to 4.2 at 6 weeks, but over half the patients had vague burning sensations in the dermatome lesioned, all of which subsided by 6 weeks.

Epidural steroid injections are also used for the palliation of spinal stenosis symptoms. Spinal stenosis presents with a variety of pain problems, with either monosegmental or unilateral pain (lateral recess stenosis) or bilateral, multisegmental pain accompanied by recurrent motor/sensory loss, often provoked by walking (neurogenic claudication) and hyperextension. Spinal stenosis may be congenital, due to spondylolisthesis, or due to arthritic proliferation of tissue and osteophytes. The diagnosis is confirmed with CT or MRI, and patients are treated with epidural injections, paravertebral root blocks, and ultimately surgery. Rivest et al.'s study of patients with radiologically confirmed spinal stenosis, who underwent a series of three ESIs, found that about 55% responded with decreased pain and improvement in function.[23]

Epidural adhesions can cause continuous pain, independent of activity, which may radiate to the limb in a mono- or multisegmental manner. Symptoms may occur after a pain-free interval immediately after surgery. Although epidural adhesions are most often associated with "failed" back surgery, they can form after a leak of proteoglycans from a herniated disc. MRI with gadolinium is the gold standard test for diagnosis. Most treatments have poor results. Surgical adhesiolysis often fails to relieve pain, as the adhesions can recur and nerve damage can result. Epidural steroid injections rarely reach the desired location due to thick granulation tissue. Hypertonic saline injections are usually of short-term benefit (only 12.5% had continued improvement after 3–6 months), and can be complicated by the development of neurological problems and cauda equina syndrome.[48,53] The most promising treatment may be SCS, as discussed further below.

There have been several recent reviews of the efficacy of ESIs. Koes compared ESIs with injections of saline, local anesthetics, and dry needling.[20] This study consisted of a review of 12 randomized clinical trials done from 1966 to 1993 with 534 patients having back pain and sciatica. The reviewed trials showed inconsistent results: six studies reported positive benefits and six studies found no benefit from ESIs. In studies with positive benefits, the effects of ESIs seemed to be of short duration only. Carette enrolled 158 patients with sciatica and radiographic evidence of a herniated disc in a randomized, double-blinded, placebo control trial comparing injections of either steroid or normal saline. The outcome measured was functional status as measured by the Oswestry scale.[201] During the first 3 months after the injection, the patients who received steroid injections had less pain and disability compared to patients who recevied placebo. However, after 3 months, there was no significant difference between the patients who received steroids and the patients who received the placebo saline. Other studies have found at least 3 months of pain relief in 60%–90% of patients after ESIs.[204,205] Evaluation of studies to assess efficacy of ESIs are complicated by reports that up to 30% of attempts to place a needle into the epidural space may be unsuccessful.[18]

A French task force in 1999 reviewed and appraised the available randomized trials for the efficacy of ESIs for low back pain and sciatica.[196] Rozenberg's group reviewed all of the relevant randomized trials published up to 1997 based on their methodological quality, results, and clinical implications. Thirteen randomized trials were discovered and were evaluated based on the study population, therapeutic intervention, the evaluation method, and data presentation/analysis. In five trials, there was pain relief within 1 month in the steroid group. In the other eight trials, there were no measurable benefits. Problems that prevent coming to a definitive conclusion include differences in the patient population, the type of steroid used, the volume of the injectate, and the number of injections given.

Selective Spinal Nerve Injections

The injection of steroid into the region of the intervertebral foramen, or near the nerve root that emerges from that foramen, is known as a selective spinal nerve root injection. Other names that are often used interchangeably are paravertebral nerve root block and transforamenal ESI, as the injectate will often flow into the spinal canal and epidural space. Figure 24–9 demonstrates fluoroscopic illustrations of paravertebral nerve root blockade, with the contrast dye in the injectate mixture providing visual confirmation of correct anatomical placement and medial fluid migration along the nerve root. These injections are used as a treatment for patients with low back pain and radicular symptoms. Radiographically, patients may have stenosis of the intervertebral foramen causing nerve root compression and pain. Also, patients who have had back surgery may have scar tissue enveloping a nerve root and causing lower extremity pain. Spinal nerve root injections can be used to deliver steroid directly to this area, especially since steroid given via the standard epidural route may not reach the area that is causing pain in these cases. Although the use of selective nerve blocks may have limited diagnostic value, as pointed out in Chapter 17, and these injections fail to predict the outcome of surgery or neuroablative procedures,[173] they play a key role in the treatment of various spinal syndromes.

Although the use of selective nerve root blockade may yield good pain relief for some patients, these injections have poor specificity, especially in terms of diagnosing the etiology of pain and in terms of predicting results from future surgery.[206] A study by North showed that even if sciatica is relieved by

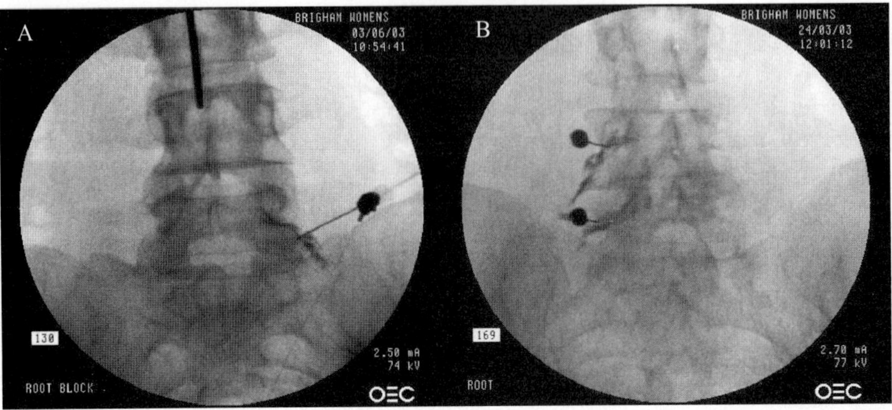

FIGURE 24–9. Paravertebral nerve root blockade. *A.* Fluoroscopic images showing lumbar paravertebral nerve root blockade of the right L-5 nerve root at the L5–S1 intervertebral foramen. A 22-gauge, 3.5 in spinal needle is directed from a paramedian approach to rest within the intervertebral foramen. Contrast dye spreads medially and this is necessary to insure proper positioning of the needle. *B.* This image shows a two level root injection at the L5 and L4 nerve roots on the right side. Again, note the spread of contrast dye medially into the epidural space.

monoradicular lumbar block, dorsal root ganglionectomy does not always provide long-term relief.[207] In addition, the results of dorsal neurotomy are poorly predicted.[208] Thus, the temporary effects of local anesthetic blocks are not maintained with ablative procedures, and diagnostic blocks often fail to predict outcomes of surgical procedures. To test the specificity of nerve blocks, North performed a series of paraspinal selective root blocks, MBB, sciatic nerve blocks, and subcutaneous control blocks in a group of 33 patients with sciatica and back pain.[206] All patients had pain for more than 6 months and three of the following four signs: limited range of motion, paraspinal tenderness, positive straight leg raise, and relief by rest. Nerve root compression was seen by imaging in 52%, neurological deficits were present in 94%, and patients with nonphysiological symptoms were excluded. The findings were that 100% of patients had relief with root blocks and sciatic blocks, and most patients reported relief with MBB. Since 25 out of 33 patients had relief from sciatic blocks even though they had a proximal pain generator, this procedure has a specificity of only 24%. Root blocks alone gave relief in only 9% of patients. The most significant association was that relief by one block yields relief by all others.

Clinical Pearl: Although the use of selective nerve root blockade may yield good pain relief for some patients, these injections have poor specificity, especially in terms of diagnosing the etiology of pain and in terms of predicting results from future surgery.

North confirmed that selective nerve root blocks are nonspecific as localizing tests, as are the other blocks that were done, since pain was relieved whether local anesthetic was given to the site of the pain generator or distally. Other studies have also shown that blocking nerves distal to the pathology can lead to pain relief.[209,210] Because of the physiology of referred pain, with branched primary afferents converging on second order neurons, blocking different inputs can have the same effect on central neurons.[211] As a result, pain can be blocked even if the actual pain generator is not blocked. Thus, a positive response to a single block lacks specificity. North suggests that if the therapeutic decision is one of low morbidity, such as RFL, then one can proceed with the ablative procedure anyway. In fact, the lack of specificity of the block may actually be an advantage, as areas outside of the pain generator that contribute to pain may be blocked beneficially. But, if the therapeutic decision to be made involves a surgically invasive procedure such as spinal fusion or laminectomy, then the risks of falsely positive blocks may be too high. Therefore, negative blocks may be of greater value, more definitively excluding the chance that surgery will be beneficial.[206] Overall, the role of diagnostic blockade should be to confirm (and not to make independently) management decisions.

Regarding the use of paravertebral selective spinal blockades therapeutically, these are used as a substitute for ESIs when clinically appropriate. For example, patients with epidural adhesions may not have an intact epidural space for steroid injection. Especially if patients have monosegmental pain, steroid can be deposited via a paravertebral approach. Clinical experience has confirmed that the efficacy of such injections may be greater. Also, selective nerve root blockade has been used for patients with lateral recess stenosis or osteophytes causing foraminal stenosis. Successful blockade depends on proper localization of the needle near the nerve root, as confirmed by fluoroscopy, paresthesia, or contrast injection. A study of 69 patients with herniated nucleus pulposus and radiculopathy reported >50% pain reduction in 75% of patients after transforamenal steroid injections.[212]

Sympathetic Blocks

Sympathetic blocks, utilized as a pain management modality since the 1940s, have been used to treat peripheral vascular disease, pain after plexus injury, postherpetic neuralgia, and "reflex sympathetic dystrophy," among other conditions.[173] If one sympathetic block relieves pain, the thinking is to perform a series of sympathetic blocks culminating with neurolysis or surgical sympathectomy. Recent reviews have pointed out that the evidence for this approach is lacking.[213]

Several limitations are present in judging the usefulness of sympathetic blocks. The physiological outcome of a sympathetic block is difficult to measure, since tests such as sweat testing, skin resistance, and skin blood flow measurement are cumbersome. Skin temperatures should rise after a sympathetic block, but the results can be variable and the temperature rise may depend on the completeness of the block.[173] For various anatomic reasons, the sympathetic block may be incomplete. Stellate blocks may miss the lower levels of the sympathetic system, the nerve of Kuntz, and the local anesthetic may fail to provide a complete blockade.[214] A common scenario is a complete Horner's syndrome but no warming of the hand. In the lumbar spine, there are contralateral pathways and multisegmental connections. A sympathetic block may not selectively block only the sympathetics, as local anesthetic may spread to the epidural space, along somatic nerves, and interrupt visceral fibers, therefore making it uncertain that pain relief is only due to a sympathectomy.[173] The technical failure rate of sympathetic blocks can approach 40%.[215]

Boas questioned the appropriate use of sympathetic blockade in light of changing ideas of pain mechanisms.[213] In understanding the etiology of neuropathic and inflammatory pain disorders, the contribution of the sympathetic nervous system needs to be reconsidered. To reflect new understandings in pain physiology, the terminology for "reflex sympathetic dystrophy" was renamed as "complex regional pain syndrome" (CRPS). Because only a questionable sympathetic contribution at the dorsal root ganglia can be ascribed to these disorders, sympathetic blocks are inappropriate in determining a clinical diagnosis for a painful condition.[213] Indeed, many patients who fulfill the clinical criteria of CRPS may have pain that does not react to a sympathetic block. On the other hand, sympathetic blocks can still be part of a balanced pain treatment strategy to activate patients to enable functional restoration. The use of sympathetic blocks in the treatment of postherpetic neuralgia has found little evidence showing their effect on long-term pain.[213] For the treatment of ischemic pain, neurolytic/thermal sympathectomies can provide about 50% improvement in long-term blood flow with decreased pain and decreased ulceration in patients with peripheral vascular disease.[216]

Sympathetic blocks for low back pain have been advocated for use in the diagnosis and treatment of ventral pain syndromes.[52] By blocking the sinuvertebral nerve, the rami communicantes, and the sympathetic trunk, pain from annular tear, vertebral compression fractures, and injury to the anterior and posterior longitudenal ligaments can be relieved. Diagnostic sympathetic blocks are difficult to achieve since the volume of local anesthetic may spread. Blockade of the sinuvertebral nerve is the optimal block for the ventral compartment, but selective block is difficult due to overflow to communicating rami and spinal nerves. Neurolytic blocks can also leak to the epidural space and somatic nerves. Radiofrequency lesions may not completely denervate the sympathetic trunk.

Intrathecal Infusion Therapy

Intrathecal opioid therapy was first provided in 1979,[217] and since then has been shown to provide analgesia for both cancer and noncancer pain with fewer side effects than equianalgesic doses of systemic opioids. Various studies have been done to determine efficacy, looking at the balance between analgesia and side effects. Outcome measures studied include patient satisfaction, the need for additional analgesic medications, improvements in activities of daily living parameters and function, quality of life, and work status.

In a retrospective analysis of 51 patients who were receiving long-term intrathecal infusions of morphine and morphine/bupivacaine for the treatment of cancer pain, both pain relief and the incidence of complications was studied.[218] Patients were taking maximal doses of systemic analgesics with inadequate pain control or intolerable side effects and had exhausted treatment with co-analgesics and antitumor therapy. Lumbar catheters were placed and tunneled subcutaneously. Patients received morphine 0.5–1 mg/mL and 17 patients also received bupivacaine 1.5–3 mg/mL. Although patients required increasing doses of morphine during the first 20 days, requirements were stable later and only slowly increased toward the end of life. Most patients continued to take variable doses of systemic morphine and co-analgesics. Of the 17 patients who had poor relief with IT morphine and required the addition of bupivacaine, 58% achieved good pain relief and only 3 had poor pain relief. The initial bupivacaine dose was 10–15 mg/day, rising to up to 31 mg/day. Side effects included nausea (21%), PDPH (10%), catheter dislodgement (8%), and local infection (2%). With bupivacaine doses of 30 mg/mL, there were no motor or sensory changes, and orthostatic hypotension was not an issue.

Clinical Pearl: Intrathecal opioid therapy was first provided in 1979, and since then has been shown to provide analgesia for both cancer and noncancer pain with fewer side effects than equianalgesic doses of systemic opioids.

A prospective study of long-term intrathecal morphine use in the management of chronic nonmalignant pain was done by Anderson.[219] Of the 40 patients who had severe nonmalignant pain unresponsive to systemic medications, 30 had successful pain relief following a trial of intrathecal morphine. These patients were implanted with intrathecal pumps, and their pain and functional status were assessed pre- and postimplant to 24 months, as were the opioid and device-related complications. Patients had a mean age of 58 +/−13 years, with a pain duration of 8 +/−9 years. Mixed pain was present in 15 of 30, neuropathic in 10 of 30, deafferentation pain in 4 of 30, and nociceptive pain in 1 of 30 patients. Previous back surgery had been performed in 47% of patients. After implant, the VAS score improved in 50% of patients, with 11 of 22 reporting at least a 25% reduction in VAS at 24 months. In addition, improvements were seen in the McGill Pain Questionaire, functional status, pain coping, and the Chronic Illness Problem Inventory. Pharmacological side effects were managed with changes in the dose of morphine, adding bupivacaine, or switching to a different opioid such as hydromorphone. Device complications requiring surgery occurred in 20% of patients.

The efficacy and complications of intrathecal therapy for nonmalignant pain were also evaluated with regards to the type of approach used (epidural/intrathecal), the drug given (opioid/opioid–bupivacaine/bupivacaine), and the type of catheter (externalized/internalized).[220] Groups were analyzed for efficacy of pain relief, failures, and the rate of technical complications. Intrathecal catheters were found to have a higher rate of satisfactory pain relief than epidural catheters (externalized: 95% vs. 42.5%) (internalized: 89% vs. 59%). There was a higher rate of treatment failure with externalized epidural catheters (59%) compared to internalized IT catheters (11%). There was a higher rate of treatment failures with internalized epidural catheters (38%) than internalized IT catheters (11%). System removal occurred in 45% of internalized epidural catheters compared to 10% of internalized IT catheters. Finally, there was a higher rate of catheter complications with epidural versus IT catheters (dislodgement: 10% vs. 4%) (leaking: 10% vs. 0.9%).

Nitescu looked at the use of continuous opioid and bupivacaine combinations in nonmalignant pain via externalized intrathecal catheters.[221] Ninety patients, 20-to 96-years-old, with pain of 0.3–50 years duration were included in the study when pain dominated their lives, other methods had failed to achieve relief, or unacceptable systemic opioid side effects occurred. Patients had mostly mixed neuropathic and nociceptive pain and received intrathecal morphine 0.5 mg/mL with bupivacaine 4.75–5 mg/mL at infusion rates of 0.2 mL/h with bolus doses of 0.1 mL, one to four times per hour. Rates were increased or decreased to give the best results. Outcomes were measured by pain intensity, pain relief, medication use, and rates of adverse effects. During the IT period (3–1706 days), 95% of patients received adequate pain relief (60%–100%). Nocturnal sleep increased from 4 to 7 hours. Nonopioid analgesic consumption was two times lower. There were no problems with gait or ambulation. Treatment failed in 29 of 85 patients, whereas 23 of 85 died (not attributable to the therapy), and 32 of 85 had good pain control. Principal side effects included bradypnea (1 patient), paresthesia (26 patients), paresis (16 patients), temporary urinary retention (34 patients), episodic hypotension (11 patients), and 5 patients attempted suicide (3 successfully).

Two other retrospective studies looked at the efficacy of intrathecal pain therapy. Paice studied 429 patients, 42% who had failed back syndrome and 31% who had cancer.[222] Pain relief was reported by physicians to be excellent in 52%, good in 42%, and poor in 5%. The mean morphine dose at 1 year was 9.2 mg/day. Improvements in activities of daily living were seen in 82% of patients, but only 28 patients returned to work. Delivery system complications occurred in 21.6% of patients, with medication complications being nausea/vomiting (25%), pruritis (13%), and decreased libido (5%). The methodologic flaws of this survey report include observer bias, reporting bias, and unknown generalizations. Winkelmuller reported on 120 noncancer patients in whom pain was reduced, 79% at their 12-month follow-up.[223] Patients' level of activity, mood, and sleep habits were improved. Most patients had mixed nociceptive/neuropathic pain after failed back surgery and had failed conservative therapies. Morphine was well tolerated, with a starting dose of 2.7 mg/day increasing 1.6–2-fold during the year, with three patients experiencing rapid dose escalation. Side effects from morphine included early nausea/vomiting, pruritis, constipation, urinary retention, and loss of libido.

Technical problems necessitated the replacement of 16.8% of pumps. Key complications were pocket infection (2 patients), CSF leak (5 patients), and desire for explant (6 patients).

Complications from intrathecal morphine are the same as with systemic morphine, and most resolve within a few days, with the exception of constipation. In Paice's study, pruritis occured 13.3% of the time and responded to antihistamine drugs.[222] Nausea and vomiting occured in 30% of opioid-naive patients and was relieved with antiemetics. Urinary retention had an incidence of 42%–80%, happening mostly in older men. Urinary retention is caused by the opioid binding to spinal opioid receptors in the sacral canal and responds to terazocin. Constipation is due to prolonged intestinal transit time and can be treated with laxatives. Decreased libido has been found in a number of patients. Opioids are known to decrease testosterone levels and decrease penile erections. Miscellaneous effects from intrathecal opioids include peripheral edema from vasopressin release from cephalad migration of the opioid in the CSF and persistent sweating, which may be due to interactions of opioids in the hypothalamus.

Technical complications associated with implantation of intrathecal delivery systems include bleeding, infection, CSF leaks, seroma formation, and mechanical problems with the pump.[224] Bleeding is rare, but uncorrected coagulopathy is a contraindication to pump placement, and cauda equina syndrome can result. Infection occurs mostly in the surgical pocket, often necessitating explant. Epidural and intrathecal infections are rare, presenting with stiff neck, fever, and meningeal stretch signs. Since low grade fever and meningeal signs may occur as a normal phenomenon in some patients after implant, if a complete blood count (CBC) and a CSF gram stain are normal, the patient can be watched expectantly. CSF leaks cause postdural puncture headaches 15–20% of the time, sometimes requiring blood patch.[225] Subcutaneious CSF hygromas are usually self-limited and resolve in 1–2 weeks. Seromas can last for several months, and are often treated symptomatically with an abdominal binder. Mechanical complications happen 8.5% of the time and include catheter breaking and kinking, as well as battery failure, pump failure, programming errors, and drug-dosing errors.[226]

Intrathecal and epidural analgesia has also been used for cardiac surgery.[227] The ability of spinal techniques to control pain and diminish the stress response associated with surgery may decrease morbidity of high-risk patients. Intrathecal and epidural analgesia can result in profound pain control, stress response attenuation, and thoracic cardiac sympathectomy, decreasing the incidence and severity of myocardial ischemia. The stress response can be inhibited by infusion of local anesthetic/opioid mixtures. Epidural and intrathecal local anesthetics can block thoracic sympathetics, increase the diameter of stenotic coronary artery segments, decrease myocardial oxygen demand, improve left ventricular function, and decrease angina.

Epidural clonidine has been found to be effective for the treatment of cancer pain.[67] Although most patients with cancer pain receive adequate analgesia from standard systemic therapies, patients with neuropathic pain may experience severe pain in spite of maximal doses of systemic or spinal opiates. In this study, 85 such patients were randomized to receive clonidine epidurally 30 mcg/h compared to placebo, with rescue doses of epidural morphine made available. Outcome was assessed by VAS scores, the McGill Pain Questionaire, and daily morphine consumption. Analgesia was successful in 45% of the clonidine patients compared to 21% of patients receiving placebo. For patients with neuropathic pain, clonidine was successful in 56% compared to 5%. Main side effects were decreased blood pressure and heart rate.

Another intrathecal therapy shown to be efficacious for the treatment of chronic pain is intrathecal baclofen. Intrathecal baclofen is used for the treatment of chronic medically intractable spasticity and rigidity in patients with spinal cord injuries, stroke, and multiple sclerosis. Increased motor tone can cause difficulty with sitting, transfers, and hygiene, and it can be painful. Standard muscle relaxants, which include dantrolene, diazepam, baclofen, and tizanidine, can cause intolerable side effects and toxicity. Intrathecal baclofen can control spasticity while preserving function and help the patient avoid destructive procedures.

The seminal study by Coffey on intrathecal baclofen reported on 93 patients screened for intrathecal baclofen.[228] Patients received a trial dose of placebo or baclofen, 50–75–100 mcg. If the Ashworth scale of spasticity decreased 2 points, and if muscle spasm was noted to decrease without intolerable side effects, a pump was implanted. Thus, 88 patients (94.6%) responded to the trial injections, and a total of 75 had a pump implanted. Patients were then followed for 19 months. No patients died during this time, and there were no neurological deficits related to baclofen. The Ashworth scale dropped from 3.9 to 1.7, and muscle spasm scores decreased from 3.1 to 1.0. The daily dose of baclofen increased from 187 to 405 mcg during the 19-month period. Six patients had "tolerance" develop, with rapidly escalating doses, managed with a 3–37-day holiday from IT baclofen. Complications included mechanical failure (3 cases), wound complications (6 cases), catheter malfunctions (22 cases), drug complications (9 cases), seizures (2 cases), respiratory depression (2 cases), and sedation (2 cases).

Spinal Cord Stimulation

Spinal cord stimulation is a modality that has been used for over 30 years, and there have been many reports on its effectiveness for certain conditions. However, prospective studies with good methodology are still lacking to prove its efficacy.[229] Although advances in technology have increased the success rate of SCS, the results depend on careful patient selection. There are four major conditions for which SCS is used: Failed back surgery with radiculopathy, angina pectoris, neuropathic pain, and peripheral vascular disease.

The most common indication for SCS in the United States is for the failed back surgery syndrome.[230] In order to be considered for this modality, patients must first exhaust medical treatment, not be surgical candidates, have psychological clearance, and exhibit pain relief with a temporary electrode trial. Patients with radicular pain and epidural fibrosis respond the best. Most studies since 1990 show 55%–80% success rates.[230] North reviewed 20 years of experience with SCS and found that 52% of patients had >50% relief of pain, 58% had reduced intake of analgesics, and most patients had increased activity levels.[231] Fiume reported 56% of patients had >50% improvement in pain, with a 55 month follow-up.[232] There was a decrease in analgesic consumption and 29% of patients returned to work. Turner reported on 39 nonrandomized trials of patients who had implantation of spinal cord stimulators for low back pain or failed back surgery syndrome.[62] Most studies were case series, with 29 reporting at least 50% pain relief as an outcome and 59% of patients achieving this outcome. At 1 year, 14 studies reported a success rate of 62%, and at 5 years, 3 studies reported a mean success rate of 53%.

Burchiel conducted a prospective multicenter study of SCS for relief of chronic back and extremity pain.[55] Data were collected on 70 patients with a 1-year follow-up, with pain, quality of life, and functional measures examined pre- and postimplant. Overall, 219 patients in six centers were recruited. All patients underwent a trial of SCS before implantation, and most patients were screened psychologically. Of the 182 patients implanted, at 1-year follow-up, data were available on 70 patients, 88% of whom had pain in the back and legs. In these patients, all pain and quality of life measures improved during the treatment year. There was improvement in the McGill Pain Questionnaire, the Oswestry Disability Questionnaire, the Sickness Impact Profile, and the Beck Depression Inventory scales. The criteria for success was determined as >50% pain relief. As such, 55% of patients had success with SCS at 1 year, although there was no influence on medication usage or work status. There was a 17% incidence of complications requiring repeat surgery.

Clinical Pearl: The most common indication for SCS in the United States is the failed back surgery syndrome.

Spinal cord stimulation has been used to treat various neuropathic pain problems, including peripheral nerve injury, CRPS, phantom limb, spinal cord lesions with segmental pain, postherpetic neuralgia, and others. Most studies have found improvements in pain, use of analgesics, and return to work.[230] Barolat evaluated patients with CRPS who had undergone sympathetic nerve blocks or sympathectomy and who had SCS performed.[233] Of the 13 patients, 10 had decreased pain and decreased swelling of the extremity. Sanchez-Ledesma reported that of 49 patients with deafferentation pain, 57% had >75% relief with SCS.[234] Studies have also found improvement with SCS in patients with CRPS or RSD/causalgia (91% improvement), phantom limb (33% better), plexus avulsion (50% better), vascular pain (73% better), and somatic pain (27% better).[230]

NERVE BLOCKS, OUTCOMES, THE LAW OF DIMINISHING RETURNS, AND PATIENT EXPECTATIONS

Ever since Bonica observed that analgesic blocks resulted in prolonged pain relief in some patients, the role of nerve blocks in pain management has been under scrutiny.[170] In spite of thousands of procedures that have been done over the past 50 years to treat chronic pain, there are few well-conducted controlled trials. Nerve blocks are often performed based on clinical intuition and not on well-studied scientific research.

In McQuay's review of outpatient services for chronic pain control, the database was searched of over 15,000 studies and 150 reviews that look at pain as an outcome.[197] Review of the literature based on methodological quality allowed conclusions to be drawn for only two neural blockade procedures: ESI and SCS. With ESI, a positive short-term effect on outcome was seen, whereas for SCS, there was a lack of evidence for a definite beneficial outcome, in spite of the fact that some studies indicate that "50% pain relief in 50% of patients at 5 years" occurs.

Since it is often difficult to identify the source of pain, Pang proposed the application of spinal pain mapping in the diagnosis of low back pain.[235] Pain mapping involves a sequence of well-organized nerve block procedures to see which nerve block yields the best results in a patient. A group of 104 patients with intractable back pain were evaluated, examined, and 39% had either CT, MRI, or EMG done. Since the diagnosis remained uncertain, and the patients failed to respond to conservative therapies, a sequence of nerve blocks was conducted. Based on the results of the blocks, the source of pain was found to be sacroiliac (6%), lumbar nerve root (20%), facet joint (24%), combined root/facet (24%), internal disc disorder (7%), facet/SI (4%), sympathetically-mediated (2%), and still unknown (13%). The authors concluded that spinal pain mapping helped them determine the etiology of low back pain in 87% of patients. This type of method needs to be scrutinized carefully in light of North's findings[206] on the general lack of specificity of nerve blocks in the diagnosis of pain.

For many patients in pain centers, there seems to be a diminution of success from each successive treatment that is instituted. Although this phenomenon may not occur when different medications are tried, when multiple nerve blocks are given, there seems to be diminishing success with each successive procedure.[236] This is yet another important factor to consider in a pain center, where treatments and options can seem to continue indefinitely, often with poor results. How does one answer the question for which patient to deny access to multiple therapies and when to stop interventions?

Finally, both patient and physician expectation may play a role in predicting the response to pain-relieving procedures.[171] In a prospective study of 46 patients, the relationship between patient and physician expectations of pain relief and subsequent pain relief was investigated. Patients were given either IV drug infusions or underwent nerve blocks, and their pre- and postprocedure pain and pain relief ratings were assessed. The study found that patient expectations did not correlate with postprocedure pain relief, while physician expectations of pain relief indeed were a predictor of pain relief ratings and changes in pain intensity. According to Galer, physicians can subtly communicate their expectations to patients, a factor which may influence patient response to nerve blocks. This type of treatment effect may be difficult to study.

As many investigators have pointed out, determining outcomes from nerve block procedures can be complicated by numerous factors that give false results.[52,170,173,206] False positive results from nerve injections can occur due to a high volume of local anesthetic spreading to sensory nerves, local anesthetic systemic absorption causing analgesia, systemic analgesic use, high volumes of local anesthetic used to anesthetize the overlying muscles and skin, physician bias, and a placebo response that may be seen in as many as 30% of patients. False negative results from a nerve injection can occur in cases of incorrect needle placement, inadequate injectate volume, traumatic technique, and patient anxiety and negative expectations. These types of variables, which affect sensitivity and specificity, should be considered in the performance of neural blockade in pain management.

Nerve blocks will continue to have a role in pain management, but practitioners need to understand their limitations. Raja points out several more confounding factors.[170] Often, the origin of nociception is not known and stimulation of adjacent nerves can cause pain. Therefore, there is a risk of misinterpreting diagnostic blocks. Changing concepts of pain mechanisms point out the hazards of diagnosing pain by sympathetic blocks, which exposes patients to further unnecessary injections. In assessing outcomes from neural blockade, there are problems with selecting appropriate pain measurement scales, avoiding observer error, accounting for the placebo effect, dealing with the bias of the patient's expectations, and issues with insuring impeccable procedural technique. Also, psychophysiological conditions such as anxiety, expectations, and learning may influence results.[170]

CONCLUSION

In order to have success in the management of pain caused by spinal syndromes, a reliable differential diagnosis must first be made. It is important to realize that because of the multisegmental innervation of the spine, complete denervation is impossible. Nonetheless, there are a variety of management options for patients who suffer from one or more of the common conditions causing pain from spinal syndromes. For some conditions, strong evidence exists to support the use of a particular neural blockade procedure, whereas for other conditions the data are incomplete. In such cases, clinicians rely on their collective clinical judgment so that patients will benefit.

Finally, there are certain patients who can be predicted to have a poor outcome from procedural approaches. Many of these will benefit from a full multidisciplinary approach. In order to better manage pain, one must also understand the role of psychosocial issues, which may perpetuate suffering, and the effectiveness of multimodal therapy and multidisciplinary treatments.

As part of a comprehensive multidisciplinary pain management program, physical modalities, acupuncture, and manual techniques and exercise may be useful for many patients with back pain. In order to provide the best results for patients, a combination of treatments is often required. Some patients can be treated simply with manual techniques, exercise prescriptions, medications, and/or neural blockade techniques. Others will require more long-term multidisciplinary management, requiring the teamwork of clinicians in a variety of specialties to provide the optimal formula for their challenging and unfortunate disease state.

SUMMARY

1. This chapter provide a comprehensive review of the minimally invasive procedures used to treat spinal pain syndromes.
2. These include spinal injection therapies, spinal neuromodulation techniques, extraspinal injection therapies, and other minimally invasive procedures for discogenic and vertebral pain syndromes.
3. The chapter also reviewed outcome studies on minimally invasive spinal procedural therapies, with a focus on facet injections, radiofrequency lesioning, epidural steroid injections, spinal nerve root injections, sympathetic blocks, intrathecal infusion therapy, and spinal cord stimulation.
4. An overview of the challenges and problems inherent in studying outcomes of neural blockade procedures have been explained.

KEY REFERENCES

Waldman SD, Winnie AP, eds. *Interventional pain management*. Philadelphia: W.B. Saunders, 1996:40, 42, 194, 292, 412–422.

Moore KL, ed. *Clinically oriented anatomy*. Baltimore, MD: Williams and Wilkins, 1980:613.

Bonica JJ, ed. *The management of pain*. Philadelphia: Lea and Febiger, 1990:1397.

Kline MT. *stereotactic radiofrequency lesions as part of the mananagement of pain*. Orlando, FL: Paul M. Deutsch Press, 1992:1–23.

Cousins MJ, Bridenbaugh PO. *Neural blockade*, 2nd ed. Philadelphia: J.B. Lippincott, 1988:253–274.

REFERENCES

1. Robecchi A, Capia R. L'idiocortisone (composto F). Prime experienze cliniche in campo reumatologica. *Minerva Med* 1952;98:1259–1263.
2. Goebert HW, Jallo SJ, Gardner WJ, Asmuth CE. Painful radiculopathy treated with epidural injections of procaine and hydrocortisone acetate: Results in 113 patients. *Anesth Analg* 1961;40:130–134.
3. McCarron FR, Wimpee MW, Hudkins PG, et al. The inflammatory effect of nucleus pulposus: A possible element in the pathogenesis of low back pain. *Spine* 1987;12:760–764.
4. Dirosa M, Calignano A, Carnuccio R, Ialenti A, Sautebin L. Multiple control of inflammation by glucocorticoids. *Agents Actions* 1985;17:284–289.
5. Saal JS, Franson RC, Dobrow R, et al. High levels of inflammatory phospholipase A-2 activity in lumbar disc herniations. *Spine* 1990;15:674–678.
6. Flower RJ, Blackwell GJ. Anti-inflammatory steroids induce biosynthesis of a phospholipase A2 inhibitor which prevents prostaglandin generation. *Nature* 1979;278:456–459.
7. Devor M, Govrin-Lippmann R, Raber P. Corticosteroids suppress ectopic neural discharges originating in experimental neuromas. *Pain* 1985;22:127–137.
8. Johansson A, Bennett GJ. Effect of local methylprednisolone on pain in a nerve injury model: A pilot study. *Reg Anesth* 1997;22:59–65.
9. Johansson A, Hao J, Sjolund B. Local corticosteroid application blocks transmission in normal nociceptive C-fibers. *Acta Anaesthesiol Scand* 1990;34:335–338.
10. Katz, J. Lumbar epidural nerve block, paramedian approach. In: *Atlas of regional anesthesia*, 2nd ed. Appleton & Lange Publishers, Norwalk, CT 1994:191.
11. Katz, J. Lumbar epidural nerve block, paramedian approach. In: *Atlas of regional anesthesia*, 2nd ed. Appleton & Lange Publishers, Norwalk, CT 1994:133.
12. Bogduk N. Back pain: Zygapophysial blocks and epidural steroids. In: Cousins MJ, Bridenbaugh PO, eds. *Neural blockade in clinical anesthesia and management of pain*, 2nd ed. Philadelphia: JB Lippincott, 1988: 935–954.
13. Lindholm R, Salenius P. Caudal, epidural administation of anaesthetics and corticoids in the treatment of low back pain. *Acta Orthop Scand* 1964;1:114.
14. Cappio M. Il trattemento idrocortisonico per via epidurale sacrale delle lombosciatalgie. *Reumatismo* 1957;9:60.
15. Carron H. The changing role of the anesthesiologist in pain management. *Reg Anesth* 1989;14:4–9.
16. Pearce J, Moll JMH. Conservative treatment and natural history of acute lumbar disc lesions. *J Neurol Neurosurg Psychiatry* 1967;30:13–17.
17. Green LN. Dexamethasone in the management of symptoms due to herniated lumbar disc. *J Neurol Neurosurg Psychiatry* 1975;38:1211–1217.
18. Saal JA, Saal JS. Non operative treatment of herniated lumbar intervertebral disc with radiculopathy: An outcome study. *Spine* 1989;14:431–437.
19. Weber J. Lumbar disc herniation: A controlled prospective study with 10 years of observation. *Spine* 1983;8:131–140.
20. Koes BW, Scholten RJ, Mens J, Bouter LM. Efficacy of epidural steroid injections for low back pain and sciatica: A systematic review of randomized clinical trials. *Pain* 1995;63:179–288.
21. Beliveau P. A comparison between epidural anesthesia with and without corticosteroid in the treatment of sciatica. *Rheumatol Phys Med* 1971;11:4–43.
22. Hopwood MG, Abram SE. Factors associated with failure of lumbar epidural steroids. *Reg Anesth* 1993; 18:238–243.
23. Rivest C, Katz JN, Ferrante FM, Jamison RN. Effects of epidural steroid injections on pain due to lumbar spinal stenosis or herniated discs: A prospective study. *Arthritis Care Res* 1998;11:291–297.
24. Albright GA. Lumbar epidural anesthesia. In: *Anesthesia in obstetrics: Maternal, fetal and neonatal aspects*. Menlo Park, CA: Addison Wesley, 1978:224–246.
25. Benzon HT, Braunschweig R, Molloy RE, et al. Postdural puncture headache in patients with chronic pain. *Anesth Analg* 1980;60:874–877.

26. Cousins MJ, Bromage PR. Epidural neural blockade. In: Cousins MJ, Bridenbaugh PO, eds. *Neural blockade in clinical anesthesia and management of pain*, 2nd ed. Philadelphia: JB Lippincott, 1988:253–360, 266.
27. Plummer JL et al. Long-term spinal administration of morphine in cancer and non-cancer pain: A retrospective study. *Pain* 1991;44:215–220.
28. Ling C, Atkinson PL, Munton CGF. Bilateral retinal haemorrhages following epidural injection. *Br J Opthalmol* 1993;77:316–317.
29. Purdy EP, Ajimal GS. Vision loss after lumbar epidural steroid injection. *Anesth Analg* 1998;86:119–122.
30. National Health and Medical Research Council (NHMRC) of the government of Australia. Canberra, ACT, Australia. 1994. *Epidural use of steroids in the management of back pain and sciatica of spinal origin*. 1994.
31. Nelson DA. Dangers from methlyprednisolone acetate therapy by intraspinal injection. *Arch Neurol* 1988;45:804–806.
32. Sehgal AD, Gardener WJ. Corticosteroids administered intradurally for relief of sciatica. *Cleve Clin J Med* 1960;27:198–201.
33. Boines GJ. Remissions in multiple sclerosis following intrathecal methylprednisolone acetate. *Del Med J* 1961;33:231–235.
34. Van Buskirk L, Poffenbarger AL, Capriles LF, et al. Treatment of multiple sclerosis with intrathecal steroids. *Neurology (Minneap)* 1964;14:595–597.
35. Cohen FL. Conus medullaris syndrome following intrathecal corticosteroid injections. *Arch Neurol* 1979;36:228–230.
36. MacKinnon SE, Hudson AR, Gentili F, et al. Peripheral nerve injection injury with steroid agents. *Plast Reconstr Surg* 1982;69:482–489.
37. Shantha TR, Evans JA. The relationship of epidural anesthesia to neural membranes and arachnoid villi. *Anesthesiology* 1976;5:543–557.
38. Abram SE, O'Connor TC. Complications associated with epidural steroid injections. *Reg Anesth* 1996;21:149–162.
39. Sehgal AD, Tweed DC, Gardner WJ, et al. Laboratory studies after intrathecal corticosteroids. *Arch Neurol* 1963;9:74–78.
40. Edmonds LC, Vance ML, Hughes JM. Morbidity from paraspinal depo corticosteroid injections for analgesia: Cushing's syndrome and adrenal suppression. *Anesth Analg* 1991;72:820–822.
41. Knight CL, Burnell JC. Systemic side effects of extradural steroids. *Anaesthesia* 1980;35:593–594.
42. Manning DC, Rowlingson JC. Back pain and the role of neural blockade. In: Cousins MJ, Bridenbaugh PO, eds. *Neural blockade in Clinical Anesthesia and Management of Pain*, 3rd ed. Philadelphia: Lippincott-Raven, 1998:879–914.
43. Smith et al. Radiofrequency neurolysis in a clinical model. *J Neurosurg* 1981;55:246–253.
44. Organ LW. Electrophysiologic principles of radiofrequency lesion making. *Appl Neurophysiol* 1976–1977; 39:139–153.
45. Shealy CN. Percutaneous radiofrequency denervation of spinal facets. *J Neurosurg* 1975;43:448–451.
46. Burton C. Percutaneous radiofrequency facet denervation. *Appl Neurophysiol* 1976–1977;39:80–86.
47. Kline MT. Clinical use of radiofrequency procedures in the treatment of disorders of the lumbar spine. In: Kline MT, ed. *Stereotactic radiofrequency lesions as part of the management of pain*. Orlando, FL: Paul M. Deutsch Press, 1992:10–14.
48. Racz, GB, Heaver JE, Raj PP. Nonsurgical management of spinal radiculopathy by the use of lysis of adhesions (neuroplasty). In: Aronoff GM, ed. *Evaluation and treatment of chronic pain*, 3rd ed. Baltimore, MD: Williams and Wilkins, 1999:533–542.
49. Kuslich SD, Ulstrom CL, Michael CJ. The tissue origin of low back pain and sciatica. *Orthop Clin North Am* 1991;22:181–187.
50. Racz GB, Heavner JE, Diede JH. Lysis of epidural adhesions utilizaing the epidural approach. In: Waldman SD, Winnie AP, eds. *Interventional pain management*. Philadelphia: Dannemiller Memorial Educational Foundation, W.B. Saunders, 1996:339–351.
51. Lewandowski EM. The efficacy of solutions used in caudal neuroplasty. *Pain Digest* 1997;7:323–330.
52. Stolker RJ, Vervest ACM, Gerbrand JG. The management of chronic pain by blockades: A review. *Pain* 1994;58:1–19.
53. Arthur J, Racz G, Heinrich R, et al. Epidural space: Identification of filling defects and lysis of adhesions in the treatment of chronic painful conditions. In: *Abstracts of the 7th World Congress on Pain*. Paris: IASP Publications, 1993.
54. Cherny NI, Portenoy RK. The management of cancer pain. *CA Cancer J Clin* 1994;44:262–303.
55. Burchiel KJ, Anderson VC, Brown FD, et al. Prospective, multicenter study of spinal cord stimulation for relief of chronic back and extremity pain. *Spine* 1996;21:2786–2794.
56. Melzack R, Wall PD. Pain mechanisms: A new theory. *Science* 1965;150:971–979.
57. Barolat G. Epidural spinal cord stimulation: Anatomical and electrical properties of the intraspinal structures relevant to spinal cord stimulation and clinical correlations. *Neuromodulation* 1998;1:63–71.
58. Roberts M, Rees H. The physiological basis of spinal cord stimulation. *Pain Rev* 1994;1:184–198.
59. Meyerson BA, Linderoth B. Mechanisms of spinal cord stimulation on neuropathic pain. *Neurol Res* 2000;22:285–292.
60. North RB, Ewend MG, Lawton MT, Kidd DH, Piantadosi S. Failed back surgery syndrome: 5-year follow-up after spinal cord stimulator implantation. *Neurosurgery* 1991;28:692–699.
61. Broseta J, Barbera J, de Vera JA, et al. Spinal cord stimulation in peripheral arterial disease: A cooperative study. *J Neurosurg* 1986;64:71–80.
62. Turner JA, Loeser JD, Bell KG. Spinal cord stimulation for chronic low back pain: A systematic literature synthesis. *Neurosurgery* 1995;37:1088–1096.
63. Burchiel K, Anderson VC, Wilson BJ, et al. Prognostic factors of spinal cord stimulation for chronic back and leg pain. *Neurosurgery* 1995;36:1101–1111.

64. Kumar K, Nath R, Wyant GM. Treatment of chronic pain by epidural spinal cord stimulation: A 10-year experience. *J Neurosurg* 1991;75:402–407.
65. De La Porte C, Van de Kelft EV. Spinal cord stimulation in failed back surgery syndrome. *Pain* 1993;52:55–61.
66. Kumar K, Wyant GM, Ekong CEU. Epidural spinal cord stimulation for relief of chronic pain. *Pain Clinic* 1986;1:91–99.
67. Eisenach JC, De Kock M, Klimscha W. ·Alpha 2-adrenergic agonists for regional anesthesia—A clinical review of clonidine (1984–1995). *Anesthesiology* 1996;85:655–674.
68. Katz, J. Lumbar epidural nerve block, paramedian approach. In: *Atlas of regional anesthesia*, 2nd ed. Appleton & Lange Publishers, Norwalk, CT 1994:183.
69. Waldman SD, Leak DW, Kennedy LD, Patt RB. Intraspinal opioid therapy. In: Patt RB, ed. *Cancer pain.* Philadelphia: JB Lippincott, 1993:285–328.
70. Blount JP, Remley KB, Yue SK, Erickson DL. Intrathecal granuloma complicating chronic spinal infusion of morphine: Report of three cases. *J Neurosurg* 1996;84(2):272–276.
71. Bejjani GK, Karim NO, Tzortzidis F. Intrathecal granuloma after implantation of a morphine pump: Case report and review of the literature. *Surg Neurol* 1997; 48(3):288–291.
72. Cabbell KL, Taren JA, Sagher O. Spinal cord compression by catheter granulomas in high-dose intrathecal morphine therapy: Case report. *Neurosurgery* 1998;42(5):1176–1181.
73. Edwards WT, DeGirolami U, Burney RG, et al. Histopathologic changes in the epidural space of the guinea pig during long-term morphine infusion. *Reg Anesth* 1986;11:14.
74. De Jong RC, Kansen PJ. A comparison of epidural catheters with or without subcutaneous injection ports for treatment of cancer pain. *Anesth Analg* 1994; 78:94–100.
75. Wang JS, Fellows DG, Vakharia S, Rosenbaum AE, Thomas PS. Epidural abscess —Early magnetic resonance imaging detection and conservative therapy. *Anesth Analg* 1996;82:1069–1071.
76. Travell JG, Simons DG. *Myofascial pain and dysfunction: The trigger point manual.* Baltimore, MD: Williams and Wilkins, 1983.
77. Garvey TA, Marks MR, Wiesel SW. A prospective, randomized, double-blind evaluation of trigger point injection therapy for low back pain. *Spine* 1989;14:962–964.
78. Hong CZ. Lidocaine injection versus dry needling to myofascial trigger points: The importance of local twitch response. *Am J Phys Med Rehabil* 1994;73:256–263.
79. Aronoff GM, Gallagher RM. Pharmacologic management of chronic pain: A review. In: Aronoff GM, ed.*Evaluation and treatment of chronic pain,* 3rd ed. Baltimore, MD: Williams and Wilkins, 1999:433–453, 450.
80. Myobloc botulinum toxin type B injectable solution. Product Information Sheet. Elan Pharmaceutical, Inc. 2000. Available at: www.elan.com/Products/neurology/myobloc. Accessed June 8, 2002.
81. Scott AB. Botulinum toxin treatment of strabismus. American Academy of Ophthalmology, Focal Points 1989: Clinical Modules for Ophthalmologists Vol VII Module 12.
82. FDA approves botox to treat frown lines. FDA Talk Paper T02-20, April 15, 2002. Available at: http://www.fda.gov/bbs/topics/ANSWERS/2002/ANS01147.html. Accessed June 8, 2002.
83. Botulinum toxin type A (parenteral-local). Medline Plus Health Information: A service of the National Library of Medicine. Micromedex, Inc. 2000. Available at: http://www.nlm.nih.gov/medlineplus/druginfo/botulinumtoxintypeaparenterall202608.html. Accessed June 15, 2002.
84. Chen R, Karp BI, Goldstein SR, Bara-Jiminez W, Yaseen Z, Hallett M. Effect of muscle activity immediately afer botulinum toxin injectin for writer's cramp. *Mov Disord* 1999;14:307–312.
85. Guyer B. Mechanism of botulinum toxin in the relief of chronic pain. *Curr Rev Pain* 1999;3:427–431.
86. Hallet M. How does botulinum toxin work. *Ann Neurol* 2000;48:7–8.
87. Botox botulinum toxin type A. Prescribing Information. Allergan Pharmaceuticals, Ltd. 2000. Available at: http://www.botox.com/index.jsp?hpandprescribing-botox. Accessed June 8, 2002.
88. Hallet M. One man's poison: Clinical applications of botulinum toxin. *New Eng J Med* 1999;341:118–120.
89. Molloy FM. Botulinum toxin (botox): Dystonia treatment. *EMedicine J* February 18, 2002;3(2). Available at: http://www.emedicine.com/neuro/topic585.htm. Accessed June 15, 2002.
90. Claus D, Druschy A, Erbguth F. Botulinum toxin: Influence on respiratory heart rate variation. *Mov Disord* 1995;10:574–579.
91. Schnider P, Brichta S, Schmied M, Auff E. Gallbladder dysfunction induced by botulinum A toxin. *Lancet* 1993;342:811—812.
92. Kedlaya D. Botulinu toxin: Overview. *Emedicine J* January 15, 2002;3(1). Available at: http://wwwemedicine.com/pmr/topic216.htm. Accessed June 15, 2002.
93. Koman LA et al. Management of cerebral palsy with botulinum-A toxin: Preliminary investigation. *J of Pediatr Orthop* 1993;13:489–495.
94. Greene P, Kang U, Fahn S, et al. Double blind, placebo controlled trial of botulinum toxin injection for the treatment of spasmodic torticollis. *Neurology* 1990;40:1213–1218.
95. Grazko MA, Polo KB, Jabbari B. Botulinum toxin A for spasticity, muscle spasms, and rigidity. *Neurology* 1995;45:712–717.
96. Foster L, Clapp L, Erickson M, Jabbari B. Botulinum toxin A and chronic low back pain: A randomized, double-blind study. *Neurology* 2001;56:1290–1293.
97. Schwarzer AC, Aprill CN, Derby R, Fortin J, Kine G, Bogduk N. The prevalence and clinical features of internal disc disruption in patients with chronic low back pain. *Spine* 1995;20:1878–1883.

98. Freemont AJ, Peacock TE, Goupille P, Hoyland JA, O'Brien J, Jayson M. Nerve ingrowth into diseased intervertebral disc in chronic back pain. *Lancet* 1997;350:178–181.
99. Coppes MH, Maranni E, Tahoma RT, Groen GI. Innervation of "painful" lumbar discs. *Spine* 1997;22:2342–2350.
100. Robert S, Eisenstein SM, Menage J, et al. Mechanoreceptors in intervertebral discs. *Spine* 1995;20:2645–2651.
101. Derby R, Eek B, Chen Y, O'Neill C, Ryan D. Intradiscal electrothermal annuloplasty (IDET): A novel approach for treating chronic discogenic back pain. *Neuromodulation* 2000;3:82–88.
102. Saal JA, Saal JS. Intradiscal electrothermal therapy for the treatment of chronic discogenic low back pain. *Oper Tech Orthop* 2000;10:271–281.
103. McGraw JK, Silber JS. Intradiscal electrothermal therapy for the treatment of discogenic back pain. *Appl Radiol* 2001;30:1–6.
104. Shah RV, Lutz GE, Lee J, Doty SB, Rodeo S. Intradiscal electrothermal therapy: A preliminary histologic study. *Arch Phys Med Rehabil* 2001;82:1230–1237.
105. Houpt J, Conner E, McFarland E. Experimental study of temperature distributions and thermal transport during radiofrequency current therapy of the intervertebral disc. *Spine* 1996;21:1808–1813.
106. Troussier B, Lebas JF, Chirossel JP, et al. Percutaneous intradiscal radio-frequency thermocoagulation: A cadaveric study. *Spine* 1995;20:1713–1718.
107. Windsor R. Radiofrequency annular denervation. Presented at the International Spinal Injection Society Third Annual Meeting, New Orleans, September 1995:23–24.
108. Salinger D. Radiofrequency lesion for internal disc disruption. *Int Spinal Injection Soc Newsl* 1997;2:10–12.
109. Saal JA, Saal JS. Intradiscal electrothermal treatment for chronic discogenic low back pain: A prospective outcome study with minimum 1-year follow-up. *Spine* 2000;25:2622–2627.
110. Saal JS, Saal JA. Management of chronic discogenic low back pain with a thermal intrediscal catheter: A preliminary report. *Spine* 2000;25:382–388.
111. Kuslich SD, Ulstrom C, Griffith S, et al. The Bagby and Kuslich method of lumbar interbody fusion: History, techniques, and 2-year follow-up results of a United States prospective, multicenter trial. *Spine* 1998;23:1267–1279.
112. Turner JA, Ersek M, Herron L. Patient outcomes after lumbar spine fusions. *JAMA* 1992;268:907–911.
113. Karasek M, Bogduk N. Twelve-month follow-up of a controlled trial of intradiscal thermal annuloplasty for back pain due to internal disc disruption. *Spine* 2000;25:2601–2607.
114. Wetzel FT, Andersson GB, Peloza JH, et al. Intradiscal electrothermal therapy (IDET) to treat discogenic low back pain: Two-year results of a multi-center prospective cohort study. Presented at the 16th Annual Meeting of the North American Spine Society, October 31–November 3, 2001.
115. Thompson KJ, Eckel T. Two-year results from the intradiscal electrothermal therapy (IDET) national registry. Presented at the 16th Annual Meeting of the North American Spine Society, October 31–November 3, 2001.
116. Saal JA, Saal JS, Wetzel FT, Thompson K, Maurer P, Hill J. IDET related complications: A multi-center study of 1675 treated patients with a review of the FDA MDR data base. Presented at the 16th Annual Meeting of the North American Spine Society, October 31–November 3, 2001.
117. Lee J, Lutz GE, Campbell D, Rodeo SA, Wright T. Stability of the lumbar spine after intradiscal electrothermal therapy. *Arch Phys Med Rehabil* 2001;82:120–122.
118. Welch WC, Gerszten PC. Alternative strategies for lumbar discectomy: Intradiscal electrothermy and nucleoplasty. *Neurosurg Focus* 2002;13(2):1–6.
119. Nucleoplasty. Sunnyvale, CA: Arthrocare, 2001. Available at: http://www.nucleoplasty.com. Accessed April 5, 2003.
120. Sharps L. Percutaneous disc decompression using nucleoplasty. Study Summary. Sunnyvale, CA: Arthrocare, 2001. Available at: http://www.nucleoplasty.com/dph/information/lewis_sharps_study_for_ISIS.pdf. Accessed April 5, 2003.
121. American Board of Interventional Pain Management. Coblation Nucleoplasty. Accessed at: www.abipm.org/coblationnucleoplasty.htm. Accessed April 5, 2003.
122. Yetkinler DN, Brandt, LL. Intervertebral disc temperature measurements during nucleoplasty and IDET procedures. Sunnyvale, CA: Arthrocare, 2001. Available at: http://www.nucleoplasty.com/dph/information/temperature_comparison_nuc_IDET.pdf. Accessed April 5, 2003.
123. Simmons JW, Nordby EJ, Hadjipavlou AG. Chemonucleolysis: The state of the art. *Eur Spine J* 2001;10:192–202.
124. Smith L. Enzyme dissolution of the nucleus pulposus in humans. *JAMA* 1964;187:137–140.
125. Alexander AH. Chemonucleolysis for lumbar disc hernation. *J Musculoskel Med* 1995;12:13–24.
126. Van de Belt H, Franssen S, Deutman R. Repeat chemonucleolysis is safe and effective. *Clinl Orthop Relat Res* 1999;363:121–125.
127. Leivseth G, Salvesen R, Hemminghytt S, Brinckmann P, Frobin W. Do human lumbar discs reconstitute after chemonucleolysis? A seven year follow-up study. *Spine* 1999;24:342–347.
128. Nordby EJ, Fraser RD, Javid MJ. Chemonucleolysis. *Spine* 1996;21:1102–1105.
129. Benoist M. 20 years of lumbar chymonucleolysis. *Press Med* 1996;25:743–745.
130. Javid MJ, Nordby EJ. Current status of chymopapain for herniated nucleus pulposus. *Neurosurg Q* 1994;4:92–101.
131. Gogan WJ, Fraser RD. Chymopapain: A 10-year, double-blind study. *Spine* 1992;17:388–394.
132. Lecuire F, Jaffar-Bandjee Z, Basso M, Sorba L, Honore M, Rebouillat J. Long-term result of lumbar disk

chemonucleolysis: An 8 to 12 year follow-up. *Rev Chire Orthopt Reparatrice de l'Appарl Mot* 1994;80:468–475.

133. Norby EJ, Wright PH. Efficacy of chymopapain in chemonucleolysis: A review. *Spine* 1994;19:2578–2583.
134. Wittenberg RH, Oppel S, Rubenthaler FA, Steffan R. Five-year results from chemonucleolysis with chymopapain or collagenase: A prospective randomized study. *Spine* 2001;26:1835–1841.
135. Poynton AR, O'Farrell DA, Mulcahy D, Corrign NT, McManus F. Chymopapain chemonucleolysis: A review of 105 cases. *J R Coll Surg Edinb* 1998;43:407–409.
136. Javid MJ. A 1- to 4-year follow-up review of treatment of sciatica using chemonucleolysis or laminectomy. *J Neurosurg* 1992;76:184–190.
137. Hadjipavlou A, Lander P, Antoniou J. The effect of chymopapain on low back pain. *Orthop Rev* 1992;21:733–738.
138. Gibson JN, Grant IC, Waddell G. The Cochrane review of surgery for lumbar disc prolapse and degenerative lumbar spondylosis. *Spine* 1999;24(17):1820–1832.
139. Riggs BL, Melton LJ. The worldwide problem of osteoporosis: Insights afforded by epidemiology. *Bone* 1995;17(5 Suppl):505S–511S.
140. Leech JA, Dulberg C, Kellie S, Pattee L, Gay J. Relationship of lung function to severity of osteoporosis in women. *Am Rev Respir Dis* 1990;141:68–71.
141. Cook DJ, Guyatt GH, Adachi JD, et al and the Multicentre Vertebral Fracture Study Group. Quality of life issues in women with vertebral fractures due to osteoporosis. *Arthritis Rheum* 1993;36:750–756.
142. Kado DM, Browner WS, Palermo L, Nevitt MC, Genant HK, Cummings SR. Vertebral fractures and mortality in older women: A prospective study. Study of Osteoporotic Fractures Research Group. *Arch Intern Med* 1999;159:1215–1220.
143. Galibert P, Deramond H, Rosat P, Le Gars D. Note preliminaire sur le traitement des angiomes vertebraux par vertebroplastie acrylique percutanee. *Neurochirurgie* 1987;233:166–168.
144. Cotten A, Boutry N, Cortet B, et al. Percutaneous vertebroplasty: State of the art. *Radiographics* 1998;18:311–320.
145. Garfin SR, Reilley MA. Minimally invasive treatment of osteoporotic vertebral body compression fractures. *Spine J* 2002;2:76–80.
146. Vertebroplasty. Massachusetts General Hospital Department of Radiology. Available at: http://massgeneralimaging.org/Vertebroplasty_Site/vertebro.html. Accessed March 2, 2002.
147. Garfin SR, Reilley MA. New technologies in spine: Kyphoplasty and vertebroplasty for the treatment of painful osteoporotic compression fractures. *Spine* 2001;26:1511–1515.
148. Martin JB, Jean B, Sugiu K, et al. Vertebroplasty: Clinical experience and follow-up results. *Bone* 1999;25(Suppl 2):11S–15S.
149. Maynard AS, Jensen ME, Schweickert PA, Marx WF, Short JG, Kallmes DF. Value of bone scan imaging in predicting pain relief from percutaneous vertebroplasty in osteoporotic vertebral 2000;21:1807–1812.
150. O'Brien JP, Simms JT, Evans AJ. Vertebroplasty in patients with severe vertebral compression fractures: A technical report. *AJNR Am J Neuroradiol* 2000;21:1555–1558.
151. Liebschner MA, Rosenberg WS, Keaveny TM. Effects of bone cement volume and distribution on vertebral stiffness after vertebroplasty. *Spine* 2001;26:1547–1554.
152. Belkoff SM, Mathis JM, Jasper LE, Deramond H. The biomechanics of vertebroplasty: The effect of cement volume on mechanical behavior. *Spine* 2001;26:1537–1541.
153. Cortet B, Cotton A, Boutry R, et al. Percutaneous vertebroplasty in the treatment of osteoporotic vertebral compression fractures: An open prospective study. *J Rheumatol* 1999;26:222–228.
154. Dean JR, Ison KT, Gishen P. The strengthening effect of percutaneous vertebroplasty. *Clin Radiol* 2000;55:471–476.
155. Cotton A, Dewatre F, Cortet B, et al. Percutaneous vertebroplasty for osteolytic metastases and myeloma: Effects of the percentage of lesion filling and the leakage of methylmethacrylate at clinical follow-up. *Radiology* 1996;200:525–530.
156. Deramond H, Wright NT, Belkoff SM. Temperature elevation caused by bone cement polymerization during vertebroplasty. *Bone* 1999;25(Suppl 2):17S–21S.
157. Watts NB, Harris ST, Genant HK. Treatment of painful osteoporotic vertebral fractures with percutaneous vertebroplasty or kyphoplasty. *Osteopor Int* 2001;12:429–437.
158. Grados F, Depriester C, Cayrolle G, Hardy N, Deramond H, Fardellone P. Long-term observations of vertebral osteoporotic fractures treated by percutaneous vertebroplasty. *Rheumatology* 2000;39:1410–1414.
159. Deramond H, Depriester C, Galibert P, Le Gars D. Percutaneous vertebroplasty with polymethylmethacrylate: Techniques, indications, and results. *Radiol Clin North Am* 1998;36:533–546.
160. Ratliff J, Nguyen T, Heiss J. Root and spinal cord compression from methylmethacrylate vertebroplasty. *Spine* 2001;26:E300–E302.
161. Hardouin P, Grados F, Cotton A, Cortet B. Should percutaneous vertebroplasty be used to treat osteoporotic fractures? An update. *Joint Bone Spine* 2001;68:216–221.
162. Levine SA, Perin LA, Hayes D, Hayes WS. An evidence-based evaluation of percutaneous vertebroplasty. *Manag Care* 2000;9:56–60.
163. Barr JD, Barr MS, Lemley TJ, McCann RM. Percutaneous vertebroplasty for pain relief and spinal stabilization. *Spine* 2000;25:923–928.
164. Weill A, Chiras J, Simon JM, Rose M, Sola-Martinez T, Enkaoua E. Spinal metastases: Indications for and results of percutaneous injection of surgical cement. *Radiology* 1996;199:241–247.
165. Ryu KS, Park CK, Kim MC, Kang JK. Dose-dependent epidural leakage of polymethlmethacrylate after percutaneous vertebroplasty in patients with osteoporotic vertebral compression fractures. *J Neurosurg* 2002;96(Suppl 1):56–61.

166. Harrington K. Major neurological complications following percutaneous vertebroplasty with polymethylmethacrylate: A case report. *J Bone Joint Surg Am* 2001;83:1070–1073.
167. Padovani B, Kasriel O, Brunner P, Peretti-Viton P. Pulmonary embolism caused by acrylic cement: A rare complication of percutaneous vertebroplasty. *Am J Neurorad* 1999;20:375–377.
168. Kaufmann TJ, Jensen ME, Schweickert PA, Marx WF, Kallmes DF. Age of fracture and clinical outcomes of percutaneous vertebroplasty. *Am J Neuroradiol* 2001;22:1860–1863.
169. Cortet B, Cotton A, Boutry N, et al. Percutaneous vertebroplasty in patients with osteolytic metastases or multiple myeloma. *Rev Rhum Engl Ed* 1997;64:177–183.
170. Raja S. Nerve blocks in the evaluation of chronic pain: A plea for caution in their use and interpretation. *Anesthesiology* 1997;86:4–6.
171. Galer BS, Schwartz L, Turner JA. Do patient and physician expectations predict response to pain-relieving procedures? *Clin J Pain* 1997;13:348–351.
172. Ellis SJ, Adams RF. The cult of the double-blind placebo-controlled trial. *Br J Clin Pract* 1997;51:36–39.
173. Hogan QH, Abram SA. Neural blockade for diagnosis and prognosis: A review. *Anesthesiology* 1997;86:216–241.
174. Goldthwait JR. The lumbosacral articulation: An explanation of many cases of lumbago, sciatica and paraplegia. *Boston Med Surg J* 1911;164:365–372.
175. Putti V. New conceptions in the pathogenesis of sciatic pain. *Lancet* 1927;2:53–60.
176. Ghormley RK. Low back pain with special reference to the articular facets, with presentation of an operative procedure. *JAMA* 1933;101:1773–1777.
177. Rees WES. Multiple bilateral subcutaneous rhizolysis of segmental nerves in the treatment of the intervertebrate disc syndrome. *Ann Gen Prac* 1971;26:126–127.
178. Shealy CN. Facet denervation in the management of back and sciatic pain. *Clin Orthop* 1976;115:157–164.
179. Bokduk N, Long DM. Percutaneous lumbar medial branch neurotomy: A modification of facet denervation. *Spine* 1980;5:193–200.
180. Jackson RP, Jacobs RR, Montesano PX. 1988 Volvo award in clinical sciences. Facet joint injection in low-back pain. A prospective statistical study. *Spine* September 1988;13(9):966–971.
181. Revel M, Poiraudeau S, Auleley G, et al. Capacity of the clinical picture to characterize low back pain relieved by facet joint anesthesia. Proposed criteria to identify patients with painful facet joints. *Spine* September 15, 1998;23(18):1972–1976.
182. Revel M, Listrat VM, Chevalier X, et al. Facet joint block for low back pain: Identifying predictors of a good response. *Arch Phys Med Rehab* 1992;73:824–828.
183. Schwarzer AC, Aprill CN, Derby R. The false-positive rate of uncontrolled diagnostic blocks of the lumbar zygapophysial joints. *Pain* August 1994;58(2):195–200.
184. Schwarzer AC, Wang SC, O'Driscoll D. The ability of computed tomography to identify a painful zygapophysial joint in patients with chronic low back pain. *Spine* April 15, 1995;20(8):907–912.
185. Dolan AL, Ryan PJ, Arden NK, et al. The value of SPECT scans in identifying back pain likely to benefit from facet joint injection. *Br J Rheumatol* 1996;35(12):1269–1273.
186. Kaplan M, Dreyfuss P, Halbrook B, Bogduk N. The ability of lumbar medial branch blocks to anesthetize the zygapophysial joint. A physiologic challenge. *Spine* 1998;23(17):1847–1852.
187. Lovely TJ, Rastogi P. The role of provocative facet blocking as a predictor of success in lumbar spine fusion. *J Spinal Disord* 1997;10:512–517.
188. Lord SM, Barnsley L, Wallis BJ, McDonald GJ, Bogduk N. Percutaneous radio-frequency neurotomy for chronic cervical zygapophysial joint pain; *NEJM* December 5, 1996;335(23):1721–1726.
189. McDonald GJ, Lord SM, Bogduk N. Long-term follow up of patients treated with cervical radiofrequency neurotomy for chronic neck pain. *Neurosurgery* 1999;45:61–68.
190. Van Suijlekom HA, Van Kleef M, Barendse GAM, Sluijter ME, Sjaastad O, Weber WEJ. Radiofrequency cervical zygapophyseal joint neurotomy for cervicogenic headache: A prospective study of 15 patients. *Funct Neurol* 1998;13(4):297–303.
191. North RB, Ham M, Zahurak M, Kidd DH. Radiofrequency lumbar facet denervation:analysis of prognostic factors. *Pain* 1994;57:77–83.
192. Raymond J, Dumas JM. Intraarticular facet block: Diagnostic test or therapeutic procedure? *Radiology* May 1984;151(2):333–336.
193. Carette S, Marcoux S, Truchon R. A controlled trial of corticosteroid injections into facet joints for chronic low back pain [see comments]. *N Engl J Med* October 3, 1991;325(14):1002–1007.
194. Bogduk N, Aprill C. On the nature of neck pain, discography and cervical zygapophyseal joint blocks. *Pain* 1993;54, 213–217.
195. Watts RW, Silagy CA. A meta-analysis on the efficacy of epidural corticosteroids in the treatment of sciatica. *Anaesth Intensive Care* 1995;23:564–569.
196. Rozenberg S, Dubourg G, Khalifa P, Paolozzi L, Maheu E, Ravaud P. Efficacy of epidural steroids in low back pain and sciatica. A critical appraisal by a French Task Force of randomized trials. Critical Analysis Group of the French Society for Rheumatology, *Rev Rhum Engl Ed* 1999;66:79–85.
197. McQuay HJ, Moore RA, Eccleston C, Morley S, Williams AC de C. Systematic review of outpatient services for chronic pain control. *Health Technol Assess* 1997;1(6):1–135.
198. Bernard TN. Lumbar discography followed by computed tomography: Refining the diagnosis of low back pain. *Spine* 1990;15:690–707.
199. Jackson RP, Cain JE, Jacobs RR, Cooper BR, McManus GE. The neuroradiographic diagnosis of lumbar herniated nucleus pulposus: I. A comparison of computed tomography (CT), myelography, CT-myelography, discography, and CT-discography. *Spine* 1989;14:1356–1361.

200. Collins CD, Stack JP, O'Connell DJ, et al. The role of discography in lumbar disc disease: A comparative study of magnetic resonance imaging and discography. *Clin Radiol* 1990;42:252–257.
201. El-Khoury GY, Ehara S, Weinstein J, et al. Epidural steroid injection: A procedure ideally performed with fluoroscopic control. *Radiology* 1988;168:554–557.
202. Van Kleef M, Spaans F, Dingemans W, Barendse GAM, Floor E, Sluijter ME. Effects and side effects of a percutaneous thermal lesion of the dorsal root ganglion in patients with cervical pain syndrome. *Pain* 1993;52:49–53.
203. Carette S, Leclaire R, Marcoux S, et al. Epidural corticosteroid injections for sciatica due to herniated nucleus pulposus. *New Engl J Med* 1997;336:1634–1650.
204. Benzon HT. Epidural steroid injections for low back pain and lumbosacral radiculopathy. *Pain* March 1986;24(3):277–295.
205. Weinstein SM, Herring SA, Derby R. Contemporary concepts in spine care. Epidural steroid injections. *Spine* August 15, 1995;20(16):1842–1846.
206. North RB, Kidd DH, Zahurak M, Piantadosi S. Specificity of diagnostic nerve blocks: A prospective, randomized study of sciatica due to lumbosacral spine disease. *Pain* 1996;65:77–85.
207. North R, Kid DH, Campbell JN, Long DM. Dorsal root ganglionectomy for failed back surgery syndrome: A five year followup study. *J Neurosurg* 1991;74:236–242.
208. Loeser JD. Dorsal rhizotomy for the relief of chronic pain. *J Neurosurg* 1972;36:745–750.
209. Xavier AV, McDanal J, Kissin I. Relief of sciatic radicular pain by sciatic nerve block. *Anesth Analg* 1988; 67:1177–1180.
210. Kissin I, Xavier AV, McDanal J. Blockade of sciatic nerve branches relieves sciatic radicular pain (letter). *Anesth Analg* 1989;69:260–269.
211. Gillette RG, Kramis RC, Roberts WJ. Characterization of spinal somatosensory neurons having receptive fields in lumbar tissues of cats. *Pain* 1993;54: 85–98.
212. Lutz GE, Vad VB, Wisneski RJ. Fluoroscopic transforaminal lumbar epidural steroids: An outcome study. *Arch Phys Med Rehabil* November 1998; 79(11): 1362–1366.
213. Boas R. Sympathetic nerve blocks: In search of a role. *Reg Anesth Pain Med* 1998;23:292–305.
214. Kirgis H, Kuntz A. Inconsistent sympathetic neural pathways. *Arch Surg* 1942;44:95–102.
215. Hogan Q, Taylor ML, Goldstein M, Stevens R, Kettler R. Success rates in producing sympathetic blockade by paratracheal injection. *Clin J Pain* 1994;10:139–145.
216. Hatangdi VS, Boas RA. Lumbar sympathectomy: A single needle technique. *Br J Anaesth* 1985;57:285–289.
217. Wang JF, Nauss LA, Thomas JE, et al. Pain relief by mtrathecally applied morphine in man.*Anesthesiology* 1979;50:149–151
218. Van Dongen RTM, Crul BJP, Bock de M. Long-term intrathecal infusion of morphine/bupivicaine mixtures in the treatment of cancer pain; a retrospective analysis of 51 cases. *Pain* 1993;55:119–123.
219. Anderson VC, Burchiel K. A prospective study of long-term intrathecal morphine in the management of chronic nonmalignant pain. *Neurosurgery*. February 1999;44(2):289–300.
220. Dahm P, Nitescu P, Appelgren L, et al. Efficacy and technical complications of long-term continuous intraspinal infusions of opioid and/or bupivacaine in refractory nonmalignant pain: A comparison between the epidural and the intrathecal approach with externalized or implanted catheters and infusion pumps. *Clin J Pain* 1998;14:4–16.
221. Nitescu P et al. Continuous infusion of opioid and bupivacaine by externalized intrathecal catheters in long-term treatment of "refractory" nonmalignant pain. *Clin J Pain* 1998;14(1):17–28.
222. Paice JA, Penn RD, Shott S. Intraspinal morphine for chronic pain: A retrospective, multicenter study. *J Pain Symptom Manage* 1996;11:71–80.
223. Winkelmuller M, Winkelmuller W. Long-term effects of continuous intrathecal opioid treatment in chronic pain of nonmalignant etiology. *J Neurosurg* 1996;85:458–467.
224. Paice JA, Winkelmuller W, Burchiel K, Racz GB, Prager JP. Clinical realities and economic considerations: Introduction. *J Pain Symptom Manage* 1997; 14(Suppl):S14–S26.
225. Krames ES. Intraspinal opioid therapy for chronic nonmalignant pain: Current practice and clinical guidelines. *J Pain Symptom Manage* June 1996;11(6): 333–352.
226. Nitescu P, Sjoberg M, Appelgren L, et al. Complications of intrathecal opioids and bupivacaine in the treatment of "refractory" cancer pain. *Clin J Pain* 1995;11:45–62.
227. Chaney MA. Intrathecal and epidural anesthesia and analgesia for cardiac surgery. *Anesth Analg* 1997; 84:1211–1221.
228. Coffey RJ, Cahill D, Steers W, et al. Intrathecal baclofen for intractable spasticity of spinal origin: Results of a long-term multicenter study. *J Neurosurg* 1993;78:226–232.
229. Ten Vaarwerk IAM, Staal MJ. Spinal cord stimulation in chronic pain syndromes. *Spinal Cord* 1998;36:671–682.
230. Staats, PS. *Spinal cord stimulation: Patient selection/patient outcomes*. Staats PS, Kazim DA, Eds. Conference Syllabus; Johns Hopkins University, Baltimore, MD, 1999.
231. North RB, Kidd DH, Zahurak M, James CS, Long DM. Spinal cord stimulation for chronic, intractable pain: Experience over two decades. *Neurosurgery* 1993;32:384–395.
232. Fiume D, Sherkat S, Callovini GH, et al. Treatment of the failed back surgery syndrome due to lumbsacral epidural fibrosis. *Acta Neurochir* 1995;64:116–118.
233. Barolat G, Schwartzman R, Woo R. Epidural spinal cord stimulation in the management of reflex sympathetic dystrophy. *Stereotact Funct Neurosurg* 1989;53:29–39.

234. Sanchez-Ledesma MJ, Garcia-March G, Diaz-Casacajo P, Gomez-Moreta J, Broseta J. Spinal cord stimulation in deafferentation pain. *Stereotact Funct Neurosurg* 1989;53:40–45.

235. Pang WW, Mok MS, Lin ML, Chang DP, Hwang MH. Application of spinal pain mapping in the diagnosis of low back pain—Analysis of 104 cases. *Acta Anaesthesiol Sin* June 1998;36(2):71–74.

236. Davies HT, Crombie IK, Brown JH, Martin C. Diminishing returns or appropriate treatment strategy?—An analysis of short-term outcomes after pain clinic treatment. *Pain* 1997;70:203–208.

CHAPTER

25

MANUAL THERAPEUTIC TECHNIQUES FOR LOW BACK SYNDROMES: AN OVERVIEW

Vladimir Janda, Philip Greenman, Leonard J. Faye, Donald R. Murphy, and Craig E. Morris

OUTLINE

OBJECTIVES

1. To provide a multidisciplinary perspective regarding manual therapeutic methods utilized in the treatment of low back disorders.
2. To define various types of manual therapeutic techniques.
3. To clarify the local versus global effects of manual therapeutic techniques.
4. To discuss varying management strategies of manual therapeutic techniques.
5. To discuss the integration of manual therapeutic techniques with other treatment approaches for low back syndromes.
6. To demonstrate the application of manual therapeutic techniques for a complex low back disorder with a theoretical case study.
7. To provide the reader with "35 Golden Rules of Manual Therapeutic Techniques."

INTRODUCTION

If low back syndromes (LBS) are old as man, then it stands to reason that the laying on of hands to relieve such maladies was probably the first method of treatment. History demonstrates that differing regions and professions have organized a broad array of such treatment strategies, which will be defined in this chapter as *manual therapeutic techniques* (MTT). These methods are commonly used for the treatment of LBS.

Prior chapters have discussed various aspects of manual techniques with regard to both assessment and treatment. This chapter will draw upon the conclusions of those evidence-based chapters and incorporate the experience of an interdisciplinary group of instructors (including medical, osteopathic, and chiropractic physicians), in manual methods, who total nearly 200 years of clinical experience, in order to provide additional commentary regarding MTT. This will include the management of a fictional case study that all agree represents a reasonable example of a patient with a complex LBS. Also, the authors have provided 35 "golden rules of MTT," which have been added at the end of the chapter.

Earlier chapters of this textbook have discussed the complexity of the neurophysiological aspects of motor control, in addition to the physical examination and the functional assessment. Manual techniques utilizing McKenzie protocols have been covered, in addition to chapters dedicated to mobilization and manipulation techniques, as well as the biomechanical effects of spinal manipulation.

Therefore, this chapter will address common aspects of MTT in an attempt to provide additional insights into this fascinating field of health care. Such insights are hoped to enlighten the reader's understanding of the potential benefit of manual techniques, while inspiring students and practitioners of this field to deeper levels of understanding and higher levels of skills. Finally, it is hoped that non-MTT clinicians would use this information to better appreciate the rationale for MTT in order to more effectively utilize this avenue for their patients' management of LBS.

Clinical Pearl: There remain a number of issues that divide varying schools of thought regarding MTT. Perhaps the competitive aspects of human nature have directed an overemphasis to these divisions, while ignoring the common principles upon which they are based.

COMMON ASPECTS OF MANUAL METHODS

Dividing Manual Techniques

MTT can be divided in many ways. For the purpose of this chapter, they will be divided into passive, semiactive, and active techniques. It should be understood that there are a number of logical ways to organize these methods.

The passive techniques include those methods in which the patient remains as inactive and relaxed as possible while treatment is rendered. In such instances, the health-care provider performs all of the work. The passive techniques can be subdivided into manipulation, mobilization, and massage.

The semiactive techniques include those methods in which the patient is actively in motion although the target region being treated is not. Meanwhile, a clinician can provide manual treatment to the target region, or the patient may perform these methods alone. An example of a semiactive procedure would include the McKenzie lumbar spine "press-up" maneuver, in which the prone patient actively extends the arms to elevate the upper torso as the abdominal and thoracolumbar region remains relaxed. This active upper body maneuver allows extension of the lumbar spine (i.e. the clinical target region) to passively occur. Manipulation and massage would be excluded from semiactive techniques.

Active techniques are those in which both the patient and the clinician expend energy and motion of or to the target region to be treated. Examples of these methods include muscle energy techniques and proprioceptive neuromuscular facilitation techniques. These methods may draw upon the neurophysiological principles of facilitation and inhibition to accelerate the response, a topic that was discussed in Chapter 23.

Joint Techniques—Defining Manipulation and Mobilization

Manipulation has been defined as mobilization that includes a thrust. This is also called a high-velocity, low-amplitude (HVLA) force, in that it is performed quickly but the force is not designed to travel deeply into the body's tissues. There are, however, other schools of thought that include nonthrust techniques that fall under the heading of manipulation. This contradiction of definitions creates difficulties in finding common ground for the field of manipulation, and ultimately requires a unified definition.

The definition of joint mobilization is less complex. This is defined as manual techniques designed to reduce tissue tone via manual application of low-velocity techniques, but typically for longer periods than for manipulation. The loads may be applied on a continuous basis or rhythmically.

Neurophysiological Aspects

The greatest misconception about MTT is that the primary response is biomechanical, when in fact it is neurophysiological. However, recent studies have helped to confirm the theoretical aspects of manual techniques that formed the basis for manual therapy professions such as osteopathy and chiropractic. It is this response that allowed early practitioners of these disciplines to theorize why patients at times noted improvements in distal body musculoskeletal regions or of splanchnic conditions. Chapters 20 and 23 discussed the neurophysiological changes that occur with manipulative techniques and also mobilization techniques.

The neurophysiological effects of MTT appear to involve the stimulation of various receptors, especially mechanoreceptors, which leads to a reflexive local inhibition and a central nervous system facilitation. A reflexive nociceptive inhibition from MTT often results in decreased pain and subsequent improvements in motor patterns and pain-related attitudes. Indeed, manual therapy practitioners have observed for centuries that patients who received manual techniques found reductions of pain and local hypertonicity while noting improved overall locomotor system function and coordination. Such results, after all, are the reasons for the popularity, longevity and growth of MTT.

With the increasing evidence-based understanding of the global neurophysiological response of MTT, other specialties will come to increasingly embrace its global therapeutic potential. Whereas those who utilize pharmacotherapeutics understand their modality is spread via the circulatory system, they should equally understand that MTT are more rapidly transmitted through the intricate neural network.

Because of the local neurophysiological response of MTT, those clinicians involved in region-specific care, such as surgical and pain medicine specialists, should come to increasingly embrace MTT specialists. This is because the MTT specialist can assist in differentiating a local syndrome that is primarily due to pathophysiology or pathoanatomy. It has been stated throughout this textbook that pathoanatomical changes poorly correlate with specific pain syndromes; MTT specialists can therefore help to rule out those conditions whose etiologies are pathophysiological in nature. This strategy should allow the surgeon of open or minimally invasive procedures to increase the success rates by isolating those cases where anatomical corrections are most appropriate.

Biomechanical Aspects

Of course, MTT also encompass a biomechanical (or structural) aspect, typically resulting in increased mobility. While this has been a main emphasis in the past, it is now becoming clear that increased mobility without adequate stability from necessary motor control results in functional instability. Therefore, it is important to appreciate the interactions between these two MTT responses, as one would expect any alterations in the neurophysiological aspects to affect the biomechanics and vice versa. A symbiotic relationship in which there is increased, controlled motion is therefore the functional goal.

Specific versus Generic Treatment

MTT can be applied in a generic fashion or can target specific tissues. The degree of specificity can vary by target region, clinician skill, and even then remains controversial as to what degree of specifity can be achieved. The authors of this chapter have found that specific techniques are at times necessary for specific conditions, while generic methods can be quite sufficient at other times. Therefore, the important point is that experts in MTT have the skill to properly determine whether a specific or a generic MTT should be applied and then have the skill to perform the appropriate procedure. Lay practitioners of MTT, such as massage therapists, must remember to appreciate the limits of their craft and be prepared to refer their clients to an MTT specialist when the complexity of the findings extends beyond their training.

The Barrier Phenomenon The barrier phenomenon was discussed in Chapter 23 in detail. Nevertheless, it should be stated here that this concept forms the diagnostic and therapeutic basis of MTT. The barrier is the first palpated resistance to any given tissue, allowing the clinician to determine the degree of tone prior to, during and following treatment. The barrier phenomenon can be used to assess all of the tissues targeted by MTT. The skills required to be mastered for finding the barrier of various tissues are quite difficult to acquire, requiring years to do so.

Targeting Specific Tissues MTT can be utilized to target general body regions, general local tissues, or specific tissues. In order to master a broad variety of methods, one must be able to utilize layer palpation to optimally isolate specific tissues. With this proficiency, the clinician can then therapeutically target tissues. Dermal tissues are easily isolated, while joints are more challenging. Myofascial tissues can and should also be targeted. This topic was discussed in detail in Chapter 23. These techniques do not aim to take joints to their end range but instead take myofascial tissues to the barrier, loading in their lines of tensioning. Because of the neurophysiological response, significant locomotor alterations can occur such as increased mobility and improved posture.

MTT are often used for the treatment of scar tissue adhesions. This is often an overlooked area of treatment; however, it has become increasingly important over the past few decades. Assessment and treatment of scar tissue is considered to be a vital aspect of any manual therapy practitioner's assessment and treatment protocols. This is because adhesive scar tissue is initially locally facilitory and, conversely, inhibitory in the chronic stage. This means that local tissues in the early stage become overactive because of the increased local tension of the scar tissue. However with time, the increased tone of the adhesive scar causes a neurological inhibition at the region, compromising functional and dynamic stability. Adhesive scar tissue can be present at the skin level or can occur in the deeper tissues, binding layers together and interfering with their independent functional duties. As locomotor system stability is dependent on afferentation, altered sensation from the adverse tone of the scar compromises the subsequent efferent response, leading to incoordination and some degree of functional instability. In such a case, a pathological scenario has developed.

Management Aspects

Management aspects of MTT require the clinician to obtain a thorough understanding of anatomy, physiology, and locomotor system pathology. While the emphasis in the past was placed on the mobilization of skin, soft tissues, and joints, recent emphasis has focused more on functional stabilization, since increased mobility without stability typically leads to increased risk of pain and injury. As such, management must always focus on ensuring that the patient establishes sufficient dynamic or functional stability to be able to control any gains made in mobility with manual techniques.

Skill Aspects

Use of MTT requires a variety of skills. These skills have been called the *clinical literacy skills*. First, clinical visual literacy was defined by Morris in Chapter 13, addressing the clinicians' increasing ability to observe significant subtleties in the patient's posture, movement, body contours, discolorations, etc. These observations are integrated into the greater clinical pool of information to establish a more comprehensive summary of locomotor system function or pathology.

Second of the clinical literacy skills is that of palpatory literacy. This was also discussed in Chapter 13 and emphasizes the importance of the clinicians' ability to gain palpatory skills in order to better assess and treat their patients.

The clinical literacy skills are important not only in the assessment and the treatment of the patient but also in the clinicians' ability to determine what changes may have occurred following treatment. Finally, the importance of these high-caliber clinical literacy skills is that they help the patient to understand and appreciate the clinicians' skills in being able to observe his or her condition. This is because the patient gains great confidence in knowing that the clinician can indeed feel what he or she is feeling or observe slight alterations in posture and movements.

The authors of this chapter would like to emphasize that no clinician in this field should ever become complacent or content with their level of proficiency. Rather, the clinical literacy skills are those that should continue to be honed over a lifetime. Despite the greatest of skill, the clinician should never be fully confident, trusting in his or her findings. Instead, he or she should always be rechecking to confirm the correctness of such observations, always remembering that locomotor system changes in tone can occur quickly, especially because of the interactive nature of the nervous system.

All practitioners of MTT must remember to avoid overreliance on subtle findings of visual and palpatory literacy, as this leads to clinical presumptuousness and error.

Clinical Pearl: Because strong inter-examiner reliability has not been established for visual or palpatory literacy, clinical literacy findings must be considered supportive of other more evidence-based observations, or utilized when those observations have proven fruitless in establishing the etiological aspects of a case.

Full-Time Vocation The authors of this chapter insist that establishing and maintaining expertise in MTT is a full-time vocation, especially in the field of manipulation. The ability to assess, diagnose, and provide appropriate, effective, and safe treatment is a professional skill that must not be taken lightly. While laypersons may at times utilize mobilization and even manipulation on family and friends because they have basic skills, it should be noted that they also have the writing skills to physically write a prescription for medication. Although safeguards are fortunately in place to protect the public from improper prescription medication sales, the analogy of this statement remains important. That is, it is the ability to determine the appropriate application, integrating the complicating clinical factors, of a therapeutic intervention that distinguishes the health-care provider from the layperson.

Diagnostic Aspects

Many clinicians fail to realize the diagnostic aspect of MTT. Such techniques can act as a type of orthopedic or neurological testing in many instances. For example, a patient who responds better to a distractive type of manipulation, but in whom a compressive type of manipulation provokes the symptoms, may suggest the presence of some type of pathoanatomical lesion. Therefore, a clinician must always take into account the biomechanical loading of therapeutic techniques utilized, while remembering that a positive, a negative, or an absent change in the patient's condition may provide invariable clinical insights into its etiology and ultimate resolution.

Trial Courses of MTT

Trial courses of medications are commonly accepted strategies in health care. This is less so when the method of treatment involves MTT. Therefore, while it may be appropriate to try a different type of medication after an initial failed trial, there is less support for a second trial of a different MTT method. Although it may not be exactly fair to compare pharmacotherapeutics and MTT, there is value in the comparison. This is because there are significant varieties in the manner, skills, and methods of clinicians who provide MTT, and patients may indeed benefit from some methods more than others in the same way they may benefit more from one medication than another.

The authors of this chapter have successfully resolved numerous complex LBS with MTT after multiple trial courses of MTT previously failed with other clinicians. Therefore, guidelines strategies that include one trial of MTT and multiple trials for medications, such as various nonsteroidal anti-inflammatory medications (NSAIDs), should rethink their policy.

Clinicians who utilize MTT in practice must bear their professional responsibilities also. This includes determining the efficacy, or lack thereof, of their treatment plans. Failed trial courses of treatment require reassessment and alteration of a different trial, referral to a different specialist, or a comanagement strategy that includes both.

Strengths and Weaknesses

All treatment methods have strengths and weaknesses. This of course holds true for MTT. While the aspects of pain reduction, local tissue relaxation, improved motor patterns, improved function, and subsequent emotional improvement (i.e. which typically occurs once one feels better) are all strong points, there are also dangers that these methods hold that must be stated.

The first is that these methods use various levels of force, and the clinician must be certain that such methods can be safely administered. These topics were previously discussed in the red flags chapter (Chapter 10) and also in the manipulation chapter (Chapter 20) of this text.

The second concern is that the benefits of MTT may provide temporary relief of a more complex underlying locomotor system dysfunction. If the clinician is unaware that such complexity is present, then an ongoing repetition of MTT sessions might ensue, providing temporary relief indefinitely without ever resolving the condition. Because the locomotor system encompasses many organ systems into a dynamically complex functional unit, many consider locomotor system assessment to be the most challenging in all of health care. Therefore, determining the true etiological aspects of a chronic pain syndrome is indeed difficult and not always successful. If the patient's symptoms and clinical presentation persists after a brief trial course of MTT, the clinician must consider this as a failed trial course and reassess the situation. Perhaps the patient is provoking the condition with some inappropriate activities. Perhaps the diagnosis is incorrect. Perhaps the wrong MTT methods are being used. Perhaps the condition is more complex and requires a more complex assessment. Perhaps referral to another type of specialist is appropriate.

The third concern involves that of patient dependence. This is perhaps the least discussed danger of MTT. Unlike dependencies on pharmacotherapeutics, there is no risk with MTT of organ morbidities. Nevertheless, the patient–clinician relationship can be extremely close, which is magnified by the hands-on nature of the treatment. The sense of touch is considered the most pleasant of the five basic senses. It is therefore important that the clinician look for any signs of patient dependence and council the patient on the importance of self-dependence as the ultimate goal of treatment. Finally, clinicians must be able to determine whether the patient has reached a plateau in their recovery and explain this to the patient so that new management strategies can be established, such as referral to another spine specialist.

Clinical Pearl: The strong emotional bond and physical benefit of MTT, even if it is temporary, can lead to emotional dependency on the treatment and provider.

INTEGRATING MTT WITH OTHER TREATMENT METHODS

Utilizing Outcome Measures

Outcome measures, as discussed in Chapter 14, are a relatively new tool in the health-care world. However, these invaluable tools have become well validated and provide a variety of measures that can allow the clinician to objectify efficacy of their treatment or lack thereof. In order for the clinician to be able to establish a measurable functional baseline at the outset of treatment and then monitor progress in an objective manner, outcome measures are simple and practical. As such, it is highly recommended that outcome measure be integrated with the overall management of the treatment of MTT.

Evidence Basis of MTT

MTT have gained the greatest degree of validated benefit for acute low back pain (LBP). Indeed, there are now a significant number of randomized controlled trials that have demonstrated the true efficacy of manipulation. Other treatments such as mobilization and massage have also been measured and have shown efficacy for acute LBS. Ongoing research has shown what manual therapy practitioners have observed for generations; MTT are effective for pain reduction and improved mobility and can be an important tool in helping to establish functional restoration.

With regard to chronic LBS, there is less quality research available supporting this approach, although this portfolio of work continues to grow. However, clinicians have again appreciated the benefit of MTT for the treatment of chronic LBS. This is not to say that they are a cure-all for this complex problem, but it does say that they are an important component of the treatment program and ultimate.

Integrating Rehabilitation

MTT must be integrated within a rehabilitation protocol for chronic cases and also for certain acute LBS. In the case of the acute LBS, if the clinician finds that the syndrome was brought on in part by deconditioning or some other combination of clinical factors that may place the patient at increased risk for recurrence, then the clinician may choose to implement a rehabilitative strategy in the management of that case. For example, the patient who is simply deconditioned may require brief instruction in home exercises with counseling stressing the importance of independent exercises to reduce risks of recurrence. In other instances, other comorbid conditions may require a more complex and supervised rehabilitation strategy. Although this management strategy has not yet been supported or refuted by evidence-based studies, the authors of this chapter recommend that such a strategy be implemented for the reduction of risk of recurrences.

Integrating Medication

The integration of MTT with medication is somewhat controversial. There are schools of thought who feel that the integration of this physical approach can result in significant benefits while others have philosophical differences that concern the risk benefit ratio of various types of drugs. The controversy of this topic will not end anytime soon.

Integrating Minimally Invasive Surgical Procedures

MTT can be used in conjunction with minimally invasive surgical procedures typically utilized in the specialty of pain medicine. These topics are covered in Chapters 17 and 24. While minimally invasive procedures can be used to provide either analgesic or anti-inflammatory agents to specific pain generators, MTT can then be used to help to bring about functional restoration by normalizing joint motion and improving myofascial balance and tone. Other minimally invasive procedures can be used to change or alter spinal morphology, such as procedures directed at the intervertebral disc. Co-management of these methods may indeed improve the overall outcome, although randomized trials have not yet been performed to confirm or refute this.

Integrating Open Surgical Methods

Following open surgical spinal procedures, scar mobilization techniques should be used as soon as the wound has sufficiently healed in order to avoid adhesive scar tissue formation. Depending on the type of surgery performed, MTT can also be utilized to reestablish joint motion and myofascial balance as a key aspect of rehabilitation. Chapter 27 discusses strategies that integrate MTT with rehabilitation for low back surgical cases.

Integrating Patient Education

MTT integrate well with the strategy of patient education, or counseling. Education is considered to be the most important aspect of treatment of locomotor system dysfunctions, in that it helps the patient to better understand his or her condition, while reducing the risk of illness behavior and inspiring him or her toward a healthier lifestyle. As previously mentioned, an exceptionally close bond is often established between MTT clinicians and their patients, which can allow the counseling to have a greater impact.

CASE STUDY

The following fictional case study is presented as an example of clinical case management using MTT.*

History

This patient is a 35-year-old woman complaining of right-sided LBP with right leg pain. This began approximately 6 months earlier and developed insidiously. The LBP is located in the area of the right sacroiliac joint, and the leg pain extends to the right buttock and down the posterolateral thigh and leg to the bottom of the foot. The most intense pain is in the right calf. Walking is the major pain-provoking activity, which begins as soon as she starts walking, and this increases as she continues. When she stops walking, the pain gets somewhat better, but she is left with a residual "throbbing." Forward flexion and standing from a seated position also increase her pain and she is generally better at rest. She describes some "tingling" in the area of her right leg pain at times, but this is inconsistent. She denies motor loss. She does note

* Any correlation with the case study of the fictional patient in this chapter and another individual is purely coincidental.

that she has had some "fever and chills" for the past month. She also notes that she has had some increased difficulty with urination recently. She states that she has experienced a slight residual leakage following her prior pregnancies, but that this incontinance has recently worsened somewhat while laughing, coughing, sneezing, or straining.

Her past medical history includes a discectomy at L4–L5 15 years ago, which resolved the right-sided L5 radiculopathy that she was experiencing at that time. She is multiparous time three, with her 2nd and 3rd delivery each requiring C-section. She related that she attends her annual gynecological visit, which was recently completed and all results found to be normal. She is hypertensive and takes a β-blocker medication for this. She had dental work performed the previous week, no other physician visits over the past 6 months, with the exception of a visit 2 weeks earlier to her family doctor regarding her present complaints. She was prescribed a trial of antibiotics and subsequently referred her for today's spine specialty consult.

She lives with her husband, considering herself very happily married, and three children (ages 12, 10, and 6), all of who are healthy. She is not employed, but rather is a homemaker for her family, which she enjoys. She smokes approximately two packs of cigarettes per day, drinks alcohol socially, and does not exercise regularly.

Review of systems reveals shortness of breath when walking long distances and recent difficulty with short-term memory. During consultation, she appears to demonstrate a low *disability-prone profile* in light of very few yellow flags.

Examination Findings

Examination revealed a well-nourished, pleasant woman who appeared in no acute distress. Blood pressure was 138/88 on the left. Temperature was 101°F. Her height was 5′6″ (1.68 m) and her weight was 128 lb (58 kg). Pulse was 88 per minute and respirations were 20 per minute.

Still upright postural evaluation from behind demonstrated an accentuated lumbar lordosis and a pronated right foot. There was a slight pelvic obliquity noted, which was lower on the right side. This obliquity appeared to improve when the patient was instructed to stand on the outsides of her feet (i.e., the fifth rays) in order to remove any potential functional leg discrepancy from an asymmetrically lower arch of the foot. This test was described in the functional assessment chapter (Chapter 13). Further inspection demonstrated mild atrophy of the right (dominant) calf. Which was 3/4″ smaller girth than the left. Review of medical records, however revealed that this atrophy was present following her prior right radiculopathy case. This emphasizes the importance of obtaining prior medical records and this finding was therefore considered clinically irrelevant. From the anterior view, inspection of the abdomen demonstrated a rounded abdomen despite the fact that she was relatively lean.

Straight-leg raise (SLR) test was positive on the right at 60 degrees for reproduction of her lower back and leg pain to the right foot. Braggard's test was also positive for reproduction of her pain, while well-leg raise test was negative at 70 degrees. Patrick's test, Gaenslen's test, and thigh thrust test were all positive for reproduction of her LBP, but not her leg pain. Extension of the lumbar spine in the prone position reproduced her LBP and leg pain and this became worse with repetition and overpressure. Flexion of the lumbar spine in the standing position reproduced her leg pain only and this worsened and peripheralized with repetition. Flexion in the supine position was not painful, even with repetition. Side glide to either side in the standing position was somewhat restricted but not painful.

Heel, toe, and tandem walking were within normal limits, as was squatting. Sensory examination to pin in the lower extremities was unremarkable. Motor strength was 5/5 bilaterally in the lower extremities. Muscle stretch reflexes were 2+ and symmetric in the knees and 2+ on the left and absent on the right in the ankles. Plantar responses were downgoing bilaterally.

Spinal palpation revealed painful joint restriction at both the sacroiliac joint and the L5–S1 zygapophyseal joint on the right. Palpation of each of these partially reproduced the patient's pain. Muscle palpation revealed diffuse tenderness, as well as specific myofascial trigger points (TrPs) in the lumbar erector spinae and right quadratus lumborum muscles, palpation of which reproduced her LBP and right buttock pain, but not her leg pain. The right piriformis muscle was nontender.

Hip extension movement pattern test revealed delayed contraction of the gluteus maximus on the right, with no deviation of the lumbar spine. It was normal on the left. Active SLR test was positive on the right for reproduction of her LBP but not her leg pain. This pain was relieved when the maneuver was performed with overpressure.

Examination of the abdomen was negative as bruit and bowel sounds were normal. There was no evidence of hernia. A transverse C-section scar was present, which was slightly reddened on the right. Dragging skin palpation across this scar demonstrated resistance consistent with an "active scar" and deeper palpation demonstrated adhesions and myofascialTrPs. On further questioning, the patient admitted that her abdominal muscles had remained weakened following her first C-section despite her attempts to strengthen them with exercises. This weakness worsened after her subsequent deliveries, so she accepted this weakness as a consequence of her pregnancies and discontinued further attempts at abdominal exercises.

Questions

1. Are there any red flags for serious or potentially life-threatening diseases?
   a. The potential red flag is the fever and elevated pulse rate, and perhaps a minor elevation of her BP. Fever in the presence of spinal pain is a sign of potential infection, and an epidural abscess is the most common spinal infection. This can lead to rapid neurological deterioration and even death, a stat MRI must be ordered in this situation, and immediate admission must be initiated if the MRI demonstrates an abscess.
2. What additional tests might be added?
   a. Additional testing might include the sitting SLR test with neck flexion, which is the slump test. Also, the Mennell lumbar springing test might be used, in which springing over the posterior joints of the prone patient's lumbar spine might isolate any sudden increase in pain. The same maneuver is then performed with the patient actively lifting his or her head and shoulders off the table with the hands behind the neck. This active extension strategy locks the posterior joints and if the spring is much less painful it is a sign that the posterior joints are pain generators. Finally an examination for any dysfunction along the closed kinematic system of locomotion, i.e., the foot, ankle, superior tibia–fibula joint, knee, hip, symphysis pubis, thoracic, costotransverse, costosternal, cervical, and temporoman dibular joint complexes. Although the current level of evidence-based research is nowhere close to establishing these etiological factors, the authors of this chapter have consistently observed that these distant sights are capable of affecting the function of the lumbopelvic region. Therefore they should be assessed for complex cases, especially if previous treatment trials directed to the symptomatic region has failed to resolve the problem.
   b. An erect posterior gravity line can be a chronic stress factor in back pain and can be detected by the toe-raise test. In this test, the patient is instructed to stand in a normal posture. Meanwhile, the examiner stands in front of the patient and places a restrictive finger on the patient's sternum. The patient is instructed to stand on tiptoes. If there is a posterior gravity line, the patient will attempt to translate the torso anteriorly (i.e., to establish a more forward center of mass) pressing against the examiner's finger. Because the forward momentum is blocked, he or she will not be able to move forward to toe raise. Johnson (Toronto-unpublished) demonstrated a relationship between posterior vertebral joint strain and those people that stood back on their heels and hyperextended their knees.
   c. The patient can also be assessed for a forward-drawn posture. This is described by Lewit as a condition in which the patient's center of mass is anterior to the midfoot, requiring additional loading to the gastrocnemius and erector spinae in order to maintain equilibrium. These patients tend to have tight, short abdominal muscles, which promote the chronicity of this posture. Because of the imbalance, additional loading is placed on the lumbopelvic region, which can ultimately lead to a pain syndrome. This can be assessed by instructing the patient to perform the opposite maneuver with the toes as demonstrated above. This time, the patient should elevate the toes to force weight bearing on the midfoot. Since the forward-drawn posture requires the patient to place his or her weight toward the forefoot, he or she would have to transition posteriorly to move the center of mass backward. This maneuver is considered positive when the patient transitions backwards in the posture as the toes elevate.
   d. Palpate the thoracolumbar junction to rule marked dysfunction. Severe dysfunction of the thoracolumbar junction has been theorized to make the angle of the roots much more obtuse and displace a root onto the convex disc as described by A. Breig in *The Biomechanics of the Central Nervous System*. In these cases the slump test may be much more sensitive than the SLR test. This diagnosis is supported by a quick reduction of symptoms following manipulation of the thoracolumbar junction.
   e. The examination should include palpatory assessment of the femoral and dorsalis pedis arteries to rule out vascular claudication. Any patient with lower extremity symptomatology should be assessed for this, but this becomes more important when there are any symptoms with walking or standing. These pulses were assessed and found to be intact bilaterally.
   f. One of the most overlooked joints associated with LBS is the hip. Ironically, it seems to be overlooked because of its anatomical proximity. Therefore, a thorough hip examination should be performed, especially after the Patrick's screening test was positive. Also,

Janda stated that the first sign of hip arthrosis was that of ipsilateral gluteus medius weakness due to arthrogenic inhibition. Therefore, the key observation occurs during visual assessment of gait. When the patient demonstrates increased lateral deviation of the ipsilateral pelvis on the weigh-bearing leg. Pain can occur second, and this can be local or referred to the pelvis or down the leg.

3. What primary pain generator(s) may be suspected?
   a. The pain generators appear to be posterior joint and lumbar nerve root stress with low backTrPs. Of course, any of these findings can cause leg pain via radicular (i.e., nerve root) or referred (i.e., TrP) or sclerotogenous (i.e., discogenic or posterior joint) origin. The more chronic the LBS, the greater likelihood that this will be some sort of combined syndrome due to the altered mechanics and secondary locomotor system compensation.
4. Are there any findings that may serve as perpetuating factors to the disorder?
   a. The elevated temperature means she is in a general adaptive response as described by Hans Selye and there would be an amplification of any local inflammation as well.
   b. There appears to be lumbopelvic functional instability because of abdominal weakness following three C-sections. This may be a primary or secondary etiological factor, or it may simply be incidental. If it is primary, it can directly interfere with symptom reduction, and so this will have to be addressed early in the treatment plan. If it is considered secondary, then this can be a part of the rehabilitation plan for functional stabilization. Although it may be incidental for the current condition, most MTT specialists would be concerned about the inhibition caused by this adhesive scar and the subsequent abdominal muscular dysfunction. Therefore, this would be addressed in the later stages of treatment to reduce risks of recurrences or future lumbopelvic conditions due to functional lumbopelvic instability. If and when treatment was indicated, scar-lysing and other myofascial MTT would be employed. These can be uncomfortable procedures, so additional patient communication is warranted, including the fact that multiple MTT and daily home self-mobilization procedures are typically necessary. Success is achieved when the redness, tenderness, and increased resistance of the scar are removed and the patient can again perform abdominal exercises as she did prior to her surgery.
   c. Pelvic obliquity was observed as a result of what appeared to be a functional short leg due to right foot pronation. A functional short leg is one in which there is skeletal symmetry, but dysfunction causing one leg to appear shorter. This can occur with dysfunctions such as pelvic torsion or unilateral foot pronation. As with an anatomical short leg, this places asymmetrical loading of the pelvis and spine and at times is considered a complication factor in locomotor dysfunction and pain syndromes. Although the literature fails to correlate a short leg with increased risk of back pain, the authors feel that this is a matter of adaptability. That is, individuals who are conditioned and young may be able to function well for decades with a leg-length asymmetry. However, as the person loses locomotor system adaptability, the asymmetrical loading factor can then come into play. If this were considered as a possible primary or secondary factor for this patient's current spinal condition, then a trial course of elevating the lower pelvis could be attempted with MTT, designed to normalize tarsal mobility and facilitate intrinsic pedal stability, a right heel left to elevate the low pelvis, or by taping the foot to provide support to the lowered right arch. If the MTT improved the foot pronation, at least temporarily, then foot exercises would be added to bolster the lowered arch. If either the heel lift or taping were found to be effective in leveling the pelvis and reducing symptoms, or if the MTT and exercises failed to provide lasting arch improvement, then the patient might be fitted for custom-fitted foot orthotics to provide ongoing tarsal support.
5. Should diagnostic imaging be ordered? If so, what imaging modality?
   a. Plain-film radiographs of the lumbosacral spine due to the risk of Red Flags to serve as an initial imaging screen. These films were performed and were essentially negative, except for moderate degenerative changes at the L4–5 level.
   b. Because of the persistent fever and low back pain, an MRI study to rule out spinal abscess would be appropriate, with and without contrast to assess for postsurgical scar formation.
   c. A request for commentary on the multifidus group of muscles, especially noting if any fatty degeneration is present. Most radiologists will not comment unless requested. Because of the prior discopathy and surgical decompression, it is assumed that such muscular wasting will be present. However, it is good to document the extent of the multifidus wasting.

6. Should any other special tests be ordered, i.e., blood work or electrodiagnostic studies?
   a. The absent Achilles reflex without muscle weakness and paraesthesia probably does not warrant an electromyography (EMG) or nerve conduction test, but does warrant close monitoring. This may be a normal variant, as was discussed in Chapter 12, or it may be due to hypertonicity of the gastrocnemius/soleus complex. A poor patient response, such as persistent or increasing neurological findings, would then warrant a neurological consultation and probable neurodiagnostic studies.
   b. Because of the recent increase in urinary frequency and persistent fever, a urinalysis would be appropriate to rule out urinary tract infection. If there were a kidney infection, this can also account for unilateral back pain, which can cause severe pain and muscle spasm (i.e., the classic kidney colic) via viscerosomatic pathways. In the early stages, the typical finding of a kidney infection includes unilateral rigidity of the posterolateral flank, with little or no spinal dysfunction except for the asymmetrical tone and altered posture. With time, a secondary spinal syndrome can occur because of altered mechanics. Hopefully, this would be accomplished by the provider to whom the patient was referred, but the clinician can never assume so and must remain vigilant for issues overlooked by another or one's self.
7. What treatment strategies should be considered if red flags are ruled out?
   a. A trial course of MTT and adjunctive measures for 2–4 weeks should be tried. The treatment plan might include modalities to reduce pain or hypertonicity and also to allow the patient to become more relaxed prior to MTT. Others may instead choose to use manual methods such as massage or mobilization methods. For example, postisometric relaxation might be quite effective in reducing the TrPs of the right quadratus lumborum and erector spinae. If the thoracolumbar junction palpated as dysfunctional, manipulation (HVLA) of this region would be attempted with the patient supine with her arms crossed over her chest and hands on opposite shoulders. If the McKenzie passive extension posture did not peripheralize her symptoms, this would be provided as a home assignment with the application of ice and a "no heat" warning. If this strategy improved function (i.e., increased mobility and decreased pain), then the patient would be instructed to perform tolerable self-mobilization exercises for home, to use a cold pack 15 minutes/hour for pain, and to slightly increase her walking, as long as it did not provoke her symptoms.
   b. One might manipulate the lumbar and pelvic joints to free any joint dysfunction. On rare occasions a lumbar support belt or a trochanteric belt is provided for short-term use. The sit/stand test is used to determine this, which is considered positive if the patient cannot rise from a chair with his or her arms crossed in front of the chest without help. If the sacroiliac joints need stabilization, a trochanter belt will make this action possible.
   c. Due to the clinical history and current presentation, neural mobilization techniques may be quite helpful and a trial course would be prudent.
   d. There is evidence to suggest sacro-iliac dysfunction as a contributing pain generator. So a trial course of mobilization and/or manipulation would be recommended.
   e. There is evidence of lumbosacral/pelvic instability, so a sensorimotor training and lumbopelvic stabilization should be instituted.
   f. Ongoing patient communication and education is very important in order to reduce the negative effects of illness behavior. Topics should include a clear understanding of "hurt versus harm" and also to anticipate some brief, tolerable increases in her symptoms as a result of the MTT, exercises and altered body mechanics.

Continuing Presentation

Because of the findings that included LBP in the presence of unresolved fever, stat MRI was ordered to rule out epidural abscess. Additional contrast studies were ordered to differentiate new disc herniation from postsurgical scar. These studies demonstrated postsurgical changes at L4–L5 but no specific nerve root scarring. There was no sign of epidural abscess or any other infectious process. Disc herniation was found at L5–S1 on the right that encroached upon, but did not contact, the S1 nerve root.

Questions

1. What type(s) of manual method(s) would be appropriate for this patient, if any?
   a. In the early stages the nerve root and posterior joints need to be protected from the forces of HVLA manipulation. Therefore, joint mobilization may be effective if it is tolerable. Any HVLA manipulation should be directed to other dysfunctional joints in the closed, kinematic system and performed in such a

manner as avoid stress to the disc and nerve root and posterior joints. Brief applications of cold packs may be helpful to provide pain relief.

2. What manual methods would be contraindicated, if any?
   a. HVLA manipulation in the lower lumbar segments may be contraindicated. Premanipulation positioning and pre-thrust testing should confirm or refute this. However, a trial course of mobilization and muscle energy procedures may be effective. Some practitioners employ intermittent, flexion distraction with success while others add intermittent traction gradually as tolerated, when the area is less inflamed to avoid the occasional crisis.
3. Would referral for co-management be appropriate? If so, what type of specialist(s) would be recommended?
   a. In this case the fever had to be assessed, as previously stated, and so comanagement may have been essential, depending on the MTT clinician's training ability to order appropriate diagnostic testing, and the subsequent test results.
   b. If the condition responds to conservative measures as outlined above, then these should be continued on a decreasing frequency as corrective exercises are introduced at the office and continued independently at home. It must be stated that the leg symptoms should supersede the low back symptoms here, so improvement would be defined as a centralization of symptoms as defined by McKenzie. This case would not be co-managed with or fully referred to a surgeon unless conservative methods proved to be ineffective.
   c. If the patient remains essentially unchanged in her leg symptoms, despite a trial of MTT, then a referral to another type of spine specialist would be appropriate. The referral might be to a neurologist, an orthopedist, or a pain medicine specialist. In such a case, the MTT provider may choose to continue comanagement of the case if it is felt that additional MTT and/or rehabilitation would be beneficial in conjunction with the additional treatment provided by the newly included specialist. For example, if the MTT and pain medicine specialist both felt that epidural injections would reduce the leg pain, then additional MTT and rehabilitation would be appropriate. However, if the MTT feels that this case would not benefit from a co-management strategy, then the referral should be made so that no further MTT would be recommended at that point. As such, the new spine specialist would assume full control of that case.
   d. If the patient's condition deteriorates despite MTT, then such treatment should be either altered or discontinued. In either case, a referral to another spine specialist would be appropriate.

Continuing Presentation

Following the application of MTT for this patient, posttreatment assessment demonstrated improved sacroiliac function, decreased TrPs of the erector spinae musculature, and a more balanced posture and gait. Subjectively, the patient noted a 25% decrease in back and leg pain. She was taught self-mobilization exercises after she demonstrated the ability to tolerably perform them well. These were designed to reduce hypertonicity and increase motion, while allowing her to start to become comfortable with the concept of safe, therapeutic activities and the benefit of independent exercise. She was warned that, because of the length (chronicity) of her condition, her symptoms would probably recur and might even be initially a little bit worse for a few days.

She was instructed to perform self-stretches, use local cold applications for 15 minutes every hour, and not to let this upset her if it occurred. If, at any time, she felt that she was having problems that seemed excessive, beyond what was described here, she was told to immediately call and discuss it. She was rescheduled for 2–4 days.

The patient returned as scheduled, noting a further decrease in her leg pain, but also stating that her back pain had increased slightly since her last visit. She also complained of a new symptom, lower mid-back pain, which began the day after the last visit. On examination, palpable joint dysfunction was noted, as was increased hypertonicity of the local paraspinal musculature.

Questions

1. What type(s) of manual method(s) would be appropriate for this patient, if any?
   a. The thoracolumbar region requires assessment, but this new symptom is not an uncommon event as the patient begins to resume more activities and alter movement patterns with prescribed exercises. As noted above, the patient was warned that symptoms could migrate a little following treatment of a chronic condition. Likewise, the increase of the right-sided low back symptoms is not an uncommon finding, as the chronic symptoms wax and wane. However, each of these regions requires

examination by the clinician to confirm that these are indeed simple flare-ups as suspected.

   b. As the patient improves, there is less concern as to contraindications and greater focus on what remaining joints and soft tissues remain dysfunctional. Once this is determined, the MTT practitioner can then choose the best technique for each given dysfunction. However, techniques that help to improve muscle balance and coordination, in addition to joint motion, such as muscle energy and proprioceptive neuromuscular facilitation (PNF) maneuvers, would be especially helpful. In addition, sensorimotor training and a functional stabilization program, as described in Chapter 28, may now be initiated as the patient starts to resume more daily activities.
   c. As the patient is provided with specific exercises to counter the assessed dysfunction, it is an excellent time to continue to counsel her regarding the importance of consistent exercise, while observing any signs of illness behavior that may need to be addressed.
2. What manual methods would be contraindicated, if any?
   a. Any technique that peripheralized the patient's symptoms during the pretest thrust would be contraindicated.
3. Would referral for co-management be appropriate? If so, what type of specialist(s) would be recommended?
   a. In this case, the patient appears to be improving with regard to her leg symptoms. In the absence of a significant increase in symptoms or the sudden appearance of red flags, the only referral might be to a rehabilitation specialist, if the MTT provider does not provide these services.

Continuing Presentation

As her condition improved, she was counseled on her risks of chronicity and the importance of learning to independently reduce these risks. Special emphasis was placed upon her deconditioning a topic she could clearly self manage. She expressed a strong desire to avoid any future back problems and was prepared to assume the responsibility for this goal. Accordingly, a functional lumbosacral stabilization program was introduced, including a variety of floor exercises. Unfortunately, she was unable to perform lumbopelvic stabilization exercises because of abdominal weakness; so specific abdominal "crunch" exercises were provided for home use. However, her inability to perform these well or gain additional abdominal stability prompted scar lysing and myofascial MTT to be employed by the clinician following appropriate patient education. She was taught self-mobilization methods for daily home care that also included cold applications for anticipated secondary edema. After 2 weeks, the tenderness from the scar was significantly reduced and she found that she could isolate and contract her abdomus rectus well for the first time in years. Therefore, the functional lumbopelvic stabilization program was resumed.

The patient noted that her mild urinary incontinence improved as her symptoms decreased and as she made gains in her functional lumbosacral stability. However, her symptoms did not fully resolve, so she was provided with additional pelvic floor exercises, including Kegel exercises, performed several times daily. These helped her to fully resolve her urinary incontinence; otherwise MTT for the pelvic floor would have been recommended. Some MTT specialists perform such treatment, while others refer the patients to clinicians who specialize in male and/or female pelvic dysfunction.

As the patient continued to improve in her condition and functional stability, she found that her final remaining symptom was that of mild right-sided LBP after walking for more than 20 minutes, which gradually worsened if she continued to walk. The previously noted right foot pronation was suspected as being clinically relevant, so a trial course of MTT and foot exercises seemed to bring some temporary improvement. Therefore, a trial course of foot taping to elevate and stabilize the arch was attempted, which brought about significant improvement for several days. Unfortunately, the symptoms recurred after the tape was removed, so the patient was fitted for orthotics. These devises resulted in the resolution of her remaining symptom of back pain with prolonged walking. She was also provided with intrinsic foot exercises in the hopes that she might gradually be able to bolster the arch of her foot and ultimately avoid the ongoing use of foot supports.

On her final visit, the patient's customized exercise program was altered to include those exercises that would provide the broadest functional benefit for her specific functional needs. She was given those for which she demonstrated a positive attitude, those that could be practically performed at home, and those that fit within her daily timetable. She was inspired to continue with this regimen despite the fact that the painful condition that initially inspired her was now past. A verbal confirmation that she would continue with her home exercises was requested and received. The patient was not rescheduled.

THE FUTURE OF MTT

Evidence-based health care appears to be the way of the future. This presents a mixed blessing for practitioners of MTT. On one side, there is growing evidence of clinical benefit from methods such as manipulation and mobilization for the treatment of LBS. However, the complexity of understanding the etiological factors of LBS and the neuromuscular changes because of MTT is extremely complex. Therefore, the authors of this chapter feel that it will require decades before sufficient understanding is gleaned to sufficiently understand these mechanisms. Once these mechanisms are better clarified, additional time and research will be required to determine the proper applications of MTT for the appropriate, evidence-based condition.

Local versus Global Treatment

At this point in history, much of MTT research regarding LBS involves manipulation. In most studies manipulation is addressed to the site of pain, i.e., the low back. The process of researching MTT for LBS in which the treatment is directed to body regions away from the low back presents an array of additional research complications. As such, there remains a paucity of available quality research regarding the efficacy of applying MTT to distant body sites in the treatment of LBS. Nevertheless, the authors of this chapter have found that treatment of other body regions such as the cervical spine, the thoracic spine, and the feet with MTT can have a profound impact on certain LBS.

The problem is that these are not generic types of cases and that the clinician must possess high levels of clinical assessment skills in order to determine dysfunction of these distant body regions and then provide correct measures.

Until such time as researchers can properly identify and isolate patients with LBS that are caused by distant body region dysfunctions and then perform randomized clinical trials on such patients, this topic will remain speculative. Nevertheless, the authors of this chapter strongly feel that many of today's patients with recurrent LBS are in need of treatment outside of the lumbopelvic region, and that sufficient clinical literacy skills will direct the clinicians to isolate these types of cases and assist their patients when other more evidence-based methods have failed.

Preventative Aspects of MTT

There is a great deal of controversy regarding whether MTT can be used as a preventative strategy for reducing LBS recurrences. The authors of this chapter feel that this is a relative issue, based upon each individual's specific risk factors for chronicity. For example, some patients who receive periodic manipulations may benefit from minor reductions of pain while being reminded to perform the home exercises, inspiring them to perform these tasks when they otherwise would not. While the only preventative strategies for recurrent LBS are education and exercise, it remains speculative whether occasional MTT may indeed be successful in reducing costs and suffering for a circumscribed group of patients. The authors of this chapter feel that ultimately there will be sufficient research to allow clinicians to be able to determine which patients would best benefit from preventative MTT and that this strategy will result in a reduction of suffering and cost associated with chronicity.

SUMMARY

1. This chapter has provided commentary regarding the opinions on MTT.
2. The observations and opinions expressed here are of multidisciplinary instructors in MTT who are aware of the current state of clinical mixed evidence regarding treatment for LBS, but who feel strongly that time and further research will lead to important advances supporting the methods described here.
3. The authors recommend that clinicians who utilize MTT, or students intending to utilize MTT, remain determined to continually improve their clinical literacy (i.e. clinical palpatory and visual) skills.
4. The authors recommend that MTT stay a breast of the most current evidence-based criteria for the management of LBS. Where appropriate, those methods should be utilized, with other MTT being integrated as supporting measures.

THE GOLDEN RULES OF MTT

1. MTT have a greater impact on the neurophysiological response than the biomechanical response. However, these two issues are functionally integrated.
2. A structural and functional diagnosis is an essential component of a total patient evaluation. The emotional, or psychosocial aspect is a subset of the functional aspect.
3. A structural diagnosis looks for altered functional capacity of the locomotor system as a reflection of the level of wellness or illness in the patient at that moment in time.
4. The structural diagnostic process evaluates the altered functional symmetry of the body, i.e., altered range of regional and joint motion. This is primarily hypomobility and altered tissue texture of the related soft tissues, namely myofascial hypertonicity and altered tissue mobility.
5. Altered findings on examination can be used prognostically, since they should show improvement when the appropriate MTT is applied. Lack of improvement should alert the clinician to use other diagnostic therapeutic interventions.

6. The appropriate application of MTT should result in the enhanced capacity of the patient to cope with the dysfunction.
7. The greater number of MTT the clinician masters, the better for the patient.
8. Most treatment affects the neural, respiratory, and circulatory functions of the patient but the outcomes depend upon the inherent capacity of the patient to get well.
9. MTT should give the patient the ability to positively affect his or her health with appropriate exercise. The patient's compliance with exercise is crucial for long-term benefit.
10. MTT must be prescribed and dosed as any other therapeutic intervention. Age and physical condition of the patient plus knowledge of other therapeutic interventions concurrently being applied to the patient will modify the type and amount of manual treatment to be given.
11. Do not initiate treatment until a working diagnosis has been established and a subsequent trial course of treatment determined. The effectiveness of this trial should be established within a few visits, assuming the patient is being properly instructed and is compliant with his or her activities between office visits.
12. The working diagnoses are usually confirmed by the response to treatment. This response includes both the patient's subjective statements and the clinician's observations based upon his or her clinical literacy skill.
13. In cases where reduced mobility is present, where patients do not demonstrate increased mobility after a few visits of MTT, the clinician should reevaluate and suspect nonmusculoskeletal conditions as the true etiology.
14. Treating the spine is like gardening rather than bricklaying. The manual therapy provider is attempting to alter the neurophysiological aspects far more than the structural aspects of the patient.
15. It is important to remember that pathology is a process and also to determine the underlying pathogenesis. It is not uncommon for too much treatment to be applied to the pathology and insufficient attention paid to the true etiological factors.
16. The motion units that are manipulated or mobilized are often performed around only one axis of rotation, whereas the restrictions may be in all the axes of rotation. Therefore the clinician must possess the skills to both assess and correct such multidimensional dysfunction.
17. Clinicians often initiate exercises too soon and the rehabilitation strategy too late. Rehabilitation begins with patient education, helping the patients to understand their condition and overcome their fears and misperceptions. Therefore, instructing the patients in the resumption of tolerably safe activities as soon as possible is a proper rehabilitation strategy.
18. In today's evidence-based world, students and clinicians must realize that manual medicine, chiropractic, and osteopathic methods are rich in observational studies and empirical reporting that demonstrate the efficacy of their procedures for complex conditions. Unfortunately, many of these methods have not yet been validated by randomized studies. This is partly because the diagnosis upon which the treatment is based is not yet globally accepted as evidence-based. Nevertheless, this is neither the fault of the patient nor the clinician but rather of the system, which must allow patients the opportunity to receive trial courses of such long-established treatments until such times as their efficacy is either proven or disproven.
19. With regard to lumbopelvic pain syndromes, there is increasing evidence that the pelvic floor is an increasingly important region from both an etiological and therapeutic perspective. The authors of this chapter believe that further research and treatment must be dedicated to add training to the assessment and treatment of the pelvic floor and that such energies will result in greater success rates in the treatment of chronic LBS.
20. Myofascial pain syndrome requires, by definition, the presence of myofascialTrPs, as noted in Chapter 9. While these were initially thought to be more of a biomechanical entity caused by overload, neurophysiological and etiological factors now appear to be more closely associated with this condition. Therefore, the authors have observed that all neuromusculoskeletal syndromes have a myofascial component as a secondary or tertiary issue, a concept they feel will be accepted with time.
21. A practitioner should attempt to apply methods of manual diagnosis that have known reliability and validity whenever possible, and avoid tests in isolation with poor reliability or validity. Therefore, a battery of tests in combination with the history still allows working diagnoses to be established.
22. All diagnoses in patients with LBS are working diagnoses that are tested with the most important diagnostic procedure, a trial course of treatment.
23. If a patient is not improving with an adequate trial of MTT, it is unlikely that "one more attempt" with the same method will be beneficial. The practitioner should have a low threshold for deciding what constitutes an "adequate trial." In most cases, some change should be seen in one to three treatments. This strategy is, of course, dependent on the patient's activities between treatments and the complexity of the case.

24. If the patient is not improving with MTT, consider four things: (a) the diagnosis is incorrect; (b) the diagnosis is partially correct but there are additional factors that have been overlooked; (c) the diagnosis is correct but the treatments applied are ineffective; and (d) there are lifestyle-related or psychosocial perpetuating factors that are interfering with progress.
25. Remember that manual diagnoses and treatment do not involve the practitioner "doing things to" a patient. They involve the interaction between the practitioner and patient, a scenario in which both parties play an active and dynamic role.
26. What the patient experiences during manual diagnosis and treatment is more important than what the practitioner is experiencing. Again, however, it is the dynamic interaction of these factors that encompasses the clinical experience.
27. The practitioner may feel that a certain finding is significant, but must always consider its significance in relation to the patient's condition, not just the practitioner's concept of "normal."
28. Any manual method that the practitioner chooses should be matched to the diagnosis or to some aspect of that diagnosis. One should not attempt to force the patient to match the MTT.
29. Every attempt should be made to provide at least one activity, perhaps an exercise, to complement the manual methods that are being used. This empowers the patient and allows him or her to further benefit from these methods by functionally or practically integrating them into the movement patterns.
30. MTT clinicians should abide by Morris's rule of "proving safety." This means that patients must "prove" the safety of more forceful MTT before they are actually performed. This means, for example, that the patients should be able to tolerate the "prethrust test," positioning and light loading in the same line of drive as the HVLA manipulation would be performed. Also, one must assess for any symptom peripheralization (i.e. increased pain/symptoms extending farther down an extremity) with this test, which would contraindicate the maneuver if positive.
31. MTT clinicians continue to grow in their understanding and appreciation of the broad spectrum of manual assessment and therapy methods. The time required to gain true expertise in these methods is long. However, students and clinicians who fail to aspire to such expertise fail to appreciate all of the potential options available that might benefit their patients.
32. Non-MTT clinicians who assess and treat LBS should continue to grow in their understanding and appreciation of MTT in order to more effectively manage these cases.
33. The key rule of clinical palpatory literacy is appreciation of the barrier phenomenon. This is the first barrier of resistance found in connective tissues. No practitioner can apply manual procedures with maximum effectiveness without an appreciation, both conceptually and from the standpoint of sensory perception of the barrier phenomenon.
34. Professor Karel Lewit of Charles University, Czech Republic, stated, "The clinician who only looks to the site of pain is lost." Chronic back disorders require global assessment to determine where the etiological dysfunction is located, which at times can be quite distant from the region of pain.
35. Janda stated that all clinicians must remember to observe the patient as a whole person, rather than as a biological entity or a regional dysfunctional challenge. It is in this context that the most comprehensive assessment and treatment plan can be established.

DEDICATION

This chapter is dedicated to the lead author, the late Professor Vladimir Janda. This was the commentary he had envisioned for years and always hoped to read. He outlined it along the lines of that vision, and we have endeavored to complete it in his sorely-missed absence. Although he is not with us to review the final product, the remaining contributors pay tribute to his insights and would like the reader to know that all attempts have been made to maintain his high standard.

PART

V

REHABILITATION OF THE LOW BACK

CHAPTER

26

REHABILITATION STRATEGIES IN LOW BACK SYNDROMES

Donald R. Murphy and Craig E. Morris

OUTLINE

OBJECTIVES

1. To explain the clinical importance of rehabilitation for patients with low back syndrome.
2. To clarify the key purposes of rehabilitation for low back patients.
3. To appreciate the importance of a "rehabilitation mind set."
4. To define typical type of rehabilitation strategies.
5. To explain when various rehabilitation strategies may be best utilized.
6. To emphasize the importance of utilizing outcome measures to monitor rehabilitation progress.
7. To discuss the effectiveness of rehabilitation for patients with low back syndromes.

INTRODUCTION

Essential to full recovery in many patients is some form of rehabilitation. Most patients, and too many clinicians, mistakenly believe that a full recovery is defined as merely the resolution of symptoms. Unfortunately, asymptomatic patients are frequently left with residual functional compromises following treatment, such as diminished strength, endurance, fear of activities, etc., that increases risk of recurrence of their supposedly "resolved" condition or sets the scene for a new condition secondary to the residual effects of the earlier problem. For these reasons, and several others that will be explained in this chapter, rehabilitation can fill a vital clinical void and greatly increase the chance of a patient's full recovery.

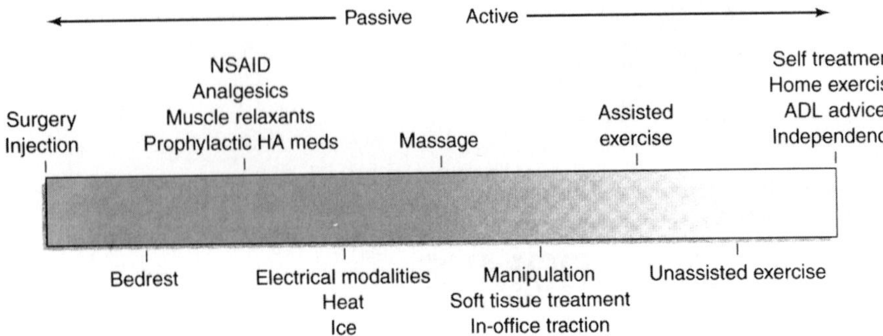

FIGURE 26–1. A conceptual model of the passive to active paradigm of rehabilitation. *(Reprinted with permission from Murphy DR. Protocols for the management of patients with cervical spine syndrome. New York: McGraw-Hill, 2000:691–700.)*

Rehabilitation literally means to return to one's habits. However, it has come to include the prevention of functional debility and the maintenance and optimization of functional ability. In a broad sense, it can be said that any procedure that helps to improve, or optimize, patient functioning can be considered rehabilitative. As such, rehabilitation begins at the clinician's initial encounter with the patient. However, for the purpose of this chapter, rehabilitation will be considered the integration of educational and exercise strategies for the promotion of functional recovery.

THE REHABILITATION MINDSET

Although only a portion of the patients who consult a conservative care clinician for a low back syndrome anticipate undergoing a rehabilitation program, the clinician must always utilize a *rehabilitation mindset* from the outset. That is, he or she must initially assess the patient in a manner that screens for the various biopsychosocial barriers to recovery in order to determine the case complexity and prioritize the methods necessary to effectively restore locomotor system function. This so-called *rehabilitation strategy* is composed of short- and long-term goals, which are dynamic in nature, being altered as the patient's condition changes. In simple cases, briefly counseling the patient on reducing the risks of an early-stage dysfunction with, for example, corrective postural and ergonomic advice may be a sufficient rehabilitation strategy.

Clinical Pearl: Rehabilitation literally means to return to one's habits. However, it has come to include the prevention of functional debility and the maintenance and optimization of functional ability.

The rehabilitation strategy typically becomes multifaceted in chronic low back syndrome cases, especially those that entail disability, a work-related injury, and or medicolegal issues (see Chapters 19 and 36). This strategy may include comanagement with one or more other specialists. In such cases, interprofessional dialogue becomes vital in order to present a consistent message to the patient and a coordinated treatment plan that is complimentary to the goals of each specialist.

Although this textbook addresses conservative management approaches to low back syndromes, this does not mean that such management necessarily ends with nonconservative measures such as surgery. Indeed, surgical options at times are welcome by the clinician and patient alike who have failed all attempts to sufficiently improve the recalcitrant case (see Chapters 34 and 35). However, once the surgical procedure has been performed and pathoanatomical issues addressed, the patient should then be returned for postsurgical rehabilitation (see Chapter 29). Once the determination for surgery is made, the rehabilitation strategy may then be to optimally presurgically condition the patient in a tolerable manner so that they require as little reconditioning postoperatively as possible. The next chapter addresses early postoperative surgical rehabilitation strategies in detail.

The rehabilitation strategy typically involves a continuum of measures or exercises that begins with rather conservative, tolerable approaches and gradually, tolerably evolves to include more demanding methods. Although the exact order of these measures may at times vary, the lead author addressed this continuum of care rehabilitation strategy,[1] which is explained in Figure 26–1.

REHABILITATION: THE FIVE BASIC PURPOSES

There are five basic purposes of rehabilitation in the patient with a low back syndrome, which are listed in Table 26–1. It is important to keep these purposes in mind when devising a rehabilitation strategy, as the approach must always have at its core those endpoints that need to be met in each individual patient. This way, one can avoid "cookbook" rehabilitation, and can focus on designing the strategy for the specific needs of each individual patient.

Optimize the Function of the Locomotor System

In Chapter 13, the functional assessment of the patient with low back syndromes was presented. This

TABLE 26–1. The Five Purposes of Spinal Rehabilitation

1. Improve the function of the locomotor system.
2. Improve automatic stabilization responses.
3. Reverse or prevent central sensitization.
4. Improve strength in key muscles and overall physical fitness.
5. Prevent or reverse ineffective illness behavior.

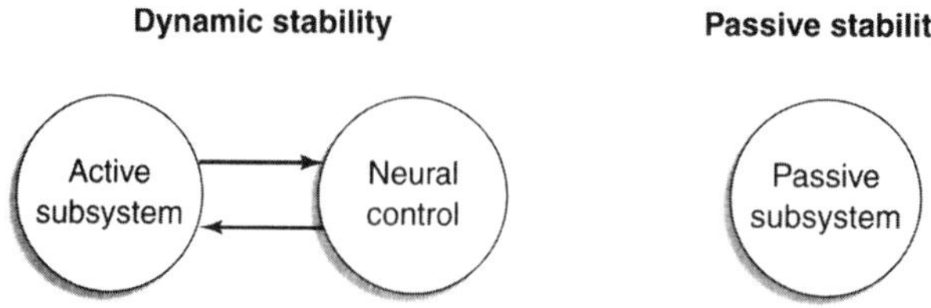

FIGURE 26–2. The interaction between the components of the dynamic stability system. *(Reprinted with permission from Murphy[5].)*

assessment allows the clinician to detect those specific functional deficits that are present in the patient that may have an impact on the perpetuation of their pain experience. These findings then determine the initial specific rehabilitation strategies that are needed to correct the dysfunction. For example, in the presence of a positive hip extension test revealing delay in the contraction of the gluteus maximus, sensorimotor training, with particular emphasis on activation of the gluteus maximus (see Chapter 23), may be one of the rehabilitation methods of choice.[2] Depending on the complexity and chronicity of the particular case, there may be many such isolated dysfunctions. For example, a patient with low back pain who was antalgic for several weeks may have developed abnormal postural compromises in the hips, pelvic region, and upper back that become automated with repetition. As each functional compromise is addressed, the clinician must observe the effects, both locally and globally, of the treament. As various dysfunctions are improved, the stage can then be set for more complex and integrative rehabilitative protocols that will be discussed later in this chapter.

Improve Automatic Stabilization Responses

It used to be thought that spinal instability involved "overstretching" of the ligaments of the spine, leading to excessive mobility as a result of the inability of the ligaments to control range of motion.[3] In recent years, however, the concept of spinal instability has changed. In fact, whether the spinal ligaments have any passive role to play in controlling intersegmental stability in the spine, known as "passive stability," has been brought into question.[4] Instead, the ligaments are now thought to be only a part of a much more complex, dynamic, and inherent spinal stabilization mechanism.

What has been termed "dynamic stability"[5–7] has recently been seen as an important function that is designed to prevent or minimize microtrauma to the spinal tissues, thus to prevent or minimize pain and injury. This concept is explored in detail in Chapter 5, and is only presented superficially here. The responses are generated by the central nervous system (CNS) to provide stability to the spine function in such a way as to occur automatically in response to (feedback mechanism) or in anticipation of ("feed-forward" mechanism) a perturbation that has the potential to cause strain to the spinal tissues.

Clinical Pearl: In recent years, however, the concept of spinal instability has changed. In fact, whether the spinal ligaments have any passive role to play in controlling intersegmental stability in the spine, known as "passive stability,"has been brought into question.

Rather than being seen as a passive function that merely controls end ranges, dynamic stability is provided by a complex system of highly coordinated actions that involve the ligamentous tissues of the spine, the spinal and pelvic muscles, and the CNS[8] (Fig. 26–2). When the spine is subjected to a perturbation, i.e., a force that has the potential to cause injury to the intersegmental tissues, this perturbation is first detected by the mechanoreceptors in the involved tissues, particularly the ligamentous receptors and the muscle spindles of the intrinsic spinal muscles (Fig. 26–3). Information with regard to the amplitude

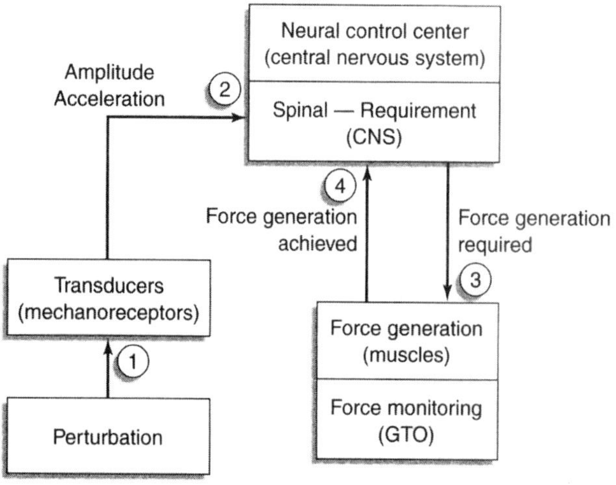

FIGURE 26–3. The mechanism of dynamic stability of the spine (see text for explanation). *(Reprinted with permission from Murphy[5].)*

and acceleration of the perturbation is transmitted by the mechanoreceptors to the CNS, which determines the degree, speed, and coordination of force generation that is required to provide stability. This information is relayed to the force generators of the spine, i.e., the muscles. The muscles generate the amount of force that they are instructed and, via the afferent input from the receptors in muscle that transmit tension feedback, primarily the golgi tendon organs, apprise the CNS as to the amount of force that was generated The CNS then determines whether the requirement for stability was met. If it was not, an adjustment is made.

It is important to note here that "the muscles" includes the "intrinsic" spinal muscles, i.e., the transverse abdominis, quadratus lumborum, internal oblique and multifidus, the pelvic floor, and abdominal diaphragm,[9–12] and the larger "extrinsic" muscles, i.e., the external oblique, rectus abdominis, and erector spinae. While it is common to make distinctions between these intrinsic and extrinsic muscles with regard to stability, any true functional distinction has recently been questioned.[13] Furthermore, there is evidence that one muscle, the multifidus, may indeed display intrinsic and extrinsic qualities, depending on whether the fibers are deep or superficial.[14] It is the harmonious activity of all the muscles that is the essential feature of stability and, while certain muscles may play a more important role in providing stability in certain tasks, and a lesser role in other tasks, no particular muscle or set of muscles should be seen as "primary stabilizers."

It has been demonstrated that these responses associated with dynamic stability do not function properly in patients with chronic low back pain (LBP),[15–21] leading to the suggestion that improper and inefficient stabilization responses may serve as a perpetuating factor in these patients. It is therefore essential that these automatic responses are detected on examination, to whatever extent possible, and corrected in rehabilitation.

Reverse or Prevent Central Sensitization

In recent years, it has become increasingly clear that central sensitization plays an important role in chronic LBP.[22–25] Central sensitization occurs as a result of acute nociceptive bombardment[26–28] or from chronic ongoing nociceptive activity.[29] Both these nociceptive phenomena can cause several changes in the CNS that lead to altered pain sensation. First, both nociceptive specific and wide dynamic range neurons in the dorsal horn can become sensitized to nociceptive input, thus responding more intensely to subsequent stimuli. But the wide dynamic range neurons have been shown to become more intensely sensitized than nociceptive-specific neurons. Wide dynamic range neurons receive input from nonnociceptive sources as well as nociceptive sources.[22] In addition, once they are sensitized, wide dynamic range neurons often will respond as intensely to nonnociceptive input as they did to the original nociceptive input, because of strengthened synaptic links with these nonnociceptive afferents that are normally benign from a pain-perspective.[30,31] This causes the CNS to misinterpret intense activity from nonnociceptive input, particularly from deep tissues such as joints, ligaments, and muscles, as being painful because of the intensity of the input. So by this mechanism, normal movement can continue to produce pain even in the absence of peripheral tissue damage or inflammation, or in the presence of low-grade peripheral tissue damage.

Bennett[29] identifies four clinical features of central sensitization: (1) the description of pain seems to be inappropriate in comparison with the degree of tissue pathology, or no tissue pathology may be discernable; (2) noxious stimuli result in a pain experience that is greater and more unpleasant than would normally be expected (i.e., hyperalgesia); (3) normally nonnoxious stimuli result in pain (i.e., allodynia); and (4) the extent of the pain boundary is greater than would be expected with acute tissue injury. It should be noted that these clinical features are strikingly similar to those that are associated with ineffective illness behavior[32,33] and it is important for the clinician to recognize the interrelationship between these phenomena. One must not assume the presence of a behavioral disorder in the presence of incongruence between the patient's description of the pain and the physical findings. Pain descriptions and behavior that are out of proportion with apparent tissue pathology or dysfunction should not be assumed to be purely of "psychosocial" origin. This assumption can have an extremely detrimental impact on the success of management, causing the clinician to search for the "psychosocial problems" that are producing chronic illness behavior, at the risk of alienating the patient, rather than directing attention to the central sensitization. Of course, central sensitization often occurs hand-in-hand with ineffective illness behavior.

Clinical Pearl: In recent years, it has become increasingly clear that central sensitization plays an important role in chronic LBP. Central sensitization occurs as a result of acute nociceptive bombardment or from chronic ongoing nociceptive activity.

It has been suggested that repetitive stimulation of the CNS with afferent input to the point of pain perception, but without producing excessive pain, can cause an adaptation response to occur.[34] This may lead to reprogramming of the dysfunctional pain pathways, decreasing the intensity of pain experienced with normal activities.[35] Clinically, this can be begun manually through the use of manipulation and other manual therapies that are believed to cause afferent impulses to be sent to the CNS,[34] and can progress to the use of stabilization and sensorimotor training and, ultimately, graded activity, in which the patient is gradually exposed to greater intensity of exercise or common activities of daily living (ADL), with increases in intensity occurring as pain tolerance increases.[36] Taking an active, exercise-based approach to patient management in the acute stage may help to prevent the development of central sensitization by repetitively exposing dorsal horn neurons to increased levels of physiological mechanoreceptive input.

Improve Strength in Key Muscles and Restore or Develop Overall Physical Fitness

Muscle strength, contrary to previous assumptions, does not play a strong role in the risk or perpetuation of LBP.[37–39] However, when returning a patient to normal work and/or personal activities that require strength, such as the injured industrial worker whose job tasks involve heavy lifting, it is sometimes necessary to restore strength in those muscles that are related to the involved tasks. In addition, clinical experience, along with some experimental evidence[40,41] suggests that those patients who are physically fit tend to handle LBP better than those who are deconditioned. Thus, it is important in some patients that specific strength training and general fitness training be instituted.

Prevent or Reverse Ineffective Illness Behavior

Behavior is of critical importance in patients with chronic LBP. Perhaps the most damaging type of behavior is fear-avoidance behavior.[42–49] Fear-avoidance behavior typically arises from the belief that "hurt equals harm," that is, that if the patient engages in an activity that provokes pain, that activity must be avoided to prevent further damage.[50] As this behavior persists, and the belief is reinforced by persistent activity-related pain, "stimulus generalization" can occur, in which fear avoidance expands to include activities that are only suspected of being potentially painful.[51]

It is essential to understand that ineffective illness behavior rarely occurs in the absence of true physical pain.[52] That is to say, patients who are engaging in illness behavior that is out of proportion to any signs tissue injury should not be assumed to be "faking it," have a primary psychological disorder, or have their symptoms purely attributed to "psychosocial problems." The behavior must be seen in the context of the entire clinical picture, and a careful and skilled search for the pain generators and underlying dysfunction that is contributing to the pain experience must be undertaken, in addition to identifying the behavioral signs that are present.

As was stated earlier, ineffective illness behavior often occurs in conjunction with central sensitization. Wide dynamic range neurons in the dorsal horn that are already sensitized by the nociceptive bombardment of the initial injury and/or by ongoing lower grade nociceptive input from dysfunction are further facilitated by attentional and behavioral processes.[53] That is to say that when increased attention is paid to nociceptive impulses, there occurs an enhancement of the process of central sensitization in the dorsal horn, thus intensifying the pain experience. In addition to this, when a patient behaves as one would when in acute pain, the behavior itself further facilitates the process of central sensitization, leading to a greater pain experience. Often, this enhancement of the pain experience then leads to further attention to the pain, and reinforcement of pain behavior, and a "viscious cycle" is created.

The authors have found that the most effective way to address both activity-related fear and central sensitization is the gradual desensitization of the patient through the introduction of movements (i.e., exercises). These activities challenge the patient's beliefs, in addition to challenging the hypersensitivity of the CNS, but not to the extent that they create a great deal of anxiety. Slowly increasing the intensity of the exercise allows for decreasing the patient's fear in a safe, controlled environment.[42]

Clinical Pearl: The authors have found that the most effective way to address both activity-related fear and central sensitization is the gradual desensitization of the patient through the introduction of movements (i.e., exercises).

TYPES OF REHABILITATION STRATEGIES AVAILABLE TO THE SPINE SPECIALIST

There are several strategies that have usefulness for certain patients in certain situations. It is important that these strategies be chosen on the basis of specific clinical indicators for their necessity, rather than being randomly applied in a "shotgun" manner. Described here are the most important methods in the rehabilitation of patients with low back syndromes.

Sensorimotor Training

Sensorimotor training is a method of exercise that involves the use of unstable surfaces on which the patient bears weight. Its purpose is to stimulate the afferent system in order to facilitate more effective motor programs for improved dynamic stability, posture, and movement patterns.

Stereotyped movement patterns are programmed into the CNS, beginning in the infant's developing locomotor system.[54] It is believed that there are certain programs for movement patterns that are inherent in the CNS and that naturally develop during the maturation process of the CNS. Other programs are created as a result of repetition. For example, gait is an inherent motor program—the individual naturally is programmed to engage in this activity. So, as the infant develops, he or she naturally moves toward developing the ability to walk, without having to be "taught" this movement pattern. On the other hand, driving a manual transmission automobile is an example of a learned motor program. The individual is not born with the program for engaging in this activity, and so must learn the activity and then form a program within the CNS through repetition, i.e., repetetively driving the vehicle. Once this program is formed, the individual no longer has to concentrate on performing the activity—he or she must simply get into the car, consult the program, and take off with very little cortical involvement. In either case, the motor program for each movement pattern is saved in an *engram* within the cerebral cortex.[54]

The maintenance of these motor programs is dependant, in part, on afferent information that arises from the receptors in the locomotor system.[55] This afferent information provides the "data" that determine the precise neural activity patterns that are involved in each specific program. It is important to note that this afferent information is presented as a whole "picture" to the CNS, rather than as a group of individual messages from each receptor.[56,57]

A motor program that is particularly important, and that is addressed with sensorimotor training, is that of postural stability.[58] Postural stability is the ability to maintain stable upright stance. This function has been shown to be impaired in some patients with chronic low back syndromes[59,60] and is believed to be an important perpetuating factor to the syndrome.

The purpose of sensorimotor training is based on the concept that motor programs can be negatively impacted by alteration of the afferent information that is arising from the periphery (i.e., outside) of the nervous tissue.[55] This can lead to the development of faulty movement patterns.[61] It has been suggested that faulty movement patterns can result from joint and muscle dysfunction, which alters the afferentation arising from the mechanoreceptors in the involved tissues.[62] So in the rehabilitation of faulty movement patterns, including dynamic instability, correction of the joint and muscle dysfunction via manual procedures (see Chapters 13, 20, and 23) may correct the faulty movement pattern, but if the motor program for the faulty pattern is well established in the CNS, the faulty movement pattern may not normalize quickly or automatically. Teaching the patients to carry out the movement themselves may lead to correct performance in the office, but this may not transfer adequately into everyday life. Sensorimotor training attempts to bypass the conscious correction of the movement patterns via a bombardment of the CNS with afferent signals to normalize the inborn motor program itself. It is hoped that this will lead to the correct carrying out of the movement pattern without the patient having to consciously focus on it.[61]

Sensorimotor training can be done using rocker boards, wobble boards, balance sandals, or virtually any unstable surface upon which a patient can stand. Depending on how much difficulty the patient has with balancing on an unstable surface, the patient will have to be started at a level that is challenging but one that he or she can handle. In many cases, this may be with the rocker board. Progression is made to the wobble board and, ultimately, to one-legged standing (Fig. 26–4). Balance sandals are also used (Figs. 26–5 and 26–6). These are sandals with hemispheres on the bottom and provide stimulation of each lower extremity separately during gait-related exercises. Instruction in proper utilization of balance (aka

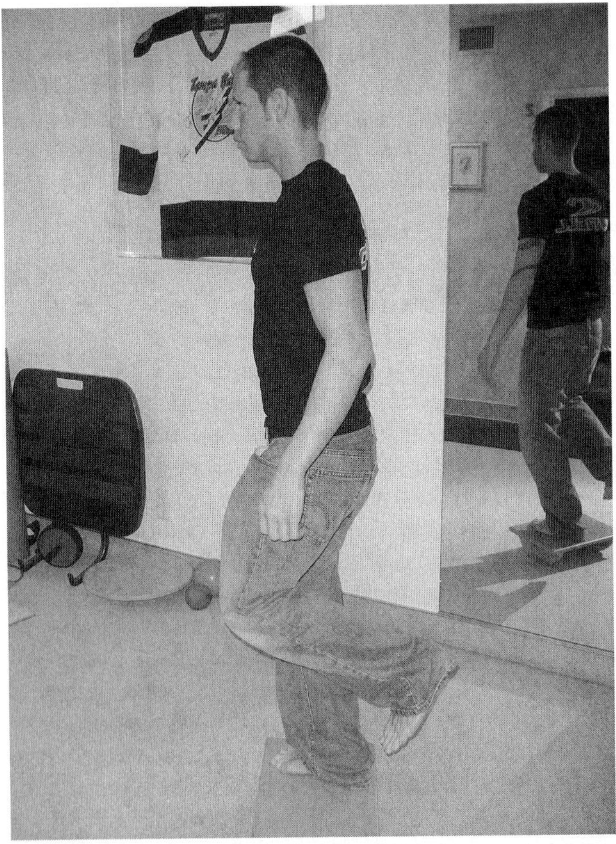

FIGURE 26–4. One-legged stand on the wobble board is an advanced strategy for integrating still upright posture into a sensorimotor training strategy.

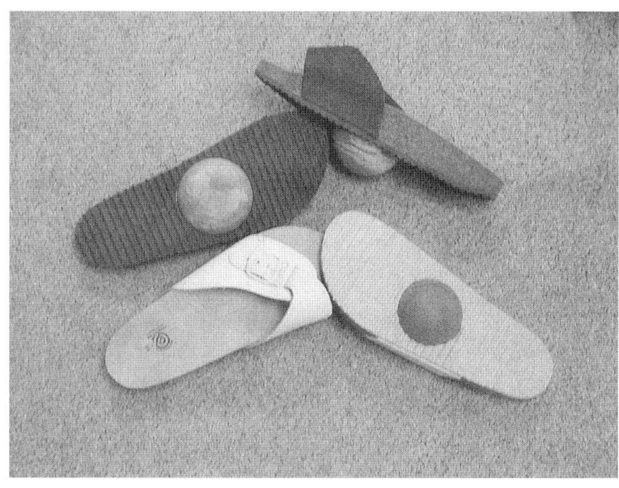

FIGURE 26–5. Photograph of balance (aka rehabilitation) sandals.

rehabilitation) sandals is discussed in detail in Chapter 28, which addresses sensorimotor training.

Stabilization Training

Stabilization training is a method by which exercises are used to alter the neurological program for stability mechanisms, so that these mechanisms occur automatically, subconsciously, and with maximum efficiency. As was discussed earlier in this chapter, and in greater detail in Chapter 5, there are natural, inborn mechanisms by which the locomotor system responds to potentially injurious perturbations. Via these inborn mechanisms, the stability system causes coactivation of those particular muscles that are best able to respond to any perturbation to which the spine may be subjected at any given time and provide protection to the spinal tissues with maximum speed and efficiency.[63–66]

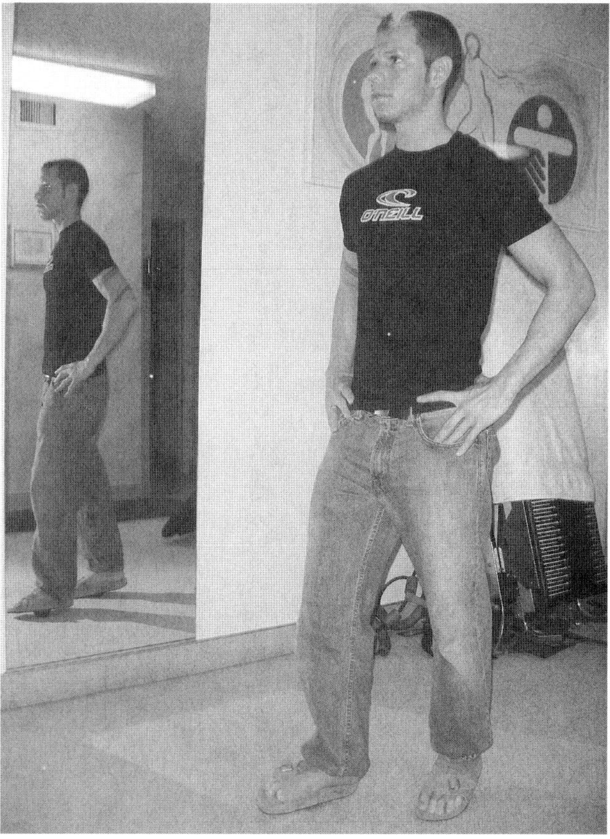

FIGURE 26–6. Use of balance (aka rehabilitation) sandals to integrate sensorimotor training with gait.

In the lumbar spine, there are a variety of muscles that are important in this regard, and which muscles play the most essential role depends on the particular activity at hand. These include the small, "intrinsic" muscles,[67,68] particularly the transverse abdominis,[69–77] multifidis,[4,78,79] quadratus lumborum,[13] diaphragm,[21,80] and pelvic floor muscles,[81] and the large "extrinsic" muscles, such as the erector spinae, rectus abdominis, external oblique, and latissimus dorsi.[14,82] For pelvic stability, the gluteus maximus and gluteus medius are particularly important,[82] in addition to the above-listed muscles. When the stability system is functioning normally, the CNS orders the precise combination of these muscles to contract at the appropriate time and with the ideal intensity to provide stability in response to a perturbation. The result of this coactivation is increased spinal stability as a result of direct effects on the intersegmental joints as well as through tension in the thoracolumbar fascia,[77,78] increase in intra-abdominal pressure,[70] and the stable transmission of forces between the upper extremity and the lower extremity.[83]

It has been demonstrated experimentally that certain muscles, specifically the transverse abdominis[19,73,84] and multifidis,[85–87] tend to become inhibited in patients with chronic LBP. Because of this, the first step in the process of training stability must be teaching the CNS to be able to identify these muscles. This ability is often lost in patients with chronic LBP.[19] So the patient must be taught to, first, consciously activate the muscles inhibited, and then to cause those muscles to provide their stabilization action while the patient moves the extremities. The expectation is that, with increasingly complex extremity movements performed while conscious cocontraction of the stability muscles is taking place, the cocontraction response will become subconscious and automatic. Therefore, the patient is first simply taught to isolate the transverse abdominis and multifidis by "drawing in" the abdomen. He or she is then taught to contract the pelvic floor muscles. Once these isolated coactivation maneuvers are mastered, and the patient is able to coactivate these muscles in the relative absence of contraction of the superficial muscles (rectus abdominis, external oblique, longissimus), the maneuvers are combined, so that the patient is coactivating the transverse abdominis, multifidis, and pelvic floor muscles. It is essential that the patient avoid breath holding and raising of the chest during these maneuvers in order to ensure proper involvement of the diaphragm.

Clinical Pearl: Stabilization training is a method by which exercises are used to alter the neurological program for stability mechanisms, so that these mechanisms occur automatically, subconsciously, and with maximum efficiency.

The patient is then started on very simple and basic extremity movements. The purpose of these movements is twofold: first, they force the stabilizing muscles to work under a light load and, second, they begin the process of forcing the cerebral cortex to focus on moving the extremities. This gradual shift of the focus from the coactivation to the extremity movements is important in encouraging the coactivation of the stabilizing muscles to become subconscious. The movements start out as a simple single extremity movement, such as raising the arm, while maintaining the coactivation of the stabilizing muscles (Fig. 26–7). The patient then progresses to raising one leg, which causes the muscles to maintain stability under a greater load than when the arm is raised. From here, progression moves to moving a single arm and leg at the same time. The arm and leg that are being moved are on opposite sides of the body (Fig. 26–8). This opposide-side extremity movement is essential, as it forces the stabilizing system to work not only under load, but also under circumstances in which the cerebral cortex must focus on the complex extremity movements. Therefore, the cortex must take focus away from the coactivation of the stabilizing muscles,

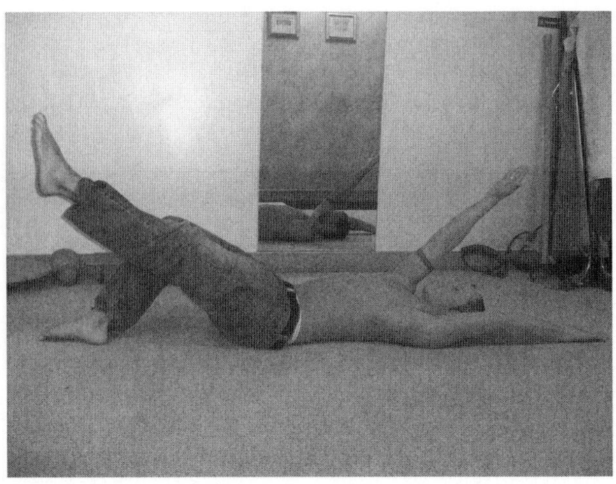

FIGURE 26–8. Raising the opposite arm and leg in the supine position.

and this coactivation is encouraged to become more subcortical. This subcortical activation of the stabilizing muscles paves the way for the response to become automatic, without the need for conscious effort on the part of the patient. Ultimately, the goal of stabilization training is to program the CNS to automatically order the correct stabilization response to a perturbation, recruiting those muscles that are made for stabilization.

From here, the exercises can involve varying positions, such as quadruped (Fig. 26–9) and the use of a gymnastic ball (Fig. 26–10), which adds further challenge to the stabilization system by forcing it to operate in the unstable environment created by the ball. Also, other important stabilizing muscles can be targeted, such as those of the pelvis (Fig. 26–11) and the scapular stabilizers (Fig. 26–12). Ultimately, the patient can be taught to recruit the stabilizing muscles during activities of daily living, particularly during

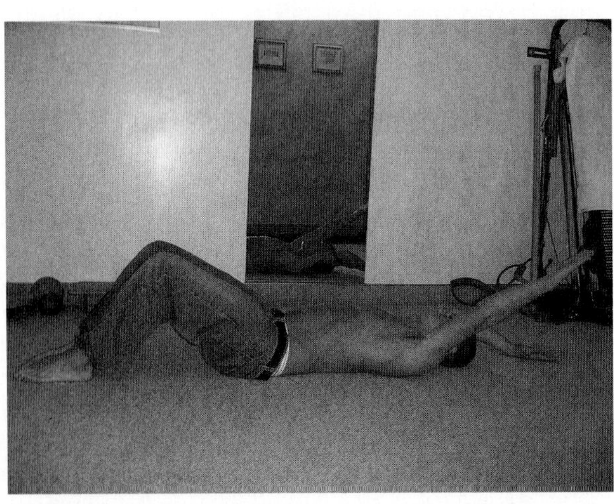

FIGURE 26–7. Single-arm raise in the supine position.

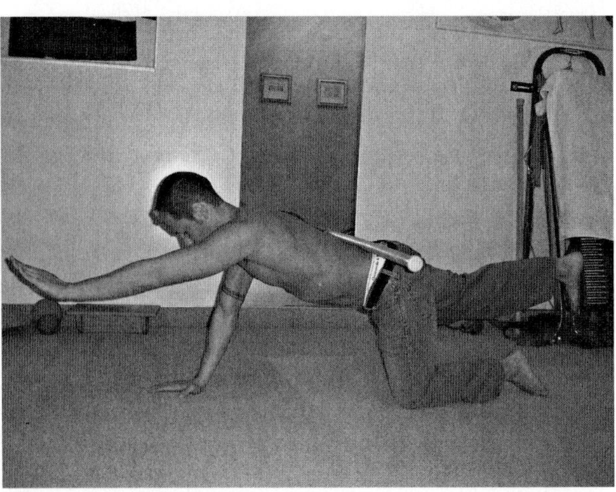

FIGURE 26–9. Raising the opposite arm and leg in the quadruped position.

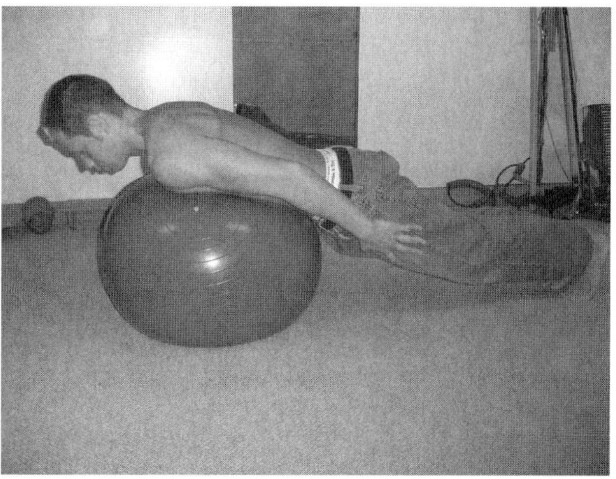

FIGURE 26–10. Prone walkout on the gymnastic ball.

activities that have the potential to cause injury such as heavy lifting.

As the patient transitions through these multipositional exercise strategies, it becomes easy to overlook the basic aspects of lumbopelvic stabilization and instead focus on new and intrigueing challenges posed by the exercises themselves. For instance, the balance challenges presented by the gymnastic ball may cause the patient to forget about the neutral pelvis. In many cases, the patient may have resumed a more stable lumbopelvic movement strategy and the continuum of exercises can proceed with minimal supervision of the postural and movement patterns. However, the clinician must avoid the assumption that all patients will follow the path of consistent lumbopelvic stability and be prepared to interrupt the continuum of more demanding exercises in order to apply a peel-back remedial exercise or two. For example, the patient who is unable to maintain the neutral pelvis during the opposite arm–leg raising phase of the quadruped exercises must be spotted and given appropriate remedial exercises until he or she gains sufficient lumbopelvic control. It is the skill of the clinician, to be able to spot the faulty movement pattern and practically correct the problem, that helps to define the clinical art of rehabilitation.

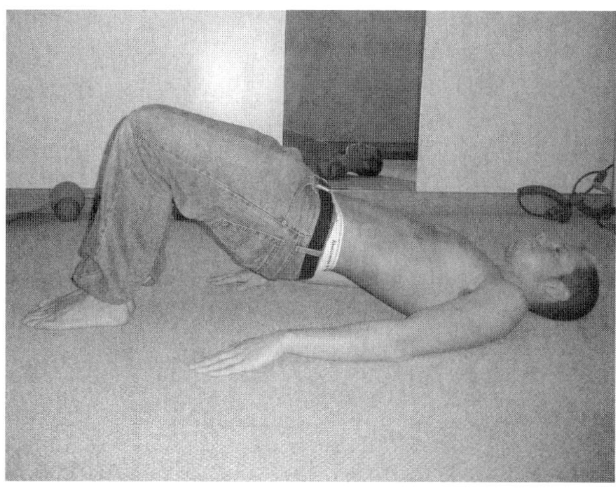

FIGURE 26–11. Supine bridge.

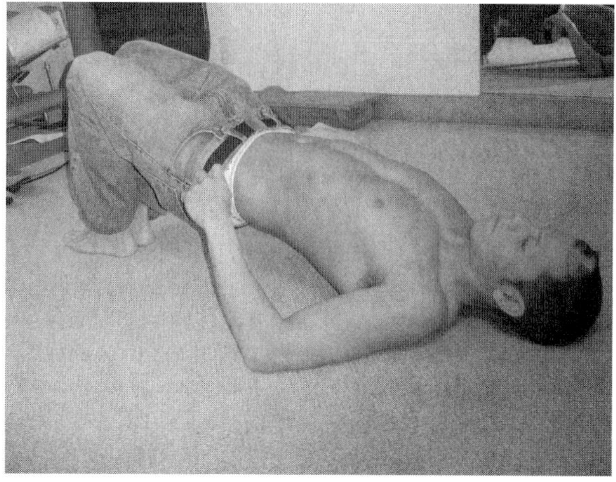

FIGURE 26–12. Supine bridge with recruitment of the scapular stabilizers.

Finally, the process incorporates the principles of stabilization into activities of daily living. In some cases, this may involve teaching the patient to gently brace the trunk muscles when lifting heavy objects.

Clinical Pearl: It is the skill of the clinician, to be able to spot the faulty movement pattern and practically correct the problem, that helps to define the clinical art of rehabilitation.

An important approach is training the patient to avoid end-range flexion loading and repetitive flexion movement, which has been shown to both be a cause of tissue injury[88–90] and to compromise the mechanism of dynamic stability.[7,91] Avoidance of end-range flexion is particularly important in the morning, when intradiscal pressure is at its highest and the disc is believed to be most vulnerable to injury. In fact, one randomized, controlled trial[92] demonstrated that patients with chronic LBP benefited from a program of morning flexion avoidance even when no other treatment was applied. The benefit was found to be long term.[93] The improvement in the patients in these studies was modest, and certainly do not support the use of this approach in isolation of the many others available to the LBP patient, but they show that end-range flexion avoidance in the morning can be an important factor in the recovery process. Avoidance of end-range flexion coupled with daily extension exercises has also been shown to prevent recurrences.[94] The "Good Morning" exercise (see Chapter 30) is an important first step in the process of training patients to bend without flexing the lumbar spine.

Isotonic Strength Training

In many cases, isotonic strength training is not necessary. During most normal activities only approximately 1%–3% of maximum voluntary contraction of the stabilizing muscles is required to maintain stability,[68] and so great strength is not necessary as long as there are efficient stabilization responses to perturbations. And it is not clear as to whether decreased strength plays a strong role in the susceptibility or perpetuation of LBP.[95] However, bed rest produces 3% loss of muscle strength per day, with likely similar losses due to the relative inactivity that is often seen after acute injuries. In those individual patients who are required to return to an occupation that involves heavy lifting after an absence due to injury, especially if bed rest was a component of their acute management, this strength loss can have a great impact on the ability to return to that heavy activity. In these cases, strength training is often helpful in preparing the patient for return to work. In addition to this, there are a number of patients in whom one of the primary problems that is perpetuating LBP is deconditioning.[96,97] That is, the patient is simply out of shape. These patients require improved physical fitness in order to get back to their normal daily activities without being limited by pain. Finally, strength training is an excellent way to provide graded activity (see later discussion) because it allows for the introduction of increasingly challenging activities in a way that is both controlled and measurable. For maximum benefit, strength training should be conducted in a motor-control environment, i.e., an environment in which a functional stabilizing system is being challenged while the large, torque-generating muscles are being trained for strength.

There are certain muscles that are particularly important to target in patients who require the return to lifting occupations. These are the large, torguegenerting muscles that are utilized in lifting. These muscles are

- Latissimus dorsi
- Rectus abdominis
- Erector spinae
- Gluteus maximus
- Quadriceps
- Hamstrings

Of course, these are not the only muscles that are used by most people during functional activities, and a general fitness program may require attention to other muscles as well, but these are the most important muscles to target from the standpoint of involvement in lifting activities.

For strength training, exercise sets of 8–12 repetitions is generally considered ideal. The number of sets that are required to produce strength gains is debated. In general, it is considered that three sets per exercise is best, although recent evidence suggests that single sets is adequate in developing both strength[98,99] and endurance.[100]

For patients who are significantly deconditioned, it is obvious that starting out with low-intensity exercise, with gradual increase as the individual's condition improves, is necessary. It is often useful at this stage to have the patient move from one exercise to the next with minimal rest between sets in order to maintain the heart rate at a target level (see later discussion).

Aerobic Training

Aerobic training is often an important part of rehabilitation, particularly in the deconditioned patient or the patient who is required to return to a physically vigorous job that requires endurance. This must be done in an environment that places minimal strain in the lower back, yet maximizes the ability to elevate the heart rate to the desired level. The use of the recumbent bicycle (Fig. 26–13) allows for this. Unlike the recumbent bicycles that are seen in many health clubs, in which the rider is sitting upright (which likely

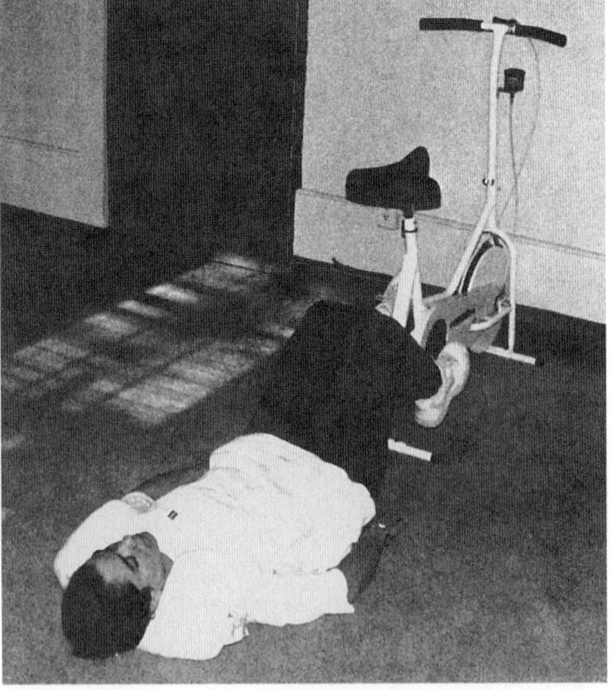

FIGURE 26–13. The recumbent bicycle. *(Reprinted with permission from Ierna GK, Murphy DR. Management of acute soft tissue injuries of the cervical spine. New York: McGraw-Hill, 2000:531–552.)*

increases, rather than decreases, intradiscal pressure), the setup shown here allows for true recumbency.

Clinical Pearl: During most normal activities only approximately 1%–3% of maximum voluntary contraction of the stabilizing muscles is required to maintain stability, and so great strength is not necessary as long as there are efficient stabilization responses to perturbations.

It is important to ensure that the patient is exercising at an aerobic level. It is generally considered that aerobic respiration is engaged in when the individual is exercising at between 60% and 80% of his or her maximum heart rate. This can be calculated by using a simple formula:

220 − patient's age − ×.6 and 220 − patient's age × .8

This estimates 60% and 80%, respectively, of the patient's maximum heart rate. The desired heart rate at which they are to be exercised should fall between these extremes. The pulse rate should be monitored periodically during the course of the aerobic exercise to ensure that the patient remains in his or her target range.

Graded Activity

In a patient with significant central sensitization and/or ineffective illness behavior, it is essential to challenge the patient's beliefs about what he or she can do, as well as to challenge the CNS to reprogram nociceptive processing. Negative beliefs about one's ability to return to normal function have been shown to directly influence behavior and, thus, disability.[101] At the same time, care must be taken when instituting exercise as it is easy to exacerbate the pain in an effort to help the patient overcome it. This only leads to discouragement and reinforcement of both fear-avoidance beliefs and central sensitization, undermining the process. Striking a proper balance between these results is a fine art, and the skill with which this balance is maintained can mean the difference between ongoing disability and the restoration of function.

Clear communication throughout the process is of the utmost importance. It must be impressed upon the patient that the overriding goal of rehabilitation is for him or her to *overcome* the low back syndrome, not necessarily *get rid of* it. One way to overcome LBP is to eliminate it completely, but that is only one way, and it is not always realistic. However, it is often realistic for the patient to be able to return to some, most, or all of his or her normal activities, occupational and recreational, in spite of the presence of pain.[102] The patient who can sincerely understand this concept is well on his or her way to recovery. But in order to do this, the patient must suspend any disbelief about his or her ability to be successful, and simply work with the clinician one step at a time. This is the essence of the graded activity approach, and when the patient and clinician are congruent with regard to this, outcomes are vastly improved.[103]

Exercise is the first step in the process of reversal of ineffective illness behavior and central sensitization. There are many purely physical benefits of exercise, such as improved stability, increased strength, improved physical fitness, etc. But, in some patients, perhaps the more powerful benefit is that exercise allows the clinician to challenge the beliefs of the patient in a relatively safe, controlled environment. While ultimately it is essential to transition the patient to the performance of ADLs, in most patients with chronic low back syndromes, these activities are those for which they have already formed a set of beliefs regarding their ability, or inability, to perform. On the other hand, exercise represents an activity that is novel, and thus most patients will not have such beliefs already formed. So exercise can be an excellent starting point in the graded activity process.[104] This is followed by the introduction of activities that mimic those in which the patient has not been able to engage because of activity intolerance. The more specific to the patient's normal activities, the better, as it allows for more specific challenge to both the patient's beliefs and fears about the activity[105] and to the body's ability to adapt to the physical rigors of the activity. Gradually, more intense activities are introduced, creating further challenge, in a controlled and relatively safe environment, to beliefs, fears, and physical capacity.

INDICATIONS FOR THE USE OF EACH REHABILITATION STRATEGY

The importance of exercise in patients with chronic LBP is well recognized, evidenced by the almost universal recommendation of exercise in many guideline documents.[106–109] What is less appreciated is the importance of applying the specific exercise approach that is most appropriate for each individual patient. The authors consider specific exercise applications for specific conditions to be of the utmost importance in applying effective rehabilitation. The question remains, how does one determine in each patient what type of exercise approach, or combination of exercise approaches, is needed?

Clinical Pearl: The authors consider specific exercise applications for specific conditions to be of the utmost importance in applying effective rehabilitation.

While the literature in this area is limited, a systematic approach to examination of the patient can allow one to make educated choices about what exercise strategies are most likely to address those specific dysfunctions that are most important in the individual patient. For example, in a patient in whom history and examination suggest that passive or dynamic instability is most prominent, but in whom central sensitization does not play a prominent role, stabilization training will be the approach of choice, and graded activity will likely be unnecessary. In another patient, faulty movement patterns related to the program for gait may be most prominent, while there may be little passive or dynamic instability. In this patient, emphasis will be placed on sensorimotor training rather than stabilization training.

There are clinical tests and historical findings that help one to decide what type of dysfunction is most prominent in each patient, and thus allow one to choose a rehabilitation strategy (or a combination of strategies) in each individual patient.

Stabilization Training

As was stated earlier, the purpose of stabilization training is to restore to normal, and ultimately maximize the efficiency of, the neurological program for automatic stability responses. Thus, the most important indication for the need for stabilization training is passive or dynamic instability.

1. Dynamic instability—as determined by hip extension movement pattern test and active straight-leg raise test.
2. Passive instability—as determined by stress radiographs.

Sensorimotor Training

1. Faulty program for gait—determined by stepping test.
2. Dynamic pelvic instability—indicated by:
   - *Hip extension movement pattern test*. Particularly with the finding of late or incomplete contraction of the gluteus maximus (see Chapter 13 for a complete description of this test and Figure 13–29 for an illustration).
   - *Active straight-leg raise test.*
   - *Hip abduction movement pattern*. Particularly any finding suggesting inhibition of the gluteus medius.
3. Postural instability—indicated by one-legged stand/ squat test and postural foot reaction test (Vele's test).

Isotonic Strength Training and Aerobic Training

1. Decrease in strength and/or endurance of the spinal extensors, particularly the multifidi—indicated by positive Sorensen's test (see Chapter 14).
2. Indicated in a patient who requires return to an occupation or important functional activity that requires significant strength and/or endurance after a relatively long layoff because of injury, as with a worker in an occupation that requires frequent lifting of heavy objects.
3. Indicated in a patient who has significant deconditioning and in whom it is felt this plays a role in interfering with recovery.

Graded Activity

Graded activity is indicated in a patient with significant activity intolerance in whom manual and exercise correction of peripheral joint and muscle dysfunction, instability, and faulty movement patterns have not improved this tolerance. It is likely that either ineffective illness behavior or marked central sensitization (or both) are involved.

Ineffective illness behavior can be detected using Waddell's nonorganic signs (see Chapter 14)[52,104] with good reliability.[110–114] Significant fear-avoidance behavior can be detected using the Fear-Avoidance Beliefs Questionnaire[115] or the Fear-Avoidance Pain Scale.[116] There currently is no way of objectively demonstrating the presence of central sensitization in a reliable, clinically useful way. However, its presence can be inferred by the presence of pain that is out of proportion to an *adequate* search for pain generators and locomotor system dysfunction that would explain it. This often requires one or more trials of treatment of possible pain generators.

It should be noted that there is some overlap with these indications, i.e., some clinical tests serve as indicators for more than one type of exercise strategy. This is because some exercise strategies, particularly stabilization training and sensorimotor training, have a certain degree of overlap in the physiological effects that they facilitate. In these cases, a certain degree of substitution can be made, although the choice of exercise strategy should be based on the overall clinical picture, rather than the results of a single test.

For example, in a patient with a positive hip extension movement pattern with delayed contraction of the gluteus maximus, rehabilitation could involve either stabilization training or sensorimotor training, or, in some cases, both. But if the patient also has deviation of the lumbar spine on hip extension (indicative of lumbar instability), the best choice of strategy may be stabilization training. On the other hand, if the patient also has a positive stepping test, sensorimotor training may be the best choice. In this way, the limited time that is available for rehabilitation is maximized and the management can be focused on those methods that have the greatest likelihood of addressing the most clinically important dysfunctions in each individual patient.

MONITORING PATIENT PROGRESS WITH OUTCOME MEASURES

In addition to functional assessment, another measure has become a vital group of tools in the rehabilitation world: outcome measures. Outcome measures provide invaluable clinical information for clinicians, patients, and third-party reviewers regarding the patient's function in such areas as symptomatology, activities of daily living, and psychosocial attitudes. When properly utilized, they provide a functional baseline at the outset of the case so that functional improvements, or lack thereof, can be objectified. Chapter 14 addressed outcome measures in great detail, while Chapter 19 discussed the psychosocial outcome measures. However, numerous chapter contributors have integrated the use of outcomes because they are now considered vital in proper case management. This is definitely true with rehabilitation.

END-STAGE REHABILITATION

It was mentioned earlier in this chapter that a rehabilitation mindset is vital for the conservative management of low back syndromes. The topic of short- and long-term goals was also broached, which should be envisioned at the initial visit. Optimal long-term goal setting is designed to establish a clear picture of the patient's work duties and activities of daily living, so that patient and clinician can together envision what is necessary to reach that endpoint. This should be compared with their restrictions at the time of the initial visit and discussed with the patient so that a comparison of restrictions and goals is mutually agreed upon from the outset.

Clinical Pearl: Optimal long-term goal setting is designed to establish a clear picture of the patient's work duties and activities of daily living, so that patient and clinician can together envision what is necessary to reach that endpoint.

As the patient progresses in their functional restoration, the long-term goals come into focus and take on the appearance of reality instead of what may have initially seemed a mirage. The rehabilitation strategy at this time must be appropriately altered to more specifically address the unique demands of the patient's work and lifestyle. These so-called end-stage rehabilitation strategies are generally composed of more complex exercises and activities that replace remedial exercises while utilizing the functional skills that such exercises returned. In addition, these complex exercises are customized toward a specific physical demand that was lost but is necessary, for example, to resume work.

End-stage training can be accomplished in many ways and has several names. In some regions, it may be called work hardening or work conditioning. In this context, the program typically mimics the patient's specific work tasks and trains them in these duties in anticipation of the patient's return to work.

End-stage training may be equally or more important outside of the workplace. Patients may have lost the ability to perform activities of daily living that significantly impacts the quality of their life and/or that of their loved ones. For example, a patient may recover the ability to lift the 30 pounds necessary to resume work, but be unable to lift an ailing, dependent family member, drive for prolonged periods, or resume their passion for gardening because of low back dysfunction. In each of these cases, end-stage rehabilitation strategies come into play.

End-stage training occurs in the sports world as athletes of various sports attempt to return to the specific demands of their game. In many cases, the clinician may discontinue the direct rehabilitation in favor of a team therapist or trainer. Because of the complexity and variation of this topic, Chapter 32 addresses end-stage training for athletes in detail.

EVIDENCE OF EFECTIVENESS OF REHABILITATION IN LOW BACK SYNDROMES

Research related to the management of patients with low back syndromes is problematic, and making clinical use of the data from research studies is even more so. This is because no two patients with a low back syndrome are alike, and in most cases the cause is multifactorial. Because of this, it is not effective to simply apply a *treatment* or even a *series of treatments* for the patient, but, rather, it is necessary to apply a *strategy* to help the patient overcome the syndrome. With the randomized, controlled trial (RCT) design, it is much easier to study a single treatment that is applied randomly to a group of patients and compare this random application to that of another treatment, to placebo, or to doing nothing, than it is to study the application of a management strategy that is particularized to each patient. With the strategic approach, each patient is treated as an individual, with attention paid to the specific dysfunctional, pathoanatomical, psychosocial, and behavioral components that are unique to that patient. Clearly, this is incompatible with the random application of an identical treatment to a series of patients.

The RCT is currently the "gold standard" in the research world, and this is currently true for the world of spinal research. The glaring weakness of such methodology for manual techniques and rehabilitation require little imagination to envision. While an RCT seems quite logical for testing medications, in which a medication and placebo can appear to be identical, the same is simply not true in other aspects of treatment such as manual techniques and rehabilitation. In research regarding manipulation, for example, how many patients would be unable to differentiate a "sham" manipulation from a true manipulation? Nevertheless, some sort of control is required to fulfill the methodological criteria. In rehabilitation, the myriad-specific complications unique to a patient, such as his or her myofascial pain components of various muscles or the attitudes regarding exercise and fear-avoidance behavior, become practically prohibitive in a large RCT. Ironically, the strength of the RCT, the approach to remove biases and provide structure, may indeed prohibit the ability to validate the dynamic approaches to rehabilitation.

Indeed, the current research literature in the area of rehabilitation in patients with low back syndromes is helpful to obtain a general idea of the efficacy of certain therapeutic approaches, but falls short when strictly applying it to determine how to manage individual patients. Nonetheless, there are a number of studies that have been helpful in evaluating the role that rehabilitation plays in low back syndrome management.

One of the topics addressed in Chapter 13 addressed the topic of false hip extension, involving poor pelvic control associated with decreased pelvofemoral motion and compensatory lumbosacral motion during gait. One of the rehabilitation topics that will be addressed involves exercises for the regaining stability of the "neutral pelvis." Elia et al. used pelvifemoral rhythm measures to prove that patients experienced with dynamic pelvic stabilization could indeed actively limit pelvic motion, while the novice group could not.[117]

In addition, spinal stabilization programs are designed to incrementally increase stability as part of their strategy. Hagins et al. demonstrated that 44 asymptomatic subjects who underwent a 4-week lumbar stabilization exercise program, with weekly intervals of reinstruction and testing, improved in their ability to perform progressively difficult lumbar stabilization exercises.[118]

There remain questions as to whether specific exercises indeed provide greater benefit than a generic exercise program. Descarreaux et al. found that a group of patients with acute and subacute back pain who underwent specific exercise prescription on the basis of the physical evaluation significantly reduced their level of pain and disability, whereas the control group did not.[119] O'Sullivan found that patients with LBP and spondylolisthesis who were given an exercise prescription that focused on specific segmental stabilization exercise had better outcomes over the short- and long-term than a control group, most of whom were managed with nonspecific, health-club-type exercise (swimming, walking, exercise in the gym).[120] So it would appear that specific exercise designed to address the particular functional deficit found in each patient is a more effect approach than a generic exercise approach.

Clinical Pearl: Indeed, the current research literature in the area of rehabilitation in patients with low back syndromes is helpful to obtain a general idea of the efficacy of certain therapeutic approaches, but falls short when strictly applying it to determine how to manage individual patients.

Chapter 5 discussed functional and anatomical compromises in trunk muscles, especially the multifidus, associated with chronic back pain. Rissanen et al. demonstrated increases in multifidus strength and reversed type 2 muscle fiber atrophy by implementing a rehabilitation program for 30 patients with chronic back pain.[121]

Which larger studies have demonstrated sufficient levels of success to support the growing interest in spinal rehabilitation? In a landmark study, Saal and Saal demonstrated a 90% good or excellent outcome and a 92% return to work rate for 64 patients with documented lumbar disc herniations, verified by computed tomography scan and electromyographic testing, who underwent a nonoperative physical rehabilitation program.[122]

Timm presented strong support for rehabilitation in yet a larger study involving 250 post-L5-laminectomy patients with residual chronic low back pain. In comparing the efficacy of groups receiving either physical agents, joint manipulation, low-tech exercise, or high-tech exercise, only the low- and high-tech exercise groups demonstrated significant improvement. Furthermore, it was concluded that low-tech exercise was more cost-effective and produced the most long-term results.[123]

While the process of establishing the efficacy of specific rehabilitation programs for specific programs is still in the early stages, perhaps the strongest evidence that progress is being made follows. Revel stated in 1995 that, "There is evidence that functional restoration programs based on graded activity may provide long-term benefits including better social and occupational outcomes."[124] However, 5 years later a group of authors that included Revel stated the following: "There is now strong evidence that functional restoration programs provide long-term benefits including better social and occupational outcomes."[125]

CONCLUSIONS

This chapter has provided an overview of rehabilitation strategies for low back syndromes. Ensuing chapters will delve into various aspects of rehabilitation in greater depth than was superficially covered in this introductory chapter. The variation among the different strategies, procedures, and techniques is immense; however, an increasing wealth of literature-based procedures is helping the rehabilitation specialist to refine their protocols. Greater international and interprofessional communication and working arrangements are providing a collage of approaches that are both complex and fascinating. Despite such dynamic and broad-based growth, the rehabilitation world accepts that the pillars of this specialty remain an emphasis on functional restoration and outcome measures.

SUMMARY

1. This chapter provided the clinical rationale for implementing rehabilitation strategies for low back syndromes.
2. Clinicians must understand that rehabilitation is a mind set, a vital aspect of an overall clinical management strategy.
3. The five basic purposes of rehabilitation, an organizational model designed to classify divisional strategies within the broad and complex field, have been presented.
4. Five therapeutic strategies of spinal rehabilitation, which will be described in greater detail in Chapter 28, have been presented.
5. A strong emphasis has been placed on utilizing outcomes measures to monitor functional progression during rehabilitation.
6. There is growing evidence in the literature to support the rationale for utilizing rehabilitation in the management of low back disorders.

REFERENCES

1. Murphy DR. The passive/active care continuum: A model for the treatment of spine related disorders. *J Neuromusculoskeletal Syst* 1996;4(1):1–7.
2. Bullock-Saxton JE, Janda V, Bullock MI. Reflex activation of gluteal muscles in walking. An approach to restoration of muscle function for patients with low back pain. *Spine* 1993;18(6):704–708.
3. Pope MH, Panjabi M. Biomechanical definitions of spinal instability. *Spine* 1985;10:255–256.
4. Solomonow M, Zhou BH, Harris M, et al. The ligamento-muscular stabilizing system of the spine. *Spine* 1998;23(23):2552–2562.
5. Murphy DR. Normal function of the cervical spine. II. Neurophysiology and stability. In: Murphy DR, ed. *Conservative management of cervical spine syndromes*. New York: McGraw-Hill, 2000:45–70.
6. Mottram S, Comerford M. Stability dysfunction and low back pain. *J Orthoped Med* 1998;20(2):13–18.
7. Solomonow M, Zhou BH, Baratta RV, Lu Y, Harris M. Biomechanics of increased exposure to lumbar injury caused by cyclic loading. Part 1. Loss of reflexive muscular stabilization. *Spine* 1999;24(23):2426–2434.
8. Panjabi MM. The stabilizing system of the spine. Part I. Function, dysfunction, adaptation and enhancement. *J Spinal Disord* 1992;5(4):383–389.
9. Hodges, PW, McKenzie, DK, Heijnen, I, Gandevia SC. Reduced contribution of the diaphragm to postural control in patients with severe chronic airflow limitation. In: *Proceedings of Annual Scientific Meeting of the Thoracic Society of Australia and New Zealand*, Melbourne, Australia, 2000:8.
10. Hodges P, Gandevia S. Changes in intra-abdominal pressure during postural and respiratory activation of the human diaphragm. *J Appl Physiol*, 2000;89(3): 967–976.
11. Hodges P, Gandevia S. Activation of the human diaphragm during a repetitive postural task. *J Physiol (London)* 2000;522:165175.
12. Hodges P, Cresswell A, Daggfeldt K, Thorstensson A. Evidence for a mechanical effect of intra-abdominal pressure on the human spine. In: *Proceedings of the 27th Annual Meeting of the International Society for the Study of the Lumbar Spine*, Adelaide, p. 262.
13. McGill S, Juker D, Kropf P. Quantitative intramuscular myoelectric activity of quadratus lumborum during a wide variety of tasks. *Clin Biomech* 1996;11(3):170–172.
14. McGill S. *Low back disorders: Evidence-based preventions and rehabilitation*. Champagne, IL: Human Kinetics, 2002.
15. Hodges PW, Richardson CA. Inefficient muscular stabilization of the lumbar spine associated with low back pain: A motor control evaluation of transversus abdominis. *Spine* 1996;21(22):2640–2650.
16. Magnusson ML, Aleksiev A, Wilder DG, et al. Unexpected load and asymmetric posture as etiologic factors in low back pain. *Eur Spine J* 1996;5:23–35.
17. Wilder DG, Aleksiev AR, Magnusson ML, et al. Muscular response to sudden load: A tool to evaluate fatigue and rehabilitation. *Spine* 1996;21(22):2628–2639.
18. Aleksiev A, Pope MH, Hooper DM, et al. Pelvic unlevelness in chronic low back pain patients—Biomechanics and EMG time-frequency analyses. *Eur J Phys Med Rehabil* 1996;6(1):3–16.
19. O'Sullivan P, Twomey L, Allison G, et al. Altered pattern of abdominal muscle activation in patients with chronic low back pain. *Aust Physiother* 1997;43:91–98.
20. Hodges PW, Richardson CA. Relationship between limb movement speed and associated contraction of trunk muscles. *Ergonomics* 1997;40:1220–1230.
21. Hodges PW, Butler JE, McKenzie DK, Gandevia SC. Contraction of the human diaphragm during rapid postural adjustments. *J Physiol* 1997;505(2):539–548.
22. Kramis RC, Roberts WJ, Gillette RG. Non-nociceptive aspects of persistent musculoskeletal pain. *J Orthop Sports Phys Ther* 1996;24:255–267.

23. Sluka KA. Pain mechanisms involved in musculoskeletal disorders. *J Orthop Sports Phys Ther* 1996; 24:240–254.
24. Flor H, Braun C, Elbert T, Birbaumer N. Extensive reorganization of primary somatosensory cortex in chronic back pain patients. *Neurosci Lett* 1997;224: 5–8.
25. Grachev ID, Fredrickson B, Apkarian V. Abnormal brain chemistry in chronic back pain: An in vivo proton magnetic resonance spectroscopy study. *Pain* 2000;89:7–18.
26. Price DD. Characteristics of second pain and flexion reflexes indicative of prolonged central summation. *Exp Neurol* 1972;37:371–387.
27. Farr M, Mathews J, Zhu DF, Ambron RT. Inflammation causes a long-term hyperexcitability in the nociceptive sensory neurons of aplysia. *Learn Mem* 1999;6:331–340.
28. Bennett RM. Emerging concepts in the neurobiology of chronic pain: Evidence of abnormal sensory processing in fibromyalgia. *Mayo Clin Proc* 1999;74:385–398.
29. Seaman DR, Winterstein JF. Dysafferentation: A novel term to describe the neuropathophysiological effects of joint complex dysfunction. A look at likely mechanisms of symptom generation. *J Manipulative Physiol Ther* 1998;21(4):267–280.
30. Mendel LM. Modifiability of spinal synapses. *Physiol Rev* 1984;64:260–324.
31. Meyer RA, Campbell JN, Raja SN. Peripheral neural mechanisms of nociception. In: Wall P, Melzack R, eds. *The textbook of pain*, 3rd ed. New York: Churchill Livingstone, 1994:13–44.
32. Waddell G, McCulloch JA, Kummel EG, Verner RTM. Non-organic physical signs in low back pain. *Spine* 1980;6:117–125.
33. Main CJ, Waddell G. Behavioral responses to examination: A reappraisal of the interpretations of "Nonorganic Signs." *Spine* 1998;23(21):2367–2371.
34. Shacklock MO. The clinical application of central pain mechanisms in manual therapy. *Aust J Physiother* 1999;45:215–221.
35. Shacklock MO. Central pain mechanisms: A new horizon in manual therapy. *Aus J Physiother* 1999;45:83–92.
36. Vlaeyen JWS, Linton SJ. Fear-avoidance and its consequences in chronic musculoskeletal pain: A state of the art. *Pain* 2000;85:317–332.
37. McGill SM. Stability: From biomechanical concept to chiropractic practice. *J Can Chiro Assoc* 1999;43(2):75–88.
38. Adams MA, Mannion AF, Dolan P. Personal risk factors for first-time low back pain. *Spine* 1999;24(23): 2497–2505.
39. Lee JH, Hoshino Y, Nakamura K, Ooi Y. Trunk muscle imbalance as a risk factor of the incidence of low back pain: A 5 year prospective study. *J Neuromusculoskeletal Syst* 1999;7(3):97–101.
40. Mayer TG, Polatin P, Smith B, et al. Spine rehabilitation: Secondary and tertiary nonoperative care. *Spine* 1995;20(18):2060–2066.
41. Gordon GA. A molecular basis for low back pain in Western industrialized cultures. *Med Hypotheses* 1990; 33:251–256.
42. Kori SH, Miller RP, Todd DD. Kinisophobia: A new view of chronic pain behavior. *Pain Manage* January/ February 1990;35–43.
43. Vlaeyen JWS, Kole-Snijders AMJ, Boeren RGB, van Eek H. Fear of movement/reinjury in chronic low back pain and its relation to behavioral performance. *Pain* 1995;62:363–372.
44. Asmundson GJG, Norton GR, Allerdings MD. Fear and avoidance in dysfunctional chronic back pain patients. *Pain* 1997;69(3):231–236.
45. Vlaeyen JWS, Crombez G. Fear of movement/(re) injury, avoidance and pain disability in chronic low back pain patients. *Man Ther* 1999;4(4):187–195.
46. Vlaeyen JWS, Seelen HAM, Peters M, et al. Fear of movement/(re)injury and muscular reactivity in chronic low back pain patients: An experimental investigation. *Pain* 1999;82(3):297–304.
47. Crombez G, Vlaeyen JWS, Heuts PHTG, Lysens R. Pain-related fear is more disabling than pain itself: Evidence on the role of pain-related fear in chronic back pain disability. *Pain* 1999;80(1,2):329–340.
48. Al-Obaidi SM, Nelson RM, A-Awadhi S, Al-Shuwaie N. The role of anticipation and fear in the persistence of avoidance behavior in patients with chronic low back pain. *Spine* 2000;25(9):1126–1131.
49. Vlaeyen JWS, Linton SJ. Fear-avoidance and its consequences in chronic musculoskeletal pain: A state of the art. *Pain* 2000;85:317–332.
50. Main CJ, Watson PJ. Psychological aspects of pain. *Man Ther* 1999;4(4):203–215.
51. Zusman M. Structure-oriented beliefs and disability due to back pain. *Aust J Physiother* 1998;44:13–20.
52. Waddell G, Main CJ. Illness behavior. In: Waddell G, ed. *The back pain revolution*. Edinburgh: Churchill Livingstone, 1998:155–172.
53. Dubner R. The effect of behavioral state on the sensory processing of nociceptive and non-nociceptive information. In: Fields HL, Besson JM, eds. *Progress in brain research*. Elsevier Science, Amsterdam 1988:213–223.
54. Kupferman I. Learning and memory. In: Kandel ER, Schwartz JH, Jessel TM, eds. *Principles of neural science*, 3rd ed. Norwalk, CT: Appleton and Lange, 1991:997–1008.
55. Gordon CR, Fletcher WA, Jones GM, Block EW. Adaptive plasticity in the control of locomotor trajectory. *Exp Brain Res* 1995;102:540–545.
56. Korr IM. The spinal cord as organizer of disease processes: Some preliminary perspectives. *J Am Osteopath Assoc* 1976;76:89–99.
57. Murphy DR. The locomotor system: Korr's primary machinery of life. *J Manipulative Physiol Ther* 1994;17(8):562–564.
58. Cordo PJ, Nashner LM. Properties of postural adjustments associated with rapid arm movements. *J Neurophysiol* 1982;47:287–302.
59. Byl NN, Sinnott PL. Variations in balance and body sway in middle aged adults: Subjects with healthy

backs compared with subjects with low back dysfunction. *Spine* 1991;16(3):325–330.

60. Mientjes MIV, Frank JS. Balance in chronic low back pain patients compared to healthy people under various conditions in upright standing. *Clin Biomech* 1999;14:710–716.
61. Janda V. Muscles and motor control in cervicogenic disorders: Assessment and management. In: Grant R, ed. *Physical therapy of the cervical and thoracic spine*. New York: Churchill Livingstone, 1994:195–216.
62. Murphy DR. Dysfunction in the cervical spine. In: Murphy DR, ed. *Conservative management of cervical spine syndromes*. New York: McGraw-Hill, 2000:71–104.
63. Bergemark A. Stability of the lumbar spine: A study in mechanical engineering. *Acta Orthop Scand* 1989; 60(Suppl 230):5–54.
64. Lavender SA, Tsuang YH, Andersson GBJ. Trunk muscle activation and cocontraction while resisting applied moments in a twisted posture. *Ergonomics* 1993;36:1145–1157.
65. Cholewicki J, Panjabi M, Khachatryan A. Stabilizing function of trunk flexor–extensor muscles around a neutral spine posture. *Spine* 1997;22(19):2207–2212.
66. Gardner-Morse M, Stokes I. The effects of abdominal muscle coactivation on lumbar spine stability. *Spine* 1998;23(1):86–92.
67. Panjabi M, Abumi K, Durenceau J, Oxland T. Spinal stability and intersegmental muscle forces: A biomechanical model. *Spine* 1989;14(2):194–200.
68. Cholewicki J, McGill S. Mechanical stability of the *in vivo* lumbar spine: Implications for injury and chronic low back pain. *Clin Biomech* 1996;11:1–15.
69. De Troyer A, Estenne M, Ninane V, et al. Transverse abdominis muscle function in humans. *J Appl Physiol* 1990;68:1010–1016.
70. Cresswell A, Grundstrom H, Thorstesson A. Observations on intra-abdominal pressure and patterns of abdominal intra-muscular activity in man. *Acta Physiol Scand* 1992;144:409–418.
71. Cresswell A, Thorstensson A. Changes in intra-abdominal pressure, trunk muscle activation and force during isokinetic lifting and lowering. *Eur J Appl Physiol* 1994;68:315–321.
72. Cresswell A, Oddsson L, Thorstensson A. The influence of sudden perturbations on trunk muscle activity and intra-abdominal pressure while standing. *Exp Brain Res* 1994;98:336–341.
73. Hodges P, Richardson CA. Inefficient muscular stabilization of the lumbar spine associated with low back pain: A motor control evaluation of transversus abdominis. *Spine* 1996;21(22):2640–2650.
74. Hodges P, Richardson CA. Relationship between limb movement speed and associated contraction of trunk muscles. *Ergonomics* 1997;40:1220–1230.
75. Pool-Goudzwaard A, Vleeming A, Stoeckart R, et al. Insufficient lumbopelvic stability: A clinical, anatomical and biomechanical approach to 'a-specific' low back pain. *Man Ther* 1998;3(1):12–20.
76. Hodges P, Richardson C. Contraction of the abdominal muscles associated with movement of the lower limb. *Phys Ther* 1997;77:132–144.
77. Hodges P. Is there a role for transversus abdominis in lumbo-pelvic stability? *Man Ther* 1999;4(2):74–86.
78. Pool-Goudzwaard A, Wilke H, Wolf S, Claes LE, Arand M, Wiesend A. Stability increase in the lumbar spine with different muscle groups. *Spine* 1995;20(2): 192–198.
79. Quint U, Wilke H, Shirazi-Adi A, et al. Importance of the intersegmental trunk muscles for the stability of the lumbar spine: A biomechanical study in vitro. *Spine* 1998;23(18):1937–1943.
80. Allison G, Kendle K, Roll S, et al. The role of the diaphragm during abdominal hollowing exercises. *Aus Physiother* 1998;44(2):95–102.
81. Hemborg B, Moritz U, Lowing H. Intra-abdominal pressure and trunk muscle activity during lifting. *Scand J Rehab Med* 1985;17:25–38.
82. Mooney V, Pozos R, Vleeming A, Gulick J, Swenski D. Coupled motion of contralateral latissimus dorsi and gluteus maximus: Its role in sacroiliac stabilization. In: Vleeming A, Mooney V, Snijders CJ, Dorman TA, Stoeckart R, eds. *Movement, stability and low back pain: The essential role of the pelvis*. New York: Churchill Livingstone, 1997:115–122.
83. Vleeming A, Pool-Goudzwaard AL, Stoekart R, van Wingerden JP, Snijders CJ. The posterior layer of the thoracolumbar fascia. Its function in load transfer from spine to legs. *Spine* 1995;20(7):753–758.
84. Evans C, Oldreive W. A study to investigate whether golfers with a history of low back pain show a reduced endurance of transversus abdominis. *J Man Manip Ther* 2000;8(4):162–174.
85. Danneels LA, Vanderstraeten GG, Cambier DC, Witvrouw EE, De Cutper HJ. CT imaging of trunk muscles in chronic low back pain patients and healthy control subjects. *Eur Spine J* 2000;9:266–272.
86. Danneels LA, et al. Differences in electromyographic activity in the multifidus muscle and the ilicostalis lumborum between healthy subjects and patients with sub-acute and chronic low back pain. *Eur Spine J* 2002;11:13–19.
87. Ng JKF, Richardson CA, Parnianpour M, Kippers V. Fatigue-related changes in torque output and electromyographic parameters of trunk muscles during isometric axial rotation exertion: An investigation in patients with back pain and in healthy subjects. *Spine* 2002;27(6):637–646.
88. Gordon SJ, Yang KH, Mayer PJ, Mace AH, Kish VL, Radin EL. Mechanism of disc rupture: A preliminary report. *Spine* 1991;16(4):450–456.
89. McGill SM. The biomechanics of low back injury: Implications on current practice in industry and the clinic. *J Biomech* 1997;30(5):465–475.
90. Simunic Di, Broom ND, Robertson PA. Biomechanical factors influencing nuclear disruption of the intervertebral disc. *Spine* 2001;26(11):1223–1230.
91. Jackson M, Solomonow M, Zhou B, Baratta RV, Harris M. Multifidus EMG and tension-relaxation recovery after prolonged static flexion. *Spine* 2001;26(7):715–723.

92. Snook SH, Webster BS, McGorry RW, et al. The reduction of chronic nonspecific low back pain through control of early morning lumbar flexion: A randomized controlled trial. *Spine* 1998;23(23):2601–2607.
93. Snook SH, Webster BS, McGorry RW. The reduction of chronic, nonspecific low back pain through the control of early morning lumbar flexion: 3 year follow up. *J Occup Rehabil* 2002;12:13–19.
94. Larsen K, Weidick F, Leboeuf-Yde C. Can passive prone extensions of the back prevent back problems? A randomized, controlled intervention trial of 314 military conscripts. *Spine* 2002;27(24):2747–2752.
95. McGill SM, Cholewicki J. Biomechanical basis for stability: An explanation to enhance clinical utility. *J Orthop Sports Phys Ther* 2001;31(2):96–100.
96. Bortz WM. The disuse syndrome. *W J Med* 1984; 141:691–694.
97. Mayer T, Gatchel R, Mayer H, et al. A prospective two-year study of functional restoration in industrial low back injury. *JAMA* 1987;258(13):1763–1767.
98. Carpinelli R, Otto R. Strength training: Single versus multiple sets. *Sports Med* 1998;26(2):73–84.
99. Hass C, Garzarella L, Hoyos D, Pollock, M. Single versus multiple sets in long-term recreational weightlifters. *Med Sci Sports Exerc* 2000;32(1):235–242.
100. Faigenbaum A, Westcott W, Loud R, Long C. The effects of different resistance training protocols on muscular strength and endurance in children. *Pediatrics* 1999;104(1):102.
101. Jensen M, Turner J, Romano JM, Lawler BK. Relationship of pain-specific beliefs to chronic pain adjustment. *Pain* 1994;57:301–309.
102. Rainville J, Ahern D, Phalen L, Childs LA, Sutherland R. The association of pain with physical activities in chronic low back pain. *Spine* 1992;17(9):1060–1064.
103. Cedraschi C, Robert J, Perrin E, et al. The role of congruence between patient and therapist in chronic low back pain patients. *J Manipulative Physiol Ther* 1996;19(4):244–249.
104. Waddell G. Rest of stay active? In: Waddell G, ed. *The back pain revolution*. Edinburgh: Churchill Livingstone, 1998:241–262.
105. Vlaeyen J, Linton SJ. Fear-avoidance and its consequences in chronic musculoskeletal pain: A state of the art. *Pain* 2000;85:317–332.
106. Clinical Standards Advisory Group. Report of CSAG Committee on Back Pain, 1994.
107. Waddell G, Feder G, McIntosh A, Lewis M, Hutchinson A for Clinical Standards Advisory Group. Low back pain evidence review. London: HMSO, 1996.
108. Waddell G, McIntosh A, Hutchinson A, Feder G, Lewis M for Clinical Standards Advisory Group. Low back pain evidence review. London: Royal College of General Practitioners, 1999.
109. Manniche C, Ankjzer-Jensen A, Olesen A, et al. Low back pain evidence review. In: *Low back pain: Frequency, management and prevention from an HTA perspective*, Danish Health Technology Assessment. London: Royal College of General Practitioners, 1999.
110. Vallfors B. Acute, subacute and chronic low back pain: Clinical symptoms, absenteeism and working environment. *Scand J Rehabil Med* 1985;11(Suppl):1–98.
111. Dzioba R, Doxey NC. A prospective investigation into the orthopedic and psychologic predictors of outcome of first lumbar surgery following industrial injury. *Spine* 1984;9:614–623.
112. Waddell G, Morris E, DiPaola MP, Bircher M, Finlayson D. A concept of illness tested as an improved basis for surgical decisions in low back disorders. *Spine* 1986;11(7):712–719.
113. Matthew B, Norris D, Hendry D, Waddell G. Artificial intelligence in the diagnosis of low back pain and sciatica. *Spine* 1988;13:168–172.
114. Ohlund C, Lindstrom I, Areksoug B, et al. Pain behavior in industrial subacute low back pain. Part I. Reliability: Concurrent and predictive validity of pain behavior assessments. *Pain* 1994;58:201–209.
115. Waddell G, Newton M, Henderson I, Sommerville D, Main C. A fear-avoidance beliefs questionnaire (FABQ)—the role of fear-avoidance beliefs in chronic low back pain and disability. *Pain* 1993;52:157–168.
116. Crowley D, Kendall N. Development and initial validation of a questionnaire for measuring fear-avoidance associated with pain: The fear-avoidance of pain scale. *J Musculoskeletal Pain* 1999;7(3):3–20.
117. Elia D, Bohannon R, Cameron D, Albro RC. Dynamic pelvic stabilization during hip flexion: A comparison study. *J Orthop Sports Phys Ther* 1996;24(1):30–36.
118. Hagins M, Adler K, Cash M, Daugherty J, Mitrani G. Effects of practice on the ability to perform lumbar stabilization exercises. *J Orthop Sports Phys Ther* 1999;29(9):546–555.
119. Descarreaux M, Normand M, Laurencelle L, et al. Evaluation of a specific home exercise program for low back pain. *J Manipulative Physiol Ther* 2002;25(8): 497–503.
120. O'Sullivan PB, Twomey LT, Allison GT. Evaluation of specific stabilizing exercise in the treatment of chronic low back pain with radiologic diagnosis of spondylolysis or spondylolisthesis. *Spine* 1997;22(24):2959–2967.
121. Rissanen A, Kalimo H, Alaranta H. Effect of intensive training on isokinetic strength and structure of lumbar muscles in patients with chronic low back pain. *Spine* 1995;20(3):333–340.
122. Saal J, Saal J. Nonoperative treatment of herniated lumbar intervertebral disc with radiculopathy. *Spine* 1989;14(4):431–437.
123. Timm K. A randomized-control study of active and passive treatments for chronic low back pain following L5 laminectomy. *J Orthop Sports Phys Ther* 1994;20(6):276–286.
124. Revel M. Rehabilitation of low back pain patients. A review. *Rev Rhum Engl Ed* January 1995;62(1):35–44.
125. Poiraudeau S, Lefevre-Colau MM, Mayoux-Benhamou MA, Revel M. Which rehabilitation for which low back pain? *Rev Prat* 2000;50(16):1779–1783.

CHAPTER

27

REHABILITATION OF THE SURGICAL LUMBAR SPINE PATIENTS

Andre Labbe, Phil Page, and Craig E. Morris

OUTLINE

OBJECTIVES

1. To discuss the importance or pre- and postoperative rehabilitation in lumbar spine patients.
2. To describe aspects of patient education during rehabilitation of the surgical lumbar patient.
3. To identify a hierarchical approach to rehabilitation of postoperative lumbar patients.
4. To discuss common lumbar spine surgeries and their implications for rehabilitation.

INTRODUCTION

One of the goals of the conservative care practitioner of low back syndromes is to resolve each patient's condition so that more dramatic procedures can be avoided. Indeed, the importance of this goal is magnified by the complexity and risk of surgical intervention.

Nevertheless, spinal surgeries are relatively commonplace in the industrialized world, often despite the best efforts of conservative care practitioners. Ironically, the conservative care clinician must be thankful for the surgeon, whose participation and procedures were avoided from the outset, for this specialist hold another option that may be vital to attain the final goal–reduction of symptoms, increase of functional abilities, and optimization of quality of life.

When the patient undergoes low back surgery, conservative management does not terminate. Postsurgical, and sometimes presurgical, management becomes a crucial strategy to restore both locomotor system function and activities of daily living.

This chapter is dedicated to the unique aspects of conservative management of the spinal surgical patient. This would include the strategies for the patient who has decided to undergo surgery, sometimes called *prehabilitation*, in addition to those who have undergone surgery. Following surgery, these unique measures will be instituted until such time as the rehabilitation approach melds into the rehabilitation approaches addressed in the previous and two ensuing chapters. It is hoped that the resumption of rehabilitation will mark the initiation of the restoration of that patient's quality of life. The manner in which this is performed—the timing, the exercises, the instruction, and the gradual introduction of manual procedures—can dramatically impact the success of the surgery and the effectiveness of the rehabilitative process.[1,2]

Prior chapters have highlighted the aspects of muscle imbalances and altered locomotor function associated with low back syndromes. Chapter 9 describes how muscle and/or muscles imbalances can be the primary or secondary generators of these conditions. These imbalances can be secondary to disease or trauma. Such conditions typically affect the afferent system and alter the function of locomotor system. Surgical techniques are another form of trauma to the spine and the clinician must realize that any preexisting muscle imbalance or motor control problem may be magnified postoperatively. These imbalances can lead to recurrent or new symptoms following surgery unless an early postoperative program to counter the risk is not employed. Therefore, early pre- and postoperative interventions designed to improve proper locomotor system firing patterns (i.e., coordination) and muscle balance are important.

Lumbar spine surgery rates are at least 40% higher in the United States, when compared to several other industrialized countries, and 5 times higher than England and Scotland.[3] Surgical intervention leaves the patient with a permanent anatomical change, and the surgery itself may in some ways be more traumatic than the original injury. Without proper rehabilitation, postsurgical trauma such as adhesive scar tissue formation, decreased tissue tolerance to stress, and an increase in tonic and phasic muscle imbalances can occur. It has been shown that over 70% of postoperative lumbar patients have residual low back pain 1–5 years postoperatively, with 12.7% of those having severe pain that required some other form of treatment to allow them to return to normal function.[4] Repeat lumbar surgery due to recurrent disc herniation occurs in 2%–19% of patients, with 74% of those occurring within 6 months following surgery.[5,6] Some surgical failures may be due to misdiagnosis or ineffective conservative treatment of a functional lesion, rather than an incidental pathoanatomical lesion. As stated in the surgical chapter (see Chapter 34), the success of the surgical procedure is contingent on proper identification and diagnosis of the problem, as well as the appropriate choice of surgical intervention.

Clinical Pearl: Repeat lumbar surgery due to recurrent disc herniation occurs in 2%–19% of patients, with 74% of those occurring within 6 months following surgery.

Some surgeons that feel that postoperative rehabilitation is unnecessary, and even contraindicated for an optimal outcome. However, a recent systematic review of rehabilitation after lumbar disc surgery suggested that there is supporting evidence for intensive exercise programs (if started about 4–6 weeks postoperatively) on short-term functional status and faster return to work.[7–10] While most of the literature surrounding rehabilitation after lumbar surgery focuses on discectomy cases, few researchers have evaluated the outcomes and efficacy of other types of lumbar surgery. As such, a gap in the literature for this topic exists that will hopefully be addressed in the future.

Clinical Pearl: A recent systematic review of rehabilitation after lumbar disc surgery suggested that there is supporting evidence for intensive exercise programs (if started about 4–6 weeks postoperatively) on short-term functional status and faster return to work.

The attitude of the surgical patient toward rehabilitation is also important. Most nonemergent surgical patients have already failed one or more conservative treatment programs and may be reasonably negative about the idea of starting another. They may be fearful that any activity may aggravate or reinjure their back. They may not understand the importance of rehabilitation once their anatomical problem, such as the disc herniation, has been repaired. These and other psychosocial barriers to recovery are addressed in detail in Chapter 19, and can limit the whole recovery process alone. Therefore, early intervention strategies must address rehabilitation in a manner that reassures the patient that he or she is not undertaking a high-risk activity. The key to success is the education of the patient on their dysfunction, the benefit of restoring such function, and how some relatively safe activities and exercises will hasten this process.

Some authors have noted that rehabilitation programs have a profoundly positive influence on the outcome of the patient with low back pain.[11,12] The ability of the patient to resume normal activities, including returning to work, is greatly improved with the use of postoperative exercises. Rehabilitation may affect the psychological deficits often associated with low back pain pre- and postoperatively. Patients who participate in a rehabilitation program often overcome the psychological hurdles of the pathology and display a more positive attitude toward their functional capacity and often "want" to return to work, play, and living a normal life.[13,14]

Clinical Pearl: Rehabilitation may affect the psychological deficits often associated with low back pain pre- and postoperatively.

PREHABILITATION

Many clinicians prescribe routinely exercise programs prior to surgical interventions, sometimes known as *prehabilitation*. The goal of a prehabilitation program is to condition the patient for surgery in the hope of facilitating the recovery period. While this approach seems reasonable and has been addressed in the literature,[15] there is no available research on the efficacy of prehabilitation for spine surgery patients.

During prehabilitation, specific exercises to improve the strength, endurance, and flexibility, which may be affected by surgery, should be prescribed. For example, posterior approaches might emphasize exercises to the multifidus and erector spinae prior to surgery to help their recovery. It is essential, of course, to avoid prehabilitation exercises that may worsen the preoperative patient's condition, such as lumbar flexion exercises that increase radicular symptoms from a disc herniation.

Sometimes, patients experience the same preoperative pain well into the postoperative rehabilitation. The etiology of such symptoms may be multifactorial. While the structural pathology may be repaired in the operating room, the "functional pathology," which may affect pain-generating structures, must also be addressed.[16] It may be helpful to identify muscles imbalance preoperatively and begin to address them before surgery. While muscle imbalance syndromes are covered in detail in Chapters 5, 9, 13, and 23, a general review of the importance of muscle balance is presented here as it relates to surgical rehabilitation.

MUSCLE BALANCE

The importance of reflex activation of the lumbopelvic musculature and its relationship to dynamic stability and function has been reported.[16–18] This topic was addressed in detail in Chapter 5 of this text. The ability of the intrinsic musulature of this region to provide supporting spinal stiffness via a coordinated increase in intraabdominal pressure was described in detail this intrinsic mechanis has been called, among others, as the "pressurized canister," the "local system" and the "core." This functional canister consists of four primary muscles: the transversus abdominis, multifidus, abdominothoracic diaphragm, and pelvic floor.[19]

Researchers have shown a delay of transverse abdominis firing in patients with chronic low back pain,[20,21] an example of disruption of the "feedforward mechanism," a strategy that allows for preemptive, stabilizing, contraction of the intrinsic musculature in anticipation of motion. Such functional pathology may indeed be as bad, if not worse, in someone who has undergone spinal surgery because of significant tissue disruption. There are no studies to date on the transverse abdominal activity in the postoperative patient, and so the effect on such muscle function remains speculative; however, it may be wise to include transversus abdominis training in both preoperative and postoperative patients.

The critical role of the multifidus in both lumbopelvic stability and following trauma was described in Chapter 5. Hides et al.[22] demonstrated multifidus atrophy after acute episodes of low back pain despite early symptom resolution. It is assumed that such dysfunction should occur with the trauma of back surgery, particularly with posterior approaches. Clinically, this may lead to increased loads on the lumbar segments and complicate postoperative rehabilitation. Therefore, prehabilitation efforts may be beneficial to optimize multifidus function so that less is necessary following surgery.

While this discussion on prehabilitation has been focused on key lumbopelvic tissues, it is important to remember the importance of a conditioning program on other systems, such as the cardiovascular system, and the associated surgical mortality and morbidity benefits that may ensue. Therefore, despite a real need for greater understanding regarding the best methods and true benefit of prehabilitation strategies, the authors feel that the current understanding of locomotor system function and dysfunction, combined with the risks of surgery from sufficient evidence to support this strategy for the presurgical spinal patient.

Clinical Pearl: Hides et al. demonstrated multifidus atrophy after acute episodes of low back pain despite early symptom resolution. It is assumed that such dysfunction should occur with the trauma of back surgery, particularly with posterior approaches.

POSTOPERATIVE REHABILITATION

Patient Education

Patient education is considered the most critical component of any postoperative rehabilitation program. It is essential that the rehabilitation professional and surgeon communicate about each individual patient in order to focus on the precise educational and functional challenges to be addressed. Most importantly, the surgeon must communicate the specific precautions associated with each patient, since even the same surgical procedure varies slightly between patients. In general, the patient should be instructed about these precautions, as well as motivated to return to some mild activities of daily living as soon as possible.

Patients should also be counseled on fear avoidance behavior, understanding the difference between "hurt and harm," learning to pace oneself, the positive and natural aspects of exercise soreness, and anticipated minor flare-ups. Special attention must be paid to fear avoidance behavior, as the success of the rehabilitation can depend on the rehabilitation specialist's proficiency in spotting and addressing this topic. The patient with fear avoidance may find any number of reasons to avoid exercise, with fear of reinjury never being mentioned. There is no generic strategy for overcoming this potential barrier to recovery. However, the important thing is that the clinician is sensitive to the patient's needs and establishes strong lines of communication so that difficult topics can be broached in an open and nonthreatening manner.

Clinical Pearl: Special attention must be paid to fear avoidance behavior, as the success of the rehabilitation can depend on the rehabilitation specialist's proficiency in spotting and addressing this topic.

Resuming Activity

Depending on the surgery, the patient may be released to light activity and some work between the second and eighth postoperative weeks. Patients undergoing minor procedures such as intradiscal electrothermal therapy and microdiscectomy will usually return to normal activity sooner than more complex surgeries such as disc replacement or fusion. Most postoperative lumbar patients can initially sustain postures for only brief periods of time, and must be able to walk and change positions intermittently throughout the day. The patient may require some form of support with sitting, standing, or driving for any period of time. Corsets or braces are sometimes used to protect healing tissue, depending on the severity of the injury and extent of instability following the surgery.

The patient is usually not allowed to drive for the first week, and even longer in the presence of any residual radicular signs. The type and seating position of a vehicle may also determine driving limitation. In some cases the vehicle may promote excessive lumbar flexion or posterior pelvic tilt, which could cause increased pain and stress to healing tissue.

Body Mechanics

Patients should be instructed in proper body mechanics in common functional activities to protect healing structures.

- Proper transfers from supine-to-sit, sit-to-stand, and mobility in bed should be taught, with precautions to prevent twisting movements.
- The patient should be taught a neutral spine position and how to perform "abdominal bracing" (co-contraction of the key lumbopelvic stabilizers, which increases spinal rigidity) when performing activities to prevent stress to the healing tissue.
- Depending on the healing incision, bathing in the shower or tub may begin after 2 weeks with precautions for avoiding flexion strategies (i.e., shaving the legs or washing the calves and feet) unless the target leg is supported on a bench or stool.

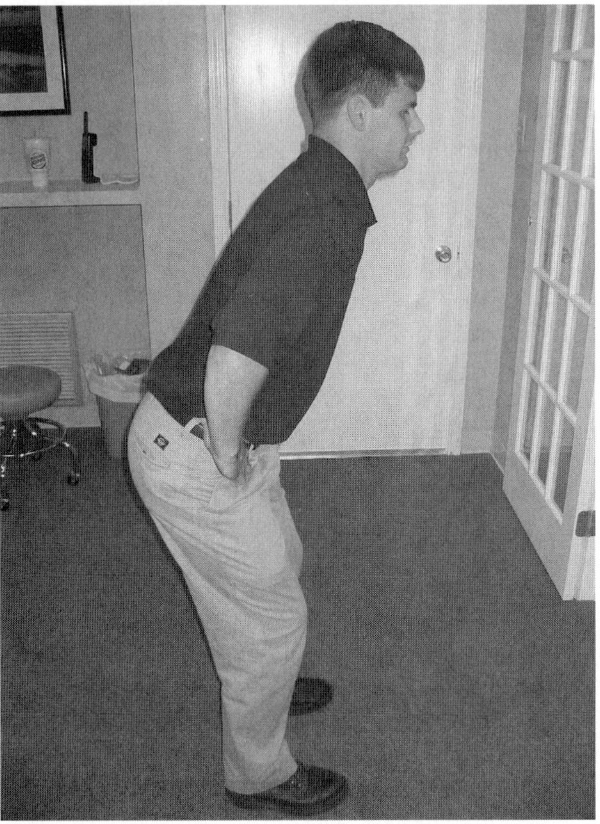

FIGURE 27–1. Performing a hip hinge during forward bending helps keep the lumbar spine in neutral and prevents a posterior tilt.

- Forward bending should be done with a hip hinge to avoid lumbar flexion (see Fig. 27–1).

Walking Activities

Depending on the extent of the procedure, walking can begin immediately. The patient should attempt to walk short distances several times daily. Their tolerance to activity will increase in relation to the amount of guarded early activity they perform. Walking will promote proper collagen formation in healing tissues and will begin activating the deep paravertebral musculature. During walking, the orientation of the lumbar zygapophyseal joints will ensure repetitive joint compression and distraction. This will stimulate mechanoreceptor input into the CNS and begin to facilitate some of the automatic postural reactions. The joint compression and rotation will also increase nutrition to the area via increased blood flow, as well as increase synovial fluid production and fibroblastic activity. The early weight bearing in the standing position may also promote increased osteoblastic activity and proper bony healing.

Clinical Pearl: During walking, the orientation of the lumbar zygapophyseal joints will ensure

repetitive joint compression and distraction. This will stimulate mechanoreceptor input into the CNS and begin to facilitate some of the automatic postural reactions.

Posture

Postural education is essential in protecting healing lumbar tissue. Educating the patient in proper sitting posture will prevent excessive load to the spine by decreasing posterior pelvic tilt while in a weight-bearing position. Postural awareness exercises such as pelvic tilts and shoulder retractions help teach the patient proper posture. Optimally, the body weight in the sitting position should be distributed into the legs and feet by keeping the spine in neutral and having the hips higher than the knees. An exercise ball may be a good option to promote proper posture in the sitting position (see Fig. 27–2).

The patient should be instructed on the following postural tips for protecting the spine:

- Do not slouch while sitting: maintain a neutral lumbar spine position.
- Utilize a lumbar roll or pillow to maintain an erect posture in sitting while at work and in the car.
- Avoid backless chairs or stadium bench seats, which promote poor posture.
- Do not sit for longer than 30 minutes without a break.
- Instruct the patient in proper sleeping postures in supine, sidelying, and prone positions. Place pillows between the legs and strategically around the lumbar spine to maintain a neutral lumbar position.
- Avoid sofas or overly soft mattresses, which are nonsupportive

Incision Site Management

Sutures may be present when the patient begins rehabilitation and the clinician must take care not to cause excessive movements or activities that would stress or open the incision sight. The clinician should also take care to monitor the sutures for excessive edema. Techniques to prevent excessive collagen formation in the area of the surgery should be used. Manual techniques of soft tissue mobilization will ensure proper collagen formation. Applying adhesive tape to the area surrounding the incision can ensure that the patient does not compromise the healing scar with early activity (see Fig. 27–3). Parallel strips placed over the

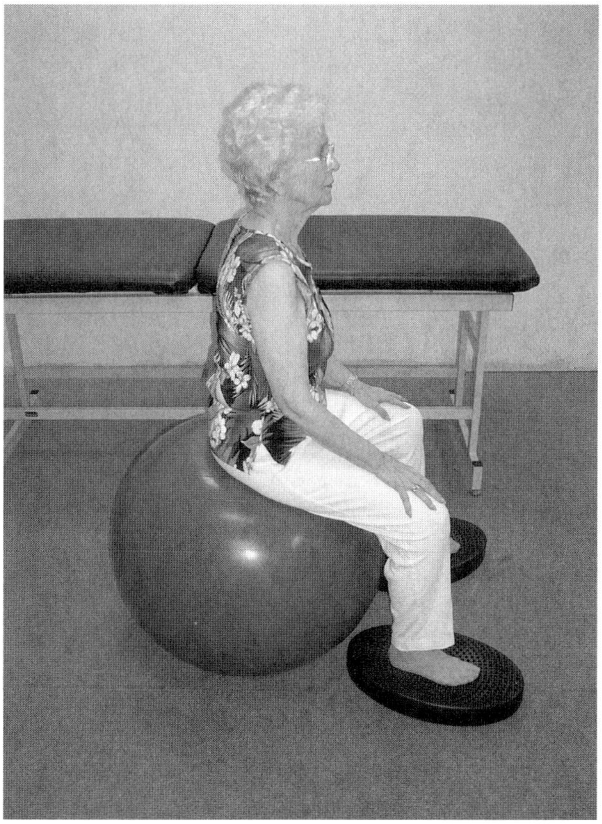

FIGURE 27–2. Sitting on an exercise ball may promote a good position for extended sitting, providing weight distribution into the legs and an anterior tilt with hips higher than knees.

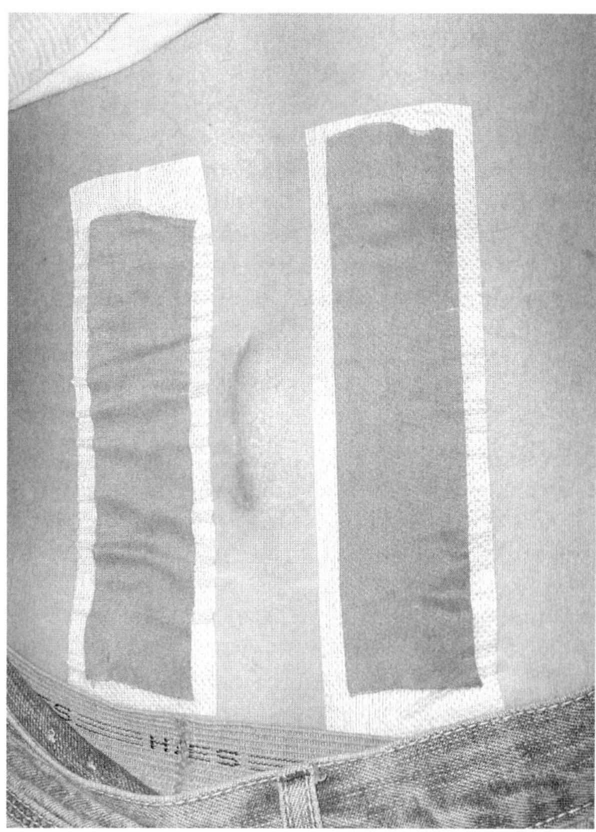

FIGURE 27–3. Tape is applied directly to the skin surrounding an incision site to increase tactile input and limit excessive movement.

longitudinal muscles may give substantial tactile and proprioceptive feedback to the patient. This increased local afferentation may facilitate the process of motor relearning in an inhibited area of localized atrophy and poor motor function, while improving control to avoid too much motion in early stages. The tape may also limit lumbar movement within safe ranges.

Clinical Pearl: Educating the patient in proper sitting posture will prevent excessive load to the spine by decreasing posterior pelvic tilt while in a weight-bearing position.

A compression bandage can decrease the amount of scar in the area. It should also be noted that the incision site should be inspected regularly for proper healing. Any signs of infection—edema, discoloration, increased skin temperature, fever, or exudates—should be seen as a possible sign of infection and reported immediately to the surgeon.

POSTOPERATIVE REHABILITATION HIERARCHY

In general, postsurgical lumbar patients should be progressed just as any other postoperative orthopedic patient. There are many factors to consider during postoperative lumbar rehabilitation, the most important of which is the extent of the repair during surgery and physical activity limitations by the surgeon. Other important factors are the preoperative condition of the patient, comorbidities, and patient motivation and compliance.

The surgeon should provide the rehabilitation professional with the specific time-based precautions of the surgery based on the procedure. For example, instructions may include "No lumbar extension for 4 weeks." Various surgeons often have different protocols for each procedure, and these may be slightly modified between different patients undergoing the same procedure. These protocols may be based on documented protocols and outcomes reported in the literature, but often are based on clinical experience. Time-based precautions are also usually based on the tissue-healing responses, such as bone repair in 6–8 weeks, ligamentous repair in 6–12 weeks, and soft-tissue healing in 2-4 weeks.

The rehabilitation professional should take these limitations into consideration when determining the appropriate rehabilitation program. Unfortunately, many postoperative protocols are rather vague, leaving the rehabilitation professional with more questions than answers to make clinical decisions. During rehabilitation, a "hierarchy" of importance may be used to assist in clinical decision making. This hierarchy consists of addressing (1) pain and tissue healing, (2) muscle balance, (3) motor control, and (4) muscular endurance in functional movement patterns.

1. *Address pain and tissue healing.* The patient must realize that some postoperative pain is to be expected, perhaps the same or more so than before surgery. He or she must be counseled regarding this issue and also must realize that an aggressive postoperative rehabilitation program has been shown in a recent study to ultimately reduce pain and improve function in 90% of the patients.[1]

   Modalities such as ice or electrical stimulation may be effectively used to control acute pain and limit the need for narcotics for pain control. While most modalities have limited benefit in managing chronic back pain, some can provide a strong afferent stimulus to dull or decrease some of the acute pain in order to facilitate exercise and increased activity levels. Some forms of electric stimulation may also promote scar healing while limiting some unwanted secondary complications such as adhesions or keloid formation.

   In addition to the incision care noted above, scar management should be addressed once the sutures are removed to decrease the possibility of secondary scar pain. Soft tissue mobilizations can be used to promote scar mobility once the incision has healed to limit adhesions, excessive muscle guarding, and myofascial pain. Tight muscles and associated scarring can limit lumbar mobility as well as reproduce preoperative pain. When addressing soft tissue problems, one must remember that a myofascial adhesion can occur at superficial, middle, and/or deep layers. Aggressive mobilization can cause discomfort, even though it may be appropriate. If necessary, the patient should be counseled in advance, in plain, understandable language as to why such a potentially painful procedure is warranted. Superficial techniques such as effleurage and petrissage are appropriate for pain reduction and superficial mobility. The deeper soft tissue mobilizing techniques, when necessary, should be used as tolerated.

   Joint mobilization may also be indicated to control pain. The clinician may not be mobilizing the surgically targeted joints, but grade 1 and 2 mobilization of local segments above and below may decrease pain. In addition, mobilizing the thoracic spine or sacroiliac joints may help to improve posture, gait, and disperse local forces from being transmitted to a healing lumbar spine.
2. *Address muscle balance.* Muscle balancing procedures were addressed in Chapter 23. However, this is a very important topic for postsurgical rehabilitation and specific topics will be addressed here for emphasis. Specific muscle function

provides a window to global functional ability. *Muscle imbalance* is defined as altered muscle length or tone between antagonistic groups. This results in faulty posture, movement patterns, and increased or asymmetrical loading of various joints and tissues, interfering with optimal spine rehabilitation outcomes.[16] An example is the relationship between the hip flexors and the gluteus maximus. In Janda's lower crossed syndrome[16] patients with chronic low back pain demonstrate a hypertonic or facilitated iliopsoas and a hypotonic or inhibited ipsilateral gluteus maximus; they also exhibit hypertonic thoracolumbar erector spinae and hypotonic rectus abdominis. This imbalance continues to place stress on the lumbar spine and associated structures that lead to pain. The lower crossed syndrome has been described in detail in the functional assessment chapter (Chapter 13). The clinician must be able to recognize such syndromes/imbalances and address them as early as possible.

Clinical Pearl: Muscle imbalance is defined as altered muscle length or tone between antagonistic groups. This results in faulty posture, movement patterns, and increased or asymmetrical loading of various joints and tissues, interfering with optimal spine rehabilitation outcomes.

The rehabilitation specialist must determine specific exercises and manual techniques to restore muscle balance depending on the cause of the imbalance. Hypertonic muscles should be restored with a number of manual procedures, such as postisometric relaxation technique.[23]

- *Hip flexors*: Iliacus and psoas muscles are often tight and facilitated in the patient with chronic back pain syndrome, and they are usually associated with gluteus maximus inhibition and weakness.[16] Tight hip flexors are associated with excessive anterior tilt and subsequent excessive stress to the lumbar spine. Hip flexors should be carefully lengthened both pre- and postoperatively without exacerbating symptoms.
- *The hamstrings*: Tight hamstrings are also associated with low back pain[24] and should be addressed before and after lumbar surgery without increasing radicular symptoms. Using an assistive device such as an elastic band can be useful in assisting patients in stretching while avoiding harmful postures or stress on healing tissue (Fig. 27–4). However, one must be careful to avoid overstretching the hamstrings if it is determined that they are preventing an increased anterior pelvic tilt.

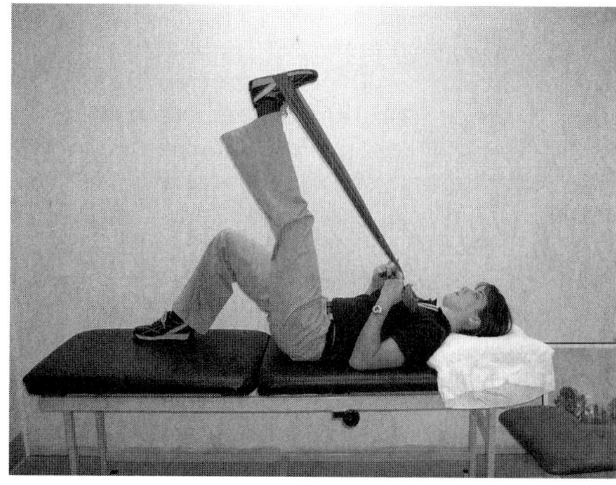

FIGURE 27–4. Using an elastic band to assist in stretching the hamstrings can help prevent excessive posterior tilt or trunk flexion.

Weak or inhibited muscles should be facilitated with specific manual techniques depending on the etiology of the imbalance. Clinically, simply stretching a tight antagonist will often reflexively restore the length of an inhibited agonist. Other techniques such as sensory motor stimulation (such as tapping, rubbing, or brushing) or proprioceptive neuromuscular facilitation procedures may be valuable in activating inhibited muscle. Once inhibited muscles have been facilitated, they can be strengthened in coordinated movement patterns. Muscles commonly inhibited in low back pain include the transverse abdominis, diaphragm, multifidus, pelvic floor, and gluteals.[16] Surgical procedures and the associated inflammation may cause or exacerbate reflexive inhibition of the phasic system muscles.

- *Transverse abdominis*: As previously noted, the transverse abdominis (TrA) is key component of the "pressurized canister" and of the postural system in general. In the case of an anterior lumbar interbody fusion, an abdominal surgical scar complicates the clinical picture. As mentioned earlier, an incision site in the abdominal musculature may inhibit the firing speed and strength of contraction of the abdominals that contribute to lumbopelvic dynamic stability. Exercises to improve activation of the TrA include "abdominal hollowing"[19]; however, exercises should quickly be progressed to more functional and reflexive activation of the TrA as it is integrated with the other trunk musculature, such as an overhead pull-over in the standing position.

- *The diaphragm*: The superior aspect of the "pressurized canister"—contraction of the diaphragm—provides a zone of stability between the ribs and the lumbopelvic region. Contractions of the TrA are directly affected by breathing patterns.[25] Therefore, evaluation and retraining of diaphragmatic respiration is an important part of lumbopelvic rehabilitation. Patients should be reminded to use this coordinated breathing pattern rather than using the accessory muscles of respiration (scalenes, sternocleidomastoid, etc.).
- *The multifidus*: The multifidus along with the erector spinae group may be compromised with a posterior approach surgical incision. It may be difficult to train these muscles directly, and so they are typically trained indirectly or reflexively. For example, simply performing an exercise such as standing elbow curls can reflexively activate the lumbar extensors (see Fig. 27–5) for lumbar stability. Abdominal hollowing exercises have been found to indirectly activate the multifidi.
- *The pelvic floor*: The pelvic floor is considered the base of the pressurized canister. Clinical signs of incontinence or poor control of urination are sometimes present early postoperatively. Strengthening exercises of the pelvic floor (such as Kegel's exercises) should be taught early in the rehabilitation process.[26] For example, the patient can perform simple activities on an exercise ball to improve pelvic floor control by simply sitting on the ball, drawing up the pelvic floor, and carefully performing anterior and posterior pelvic tilts. It is important for clinicians to include these exercises for females and males, both pre- and postoperatively.
- *Gluteal muscles*: The gluteal muscles (gluteus maximus and medius) tend to be inhibited and weak in patients with chronic low back pain.[16] Facilitation of the gluteus maximus and medius is important for restoring normal trunk muscle balance and lumbopelvic stability. Thera-Band kicks (hip abduction and extension) can be used (see Fig. 27–6) to strengthen both the kicking leg and the stance leg, as well as to promote lumbar stabilization.

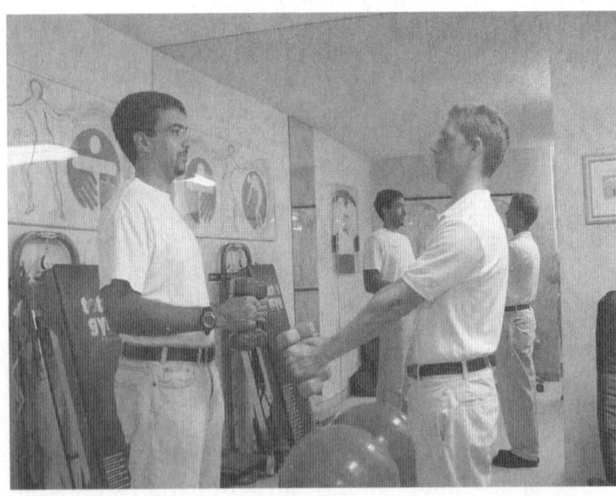

FIGURE 27–5. Exercise continuum: Performing an elbow curl with dumbbells in standing, as demonstrated by the person on the left, can reflexively activate lumbar extensors to counteract the forward bending moment created during the resistance exercise. The person on the right demonstrates a more demanding, longer lever, maneuver in which the elbows remain extended as the dumbbells are elevated using a shoulder flexion strategy.

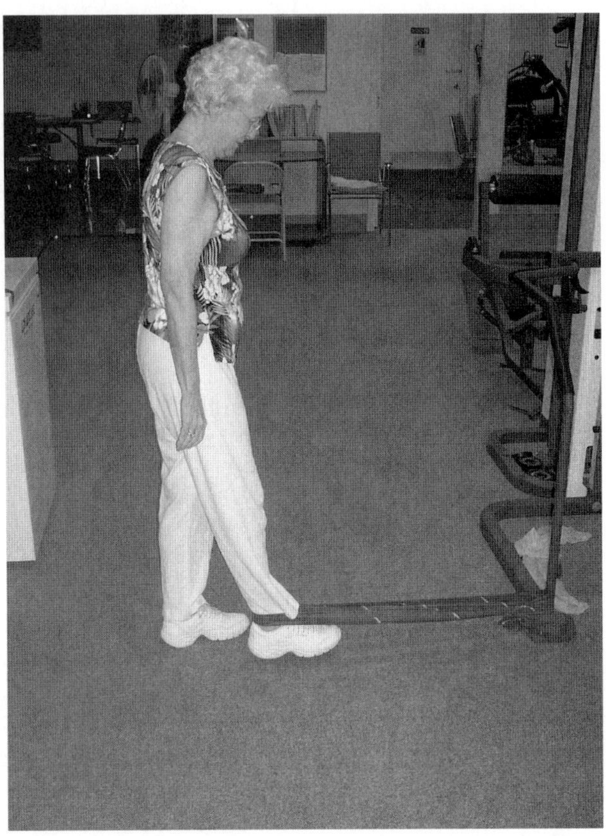

FIGURE 27–6. Thera-Band kicks help strengthen the kicking leg, as well as the stance leg, and reflexively activate trunk stabilization.

3. *Address motor control.* Optimal motor control affords humans the ability to perform voluntary, coordinated, and purposeful movements. Proper motor control is essential in lumbopelvic stability and functional movements. Once muscle balance has been addressed, the sensorimotor system should be addressed. Sensorimotor training (SMT) is covered in detail in the next chapter. Briefly, however, SMT facilitates the processing of afferent

impulses and the efferent response. Afferent routes include proprioceptive information from muscular receptors and joint mechanoreceptors. Proprioceptive information is processed within the CNS along with other afferent impulses such as visual, vestibular, and cognitive information.

The postsurgical back patient may have impaired proprioception, which may affect the sensorimotor function.[16] Too often, clinicians emphasize strength rather than motor control. During therapeutic exercise, the quality of movement should be emphasized rather than the quantity of the exercises. Fortunately, the rehabilitation specialist can begin affecting this system early in the postoperative phase, without compromising the patient's pain or healing ability.[27] Balance training with labile surfaces such as wobble and rocker boards, balance sandals, and foam surfaces have been shown to improve muscle activation of the lumbar and lower extremity regions indirectly.[28,29] Janda described a systematic approach to rehabilitation of the sensorimotor system, called sensorimotor training (SMT), which has been clinically useful in the rehabilitation of both operative and nonoperative low back patients.[27]

Clinical Pearl: The postsurgical back patient may have impaired proprioception, which may affect the sensorimotor function. Too often, clinicians emphasize strength rather than motor control.

SMT progressively increases proprioceptive input into the CNS and stimulates subcortical pathways to facilitate coordinated movement patterns. There are three major areas of proprioceptive input into the CNS: the cervical spine,[30] the sacroiliac joint,[24] and the soles of the feet.[31] Therefore, a key postsurgical rehabilitative strategy is to stimulate these areas to promote early postural and functional stability. These areas can be stimulated through manual mobilization, tactile stimulation, and proper positioning during exercise.

4. *Improve muscular endurance during functional movement patterns.* Therapeutic exercise should be gradually progressed to incorporate more whole-body functional movement patterns as healing progresses. For example, a lifting simulation with resistance helps strengthen the entire kinetic chain from the feet to the cervical spine. Multiplanar activities can help stimulate functional activities at home or work. The patient should be taught to control the lumbopelvic region during all activities. Patients should also progress to regular cardiovascular exercises (such as walking, biking, or swimming) for at least 30 minutes on most days of the week.

AQUATIC REHABILITATION

Aquatic exercises may be an excellent option to integrate into postsurgical rehabilitation patients. Underwater exercise provides an excellent environment to unload healing tissues and to stimulate stabilizing reactions. Aquatic exercise can be easily integrated with land-based rehabilitation throughout the process. Very early postoperative aquatic exercise should be avoided until the suture site is well healed to prevent the risk of infection.

Early aquatic exercises can incorporate unloaded walking in waist-deep water. The water also provides a resistant force to walking which may be beneficial from a cardiovascular, endurance, and strengthening perspective. By using other aquatic exercise tools such as hand bars or kick rollers, patients can begin to perform gentle stabilization exercises by supporting the extremities. Resistance devices such as Aquafins can be used to add drag resistance to extremity movements to facilitate lumbar stabilization (see Fig. 27–7). Aquabelts at the waist can also be used to support the body during deep-water exercises to facilitate endurance-type deep-water running.

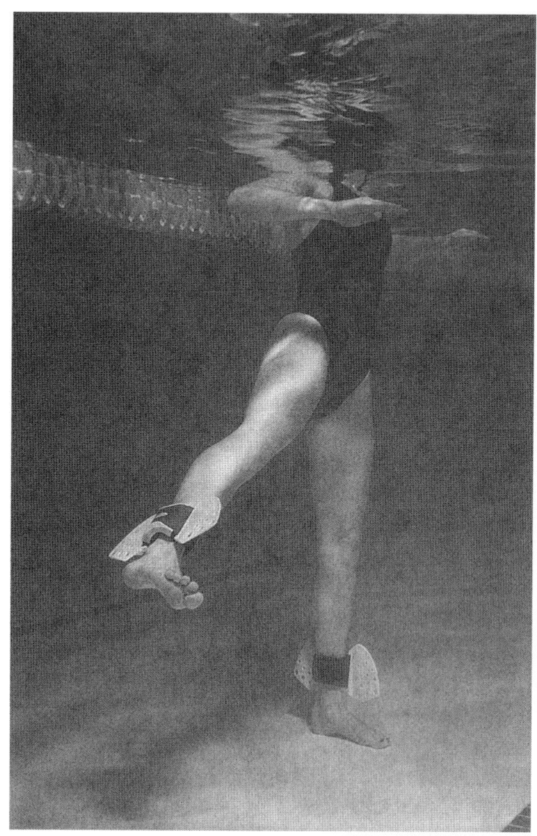

FIGURE 27–7. Using Aquafins can add resistance to extremity movements in the water to improve conditioning in an unloaded environment.

COMMON SURGICAL PROCEDURES AND IMPLICATIONS FOR REHABILITATION

Unfortunately, there is very little literature on specific protocols and outcomes of rehabilitation after lumbar surgeries. In Chapter 34, spinal surgeons will discuss lumbar surgical strategies and protocols in detail. While many rehabilitation techniques are similar between different surgeries, this chapter will briefly address the rehabilitation considerations of each of the common surgeries.

It is important that clinicians approach rehabilitation with the four-part hierarchy in mind for any surgical procedure. As stated earlier, communication between the surgeon and the rehabilitation specialist is essential. Ultimately, the surgeon should dictate the precautions and limitations for each case. The rehabilitation specialist should keep the surgeon informed of any unexpected adverse changes in symptoms, as well as their progress toward rehabilitation goals. Since every patient progresses differently, this communication is essential to ensure the best outcome.

Progression of the rehabilitation is based on the type and amount of tissue healing. For example, bony repairs such as fusions may require more than 6 months to heal before vigorous end-stage rehabilitation is initiated. Less complex surgery, such as microdiscectomy, may not significantly restrict physical activity.

Discectomy

Most literature on postsurgical lumbar rehabilitation has involved discectomy.[7–12] Ostelo et al.,[10] after a systematic review, concluded that postoperative rehabilitation after disc surgery was both safe and effective. Since lumbar discectomy has relatively low tissue morbidity, patients are generally advised to resume normal activities without excessive stress to the incision site. Increased walking, within tolerable limits, should be stressed in order to reduce the effects of deconditioning. Once the incision has sufficiently healed, scar mobilization and adhesion-lysing techniques should be employed. Abdominal hollowing protocols and sensorimotor training, utilizing balance sandals, rocker boards, and trampolines, should then ensue. Joint mobilization techniques away from the surgical site may assist in overall increases in early postsurgical mobility. Because a posterior approach is used, strengthening of the multifidus and lumbar extensors should be emphasized once the patient is capable of tolerating such exercise. A "symptoms-limited" progression is generally employed, meaning that patients are allowed to progress their rehabilitation as long as they do not increase pain or radicular symptoms.

Intradiscal Electrothermal Therapy

Intradiscal electrothermal therapy (IDET) remains a popular alternative to fusion. It is a minimally invasive procedure that has been thoroughly explained in Chapter 24. Because it involves heating the posterior annulus fibrosus, the patient is provided with a very rigid brace and is not allowed to initiate any structured postsurgical rehabilitation for at least 6 weeks. Once the rehabilitation is initiated, abdominal hollowing and unloaded water exercises can be initiated. Sensorimotor training can be later introduced in preparation to a lumbopelvic stabilization program. In general, a symptoms-limited progression should be used, although the physician should inform the rehabilitation specialist of precautions prior to the start of rehabilitation.

Stenosis Surgery

Surgical treatment for stenosis is usually associated with single or multilevel laminectomy and the hypertrophied ligamentum flavum. The surgical exploration is typically greater than a discectomy, and so longer postsurgical precautions may be implemented, particularly to avoid extension. A larger incision means greater risk of adhesive scar formation, and so manual techniques are emphasized to avoid adhesions. Once the surgeon releases the patient for more active rehabilitation, water exercises and abdominal hollowing can be initiated. Because of the subsequent change in arthro- and osteokinematics, restoration of dynamic stabilization should be the main focus of rehabilitation in order to reduce the risk of a subsequent fusion. These stabilization exercises should focus on activating the "pressurized canister" muscles mentioned earlier, in addition to sensorimotor training.

Posterolateral Fusion

A posterolateral fusion requires a posterior approach and significant surgical exploration, in addition to the decortication of the lamina and transverse processes of the levels being fused. This operation leaves a fused segment with minimal or no disc movement, and in most cases a full discectomy is done to limit any residual discogenic pain. Any fusion surgery will have significantly more morbidity and activity restrictions to allow for bony healing, which may take 6 weeks to 6 months, depending on the extent of the fusion. An even larger incision means greater risk of adhesive scar formation, and so manual scar-lysing techniques are emphasized. Once the surgeon releases the patient for more active rehabilitation, which typically occurs when the fusion is solid, water exercises and abdominal hollowing can be initiated. It is important to note that patients with fusions must emphasize dynamic stabilization activities of the other nonfused segments to prevent hypermobility at segments above and below the fusion. Sensorimotor training may be very effective in these patients.

Anterior and Posterior Interbody Fusions

The anterior interbody fusion usually requires an abdominal retroperitoneal approach. Therefore, the entry is between the peritoneal wall on one side and the TrA on the other. This anterior approach requires incision and exploration of the abdominal wall and musculature and blunt dissection of the psoas muscles on the anterior aspect of the lumbar spine. The disc removal occurs with filling of the space with bone graft or metallic cages. The posterior interbody fusion avoids the peritoneal approach and is usually associated with a laminectomy as well as the discectomy and replacement of the disc. These two approaches require the same rehabilitation considerations as mentioned in the posterior approach above, but the main difference is with the anterior approach. An anterior approach may compromise abdominal function and inhibit the rest of the "pressurized canister" from the associated swelling because of the morbidity of the approach. Abdominal scar-lysing techniques and abdominal hollowing measures are therefore even more important for these cases.

CONCLUSION

Postoperative rehabilitation of the lumbar spine presents many challenges for the rehabilitation specialist. Because of the number of factors associated with their outcomes, clinicians should implement an individualized rehabilitation strategy for each patient. A "hierarchical" approach to postsurgical rehabilitation, as described above, can nevertheless be implemented within the time-based parameters of the surgeon. This progression involves addressing pain and tissue healing first, then addressing muscular balance, then motor control issues, and finally to increasing endurance in coordinated movement patterns. Patient education continues throughout the entire postsurgical period, in preparation for more demanding functional restoration strategies once the patient is ready.

Although there is supporting research for postoperative rehabilitation, more broad-based and procedure-specific literature will provide clearer guidelines as surgical technologies and rehabilitation strategies become more refined.

This chapter presented a clinical strategy for rehabilitation specialists to utilize in directing the postsurgical spinal patient's early resumption of locomotor system function. This phase of rehabilitation can be pivotal in determining the degree of successful rehabilitation ultimately attained. Once this phase is completed, the stage is set for more challenging protocols, as explained in the preceding and ensuing rehabilitation chapters.

SUMMARY

1. When the patient undergoes surgery, conservative management does not terminate.
2. Surgical techniques are another form of trauma to the spine and the clinician must realize that any preexisting muscle imbalance or motor control problem may be magnified postoperatively.
3. Early pre- and postoperative interventions designed to improve proper locomotor system firing patterns (i.e., coordination) and muscle balance are important.
4. Without proper rehabilitation, postsurgical trauma such as adhesive scar tissue formation, decreased tissue tolerance to stress, and an increase in tonic and phasic muscle imbalances can occur.
5. The key to success is the education of the patients on their dysfunction, the benefit of restoring such function, and how some relatively safe activities and exercises will hasten this process.
6. While the structural pathology may be repaired in the operating room, the "functional pathology," which may affect pain-generating structures, must be addressed.
7. Researchers have shown a delay of transverse abdominis firing in patients with chronic low back pain,[28] an example of disruption of the "feed-forward mechanism" of the CNS.
8. Despite a real need for greater understanding regarding the best methods and true benefit of prehabilitation, the authors feel that the current understanding of locomotor system function and dysfunction combined with the risks of surgery forms sufficient evidence to support this strategy of the presurgical spinal patient.
9. Patient education is considered the most critical component of any postoperative rehabilitation program.
10. Patients should be instructed in proper body mechanics in common functional activities to protect healing structures.
11. There are many factors to consider during postoperative lumbar rehabilitation, the most important of which is the extent of the repair during surgery and physical activity limitations by the surgeon.
12. Tight muscles and associated scarring can limit lumbar mobility as well as reproduce preoperative pain.
13. Muscle imbalances result in faulty posture, movement patterns, and increased or asymmetrical loading of various joints and tissues, interfering with optimal spin rehabilitation outcomes.

14. Hypertonic muscles should be restored with a number of manual procedures, such as postisometric relaxation technique.
15. Surgical procedures and the associated inflammation may cause or exacerbate reflexive inhibition of the phasic system muscles.
16. The transverse abdominis is an important part of the "pressurized canister" and of the postural system in general.
17. Evaluation and retraining of the diaphragmatic respiration is an important part of lumbopelvic rehabilitation.
18. Abdominal hollowing exercises have been found to indirectly activate the multifidi.
19. The pelvic floor exercises should be taught early in the rehabilitation process.
20. Proper motor control is essential in lumbopelvic stability and functional movements.
21. Sensorimotor training progressively increases proprioceptive input into the CNS and stimulates subcortical pathways to facilitate coordinated movement patterns.
22. Underwater exercise provides an excellent environment to unload healing tissues and to stimulate stabilizing reactions.

REFERENCES

1. Carragee EJ, Han MY, Yang B, et al. Activity restrictions after posterior lumbar diskectomy. A prospective study of outcomes in 152 cases with no postoperative restrictions. *Spine* 1999;24(22):2346–2351.
2. Watkins RG. Lumbar disc injury in the athelete. *Clini Sports Med* January 2002;21(viii):147–165.
3. Cherkin DC, Deyo R, Loeser JD, et al. An international comparison of back surgery rates. *Spine* 1994 Jun;1(11):1201–1206.
4. Yorimitsu E, Chiba K, Toyama Y, Hirabayashi K. Long-term outcomes of standard discectomy for lumbar disc herniation: A follow-up study of more than 10 years. *Spine* March 15, 2001;26(6):652-657.
5. Cassisi JE, Rbinson ME, O'Connor P, MacMillan M. Trunk strength and lumbar paraspinal muscle activity during isometric exercise in chronic low back pain. *Spine* 1993;18:245–251.
6. Roy SH, DeLuca DL, Casavant DA. Lumbar muscle fatigue and chronic lower back pain. *Spine* 1989;14:992–1001.
7. Manniche C. Assessment and exercise in low back pain: With special reference to the management of pain and disability following first-time disc surgery. *Dan Med Bull* 1995;42:301–313.
8. Manniche C. Clinical benefit of intensive dynamic exercise for low back pain. *Scand J Med Sci Sports* 1996;6: 82–87.
9. Carragee EJ, Helms E, O'Sullivan G. Are postoperative activity restrictions necessary after posterior lumbar discectomy? *Spine* 1996;21:1893–1897.
10. Ostello RW, de Vet HC, Waddell G, Kerckhoffs MR, Leffers P, van Tulder MW. Rehabilitation after lumbar disc surgery. *Cochrane Database Syst Trev* 2002;2:C003007.
11. Danielsen JM, Johnson R, Kibsgaard SK, Hellevik E. Early aggressive exercise for postoperative rehabilitation after discectomy. *Spine* 2000;25(8):1015–1020.
12. Dolan P, Greenfield K, Nelson RJ, Nelson IW. Can exercise therapy improve outcome of microdiscectomy? *Spine* 2000;25:1523–1532.
13. Kjelby-Wendt G, Styf J. Early active training after lumbar discectomy. A prospective, randomized, and controlled study of psychometric assessment in 50 patients. *J Spine Disord Tech* 2000;72(5):518–524.
14. Palmer S. Outpatient minimally invasive lumbar paramedian microdiscectomy. Program and Abstracts for the 69th Annual Meeting of the American Association of Neurological Surgeons, Toronto, Ontario, Canada, April 21–26, 2001.
15. Ditmyer MM, Topp R, Pifer M. Prehabilitation in preparation for orthopaedic surgery. *Orthop Nurs* September–October 2002;21(5):43–51.
16. Janda, V. Muscles and motor control in low back pain: Assessment and management. In: Twomey LT, ed. *Physical therapy of the low back*. New York: Churchill Livingstone, 1987:253–278.
17. Hodges PW, Richardson CA. Contraction of the abdominal muscles associated with movement of the lower limb. *Phys Ther* 1997;77:132–144.
18. Hodges PW, Richardson CA. Feedforward contraction of transversus abdominis is not influenced by the direction of arm movement. *Exp Brain Res* 1997;114:362–370.
19. Richardson C, Jull G, Hodges P, Hides J. *Therapeutic exercise for lumbopelvic stabilization*, 2nd ed. Edinburgh: Churchill Livingstone, 2004.
20. Richardson C, Snijders CJ, Hides JA, Damen L, Pas MS, Storm J. The relationship between the transverse abdominis muscles, sacroiliac joint mechanics, and low back pain. *Spine* 2002;27(4):399–405.
21. Hodges PW, Richardson CA. Delayed postural contraction of transversus abdominis in low back pain associated with movement of the lower limbs. *J Spinal Disord* 1998;11:46–56.
22. Hides JA, Richardson CA, Jull GA. Multifidus muscle recovery is not automatic following resolution of acute first episode low back pain. *Spine* 1996;21:2763–2769.
23. Lewit K, Simons DG. Myofascial pain: Relief of post-isometric relaxation. *Archiv Phys Med Rehabil* 1984; 65(8):452–456.
24. Hinoki M, Ushio N. Lumbosacral proprioceptive reflexes in body equilibrium. *Acta Otalaryngol* 1975; 330(Suppl):197–210.
25. Hodges PW, Gandevia SC, Richardson CA. Contractions of specific abdominal muscles in postural tasks are affected by respiratory maneuvers. *J Appl Physiol* 1997; 83:753–760.
26. Carriere B. *Fitness for the Pelvic Floor*. Stuttgart: Thieme, 2002.

27. Janda V. Sensory motor stimulation. In: Liebenson C, ed. *Rehabilitation of the spine*. Baltimore: Williams & Wilkins, 1996:319–328.
28. Bullock Saxton J, Janda V, Bullock M. Reflex activation of the gluteal muscles in walking with balance shoes: An approach to restoration of function for chronic low back pain patients. *Spine* 1993;18(6):704–708.
29. Heitkamp HC, Horstmann T, Mayer F, Willer J, Dickhuth HH. Gain in strength and muscular balance after balance training. *Int J Sports Med* 2001;22:285–290.
30. Abrahams VC. The physiology of neck muscles. Their role in head movement and maintenance of posture. *Can J Physiol Pharmacol* 1977;55:332–338.
31. Freeman MA, Wyke B. Articular contributions to limb muscle reflexes. The effects of partial neurotomy of the knee-joint on postural reflexes. *Br J Surg* 1966 Jan; 53(1):61–68.

CHAPTER

28

LUMBOPELVIC SENSORIMOTOR TRAINING AND FUNCTIONAL STABILIZATION

Donald R. Murphy and Craig E. Morris

OUTLINE

OBJECTIVES

1. To provide the clinical rationale for implementing sensorimotor training in the rehabilitation of low back disorders.
2. To describe in detail commonly utilized strategies for sensorimotor training of low back syndromes.
3. To provide the clinical rationale for performing lumpopelvic stabilization as part of a comprehensive rehabilitation plan.
4. To describe commonly utilized lumpopelvic stabilization strategies.
5. To describe how the methods explained here can be organized in a set of "Tracks".
6. To provide additional strategies for the effective management of the rehabilitation methods described in this chapter.

INTRODUCTION

Previous chapters have provided a basis for the importance and rationale for rehabilitation protocols in the management of low back syndromes. *Sensorimotor training* and *spinal stabilization,* with a specific emphasis on *lumbopelvic stabilization,* were introduced in the previous two chapters, but will now be covered in depth. The purpose of sensorimotor training and spinal stabilization is to improve key areas of locomotor system function that have been determined to be contributing to the perpetuation of each patient's low back syndrome.

The rationale, underlying principles, indications, and evidence of effectiveness were discussed in detail in Chapter 24. Briefly, it was explained that chronic pain syndromes are associated with altered neural afferentation. Specifically, compromised proprioception reduces the quality of incoming neural data from the periphery to the central nervous system. Without this requisite information, the efferent motor system becomes subsequently hindered in performing optimally coordinated, fine movement. The result of this may be a slowed speed of muscle contraction and poorly timed co-contraction between antagonistic muscles, leading to dynamic instability. Dynamic instability places increased loading on the joints and tendons, promoting painful chronicity and interfering with recovery.

Dynamic instability is just one type of faulty movement pattern that can result from compromised afferent input. Other movement patterns, as has been discussed in previous chapters, are also believed to become dysfunctional. With time and repetition, these dysfunctional movements become learned or "stereotyped." Neurologically, such learned movement patterns are called motor engrams. These engrams are initially established, under typical physiological circumstances, in the maturing locomotor system in the early years of life, as the individual's control of this system evolves from lying to crawling to kneeling to bipedal stances. However, with repetition and time, faulty or pathological motor engrams are believed to *supersede* the original physiological engrams. This is an important concept, in that the initial engrams are not erased or forgotton as new faulty engrams emerge. If this is so, then sensorimotor training and spinal stabilization is not to initiate new motor engrams, but rather reestablish the initial, learned patterns deeply embedded in the CNS.

Sensorimotor training is a clinical strategy designed to rectify faulty afferentation, thereby allowing the efferent motor system to improve efficiency via improved proprioception. As afferentation is normalized with sensorimotor training, along with other previously mentioned methods such as correcting joint, soft tissue, and emotional factors, spinal stabilization strategies can then be more effectively introduced. In this chapter, the specific techniques of application for these methods are presented.

SENSORIMOTOR TRAINING

Human locomotion is, simply stated, composed of bipedal ambulation over a stable surface. As muscle system function is improved by resistance challenges (weights, elastic bands, etc.), somatosensory system function can be challenged in the same manner by trying to maintain balance on labile surfaces. Sensorimotor training is a method that uses these unstable surfaces, most commonly in the form of rocker boards, wobble boards, and balance sandals, to create an afferent bombardment of the somatosensory system in the attempt to normalize stereotyped movement patterns.

Once joint mobility and muscle tone have been normalized, Janda[1] advocated starting the process by training the patient to "make a small foot," which he stated facilitates global somatosensory function. This involves teaching the patient to tense the intrinsic muscles, particularly the quadratus plantae, adductor hallucis, interossei, and lumbricals, of the foot by attempting to make the foot shorter and narrower (Fig. 28–1). It is important that the long muscles of the foot, the flexor digitorum and hallucis muscles, do not substitute. When this faulty motion occurs, the foot takes a "hammer toe" appearance (Fig. 28–2). Once the ability to make a small foot is established, Janda suggested

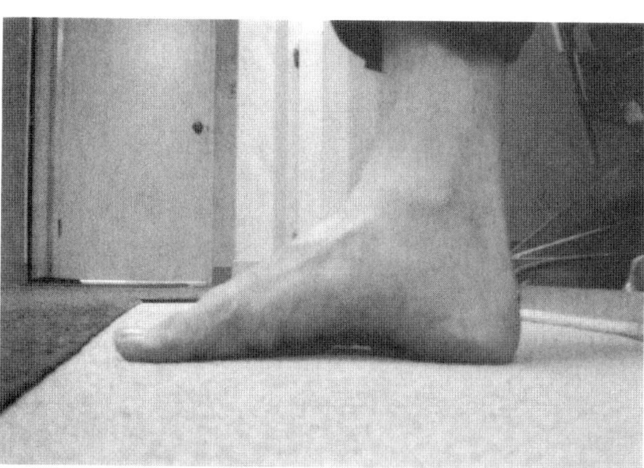

FIGURE 28–1. The small foot.

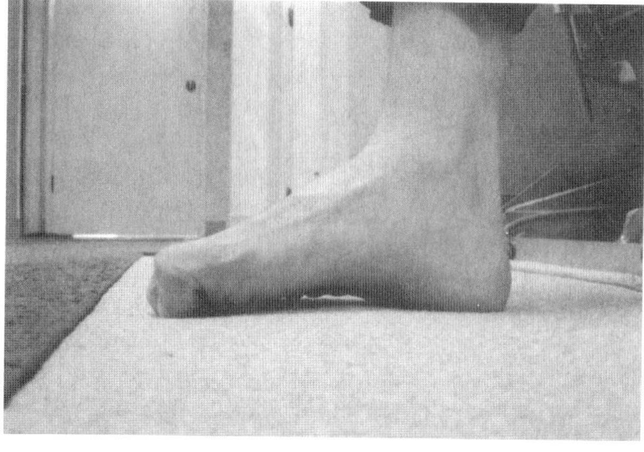

FIGURE 28–2. Incorrect technique in making a small foot.

that the patient be instructed to maintain it during all exercises that they will be performing, which he stated magnifies the neurological stimulation of each exercise.

The patient is then started on one of the unstable surface devices. It is important to start the patient on the device that challenges their balance, but is sufficiently comfortable in order to securely maintain their stance without having to raise the arms or hold on to an external object for balance. It is desirable to progress the patient as quickly as possible, which often means multiple visits over a brief period and a home training program. Aggressive treatment scheduling can speed somatosensory optimization because this is where maximum afferent stimulation can be achieved, likely producing maximum results.

Rocker Board

A beginning level of stimulation and challenge to the CNS can be introduced through the use of the rocker board, which is designed to present a labile surface in a single plane (Fig. 28–3). In preparation for the patient on the rocker board (or any labile surface training),

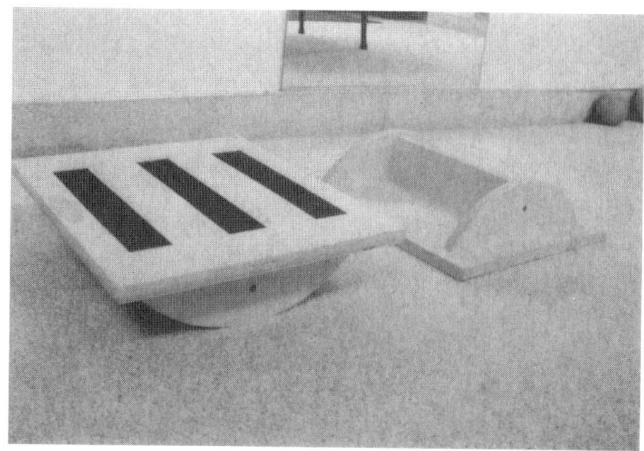

FIGURE 28–3. The rocker board.

the clinician should routinely "spot" (i.e. remain close to the patient with arms autstretched in order to assist in case of lost balance.) the patient. The clinician should stand with a stable stance close to the patient. The clinician's arms should be extended in order to catch the patient in case of a fall. The nervous patients may feel more secure with the knowledge that they are being protected, reducing anxiety and allowing them to perform labile surface training more effectively.

Clinical Pearl: As muscle system function is improved by resistance challenges (weights, elastic bands, etc.), somatosensory system function can be challenged in the same manner by trying to maintain balance on labile surfaces.

The patient first stands on the rocker board in a position such that the plane of instability of the board is "front to back" (Fig. 28–4). As previously stated, the patient is instructed to always establish a bilateral "small foot" stance, the basic position recommended for all standing somatosensory training protocols. The patient is then asked to maintain a balanced, erect ("Alexandrian") posture by instructing him or her to visualize a helium balloon attached to the posterosuperior portion of the head. This essentially causes the head to move superiorward and causes the neck to become longer.[2] The patient is then instructed to visualize his or her shoulders expanding outward and becoming wider. Finally, the patient is instructed to visualize his or her legs expanding away from the body toward the floor. The patient is told to maintain quiet, balanced stance in this position, making certain to keep the surface of the board horizontal and still.

Once the patient is able to maintain a quiet stance, the board is turned 90 degrees so that the plane of instability is left to right, or along the transverse plane (Fig. 28–5). As the patient becomes expert in maintaining quiet stance in this position, the board can be rotated 45 degrees so he or she can stand on the board in

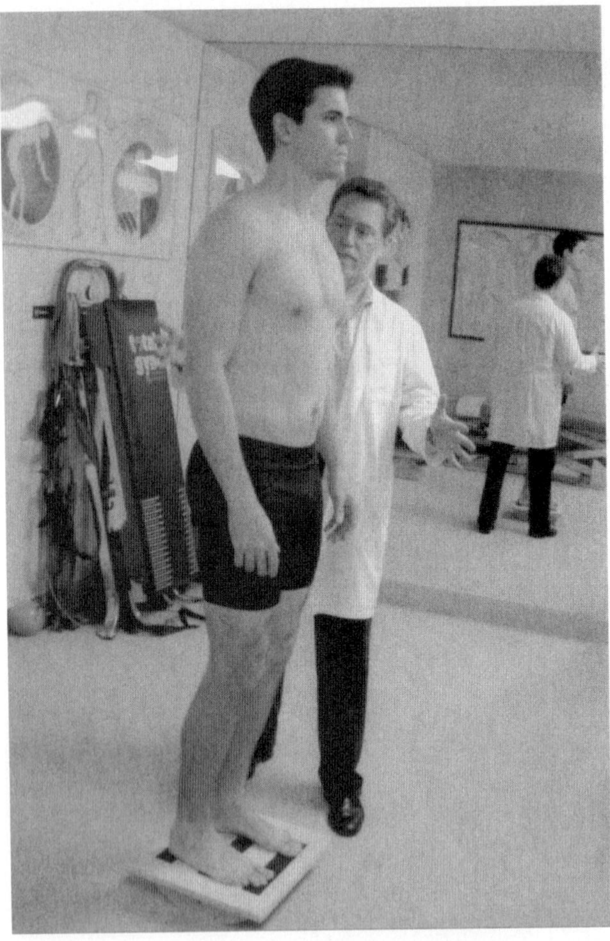

FIGURE 28–4. Two-legged stand on the rocker board with the board placed such that it is unstable from front to back. The clinician should always "spot" (i.e. remain close, prepared to assist if necessary) the patient to protect against injury from falling and to provide extra confidence for the patient who is afraid of falling.

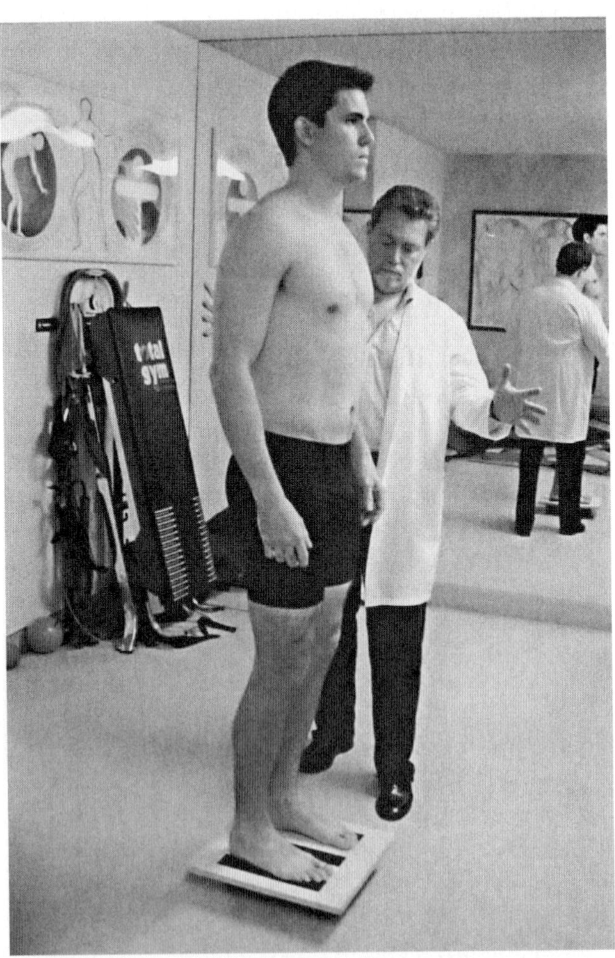

FIGURE 28–5. Two-legged stand on the rocker board with the board placed such that it is unstable from left to right.

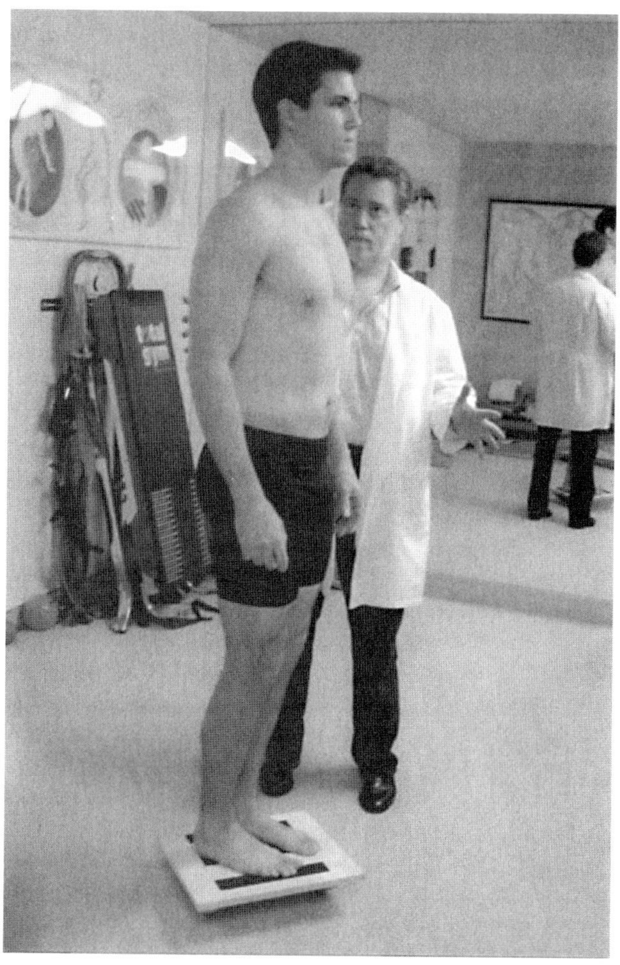

FIGURE 28–6. Two-legged stand on the rocker board with the board in the oblique position.

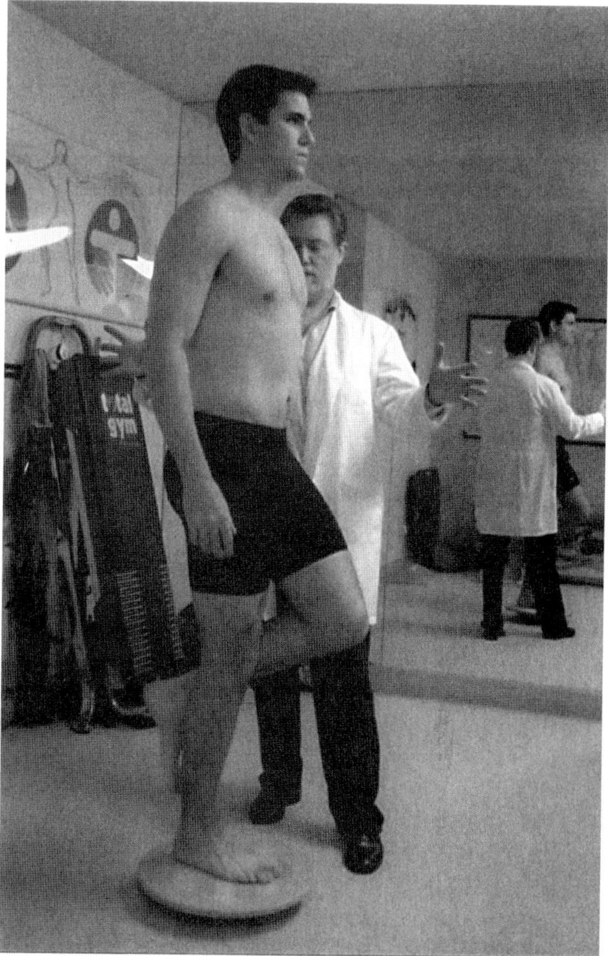

FIGURE 28–7. One-legged stand on the wobble board.

an oblique position (Fig. 28–6). Maintaining the small foot and postural set are recurrently emphasized.

As soon as the patient becomes comfortable on both feet, he or she is progressed to standing on one foot on the board.

Wobble Board

Mastery of the rocker board allows the patient to progress to the wobble board. This is a board that is rounded on the bottom and thus is unstable in all directions. This allows facilitation of postural reflexes in 360 degrees. As with quiet standing on the rocker board, here also the patient is instructed to maintain a small foot and Alexandrian posture. Again, the patient should be progressed as quickly as possible as with the uniplanar rocket board, being able to stand on one foot on the wobble board (Fig. 28–7)

Perturbations

After the ability to maintain a quiet stance has been established, perturbations can be introduced. Perturbations are small, sudden pushes from the clinician to the balancing patient's torso. These forces stimulate the CNS by upsetting equilibrium, facilitating automatic postural reactions.[1] Perturbations are important in the integration of long-loop reactions from the CNS. In normal quiet stance on a rocker or wobble board, a condition in which destabilizing forces are small in amplitude, the monosynaptic stretch reflex of the ankle muscles is adequate to correct deviations. Perturbations, in contrast, create larger amplitude disturbances, requiring more neurologically complex reactions that involve higher centers, thus producing a greater CNS response.[3]

Winter[4,5] has shown that there are two types of perturbations, each of which causes a different response from the postural stability system. External perturbations are forces acting on the body from the outside that produce *reactive* responses, based on the detection of the perturbation by the visual, vestibular, and somatosensory systems and the subsequent stabilization reaction by the CNS. Internal perturbations are forces acting on the body from within, as a result of voluntary movements, which produce *proactive* responses designed to maintain stability in anticipation of the disruption expected as a result of the movement.

Perturbations can be introduced to the body in a variety of ways, and specific responses can be elicited in the locomotor system depending on the type, direction, and location of the imposed perturbation. External perturbations can be applied in two forms: A force directed to a certain body part or a force directed to the board itself. The former stimulates a reactive stabilization response that occurs in an above–down sequence,[4–6] that is, the cervical stabilizers react first, followed by the trunk and pelvic stabilizers. The latter stimulates a reactive response that occurs in a down–up sequence and primarily relies on an ankle strategy.[4–6] In sensorimotor training of patients with low back syndromes, in which the improvement of postural stability responses and movement patterns is the aim, the perturbations directed to the body should be emphasized, as those directed to the board are less effective in eliciting spinal stabilization responses and are more appropriate for rehabilitation of ankle instability.

Varying the placement and direction of the external perturbations allows the specific facilitation of certain muscles on which the clinician may desire to place emphasis. It has been shown that immediate response is seen in the muscles near the placement of the perturbation, in addition to the above–down muscle activation pattern.[4] The clinician's hands can provide the perturbations, as this allows for control of the magnitude, frequency, and direction of the perturbation.

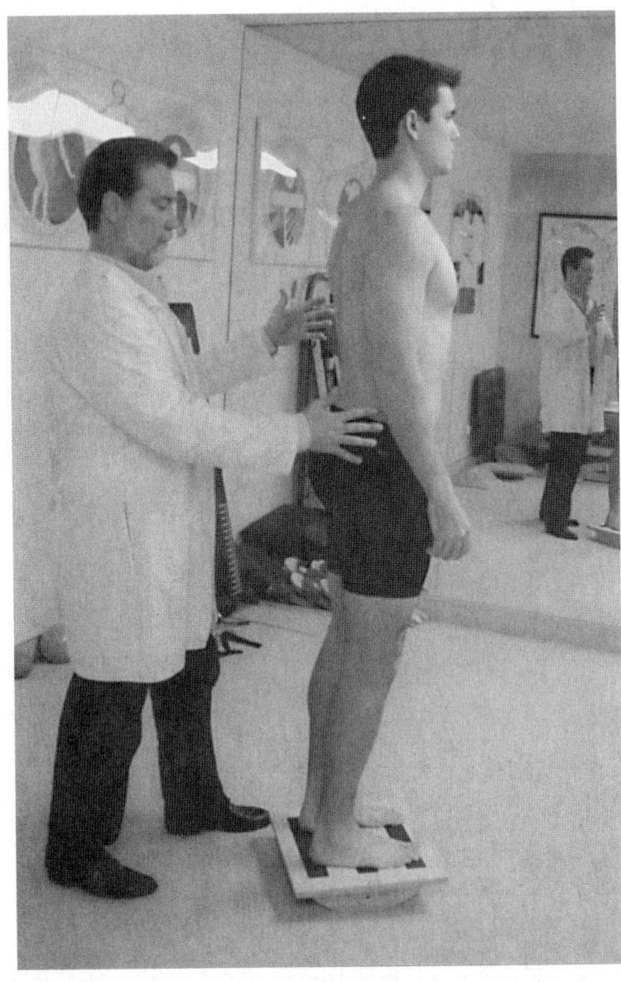

FIGURE 28–8. Applying perturbations to facilitate stabilization responses in the deep cervical flexors.

Clinical Pearl: Perturbations are small, sudden pushes from the clinician to the balancing patient's torso. These forces stimulate the CNS by upsetting equilibrium, facilitating automatic postural reactions.[1] Perturbations are important in the integration of long-loop reactions from the CNS.

Perturbations of the upper thoracic spine facilitate the deep cervical flexurs (Fig. 28–8). This causes a tendency for the chin to poke into protraction, thus forcing the deep cervical flexors to counteract this in maintaining a neutral head posture.

Perturbations appied to the lumbosacral region facilitate the deep abdominal stabilizers (Fig. 28–9). Pushes to the lumbopelvic region initially typically create an increased lumbar lordosis and anterior tilt. The stabilizers of the trunk reflexively counteract this to maintaina neutral posture.

Perturbations applied to the anterior aspect of the pelvis facilitate the gluteus maximus (Fig. 28–10). The posterior thrust creates a tendency to cause hip flexion. Finally, the gluteus medius is facilitated by applying the perturbation in a lateral to medial direction to the opposite hip (Fig. 28–11). This is best performed/done in the one-legged stance position, which creates a tendency toward an ipsilateral pelvic shift.

Internal perturbations can be introduced via body movements. This is most easily carried out through the movement of the upper extremities (Fig. 28–12). Internal perturbations can be initiated by instructing the patient to raise their arms overhead and back down again. This, as stated earlier, creates anticipatory reactions in the CNS, which facilitate stabilization responses that precede the actual movement, known as the "feedforward mechanism." Both internal and external perturbations can be stimulated in sequence by throwing an object such as a basketball or medicine ball to and from the patient (Fig. 28–13). This can also be done with the use of a Body Blade®, which the patient shakes while maintaining stability of the board (Fig. 28–14).

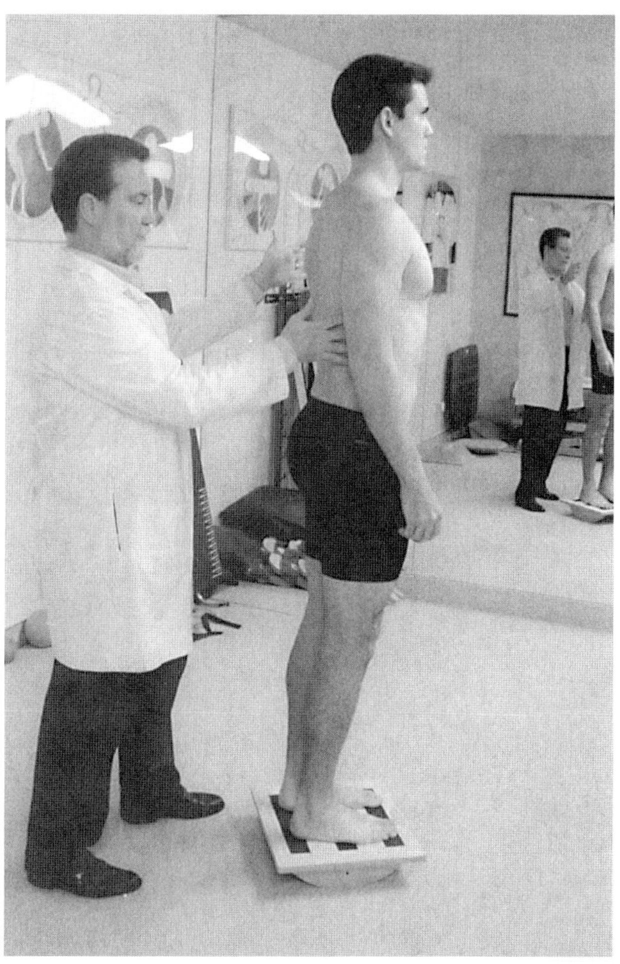

FIGURE 28–9. Applying perturbations to facilitate stabilization responses in the deep abdominal muscles.

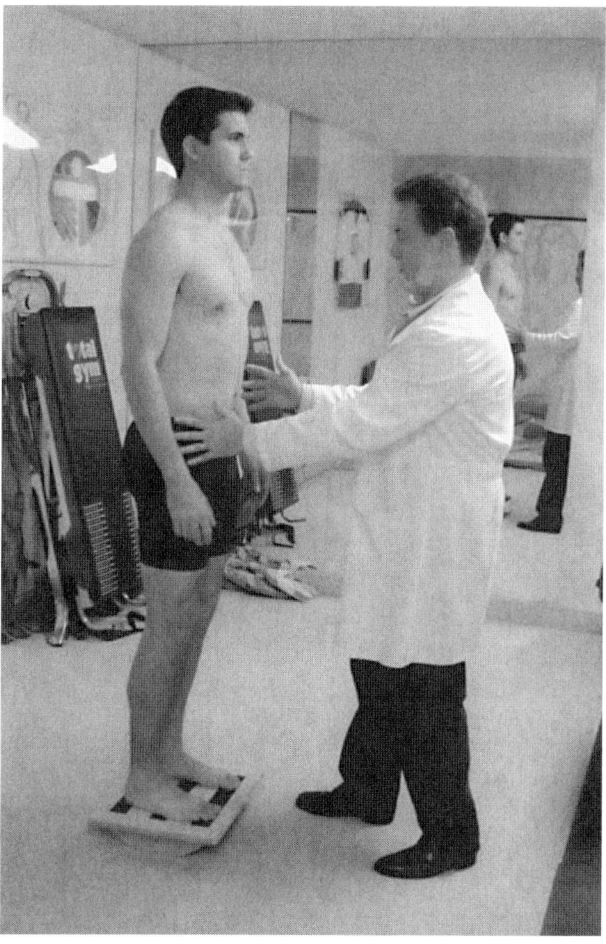

FIGURE 28–10. Applying perturbations to facilitate stabilization responses in the gluteus maximus.

Balance Sandals

Balance sandals, also called rehabilitation sandals, were invented by Janda to integrate proprioceptive training with gait and remain the only devices proven to do so.[7] These are less commonly utilized than static proprioceptive devices such as rocker boards despite their practicality and effectiveness, perhaps because of limited knowledge regarding their literature base and limited access to the European-manufactured devices in the past. Balance sandals are rigid, cork-soled devices that have a centrally placed, hard rubber hemisphere on the bottom of each (Fig. 28–15).

The barefoot patient, after being reminded to establish a small foot bilaterally and an Alexandrian posture, is instructed to slowly engage in a marching action and is carefully instructed in proper form (Fig. 28–16). It is important that the movement be isolated to the hips, knees, and ankle and that hiking of the iliac crests be avoided (Fig. 28–17). The feet, when contacting the floor, should be neutral with respect to dorsi- and plantar flexion.

Once the patient has mastered the marching form without wearing sandals, he or she is then instructed to do the same with shoes on their feet (Fig. 28–18). The same marching form that was used without shoes must be followed. The patient begins with marching in place and progresses to slowly moving forward, then backward. The patient must avoid touching the edges of the sandal with the floor. Because only the middle portion of the gait cycle bears weight on the midfoot, the sandal is designed for very short steps so the midfoot remains over the rubber hemisphere. Once the patient masters these movements, performed slowly and smoothly, lateral steps (sidesteps) are then introduced.

Janda cautioned against continuous use of balances sandals for more than 2–3 minutes at a time, warning that they provide an "afferent barrage" and rapid exhaustion. Instead, he strongly recommended several brief repetitions throughout the day for patients to improve and then maintain optimal proprioceptive input.

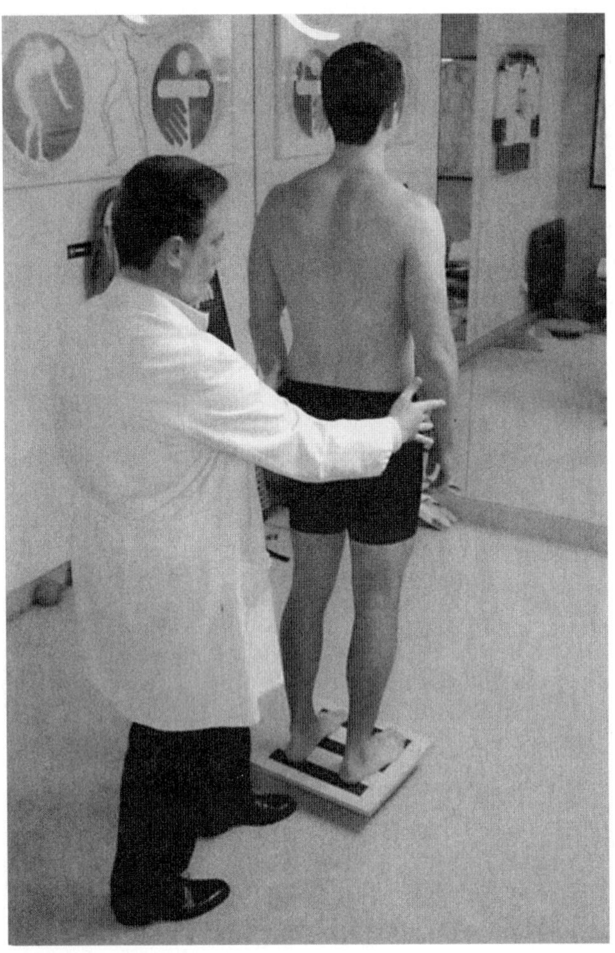

FIGURE 28–11. Applying perturbations to facilitate stabilization responses in the gluteus medius.

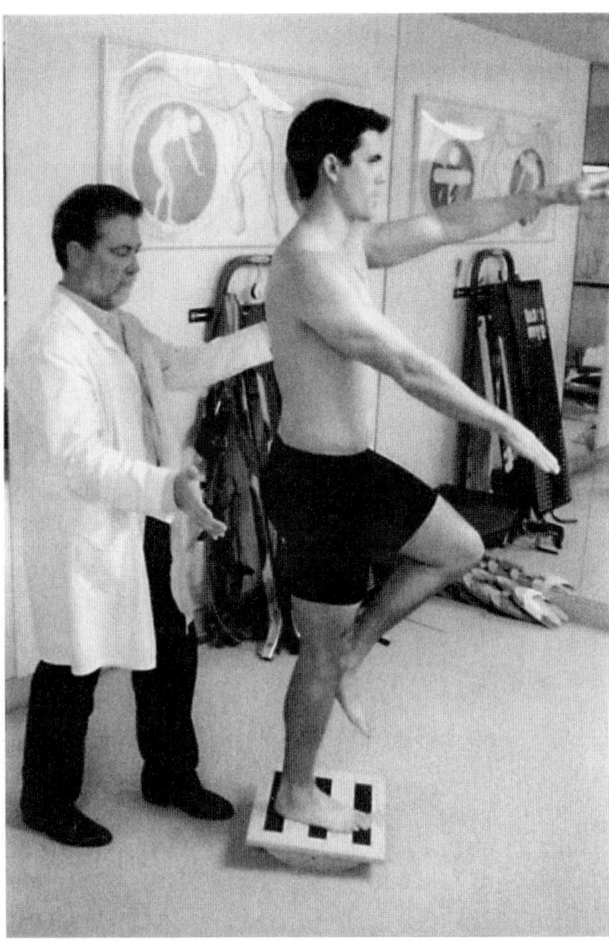

FIGURE 28–12. Facilitating proactive stabilization responses to internal perturbation.

Clinical Pearl: Balance sandals, also called rehabilitation sandals, were invented by Janda to integrate proprioceptive training with gait and remain the only devices proven to do so.

Perturbations can be introduced while the patient is marching with the shoes via the use of pushes (external perturbations) and arm movements (internal perturbations) (Figs. 28–19 and 28–20).

Long-term Use of Sensorimotor Training Devices

Chapter 13 discussed in detail the maturation and decline of the locomotor system. It was noted that one of the first aspects of this decline occurred with reduced balance secondary to proprioceptive compromise. The sensorimotor devices previously mentioned in this chapter can be utilized to maintain optimized sensorimotor function in addition to restoring sensorimotor function as part of rehabilitation strategy.

By utilizing tools like the balance sandals and rocker board, the proprioceptive challenges logically help to maintain improved balance, helping o slow the locomotor system's degenerative process and prolonging bipedalism. If this is so, then these devices should reasonably be integrated within the patient's regular exercise program as part of an overall health maintenance plan.

There is one great drawback for implementing sensorimotor devices such as balance sandals into one's exercise routine. These disciplined individuals are accustomed to enjoying the exercise "rush", an endorphin release that accompanies cardiovascular exercise and becomes associated with successfully accomplishing an athletic challenge. Because the sensorimotor devices fail to provide such a "rush", individuals must overcome this letdown and nevertheless utilize these devices because of their intellectual understading of the benefit.

While there are a number of sensorimotor challenges involved with many different types of exercises, including activities that integrate running and

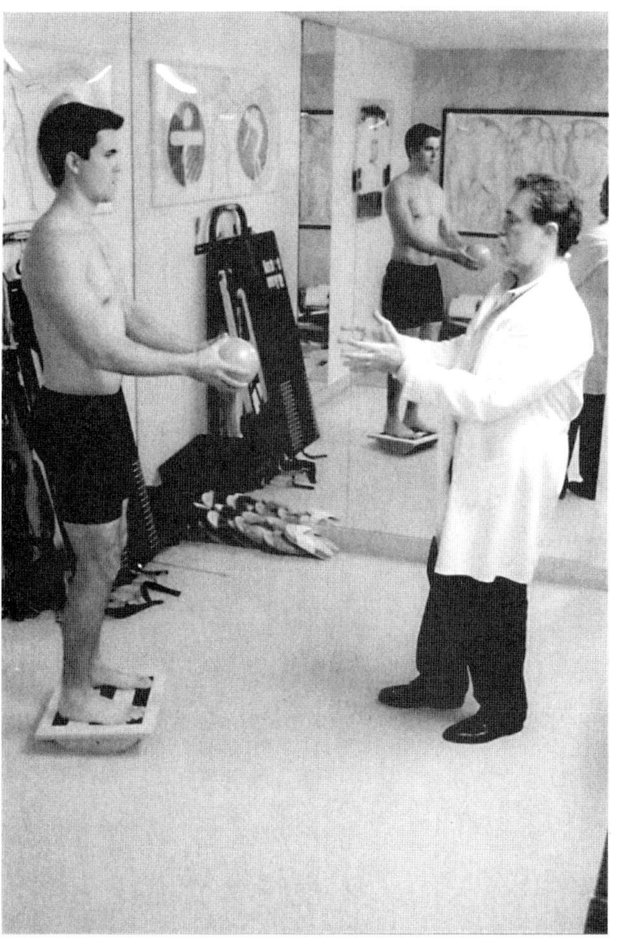

FIGURE 28–13. Facilitating reactive and proactive responses; playing catch with a medicine ball.

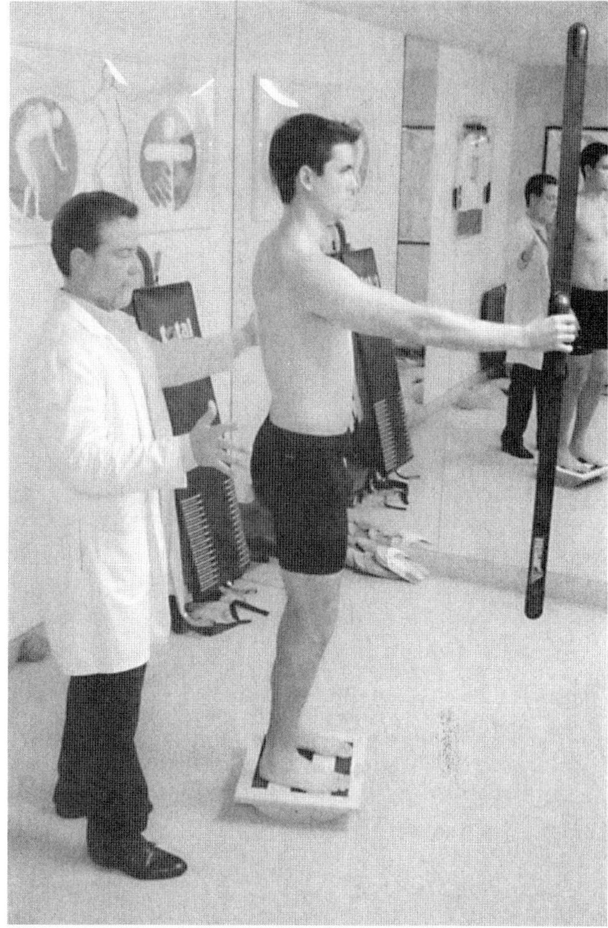

FIGURE 28–14. Using the Body Blade® to facilitate trunk stabilization responses.

jumping, the authors of this chapter recommend that sensorimotor devices be utilized on a regular lifetime basis for those individuals interested in optimal locomotor system longevity. Bullock-Saxton and Janda emphasized the unique benefit of the balance sandals, because these tools specifically provide sensorimotor stimulus during that all important aspect of locomotor function known as bipedal gait.[7]

Advanced Sensorimotor Progressions

The number of variations that can be introduced to increasingly challenge and train sensorimotor function is limited only by the clinician's imagination. Common progressions include variations of the following:

1. Full cervical extension, which challenges the labyrinthine system and perhaps the proprioceptive input from the upper cervical spine.
2. Closing the eyes, which disrupts the visual afferentation.
3. Transitioning from a soft (carpeted or padded) surface to a hard surface, which reduces stability of the sensorimotor training devices.
4. Throwing and catching a ball, being certain that the arc passes above eye level and forcing the patient to follow this with their eyes. This reduces

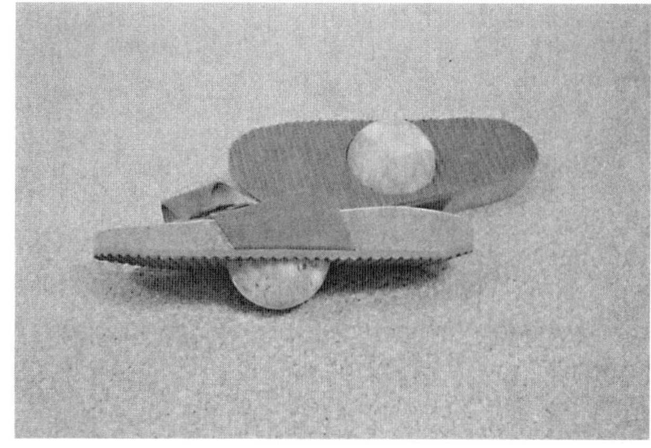

FIGURE 28–15. Balance sandals.

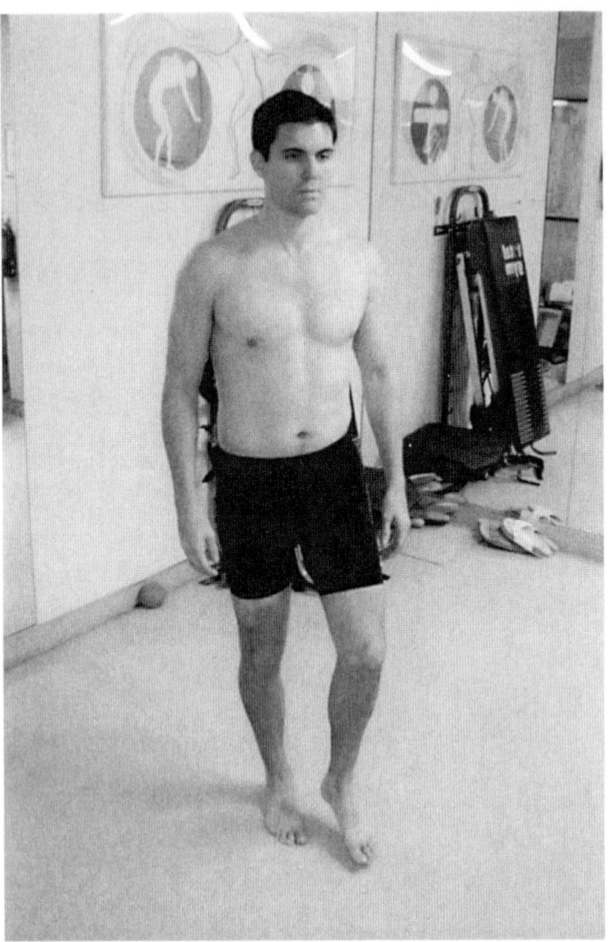

FIGURE 28–16. Proper form for marching in preparation for use of the balance sandals. Note that the hips remain level.

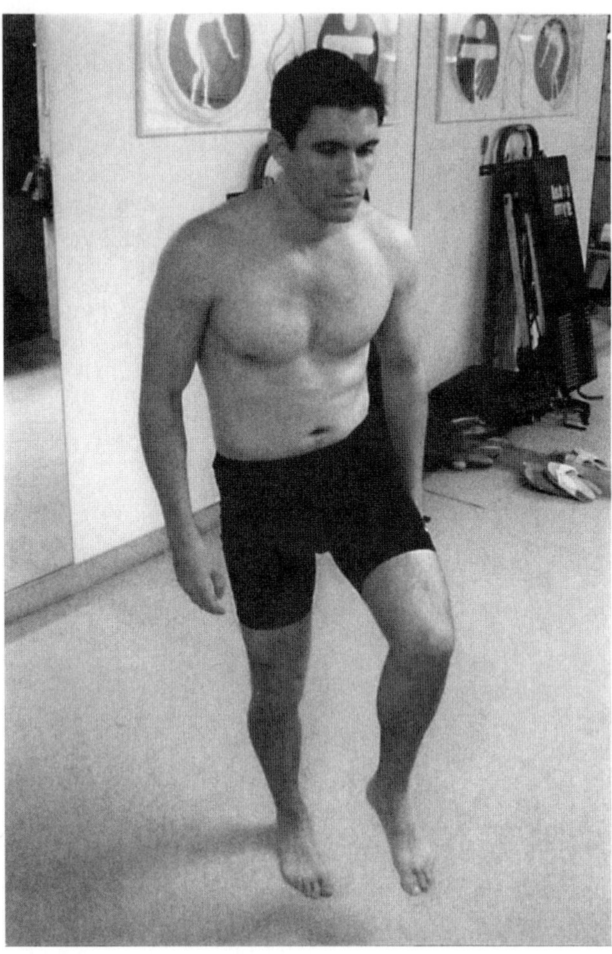

FIGURE 28–17. Improper form for marching.

visually assisted balance strategies while hand–eye coordination challenges are iniated.

5. Transitioning from an extended knee to a bent knee, which is believed to reduce proprioceptive inflow from the musculotendinous knee stabilizers.
6. Transitioning from two feet to one foot, reducing the proprioceptive input from the lower extremities and sacroiliac joints while causing unipedal body imbalance.

WHEN TO INITIATE SENSORIMOTOR TRAINING

Sensorimotor training is not typically used for the acute or subacute stage of a back syndrome. In these stages, faulty movements and postures have not had sufficient time to become stereotyped and the goal is to relieve pain before this occurs. Therefore, it is the chronic stage for which sensorimotor training is most commonly used.

Clinical Pearl: Sensorimotor training is a clinical strategy designed to rectify faulty afferentation, thereby allowing the efferent motor system to improve efficiency via improved proprioception.

Of course, in the above paragragh it is presupposed that the presenting patient has no other chronic syndrome or dysfunction (i.e., faulty posture) that would complicate the acute or subacute stage case. Often, there is an underlying dysfunction from an old injury or postural compromise, which may or may not be asymptomatic. In addition, it may have initiated in the low back or may secondarily affect the back, as can occur in lower extremity problems, for example.

In addition to determining the correct stage of the patient's condition or dysfunction, determining the optimal timing for sensorimotor training within the office visit can be helpful. While supporting literature on this topic is lacking, the authors have found such training works best directly after manual techniques have been employed. This may be because techniques that normalize joint mobility and muscle tone briefly alter proprioceptive homeostatis. Lewit stated that manipulation creates a brief period of latent hypermobility. Chapter 21 discusses in detail the

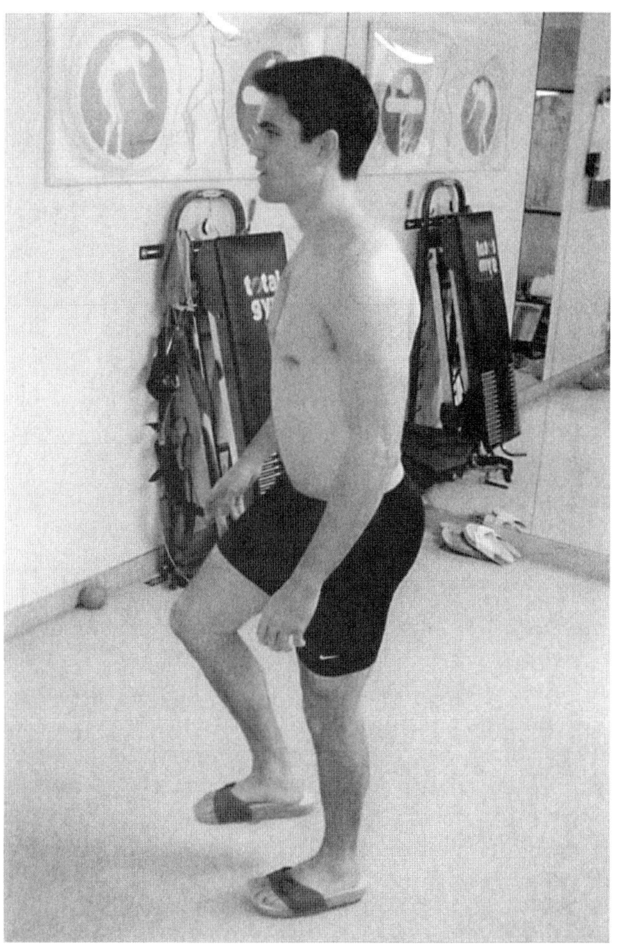

FIGURE 28–18. Marching while wearing balance shoes.

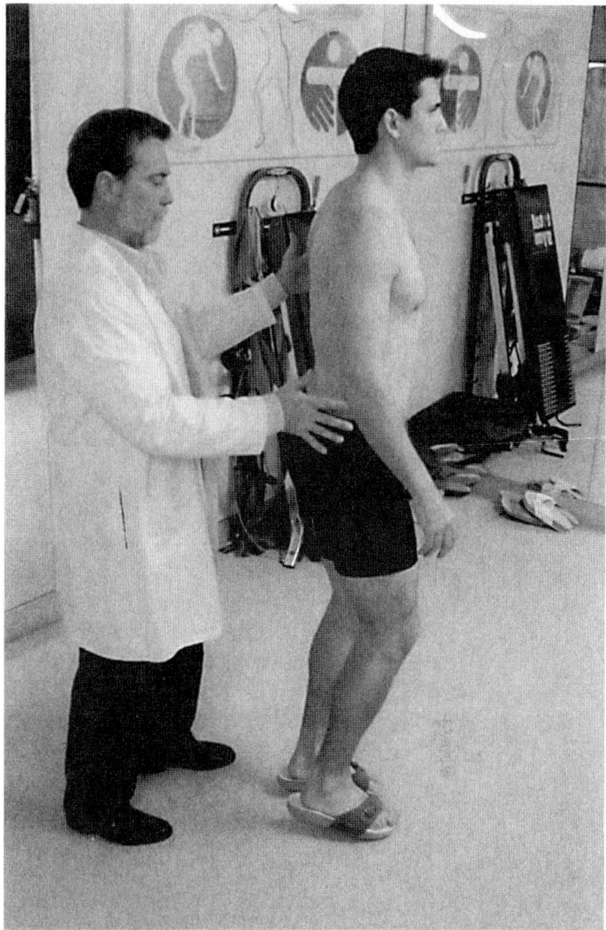

FIGURE 28–19. External perturbations with balance shoes.

neurological and biomechanical sequelae associated with joint manipulation. The same holds true for other manual techniques, which may briefly alter the proprioceptive homeostasis as joint mobility and tissue tone changes and mechanoreceptor afferentation changes provoke adaptation of the alpha and gamma motor systems.

These reasons have led the authors to recommend that sensorimotor training be utilized following such manual techniques at this point in the office visit, a point in which the locomotor system is believed to be quite amenable to.

SPINAL STABILIZATION

As was detailed in Chapters 5 and 26, spinal stability requires a harmonious pattern of contraction of muscles, the intensity and specific muscular involvement of which depends on the particular activity in which the individual engages. Stability of the intervertebral segments is believed to be primarily provided by the intrinsic, or local, muscles such as the transverse abdominis (TrA), multifidus (MULT), and quadratus lumborum (QL), while the larger, more superficial muscles, such as the rectus abdominis (RA), external obliques (EO), and erector spinae (ES), provide some additional stiffness to the spine as a whole. Because the TrA and MULT apparently easily become inhibited, the first stage in spinal stabilization involves an attempt at selective activation of these muscles. The purpose of this is to ensure, to the greatest extent possible, that these muscles are optimally participating in the ensuing exercises in which the patient engages. In order for these muscles to participate as required, the CNS must be to localize these muscles. It must be emphasized, however, that optimal spinal stability requires harmonious coactivation of all lumbopelvic, not just the intrinsic muscles.

THE ABDOMINAL BRACE

The abdominal brace is a maneuver with which the patient is taught to co-contract the TrA and MULT. The patient lies supine with the knees and hip flexed and is told to exhale and slightly "draw in"[8] the navel toward the spine. It is important that the patient does

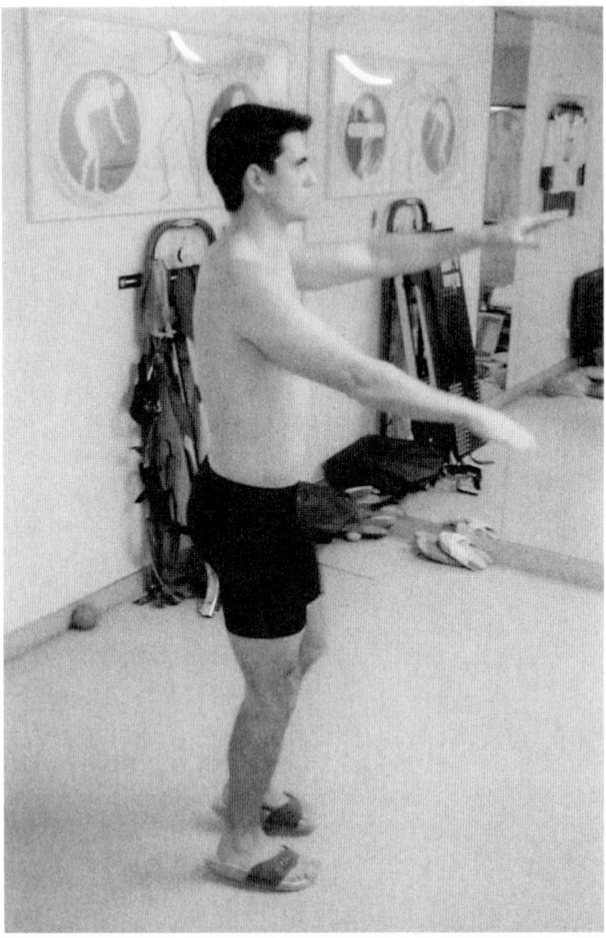

FIGURE 28–20. Internal perturbations with balance shoes.

not attempt to create a large "hollow" of the abdomen (Fig. 28–21). This "hollowing" maneuver will likely involve virtually no trunk muscle activity, but instead will involve inhibition of the diaphragm and/or contraction of the accessory muscles of respiration. It is also important that the patient does not perform a "pelvic tilt" or press the lumbar spine into the floor, which will engage the RA rather than the TrA and MULT.

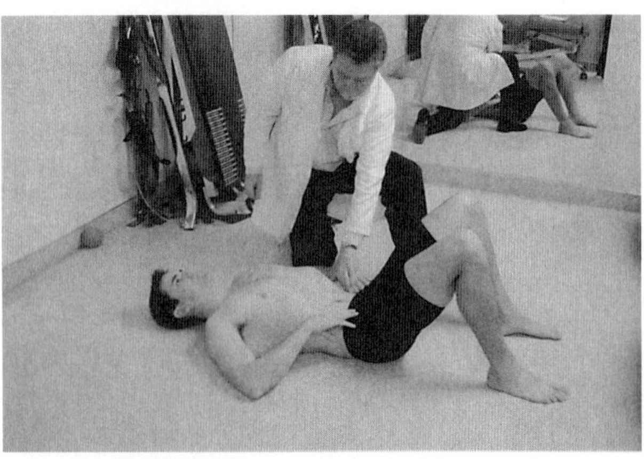

FIGURE 28–21. Creating a faulty large abdominal "hollow".

The proper contraction of the TrA can be palpated by the practitioner placing the thumbs just medial and inferior to the anterior superior iliac spines (Fig. 28–22). A light, deep contraction of the TrA should be felt, as opposed to the early and more superficial contraction that would represent the external oblique. Also, a protruding abdomen and/or flattening rib cage during the performance of the abdominal brace suggest substitution of the RA for the TrA.[9]

The MULT should also be palpated to be sure that these key muscles are taking part in the bracing maneuver. This can be done with the patient lying prone. The clinician's palpating fingers should be placed on either side of the lumbar spinous processes, in the vacinity of the MULT muscles (Fig. 28–23). The palpation should be deep, as it is the deep fibers of the MULT that are of interest in segmental stabilization.[9] The patient is asked to perform the abdominal brace, and the clinician palpates the contraction of the MULT. Improper recruitment of MULT will be represented by the lack of a deep muscle contraction. One may also find a quick, superficial tension developing, which would likely represent either recruitment of the superficial fascicles of the MULT only or tension in the descending tendon of the thoracic ES.[9] Each segment of the lumbar spine should therefore be palpated.

If improper contraction of the MULT is detected, the patient should be instructed for contraction of these muscles. This can be done by having the patient attempt to gently "swell" or "tense" those muscles while the clinician palpates the muscles for tactile cue.[9] It is important the patient be instructed to avoid moving the spine or pelvis during this maneuver, which would suggest contraction of superficial global muscles instead of intrinsic stabilizers

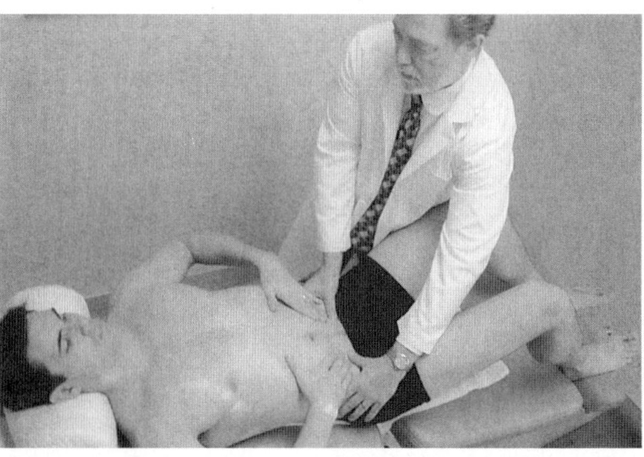

FIGURE 28–22. Palpation of the transverse abdominis. Note the patient palpates along with the clinician in order to establish kinesthetic awareness of TrA activation.

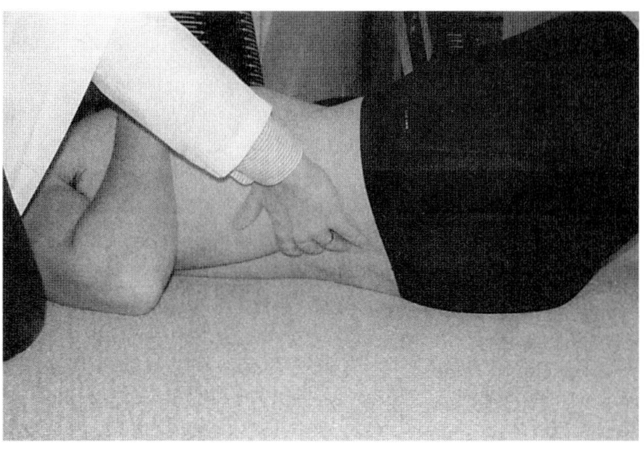

FIGURE 28–23. Palpation of the multifidis.

Clinical Pearl: The abdominal brace is a maneuver with which the patient is taught to co-contract the TrA and MULT.

In addition to this, the patient should be taught to activate the pelvic floor muscles, which also play a role in spine stability[10–12] and are neurophysiologically related to the TrA and MULT, as these muscles typically co-contract when either are consciously activated.[13] In fact, often one will encounter a patient who has difficulty in activating the TrA and MULT with the abdominal brace maneuver. In these cases, it is helpful to have the patient contract the abdominal floor muscles while the clinician palpates the TrA and MULT. This frequently causes activation of the deep spinal stabilizers and allows the CNS to "find" the TrA and MULT so that the patient can learn to activate these muscles voluntarily with the abdominal brace.

Having the patient tense these muscles as if he or she were urinating, repetitively initiating and interrupting the flow can activate the pelvic floor muscles. For men, another cue would be to have him simply elevate his scrotum, drawing it inward toward his diaphragm. This must be done gently to avoid activation of the RA and external obliques. As with abdominal brace, the TrA and MULT can be palpated to ensure proper activation of these muscles.

Another method that can be used to facilitate TrA and MULT co-contraction is to have the patient perform the abdominal brace in the quadruped position. It is thought that the weight of the viscera elicits a stretch reflex in the TrA and makes it easier to activate this muscle.[9]

Training the patient in the proper abdominal brace is an essential first step in the process of spinal stabilization training, and the necessary time must be taken to ensure that the patient is properly engaging the TrA and MULT along with the pelvic floor muscles. It is also important that the patient be able to breath normally while holding the abdominal brace and pelvic floor contraction, as the diaphragm is believed to play a role in spine stability[10,14] and holding the breath tends to cause the recruitment of RA in maintaining the brace.[15,16] There is no sense in moving on to other exercises unless the patient has demonstrated that he or she can perform a proper abdominal brace and pelvic floor activation while breathing normally. Moving on too quickly will run the risk of encouraging the tendency to leave the TrA and MULT out of the functional picture in favor of the large muscles when training stability. It is motor control that is being trained in spinal stabilization and this must be kept in mind at all times.

It must again be emphasized that the large, multisegmental muscles (ES, RA, EO) are important for spine stability and must take part in the training process. However, because the intrinsic muscles (TrA, MULT) tend to become inhibited frequently in patients with LBP,[17–19] one must make sure these muscles are appropriately participating in stabilization exercises. For this reason, meticulous attention to teaching the establishment and maintenance of the co-contraction of the TrA and MULT with the abdominal brace is essential before continuing the training process.

THE PRESSURE BIOFEEDBACK UNIT

Many clinicians involved with lumbopelvic stabilization training use the pressure biofeedback unit in both clinical application and in research. This unit, a modified sphygmomanometer, is useful in ensuring proper "drawing in" of the abdomen when the patient performs an abdominal brace.[6,8] While palpation of the TrA and MULT is effective for the clinician to be sure that the patient is appropriately co-contracting the desired muscles, the pressure biofeedback unit can be used by clinician and patient to monitor undesirable movement of the lumbar spine, particularly during limb movements. Its use will not be further discussed in this chapter, but can be found elsewhere.[6,8]

THE FLOOR STABILIZATION EXERCISES

Once the abdominal brace is mastered, the patient is progressed to floor exercises in which he or she, starting with simple extremity movements performed while holding the abdominal brace, is trained to maintain co-contraction of the TrA and MULT while the CNS is involved in moving the extremities. The purpose of these extremity movements is twofold. The first is to put the spine under a load against which the stability system must maintain control. This involves the maintenance of the co-contraction of the TrA and

MULT for intersegmental stability along with contraction of the larger muscles (RA, EO, ES) to maintain rigidity of the spine as a whole.[20] The second purpose is to start the process of involving the CNS in extremity movements so that the co-contraction of the TrA and MULT once again becomes automatic.

It is essential that the patient maintain the abdominal brace during each exercise. It is also essential that the patient maintain a neutral posture of the spine during these exercises. As was discussed in Chapter 26, the deep segmental stabilizing muscles do not function in isolation from the global muscles. Rather, all these trunk muscles work together in maintaining spinal stability. So, while it is important that the patient maintain co-contraction of the segmental stabilizers, which tend to easily become inhibited, the introduction of extremity movements involves co-contraction of the superficial muscles, as these muscles naturally co-contract with the segmental stabilizers to maintain stiffness of the spine as a whole during normal activity.[21] So activity in the deep segmental stabilizers serves to maintain the intervertebral neutral zones and the activity in the global stabilizers serves to maintain neutral posture of the spine and pelvis as a whole during movements of the extremities. This coordinated activity pattern is of paramount importance in training spine stability.

For convenience, the exercises are organized along tracks. These tracks are not meant to be followed in a "cookbook" fashion, but, rather, are designed to organize the exercises so that the clinician can choose those tracks and specific exercises that are best suited to each patient. In general, it is important that the patient develops the ability to perform each exercise with good motor control before moving on to the next exercise.

Clinical Pearl: For convenience, the exercises are organized along tracks. These tracks are not meant to be followed in a "cookbook" fashion, but, rather, are designed to organize the exercises so that the clinician can choose those tracks and specific exercises that are best suited to each patient.

It should be noted that for all supine exercises in which the arms are not active, a useful option is to have the patient externally rotate the arms, open the fingers as wide as possible, and press the arms against the floor. The purpose of this is activating the middle and lower trapezii to integrate scapular stabilization into the exercise.

The Hook-Lying Position

This is one of the keypositions for lumbopelvic stabilization exercises. The patient is supine, with hips flexed at approximately 45 degrees, knees flexed at 90 degrees, and both feet resting on the floor. If viewed from the side, the patient looks the shape of a hook, hence the popular name in the United States. It is also called the crook-lying position in other English-speaking countries.

Supine Pelvic Tilt Track

This track is initially designed to teach the patient to reestablish the basic kinesthetic ability to isolate and control the four key superficial muscles of lumbopelvic rigidity. These include the abdominis rectus, gluteus maximus, iliopsoas, and thoracolumbar erector spinae. The second goal is to establish co-contraction of the synergists that perform an optimal anterior pelvic tilt and then those that establish the posterior tilt. Once these skills are mastered, the patient is taught to find and then stabilize the *neutral spine*. Finally, diaphragmatic respiration is integrated into the stabilized neutral spine. This track establishes the basic motor skills for dynamic stability while integrating respiration. There are eight specific exercises of this track, which are all performed in the hook-lying position.

The Anterior Tilt This is the first of the three key positions of the pelvic tilt track. In order to provide optimal direction and instruction, the clinician should explain this and also what defines an anterior, or front (to simplify medical jargon for the patient), pelvic tilt. The reference point for tilting is the anterior superior spine, so the patient's fingers are placed here. As the anterior superior iliac spine (ASIS) tilts forward, a forward tilt is performed. Conversely, as the patient's ASIS tilts posteriorly, a "back tilt" is performed.

Exercise 1. Anterior Tilt Part A: Activation of the Erector Spinae The patient is in the hook-lying position and is instructed to tilt the pelvis forward by contracting the muscles of the low back. Another instuction may be to sway the back forward, which the patient should realize also causes a front tilt. Because these muscles, the erectoe spinae, typically exhibit the best control of the four key lumbopelvic stabilizers, they provide an optimal entry or initial exercise. Patients are comfortable isolating these muscles, laying a foundation of confidence and relaxation in preparation for more difficult exercises.

As the patients performs the front tilt using only the erectors spinae, they are informed this is only a partial front tilt, but helps to form an optimal front tilt.

Exercise 2. Anterior Tilt Part B: Activation of the Hip Flexors The patient is in the hook-lying position and is instructed to tilt the pelvis forward again, this time using the hip flexors. This task is typically more difficult to perform than the previous one because the hip flexors are more difficult to kinesthetically isolate.

A practical way of having the patients isolate the hip flexors is to instruct them to lift their feet an inch off the floor. As they do this, they should be made aware that their pelvis simultaneously tilted forward. They should palpate their hip flexors contracting in the lower abdomen as they begin to improve the kinesthetic awareness of this muscle group. With time and practice, they will be able to contract the hip flexors without having to think about lifting the feet. They should also be made aware that contraction of the hip flexors provides a partial front tilt, rather than a full optimal front tilt.

Exercise 3. The Optimal or Full Anterior Tilt: Co-Contraction of Anterior Tilt Once the patient is skilled at isolating the two muscle groups responsible for front pelvic tilting, he or she is instructed to contract both, or co-contract, the erector spinae and iliopsoas to perform a full or optimal front tilt. The patient remains in a hook-lying position for the full front tilt. The patient should be able to feel that this full front tilt rocks the pelvis farther forward than either of the partial front tilts.

Once the patients have mastered the three anterior tilt exercises, they are ready for the posterior tilt exercises.

Exercise 4. Posterior Tilt Part D: Activation of the Rectus abdominis The patient is in the hook-lying position and is instructed to flatten the back or tilt the pelvis back by contracting rectus abdominis, which is also called in lay terms as the "six-pack muscle." If this is difficult for the patient to understand or perform, it can be explained that this is the muscle one uses while performing a crunch-style sit-up exercise.

The patient kinesthetically isolates and contracts the rectus abdominis and should be made aware that he or she is performing a partial posterior, or back, tilt. The patient's ability to isolate and contract the recus abdominis will improve with repetition.

Exercise 5. Posterior Tilt Part D: Activation of the Gluteus Maximus The patient is in the hook-lying position and is instructed to squeeze the buttocks to perform a partial back, or posterior, pelvic tilt. Many patients with poor lumbopelvic stability have difficulty isolating and contracting the gluteus maximus. If this is a problem, a practical tip is to instruct the patient to keep the pelvis resting on the floor while squeezing the buttocks muscles and rolling the tailbone (i.e., coccyx) up away from the floor. This has proven too be a strong visual tip for patients and often facilitates the learning of this skill. A word of warning here: patients frequently have one gluteus maximus that is less functional (inhibited and/or weaker) than the other. Therefore, it is important to check both muscles to confirm sufficient and equal bilateral contraction.

The patient will master this skill with repetition and should be made aware that he or she is again performing only a partial pelvic tilt by only contrcting the gluteus maxaimus.

Exercise 6. Co-Contraction of Posterior Tilt Once the patient has mastered the initial two partial tilt exercises, he or she is ready for the optimal posterior tilt. The patient takes the hook-lying position and is now instructed to perform an optimal, or full, back tilt by contracting, or co-contracting, both the rectus abdominis and gluteus maximus.

The patient should be aware that this co-contracted back tilt provides a more compete back tilt than the previous two exercises and that the spine is more rigid with this co-contraction. Once the optimal front and back tilts are mastered, the patient isready to learn the neutral pelvis.

Note: As in most areas of health care, various preferences regarding the importance of certain stabilization tracks come into play. Some schools of thought are concerned that focus on the pelvic tracks as described above may become confused with William's exercise strategies that emphasized the posterior tilt. This is certainly not the case, because these focus on kinesthetic awareness of the posterior tilt as a means to control the neutral pelvis. Of course, if the patient demonstrates the capacity to control the global muscles associated with the posterior tilt, then the topic is elementary as the patient simply moves to the next track of exercises.

Exercise 7. Establishing the Neutral Pelvis The purpose of learning the front and back pelvic tilts is to isolate the four key muscle groups mentioned above in order to establish better control to find and maintain the neutral pelvis. The neutral pelvis can be found halfway between the front and back tilt. The neutral pelvis is a position that allows the spine to accommodate increased loading without trauma that can occur at end-range positions.

The patient takes the hook-lying position and is instructed to perform a full front and back pelvic tilt. With these end-range positions kinesthetically established, the patient is then instructed to find the halfway position between the two and to contract what are believed to be the four of the key global lumbopelvic muscles (erector spinae, iliopsoas, rectus abdominis, and gluteus maximus) to make the spine rigid in this neutral position.

With repetition, the patient will be able to find and hold the neutral pelvis, which forms the basic lumbopelvic postural strategy for most stabilization exercises. Remember, the underlying premise for these exercises is to counter the effect that the low back has lost its ability to maintain dynamic stability during various activities and becomes painful or traumatized by end-range motion overload. Reestablishing the neutral spine and pelvis allows the patient to again learn to maintain the lumbopelvic region in the safe, neutral range during various activities.

Clinical Pearl: The neutral pelvis is a position that allows the spine to accommodate increased loading without trauma that can occur at end-range positions.

Exercise 8. Integrating Abdominal Bracing and Respiration with the Neutral Pelvis Once remedial intrinsic exercises are mastered, such as abdominal bracing, pelvic floor elevation, and diaphragmatic respiration, these should repetitively be reintroduced into more advanced exercises as the patient graduates to higher levels of dynamic stability. Those specific activities that were the most difficult for the patient to learn should be the ones that are most frequently integrated with new exercises.

Pelvic Tilt Track Summary By the time the patient masters the supine lumbopelvic tilt track, he or she has reestablished the basics of lumbopelvic dynamic stability. That is, the patient has learned to co-contract the muscles of the "pressurized canister," to co-contract the key lumbopelvic stabilizing muscle groups, and to kinesthetically establish the neutral pelvis and spine. Furthermore, completion of the pelvic tilt track allows one to graduate to more advaced stabilization tracks.

Dead Bug Track

This track is designed to place focus on the abdominal muscles in stabilization. It does this by employing the extremities as long levers, adding additional challenge to maintaining the neutral pelvis to improve lumbopelvic control.

Exercise 1. Single Arm Raise The patient is in the hook-lying position with the arms held straight up so that the fingers are pointing toward the ceiling (Fig. 28–24). The patient establishes the abdominal brace. He or she is then instructed to slowly raise one arm overhead (Fig. 28–25) and then back to the starting point. This is repeated with the other arm. It is essential that the abdominal brace and neutral spine posture be maintained throughout the exercise.

Exercise 2. Double Arm Raise The patient is in the hook-lying position with the arms held straight up so that the fingers are pointing toward the ceiling (Fig. 28–24). The patient establishes the abdominal brace. He or she is then instructed to slowly raise both arms overhead (Fig. 28–26) and then back to the starting point. It is essential that the abdominal brace and neutral spine posture be maintained throughout the exercise.

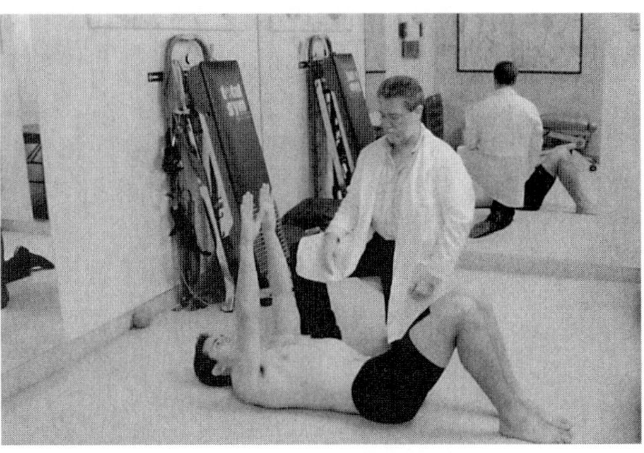

FIGURE 28–24. The hook-lying position with the fingers pointed toward the ceiling.

Exercise 3. Single Leg Raise The patient is in the hook-lying position and establishes the abdominal brace (Fig. 28–27). The patient is instructed to slowly raise one leg by flexing at the hip to 90 degrees (Fig. 28–28), and then return the leg to the starting point. This is repeated with the other leg. It is essential that the abdominal brace and neutral spine posture be maintained throughout the exercise.

Exercise 4. Single Leg Extension The patient is in the hook-lying position and establishes the abdominal brace (Fig. 28–27). The patient is instructed to slowly extend one knee (Fig. 28–29) and then return the leg to the starting point. This is repeated with the other leg. It is essential that the abdominal brace and neutral spine posture be maintained throughout the exercise.

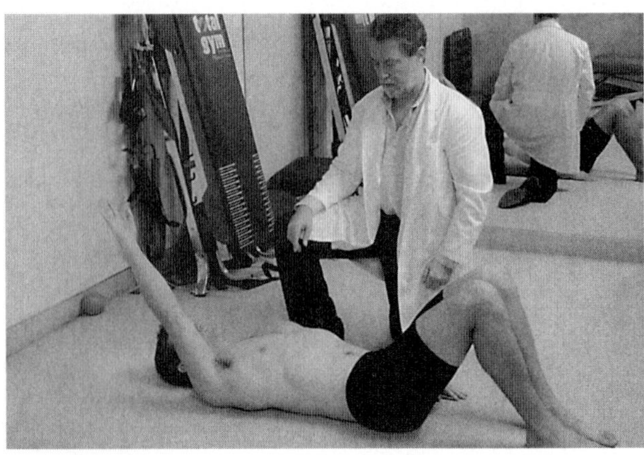

FIGURE 28–25. Supine single arm raise.

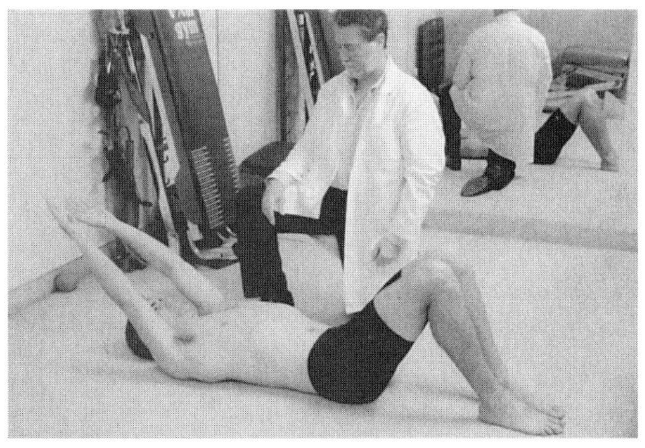

FIGURE 28–26. Supine double arm raise.

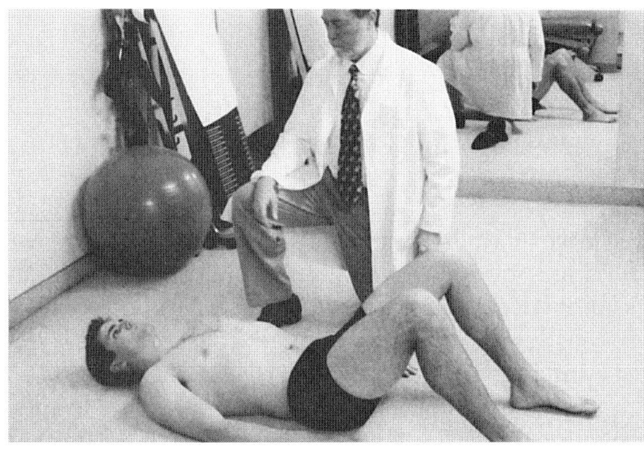

FIGURE 28–27. The hook-lying position.

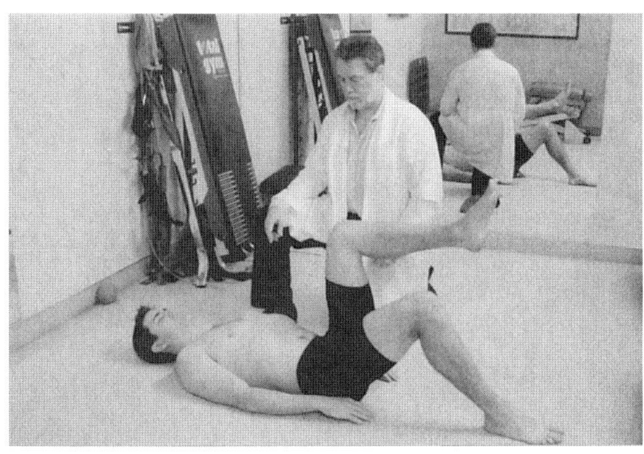

FIGURE 28–28. Supine single leg raise.

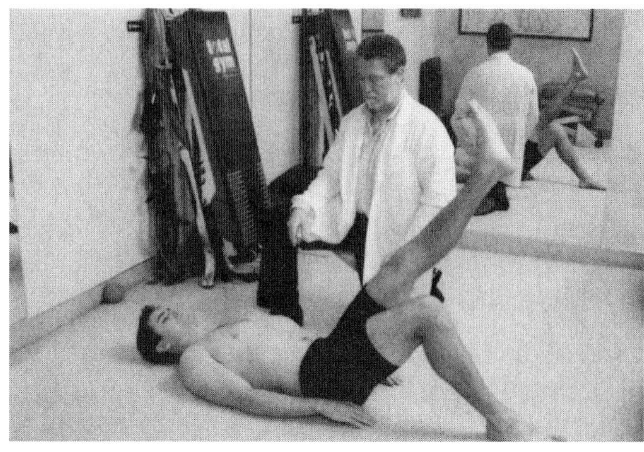

FIGURE 28–29. Supine single leg extension.

Exercise 5. Single Arm and Leg Raise The patient is in the hook-lying position with the arms held straight up so that the fingers are pointing toward the ceiling (Fig. 28–24). The patient establishes the abdominal brace. He or she is then instructed to raise one arm while also raising the opposite leg (Fig. 28–30). This engages the cerebral cortex in the complex activity of opposite-side extremity movement in the attempt to allow the co-contraction of the stabilizing muscles to become more subconscious. This is repeated with the other arm and leg. It is essential that the abdominal brace and neutral spine posture be maintained throughout the exercise.

Exercise 6. Supine Alternating Leg Movements The patient lies supine with both hips and knees flexed to 90 degrees so that the feet are off the floor (Fig. 28–31). The patient establishes the abdominal brace, and is then instructed to slowly extend one leg straight out and then return the leg to the starting point. This is repeated with the other leg. It is essential that the abdominal brace and neutral spine posture be maintained throughout the exercise. If the patient has difficulty maintaining the abdominal brace and neutral

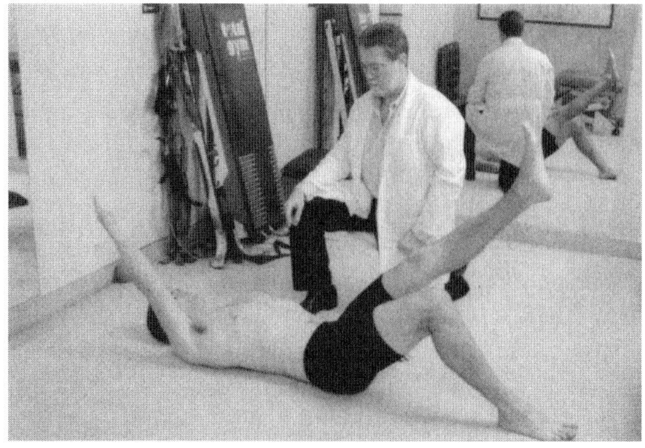

FIGURE 28–30. Supine single arm and leg raise.

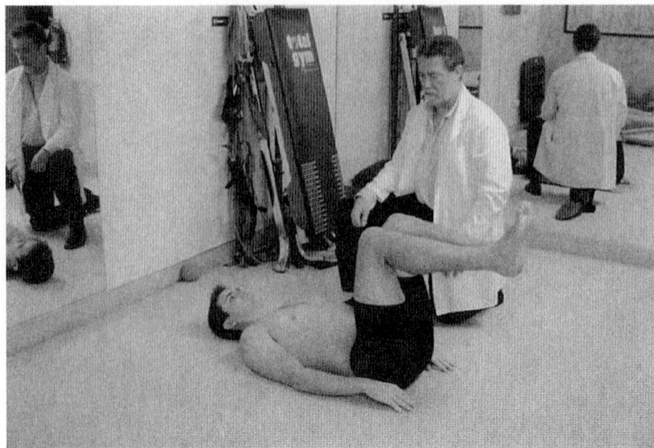

FIGURE 28–31. Position in preparation for supine alternating leg movements.

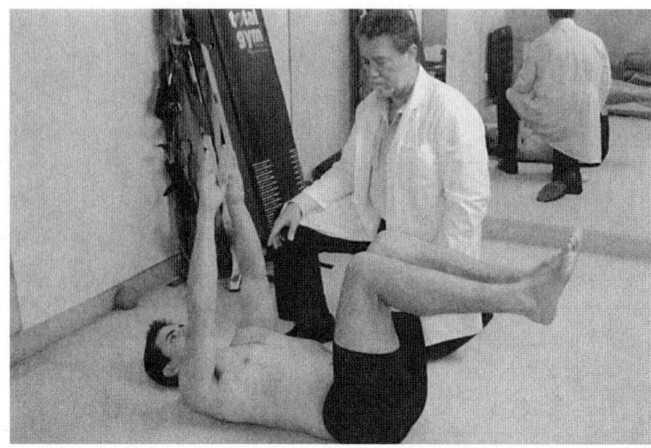

FIGURE 28–33. Position in preparation for the dead (aka dying) bug.

spine posture during the exercise, a "peel-back" strategy could be implemented in which the patient moves the leg outward and upward (Fig. 28–32). The higher the patient elevates the leg, the easier is the exercise becomes, as more weight is transferred down the shaft of the leg to the pelvis. As the patient gains motor control, the leg can be lowered during the exercise.

Exercise 7. Dead Bug The patient lies supine with both hips and knees flexed to 90 degrees so that the feet are off the floor. The arms are extended so that the fingers are pointing toward the ceiling (Fig. 28–33). The patient establishes the abdominal brace, and is then instructed to slowly extend one leg straight out while moving the opposite arm overhead (Fig. 28–34). The arm and leg return to the starting point and the movement is repeated with the other arm and leg. It is essential that the abdominal brace and neutral spine posture be maintained throughout the exercise.

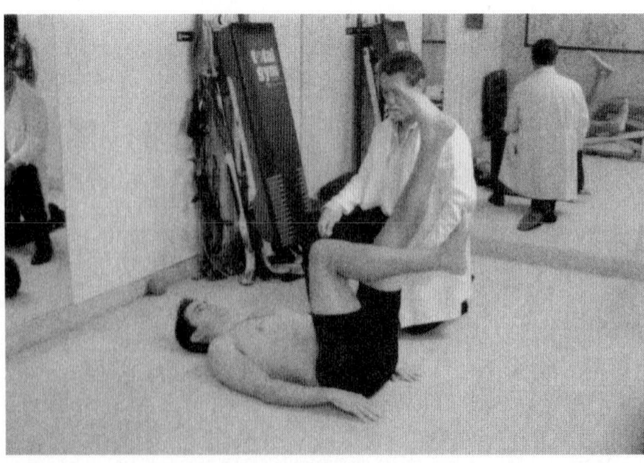

FIGURE 28–32. Supine "peel-back" alternating leg movements.

Note: There are variations of both the name and approaches for the "dead bug" maneuver. The second author prefers to call this exercise the "dying bug," because dead bugs do not move of their own volition! Some clinicians prefer to have the patient elevate both ipsilateral extremities simultaneously instead of contralateral limbs because this more closely recreates the cross-crawl mechanism, a key transitional movement of the developing locomotor system. In addition, the ipsilateral loading creates additional torsion to the stabilizing abdominal brace, increasing the challenge. It is recommended to follow the initial description of this exercise as described above, which is probably the most universally accepted approach. The cross-crawl motion may be used as a practical peel-back strategy for difficult cases. However, as there is no final authority on these exercises, it is up to the clinician to dynamically determine the corrective exercise(s) to fit the selective lumbopelvic dysfunction. Once expertise in this area is accomplished, the variety of and rationale for the various exercises is limited only by the imagination of the clinician.

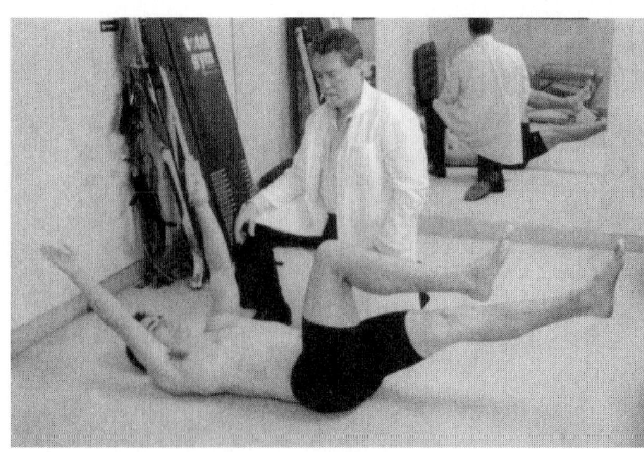

FIGURE 28–34. The dead (aka dying) bug.

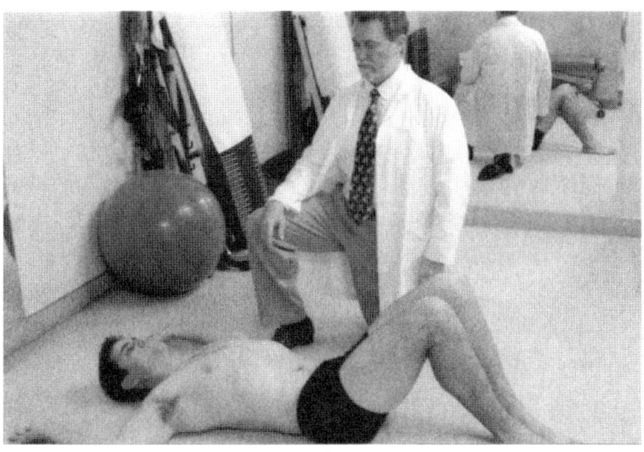

FIGURE 28–35. Position in preparation for supine pelvic rotation with the feet on the floor.

Exercise 8. Supine Pelvic Rotation with the Feet on the Floor The patient is in the hook-lying position and establishes the abdominal brace (Fig. 28–27). The arms are abducted and externally rotated, with the fingers splayed (Fig. 28–35). The patient is instructed to slowly rotate the legs to the left so that the knees move to approximately halfway to the floor (Fig. 28–36). The legs return to neutral and the movement is repeated to the right. It is essential that the abdominal brace and neutral spine posture be maintained throughout the exercise.

Clinical Pearl: There are variations of both the name and approaches for the dead bug maneuver. It is recommended to follow the initial description of this exercise as described above, which is probably the most universally accepted approach.

Exercise 9. Supine Pelvic Rotation with the Feet Off the Floor The patient lies supine with both hips and knees flexed to 90 degrees so that the feet are off the floor (Fig. 28–37). The arms are abducted and externally rotated,

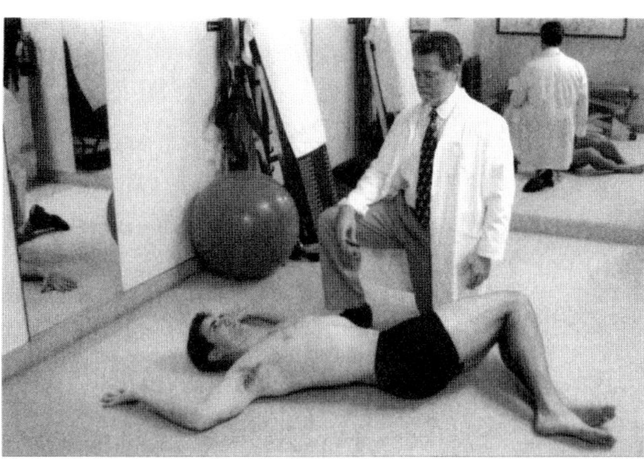

FIGURE 28–36. Supine pelvic rotation with the feet on the floor.

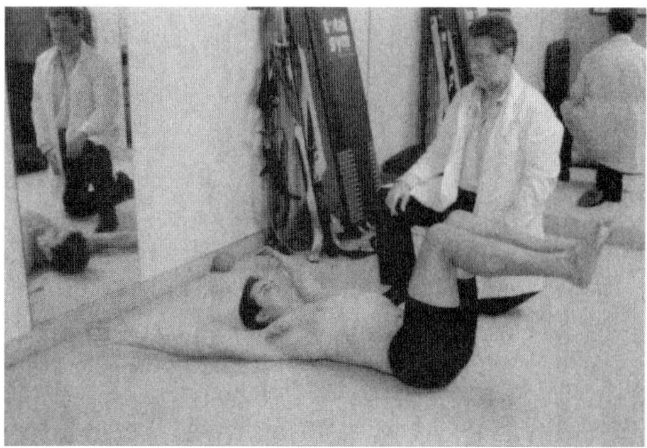

FIGURE 28–37. Position in preparation for supine pelvic rotation with feet off the floor.

with the fingers splayed. The patient is instructed to slowly rotate the legs to the left 45 degrees so they move half way to the floor (Fig. 28–38). The legs return to the neutral position and the movement is repeated to the right. It is essential that the abdominal brace and neutral spine posture be maintained throughout the exercise.

This exercise can be made more difficult by having the patient straighten the knees before performing the movement.

Exercise 10. Curl Ups The patient is in the hook-lying position, except that one leg is extended on the floor. The arms are crossed over the chest (Fig. 28–39). The patient establishes the abdominal brace, and is then instructed to slowly raise the head and shoulders off the floor without flexing at the hips (Fig. 28–40). The patient returns to neutral and repeats. It is essential that the abdominal brace be maintained throughout the exercise.

If the patient has back pain with this exercise, a "peel-back" exercise can be implemented in which the

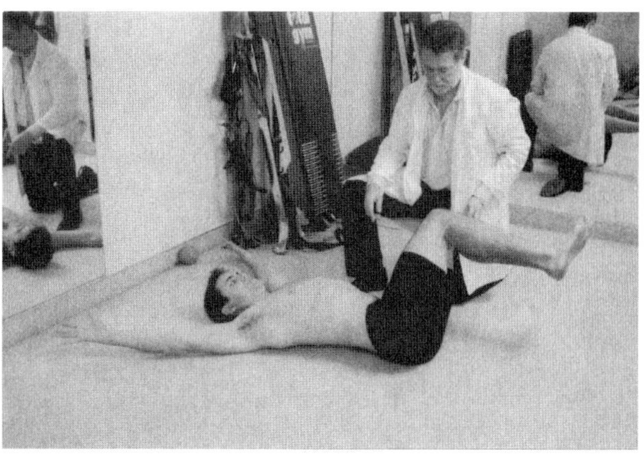

FIGURE 28–38. Supine pelvic rotation with feet off the floor.

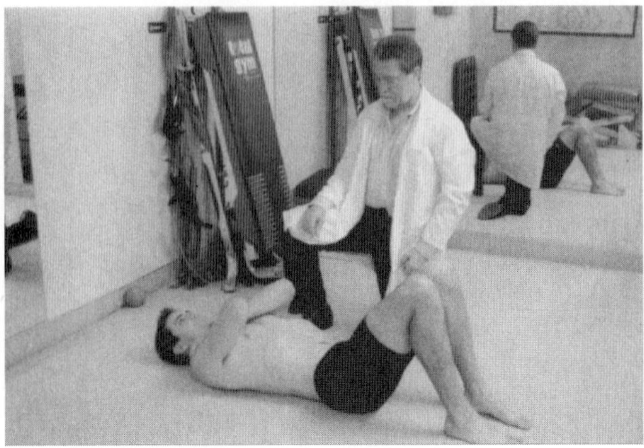

FIGURE 28–39. Position in preparation for curl up.

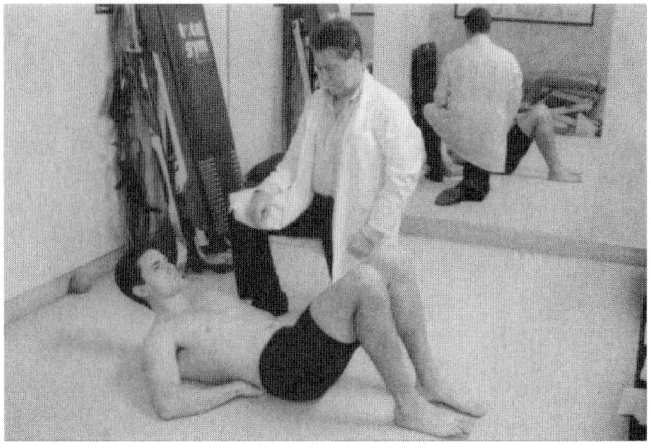

FIGURE 28–41. Curl up with helds under the lumbar spine for support.

patient places the hands under the lumbar spine for support (Fig. 28–41). Conversely, an advanced level of exercise can be implemented in which the patient clasps the hands behind the head (Fig. 28–42). It is important, however, that a neutral posture of the cervical spine be maintained, and that the patient avoids pulling the cervical spine into flexion with the clasped hands or "poking" the chin toward the ceiling.

Exercise 10. Side Bridge Made popular by McGill, the purpose of the side bridge is to target, in addition to other key trunk muscles, the quadratus lumborum.[22] It has been shown to create minimal amounts of intradiscal loading, making it a relatively safe entry-level exercise. The patient is instructed to lie on the side, propped up on one elbow, and with the knees bent to 90 degrees (Fig. 28–43). The up-side hand is placed on the downside shoulder for support. The patient establishes the abdominal brace. The patient is then instructed to raise the pelvis upward to a bridge position (Fig. 28–44), and then lower to the floor. It is essential that the abdominal brace and neutral spine posture be maintained throughout the exercise. It is also important to elevate only the pelvis to the point that the torso is straight rather, as further elevation dramatically increases the biomechanical loading and the risk. This is repeated on the other side.

If the patient cannot perform this exercise, a "peel-back" level can be utilized by having the patient place the up-side hand on the floor to assist in raising the pelvis (Fig. 28–45). The patient should be instructed to use this hand as little as possible. Another option is to place a pillow under the patient's pelvis, reducing the initial load at lift-off, as the pelvis is already partially elevated, and reducing the distance to the elevated position.

A more advanced level of this exercise is to have the patient perform it with the knees extended, which provides a longer lever (Fig. 28–46). Further advancement can be made by having the patient roll from one elbow over to the other without losing the abdominal brace and neutral spine position, the so-called "victory roll" because of the level of skill it requires (Fig. 28–47*A* and 28–47*B*).

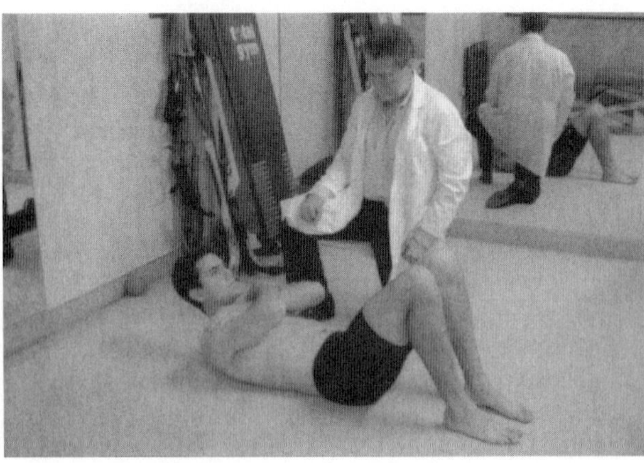

FIGURE 28–40. Curl up.

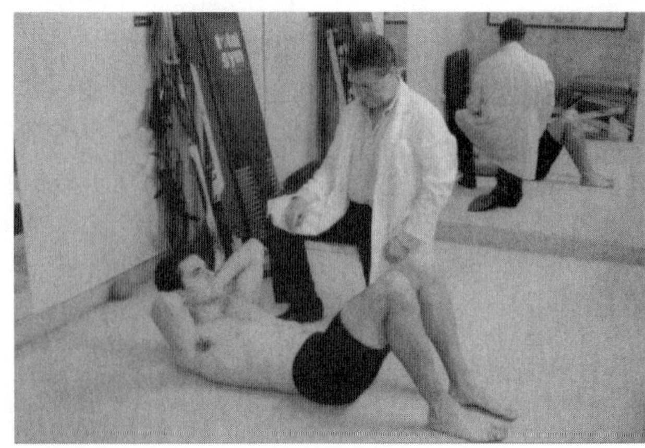

FIGURE 28–42. Curl up with hands folded behind head.

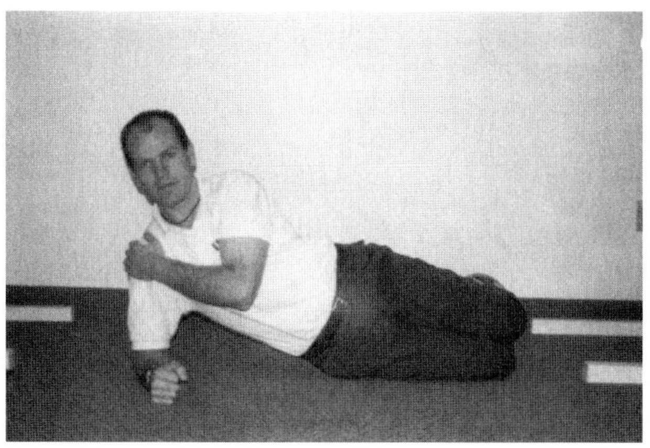

FIGURE 28–43. Position in preparation for the side bridge.

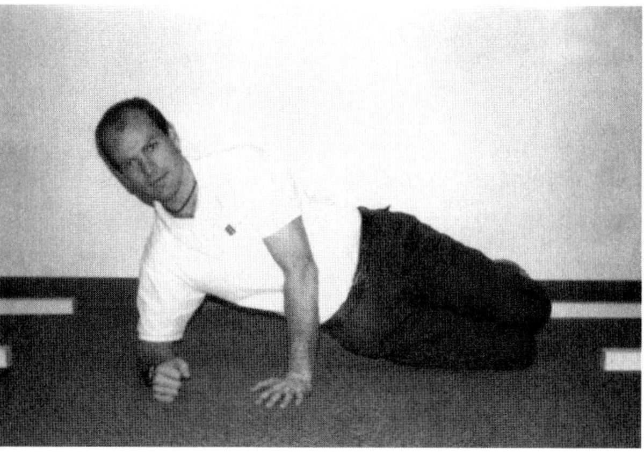

FIGURE 28–45. Peel-back level for the side bridge with the hand on the floor.

Bridge Track

This track is designed to place focus on the gluteus maximus in training, but it has also been shown to activate the MULT.[23] In addition, the patient is required to maintain a neutral spine by isometrically contracting the rectus abdominis and erector spinae, concentrically contracting the gluteus maximus, which would theoretically eccentrically contract the hip flexors. When discussed in this contex, the increasing neurophysiological complexity of the bridge track strategy becomes clear.

Exercise 1. Bridge The patient is in the hook-lying position and is instructed to establish and maintain the abdominal brace and neutral pelvis (Fig. 28–27). If the patient has problems with hamstring cramping, or if the clinician wants to facilitate gluteus maximus activation during the bridge, he or she can bring the feet closer to the buttocks, inhibiting the hamstring activity. The patient is instructed to slowly raise the pelvis off the floor as high as possible while continuing to maintain the neutral pelvis (Fig. 28–48). This is at times quite difficult for the patient with poor lumbopelvic control, and they often unknowingly lose the neutral pelvis by establishing an anterior pelvic tilt (with lumbar extension) or, less frequently, a posterior tilt (with lumbar flexion). If the patient loses the neutral pelvis, then the bridge is interupted and the patient begins again. It is essential that the abdominal brace and neutral spine posture be maintained throughout the exercise. If the patient can control the neutral pelvis only to the halfway level of elevation, for example, then they can take this exercise home with the instruction that they perform it only in this functional range.

Exercise 2. Bridge with a Strap The purpose of this exercise is to place particular emphasis on the gluteus medius and minimus. The patient is again in the hook-lying position, but with a strap or belt around the distal thighs (Fig. 28–49). The patient is instructed to establish the abdominal brace and then to slowly raise the pelvis off the floor as high as possible without

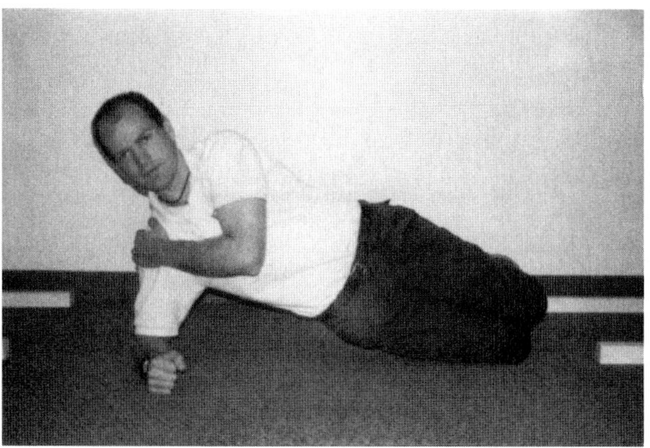

FIGURE 28–44. Side bridge.

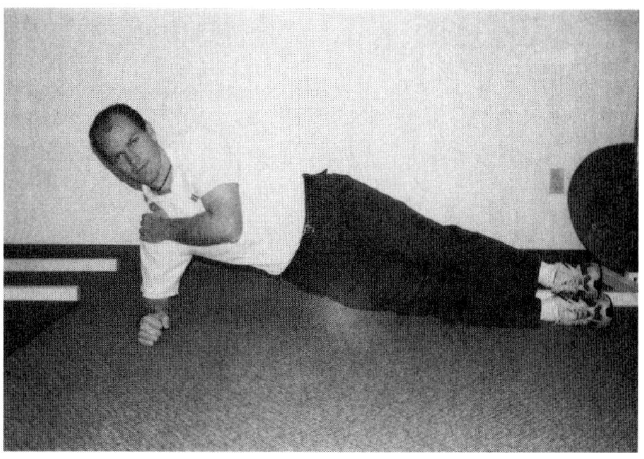

FIGURE 28–46. Advanced level of the side bridge.

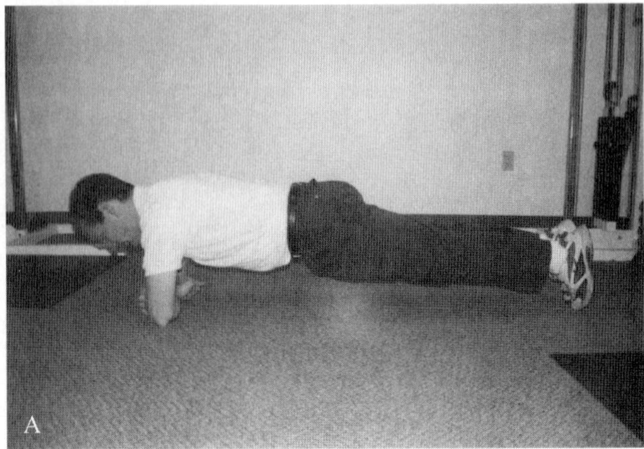

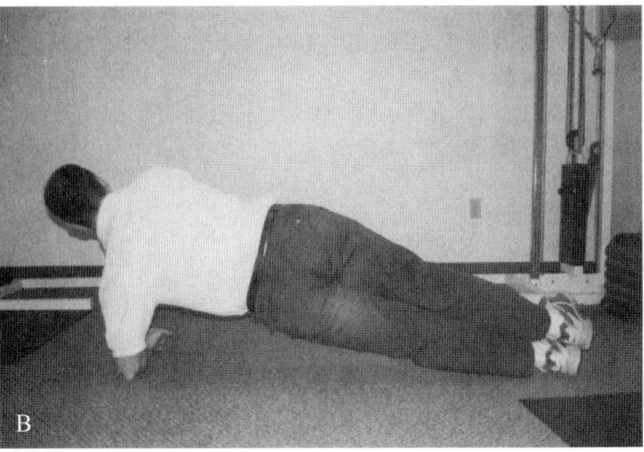

FIGURE 28–47. A and B. Body rotation from one side bridge to the other.

losing the neutral pelvis, which typically occurs by extending the lumbar spine (Fig. 28–50). The patient returns to neutral and repeats. It is essential that the abdominal brace and neutral spine posture be maintained throughout the exercise.

Exercise 3. Bridge with Heel Raises The patient is in the hook-lying position and is instructed to establish the abdominal brace (Fig. 28–27). The challenge is increased as the patient maintains the neutral pelvis, simultaniously coordinating ankle flexion and increased balance challenges presented by motion and the smaller pedal base. The patient is instructed to bring the heels close to the buttocks, slowly raise the pelvis off the floor as high as possible without flexing or extending the lumbar spine (Fig. 28–48). From this position, the patient is instructed to slowly raise one heel, then return it to the floor, followed by the same movement with the other heel (Fig. 28–51). This is repeated. It is essential that the abdominal brace and neutral spine posture be maintained throughout the exercise.

Exercise 4. Bridge with Steps The patient is in the hook-lying position and is instructed to establish the abdominal brace (Fig. 28–27). It further challenges the patient by challenging the lateral hip stabilizers (gluteus medius and mimimus) and also balance as he or she assumes a three-point stance. The patient is instructed to bring the heels close to the buttocks, slowly raise the pelvis off the floor as high as possible without flexing or extending the lumbar spine (Fig. 28–48). From this position, the patient is instructed to raise one foot off the floor (Fig. 28–52), then return it to the floor, followed by the same movement with the other foot. It is important to understand that the lateral hip stabilizers being activated are on the same side (ipsilateral) as the stabilizing leg, but that failure to adequately stabilize will be reflected as the contralateral hip drops. For example, a patient who elevates the left foot in this maneuver will activate the right hip lateral stabilizers and failure to do so is detected as the left hip drops.

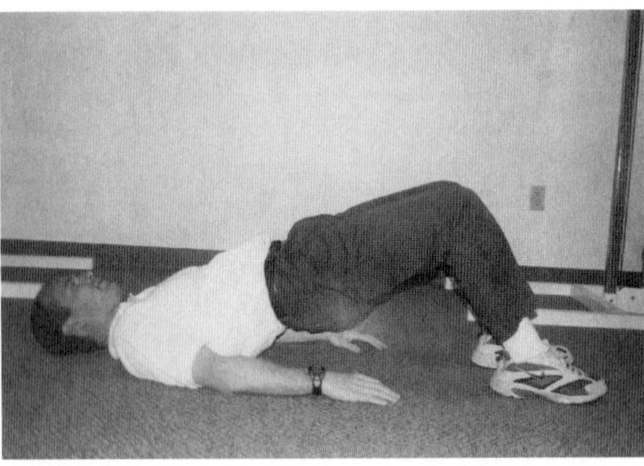

FIGURE 28–48. The bridge.

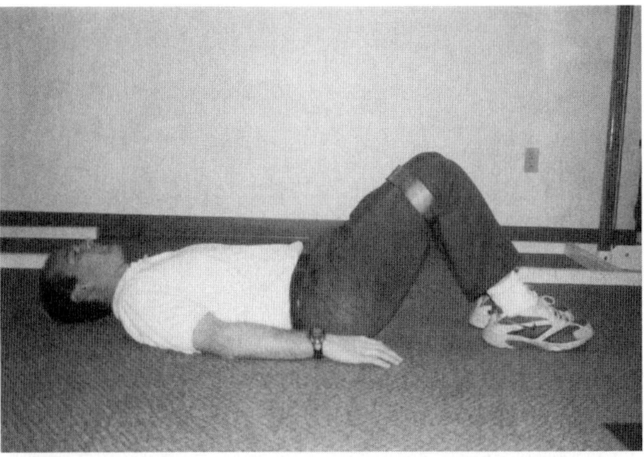

FIGURE 28–49. Position in preparation for the bridge with strap.

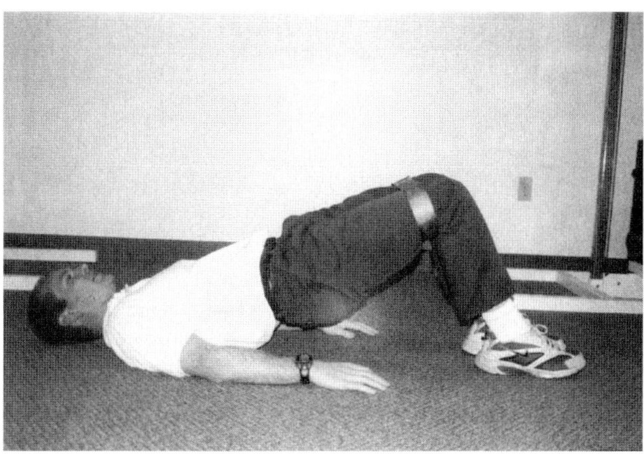

FIGURE 28–50. Bridge with strap.

Clinical Pearl: Made popular by McGill, the purpose of the side bridge is to target, in addition to other key trunk muscles, the quadratus lumborum.

Exposing an inhibited lateral hip stabilizer is common in patients with poor lumbopelvic stability. When found a peel-back, or remedial, exercise is necessary to allow the patient to "catch up," with specific gluteus medius/minimus exercises. Another strategy is to simply have the patient bring the knees and feet together, reducing the lateral loading to either hip. If the pelvis remains level, then this is repeated to improve lateral pelvic stability and the feet can gradually be placed wider apart as stability improves.

Once the patient is able to perform typical bridge with steps it is repeated. It is essential that the abdominal brace and neutral spine posture be maintained throughout the exercise.

Exercise 5. Bridge with Leg Extension The patient is in the hook-lying position and is instructed to establish the abdominal brace (Fig. 28–27). The patient is instructed to slowly raise the pelvis off the floor as high as possible without flexing or extending the lumbar spine (Fig. 28–48). From this position, the patient is instructed to extend one leg straight out (Fig. 28–53), then return it to the floor, followed by the same movement with the other leg. This strategy provides a longer lever, challenging the neutral pelvis and lateral hip stabilizers with the increased load. Once the patient demonstrates he or she can perform this procedure well, it is repeated to gain expertise. It is essential that the abdominal brace and neutral spine posture be maintained throughout the exercise.

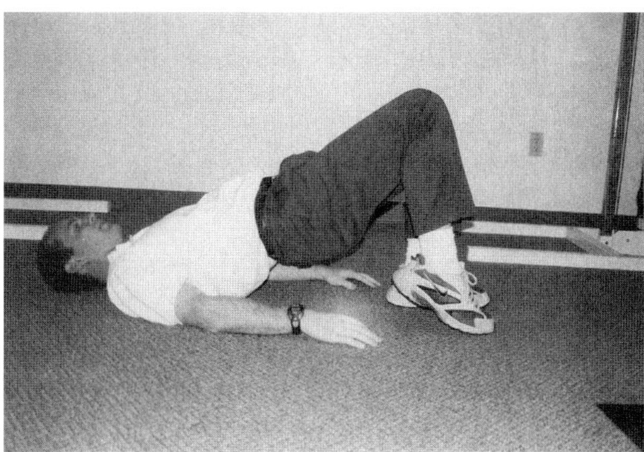

FIGURE 28–51. Bridge with heel raises.

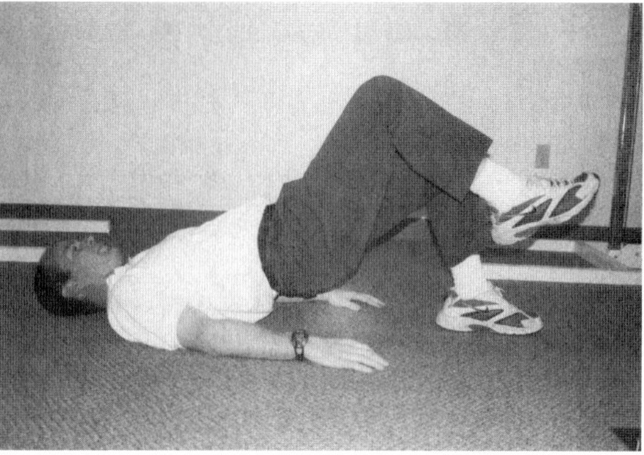

FIGURE 28–52. Bridge with steps.

Exercise 6. One Leg Bridge This is an advanced level and many patients will not require this exercise. The patient is in the hook-lying position and is instructed to establish the abdominal brace (Fig. 28–27). The patient is instructed to bring the heels close to the buttocks, slowly raise the pelvis off the floor as high as possible without flexing or extending the lumbar spine (Fig. 28–48). From this position, the patient is instructed to extend one leg straight out (Fig. 28–54*A*). The patient is then instructed to slowly lower the pelvis 1–2 in (4–5 cm) toward the floor

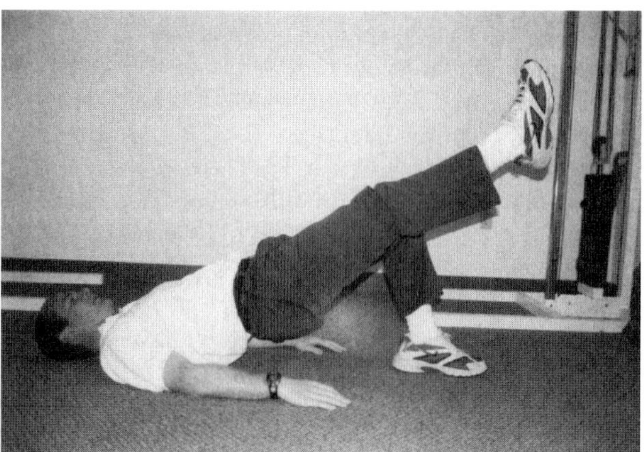

FIGURE 28–53. Bridge with leg extension.

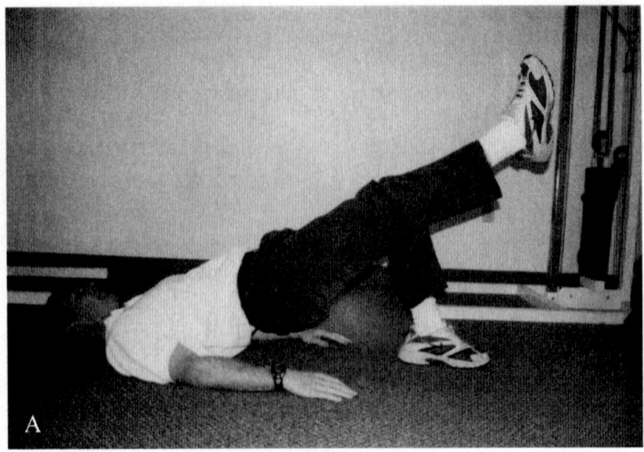

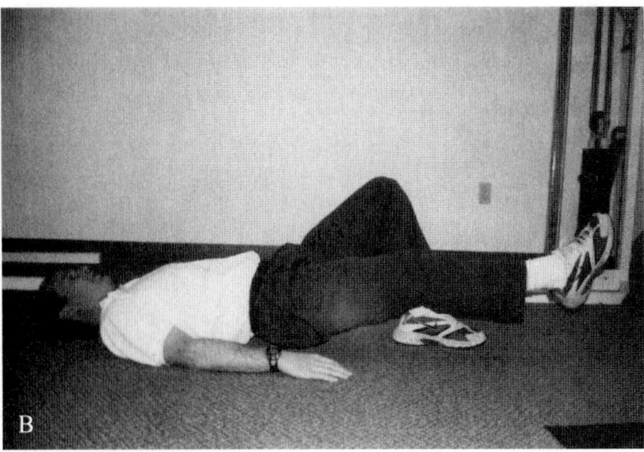

FIGURE 28–54. A and B. One leg bridge.

(Fig. 28–54*B*), then again elevate the pelvis, essentially performing a unilateral "glut squeeze," in a return to the bridge position. This is repeated. The same exercise is then performed with the other leg. It is essential that the abdominal brace and neutral spine posture be maintained throughout the exercise.

Quadruped Track

The quadruped track is designed to place particular focus on the multifidis in a low-load environment.[24] It provides a new opportunity for the patient to establish and maintain a neutral pelvis with a host of various loading and balancing strategies. In addition, the lumbopelvic region is away from the floor, reducing stabilizing torso weight bearing, exteroception and mechanoreception as the patient advances toward more elevated postural strategies. Finally, the load bearing is now placed on the extremities, requiring increased proximal stability and balancing challenges.

Exercise 1. Quadruped Cat-Cow This is an entry-level maneuver designed to demonstrate to the patient that they can perform an anterior and posterior tilt in positions beyond supine. It also can act as a maneuver to counteract fear avoidance behavior as the patient gains confidence in restoring movement following, for example, a painful back episode. The patient is instructed to position him or herself on hands and knees, also known as the quadruped position. (Or else, may bear weight on the fists in case of painful wrists and a soft surface such as padding in case of painful knees.) The patient's head is positioned in a neutral position, and he or she is instructed to look in a fixed manner stright down at the floor.

The patient is then instructed to sway the back, lowering the umbilicus toward the floor in a maneuver similar to a "sway-backed" cow. This essentially increased the spinal lordosis and creates an anterior pelvic tilt. The patient is taught that this is the same front pelvic tilt previously mastered while lying on the back. The patient is then told to raise or elevate the back toward the ceiling, in a manner similar to a hissing cat. Such analogies help to allow the patient to relate to and better remember the maneuver during this critical time in the stabilization process.

The patient is then taught to incorporate diaphragmatic respiration with the cat-cow exercise: inhaling during the "cow" and exhaling during the "cat". Once this is mastered, the patient is instructed to establish a neutral spine and abdominal brace, setting the stage for the rest of the quadruped track.

Exercise 2. Quadruped Single Arm Raise The patient is in the quadruped position (Fig. 28–55) and is instructed to establish the abdominal brace and neutral spine. The patient is then instructed to slowly raise one arm overhead (Fig. 28–56), then lower it back to the floor. This is repeated with the other arm. It is essential that the abdominal brace and neutral spine posture be maintained throughout the exercise.

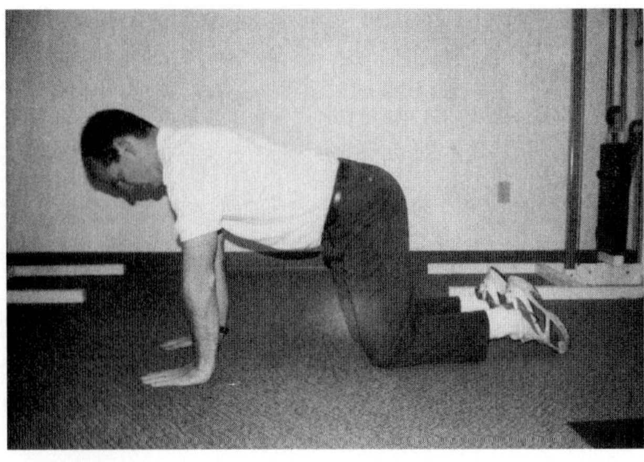

FIGURE 28–55. The quadruped position.

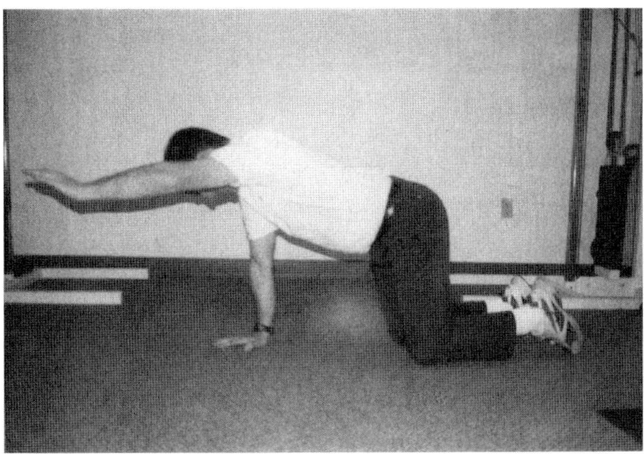

FIGURE 28–56. Quadruped single arm raise.

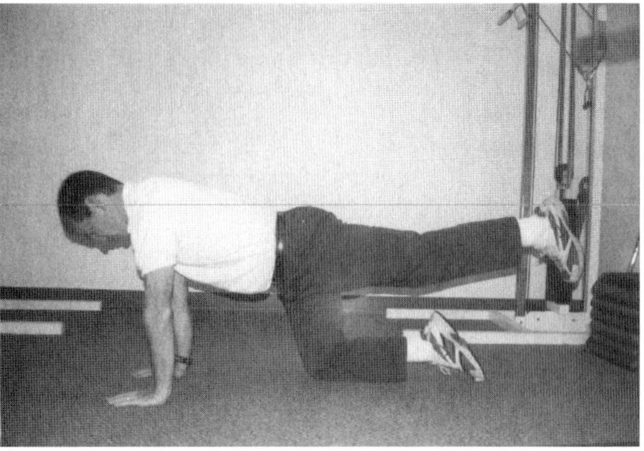

FIGURE 28–58. Quadruped single leg raise.

Exercise 3. Quadruped Single Leg Drag The patient is in the quadruped position (Fig. 28–55) and is instructed to establish the abdominal brace and neutral spine. The patient is then instructed to slowly move one leg straight out behind without raising the foot from the floor (Fig. 28–57), then move the leg back to the starting point. This is repeated with the other leg. It is essential that the abdominal brace and neutral spine posture be maintained throughout the exercise.

Exercise 4. Quadruped Single Leg Raise The patient is in the quadruped position (Fig. 28–55) and is instructed to establish the abdominal brace and neutral spine. The patient is then instructed to slowly raise one leg straight out behind with a minimum of movement of the pelvis or shift of weight to the weight-bearing leg (Fig. 28–58), then lower it back to the floor. This is then repeated with the other leg. It is essential that the abdominal brace and neutral spine posture be maintained throughout the exercise.

Exercise 5. Quadruped Cross-Crawl The patient is in the quadruped position (Fig. 28–55) and is instructed to establish the abdominal brace and neutral spine. The patient is then instructed to slowly raise one arm overhead while at the same time raising the opposite leg straight out behind with a minimum of movement of the pelvis or shift of weight to the weight-bearing leg (Fig. 28–59). The patient then lowers the arm and leg back to the floor. This is repeated with the other arm and leg. It is essential that the abdominal brace and neutral spine posture be maintained throughout the exercise.

Prone Track

The prone track is designed to place particular emphasis on the multifidis and erector spinae muscles. It creates a greater activation of the multifidi than does the quadruped track, but also places the spine under greater loads,[24] so it should be reserved for later in the stabilization program and, generally, the patient should have mastered the quadruped track before moving on to the prone track. Also, as with all the exercises provided here, this track should only be given if the patient can perform the exercises without pain.

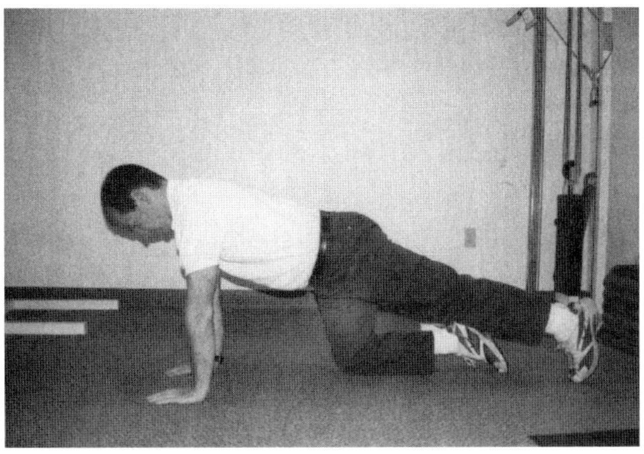

FIGURE 28–57. Quadruped single leg drag.

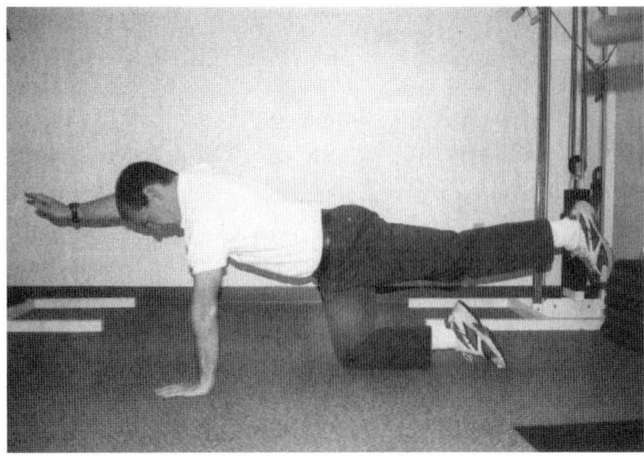

FIGURE 28–59. Quadruped cross-crawl.

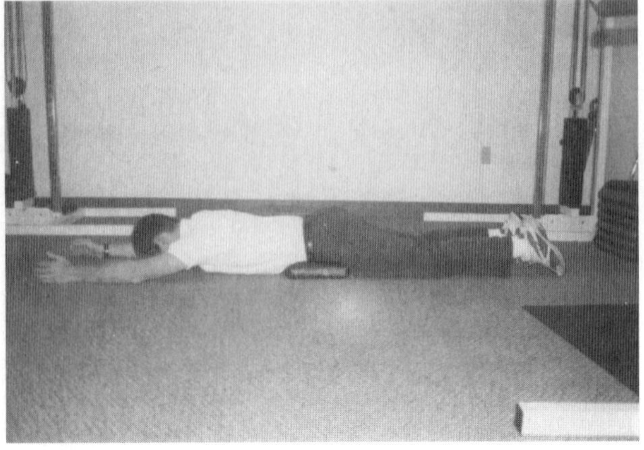

FIGURE 28–60. The prone position with pillow under the abdomen.

Exercise 1. Prone Single Arm Raise The patient is in the prone position with a small pillow under the pelvis and is instructed to establish the abdominal brace (Fig. 28–60). The patient is then instructed to raise one arm off the floor (Fig. 28–61) and then lower it back to the floor. This is repeated with the other arm. It is essential that the abdominal brace and neutral spine posture be maintained throughout the exercise.

Exercise 2. Prone Single Leg Raise The patient is in the prone position with a small pillow under the pelvis and is instructed to establish the abdominal brace (Fig. 28–60). The patient is then instructed to raise one leg off the floor (Fig. 28–62), and then lower it back to the floor. This is repeated with the other leg. It is essential that the abdominal brace and neutral spine posture be maintained throughout the exercise. The lumbar spine must be watched carefully for deviation (i.e., pivoting at the lumbosacral junction or "false hip extension") during the maneuver. If deviation occurs in spite of the maintenance of the abdominal brace, the patient is not yet ready for this exercise.

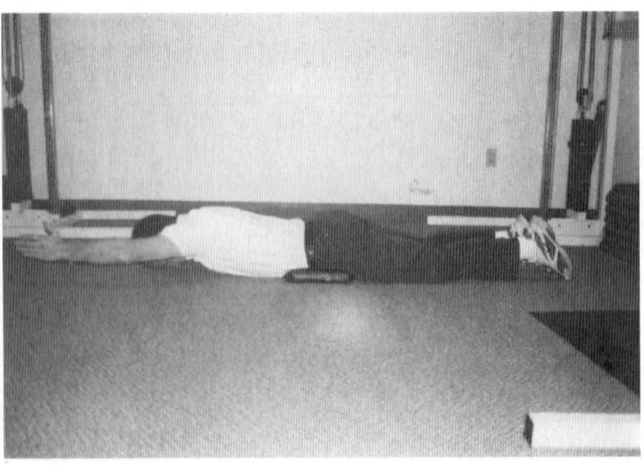

FIGURE 28–61. Prone single arm raise.

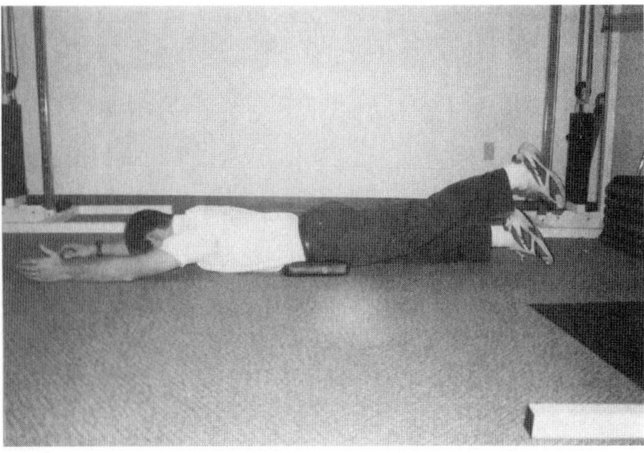

FIGURE 28–62. Prone single leg raise.

Exercise 3. Prone Single Arm and Leg Raise The patient is in the prone position with a small pillow under the pelvis and is instructed to establish the abdominal brace (Fig. 28–60). The patient is then instructed to raise one arm off the floor at the same time as raising the opposite leg off the floor (Fig. 28–63), Followed by lowering these extremities back to the floor. This is repeated with the other arm and leg. It is essential that the abdominal brace and neutral spine posture be maintained throughout the exercise. The lumbar spine must be watched carefully for deviation during the maneuver. If deviation occurs in spite of the maintenance of the abdominal brace, the patient is not yet ready for this exercise.

Kneel Ups

Kneel up exercises provide a transition strategy between floor exercises and standing, while continuing to emphasize the basic tenets of dynamic lumbopelvic stabilization, the neutral spine, and abdominal bracing. While resting on the heels in an upright position and hands placed on the hips, the patient establishes a neutral pelvis and abdominal brace. The patient is

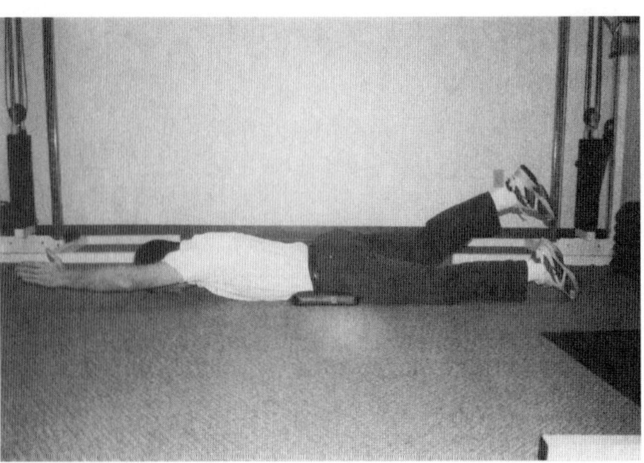

FIGURE 28–63. Prone opposite arm and leg raise.

then instructed to slowly elevate him or herself to an upright kneeling position (with the knees now positioned at 90 degrees). The patient is then instructed to lower back down to the heels while being careful to maintain their neutral spine and abdominal brace. This exercise places a great deal of load on the quadraceps musculature and also on the knees, so prescreening the patient to ensure the safety of the exercise is crucial. The clinician must ensure that the patient does not lean forward as he or she raises, being certain that a neutral pelvis and erect posture is maintained. As the patient lowers, there should be resting between repetitions. The patient should therefore again elevate up to the upright kneeling posture as soon as their buttocks touches their heels.

Standing Exercise

Good Morning Exercise The purpose of the good morning exercise is to train the coordinated action of the crossed "slings" (i.e., a continuum of muscles that establish a functional or kinetic chain) that consist of the latissimus dorsi, erector spinae, multifidis, gluteus maximus, and hamstrings and the transference of force between the upper and lower body through the thoracolumbar fascia.[25] The patient is standing and is instructed to establish the abdominal brace and the neutral spine (Fig. 28–64). The patient is instructed to bend forward by flexing at the hips, *not* at the lumbar spine. This flexion should be carried out as far as possible without flexing the lumbar spine (Fig. 28–65). The movement is stopped at the point at which the lumbar spine begins to flex. The patient returns to the upright position. It is essential that the abdominal brace and neutral spine posture be maintained throughout the exercise.

Clinical Pearl: The purpose of the good morning exercise is to train the coordinated action of the crossed "slings" (i.e., a continuum of muscles that establish a functional or kinetic chain) that consist of the latissimus dorsi, erector spinae, multifidis, gluteus maximus, and hamstrings and the transfer of force between the upper and lower body through the thoracolumbar fascia.

Further training can be elicited by having the patient hold dumbbells during the movement.

Advanced Level of Good Morning Exercise The next step from the good morning exercise in training the latissimus-erector spinae-multifidi-gluteus maximus-hamstring slings can be made employing a Roman chair or similar device. The patient lies prone on a platform that it tilted approximately 45 degrees. The platform should be positioned such that the superior-most portion on the patient's body is placed at the hip joint, that is, the pelvis should be unsupported so that the patient can flex at the hip. The arms should hang straight down toward the floor.

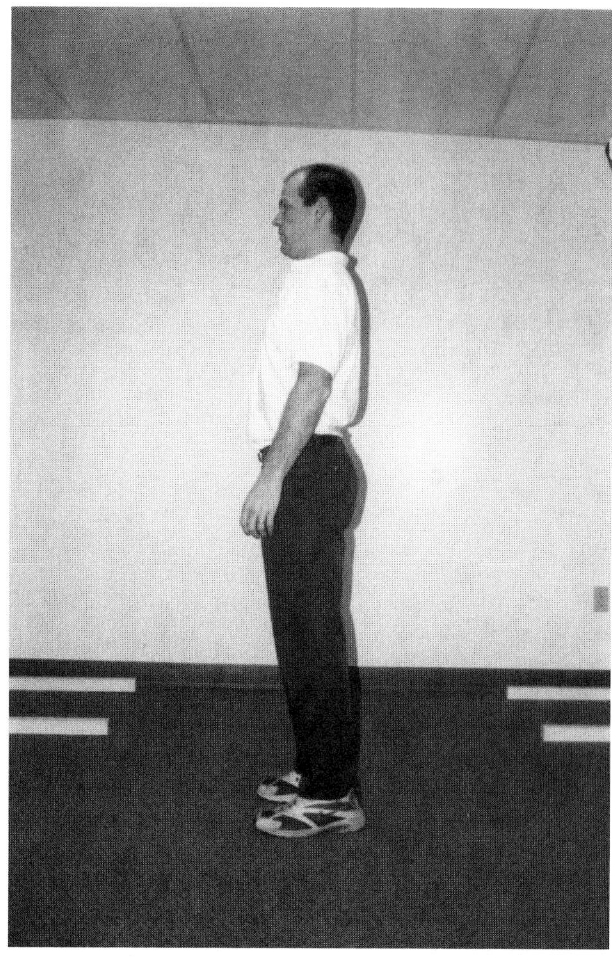

FIGURE 28–64. Starting position for the good morning exercise.

While maintaining a neutral spine, the patient flexes at the hips, moving toward the floor as low as possible without flexing the lumbar spine (Fig. 28–66*A* and 28–66*B*). It is essential that the movement occurs only at the hip, rather than at the lumbar spine, and that the lumbar spine remains neutral. The patient then rises back to the starting point. Load, and greater activation of the latissimus dorsi, can be added by having the patient perform the exercise by holding dumbbells.

Lunge Exercises

The purpose of the lunge is to train the patient to maintain a neutral spine while taking a step, challenging one's balance and stressing the lower extremities, which is another logical remedial exercise in preparation of more stable bipedal ambulation. While standing with an upright posture, the patient establishes an abdominal brace and neutral pelvis (Fig. 28–67).

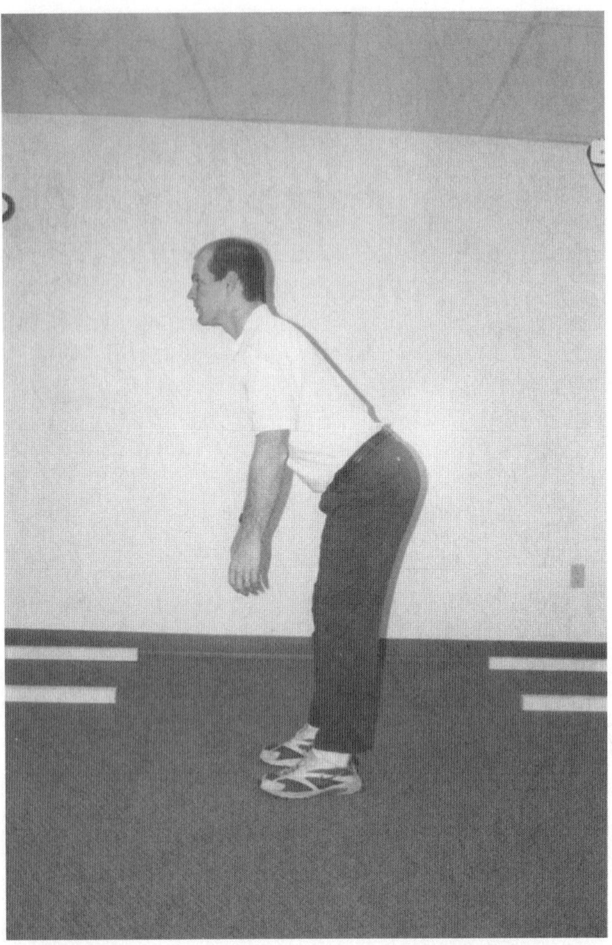

FIGURE 28–65. The good morning exercise. Note that the flexion movement is occurring at the hips rather than at the lumbar spine.

The patient is instructed to take a step forward and lower him or herself so that the knee of their trailing leg lowers to touch, but not bear weight on, the floor (Fig. 28–68). The patient is allowed to lower only to a point where stability is maintained. Therefore, any wobbling of the pelvis or torso would be considered too low to maintain stability and the patient would be restricted from lowering him or herself so far. The patient is also instructed to avoid allowing the forward knee to move in front of the forward foot, which requires the patient to maintain more weight on the trailing leg. The patient then raises to an upright position, stepping back with the forward leg to again resume an upright posture. This exercise is then repeated with the opposite leg.

Side Step Exercises

This is a very important and practical remedial standing exercise, designed to strengthen the gluteus medius and minimus. An elastic band is placed around the ankles so that the tension point of the band begins at about 12–15 in. The patient internally rotates both feet about 45 degrees, keeping the knees extended as much as possible (Fig. 28–69). The patient is instructed to brace the abdomen and establish a neutral pelvis. In this somewhat awkward position, the patient is instructed to walk sideways for about 20–30 ft before reversing direction (Fig. 28–70). This is an excellent training exercise, which can be increased with more repetitions and/or more resistive bands.

Lateral Wall Ball

This exercises the same components of stabilization training as the previous exercise. It must be remembered that isometric contraction of these muscles, when bearing weight on the ipsilateral leg, causes the pelvis to deviate to the contralateral side and also causes elevation and slight anterior movement of the contralateral pelvis. For example, bearing weight on the right leg and contracting the right gluteus medius and minimus will cause the pelvis to move to the left and slightly forward, while elevating the left hemipelvis. With this in mind, the exercise is performed with the gym ball placed between the wall and the

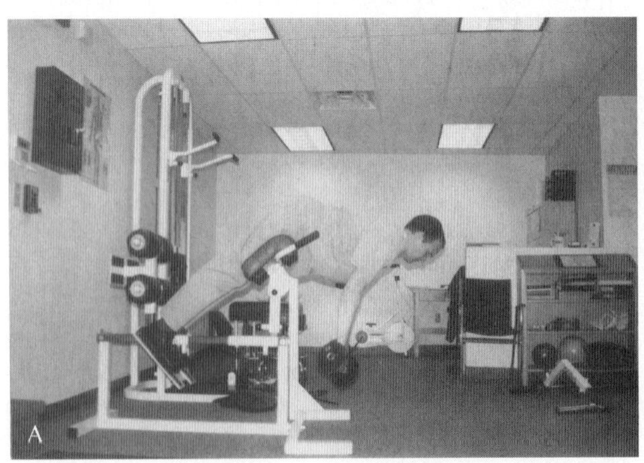

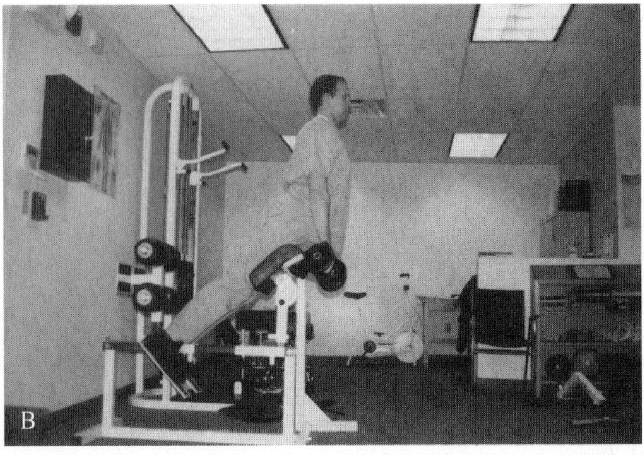

FIGURE 28–66. Advanced level of good morning exercise.

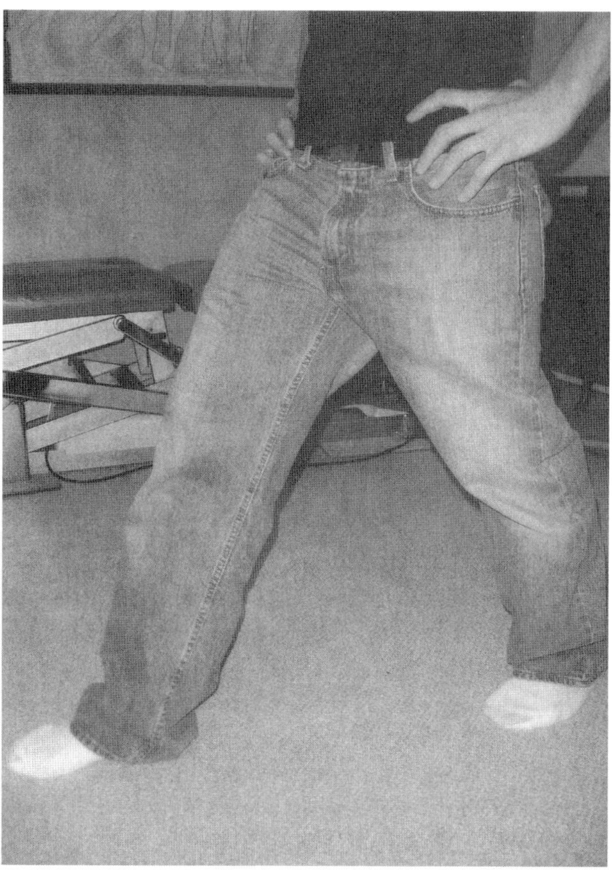

FIGURE 28–67. Starting position for lunges.

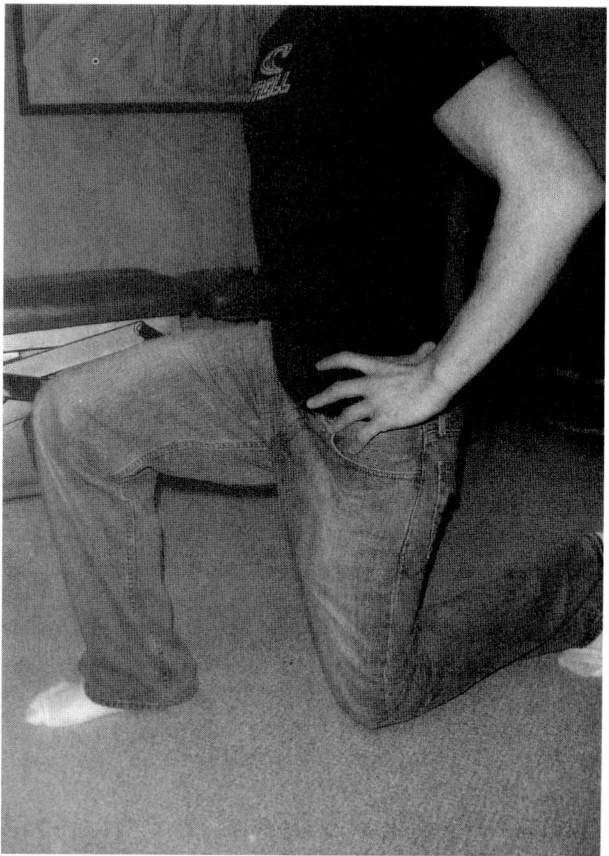

FIGURE 28–68. Lunge.

patient's left hip. Placement of the ball should be slightly anterand superior of the greater trochanter. The patient is instructed to maintain abdominal brace, establish a neutral spine, and contract the hip only in order to push their pelvis into the ball. The patient is told to push slightly forward into the ball, while also trying to slightly elevate the ball also, and then return to the neutral one-legged stance and repeat the exercise.

Roman Chair

The Roman chair is a very practical exercise tool that has grown in popularity with increasing understanding of lumbopelvic stability. While it can be utilized in a multitude of ways to isolate and exercise numerous muscles, two of the most practical approaches will be explained here. Hopefully, the explanation of these techniques will allow the clinician to undersand the fundamentals of the device in order to alter an exercise for the customized demands of the patient.

The Roman chair is essentially a device that allows the patient to establish a horizontal position above the floor, which requires the locomotor system to actively maintain a horizontal posture and simultaneously allows for movement that would be restricted while lying on the floor. The apparatus is composed of a metal base with two rising metal pillars approximately 30 in (75 cm) tall, one with a padded platform at the top for resting the pelvis and the other with a padded roll under which the feet are placed. Because there is no support available above, or rostral to, the pelvis, the upper half of the body subsequently becomes the load that the lumbopelvic stabilizing system must counteract.

Prone Roman Chair Position By instructing the patient to place the anterior pelvis on the Roman chair and tucking heels under the roll, he or she is made to establish a prone position, which challenges the erector spinae, glutus maximus, and hamstrings (see Chapter 35, Fig. 35–4). By instructing the patient to simultaneously creat abdominal hollow and focus on diaphragmatic respiration, facilitation of coordination of the intrinsic and global muscles may indeed occur. Also, the clinician may want the patient to focus on contracting the gluteus maximi, as these extensors tend toward inhibition and/or weakness.

As with other tracks, the prone Roman chair position can begin with an isometric horizontal position with the arms placed along the patient's side. The arms become important tools in altering the load of the

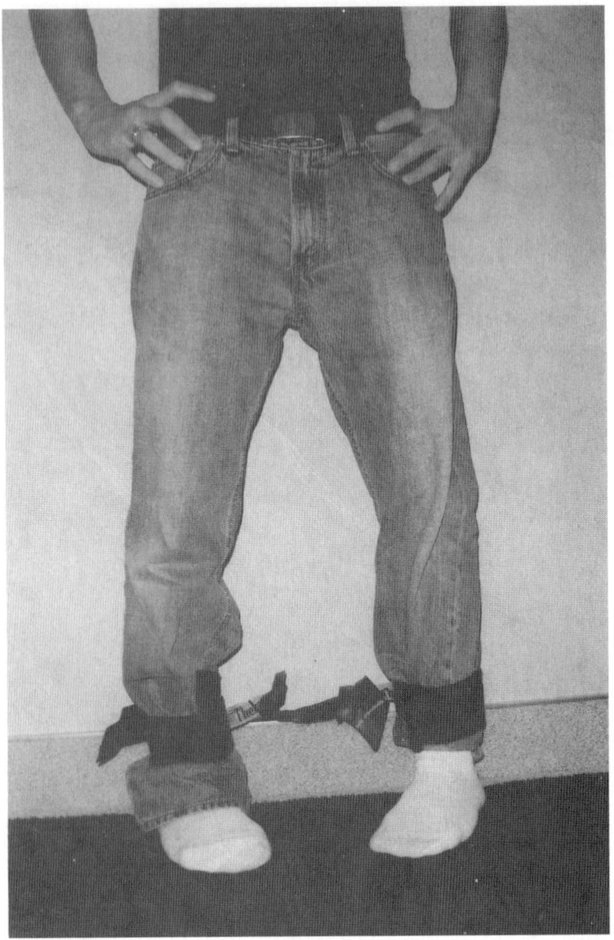

FIGURE 28–69. Start position for side step exercise.

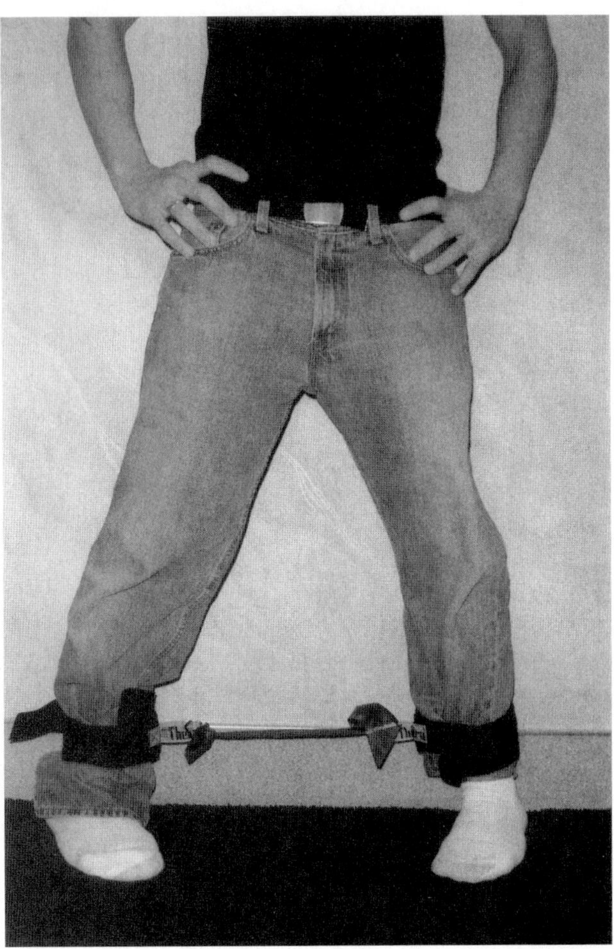

FIGURE 28–70. Side steps exercise.

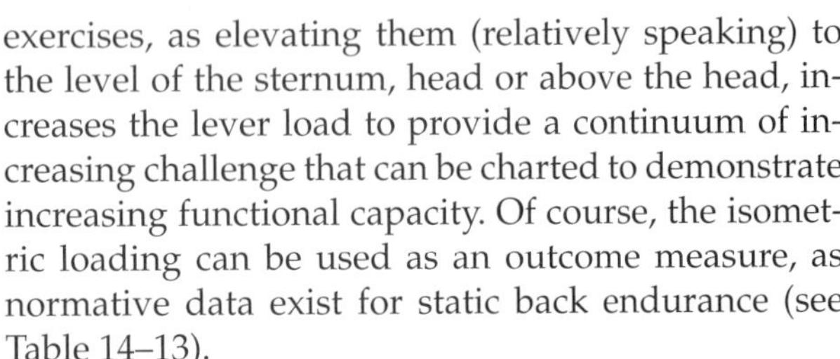

exercises, as elevating them (relatively speaking) to the level of the sternum, head or above the head, increases the lever load to provide a continuum of increasing challenge that can be charted to demonstrate increasing functional capacity. Of course, the isometric loading can be used as an outcome measure, as normative data exist for static back endurance (see Table 14–13).

In addition to maintaining an isometric, or static, horizontal position, the Roman chair allows for concentric and eccentric posterior chain loading as the prone torso is free to move toward or away from the floor. Eccentric loading occurs as the patient slowly lowers himself or herself toward the floor, while concentric loading occurs as they return to the horizontal postion. Two strategies for elevation are commonly used: either a serpentine manner (in which extension occurs first in the upper torso and then segmentally in a caudalward order with the lumbosacral junction being the final spinal joint) or a more general manner (in which the entire torso more or less moves simultaneously into extension).

It is important to prophylactically avoid hyperextension while performing the prone Roman chair extension maneuvers.

Side-Lying Roman Chair It was previously stated that the quadratus lumborum have become increasingly important target muscles as part of a complete rehabilitation program.[22] By placing the patients on their side (that is, resting their hip region on the padded pelvic support, their lateral ankle from the upper leg and medial ankle from the lower leg hooked under the foot roll) on the Roman chair, the clinician establishes an exercise continuum from the side bridges that were described earlier in this chapter (see also Chapter 30, Fig. 30–4). Of course, the quadratus lumborum is not the only musculature involved in this maneuver, but is the major muscle targeted.

Clinical Pearl: The Roman chair is essentially a device that allows patient establish a horizontal position above the floor, which requires the locomotor system to actively maintain a horizontal posture and

simultaneously allows for movement that would be restricted while lying on the floor.

As with the prone Roman chair exercises, a static or isometric side-lying position can be used in addition to concentric and eccentric maneuvers. Positions of the arms can again decrease or increase the mechanical load and alter the challenge. It must be remembered that instructing the side-lying patient to slowly lower him or herself toward the floor creates an eccentric load of the upper quadratus lumborum. That is, the patient lying on their left side loads the right quadratus lumborum: eccentrically as they move lower and concentrically as they move higher.

It is important to prophylactically to avoid elevating the patient above the horizontal position in the side-lying Roman chair exercise.

Additional Roman Chair Options Other strategies for utilizing a Roman chair Track can also be practically implemented (see Chapter 30, Fig. 30–3). Of course, simply quantatively measuring a static endurance by time can be performed, as would be the number of repetitions performed. In keeping with the general rehabilitation strategy of this text, the qualitative aspects of these exercises should also be scrutinized. For example, it is important to ensure that the patient indeed maintains a true horizontal position during a static endurance test, and that no gradual lowering occurs. One method to avoid this is to have a wall mirror nearby so that the patients can self-monitor their position. Another tool that can be of help is the tubular, wooden rehabilitation stick, which, when placed on the horizontal patient will begin to roll as he or she loses that horizantal posture.

Another Roman chair strategy that has arisen over the past few years is the variable angle Roman chair (VARC). This tool allows the patient to gradually increase the angle of their posture, transitioning from vertical to horizontal, and allowing for a graded and measurable increase in lumbopelvic loading. Another strong advantage to the VARC is that it may reduce the risk of exacerbation by avoiding the sudden, and perhaps unanticipated overload of the horizontal position. One VARC device known as the Backstrong®, allows for postural changes in 15 degrees increments.

LABILE SURFACE LUMBOPELVIC TRAINING

One of the great advances in the area of lumbopelvic training has been the inclusion of a transition from exercising on a stable surface to that of an unstable, or labile, surface. Whatever challenges arise from a stable floor exercise will be magnified on with labile strategies, which require greater stability and balance. The most commonly used labile surface device for dynamic lumbopelvic stabilization is the gym ball, also known by the misnomer Swiss Ball (because it was not devised in Switzerland).

Gym Ball Exercises

The gym ball can be used to place the patient in an unstable environment to perform exercises. The purpose of this is to further challenge the stability system. Many patients will not require this level of training, but those in whom it is particularly challenging to restore normal stability or who are interested in high levels of function, such as athletes, may benefit from using the gym ball. The gym ball can also be an excellent fitness tool. While there are a multitude of gym ball exercises for lumbopelvic stabilization training, some of the more common maneuvers are mentioned here.

Prone Walkout Track

The purpose of the prone walkout track is to place emphasis on the abdominal muscles in an unstable environment as the patient "walk" on his or her hands. In addition, the scapular stabilizers are also challenged in this exercise as the torso level while the patients alternately place weight on each hand as they "walk."

Exercise 1. Static Hold The patient hand walks out on the gym ball in the prone position and is instructed to maintain abdominal brace (Fig. 28–71). It is important that the patient maintain normal scapular stability with the scapulae held firmly against the thoracic cage. The patient must be watched closely, as he or she holds this position, for any loss of stability, represented by chin poke, rising or winging of the scapulae, movement of the lumbar spine, loss of abdominal brace, or shaking. The exercise ends at the point at which any of these changes occur. The exercise is progressed up to 30 seconds.

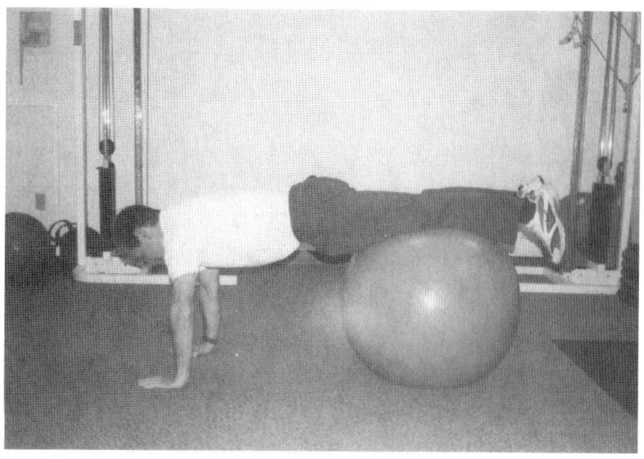

FIGURE 28–71. Prone walkout position.

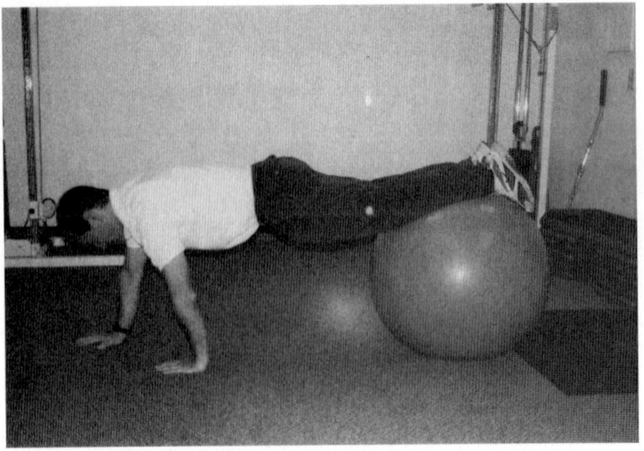

FIGURE 28–72. Walking back.

Exercise 2. Walkouts The patient walks out on the gym ball in the prone position while maintaining the abdominal brace (Fig. 28–71). The patient then walks back to the starting position, without losing stability (Fig. 28–72), and then walks out again. The patient must be careful to maintain a level pelvis, avoiding any hip elevation while taking a step.

Exercise 3. Double Arm Elevation The patient walks out on the gym ball in the prone position and is instructed to maintain an abdominal brace (Fig. 28–66). The patient is then instructed to slowly move backward on the ball by extending the arms overhead (Fig. 28–73). It is important that the clinician watch to be sure that the patient maintains the abdominal brace, a level and stable pelvis, and scapular position. The patient then returns to the static hold position.

Exercise 4. Walkout Crunches The patient walks out on the gym ball in the prone position and is instructed to maintain an abdominal brace (Fig. 28–66). The patient is instructed to flex the lumbar spine by approximating the pubic symphysis to the xiphoid process while maintaining the abdominal brace (Fig. 28–74). It is important that the clinician watch to be sure that the patient maintains the abdominal brace and scapular position as they do this. The patient then returns to the static hold position.

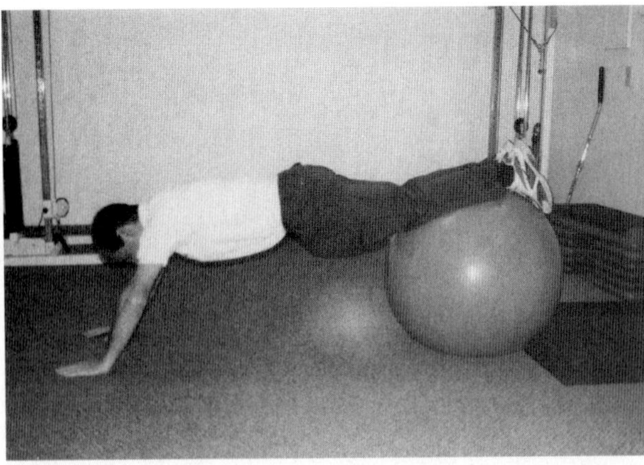

FIGURE 28–73. Double arm elevation in the prone walkout position.

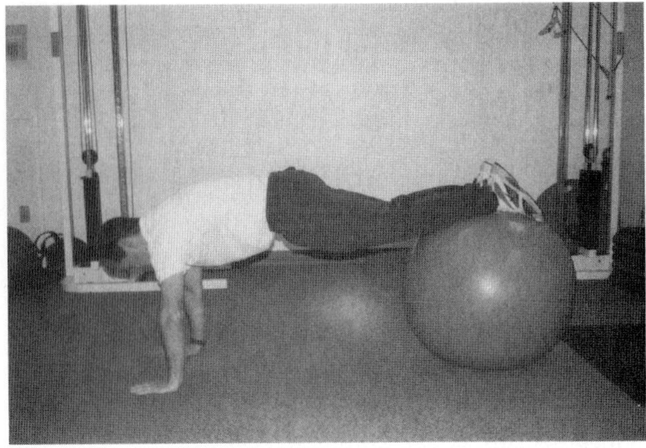

FIGURE 28–74. Walkout crunches.

For increased difficulty in the prone walkout track, the patient should move out farther on the ball so that the ball is lower on the legs (Fig. 28–75). To increase the stimulus for stabilization response, all of these exercises can be performed with the hands balancing on a duck walker (Fig. 28–76).

Rhythmic stabilization can be applied in the prone walkout track for facilitation of specific stabilization responses. Rythmic stabilization challenges are repetitive manual challenges that the clinician applies to facilitate a certain muscle. The challenge is applied rhythmically in a crescendo–decrescendo fashion, such that the clinician gradually increases it to a peak over 1–2 seconds, followed by a gradual decrease over 1–2 seconds. The peak pressure that is exerted by the clinician is determined by how much pressure the patient can resist without giving way or falling into a

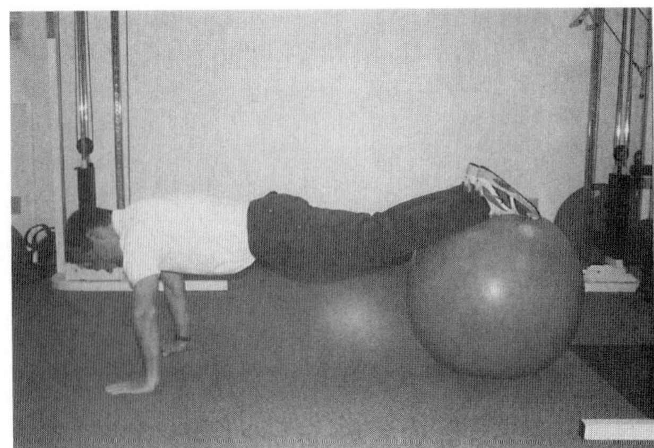

FIGURE 28–75. Advanced level of the prone walkout position.

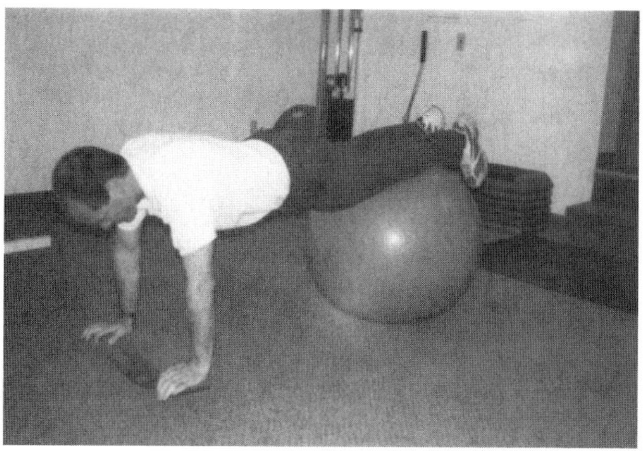

FIGURE 28–76. The use of the duck walker in prone walkout exercises.

faulty recruitment pattern. The rhythmic contractions are repeated 5–10 times, usually followed by a series of short, quick bursts. These are designed to improve reaction time in the neuromuscular circuit. This topic, including the neurophysiological basis, was discussed in detail in Chapter 5 (Fig. 28–77).

Bridge Track

The purpose of the bridge track is to place emphasis on the gluteus maximus and MULT in an unstable environment.

Exercise 1. Bridges The patient is supine on the gym ball with the thoracic spine in contact with the ball (Fig. 28–78). The patient is instructed to establish a neutral spine and slowly raise the pelvis as high as possible without flexing or extending the lumbar spine (Fig. 28–79). The patient returns to the starting point and repeats. Again, it is essential that the abdominal brace and neutral spine posture be maintained throughout the exercise.

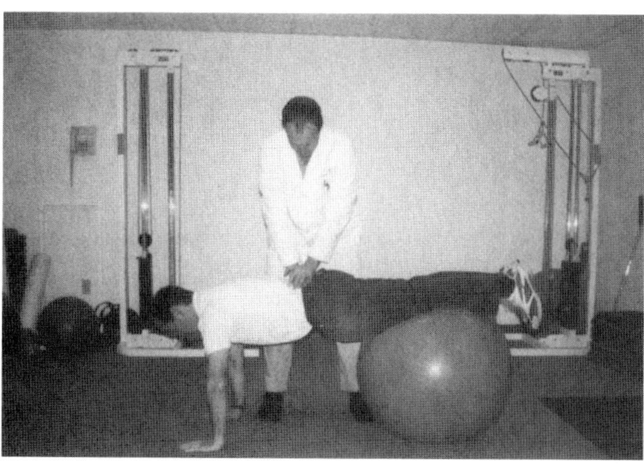

FIGURE 28–77. The use of rhythmic stabilization in the prone walkout position.

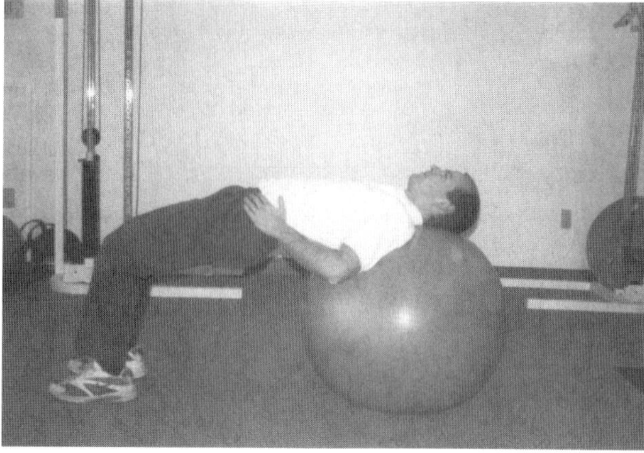

FIGURE 28–78. Preparation position for bridges on the gym ball.

Clinical Pearl: Rhythmic stabilization can be applied in the prone walkout track for facilitation of specific stabilization responses. Rythmic stabilization challenges are repetitive manual challenges that the clinician applies to facilitate a certain muscle.

Exercise 2. Bridge with a Strap The purpose of this exercise is to place particular emphasis on the gluteus medius and minimus. The patient is supine on the gym ball with the thoracic spine in contact with the ball, but with a strap or belt around the distal thighs (Fig. 28–80). The patient is instructed to establish the abdominal brace and neutral pelvis and then to slowly raise the pelvis as high as possible without flexing or extending the lumbar spine (Fig. 28–81). The patient returns to the starting point and repeats. It is essential that the abdominal brace and neutral spine posture be maintained throughout the exercise.

Exercise 3. Bridge with Heel Raises The patient is supine on the gym ball with the thoracic spine in contact

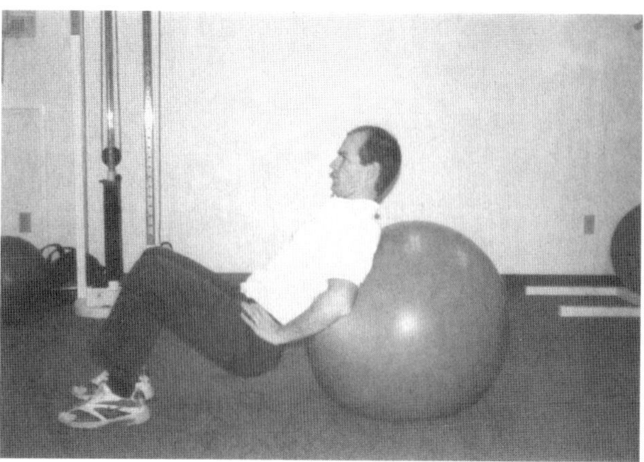

FIGURE 28–79. Bridge on the gym ball.

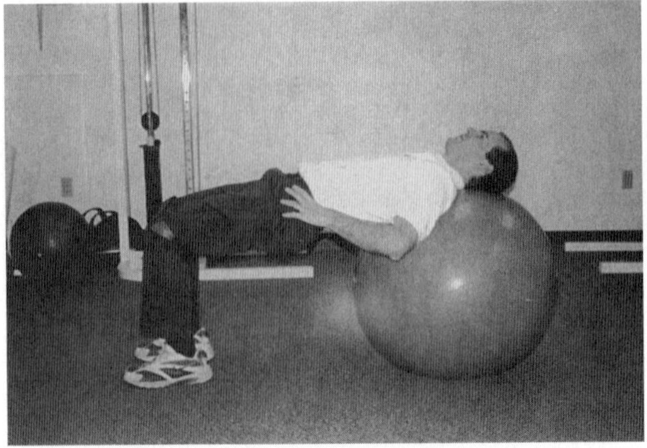

FIGURE 28–80. Preparation position for bridge with strap on the gym ball.

with the ball and is instructed to establish the abdominal brace. The patient is instructed to slowly raise the pelvis as high as possible without extending the lumbar spine. From this position, the patient is instructed to slowly raise one heel (Fig. 28–82), and then return it to the floor, followed by the same movement with the other heel. This is repeated. It is essential that the abdominal brace and neutral spine posture be maintained throughout the exercise.

Exercise 4. Bridge with Steps The patient is supine on the gym ball with the thoracic spine in contact with the ball and is instructed to establish the neutral pelvis and abdominal brace (Fig. 28–78). The patient is instructed to slowly raise the pelvis as high as possible without extending the lumbar spine. From this position, the patient is instructed to raise one foot off the floor approximately 1–2 inches (2–5 cm) (Fig. 28–83), and then return it to the floor, followed by the same movement with the other foot. This is repeated. It is essential that the abdominal brace, the level pelvis, and neutral spine posture be maintained throughout the exercise.

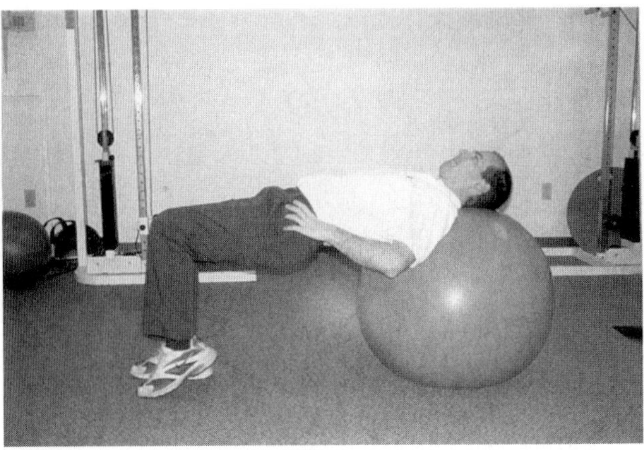

FIGURE 28–82. Bridge with heel raises on the gym ball.

Exercise 5. Bridge with Leg Extension The patient is supine on the gym ball with the thoracic spine in contact with the ball and is instructed to establish the abdominal brace (Fig. 28–78). The patient is instructed to slowly raise the pelvis as high as possible without flexing or extending the lumbar spine. From this position, the patient is instructed to extend one leg straight out (i.e., horizontally) (Fig. 28–84), then return it to the floor, followed by the same movement with the other leg. This is repeated. It is essential that the abdominal brace, level pelvis, and neutral spine posture be maintained throughout the exercise.

Exercise 6. One Leg Bridge This is an advanced level and many patients will not require, nor be able to perform, this exercise. The patient is supine on the gym ball with the thoracic spine in contact with the ball and is instructed to establish the abdominal brace (Fig. 28–78). The patient is instructed to slowly raise the pelvis as high as possible without extending the

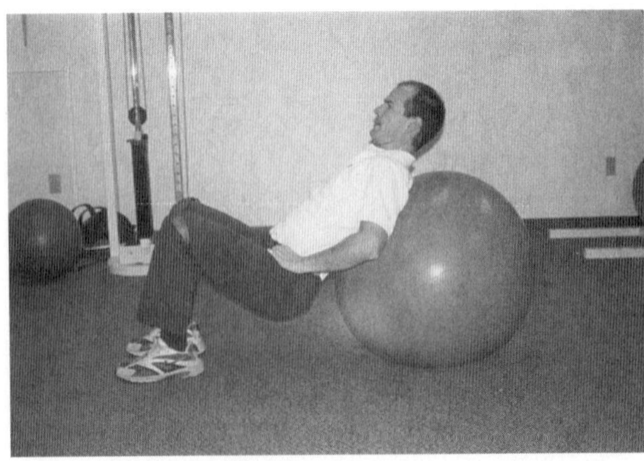

FIGURE 28–81. Bridge with strap on the gym ball.

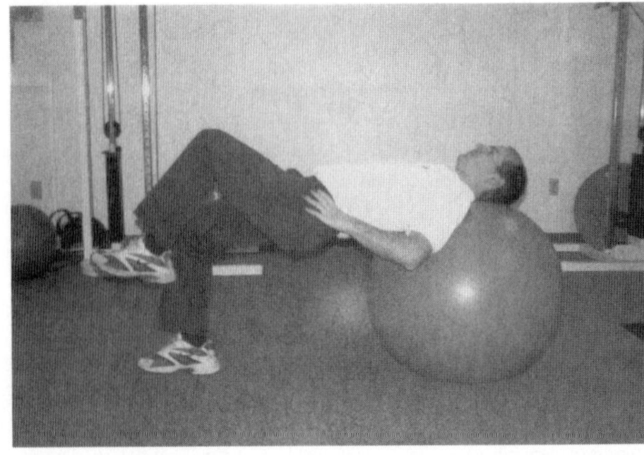

FIGURE 28–83. Bridge with steps on the gym ball.

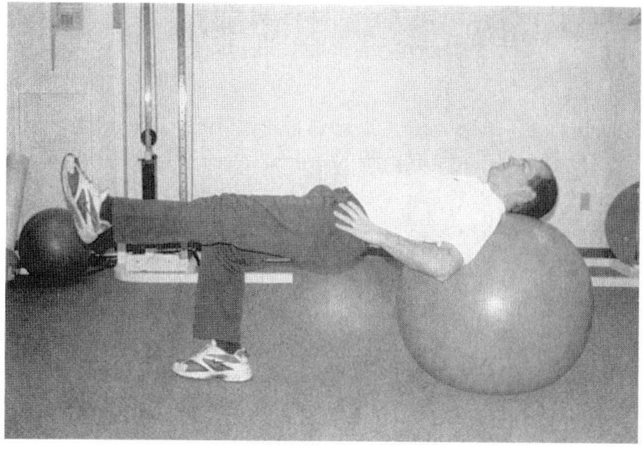

FIGURE 28–84. Bridge with leg extension on the gym ball.

lumbar spine. From this position, the patient is instructed to extend one leg straight out and slowly lower the pelvis toward the floor (Fig. 28–85), and then return to the bridge position. This is repeated. The same exercise is then performed with the other leg. It is essential that the abdominal brace and neutral spine posture be maintained throughout the exercise.

Floor Bridge Track (Using the Gym Ball)

These exercises are performed in the floor bridge position using a small gym ball.

Exercise 1. Floor Bridges The patient is supine with the legs on the gym ball. The arms are at the patient's sides, with the hands turned out (supinated), the fingers wide and the thumbs against the floor (Fig. 28–86). The patient is instructed to perform an abdominal brace and slowly raise the pelvis into a bridge position (Fig. 28–87). The patient then lowers back to the floor. It is essential that the abdominal brace and neutral spine posture be maintained throughout the exercise.

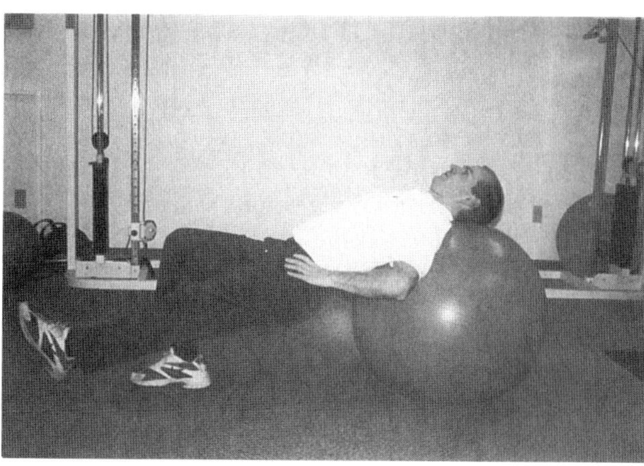

FIGURE 28–85. One leg bridge on the gym ball.

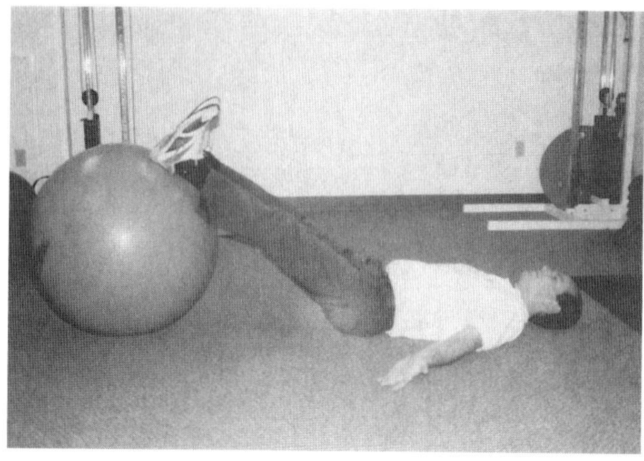

FIGURE 28–86. Preparation position for floor bridges on the gym ball.

Exercise 2. Single Leg Raise The arms are at the patient's sides, with the hands turned out, the fingers wide, and the thumbs against the floor. The patient is instructed to perform an abdominal brace and slowly raise the pelvis into a bridge position. While maintaining the abdominal brace and using the arms for lateral stability on the floor, the patient raises one leg into the air (Fig. 28–88). This leg is lowered back to the ball and the process is repeated with the other leg. It is essential that the abdominal brace and neutral spine posture be maintained throughout the exercise.

Wall Ball Squats

Exercise 1. Two-Legged Squat This exercise represents an excellent example of an advanced-level exercise, challenging balance, abdominal bracing, balance, strength, and endurance while in an upright position. The patient is instructed to place a gym ball behind their low back, pinning it between their back and a wall. Then slightly walk away from the wall, with both feet finishing about 18 in farther away from the wall. The patient then braces the abdomen and places the

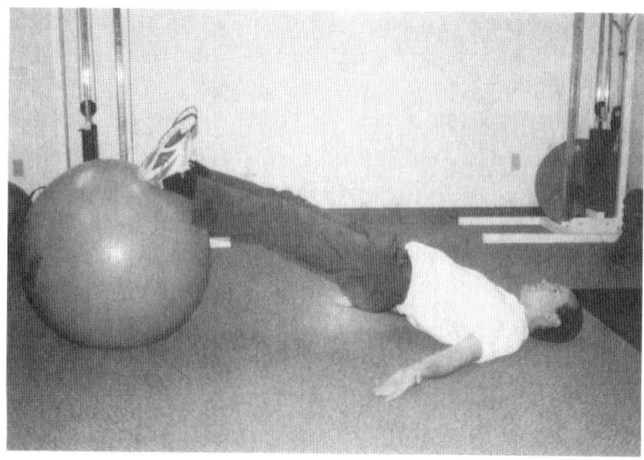

FIGURE 28–87. Floor bridges on the gym ball.

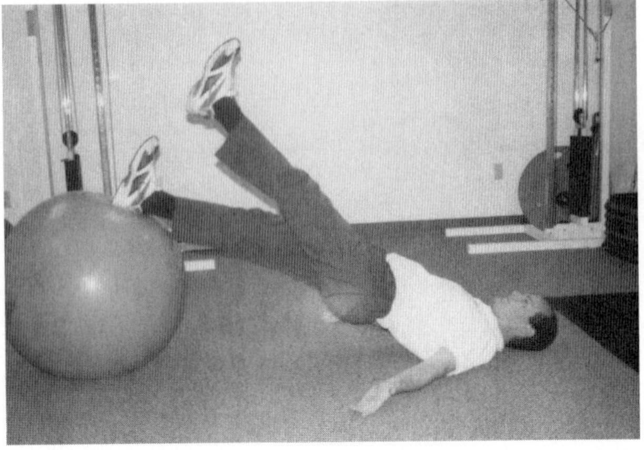

FIGURE 28–88. Single leg raise in the floor bridge position.

spine in the neutral position. While in this position, the patient then performs a squat exercise, rolling down the ball until both the knees form a 90-degree angle in flexion (Fig. 28–89). The knees should not end up in front of the feet, but rather over them. The patient is then instructed to straighten back up, being careful not to compromise the abdominal brace or the neutral spine. The exercise is then repeated.

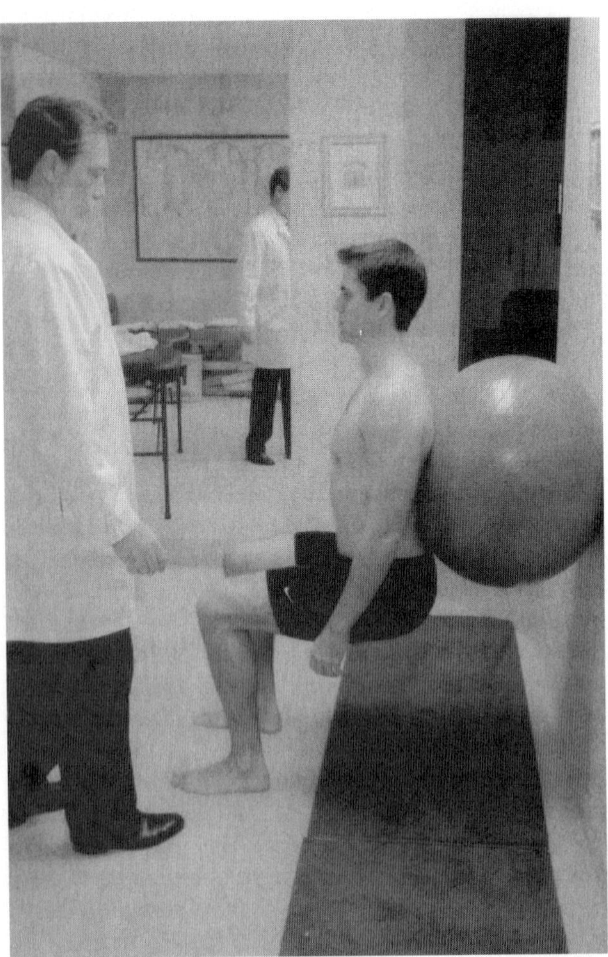

FIGURE 28–89. Two-legged wall ball squat.

Exercise 2. Single-Leg Wall Squat This exercise represents a more advanced level exercise than one mentioned above, increasing the challenges of balance, abdominal bracing, balance, strength, and endurance while in an upright position. The patient is instructed to place a gym ball behind the low back, pinning it between the back and a wall, and then step forward about 18 in with one leg, which becomes the exercise target leg. The patient then braces the abdomen and places the spine in the neutral position. While in this position, the patient performs a one-legged squat exercise, rolling down the ball until the knee forms a 90-degree angle in flexion (Fig. 28–90). The knee of the target leg should not end up in front of the foot, but rather over it. The patient is then instructed to straighten back up, being careful not to compromise the abdominal brace or the neutral spine. The exercise is then repeated with the same leg until fatigue before repeating with the opposite leg.

REHABILITATION MANAGEMENT STRATEGIES

"Hurt versus Harm"

Rehabilitation, like all other aspects of health care, is based on the old Latin adage "Primum Non Nocere" ("First of all, do no harm"). Because the target patients for sensorimotor training and dynamic lumbopelvic stabilization are chronic patients, this rule becomes particularly important. Therefore, the importance of strategies to minimize risk and maximize the effectiveness cannot be overemphasized.

Patients must be taught the difference between hurt versus harm. That is, hurt is defined as something that causes pain, while harm is something that causes further injury. In the acute stage of an injury, the difference beween these two topics is very little, and at times perhaps negligible. As such, the acute patient can be instructed to do essentially what comes natural, avoid pain-provoking activities. However, the complications associated with chronicity separate the terms by definition and require a strategy that appears to exactly contradict that of the acute case: perform activities that produce pain! Of course, there are additional rules that come into play. The pain produced must be controllably tolerable and the exercises must respect the mechanical vulnerabilities of the patient. For example, if the patient can reduce the pain from an exercise program by rest, cold or hot applications, or medication, to a tolerable level, then the exercises can be performed. Conversely, if the symptoms provoked by the exercises are intolerable, then they must be discontinued or altered in place of a more

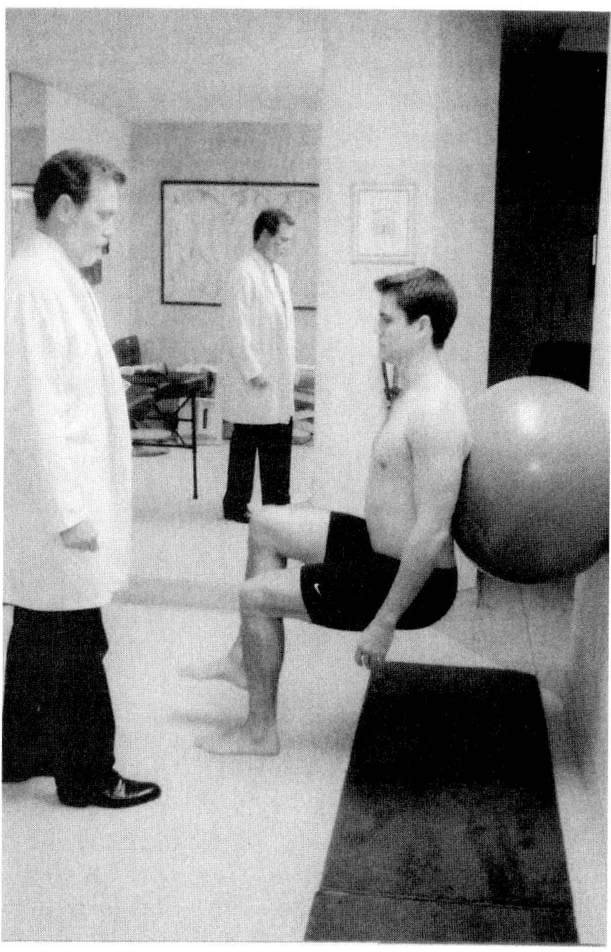

FIGURE 28–90. Single-leg wall ball squat.

effective strategy. It is important, however, for the clinician to carefully determine whether movement intolerability is related to a true inability of the patient to perform the movement, or to fear-avoidance, that is, unwillingness to try to perform the movement for fear of injury. The former should be respected, the latter gently challenged.

Clinical Pearl: Patients must be taught the difference between hurt versus harm. That is, hurt is defined as something that causes pain, while harm is something that causes further injury. In the acute stage of an injury, the difference beween these two topics is very little, and at times perhaps negligible.

In an example of a functional contraindication of an exercise, a patient with a McKenzie posterior derangement category 6 (with pain down the leg; see Chapters 15 and 22) should avoid a supine bridge with a posterior tilt (i.e., loading the posterior disc), especially if these increased the leg symptoms (or peripheralized). Later, as the radiating pain disappears to a posterior derangement, category 1, for example, posterior pelvic tilts may be reintroduced if there is no peripheralization.

The chronic patient must have a clear understanding of hurt versus harm *before* initiating the exercise program in order to come to accept this different concept and anticipate the ensuing increase in pain.

Determining Home Exercises

The various types and indications for sensorimotor and lumbopelvic stabilization training have been explained. However, it is also important to establish the correct level of difficulty among each exercise track, the number of repetitions per set and the number of sets to be performed daily. Finally, the number of exercises to be performed daily must also be established.

To establish the proper degree of difficulty of a specific exercise track, one must start at the lowest level or least demanding exercise. The patient must then demonstrate a complete command of each level within the track, until a level of challenge arises that cannot be mastered. For example, the patient demonstrates complete control of the initial exercises of the quadruped track, before finding difficulty with Exercise 4 (quadruped single leg raise). If the patient can correctly raise the leg half way before improperly extending at the lumbosacral junction (i.e., false hip extension), then it must be determined whether the patient is *kinesthetically aware* of exactly when he or she loses the neutral spine. If aware, then this exercise can be prescribed for home, with the specific instruction that the leg should be raised only to the level where the neutral spine is maintained. Because the goal is to reestablish control, the emphasis of these exercises must be quality of the movement pattern. If the patient is unaware of when they lose lumbopelvic control, then they cannot take this exercise home and should be given the next less demanding maneuver in the same track or move to another track.

The number of repetitions and sets of an exercise depends on the difficulty and conditioning of the patient. With marked difficulty in proper form of a task and severe deconditioning, for example, only a few repetitions may be in order before fatigue and faulty movement patterns arise. Generally speaking, the number of repetitions in a set can vary from 5 to 15 and the number of sets from one to three.

The number of exercises depends on the patient's conditioning, motivation, discipline, and time. In general, five exercises is the recommended maximum for the average patient, as more tend to be forgotton or the patient feels overburdened and is prone to discouragement. Of course, high-level athletes and others with more discipline or motivation can handle a few more exercises.

As the patient masters the quality of an exercise, the number of repetitions can be increased until, with repetition, it is appropriate to move to the next level of difficulty.

Reviewing and Correcting Exercises

Once home exercises are prescribed, the clinician must be ensure that they are being well performed with prescribed regularity. Reviewing each exercise for quality with each visit does this. Lewit states, "The capacity of a patient to ruin an exercise knows no bounds!" It is not uncommon for a patient to require correction in the performance of an exercise once or even twice before they truly execute it well. Furthermore, if the patients understand in advance they will be tested with each visit on the quality of each chore, they tend to be more consistent with the exercises in preparation for close scrutiny.

Patient Motivation

Unfortunately, not all patients are well coordinated. At times, some will also become tense when attempting to implement a rather simple exercise. Still others may be having difficulty overcoming fear-avoidance behavior, which is all too common in chronic patients.

In such cases, the clinician must be sensitive to the concerns of the patient, which are often unspoken but expressed by a change in attitude and demeanor. If left undetected, patients may indeed start to resent the clinician for exposing their inabilities. They can become discouraged regarding the entire rehabilitation program despite an optimal assessment and treatment program and drop out, to their detriment. Therefore the clinician must anticipate the patient's difficulties and direct him or her to a different or simpler exersice, one that they can succeed with and feel positive about. The clinician at these times must also act as a cheerleader, encouraging the patient's attempts and congratulating their successes, however minimal they may be.

Advanced Exercises

If one accepts the earlier recommendation regarding repetitions, sets, and number of exercises, then the continuum of these chores should evolve toward more complex movements integrating a a combination of simple exercises. As such, the limit of five exercises with time may integrate skills of 10 or 15 basic exercises. This advancement should then continue toward exercises that mimic work, sport, and everyday activities.

Measuring Progress

As has been demonstrated, sensorimotor training and lumbopelvic rehabilitation can be performed in a quite simple and brief manner or in an exceedingly complex, arduous, and prolonged approach. The more prolonged the rehabilitation, the greater the necessity of proving its clinical merit and justifying continuing rehabilitation.

How does one justify a prolonged course of care? The answer to this question is to use outcome measures to document case progress. Chapter 14 addressed outcome measures in detail, but many other chapters have also integrated outcomes tools into their approach because these are considered state-of-the-art standards of practice. In addition to those validated measures previously discussed, charting the patient's improvement in sensorimotor training and lumbopelvic stabilization can provide supporting documentation.

By increasing repetitions, increasing the level of difficulty of a specific track, and improving the quality of a movement patterns, the clinician's charting of this functional restoration can be imperative in clarifying this fact to the patient, clinicians, and third-party reviewers. This can be a strong motivator to patients, clinicians, and administrators alike that such care was strategically invaluable in the patient's recovery.

Clinical Pearl: Chapter 14 addressed outcome measures in detail, but many other chapters have also integrated outcomes tools into their approach because these are considered state-of-the-art standards of practice. In addition to those validated measures previously discussed, charting the patient's improvement in sensorimotor training and lumbopelvic stabilization can provide supporting documentation.

CONCLUSION

The purpose of this chapter was to present specific sensorimotor training and spinal stabilization exercises that are designed to improve locomotor system function and stability. Although the number of exercises that can be incorporated into any particular patient's rehabilitation strategy is virtually infinite, an attempt was made here to provide a concise, focused, and streamlined approach to providing the patient with those exercises that are likely to be most beneficial.

It is important to note that not all patients will require all exercises, and the specific rehabilitation strategy should be tailored to each particular patient's needs. For example, if the primary problem is pelvic instability (as detected by the active straight leg raise test and inhibited gluteal function on the hip extension and abduction tests) one might want to place most emphasis on the bridge track and good morning exercises. If the primary problem is lumbar instability (as detected by deviation of the lumbar spine on hip extension test, or is otherwise suspected), one might want to place particular emphasis on the dead bug, quadruped, and prone tracks. On the other hand, if the primary problem is determined to be faulty program for gait (as evidenced by a positive stepping test), sensorimotor training may be the rehabilitation method of choice. Of course, some patients will have a combination of factors involved, and will require a combined rehabilitation approach. Just as lumbopelvic stability is dynamic and complex, so must be the clinician's strategy rehabilitation strategy.

SUMMARY

1. The complete rehabilitation of the patient requires attention to those specific areas of dysfunction that are most relevant to the patient's particular low back syndrome with a systematic, focused approach whose results can be monitored and measured.
2. As was discussed, sensitivity of the patient's needs and concerns must be emphasized, as excellent clinical skills in the absence of appreciating the patient's psychosocial issues can abruptly end an optimal rehabilitation program.
3. In the end, clinical understanding, strategic planning, careful patient counseling, and enthusiastic encouragement encompass the art of clinical rehabilitation. These rehabilitation chapters provide the clinician with such an approach.

REFERENCES

1. Janda J, Va Vrova M. Sensorimotor training. In: Liebenson CS, ed. *Rehabilitation of the spine: A practitioner's manual*. Baltimore, MD: Williams and Wilkins, 1996:319–328.
2. Gelb M. *Body learning*. New York: Henry Holt and Company, 1981.
3. Davidoff RA. Skeletal muscle tone and the misunderstood stretch reflex. *Neurology* 1992;42:951–963.
4. Winter DA. *ABC of balance during walking and standing*. Waterloo, Ontario: Waterloo Biomechanics, 1995.
5. Winter DA. Human balance and posture control during standing and walking. *Gait Posture* 1995;3:193–214.
6. Prince F, Winter DA, Stergiou P, Walt SE. Anticipatory control of upper body balance during human locomotion. *Gait Posture* 1994;2:19–25.
7. Bullock-Saxton JE, Janda V, Bullock MI. Reflex activation of gluteal muscles in walking. *Spine* 1993;18:704.
8. Richardson CA, Jull GA. Muscle control—Pain control. What exercises would you prescribe? *Man Ther* 1995;1:2–10.
9. Richardson C, Hodges P, Hides J. Therapeutic exercise for lumbopelvic stabilization. A motor control approach for the treatment and prevention of low back pain. Edinburgh. Churchill-Livingstone. 2004.
10. Hemborg B, Moritz U, Lowing H. Intra-abdominal pressure and trunk muscle activity during lifting. *Scand J Rehab Med* 1985;17:25–38.
11. Hodges PW. Is there a role for transversus abdominis in lumbo-pelvic stability? *Man Ther.* 1999;4(2):74–86.
12. O'Sullivan PB. Lumbar segmental 'instability': Clinical presentation and specific stabilizing exercise management. *Man Ther* 2000;5(1):2–12.
13. Sapsford RR, Hodges PW. Contraction of the pelvic floor muscles during abdominal maneuvers. *Arch Phys Med Rehabil* 2001;82:1081–1088.
14. Hodges PW, Butler JE, McKenzie DK, Gandevia SC. Contraction of the human diaphragm during rapid postural adjustments. *J Physiol* 1997;505(2):539–548.
15. De Troyer A, Estenne M, Ninane V, et al. Transverse abdominis muscle function in humans. *J Appl Physiol* 1990;68:1010–1016.
16. Puckree T, Cerny F, Bishop B. Abdominal motor unit activity during respiratory and nonrespiratory tasks. *J Appl Physiol* 1998;84:1707–1715.
17. Hides JA, Stokes MJ, Saide M, Jull GA, Cooper DH. Evidence of lumbar multifidis muscle wasting ipsilateral to symptoms in patients with acute/subacute low back pain. *Spine* 1994;19(2):165–172.
18. Hides JA, Richardson CA, Jull GA. Multifidis muscle recovery is not automatic after resolution of acute, first-episode low back pain. *Spine* 1996;21(23):2763–2769.
19. Hodges PW, Richardson CA. Inefficient muscular stabilization of the lumbar spine associated with low back pain: a motor control evaluation of transversus abdominis. *Spine* 1996;21(22):2640–2650.
20. Comerford MJ, Mottram SL. Movement and stability dysfunction—Contemporary developments. *Manual Ther* 2001;6(1):15–26.
21. Cholewicki J, Panjabi M, Khachatryan A. Stabilizing function of trunk flexor-extensor muscles around a neutral spine posture. *Spine* 1997;22(19):2207–2212.
22. McGill SM. Low back exercises: Evidence for improving exercise regimens. *Phys Ther* 1998;78(7):754–765.
23. Arokoski JP, Valta T, Airaksinen O, Kankaanpaa M. Back and abdominal muscle function during stabilization exercise. *Arch Phys Med Rehabil* 2001;82:1089–1098.
24. Callaghan JP, Gunning JL, McGill SM. The relationship between lumbar spine load and muscle activity during extensor exercises. *Phys Ther* 1998;78(1):8–18.
25. Vleeming A, Snijders CJ, Stoeckart R, Mens JMA. The role of the sacroiliac joints in coupling between the spine, pelvis, legs and arms. In: Vleeming A, Mooney V, Dorman T, Snijders C, Stoeckart R, eds. *Movement, stability and low back pain: The essential role of the pelvis.* New York: Churchill Livingstone, 1997: 53–72.

CHAPTER

29

CLINICAL MANAGEMENT OF ATHLETES WITH LOW BACK SYNDROMES

Steven Z. George, Anthony Delitto, and Richard C. Lehman

OUTLINE

OBJECTIVES

1. Understand how the treatment based classification model is appropriate for conservative management of low back syndromes among athletes.
2. Identify yellow and red flags that are relevant for assessment in athletes.
3. Describe the primary components of treatment based classification.
4. Understand treatment philosophies for patients in Stage I, Stage II, and Stage III.
5. Distinguish between specific treatment choices available for patients in Stage I.
6. Describe how patients progress from Stage I to Stage III treatments.
7. Review sample case scenarios designed to demonstrate the practical application of the treatment based classification model for a variety of athletes with differing clinical presentations.

INTRODUCTION

This chapter highlights the use of a treatment-based classification system for the evaluation and treatment of the athlete with low back pain with or without radiating signs or symptoms. The classification system is appropriate for use by clinicians because it considers the presence of pathology and the influence of psychological factors, which may indicate referral to other health-care professionals. In addition, the classification system stages the severity of the disease process and provides matched treatment on the basis of the athlete's clinical presentation. For each level of classification, guidelines that the clinician uses to make decisions are discussed. In addition, four clinical scenarios using treatment-based classification are presented.

Low back pain (LBP) is a common experience for the general population and, unfortunately, athletes are not immune to the effects of LBP.[1] The elite athlete losing significant playing time because of a back injury is a familiar, but anecdotal story. A brief review of the literature indicates that LBP is a common cause of limited play and practice time for a variety of sports including rowing,[2] swimming,[3,4] gymnastics,[3,5,6] football,[7,8] weightlifing,[9,10] racquet sports,[11] and triathlon.[12] In addition to affecting many different types of sports, LBP is found at all levels of athletics.[13–16] Therefore, clinicians working with athletes should be familiar with the evaluation and treatment of LBP.

The majority of athletes with low back injuries are likely to have pain from a benign source.[16] These athletes will be expected to respond well to conservative treatment and return to their sport in a timely manner. A minority of athletes, however, may experience pain from a different source (i.e., spinal stress fracture or nerve root compression).[17–21] In these cases management other than conservative treatment may be indicated. The clinician evaluating athletes with low back pain for consideration of conservative treatment must be able to effectively distinguish between these two scenarios.[16]

After ruling out serious pathology ("red flags") and determining that an athlete is an appropriate candidate for conservative treatment, additional decisions must be made. For example, the clinician must consider the severity and complexity of the condition. The clinician cannot be expected to manage the athlete with mild disability from low back pain in the same manner as the athlete with major disability from low back pain. After the severity and complexity are considered, a treatment that is specific to the athlete must be employed. In making these decisions, the clinician must consider factors that are unique to the athlete's clinical presentation.

Clinical Pearl: To properly manage low back pain, clinicians must consider the appropriateness of conservative management, the severity of the condition, and clinical factors that are unique to the athlete.

Delitto et al.[22] have proposed a treatment-based classification (TBC) system for the management of low back pain. This system provides a framework for clinicians to determine whether a patient is appropriate for conservative management, to determine the severity of the disease, and to apply a specific, matched treatment for patients with acute low back pain (Fig. 29–1). Furthermore, this model establishes criteria that can be used to categorize the progression of recovery, allowing both clinician and patient an opportunity to appreciate one's improvement. The clinician makes these decisions using historical information, self-report questionnaires, and clinical examination findings. The purpose of this chapter is to discuss the evaluation and treatment of the athlete using the TBC system.[22]

Clinical Pearl: Treatment-based classification considers the appropriateness of conservative management, the severity of the condition, and clinical factors unique to the patient when determining treatment for an athlete with low back pain.

FIRST-ORDER CLASSIFICATION: IS CONSERVATIVE TREATMENT APPROPRIATE?

The question to be answered during first-order classification is "Is this athlete appropriate for conservative treatment?" The primary concern at this level of classification is the identification of situations that require the clinician to consult with other health-care professionals. This question can be answered during the initial history and clinical examination by recognizing signs of serious pathology that may or may not be musculoskeletal in nature ("red flags") or that are often misdiagnosed in athletes. Examples of such pathology were covered in great detail in Chapter 10, but may include Scheuermann's disease in the adolescent, lumbar fractures, congenital defects, spondolytic defects, neurocompressive disorders, referred pain from visceral disorders, infection, and metastatic diseases.[4,16,18,20,21] For athletes, another concern at this level of classification is the identification of psychological factors that may be negatively influencing the rehabilitation.

In TBC, athletes are screened for the presence of red flags by using a medical questionnaire, a disability questionnaire, and a pain intensity scale.[22,23] Outcome measures were already addressed in detail in Chapter 14, but those that pertain to the TBC model will be explained for the convenience of the reader. The clinician then reviews these forms so that any issues can be further discussed with the athlete during the examination. The questionnaire includes questions that are intended to identify serious pathology that is not musculoskeletal in origin. These questions focus on unexplained weight loss, history of cancer, night pain, history of immunosuppression, vascular insufficiency, and alterations of bowel and bladder function.[24,25] Any positive response on this questionnaire should be reviewed with the athlete and, if appropriate, a full screening of the body system in question should be performed.[22]

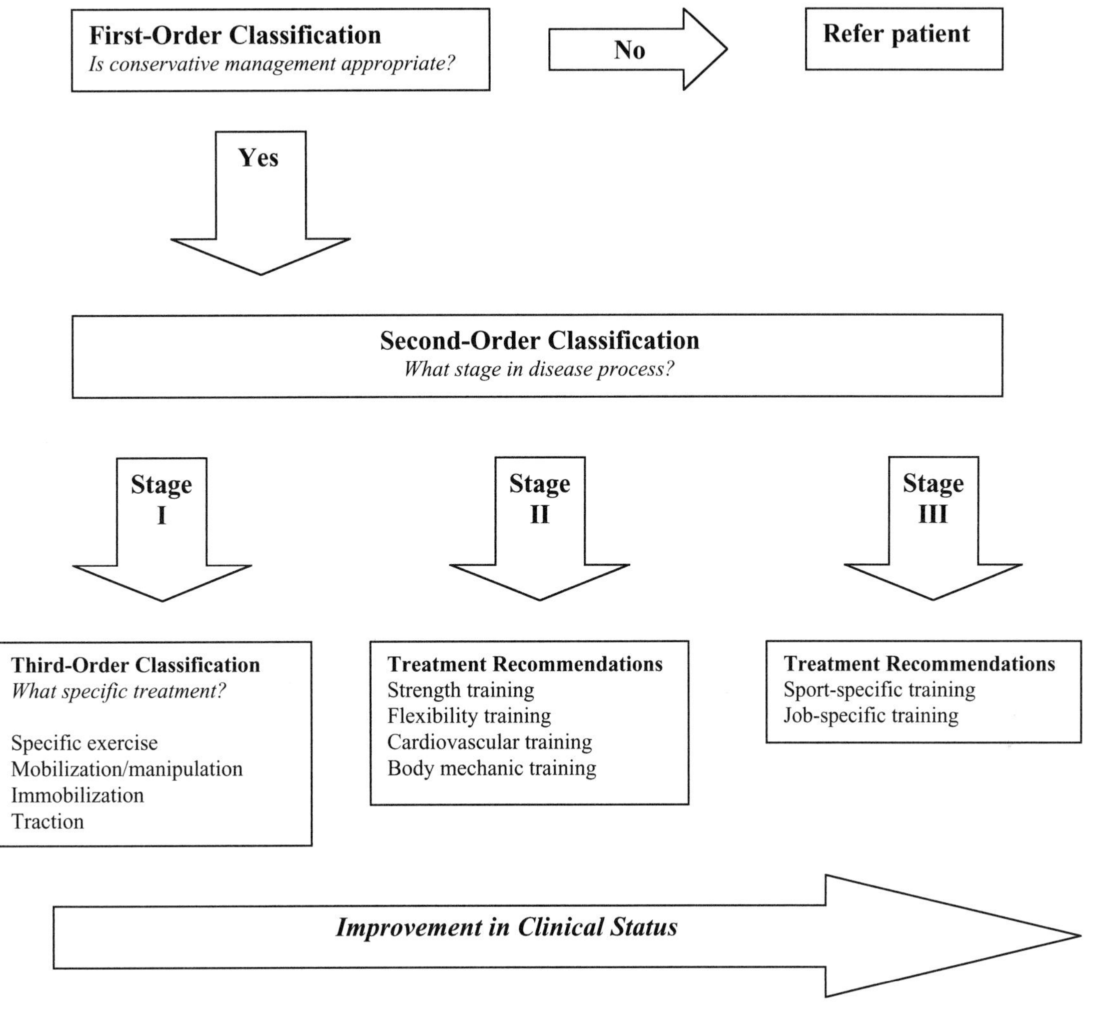

FIGURE 29–1. Overview of treatment-based classification system.

The Oswestry Disability Questionnaire (ODQ)[26,27] and the pain intensity scale are also used to screen athletes for the presence of serious pathology. For the ODQ, athletes rate their function in 10 different areas by using a 0–5 scoring system. The total score is then expressed as a percentage, with 100% indicating total disability and 0% indicating no disability.[26,27] In the absence of magnified illness behavior, ODQ scores greater than 75% raise the suspicion that serious pathology may be present.[22] For the pain intensity scale, an 11-point numeric pain rating (NPR) scale is used, in which an athlete rates pain intensity from 0 to 10 in three different situations. The first situation is the athlete's present pain, the second situation is his or her best pain rating in the last 24 hours, and the third situation is his or her worst pain rating in the last 24 hours. Since mechanical LBP is often associated with postures that reduce pain intensity, very high levels of pain (8–10) in all three conditions also increase the suspicion of serious pathology.[22]

In addition to considering the presence of serious pathology, the clinician evaluating athletes with LBP must be aware of situations that are unique to athletes. A high level of suspicion for pars interarticularis pathology is appropriate for athletes involved in sports involving frequent collisions, loading of the lumbar spine in hyperextension, or repetitive, combined extension and rotation movements of the lumbar spine (i.e., gymnastics, ballet, football, diving, lacrosse, soccer, or hockey).[28–30] Because stress reaction is often not detected during radiographic examination, additional diagnostic testing is often indicated to decrease the suspicion of pars interarticularis pathology.[28,29] In addition to lumbar spine defects, Featherstone[17] recommends the evaluation of sacral stress fracture through magnetic resonance imaging in athletes with persistent LBP. Special attention should be given to the adolescent and younger athlete. Micheli recommends that a high level of suspicion should be maintained in order to diagnose stress fractures and spondolytic defects in these athletes.[6] To ensure proper evaluation of these defects, Libson[20] suggests the use of oblique lumbar spine views. In order to detect rare conditions that may mimic LBP, Watkins and Dillen[16] recommend bone scans in adolescent athletes having significant LBP for more than 3 weeks.

Clinical Pearl: An athlete with an Oswestry score of 80% and consistent 8–10/10 pain intensity ratings would not be considered a candidate for conservative management until further testing ruled out medical or lumbar pathology.

The evaluating clinician must also consider the influence that psychological factors have in the athlete recovering from acute low back injury.[31–34] The literature has demonstrated that psychological factors like fear-avoidance beliefs and coping strategy may prolong the recovery time from low back injury in general practice and work-related patient populations.[35,36] Several authors have hypothesized that these, and other, psychological factors like anxiety and/or depression may play similar roles in the athletic population.[31,32,34] For example, Nideffer[34] proposed that fear of reinjury at times elicits a cycle of physical and psychological sequelae that prolongs the recovery time of an athlete with a low back injury.

Clinicians evaluating athletes with low back injury who have an interest in screening patients for such psychological factors should use established self-report measures. Some modification of the self-report measures may be necessary. For example, a clinician interested in determining whether fear of reinjury was affecting an athlete's rehabilitation could use the Fear-Avoidance Beliefs Questionnaire (FABQ).[37] The FABQ measures fear-avoidance beliefs after low back injury in two different life domains: physical activity and work.[37] It was originally intended to measure fear avoidance from low back injury in general practice and work-related populations, but a modified version was used in a study of patients with cervical spine pain.[38] To modify the FABQ for use with athletes, the authors suggest having the athlete substitute his or her sport for FABQ questions that relate to beliefs about work. Unfortunately, this type of approach has not been validated in the scientific literature. However, this practical measure must suffice until validated sport-specific measures become available.

Clinical Pearl: Psychological variables that have the potential to prolonged recovery from a low back injury include fear avoidance, fear of pain, anxiety, coping strategies, and depression.

Signs of serious systemic pathology, indications of lumbar pathology, and psychological influences all need to be considered by the clinician when evaluating an athlete for consideration of conservative management of low back pain syndromes. When signs of serious pathology are present, the clinician should consider the appropriate referral for additional diagnostic testing before a definite decision regarding conservative management is made. If the clinician suspects that psychological factors are confounding the recovery process, a referral to a sports psychologist for case comanagement should be considered.[33] Because this approach to conservative management encourages interaction with and referral to other health-care professionals, it helps to ensure that the athlete is appropriately managed.

SECOND-ORDER CLASSIFICATION: DETERMINING CHRONICITY

The question to be answered during second-order classification is "What stage in the disease process is this athlete?" This is accomplished by determining the severity of the LBP, which traditionally involves measuring the duration of time that the athlete has been experiencing his or her symptoms. However, other factors are used to determine the severity of the athlete's LBP when using TBC. For example, the severity of LBP is based on the athlete's ability or inability to perform basic and advanced functional activities, and the amount of self-reported disability (via ODQ score) that the athlete is experiencing. Using these criteria, *there are three possible treatment stages during second-order classification in which the athlete can be subcategorized:* Stage I, Stage II, and Stage III.

Clinical Pearl: The decision of whether an athlete is appropriate for Stage I, Stage II, or Stage III treatment is *not entirely based* on how long the athlete has been experiencing the symptoms. Instead, it is based on sitting, standing, and walking tolerance, ODQ score, and limitations in his or her sport.

Athletes with noticeable limitations from LBP in basic functional activities are considered appropriate for Stage I treatment.[22] For example, an athlete would be treated with Stage I treatment principles if he or she was unable to perform any one of the following activities because of LBP: stand for 15 minutes, sit for 30 minutes, or walk one fourth of a mile. In the authors' clinical experience, these athletes are expected to have an ODQ score that ranges between 40% and 60%.

Clinical Pearl: The primary treatment goal of Stage I is pain modulation.

Athletes are considered appropriate for Stage II treatment when they exceed the requirements of

Stage I, but still have limitations in performing daily activities that are more advanced than standing, sitting, and walking.[22] For example, an athlete would be treated with Stage II treatment principles if he or she could stand for 30 minutes, sit for an hour, walk for three fourths of a mile, but could not jog because of LBP. In the authors' clinical experience, these athletes are expected to have an ODQ score that ranges between 20% and 40%. It should be noted that the athlete with LBP may progress from Stage I to Stage II with treatment, or the athlete may have symptoms that are consistent with Stage II during the initial examination session. The primary goal of Stage II treatment is to address physical impairment that is contributing to the athlete's LBP. In Stage II, pain modulation continues to be a goal of treatment, but it is considered a secondary treatment goal in this stage. Stage II treatment is geared toward the athlete's specific physical impairments detected during the athlete's physical examination.

Recommendations for Stage II treatment include strength training, flexibility training, aerobic training, and postural/body mechanics training. Typically, TBC does not provide specific recommendations for Stage II treatment; however, one of the authors (S.Z.G.) has recently described a possible exception to this guideline. One case report that has been published highlights the identification of adverse neural tension in patients who were appropriate for Stage II treatment and another case report describes symptom outcomes for six consecutive patients who were treated with an adverse neural tension technique (slump stretching).[39,40] An example of such a case is provided in clinical scenario #4 at the end of this chapter. In these case reports the author hypothesizes that, just as there are for Stage I treatment, there may be subgroups of patients classified for Stage II treatment who are appropriate for specific treatment.

Clinical Pearl: The primary treatment goal of Stage II is to address physical impairment that may be related to the development of low back pain. Pain modulation is a secondary treatment goal in Stage II.

Athletes are considered appropriate for Stage III treatment when they *can perform all basic functional activities, a majority of advanced functional activities*, but are *not able to resume full participation in their sport*.[22] For example, an athlete would be treated with Stage III principles if he or she no longer noted limitations in standing, sitting, or walking, was able to jog for up to 45 minutes, but could not return to basketball. Stage III treatment principles are also appropriate for athletes with minimal disability from LBP, but who continue to have recurrent episodes of LBP. In the authors' clinical experience, athletes appropriate for Stage III treatment are relatively asymptomatic and are expected to have an ODQ that is below 20%. The treatment goal for athletes in Stage III is to return to full athletic participation and to prevent future recurrence of LBP. This is accomplished through trunk strengthening exercises, functional training, and sport-specific training. The authors believe that Stage III treatment represents the most important component of managing the athlete because it results in the athlete returning to sport and instructs the athlete in an exercise program that may prevent future episodes of LBP. Important components of Stage III treatment are discussed in more detail in other chapters of this textbook, including the next chapter on sport-specific training for the elite athlete and a chapter discussing lumbar stabilization exercises (Chapter 28).

Clinical Pearl: The primary treatment goal of Stage III is to return the athlete to full participation.

Before discussing third-order classification, there are two relevant issues that must be addressed when using TBC to determine the severity of LBP. The first issue is that TBC should be viewed as a model to provide general treatment guidelines based on the severity of LBP. Although discrete stages (i.e., Stage I, Stage II, Stage III) are presented in TBC, the authors acknowledge that the transition from a more severe state of LBP to that of a less severe state most likely occurs on a continuum. As a result, when evaluating and treating athletes with LBP, the clinician can expect to observe overlap between the stages. However, the utilization of these stages remains clinically relevant because it allows the clinician to make treatment decisions and set goals that are appropriate for the severity of the athlete's LBP. The second issue has to do with what appears to be a measurement limitation for the ODQ. In the authors' experience, the ODQ is of most assistance in documenting disability in Stage I and Stage II. Athletes in Stage III will often have very low ODQ scores, but still not be able to return to their sport. The reason for this is that the ODQ is designed to measure restrictions in *typical* activities of daily living (ADL) and is probably not sufficiently sensitive in rating disability among individuals who return to activities with a high physical demand.

THIRD-ORDER CLASSIFICATION: SPECIFIC TREATMENT FOR THE ACUTE CONDITION

Third-order classification is reserved for athletes who are appropriate for Stage I treatment. The question to be answered at this level of classification is "What specific treatment is most appropriate for this athlete?" This question is best answered by having the clinician

TABLE 29–1. Summary of Treatment-Based Classification System

Classification	Key Examination Findings	Recommended Treatment
Extension syndrome*	Flexion activities increase pain	Extension exercises
	Status improves with extension testing	Restriction of flexion activities
	Status worsens with flexion testing	
Flexion syndrome*	Extension activities increase pain	Flexion exercises
	Status improves with flexion testing	Restriction of extension activities
	Status worsens with extension testing	
Mobilization syndrome (lumbar)	Local, unilateral low back pain	Mobilization techniques
	Patterned, restricted range of motion	Manipulation techniques
Moblization syndrome (sacroiliac)	Local pain at PSIS†	Mobilization techniques
	Positive sacroiliac tests	Manipulation techniques
Immobilization syndrome	Frequent episodes of low back pain	Avoidance of sustained posture
	Increased pain with static posture	Trunk–strengthening exercises
Lateral shift syndrome	Visible deformity	Pelvic translocation exercises
	Unilateral side bending restriction	Extension exercises
Traction syndrome	Radicular symptoms	Mechanical traction
	Status worsens with lumbar movements	Auto-traction

*Adapted from principles originally described by McKenzie.[42]

†PSIS: Posterior superior iliac spine.

Source: From Delitto et al.[22]

form an initial hypothesis as to what kind of treatment the patient would most likely benefit from.[41] Examination findings then may influence the clinician to alter the working diagnosis.[41]

Components of the clinical examination used to formulate and test treatment hypotheses include the patient history, the observation of posture, the assessment of pelvic landmarks, and the examination of lumbar movements.[22] The clinician identifies clusters of key examination findings that are unique to the appropriate treatment classification. Refer to Table 29–1 for a list of Stage I treatment syndromes and the corresponding key examination findings.

Seven individual treatment classifications, divided into four categories, have been described by Delitto et al. (Fig. 29–2).[22,43] The first treatment classification is specific exercise, containing the extension syndrome and flexion syndrome. The specific exercise classification is based on and modified from examination and treatment principles first described by McKenzie.[42] Chapters 15 and 22 address McKenzie assessment and treatment protocols in detail. Athletes appropriate for this treatment category frequently note a postural preference and often have symptoms radiating into the lower extremity. Age is also an important consideration in this treatment classification. Younger (below 40) athletes should be considered more likely to be extension syndrome candidates, athletes between the ages of 40 and 55 are not believed to have a specific exercise preference, and older athletes (over 55) should be considered more likely to be flexion syndrome candidates.[43]

The key examination finding that confirms the specific exercise treatment classification is the ability of the athlete to reduce symptoms from the extremity (improve or centralize[42]) or increase symptoms along the extremity (worsen or peripheralize) by performing repeated lumbar movements.[22,42] This treatment

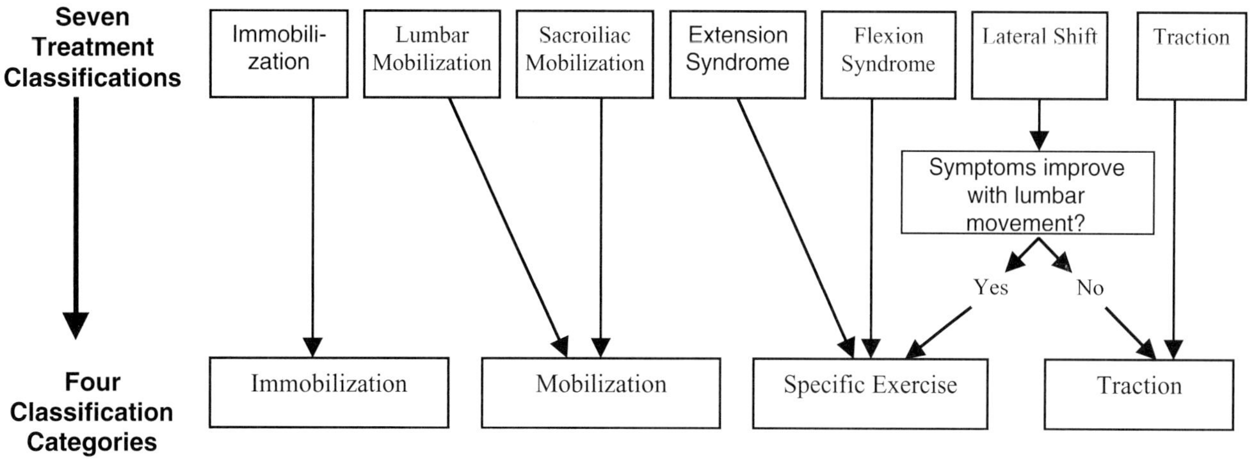

FIGURE 29–2. Original seven treatment classifications divided into four treatment categories. *(From Delitto et al.[22] and Fritz and George.[43])*

classification also consists of patients who were originally classified for lateral shift treatment and were able to improve their symptoms with lumbar movements. The lumbar movement associated with improvement is reinforced through therapeutic exercise. The lumbar movement associated with a worsening of symptoms is discouraged through education or bracing.

Clinical Pearl: Athletes appropriate for specific exercise tend to have symptoms radiating into their lower extremity, a postural preference (i.e., prefer sitting or standing), and are able to improve their symptoms with repeated or sustained lumbar movements (i.e., flexion or extension).

The second treatment classification is *mobilization*, containing sacroiliac mobilization and lumbar mobilization. Athletes in this treatment classification typically have symptoms that are unilateral and localized to the low back or sacroiliac region. The key examination findings for the sacroiliac mobilization treatment syndrome are based on pelvic landmark testing and sacroiliac tests. If the clinician notes multiple positive findings during these tests, then sacroiliac mobilization is confirmed as the appropriate treatment. Treatment consists of a sacroiliac manipulation/mobilization technique, which is typically followed by lumbar range of motion exercises. Sacroiliac manipulation techniques are discussed in detail in Chapter 20.

The key examination finding for the lumbar mobilization treatment classification is the presence of an *opening* or *closing lumbar movement pattern* in a patient with unilaterally dominant pain. An *opening pattern* is consistent with limited lumbar flexion and limited lumbar side bending in the opposite direction of the side of pain. An example of an opening pattern would be a patient with left-sided low back pain who is restricted in lumbar flexion and right lumbar side bending. A *closing pattern* is consistent with limited lumbar extension and limited lumbar side bending in the same direction of the side of pain. After the movement pattern is detected, the clinician confirms the location of the limitation through passive intervertebral joint testing. Treatment consists of the appropriate lumbar mobilization/manipulation technique (i.e., closing mobilization technique for a closing pattern), which is typically followed by active lumbar range of motion exercises. The appropriate lumbar mobilization/manipulation techniques are discussed in detail in Chapters 20, 24, and 26.

When determining whether an athlete is appropriate for mobilization/manipulation for low back pain, contraindications of manual techniques must be considered. In the athletic population, contraindications for these techniques include signs/symptoms of spinal fracture, unstable spondylolisthesis, loss of bone density, or lumbar segmental instability.[44] Further discussion of contraindications for manual therapy techniques is found in Chapter 31.

Clinical Pearl: Athletes appropriate for mobilization/manipulation tend to have unilateral symptoms local to the low back, have distinct movement patterns (i.e., opening or closing), or have unique findings for special tests (sacroiliac test battery).

The third treatment classification is *immobilization*. Athletes in this treatment category typically have a history of frequent episodes of low back pain, often from minimal spinal perturbations. In addition, a history of increased pain with prolonged static postures is associated with this treatment syndrome. Key examination findings that help to confirm the immobilization classification are the presence of a painful arc of motion during lumbar motion testing and a positive response to the segmental instability test. Treatment initially focuses on the avoidance of end-range spinal postures through education and bracing. Later, trunk strengthening exercises and motor control exercises are prescribed for this treatment classification.

Clinical Pearl: Athletes appropriate for immobilization treatment tend to have frequent episodes of low back pain, increased symptoms with static postures, and key examination findings (segmental instability test and painful arc).

The fourth treatment and final classification is *traction*. Athletes in this treatment category will have symptoms radiating into the lower extremity and are expected to have higher amounts of self-reported disability (i.e., ODQ scores above 50%). The key examination finding that confirms the traction classification is that the athlete is not able to improve (centralize) his or her symptoms with any lumbar movements. In fact, the athlete may experience a worsening of the symptoms with most lumbar movements. This treatment category also includes athletes with lateral shift deformities who are unable to improve their symptoms with shift correction and lumbar movements. Treatment for the traction classification consists of intermittent mechanical traction or autotraction. During treatment, the clinician must carefully monitor the athlete's neurological status through reflex, strength, and sensory testing. Any deterioration in neurological status should be communicated so that the appropriate medical and/or surgical decisions can be promptly made.

Clinical Pearl: Athletes appropriate for traction treatment tend to have severe symptoms that radiate into their lower extremity, high self-reports of disability by ODQ score, and are not able to centralize their symptoms with lumbar movements.

CLINICAL SCENARIOS

The management of an athlete using TBC will be highlighted in four clinical scenarios. Because acute injuries are thought to be of common occurrence in athletic populations,[12,14] the first two scenarios demonstrate how the appropriate Stage I treatment is determined. The third scenario provides the rationale used to determine a Stage II and Stage III exercise prescription for an athlete with recurring low back pain and suspected lumbar segmental instability. The fourth scenario describes the identification and treatment of an athlete with "adverse neural tension" within the TBC system. In the first two clinical scenarios, information will be reviewed that helped the clinician determine the appropriateness of conservative management (first-order classification) and chronicity (second-order classification). In the last two clinical scenarios, an assumption can be made that conservative management has already been determined to be appropriate by the clinician and only decision making regarding second-order classification will be reviewed.

Scenario #1

This athlete is a 20-year-old female tennis player without any previous episodes of low back pain. She noted in her history that she experienced a sudden onset of low back pain 5 days prior to the visit, which occurred on the tennis court while reaching for an opponent's drop shot. She initially treated her back pain with ice and rest, but the pain worsened over the ensuing 5 days, prompting her to present for treatment. She noted that her sitting time was limited to about 10 minutes, her standing time to 5 minutes, and her walking time to 20 minutes (which she estimates to be three fourths of a mile). She denied any prior episodes of low back pain or a significant past medical history (including no red flags on medical questionnaire). Her initial ODQ score was 42% and Figure 29–3 describes the anatomical location of this athlete's symptoms. Her pain intensity ratings over the previous 24 hours were 5/10 (at present), 8/10 (at worst), and 3/10 (at best).

First-Order Classification The clinician determined that this patient was appropriate for conservative management because she had a specific onset mechanism, lacked any red flags, and had a pain intensity pattern consistent with mechanical pain.

Second-Order Classification The clinician determined that this patient was appropriate for Stage I treatment because she had an ODQ score that exceeded 40% and her functional limitations in sitting and standing were consistent with the Stage I treatment parameters.

Third-Order Classification The clinician's initial hypothesis was that this patient was appropriate for the mobilization classification. This decision was based on two factors: the symptoms were local to her low back and her first episode of low back pain. To test his initial theory, the clinician focused the clinical examination on the athlete's response to lumbar movements, pelvic landmark tests, and sacroiliac tests. During the single lumbar movement testing, the clinician detected a decrease in lumbar flexion, but did not detect an opening or closing pattern with the side bending movements.

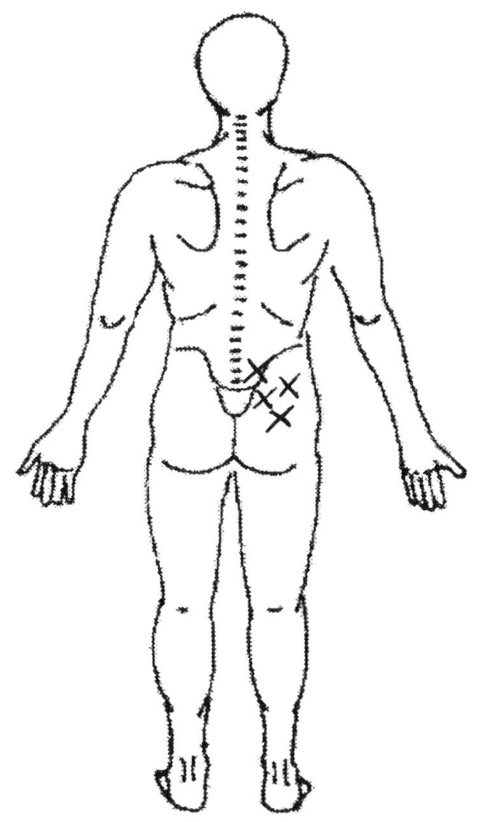

FIGURE 29–3. Pain diagram depicting location of symptoms for scenario #1. The "X" used by the athlete corresponds with a burning symptom descriptor.

During the lumbar movement testing the clinician also noted that the athlete could not improve or worsen her symptoms with repeated lumbar movements. He detected elevated posterior superior iliac spine (PSIS) on the right side and also detected positive seated lumbar flexion and standing lumbar flexion tests. With this information, the clinician felt that the mobilization classification was confirmed and that sacroiliac mobilization was the most appropriate treatment. This was because of the lack of a lumbar movement pattern and the presence of positive sacroiliac joint tests.

Clinical Pearl: Sacroiliac tests are inherently unreliable, and therefore, a group of the tests should be used when confirming the presence of sacroiliac joint dysfunction.

Treatment The clinician decided to initiate treatment by performing a sacroiliac joint manipulation. After the manipulation was performed, the athlete's pain intensity and lumbar range of motion were reassessed by the clinician. The athlete noted a slight decrease in pain intensity and the clinician observed an improvement in lumbar flexion range of motion. At this point, the athlete was prescribed lumbar range of motion exercise for her home program and instructed to return to the clinic in 2 days.

When the athlete returned to the clinic, she noted a continued improvement in symptoms, but was hesitant to return to practice, even at modified intensity. Her ODQ had improved slightly to 35% and her pain intensity ratings were decreased to 4/10 (at present), 6/19 (at worst), and 1/10 (at best).

Reevaluation for Psychosocial Factors The clinician then suspected that fear of reinjury/fear avoidance was contributing to this athlete's clinical presentation and measured the level of fear with the Fear-Avoidance Beliefs Questionnaire (FABQ).[37] On the FABQ, higher scores indicate higher levels of fear-avoidance and this athlete scored a 20 out of a possible 24 on the physical activity scale and a 34 out of 42 on the work scale (which the patient answered in the context of her sport). What constitutes an "excessive amount" of fear avoidance for athletes with low back injury has not been established in the scientific literature, but in the authors' clinical experiences, these scores were sufficient to warrant clinical action.

Treatment Modification To address the "excessive" fear-avoidance beliefs, the clinician decided to implement two strategies. The first strategy was specific, unambiguous patient education that a low back injury is only temporarily disabling in the vast majority of cases and that avoiding activity is actually detrimental to recovery.[45] The clinician educated the athlete by issuing her a pamphlet that has reduced fear-avoidance beliefs in a previous clinical trial.[46] Then, the clinician reinforced the pamphlet's message in subsequent clinical sessions. The second strategy was the addition of a graded exercise program to the athlete's exercise prescription.[45,47] The clinician accomplished this by adding treadmill jogging to the exercise prescription and used *quota-based criteria*, instead of pain-based criteria, to progress the patient's exercise intensity and duration during subsequent clinical sessions.

In a quota-based exercise program, the athlete works toward a predetermined exercise dosage, which is increased each time the athlete meets the predetermined dosage and is *not* influenced by a change in pain intensity. For example, this athlete was started on treadmill ambulation for 10 minutes at 4 mph. The athlete completed 10 minutes, but noted an increase of low back pain from 4/10 intensity to 6/10 intensity. Because this increase in intensity was not associated with any clinical signs of deterioration (i.e., weakness, reflex change, or sensory loss in the lower extremities), the exercise dosage was increased to 12 minutes at 4 mph for the next treatment session. Throughout the treatment sessions, any decisions regarding the exercise prescription were made on similar exercise quota-based principles.

Clinical Pearl: Graded exercise (using quota-based criteria) can be a useful treatment supplement when treating a patient with elevated fear-avoidance beliefs because it shifts the focus of treatment to improving activity tolerance.

Outcome After 3 weeks of this treatment, the athlete expressed more confidence and was reevaluated for return to sport. At this point, her ODQ score of 12% represented a clinically significant improvement from the initial evaluation session.[48] Her pain intensity ratings were improved to 1/10 (at present), 2/10 (at worst), and 0/10 (at best). The clinician also readministered the FABQ and the athlete scored considerably lower, 10 out of 24 on the physical activity scale and 18 out of 42 on the work scale. This information, with an improvement in lumbar range of motion and pain intensity, allowed the clinician to comfortably discharge the athlete for return to sport. It should be noted that if the fear-avoidance beliefs persisted and the athlete had difficulty returning to sport, she would have been referred to a sports psychologist for a more thorough psychological evaluation. Then, the athlete would have been comanaged with the sports psychologist until she was able to successfully return to sport.

Scenario #2

The second clinical scenario involves an 18-year-old male high school football player who experienced a sudden onset of symptoms after a tackling drill in which he was forced into a flexed position. He reports that the low back pain radiates into his lower extremity, but does not go below his knee (Fig. 29–4). He notes that his sitting time is limited to 10 minutes, but can stand and walk for up to 1 hour without a change in his symptoms. In addition, he notes that he has less leg pain when standing but his low back pain remains the same. The athlete notes that he has had two or three episodes of low back pain in the past, but none that limited his activity this severely or that included leg pain. His past medical history is significant only for exercise-induced asthma and he does not report any red flags on his medical questionnaire. His initial ODQ score was 64% and his pain intensity ratings are 7/10 (at present), 9/10 (at worst), 5/10 (at best).

First-Order Classification The clinician determined that this athlete was appropriate for conservative management because the athlete had a definite onset mechanism for low back pain and a pain intensity pattern consistent with mechanical low back pain. The clinician did have some concern that this patient may be exhibiting signs (i.e., radicular symptoms and high self-report of disability on ODQ) consistent with a neurocompressive disorder that might require a surgical consultation. However, only weakness of the great-toe extensor (rated 4/5 on the involved side) was observed when motor, reflex, and sensory testing was performed.

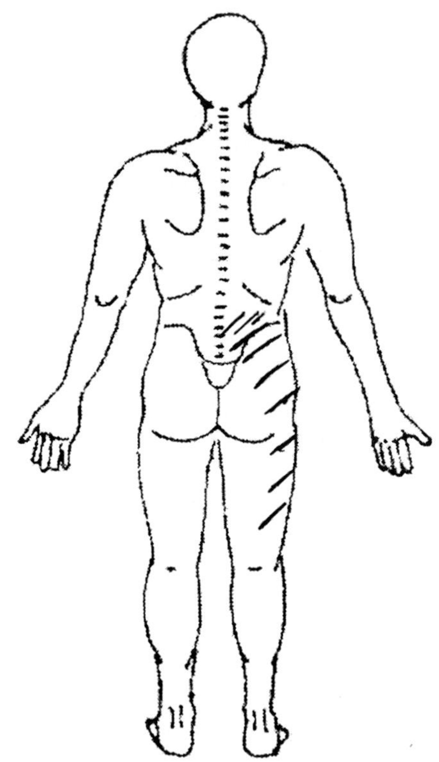

FIGURE 29–4. Pain diagram depicting location of symptoms for scenario #2. The "/" used by the athlete corresponds with a stabbing symptom descriptor.

Clinical Pearl: For this athlete, a neurological examination was necessary during first-order classification because of the high self-report of disability and the presence of symptoms radiating into the lower extremity.

Second-Order Classification The clinician determined that this athlete was appropriate for Stage I treatment because of the functional limitation in sitting and the ODQ score that exceeded 40%.

Third-Order Classification The clinician's initial hypothesis was that this athlete would be most appropriate for extension classification within the specific exercise category. This theory was based on the following factors: the presence of symptoms in the lower extremity, the athlete's postural preference, and the athlete's age. The clinician decided to focus the clinical examination on pelvic landmark testing and lumbar movements. The clinician did not detect any asymmetries during pelvic landmark testing. With single lumbar movement testing, the clinician detected a significant limitation in flexion and extension. With repeated lumbar movement testing, the athlete was unable to improve his symptoms with flexion or extension. During repeated flexion, the athlete noted that the symptoms went below his knee after the fifth repetition. Another neurological examination revealed no change in motor, reflex, and sensory findings, and additional repeated lumbar movements were not performed.

The clinician decided to alter the initial treatment classification of extension and classified this athlete for traction treatment because of the clinical examination results. This change in treatment classification was made because the athlete could not improve his symptoms with lumbar movements. The clinician decided to use the results of the neurological examination (weakness in the great-toe extensor) to monitor this athlete's response to treatment. The clinician decided that treatment would consist of intermittent lumbar traction, and that without improvement in neurological status within 1 week, the athlete would be referred for surgical consultation and appropriate diagnostic testing.

Clinical Pearl: The key finding that led this clinician to traction treatment was the inability to centralize this athlete's symptoms with lumbar movements.

Treatment After 1 week of four sessions of intermittent traction, the athlete noted a 10-minute improvement in his sitting tolerance. The clinician reevaluated the athlete's neurological status and found that his great-toe extensor strength had improved by a muscle grade to 5/5. The clinician decided to delay the referral to the neurologist and continue intermittent lumbar traction for another week. After an additional week of traction, the athlete noted an additional-10 minute improvement in sitting tolerance and his ODQ score had decreased to 44%. During the reevaluation, it was observed that lumbar extension movements improved the athlete's status by centralizing his symptoms from his posterior thigh to his buttock. At this point, the clinician decided that the athlete would no longer benefit from intermittent lumbar traction and prescribed a lumbar extension protocol for the patient to perform outside of the clinic.

Progression to Stage II and Outcome After a second week, the athlete was evaluated again and continued to show improvement as his standing, sitting, and walking tolerance all had improved. His symptoms had not radiated into his leg during the past 3 days and his ODQ score was 28%. At this point, the clinician felt the athlete was appropriate to begin Stage II treatment principles and began flexibility, strength, and aerobic training with the athlete. After 3 weeks of Stage II treatment, the athlete complained of mild low back pain, with pain intensity ratings of 2/10 (at present), 3/10 (at worst), and 1/10 (at best). He no longer had sitting limitations and was able to jog 2 miles without an increase in his low back pain. The athlete also demonstrated full lumbar range of motion, which did not worsen his low back pain, and his ODQ score was 8%. At this point, the athlete was discharged and cleared to resume practice with his team, under the supervision of the trainer.

Scenario #3

The third clinical scenario involved a 28-year-old dancer with recurrent episodes of low back pain that seemed to be increasing in frequency over a 2-year period. The present episode started about 2 weeks ago after practice. She complained of mild to moderate low back pain (pain intensity ratings ranging from 2/10 to 4/10), did not have limitations with sitting, standing, or walking, and had an ODQ score of 18%. The athlete had not completed a full practice session since this recent onset of pain.

Second-Order Classification The clinician decided this athlete was appropriate for Stage II treatment because of the athlete's ability to perform basic functional activities (sitting, standing, and walking) and "low" ODQ score.

Treatment Rationale During the physical examination, the clinician detected several potential clinical signs of lumbar dynamic instability (i.e., history of recurrent episodes, painful arc in lumbar flexion, and positive segmental instability test). Therefore, the clinician hypothesized that this patient had a component of dynamic lumbar instability and decided to focus the Stage II treatment on trunk strengthening exercises. In selecting an exercise prescription for trunk strengthening, the clinician must consider several factors including the amount of lumbar compressive forces generated by the exercise, the amount of lumbar shear forces generated by the exercise, that the appropriate muscle groups are targeted, and that the parameters of the exercise prescription are appropriate.[49,50]

Clinicians should prescribe trunk strengthening exercises that generate minimal lumbar compressive and lumbar shear forces.[50] For example, McGill[51–53] has suggested that bent and straight-knee curl-ups are to be avoided because of the excessive compressive and shear forces generated. In addition, excessive compressive forces may be generated with exercises that emphasize the lumbar erector spinae muscles.[54,55] The clinician should prescribe trunk strengthening exercises that activate muscles that stabilize the spine. A consensus has not been reached, but evidence in the literature exists supporting the role of the transversus abdominis,[56,57] the oblique abdominals,[56] the multifidus,[56,58] the erector spinae,[54] and the quadratus lumborum[59] as spinal stabilizers. Lastly, the clinician must consider the manner in which the trunk muscles are trained. A recent review indicates that more evidence exists for exercise prescription that trains trunk muscles for endurance parameters rather than strength parameters.[50]

In this scenario, the clinician decided to initiate trunk endurance and strengthening by training the athlete's transversus abdominis, oblique abdominals, multifidi, and erector spinae muscle groups. A randomized trial reported that patients with chronic LBP performing exercises similar to these had less pain and disability at short-term (10 weeks) and long-term (30 months) follow-up periods.[56] In addition, the authors of this chapter hypothesize that performance of trunk strengthening exercises is an important component in preventing recurrence of LBP. The clinician selected exercises that have been documented in the literature as generating acceptable amounts of lumbar compressive forces. The clinician selected exercise parameters that had the athlete perform high repetition, low-load tasks on a daily basis. As the athlete with suspected dynamic instability progresses through a rehabilitation program (i.e., to Stage III), it has been proposed that the motor control system should also be trained.[57,60] One way to do this is to perform the trunk strengthening exercises during sport-specific activities or on unstable surfaces. These and other issues related to Stage III exercise prescriptions are covered in more detail in this textbook: training the elite athlete (Chapter 30) and lumbar stabilization (Chapter 28).

Clinical Pearl: Recent evidence suggests that dynamic stabilization exercise programs should target the transversus abdominis, the oblique abdominals, the multifidus, the erector spinae, and the quadratus lumborum muscles.

Outcome After completing 4 weeks of the trunk endurance and strengthening training program, the dancer noted an improvement in pain intensity (ranging from 0/10 to 2/10) and self-report of disability (ODQ score of 8%). In addition, the dancer was able to complete two full practice sessions in the last week. The dancer was then discharged from therapy, resumed a full practice schedule, and continued the trunk endurance and strengthening program as part of a home exercise program.

Scenario #4

The fourth clinical scenario involved a 39-year-old female recreational runner complaining of long-standing low back and posterior thigh pain. The athlete noted that the problem started after tearing a

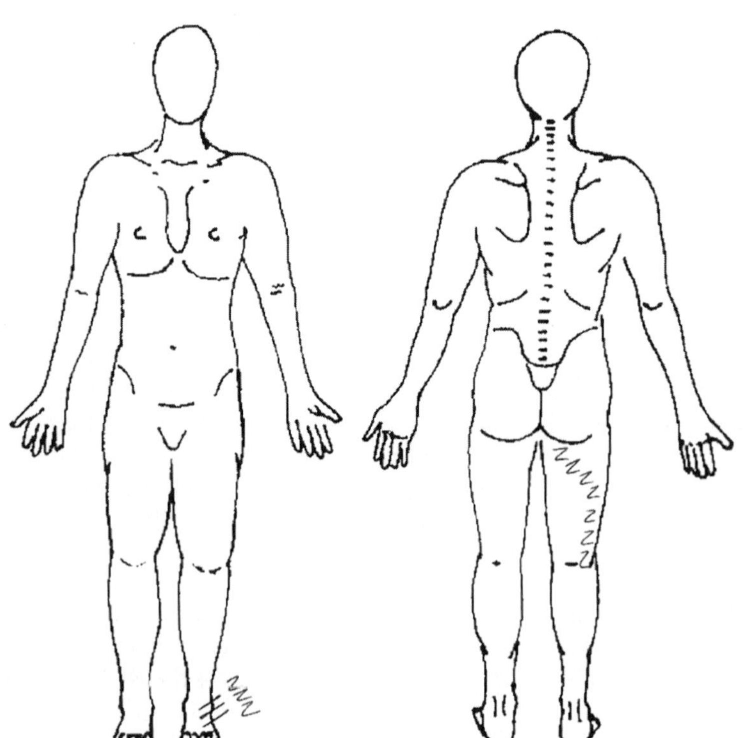

FIGURE 29–5. Pain diagram depicting location of symptoms for scenario #4.

hamstring muscle while in the weight room approximately 2 years before. Since then, she has experienced ongoing symptoms in her low back and posterior thigh that have been resistant to various treatment approaches used by practitioners of conservative treatment, joint manipulation, passive modalities, massage, strength training, flexibility training, NSAIDs, steroid injections, and bed rest. She did not have any limitations in sitting, standing, or walking but could not run for longer than 10 minutes because of the pain. Her pain intensity ratings were 7/10 (at present), 9/10 (at worst), and 5/10 (at best). Her ODQ score is 25% and Figure 29–5 describes the anatomical location of her symptoms.

Second-Order Classification The clinician decided that this athlete is appropriate for Stage II treatment because she had no problems with sitting, standing, and walking, but continued to have low levels of self-reported disability. However, in order to confirm that hypothesis, the clinician wanted to assess the athlete's neurological status and symptom response to repeated lumbar movements to rule out the possibility of using Stage I treatment principles. For this athlete, no neurological deficits were noted with motor, reflex, and sensory testing. Repeated lumbar movements did not centralize or worsen the athlete's symptoms. Therefore, despite the pain radiating into the athlete's lower extremity, the clinician felt this patient was appropriate for Stage II treatment principles.

Treatment In TBC, specific treatment categories have not been described for Stage II athletes and treatment is guided by the results of the physical examination. In this athlete's case the clinician wanted to assess the hamstring musculature and the presence of adverse neural tension for treatment options. In this athlete, length and strength testing of the hamstring muscle group did not provoke the patient's symptoms and only mildly differed from the uninvolved side. However, the slump test (Table 29–2), which is believed to stress nervous structures associated with sciatic nerve, was positive and the clinician decided to treat for adverse neural tension.

The athlete was then treated two times a week for the next 4 weeks using a protocol integrating the use of "sliders."[61] In this treatment protocol, the athlete warmed up for 5–10 minutes on a stationary bicycle. Then, the therapist manually stretched the patient using two separate techniques. The first technique was to perform a slump stretch with clinician overpressure into flexion at the cervical, thoracic, and lumbar spines, and into extension at the knee and dorsiflexion at the ankle. The second technique was to perform a straight-leg raise stretch with clinician overpressure into hip flexion, knee extension, and ankle dorsiflexion. Each stretch was performed as a sustained mobilization technique at end range of tissue resistance (grade IV), with the hold lasting 30 seconds and repeated five to seven times. The patient performed exercises that mimicked the techniques as part of her daily home exercise program.

TABLE 29–2. Description of Slump Test

Order	Summary
1	The athlete was asked to sit with erect sitting posture, knees at 90 degrees of flexion and the popliteal surface in contact with the treatment surface.
2	The athlete was asked to relax shoulders and lower back. The clinician maintained cervical spine in a neutral position and applied overpressure to thoracic and lumbar spines into flexion.
3	Maintaining the position described in step 2, the athlete was asked to tuck "chin to chest" and the clinician added overpressure to cervical spine into flexion.
4	The clinician continued to add overpressure, maintaining the fully flexed position, and the athlete actively extended the knee.
5	The clinician maintained overpressure from step 4 and the athlete actively dorsiflexed the ankle while maintaining the knee in extension.
6	Overpressure at the cervical spine was released and the athlete extended the neck to return to neutral cervical spine position.

Source: From Butler.[61]

Clinical Pearl: When the clinician reached the end range of tissue resistance, the patient's symptoms were expected to be reproduced with these manual stretching techniques.

Outcome After 4 weeks of treatment and home exercise program (no other techniques were performed), the athlete noted significant improvements in symptom intensity and the symptoms no longer radiated into the lower extremity. She was able to run for 30 minutes at which point she was experiencing mild symptom intensity that did not prevent her from finishing her goal of 45 minutes. Her self-report of disability was improved as her ODQ score decreased to 6%. At this point, she was discharged to her home exercise program consisting of stretches that mimicked the techniques used in the clinic. One month later, the athlete called the clinic to report that she had no symptoms and had increased her running time to 50 minutes without incident.

SUMMARY

1. This chapter outlined the evaluation of an athlete experiencing LBP with and without radicular symptoms using the classification system proposed by Delitto et al.
2. For outpatient orthopedic practice, evidence in the literature is available documenting the reliability[43] and the relative effectiveness of treatment guided by TBC.[62–64]
3. This classification system provides a useful framework for the clinician to evaluate athletes with LBP because it considers the appropriateness of conservative treatment by investigating the presence of serious pathology, lumbar pathology, and psychological factors.
4. In addition, the TBC classification system considers the severity of the disease process and provides matched treatment based on the athlete's clinical presentation.
5. When treating athletes with episodes of acute LBP with and without radicular symptoms, pain modulation and return to daily function are the primary treatment goals.
6. When treating athletes with episodes of chronic LBP, return to sport and prevention of recurrence are the primary treatment goals.

REFERENCES

1. Croteau LL. Managing sports-related low back pain. *Nurse Pract Forum* 1996;7:141–147.
2. Reid DA, McNair PJ. Factors contributing to low back pain in rowers. *Br J Sports Med* 2000;34:321–322.
3. Goldstein JD, Berger PE, Windler GE, Jackson DW. Spine injuries in gymnasts and swimmers. An epidemiologic investigation. *Am J Sports Med* 1991;19:463–468.
4. Wilson FD, Lindseth RE. The adolescent "swimmer's back." *Am J Sports Med* 1982;10:174–176.
5. Sward L. The thoracolumbar spine in young elite athletes. Current concepts on the effects of physical training. *Sports Med* 1992;13:357–364.
6. Micheli LJ. Back injuries in gymnastics. *Clin Sports Med* 1985;4:85–93.
7. Halpern B, Thompson N, Curl WW, Andrews JR, Hunter SC, Boring JR. High school football injuries: Identifying the risk factors. *Am J Sports Med* 1987; 15:316–320.
8. Thompson N, Halpern B, Curl WW, et al. High school football injuries: Evaluation. *Am J Sports Med* 1987;15: 117–124.
9. Aggrawal ND, Kaur R, Kumar S. A study of changes in weight lifters and other athletes. *Br J Sports Med* 1979;13:58–61.
10. Risser WL. Musculoskeletal injuries caused by weight training. Guidelines for prevention. *Clin Pediatr (Phila)* 1990;29:305–310.
11. Chard MD, Lachman SM. Racquet sports—patterns of injury presenting to a sports injury clinic. *Br J Sports Med* 1987;21:150–153.
12. Manninen JS, Kallinen M. Low back pain and other overuse injuries in a group of Japanese triathletes. *Br J Sports Med* 1996;30:134–139.
13. Micheli LJ. Sports injuries in children and adolescents. Questions and controversies. *Clin Sports Med* 1995;14:727–745.
14. Keene JS, Albert MJ, Springer SL. Back injuries in college athletes. *J Spinal Disord* 1986;2:190–195.
15. Davies JE. The spine in sport—Injuries, prevention and treatment. *Br J Sports Med* 1980;14:18–21.
16. Watkins RG, Dillin WM. *Lumbar spine injuries*. In: Fu FF, Stone DA, eds. Sports injuries: Mechanisms, prevention, treatment, 1st ed. Baltimore, MD: Williams & Wilkins, 1994:877–894.
17. Featherstone T. Magnetic resonance imaging in the diagnosis of sacral stress fracture. *Br J Sports Med* 1999; 33:276–277.
18. Garces GL, Gonzalez-Montoro I, Rasines JL, Santonja F. Early diagnosis of stress fracture of the lumbar spine in athletes. *Int Orthop* 1999;23:213–215.
19. Kujala UM, Kinnunen J, Helenius P, Orava S, Taavitsainen M, Karaharju E. Prolonged low-back pain in young athletes: A prospective case series study of findings and prognosis. *Eur Spine J* 1999;8:480–484.
20. Libson E, Bloom RA, Dinari G, Robin GC. Oblique lumbar spine radiographs: Importance in young patients. *Radiology* 1984;151:89–90.
21. Brukner P, Bradshaw C, Khan KM, White S, Crossley K. Stress fractures: A review of 180 cases. *Clin J Sport Med* 1996;6:85–89.
22. Delitto A, Erhard RE, and Bowling RW. A treatment-based classification approach to low back syndrome: Identifying and staging patients for conservative treatment. *Phys Ther* 1995;75:470–485.
23. Fritz JM. Use of a classification approach to the treatment of 3 patients with low back syndrome. *Phys Ther* 1998;78:766–777.
24. Bigos S, Bowyer O, Braen G. *Acute low back problems in adults.* Clinical Practice Guideline No. 14 Rockville, MD: Agency for Health Care Policy and Research, Public Health Service, US Department of Health and Human Services, 1994.
25. Wipf JE, Deyo RA. Low back pain. *Med Clin North Am* 1995;79:231–246.
26. Fairbank JC, Couper J, Davies JB, O'Brien JP. The Oswestry low back pain disability questionnaire. *Physiotherapy* 1980;66:271–273.
27. Fairbank JC, Pynsent PB. The Oswestry disability index. *Spine* 2000;25:2940–2953.
28. Bellah RD, Summerville DA, Treves ST, Micheli LJ. Low-back pain in adolescent athletes: Detection of stress injury to the pars interarticularis with SPECT. *Radiology* 1991;180:509–512.
29. Weir MR, Smith DS. Stress reaction of the pars interarticularis leading to spondylolysis. A cause of adolescent low back pain. *J Adolesc Health Care* 1989;10:573 577.
30. Fehlandt AF Jr, Micheli LJ. Lumbar facet stress fracture in a ballet dancer. *Spine* 1993;18:2537–2359.

31. Ahern DK, Lohr BA. Psychosocial factors in sports injury rehabilitation. *Clin Sports Med* 1997;16:755–768.
32. Crossman J. Psychological rehabilitation from sports injuries. *Sports Med* 1997;23:333–339.
33. Hemmings B, Povey L. Views of chartered physiotherapists on the psychological content of their practice: A preliminary study in the United Kingdom. *Br J Sports Med* 2002;36:61–64.
34. Nideffer RM. The injured athlete: Psychological factors in treatment. *Orthop Clin North Am* 1993;14:373–385.
35. Fritz JM, George S, Delitto A. The role of fear avoidance beliefs in acute low back pain: Relationships with current and future disability and work status. *Pain* 2001;94:7–15.
36. Burton AK, Tillotson KM, Main CJ, Hollis S. Psychosocial predictors of outcome in acute and subchronic low back trouble. *Spine* 1995;20:722–728.
37. Waddell G, Newton M, Henderson I, Somerville D, Main CJ. A Fear-Avoidance Beliefs Questionnaire (FABQ) and the role of fear-avoidance beliefs in chronic low back pain and disability. *Pain* 1993;52:157–168.
38. George SZ, Fritz JM, Erhard RE. The comparison of fear avoidance beliefs in patients with cervical pain and patients with lumbar pain. *Spine* 2001;26:2139–2145.
39. George SZ. Characteristics of patients with lower extremity symptoms treated with slump stretching: A case series. *J Orthop Sports Phys Ther* 2002;32:391–398.
40. George SZ. Differential diagnosis and treatment for a patient with lower extremity symptoms. *J Orthop Sports Phys Ther* 2000;30:468–472.
41. Delitto A, Snyder-Mackler L. The diagnostic process: Examples in orthopedic physical therapy. *Phys Ther* 1995;75:203–211.
42. McKenzie RA. *The lumbar spine: Mechanical diagnosis and therapy.* Waikanaie, New Zealand: Spinal Publications Limited, 1989.
43. Fritz JM, George S. The use of a classification approach to identify subgroups of patients with acute low back pain. Interrater reliability and short-term treatment outcomes. *Spine* 2000;25:106–114.
44. Grieve GP. *Mobilisation of the spine. A primary handbook of clinical method*, 5th ed. London, UK: Churchill Livingstone, 1991.
45. Vlaeyen JW, Linton SJ. Fear-avoidance and its consequences in chronic musculoskeletal pain: A state of the art. *Pain* 2000;85:317–332.
46. Burton AK, Waddell G, Tillotson KM, Summerton N. Information and advice to patients with back pain can have a positive effect. A randomized controlled trial of a novel educational booklet in primary care. *Spine* 1999;24:2484–2491.
47. Lindstrom I, Ohlund C, Eek C, et al. The effect of graded activity on patients with subacute low back pain: A randomized prospective clinical study with an operant-conditioning behavioral approach. *Phys Ther* 1992;72:279–290.
48. Fritz JM, Irrgang JJ. A comparison of a modified Oswestry Low Back Pain Disability Questionnaire and the Quebec Back Pain Disability Scale. *Phys Ther* 2001;81:776–788.
49. Fritz JM, Erhard RE, Hagen BF. Segmental instability of the lumbar spine. *Phys Ther* 1998;78:889–896.
50. McGill SM. Low back exercises: Evidence for improving exercise regimens. *Phys Ther* 1998;78:754–765.
51. Axler CT, McGill SM. Low back loads over a variety of abdominal exercises: Searching for the safest abdominal challenge. *Med Sci Sports Exerc* 1997;29:804–811.
52. McGill SM. Distribution of tissue loads in the low back during a variety of daily and rehabilitation tasks. *J Rehabil Res Dev* 1997;34:448–458.
53. McGill SM. The mechanics of torso flexion: Situps and standing dynamic flexion manoeuvres. *Clin Biomech (Bristol, Avon)* 1995;10:184–192.
54. Callaghan JP, Gunning JL, McGill SM. The relationship between lumbar spine load and muscle activity during extensor exercises. *Phys Ther* 1998;78:8–18.
55. Callaghan JP, McGill SM. Muscle activity and low back loads under external shear and compressive loading. *Spine* 1995;20:992–998.
56. O'Sullivan PB, Phyty GD, Twomey LT, Allison GT. Evaluation of specific stabilizing exercise in the treatment of chronic low back pain with radiologic diagnosis of spondylolysis or spondylolisthesis. *Spine* 1997; 22:2959–2967.
57. O'Sullivan PB, Twomey L, Allison GT. Altered abdominal muscle recruitment in patients with chronic back pain following a specific exercise intervention. *J Orthop Sports Phys Ther* 1998;27:114–124.
58. Hides JA, Richardson CA, Jull GA. Multifidus muscle recovery is not automatic after resolution of acute, first-episode low back pain. *Spine* 1996;21:2763–2769.
59. McGill S, Juker D, Kropf P. Quantitative intramuscular myoelectric activity of quadratus lumborum during a wide variety of tasks. *Clin Biomech (Bristol, Avon)* 1996;11:170–172.
60. Luoto S, Taimela S, Hurri H, Aalto H, Pyykko I, Alaranta H. Psychomotor speed and postural control in chronic low back pain patients A controlled follow-up study. *Spine* 1996;21:2621–2627.
61. Butler DS. *Mobilisation of the nervous system*, 1st ed. Melbourne, Australia: Churchill Livingstone, 1991.
62. Delitto A, Cibulka MT, Erhard RE, Bowling RW, Tenhula JA. Evidence for use of an extension-mobilization category in acute low back syndrome: A prescriptive validation pilot study. *Phys Ther* 1993;73:216–222.
63. Erhard RE, Delitto A, Cibulka MT. Relative effectiveness of an extension program and a combined program of manipulation and flexion and extension exercises in patients with acute low back syndrome. *Phys Ther* 1994;74:1093–1100.
64. Fritz JM, Delitto A, Erhard RE. Comparison of a classification based approach to physical therapy and therapy based on the AHCPR clinical practice guidelines for patients with acute low back pain: A randomized clinical trial. *Spine* (in review).

CHAPTER

30

CLINICAL MANAGEMENT OF ELITE ATHLETES WITH LOW BACK SYNDROMES

Richard Lehman, Craig E. Morris, Scott Rose, and Greg Roskopf

OUTLINE

OBJECTIVES

1. Demonstrate the circumstances that make elite athletes with back syndromes uniquely challenging.
2. Outline typical sport-specific mechanisms of injury and briefly recommend common clinical management strategies.
3. Describe the critical timing of the continuum of care from passive to active care for the elite athlete.
4. Describe psychosocial complexities and counseling/management strategies that come into play with elite athletes.
5. Describe in detail sport-specific physical demands and how the understanding of this plays into high-end training.
6. Provide examples of end-range sport-specific training (e.g., proprioceptive, stabilization, plyometrics, weight, and coupled) protocols.
7. Provide suggestions for the prevention of low back injuries for the athlete.

INTRODUCTION

The previous chapter addressed clinical management of back injuries in athletes. While it provides an excellent general overview for treatment, it does not specifically cover an important subgroup among this patient population: the elite athlete recovering from a back-related syndrome. These are the gifted individuals who are seeking more than just symptom resolution and an opportunity to resume an athletic pastime. Indeed, they are focused on the resumption of high-level competitive skills, to be tested against other such similarly gifted and motivated athletes on the field of play.

What are the unique aspects of clinical management for this type of patient? What special understanding is helpful in counseling them and managing their case? What special rehabilitation strategies should be employed and when? Are there sport-specific stereotypical personality traits that, once appreciated, can assist in case management? If they are involved in professional team sports, what influence does the team have on the recuperative process? What types of co-management strategies with other clinicians are helpful?

There has been much written about spinal sports injuries in general. For example, back injuries are estimated to occur in 10%–15% of all sports participants.[1,2] However, much of what has been written regarding injuries in specific sports is anecdotal, and the available literature becomes quite limited as discussion focuses on the elite athletes within their specific sport.

The contributors to this chapter combine several decades of experience in the assessment, treatment, and rehabilitation of elite athletes in a variety of sports at the amateur, collegiate, Olympic, and professional level. The lead author (R.L.) served, or currently serves, as medical director for a number of professional teams in different sports and also as a co-owner of a major professional sports franchise. Hopefully, such combined experience will provide valuable insights into the clinical management of the elite athlete during those periods when a dearth of evidence-based treatment defines the current state of understanding.

BACKGROUND

The majority of back injuries are self-limiting in patients 18 years and older; however, because of the strain that athletes place on their musculoskeletal systems, these injuries can linger.[3] These injuries can preclude the athlete's return to sport, resulting not only in physical and emotional concerns, but also in financial repercussions. Financial repercussions come into play when a sports injury interferes with one's ability to perform his or her work duties. In the case of the highly paid professional athlete, such pecuniary consequences are obviously magnified. In the case of the renowned athlete, socioeconomic sequelae may come into play. Depending on the notoriety of the athletes, the popularity of their sport, their strategic importance to their team, the regional nature the team represents, and the enthusiasm of their fan base, the socioeconomic pressures of injury prevention, early intervention, and appropriate rehabilitation strategies become magnified to ensure that the athletes are available to perform at their optimal level of competition.

Elite Athletes Defined

Defining the elite athlete is no easy task. One may use the measuring stick of being a professional athlete, but this classification appears to have several weaknesses. For example, there are many sports around the globe that are not professionally organized, and amateur organizations may represent the highest level of skill for that particular sport. In addition, promising young athletes who are not yet, but one day may be, professional athletes could certainly be considered elite (or pre-elite). There may also be athletes who, for various geopolitical reasons, are unable to compete at the very highest level of global competition. Of course, gender-based barriers still exist in the world of sports, providing another problem in establishing the requisite definition. Finally, there are sports that hold the Olympic games as the highest level of their competition, requiring a standard of skill that only a subset of the athletes in that sport can attain. Therefore, this chapter will practically define the elite athlete as one who competes at or near the highest level of available competition within the parameters of their age, sport, gender, and geopolitical environment.

The Unique Elite Athlete

In order to appreciate the challenges presented with the injured elite athlete, it becomes necessary to understand a little about what makes them unique in athletics and outstanding in their chosen field of sport. From the horseracing jockey to the basketball center to the sumo wrestler, no specific body type or even degree of leanness becomes a prerequisite to belong to this select group. What common aspects do they share? In a time when stereotyping may be unpopular, the authors have observed the following *generally* shared traits among elite athletes:

1. Elite athletes generally share a remarkable degree of determination and discipline, at least regarding their sport. For example, they are the individuals one might see jogging in the rain, swimming in a frigid ocean during the winter, bicycling in the desert during a searing summer day, or shooting

pucks at a goal in the dark on a frozen pond long after the other teammates went home.

2. Elite athletes tend to carry a burning passion for their sport. Stories are legion regarding various sports heroes who endured incredible hardship to play their beloved game. They often continue their involvement by coaching, scouting, or administrating their sport following their playing days in order to remain close to the environment.
3. Elite athletes generally love the thrill of competition. When they are away from their sport, perhaps during an off-season, they tend to play other sports with an astonishingly competitive zeal.
4. Elite athletes seem to have the capacity for amazing degrees of focus. From the golfer putting for a victory in front of a packed gallery to the batter who hits the clinching home run in the World Series, these individuals concentrate and perform well under circumstances where the average person or athlete cannot. Indeed, they tend to relax and improve their skills in such situations, looking for, perhaps insisting on, the opportunity to excel. Recent research demonstrates that elite athletes indeed have different levels of neurophysiological function than the mediocre athlete. High-level golfers showed much lower levels of neural activity than moderate golfers when imagining their golf swing during functional magnetic resonance imaging (MRI).[4]
5. The elite athlete can be extremely demanding, much more so than their less athletic counterparts. They realize that each day without training or competition can compromise their skill level and endanger their competitiveness. This demanding nature does not diminish with time and continued success. The great athlete, in the early part of his or her career, is willing to compromise. Basically this means that the athlete is happy to be in the position of success and unwilling compromise is not a driving factor. However, with continued success comes notoriety and increased expectations. Increased notoriety brings celebrity status, causing a transition in focus and determination and a diminished capacity for compromise.
6. While one of the clinician's greatest challenges may be to motivate most patients to perform exercise, the opposite challenge often occurs with the elite athlete. These uniquely driven individuals are at risk of early activity or exercises resumption or even overtraining syndrome (to be discussed later). Resumption of activities too soon can undermine the recovery process, as does overly aggressive exercise.

In summary, the physician who takes care of these athletes must understand their psyche, their drive, the pressures and expectations placed upon them, their competitive spirit, and demanding nature. The clinician must anticipate these traits, personalize them to the specific individual, and establish a strategy that capitalizes on such characteristics.

Clinical Pearl: High-level golfers showed much lower levels of neural activity than moderate golfers when imagining their golf swing during functional MRI.

SPINAL INJURIES

There are no established injury-prone profiles for athletes. Only competition anxiety has been associated with injury occurrence.[5] However, the greatest risk of low back injury for the athlete lies in the area of recurrence. In a large ($N = 679$) prospective study, Greene et al. demonstrated a threefold greater risk of college athletes with a history of prior low back injury than among those with no such history.[6]

Clinical Pearl: The greatest risk of low back injury for the athlete lies in the area of recurrence.

Back injuries in elite athletes are minimally related to back injuries in the general public. They at least compromise their performance and, in the worst cases, are career-ending. For example, financial losses to professional sports franchises based on back injuries can be staggering. Each athlete represents a significant investment and an acknowledged risk by the organization. The injured athlete, disabled with back pain, represents costs that include treatment and perhaps lost revenues if the team's competitiveness is compromised. Injuries can indeed ravage teams, interfering with their competing in lucrative postseason competitions. The majority of back injuries are self-limiting. Most of these injuries are soft tissue injuries and are due to musculoskeletal overload or imbalance. The authors in this textbook have addressed the epidemiological aspects of back syndromes in the adult population. The stereo typical aspects of back-related disability, including deconditioning and job dissatisfaction, generally do not apply to the elite athlete subgroup. Instead, the disability-related factors are more often related to over-training and performance anxiety involving a sport in which they are passionately involved. These injuries have many facets: (1) They preclude the athlete's return to sports, resulting in emotional and physical concerns; (2) There are financial ramifications. Financial pressures create an emotional situation that places further stress on the inability to resolve low back pain and low back injury; (3) Sports such as football and ice hockey have created pressure to become bigger, stronger, and faster. Low back biomechanics and functional stability is well addressed in Chapters 4 and 5, and these issues may be magnified in such instances. Conditioning standards, including endurance and strength aspects, have increased over the years in elite athletes, perhaps more so than the adaptive anatomical properties of the involved, loaded tissues.

SPORT-SPECIFIC BACK INJURIES

Injuries in elite athletes are frequently sport-specific. The loads, skills, and stresses required are unique to each sport, and perhaps unique to each position within that sport. For example, the demands placed upon the ice hockey goalie are quite different from the ice hockey forward. Gymnasts commonly have extension overload in their lower lumbar spine and thoracic spine. Sprinters and hockey players tend toward flexion overload, with tight hip flexors and anterior/posterior imbalance. Baseball players and javelin throwers have torsional stress in the lumbar spine and rib cage. Stereotypical injuries for various sports are discussed in greater detail later in the chapter.

Despite the presence of sport-specific risk factors, each injured player may nevertheless have unique circumstances that require individual attention for both assessment and treatment. It is imperative to understand the sport, the sport-specific position and the common imbalances, and prior injuries and treatment patterns that are required for every sport, for this understanding can lead to clinical shortcuts. It is always preferable to view the athlete either on videotape or in person performing his or her specific activity. For example, the lead author commonly watches videotape, preferably with slow motion footage, in sports injuries, to review both the mechanism of injury and the common movement patterns performed during the specific athletic function. Typical injuries encountered in various sports will be addressed below.

Clinical Pearl: Despite the presence of sport-specific risk factors, each injured player may nevertheless have unique circumstances that require individual attention for both assessment and treatment.

CONTRASTING SYNDROMES: DECONDITIONING AND OVERTRAINING

An excellent example of the extreme nature of the management of athletes involves the two contrasting syndromes known as deconditioning and overtraining. The elite athlete is at increased risk of each scenario and the clinician must be diligent to guard against the presence of each.

Deconditioning Syndrome

One of the primary concerns of an athlete who experiences low back injury is that he or she becomes deconditioned during the early stages of rehabilitation. Deconditioning appears to quickly affect exercise performance in some athletes. How soon can these effects occur? In one study, endurance athletes, strength athletes, and a sedentary control group were subjected to a brief period of bed rest.[7] The endurance group demonstrated a measurable reduction exercises performance (reduced oxygen uptake and decreased lactate thresholds) and modifications in neurohormonal response (earlier increase in norepinephrine and attenuated increase in human growth hormone) following only 3 days of bed rest, while the other two groups demonstrated no significant changes. Two weeks of bed rest was found to effect thermoregulatory function during exercise.[8] What changes occur in elite athletes who substantially reduce their training regimen, but not to the extreme of bed rest? Maron et al. demonstrated that there was an average loss of left cardiac ventricular septal wall thickness (from 15.8 mm to 10.5 mm) among six 1988 Seoul Olympians (rowers and canoeists) who volunteered to significantly reduce their training for a mean of 13 weeks.[9]

In order to maximize the effects of the rehabilitation process and reduce the deleterious affects of deconditioning, the rehabilitation specialist must be creative in ways to continue to condition the athlete during the acute phase of a back injury. The athlete may need to completely unload the spine by performing cardiovascular training on a stationary cycle in a supine position (see Fig. 30–1). A lumbar roll can be placed under the low back to provide additional support. This position approach holds an additional

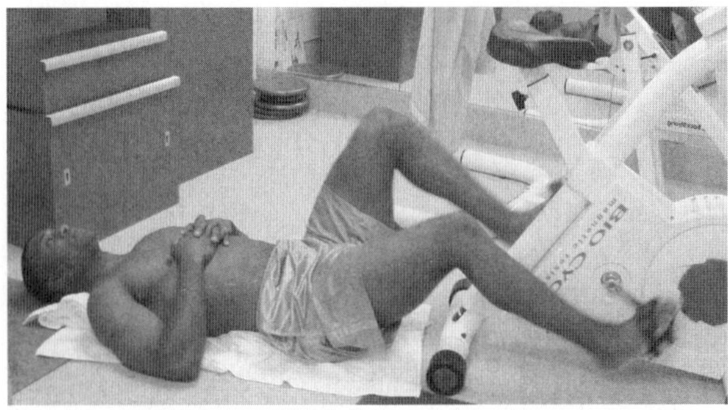

FIGURE 30–1. Avoiding deconditioning. Placing the athlete behind a stationary bicycle in a supine position effectively promotes cardiovascular conditioning with minimal loading to the low back. Upper extremity resistance training utilizing, for example, dumbbells can provide additional benefit.

benefit in that the arms remain free to perform various types of simultaneous exercise.

Another strategy to avoid deconditioning in the early and middle stages of injury involves the use of pool therapy, which protects against gravitational overload. This topic is discussed in Chapter 27.

As his or her condition improves, the athlete can progress into an upright position by sitting on the stationary bike. As the athlete becomes more comfortable with gravitational forces and maintenance of postural alignment, the athlete can continue to progress, for example, to retro walking on the treadmill. By walking backwards on a treadmill, the athlete can begin to train the body to respond to ground reaction forces, while minimizing the stresses being transferred into the low back. Retro walking on the treadmill helps to minimize the vertical forces being transmitted up through the spine.

Overtraining Syndrome

Despite receiving much attention in the literature and press, *overtraining syndrome* (OTS) remains an elusive and confusing subject. It can simply be described as an imbalance between an athlete's training and his or her recovery,[10] a scenario in which there is a decrease in physical performance despite heavy training. OTS has also been referred to in the literature as *staleness syndrome.*[11] One study found that 37% of a large group ($N = 272$) of young elite athletes reported experiencing the symptoms of staleness syndrome at least once.[11]

OTS appears to be, at least in part, a neuroendocrine disorder,[12] perhaps of a dysfunctional hypothalamic–pituitary axis response.[10] OTS-related hemorheological responses, such as mild plasma hyperviscosity and erythrocytic hyperaggregability, have also been found.[13] Finally, OTS athletes demonstrated diminished intramuscular utilization of carbohydrates with decreased maximum anaerobic lactic acid energy supply during short-endurance "stress tests" (110% of the individual anaerobic threshold until volitional exhaustion).[14]

The classic statement is that the athlete experiencing OTS has the feeling of "heavy legs," even after reasonable rest periods, a statement that has been noted in multiple languages involving several sports.[13,15] Perhaps the other early signs may be psychological in nature, as athletes tend to have sleep disorders and depression.[15] This may, however, be tied to other stressors, such as heavy training determined by the athlete as monotonous,[16] or by a less-than-positive relationship with the coach.[11,17]

Clinical Pearl: The classic statement is that the athlete experiencing OTS has the feeling of "heavy legs,"even after reasonable rest periods, a statement that has been noted in multiple languages involving several sports.

OTS has been discussed as an increased risk factor for athletic injury[17,18] although this is yet to be proven. In any case, there does appear to be sufficient evidence to appreciate the overall performance risks involved. Therefore, how does one determine the presence of OTS and what can be done for the condition?

Despite what appears to be a plethora of recent clinical interest in OTS, there has been little, if any, advances in effective tools available regarding its diagnosis.[15,19] Kentta and Hassmen suggested that failure to fully recover within 72 hours presumes the athlete has overtrained.[20] However, the clinical team and coaches must be sensitive to the status of their athletes, regarding their emotional and physical conditioning. It would appear that a combination of an athlete's mood changes, sleep problems, a feeling of "heavy legs," undergoing a heavy exercise schedule, resuming training while still very fatigued, and poor relationship with the coach (or perhaps other close authority figure) should provide adequate information to arrive at the diagnosis. While prolonged rest may be counterproductive and cause some deconditioning, a reasonably reduced physical training program with longer rest periods and improved interpersonal communication appear to be the answer to this potential problem.[11,21] Another strategy that may be integrated with others is that of periodization, which is discussed later in the chapter.

Burnout Syndrome

Burnout syndrome appears to have many similar traits with OTS. Athletes with this scenario are typically involved in a similar heavy training program and have parallel symptoms. The difference with burnout syndrome is that the athletes with this syndrome lose their motivation for training.[11] The lead authors (R.L. and C.M.) find that athletes at high risk for burnout are those pre-elite juniors and are involved in non-team sports (discussed later in the chapter), such as tennis, figure skating, and gymnastics. Emotional immaturity is often a factor as this often appears during adolescence.

Another additional stress factor for this group may be that their season lasts virtually all year, providing little, if any, time away from the rigors involved with their sport. Conversely, team sports typically have a regular season and a relatively lengthy off-season, providing a physical and emotional respite. Many gifted teenagers experiencing burnout simply quit their sport. The clinician who understands and anticipates burnout can have a major impact in helping to maintain the athletes' interest and enthusiasm and allow their continued participation.[21]

THE DYNAMIC NATURE OF SPORTS MEDICINE

In evaluating the lumbar spine in athletic injuries, there is no "cookbook" approach. How does one develop the clinical tools to effectively work in this dynamic field? The sports medicine clinician must have a clear understanding of the biomechanical, anatomical, psychological, and functional challenges associated with the sport and then progress watching the sport either live or on tape. The greater the understanding of the individual sport, the better insights can be developed as clinical tools for the specialist.

As previously mentioned, the authors have encountered stereotypical types of sport-specific injuries. Some of the risks in various sports have been addressed in the literature and are duly referenced, while others are empirical and should be integrated with this understanding. Injuries associated with the following popular sports are presented below.

Gymnastics

Gymnastics is considered a high-risk sport for the development of a back syndrome.[22] Thirteen percent of gymnastic injuries are to the spine and trunk.[23] The majority of these injuries seem to occur during practice and training.[24]

In elite gymnasts, most of the activities that are deleterious to the spine are extension injuries. Pars defects and muscle strain injuries are common. In one study, 86% of a group of elite rhythmic gymnasts reported back pain.[25] These athletes need to be examined very carefully and clinicians must separate hyperflexion and hyperextension injuries. The patient is generally not aware of a grade 1 pars defect. In a grade 2 defect there is a vertical sacrum and a loss of hip extension, as well as tightness in the hamstrings, which limits sports participation.[3]

Pelvic stress fractures have been well documented among gymnasts.[26] Athletes with marked or persistent back pain are typically referred for bone scan (scintigraphy) and MRI to rule out occult stress fracture. Facet injuries in older gymnasts are common and these athletes have classic facet-type complaints (see Chapter 8). One risk factor in female gymnasts is their excessive flexibility combined with their extensive training regimen. Nadler et al., in a prospective study, demonstrated that the highest incidence of low back pain occurred in females who demonstrated hypermobility or overuse when compared with less flexible athletes and those with measured leg discrepancy.[27]

Male gymnasts are also at increased risk of back syndromes. Sward et al. demonstrated that significantly greater incidence and severity of back pain occurred in this group compared to male wrestlers, tennis players, and soccer players.[28]

Gymnasts usually have excessive flexibility and *relatively* limited strength. The lead author feels their strength/flexibility ratio is diminished, creating lumbar region end-range mobility overload. They also tend to have anterior/posterior muscular imbalance at the level of the shoulder and lumbopelvic regions, creating a postural imbalance (upper and lower crossed syndromes; see Chapter 13).

Treatment and rehabilitation of gymnastics injuries should be a continuum. Sensorimotor and lumbopelvic (including intrinsic and extrinsic; see Chapter 29) training and core (intrinsic trunk) training provide an important functional base prior to returning to the gym. The authors recommend the trainers and coaches integrate a tumble track and specific body positioning to reeducate the athletes to avoid activities that may overload their back. This is an extremely important concept, as athletes must understand how they were injured in order to more effectively avoid recurrences.

There are basically two seasons in gymnastics. The first season begins when the athlete develops new skills and the second season begins when the actual competition commences. Because of this dual season, gymnasts have a very short off-season and continual pressure for progression of more advanced skills. These translate into increased stress, both emotional and physical. The clinician must therefore be sensitive to OTS or burnout syndrome (which was previously discussed). This has to be understood and the athlete needs to be counseled as such. The authors feel that the psychological aspects are more important in the care of gymnasts than of any other athlete. Their level of success and their expectations need to be carefully monitored. The interaction between counselor, parents, clinician, coach, and athlete is extremely important.

Golf

Low back pain in golfers is not uncommon. Up to 90% of amateur and professional golfers total injuries are cervical or lumbar spine related.[29] Asymmetrical torsional stresses associated with the golf swing are believed to be a key etiological factor. Interestingly, one study attributed no increased risk of disc herniation to golf.[30]

Little time swinging a golf club teaches one that this maneuver is indeed complex. Increasing understanding teaches one that each golfer's swing is unique. The lead author finds that there is a difference between golfers and other athletes, in that low back torsional stress occurs in golfers when their swing is efficient, fluid, and correct. The concept may be difficult to understand. It is impossible to "unload the lumbar spine" in an appropriate golf swing because in the elite golfer, the appropriate golf swing creates spinal torque. Golfers tend to have strong lumbar extensors, but show imbalance in lateral flexors and rotators of the spine. Therefore, assessing and addressing lumbopelvic muscular imbalance is recommended.[31] Because the golfing position is hip-flexed, tight hip flexors and weak abdominal strength are understandable. As such, corrective stretching and strengthening strategies need to be very delineated.

Clinical Pearl: Up to 90% of amateur and professional golfers total injuries are cervical or lumbar spine related. Asymmetrical torsional stresses associated with the golf swing are believed to be a key etiological factor.

It is imperative to imitate each elite golfer's golf swing to understand the torque being placed at the level of the ankles, knees, hips, lumbar spine, mid back, and shoulders. Again, the authors prefer to review a videotape of the swing. The processes of the back swing and follow-through are evaluated. Postural knee imbalances and shoulder positioning are evaluated. Proprioceptive feedback while striking the ball is important. When this evaluation is completed, pelvic imbalance needs to be closely followed and a pattern of hip flexor tightness, mid trunk weakness, and torsional overload at the facet joints is generally identified.

Because of the ballistic asymmetrical trunk rotation in a flexed position, even the elite golfer's refined swing subjects the spine to torsional overload.

Football (American Rules)

Football is considered a high-risk sport for back syndromes.[20] Up to 50% of football linemen suffer a disabling back injury at one point in their career.[32] Interior linemen commonly have stress fractures of the spine and require complete resolution to be able to return to their sport.[32,33]

Typical injuries include pars defects, vertebral fractures, and disc injuries.[22,32] These may be due to flexion overload, extension overload, or to contact/collision injuries.[22,34]

Interestingly, the greatest risk of disc herniation may be attributable as much or more to training for football, specifically weight lifting, rather than to playing the sport itself.[35] If true, the contradiction in risk of disc injury between the competitive weight lifter, as discussed below, and the football player who is weight lifting suggests that technique may be an important risk factor. While the training program for the weight lifter may emphasize effective lifting techniques, the football training may emphasize effective football techniques more so than safe weight-lifting methods.

Clinical Pearl: Typical injuries include pars defects, vertebral fractures, and disc injuries. These may be due to flexion overload, extension overload, or to contact/collision injuries.

The majority of football injuries seem to occur during practice and training.[24] Because of the above-noted risk factors, Gerbino and d'Hemecourt found football players to be at increased risk of degenerative spinal disease compared to the general population.[34]

Soccer (Futbol)

Soccer players appear to be at increased risk for low back pain. This seems to be true for both young and older athletes.

Low back pain was the third most prevalent injury (14%) among a large group ($N = 496$) of young male soccer players, behind knee (26%) and ankle injuries (23%).[36]

Another study demonstrated that former soccer players have a higher level of low back pain compared to shooters and long distance runners, although there was no difference in frequency of pain.[37]

Lumbar disc herniations have been documented among soccer players, with one study noting a higher frequency than among basketball, tennis, and handball athletes.[38]

Pubic stress fractures are also well documented in soccer players, probably more so than in any other sport.[26,39] Stress fractures also have been reported at the ischial tuberosity, anterior superior iliac spine (ASIS), and anterior inferior iliac spine (AIIS).[26]

Painful insertion of the adductors at the pubic bone, defined in the literature by names such as pubalgia, pubialgia, traumatic osteitis pubis, pubic pain syndrome, and gracilis syndrome, among soccer players are also well documented.[40–42]

Baseball and Softball

Baseball and softball players tend develop trunk overload because of throwing and batting. This overload is generally asymmetrical unless the player is a switch-hitter (i.e., bats both left- and right-handed). The overload is generally rotational combined with either flexion or extension, increasing the risk of back injury. Injuries due to lumbar instability have been noted among softball players.[17]

Conte et al. noted that among Major League Baseball players, the number of players and the number of player days on the disabled list have increased over an 11-year period.[43] There was no known reason for this increase, although the authors reasonably determined that such a trend deserves further attention.

One study found that injuries arise in baseball almost equally during practice (46%) and in games

(54%), with 15% of the injuries occurring in the low back.[44]

Clinical Pearl: Among Major League Baseball players, the number of players and the number of player days on the disabled list have increased over an 11-year period.

Shaffer et al. used electromyographic studies to analyze the baseball swing.[45] They concluded that the maintained, high-level muscle activity in the trunk muscles underlines the importance of back, abdominal, and rotational exercises.

Weight Lifting

Weight lifting is considered a high-risk sport for low back syndromes.[22] Back injuries are responsible for 30%–50% of injuries in weight lifters occurring at a rate of 0.43 injuries per 1000 hours of lifting.[22,30,46,47,48] In one study, weight lifters sustained far more low back injuries than did power lifters.[45]

Interesting research results have surfaced over the past few years regarding weight lifting. At first glance, these findings may appear to be contradictory. In one strong study, weight lifters have not been found to have an increased rate of disc herniation.[30] However, a significant decrease in disc height was present in retired weight lifters compared to retired wrestlers and a control group.[49]

Perhaps there may be issues to be learned from these results. First, the brief nature of the lifting maneuver requires anaerobic energy utilization, reducing the risk of injury due to fatigue occurring in sports requiring prolonged, global energy expenditure.[50] Also, competitive weight lifters may better appreciate the spinal risks involved with lifting extraordinarily heavy weight, more so than an athlete skilled in another sport who lifts for strength training. Therefore, a heavy emphasis would be placed on proper mechanics by the competition weight lifter for the sake of safety, with the added benefit of greater lifting capacity while using such techniques. Hence, optimized mechanics provides a double incentive for the competition weight lifter by increasing safety and chances of success in the sport.

Given these assumptions, it would seem logical that weight lifters would have less chance of disc herniation because of decreased fatigue and their focus on optimal lifting mechanics. Of course, continuing to lift for years, perhaps decades, may then have a cumulative effect on the low back, culminating in diminished disc height as noted above.

Basketball

Basketball players commonly develop low back syndromes, although far less frequently than injuries to the knees and ankles.[51,52] Meeuwisse et al. found that injuries occur more often during games than during practice and that centers tend to have the greatest frequency of injury.[53]

Disc herniations have been documented among basketball players.[38] Compared with other popular sports, relatively little has been written about spinal injuries in this group.

Tennis

Tennis players do not appear to develop low back syndromes more frequently than the general public.[54] However, the back problems they encounter may be due to asymmetrical trunk rotation, lateral flexion, and extension, in addition to weak trunk flexors, as occurring with the serve and overhead strokes.[55,56] Asymmetrical trunk loading may also account for increased prevalence of mild scoliosis among tennis players.[57]

More than most sports, tennis technique appears to be vital in injury prevention, including low back injury.[56,58]

Track and Field

No topic comprises such disparate physical requirements as the group of individual sports that fall under this heading. From the javelin throw to the marathon, from pole vaulting to the high jump, the variety of injuries that can lead to low back syndromes is immense, far too detailed for this brief overview. Nevertheless, a few common issues can be addressed that may help to demonstrate how low back syndromes affect this group of athletes. For example, Aggrawal et al. found a higher incidence of backache among track and field athletes than among weight lifters.[59]

Information also exists among select track and field subgroups. For example, quite a lot has been written about the high incidence of spondylolysis and spondylolisthesis among javelin throwers,[60,61] while pole vaulting has received less attention on this topic.[62] The asymmetrical, dynamic spinal loading of throwing the javelin appears to be associated with an increased incidence of mild scoliosis.[55]

Track and field runners are not exempt from low back syndromes. Reports of injuries include sacral stress fracture,[63,64] pelvic stress fractures,[26] and herniated discs.[65]

Clinical Pearl: Quite a lot has been written about the high incidence of spondylolysis and spondylolisthesis among javelin throwers, while pole vaulting has received less attention on this topic.

Swimming

Back pain in swimmers is not very common.[22] It is generally seen because of a mechanical imbalance of the hips and sacroiliac joints. These athletes commonly have great trunk strength based on training and rarely develop low back problems.

Previous sports involving hyperextension and rotational loading were associated with pars fracture, with adolescence being the age of greatest risk.[62] Diving appears to fit into this high-risk group.[62] In addition to divers, others at risk for spondylolysis are butterfly and breaststroke swimmers.[66]

Ice Hockey

Lumbopelvic injuries are common among ice hockey players. One multiregional study found that 25% of all ice hockey games missed because of injury were from lumbopelvic injury (15% groin and 10% back).[67]

Being the fastest of all team sports, collision injuries in ice hockey are common.[68] Checking from behind has been isolated as a key risk factor, and one study demonstrated a reduction in neck and back injuries once a "back checking" rule was introduced.[69] However, injury rates among males and females were found to be quite similar, despite the fact that intentional body checking is prohibited among females.[70]

Ice hockey injuries occur during game situations (i.e., either actual competition or during intrasquad games) far more often than during training situations, with one study measuring greater than a 20:1 ratio.[71] Goalies appear to be at least risks for injury, while forwards have the greatest risk during practice and defensemen during game situations.[72]

Clinical Pearl: Ice hockey injuries occur during game situations (i.e., either actual competition or during intrasquad games) far more often than during training situations, with one study measuring greater than a 20:1 ratio.

Maintaining one's balance in a contact sport played on ice is of paramount importance. Stability is maximized by lowering one's center of gravity with partial hip and knee flexion, while maintaining an erect upper torso via thoracolumbar extension (the so-called *hockey posture*). While this strategy allows for optimal bipedal stability on the ice, there are distinct disadvantages due to altered postural mechanics and uniquely increased risks of injury. The hockey posture tends to create a chronic hypertonicity of the iliopsoas, single-joint hip adductors, rectus femoris, hamstrings, tensor fascia lata (TFL)/iliotibial band, piriformis, and thoracolumbar erector spinae. In contrast, a relative weakness occurs in the abdominals, gluteals (maximi, medii, and minimi), and the lumbosacral erector spinae. Janda described this postural imbalance as the "lower crossed syndrome," which is discussed in Chapter 13. Also discussed is the limited resultant hip extensibility and subsequent "false hip extension" involving increased lumbosacral sagittal motion. For example, professional ice hockey players were found to have significantly decreased mean hip extension compared to age-matched controls.[73]

In addition to the risks associated with high-velocity contact and postural stresses, the asymmetrical rotatory loads placed upon the hockey player while striking the puck (i.e., "slapshot") are similar to those discussed with baseball batting and javelin throwing.

Another risk factor to be addressed for the ice hockey player is that of fatigue. Hockey forwards and defensemen play recurrent shifts entailing a redundant routine of ice skating sprints for 30–80 seconds separated by 3- or 4-minute rests. This is performed 30 or more times per game, increasing the risk of fatigue-related injury.

Smith et al. demonstrated significant predictability for hockey injuries due to increased measures of low vigor and high fatigue among high school athletes.[74]

Despite the relatively detailed information regarding the causative aspects, there is a relative paucity of literature detailing specific types of hockey injuries. One study discusses sacroiliac dysfunction and adductor strains as common injuries.[70] The significant loading of the single-joint adductors and subsequent injury has been highlighted in the literature.[74,75] Pars fractures during adolescence have also been discussed.[62] Nevertheless, the lead authors (R.L. and C.M.) commonly encounter iliopsoas and lower abdominal strains or tears. Less often, facet syndrome, disc injuries, and sacroiliac dysfunction are encountered.

In a recent study, a successful prevention strategy for ice hockey players was described by Tyler et al.,[76] in which a strengthening program of the hip adductors effectively reduced the frequency of adductor strains (11 incidents in 2 years was reduced to 3 incidents during the same period). Such reports provide valuable insights into the preventative aspects of elite athletes in sports with similar risks, an incentive for other sports medicine teams to initiate and report on innovative preventative programs.

Volleyball

These athletes tend to develop overuse injuries, with the low back as the most common problem (19%) among elite beach volleyball players.[77]

Lower back injury rates (11%) have been noted in regular (i.e., playing on a hard surface rather than on sand) volleyball, although this statistic appears to be qualified because of the dramatic increase in ankle injuries on the hard surface. A second study found 14.2% of injuries occurring in the back, with female athletes demonstrating a higher incidence of overall injury.

In a study that emphasizes the importance of proper sport-specific training and skills, Bartolozzi et al. demonstrated a dramatic increase in intervertebral disc lesions (degeneration, bulging, and herniation) on MRI among volleyball players who trained improperly compared to those who trained using proper protocols (21%).[78]

Sacral stress fracture has been reported among volleyball players. Although considered quite rare, it does demonstrate the dynamic spinal extension associated with this sport.[63]

The "spiking" maneuver of the volleyball player tends to create asymmetrical extension, lateral flexion, and rotational overload of the trunk. The lead authors observe thoracolumbar pain in this group.

Clinical Pearl: Sacral stress fracture has been reported among volleyball players. Although considered quite rare, it does demonstrate the dynamic spinal extension associated with this sport.

SUMMARY OF SPORT-SPECIFIC INJURIES

A significant distinction exists between the volume and quality of scientific literature regarding athletic low back syndromes and the popularity and mass appeal of the sports discussed. The research has merely started to understand the etiological aspects of each sport and subdivisions therein. Finally, some questions must be asked regarding the quality of many of the papers regarding sport-specific injuries. For example, one paper discussed low back injuries among soccer, basketball, field athletics, tennis, and handball athletes, later noting that one of the tennis players was actually injured while skiing.[38] To be more specific, should an injury of a football player injured during weight training be considered a football injury, a weighlifting injury, or perhaps fall under a third category, such as football cross-training injury? Researchers must be cautious regarding their reporting of individual injuries and clinicians must be equally diligent in screening for confounding issues that would reduce research reliability before utilizing the results in their sports programs.

Nevertheless, some distinctions can be noted among the sports that suggest patterns for clinical management. For example, in some sports, such as hockey, injuries tend to occur more during competition, while in others, such as in gymnastics, they occur during practice. Some injuries tend toward posterior arch injury, such as in gymnastics, while others tend toward pubic avulsion fracture, such as in soccer. There is some evidence that proper training regimens and psychosocial factors can reduce injury rates. Furthermore, emphasizing proper techniques and skills also accomplishes these goals while improving performance. It therefore behooves the medical team member to gain a great deal of knowledge in the sport, or sports, he or she oversees. The majority of the necessary understanding far exceeds what has been described above. Nevertheless, an understanding of what the literature has proven, what is suggested, and what has been disproven is required knowledge and forms a cornerstone for management.

INDIVIDUAL VERSUS TEAM SPORTS

Various sports can be divided into three categories: (1) individual sports, such as singles tennis and golf; (2) team sports, such as baseball, football, soccer, or hockey; and (3) semi-team sports, in which the athlete is part of a team, but competes on an individual basis, such as gymnastics and also track and field (except for the relay races).

Psychosocial strategies for elite athletic rehabilitation can be tempered depending on which of the above categories the athlete is involved. Indeed, research suggests that athletes involved in team sports typically establish more effective coping strategies and require greater degrees of social support from teammates than athletes involved in individual sports.[79,80]

A great deal of pressure can be applied by one's teammates to return to team sports, which may be helpful or harmful. This places another element of complexity in managing the injured team sport athlete. Because of this additional stress and the athlete's emotional need to fulfill his or her responsibility, decisions may be made by the athlete that are not medically directed well. It is very important for the medical and coaching team to clearly understand the situation both physically and socially in returning the athlete to his or her previous sports activities. The athlete who returns to training and competition too soon and plays in excessive pain tends to develop faulty movement patterns, reducing his or her skill level and increasing the risk of recurrent or subsequent injury. In cases where the player seems too anxious to resume training or competition following a significant injury (possibly because of social pressures from teammates, for example), the authors recommend the athlete be removed from the specific environment. The authors generally isolate the athlete in an off-site training program with a specialist in functional restoration. It is important for the sports medicine team to identify potential problem areas such as these, move swiftly to resolve the issue, and communicate often.

MANAGEMENT STRATEGIES

Treatment and management strategies for low back syndromes are discussed in other chapters. However, a few strategies will be addressed here that pertain specifically to this chapter.

Stretching Strategies

Pre- and postexercise stretching remains one of the universal hallowed traditions in the sports world. However, in a time of increasing curiosity and clinical scrutiny, no approach goes unchallenged.

The anecdotal rationale for pregame stretching has been to increase mobility and lengthen soft tissues in order to improve performance and reduce the risk of injury. The anecdotal rationale for postgame stretching was to reduce the risk of muscle soreness.

Two recent systematic reviews of stretching failed to support the value of stretching in the reduction of injury,[81,82] one of which also noted that pre- or postexercise stretching does not reduce the risk of soreness.[81] Finally, a review of the literature also found insufficient evidence to determine the effects of stretching on sports performance.[81]

To date, no method has demonstrated strong scientific evidence of efficacious prevention or treatment of delayed onset muscle soreness, commonly accepted as the result of muscle damage occurring in the early stages of exposure to eccentric muscle exercise.[83]

Clinical Pearl: Two recent systematic reviews of stretching failed to support the value of stretching in the reduction of injury, one of which also noted that pre- or postexercise stretching does not reduce the risk of soreness.

Complications from Therapeutic Modalities

Therapeutic modalities are also tools commonly used in the treatment of musculoskeletal injuries, and this is certainly true in the sports world. A recent large ($N = 905$) survey of athletic trainers by Nadler et al. surprisingly found that cryotherapy accounted for the greatest percentage of complications (42%), followed by electrical stimulation (29%) and therapeutic heat (7%).[84]

Disc Surgery Among Elite Athletes

Conservative management of disc injuries has been proven to have a high rate of success in the general population.[85] Nevertheless, surgical intervention is at times needed when nonoperative measures fail. Wang et al. reported that 9 out of 14 elite athletes with a mean age of 20.7 years successfully returned to sports.[86] Mochida et al. compared 30 elite athletes who underwent percutaneous nucleotomy with 42 nonathletes who underwent the same procedure. Interestingly, the athletes had poorer outcomes, which the authors attributed largely to the athletes' early return to vigorous sports activity.[87] As stated earlier in this chapter, the challenge with the athlete, in contrast with the nonathlete, can be trying to halt their premature training in order for proper healing and a structured rehabilitation program to be performed. In a larger and more recent study, Watkins et al. reported on 60 cases in which professional and Olympic athletes underwent microscopic lumbar discectomy.[88] All but seven of these athletes returned to sport, with the average postsurgical time of 5.2 months. The authors of this study emphasized the importance of a complete trunk stabilization rehabilitation program in the success of these cases.

Pregame Warm-Ups

Another common event is the pregame warm-up. This is designed to increase circulation, loosen muscles, increase flexibility, and prepare the player for the upcoming contest. A recent study brought to light a potential problem with some of the athletesinvolved in pre-game warm-up—those who participate in the warm-up but do not play at the beginning of the game. Ironically, Green et al. found that college volleyball players who returned to the bench after the pregame warm-up demonstrated greater spinal stiffness 30 minutes later than before they warmed up.[89] This suggests that the player would have entered the game with less stiffness if he or she had not warmed up at all, requiring a rethinking of the whole strategy for participants who do not start the game.

Periodization Strategies

Periodization is a method of training an individual to increase maximum performance while reducing the risk of overtraining by varying exercises, intensity, and volume of exercise.[90] Periodization strategies are widely used in the National Football League.[91] They have been used by collegiate women tennis players[92] and by collegiate strength and conditioning coaches.[93]

Restoring Dynamic Stability

Chapter 5 discussed in detail many of the functional aspects of lumbosacral stability. Much remains to be learned regarding this challenging complex topic. Later chapters discussed the importance of this concept in varying degrees and the chapters on rehabilitation demonstrate strategies to restore such function.

It is well established that spinal region pain disrupts the lumbosacral stability and this is also true for athletic injuries.[94] Indeed, factors such as hip muscle imbalance,[95] prior injury to the lower extremities,[96] and prior history of low back pain[97] have all demonstrated measurable dysfunction despite the athlete's asymptomatic presentation. While the exact etiology of post-injury spinal dysfunction appears to be multivariate and poorly understood, an emphasis on restoring and optimizing motor control of stability must occur in the early stages of rehabilitation. Strategies must then be established to integrate these basic functional approaches with other trunk muscular functions, such as respiration.[98] Once this is established, exercises coordinating these activities with extrinsic trunk function (i.e., locally) and then along the kinetic chain (i.e., globally) become appropriate.

A word of caution becomes necessary at this point. The authors have witnessed athletes who were provided inadequate rehabilitation programs and were left with faulty movement and postural patterns, compromising their athletic skills and increasing their risk of injury. In order to perform at the elite level, the athlete must be dynamically stable, capable of withstanding the forces that are transmitted through the body at high levels of competition. The rehabilitation specialist must therefore possess the skill to assess and correct faulty movement patterns of the injured athlete.

Clinical Pearl: While the exact etiology of post-injury spinal dysfunction appears to be multivariate and poorly understood, an emphasis on restoring and optimizing motor control of stability must occur in the early stages of rehabilitation. Strategies must then be established to integrate these basic functional approaches with other trunk muscular functions, such as respiration.

Pregame Facilitation Techniques

As previously noted, stretching prior to athletic participation may inhibit the force output capabilities of a muscle. This, in turn, can negatively affect performance levels while increasing the risk of injury. Kreighbaum and Barthels recognized that flexibility must be accompanied by periarticular ligamentous and muscular stability.[99] This is especially important prior to athletic participation. In order to ensure that joint stability is not sacrificed in attempts to increase joint mobility, athletes are using various alternative techniques for precompetition warm-up routines. Richardson and Sims demonstrated that the shortened range of muscle length is the most critical in establishing the sensitivity and optimal functional capacity of the sensory feedback system of the muscle[100] (see Figs. 30–7 and 30–8). Thus, the performance of low-load continuous muscle contraction in the muscle's shortened range can be used to enhance the ability of a muscle to stabilize joints, creating maximum muscle stiffness.[101] Muscle activation techniques (MAT) include a pregame facilitation technique that utilizes the performance of isometrics in extreme ranges (shortened positions) of motion in order to increase mobility while maintaining joint stability.

Masamoto et al. demonstrated that plyometric exercise (double-leg tuck jumps and depth jumps) 30 seconds prior to a squat lift increased the maximum performance capacity of tested male athletes.[102]

A final pregame facilitation approach involves sensorimotor training. Bullock-Saxton et al. demonstrated that there was a measurably significant increase in the speed of contraction of the gluteals following a brief period of walking on balance sandals[103] (see Figure 30–2). These devices are composed of a cork-bottomed sandal with a hard rubber hemisphere glued to the sole from below at the midpoint, strategically below the mid-foot. Maintaining one's balance is no easy maneuver, especially in the early stage of training, providing an additional labyrinthine challenge. These simple devices, requiring only 2–3 minutes, provide increased locomotor stability via increased speed of contraction, improved balance, and shortened reaction rates prior to competition (see Fig. 30–2).

Four-Stage Strategy

Sport-specific training to return to athletic competition following a low back syndrome requires four stages (adapted from Cooke et al.).[104] It may be helpful to review the treatment strategies of athletic back injuries presented in the previous chapter as a precursor to this approach.

Stage I: Mobilization of the Spine. This stage begins when the athlete has resumed a near-pain-free full

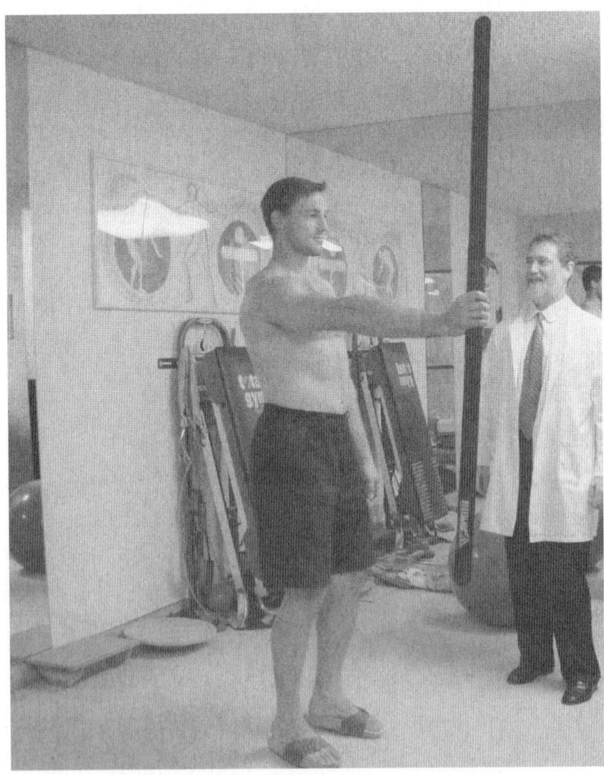

FIGURE 30–2. Sensorimotor training, utilizing balance sandals here, improves balance and muscular speed of contraction, while the Body Blade® integrates core and upper quarter resistance training. The combination provides improved neutral spine dynamic stability.

range of motion. He or she is ready for the introduction of neutral spine training, low-level sport-specific agility exercises, early restoration of adequate torso muscle strength, and endurance and control to prevent injury. This is accomplished through manual procedures, and early range of motion exercises with minimal resistance. As previously stated, unloaded endurance training, such as supine stationary bicycling or pool aerobics, should have been ongoing to reduce the affects of deconditioning.

Stage II: Stabilization of the Lumbar Spine. The goals of stabilization are to gain dynamic control of segmental spine and kinetic chain forces and minimize repetitive motion segment injury to decrease chance of acute dynamic overload. This is accomplished by co-contracting the extrinsic abdominals and trunk extensors, along with the hip flexors and extensors so that functional activities can occur while protecting the injured segment. A sensorimotor training program may be very useful at this point. Lumbopelvic floor exercises are important in this phase. As stated earlier, special emphasis must be placed on improving dynamic motor patterns, optimizing postural and ambulatory loading. These topics are discussed in detail in Chapters 28 and 29. Isometrics and low-impact aerobics are also used at the later part of this stage having the athlete co-contract his abdominals and extensors while participating in conditioning and mildly jarring activities.

Stage III: Isotonic Exercising and Sport-Specific Exercises. This stage focuses on isotonic exercising and sport-specific exercises to increase endurance and skill. This includes increasingly jarring activities that require quicker anticipation or response times. This also includes machines and free weights using the large muscles first, including the legs, and progressing to small muscles. The proper starting position is that of a neutral spine that is maintained throughout a progression toward heavy exercise. Increasing cardiovascular fitness is also important to this stage, with an emphasis toward the specific demands of the sport. For example, a hockey player or sprinter may exercise for shorter, slightly more intense periods, while the marathoner and basketball player may pace themselves for longer periods. However, heavy end-range loading, such as heavy squats, overhead pressing, and unsupported, bent-over rows should be avoided in this stage. It is important for the rehabilitation team to remember the athlete's mechanism of injury, faulty motor patterns, and sport-specific risk factors (e.g., the pars fracture athlete in a sport prone to lumbar hyperextension) and place a special emphasis on training patterns that overcome these issues, in addition to post-injury residuals (e.g., the disc injury that left the patient with weak back extensors). This is a critical stage, because the athlete is beginning to resume low-level, sport-specific activities, is feeling much better, and gaining confidence and anticipation about returning to competition. There may be additional anxiety and illness behavior associated with the trauma of the injury, the psychosocial stresses, in addition to individual and team expectations. The medical team must be sensitive to the multivariate and seemingly contradictory emotional aspects. Integration of a sports psychologist into the team, if not already included, can be prudent.

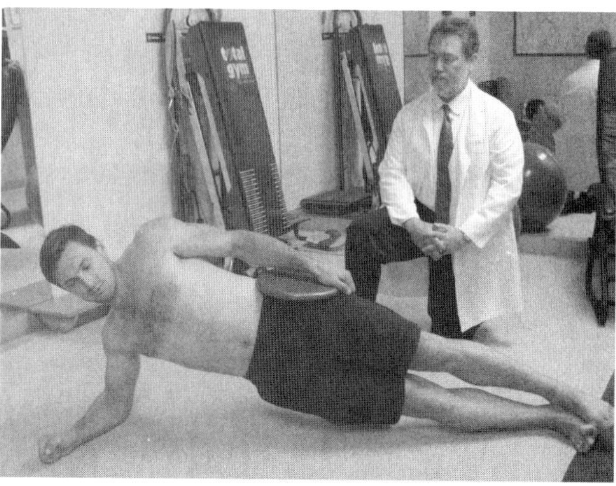

FIGURE 30–3. An advanced level side bridge strategy is used by increasing the lever load with the patient extending the legs and placing a weight on the pelvis.

Stage IV: Sport-Specific Agility and Training Drills. These are performed providing that significant dynamic stabilization and adequate muscle strength and endurance have been achieved (Figures 30–3, 30–4, 30–5, 30–6, 30–7 and 30–8). As the athlete demonstrates sufficient physical and emotional capacity to

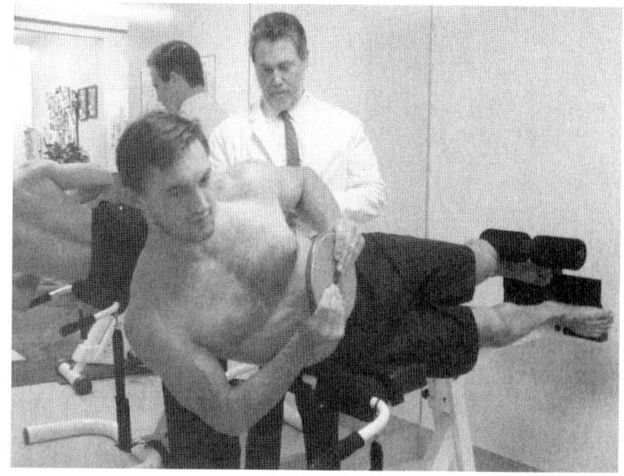

FIGURE 30–4. A further increase in lateral chain loading can be used with the side-lying Roman chair, which leaves the torso unsupported. Here, the patient moves beyond the neutral pelvis strategy and integrates concentric and eccentric loading with the additional resistance of a 25-lb (11-kg) weight.

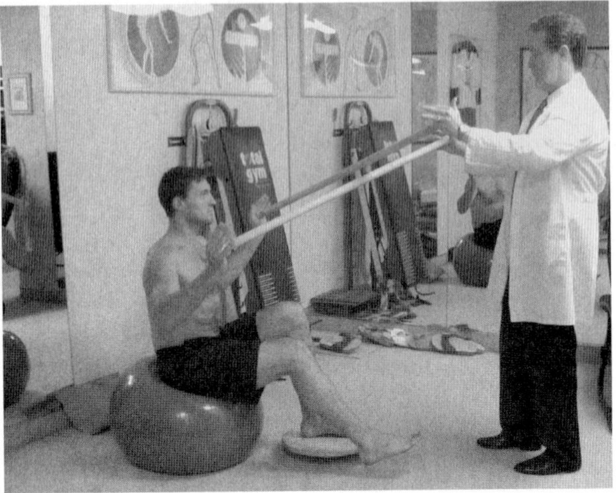

FIGURE 30–5. The challenge increases as the athlete is instructed to maintain a neutral spine despite bearing his weight on an unstable gym ball and rocker board under one of his feet. He is challenged to maintain both arms in an outstretched position, holding his posture despite sudden, asymmetrical loads from the clinician via the rehabilitation sticks.

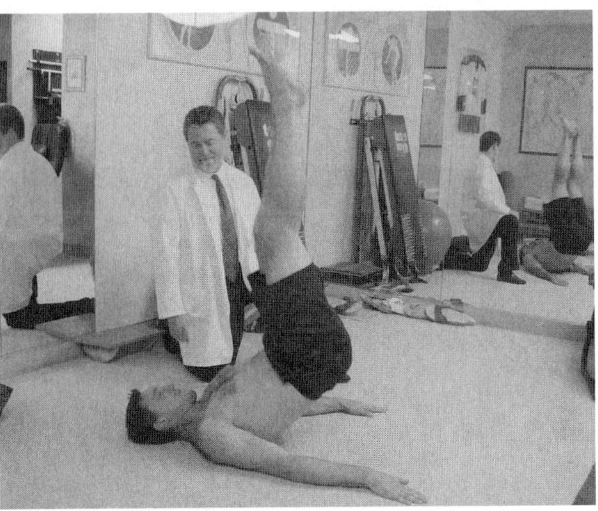

FIGURE 30–7. Leg-ups are advanced exercises that challenge the intrinsic stabilizers in addition to the torso flexors initially and torso extensors later. Because of the significant loading involved in elevating the entire lower body weight, perhaps especially to the intervertebral discs, the athlete must demonstrate extreme dynamic lumbosacral stability before this maneuver is attempted.

resume his or her sport, a critical stage of the rehabilitative process occurs. This is the organized transition back into that sport as quickly and practically as possible. In order optimize the chances of success, the authors highly recommend manual facilitory techniques, such as those demonstrated in Figures 30–9 and 30–10, as a means of improving locomotor system coordination during the pre-game/warm-up period. Meanwhile, structured administrative coordination must also occur to smooth the process. *It is important for the clinical and coaching team to work together during stage IV, as optimization of body mechanics and sport-specific patterns become integrated* (see Fig. 30–11). Such strategic teamwork by the staff can reduce the risk of injury recurrence and increase skills by providing feedback to avoid faulty postures and bad habits.

Clinical Pearl: It is important for the clinical and coaching team to work together during stage IV, as optimization of body mechanics and sport-specific patterns become integrated. Such strategic

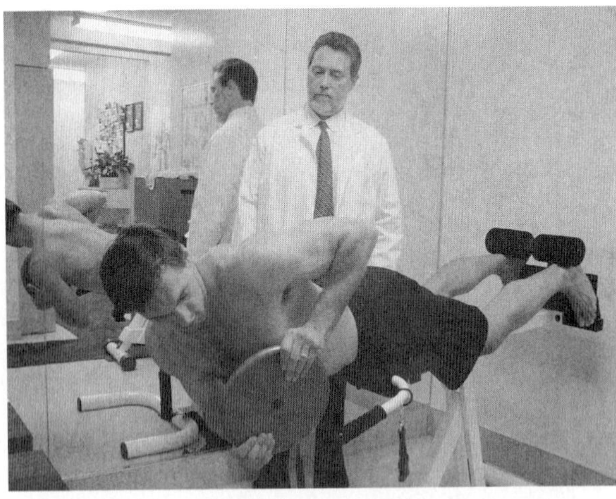

FIGURE 30–6. Advanced Roman chair exercise strategies can integrate core (intrinsic) and posterior kinetic chain training along with sport-specific motions. Here, this professional hockey player recreates slapshot mechanics by adding trunk rotation maneuvers while holding a 25-lb (11-kg) weight.

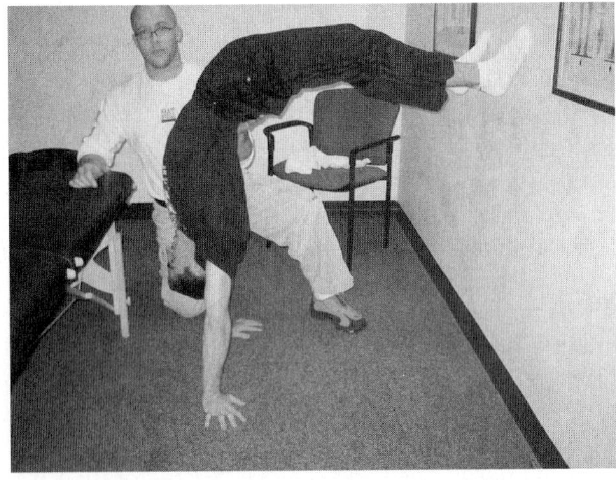

FIGURE 30–8. Gymnasts are at increased risk of end-range spinal injury due in part to their hypermobility. Here, this Olympic caliber gymnast performs a unique closed chain maneuver that requires marked upper body strength, maintaining dynamic joint stability despite lumbar extensibility far beyond the average range.

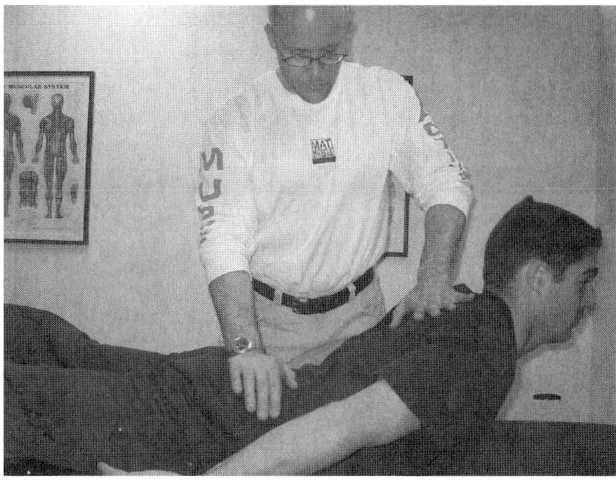

FIGURE 30–9. Muscular facilitation techniques directly prior to competition can improve dynamic spinal stability, optimizing locomotor control while reducing the risk of injury. Here, the thoracolumbar erector spinae are facilitated while this hypermobile athlete maintains partial spinal extension.

teamwork by the staff can reduce the risk of injury recurrence and increase skills by providing feedback to avoid faulty postures and bad habits.

The neutral spine remains an important strategy during the early part of this phase. Each of the components of sport is practiced in this position with predictable and unpredictable challenges, or perturbations. For example, a football player will hold a lumbar neutral position while hitting a tackling sled (i.e., predictable) when taking a "blindsided hit" (i.e., unpredictable). In the later portion of this stage, the athlete must then evolve beyond the mastered neutral

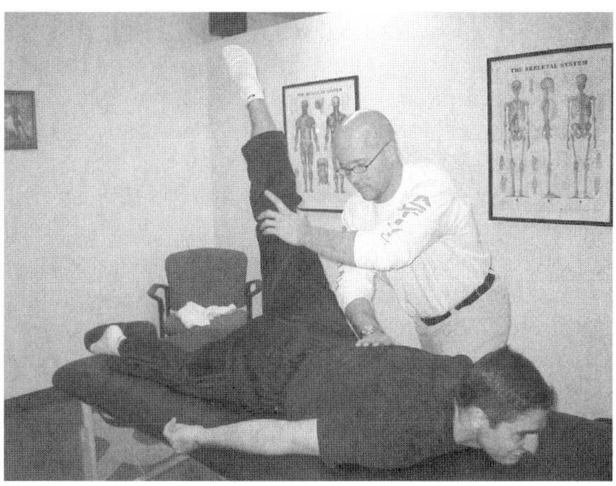

FIGURE 30–10. Precompetition stabilization of the periphery via muscular facilitation techniques should occur following muscle lengthening procedures and trunk stabilization. Here the gymnast maintains hip extension while the trainer provides facilitory, loading methods.

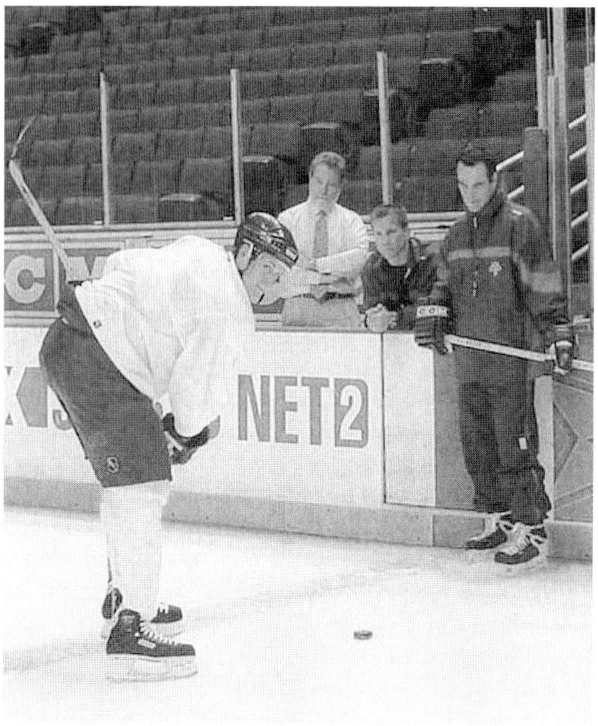

FIGURE 30–11. Critical teamwork. As the athlete transitions back to competition-level sport, clinical and coaching staff teamwork focusing on optimal biomechanics and sport-specific skills can mean the difference between a successful return or a failed recurrence of symptoms. Here, the coach, trainer, and team doctor critically review the athlete.

lumbar position as they reestablish a greater range of safe, dynamically stable motion. Aerobic activities are also included in advanced programs. A functional progression should be used to increase the difficulty and stress of the exercises and plyometric challenges should also be introduced. Exercises should be used to incorporate trunk control and stability until the athlete is ready to resume team practice.

CASE STUDIES

The following fictional case studies involve a variety of athletes who have already been deemed appropriate for rehabilitation elite athletic retraining. These cases are different from the general population in that they may now test very well on standardized scoring measures of basic function used for patients with back pain. In these circumstances, the general population would probably be at or near discharge and expected to resume to regular activity and hopefully independently maintain a home exercise program.

Elite athletes, however, are just getting started in preparation for the extremes of physical forces encountered as they return to their sport. The sports medicine team now has to be acutely aware of the rigors placed on these athletes in daily competition and be aware of the external forces that will now occur.

Case Study #1

Cameron is a 16-year-old male high school pre-elite interior lineman playing American football who sustained an injury to the pars (bilateral fractures at L5 level) from an extension overload while push blocking. The pars defect was detected radiographically and monitored by periodic bone scans (scintigraphy). There was no evidence of anterior body slippage (spondylolisthesis). The acute stage was treated with a back brace and reduced axial loading and motion. Once healing occurred, typically requiring about 3 months, an aggressive rehabilitation program was started, limiting extension. He was taught about the nature of his injury and the importance of avoiding extension overloading during the rehabilitative process. He was very anxious about returning to the field of play to help his team and to increase his chances for a college football scholarship. Because of these concerns, his parents and coach were brought together for a counseling session with the trainer and team doctor regarding the risks of overly aggressive rehabilitation. He was still growing, so the risks of reinjury at the secondary growth center along the posterior arch remained increased. Once stages I, II, and III were completed, Cameron was transitioned to moderate and then heavy weight lifting. He was monitored for increased pain or loss of lumbopelvic stability while performing these tasks (i.e., avoid extreme spinal lordosing during bench or incline presses). He graduated from the stationary bike to aerobics on grass surfaces and had no pain with sprints or 1/4 to 1/2 mile runs.

Cameron was then ready for sport-specific training. Sprints out of a "cage," which do not allow the athlete to stand up immediately and require a low center of gravity, are helpful. This becomes as important or more important in the cardiovascular conditioning of the athlete than running on grass. The typical "run" for a lineman is only 3–5 yards unless he is releasing from a block to pick up another block downfield. He must remain semicrouched to maintain a low center of gravity, regardless of his specific tasks for each play. Cameron started sport-specific agility drills before the lower body plyometric movements were completed to improve proprioception and locomotor coordination. To integrate sport-specific upper body plyometrics, he was instructed to dive forward, catching himself with his arms (e.g., a push-up position) in a controlled manner and then rolling to one side (log roll) to quickly assume an upright position and tackle a dummy several yards away. He was reminded to integrate the neutral spine strategy that he was taught and gradually became slightly less lordotic in his postural strategies during practice.

Cameron used these skills during blind trunk stability challenges, designed to "shuck" (i.e., block and push away) teammates from the front and at angles. He used these skills in a pass blocking position with his feet pumping and running in place while he is struck with handheld blocking dummies from various angles to compromise his center of gravity. This would be performed at many angles and many of those would not be in his visual field (i.e., blindsided hits), which is common in football. This type of activity in a controlled sense helped the sports medicine team and Cameron develop confidence in his ability to take a blow from any angle, suspected or not, without the loss of balance or stabilization of the previously injured area. He was then ready to return to full contact practice with the team.

Case Study #2

Jana is a 22-year-old female Olympic caliber freestyle swimmer in relay and solo events. She injured her right sacroiliac joint coming from a flexed position off the block ballistically and diving into the water. Stages I, II, and III are complete at this time and the sacroiliac joint appears to be stable. Special considerations in this injury are the fact that the sport is primarily performed in a horizontal and gravity "neutral" position. This means that getting back to sport for cardiovascular work can usually be done much earlier as getting horizontal in the water can sometimes be less irritating for the athlete than cardiovascular work on land.

It should be noted that manual techniques to normalize sacroiliac motion were important in the early stages of this case (see Chapters 20 and 23). Also, a core-training program to activate the intrinsic musculature was considered vital. This included exercises to activate the pelvic floor. The intrinsic muscles have been found to be important in dynamic stability ("force closure") of the sacroiliac joint, as discussed in Chapters 4 and 9.

Another special consideration is that this sport is rotational in nature. This athlete must start with rotational strengthening as soon as possible along with intense lower trap and shoulder retractor strengthening. Strengthening of the latissimus not only improves the mechanics of her stroke, but also helps to stabilize the back because of the attachment to the lumbar fascia and iliac crest, providing a rigid mechanical muscular support for the posterior spine.

Jana was allowed back in the pool quite early because of the gravity neutral spinal unloading. In addition, additional land-based exercises were performed to help stabilize her back to return her to a competitive level. Standing resistance band rotations were initiated, moving in a diagonal position from her shoulder closest to the resistive bands, continuing across her body caudally to the contralateral hip. Other land exercises included standing back-to-back trunk rotations with the clinical team member while passing a medicine ball from one to the other going both clockwise and counterclockwise in successively faster rotations. Adding breathing exercises (quick breaths in and slow four to eight count breaths out depending on the swimmers stroke) further prepares their cardiovascular system for return to competition.

The swimmer's block start posed another problem. This placed Jana in a flexed position, one that is traditionally related to an "unprotected" position of the spine. Forced extension to facilitate water entry increases stress in her spine. This also replicated the injury activity and caused the sports medicine team to approach her training with additional caution. She was given Roman chair exercises, performed in the prone position with a neutral spine, in order to improve strength and endurance to the posterior kinetic chain. To train for this part of the sport, Jana was started with plyometric jump-off blocks with solid landing in a squatted position. After that was mastered, a high jump was added immediately after the landing so that the athlete would jump off a 2-ft high box, land in a squat, and immediately jump as high as possible toward the ceiling. The next step was to replace the high jump with a long jump to further replicate the position of exploding off the block. When she could land from a 2-ft box and propel herself into an immediate long jump without pain, the athlete was allowed to restart her block starts at submaximal effort and work back up to full explosive effort off the block. Once accomplished at full effort, the swimmer was returned to sport. Similar approaches of the land-based exercises can be used for other rotational sports such as golf and tennis or baseball with a concentration on the spinal rotational stabilizers.

Case Study #3

Chris is a 28-year-old professional hockey defenseman who sustained a mechanical dysfunction of the lumbar spine including facet syndrome and joint dysfunction. This occurred when he was checked in the back while experiencing his third acute episode of low back pain over a 1-year period. Stages I, II, and III were successfully completed and he was essentially pain-free.

Training for hockey players (and many other sports as well) depends a lot on the position of the player. Defensemen are more stoutly built and are required to do much of their sport while skating backwards. The defenseman must have rotatory trunk stability for a powerful slapshot from the blue line.

The forward-drawn, hip-flexed posture of the ice hockey player was discussed earlier in the chapter, as were the typical associated injuries. There was also additional concern because of the recurrent nature of the symptoms. To address the postural imbalances associated with this sport, a variety of manual joint and muscle balancing techniques were used to improve joint mobility and establish a more neutral posture. Sensorimotor training was integrated with the use of balance sandals and rocker boards, followed by a lumbopelvic stabilization program. Prone Roman chair exercises were introduced to increase posterior kinetic chain endurance and strength.

For Chris, it was important to return to skating motions for proper muscle development and also for the rigorous conditioning that faces the athlete. Use of a slideboard to mimic the motion of skating is imperative as joint dysfunction. Some postexercise soreness of back musculature and of the legs is typical. Use of the slideboard allows the sports medicine team to evaluate his form. This would otherwise be very difficult and can be controlled, allowing early cardiovascular work and locomotor training. It is important to remember that all of the core and stabilization techniques are followed through to this phase and it is the responsibility of the management team to oversee the athlete for competency in performing trunk motor training.

As Chris reconditioned his legs in the early stages of using the slideboard, he was challenged to enhance single-leg stance while rotating his body for a slapshot. This was performed by having him stand on a "wobble board," balance sandals, or roll of foam along the plane of the foot. He was then given a hockey stick with resistive bands and was instructed to practice a "slapshot" motion against the resistance of the bands. This does not simulate the push-off of the final phase of the shot, but is a good preparatory activity. Once this was accomplished, the stick activity was added while using the slideboard with small lateral strides so that the clinician behind the player could provide resistance with elastic tubing. The timing was coordinated with the push-off from the side of the slideboard to further simulate the actual shot. Because a defender must skate backwards and use his stick to "check" forwards, he places himself in an awkward position. His legs move to skate backward, his spine is trying to stabilize the trunk while rotating and performing an extension moment as he checks the oncoming player. To simulate this, Chris used the resistive bands or the slideboard while stabilizing himself in spinal extension.

Other land-based strengthening of the upper body in terms of weight lifting were added, as defenders require the strength necessary for stopping the advancing opponents. Upper body exercises used in traditional settings were added at this time with the same precautions listed earlier. The bulk of the defender's cardiovascular work was provided earlier by supine stationary bicycling and the slideboard, but backwards skating can only be truly simulated by performing that maneuver. Once the above tasks were mastered and Chris was capable of performing force displacement against resistance drills, he was returned to the ice for skating.

On-ice cardiovascular drills were then reinstituted. Backwards skating at 45-degree angles back over each shoulder were used by the training members to get the defender used to rapidly having to change directions (further stressing the rotational stability of the spine). Slapshots were then performed on the ice and after successful completion of backwards skating and shooting. He was challenged in keeping his balance while on skates in a controlled ice activity. He was "nudged" by players surrounding him from various angles where some, at least, were not in his visual field. After successfully passing this final test, the defender was put back into full practice in a nonchecking environment until he could keep up with the other players and then returned to full contact.

Case Study #4

Andrei is a 27-year-old male hockey goalie with a lumbar disc syndrome, with pain initially extending into the right buttock to his knee. He first experienced pain while at the goal during an off-season pickup game. This occurred when he was bent forward and another player unexpectedly fell on his back. A lumbar MRI revealed a right-sided L4–L5 disc bulge of 3–4 mm. Neurological testing, including reflex, sensory, motor, and electrodiagnostic testing were negative for the lower extremities. A multifaceted approach of manual and rehabilitative procedures can be quite effective in such cases,[105] and such a method was used following McKenzie protocols. He responded well to a McKenzie protocol for posterior derangement as explained in Chapter 22, in addition to various manual procedures including manipulation, mobilization, and muscle balancing techniques. Chris responded well, completing stages I and II, and was ready for sport-specific training.

The physical demands of the ice hockey goalie and defenseman are quite different, providing an excellent example of how different rehabilitation strategies may be required within the same sport. In contrast to a defenseman, balanced quickness in conjunction with controlled hypermobility and heightened hand/eye coordination are paramount for the goalie. While the defenseman must perform repetitive on-ice sprints between brief, seated rest periods, the goalie remains on the ice for the entire game. The goalie does not perform such sprints, but maintains a crouched position for prolonged periods, along with sudden, imbalanced, contorted, ballistic moves involving multiple extremities in order to protect the goal.

Rehabilitation for Andrei included significant muscle balancing techniques to improve sport-specific postural imbalances. Additional work was included to stabilize the intrinsic torso muscles and coordinate this with diaphragmatic respiration. Training was performed with a bias toward extension in an effort to reduce posterior spinal loading. To work on stability, proprioception, and hand/eye coordination, he was placed in balance sandals with a goalie stick in one hand along with a blocker and a glove in the other hand. He was instructed to swing the arms alternatively while balancing on one foot to get used to swinging the weight of the stick and blocker and glove. This was advanced to faster motions to where the player was asked to assume this position and block rubber balls thrown at him. This exercise was performed on each leg. The same type of exercise was performed while in a side-facing position on one knee, the opposite foot and one hand being in contact with the floor. The free hand was used to stop projectiles of progressively smaller objects that were thrown at him. Eventually, an actual indoor stick and puck were used to progressively fire faster and faster shots at the goalie in pads to sharpen hand/eye coordination.

Being able to "flop" and get back up is something that the goalie must master. Andrei found that this activity, along with splayed extremities and hip flexion, caused a mild recurrence of local back pain, so the drills were temporarily discontinued. It was felt that Andrei was flexing at the lumbosacral junction also and did not yet have sufficient lumbopelvic control, requiring a "peel back" strategy. Further core and lumbopelvic training, sensorimotor training, land-based weight training, and slideboard training was reinstituted for four more days. Increasingly demanding combinations of these procedures were enacted, including perturbation strategies and gym ball activities to further optimize lumbopelvic stabilization. Another trial of "flop" maneuvers was attempted, which did not reproduce pain, allowing the rehabilitation continuum to proceed.

The next step was to initiate quick, scrambling motions in awkward positions not only with extremity movements as listed above, but also with impact on the supporting surface. Andrei was properly padded and instructed to throw himself to the ground in a prone manner, catching himself with his arms (i.e., push-up position). He then had to quickly flip to his back, then to his side, and then the other side. He was then instructed to perform the same maneuvers while assuming a goalie's crouched position before repeating this maneuver. This strategy allows a goalie to reestablish the locomotor stability from the stable ground prior to the slippery ice. This technique was later used on the ice and in skates as the last check before successfully returning this player to active practice.

SUMMARY

1. This chapter provided a brief insight into the current issues confronting health-care providers who are involved in the management of low back syndromes of elite athletes.
2. While each subgroup of patients present with their own unique complications, the authors feel that this subgroup is one of the most challenging.
3. Ironically, this collection of overachievers can at times be terribly frustrating to assist, while being quite rewarding in the majority of cases.
4. Hopefully, further research will help to provide more concrete answers regarding sport-specific etiological factors to injuries, in addition to providing insights in more effective treatment protocols in the future.

The authors would like to thank the following professional ice hockey players for their assistance in serving as models for this chapter. Mr. Andrei Zyuzin, Mr. Kevin Weekes, and Mr. Branislav Mezei. Also, the authors would like to thank Mr. John Tortarella and David Boyer and the Florida Panthers, Ice Hockey Team (NHL) for their assistance with photograph Figure 30–11.

REFERENCES

1. Hubbard DD. Injuries to the spine in children and adolescents. *CIRN Orthoped* 1974;100(0):56–65.
2. Merbs C. Incomplete spondylolysis and healing. *Spine* 1995;20(21):2328–2334.
3. Micheli LJ. Low back pain in the adolescent: Differential diagnosis. *Am J Sports Med* November/December 1979;7(6):362–364.
4. Ross JS, Tkach J, Ruggieri PM, Lieber M, Lapresto E. The mind's eye: Functional MR imaging evaluation of golf motor imagery. *Am J Neuroradiol* June/July 2003;24(6):1036–1044.
5. Junge A. The influence of psychological factors on sports injuries. Review of the literature. *AM J Sports Med* 2000;28(Suppl 5):S10–S15.
6. Greene HS, Cholewicki J, Galloway MT, Nguyen CV, Radebold A. A history of low back injury is a risk factor for recurrent back injuries in varsity athletes. *Am J Sports Med* November/December 2001;29(6):795–800.
7. Smorawinski J, Nazar K, Kaciuba-Uscilko H, et al. Effects of 3-day bed rest on physiological responses to graded exercise in athletes and sedentary men. *J Appl Physiol* 2001;91:249–257.
8. Greanleaf JE, Reese RD. Exercise thermoregulation after 14 days of bed rest. *J Appl Physiol* 1980;48:72–78.
9. Maron BJ, Pellicia A, Sparato A, Granata M. Reduction in left ventricular wall thickness after deconditioning in highly trained Olympic athletes. *Br Heart J* February 1993;69(2):125–128.
10. Meeusen R, Piacentini MF, Busschaert B, Buyse L, De Schutter G, Stray-Gunderson J. Hormonal responses in athletes: The use of a two bout exercise protocol to detect subtle differences in (over)training status. *Eur J Appl Physiol* 2004 Mar; 91(2–3):140–146.
11. Kentta G, Hassmen P, Raglin JS. Training practices and overtraining syndrome in Swedish age-group athletes. *Int J Sports Med* August 2001;22(6):460–465.
12. Pearce PZ. A practical approach to the overtraining syndrome. *Curr Sports Med Rep* June 2002;1(3):179–183.
13. Varlet-Marie E, Gaudard A, Mercier J, Bressolle F, Brun JF. Is the feeling of heavy legs in overtrained athletes related to impaired hemorheology? *Clin Hemorheol Microcirc* 2003;28(3):151–159.
14. Urhausen A, Gabriel HH, Weiler B, Kindermann W. Ergometric and psychological findings during overtraining: A long-term follow-up study in endurance athletes. *Int J Sports Med* February 1998;19(2):114–120.
15. Unterhausen A, Kindermann W. Diagnosis of overtraining: What tools do we have? *Sports Med* 2002; 32(2):95–102.
16. Foster C. Monitoring training in athletes with reference to overtraining syndrome. *Med Sci Sports Exerc* July 1998;30(7):1164–1168.
17. Meyers MC, Brown BR, Bloom JA. Fast pitch softball injuries. *Sports Med* 2001;31(1):61–73.
18. Small E. Chronic musculoskeletal pain in young athletes. *Pediatr Clin North Am* June 2002;49(3):vii, 655–662.
19. Armstrong LE, VanHeest JL. The unknown mechanism of the overtraining syndrome: Clues from depression and psychoneuroimmunology. *Sports Med* 2002:32(3):185–209.
20. Kentta G, Hassmen P. Overtraining and recovery. A conceptual model. *Sports Med* July 1998;26(1):1–16.
21. Anthony J. Psychologic aspects of exercise. *Clin J Sport Med* January 1991;10(1):171–180.
22. Alexander MJ. Biomechanical aspects of lumbar spine injuries: A review. *Can J Appl Sport Sci* March 1985; 10(1):1–20.
23. Garrick JG, Requa RK. Epidemiology of women's gymnastic injuries. *Am J Sport Med* 1980;8:261–264.
24. Keene JS, Albert MJ, Springer SL, Drummond DS, Clancy WG Jr. Back injuries in college athletes. *J Spinal Disord* September 1989;2(3):190–195.
25. Hutchinson MR. Low back pain in elite rhythmic gymnasts. *Med Sci Sports Exerc* November 1999;31(11): 1686–1688.
26. Rossi F, Dragoni S. Acute avulsion fractures of the pelvis in adolescent competitive athletes: Prevalence, location and sports distribution of 203 cases collected. *Skeletal Radiol* March 2001;30(3):127–131.
27. Nadler SF, Wu KD, Galski T, Feinberg JH. Low back pain in college athletes. A prospective study correlating lower extremity overuse or acquired ligamentous

laxity with low back pain. *Spine* April 1998;23(7): 828–833.
28. Sward L, Hellstrom M, Jacobsoson B, Peterson L. Back pain and radiologic changes in the thoracolumbar spine of athletes. *Spine* February 1990;15(2):124–129.
29. Duda M. Golfers use exercise to get back into the swing. *Phys Sports Med* 1989;17:109–113.
30. Mundt DJ, Kelsey JL, Golden AL, et al. An epidemiologic study of sports and weight lifting as possible risk factors for herniated cervical and lumbar discs. The Northeast Collaborative Group on Low Back Pain. *Am J Sports Med* November/December 1993;21(6): 854–860.
31. Weishaupft P, Obermuller R, Hofmann A. Spine stabilizing muscles in golfers. *Sportverletz Sportschaden* June 2000;14(2):55–58.
32. Mannor DA, Lindenfeld TN. Spinal process apophysitis mimics spondylolysis. Case reports. *Am J Sports Med* March/April 2000;28(2):257–260.
33. Gatt CJ Jr, Hosea TM, Palumbo RC, et al. Impact loading of lumbar spine during football blocking. *Am J Sports Med* 1997;25:317–320.
34. Gerbino PG, d'Hemecourt PA. Does football cause an increase in degenerative disease of the lumbar spine? *Curr Sports Med Rep* February 2002;1(1):47–51.
35. Day AL, Friedman WA, Indelicato PA. Observations on the treatment of lumbar disk disease in college football players. *Am J Sports Med* January/February 1987;m15(1):72–75.
36. Schmidt-Olsen S, Jorgenson U, Kaalund S, Sorenson J. Injuries among young soccer players. *Am J Sports Med* May/June 1991;19(3):273–275.
37. Raty HP, Kujala UM, Videman T, et al. Lifetime musculoskeletal symptoms and injuries among former elite male athletes. *Int J Sports Med* November 1997; 18(8):625–632.
38. Kovacs D, Negovetic L, Vukic M, Klanfar Z, Jajic Z. Surgical treatment of lumbar disc hernias in athletes. *Reumatizam* 1998;46(1):35–41.
39. Iwamoto J, Takeda T. Stress fractures in athletes: Review of 196 cases. *J Orthop Sci* 2003;8(3):273–278.
40. Zetoun F, Frot B, Sterin P, Tubiana JM. Pubalgia in sportsmen. *Ann Radiol (Paris)* 1995;38(5):244–254.
41. Le Jeune JJ, Rochcongear P, Vazelle F, Bernard AM, Hery JY, Ramee A. Pubic pain syndrome in sportsmen: Comparison of radiographic and scintigraphic findings. *Eur J Nucl Med* 1984;9(6):250–253.
42. Wiley JJ. Traumatic osteitit pubis: The gracilis syndrome. *Am J Sports Med* September/October 1983; 11(5):360–363.
43. Conte S, Requa RK, Garrick JG. Disability days in major league baseball. *Am J Sports Med* July/August 2001;29(4):431–436.
44. McFarland EG, Wasik M. Epidemiology of collegiate baseball injuries. *Clin J Sport Med* 1998;8(1):10–13.
45. Shaffer B, Jobe FW, Pink M, Perry J. Baseball batting: An electromyelographical study. *Clin Orthop* July 1993;(292):285–293.
46. Brown EW, Kimball RG. Medical history associated with adolescent power lifting. *Pediatrics* 1983;72: 636–644.
47. Raske A, Norlin R. Injury incidence and prevalence among elite weight and power lifters. *Am J Sports Med* March/April 2002;30(2):248–256.
48. Keeves RK, Laskowski ER, Smith J. Weight training injuries. Part 2. Diagnosing and managing chronic conditions. *Physician Sports Med* 1998;26(3):54–63, 73.
49. Granhed H, Morelli B. Low back pain among retired wrestlers and heavy weightlifters. *Am J Sports Med* September/October 1988;16(5):530–533.
50. Zajac A, Waskiewicz Z, Pilis W. Anaerobic power, creatin kinase activity, lactate concentration and acid–base equilibrium changes following bouts of exhaustive strength exercises. *J Strength Cond Res* August 2001;15(3):357–361.
51. Henry JH, Lareau B, Neigut D. The injury rate in professional basketball. *Am J Sports Med* January/February 1982;10(1):16–18.
52. Hickey GJ, Fricker PA, McDonald WA. Injuries of elite female basketball players over a 6-year period. *Clin J Sport Med* October 1997;7(4):252–256.
53. Meeuwisse WH, Sellmer R, Hagel BE. Rates and risks of injury during intercollegiate basketball. *Am J Sports Med* May/June 2003;31(3):379–385.
54. Saraux A, Guillodo Y, Devauchelle V, Allain J, Guedes C, Le Goff P. Are tennis players at increased risk for low back pain and sciatica? *Rev Rhum Engl Ed* March 1999;66(3):143–145.
55. Sward L, Svensson M, Zetterberg C. Isometric muscle strength and quantitative electromyography of back muscles in wrestlers and tennis players. *Am J Sports Med* July/August 1990;18(4):382–386.
56. Elliot BC. Biomechanics of the serve in tennis. A biomedical perpective. *Sports Med* November 1988; 6(5):285–294.
57. Sward L. The thoracolumbar spine in young elite athletes. Current concepts on the effects of physical training. *Sports Med* May 1992;13(5):357–364.
58. Kulund DN, McCue FC III, Rockwell DA, Gieck JH. Tennis injuries: Prevention and treatment. A review. *Am J Sports Med* July/August 1979;7(4):249–253.
59. Aggrawal ND, Kaur R, Kumar S, Wathur DN. A study of changes in the spine in weight lifters and other athletes. *Br J Sports Med* June 1979;13(2):58–61.
60. Hasler C, Dick W. Spondylolysis and spondylolisthesis during growth. *Orthopade* January 2002;31(1): 78–87.
61. Schmitt H, Brocai DR, Carstens C. Long-term review of the lumbar spine in javelin throwers. *J Bone Joint Surg Br* April 2001;83(3):324–327.
62. Stress reaction of the pars interarticularis leading to spondylolysis. A cause of adolescent low back pain. *J Adolesc Health Care* November 1989;10(6):573–577.
63. Shah MK, Stewert GW. Sacral stress fractures: An unusual cause of low back pain in an athlete. *Spine* February 15, 2002;27(4):E104–E108.
64. Major NM, Helms CA. Sacral stress fractures in long-distance runners. *AJR Am J Roentgenol* March 2000; 174(3):727–729.
65. Guten G. Herniated lumbar disk associated with running. A review of 10 cases. *Am J Sports Med* May/June 1981;9(3):155–159.

66. Nyska M, Constantini N, Cale-Benzoor M, Back Z, Kahn G, Mann G. Spondylolysis as a cause of low back pain in swimmers. *Int J Sports Med* July 2000;21(5): 375–379.
67. Biasca N, Simmen HP, Bartolozzi AR, Trenz O. Review of typical ice hockey injuries. Survey of the North American NHL and Hockey Canada versus European Leagues. *Unfallchirurg* May 1995;98(5):283–288.
68. Groger A. Ten years of ice hockey-related-injuries in the German Ice Hockey Federation—A ten year prospective study/523 International Games. *Sportverletz Sportschaden* December 2001;15(4):82–86.
69. Warson RC, Singer CD, Sproule JR. Checking from behind in ice hockey: A study of injury and penalty data in the Ontario Athletic Association Hockey League. *Clin J Sport Med* April 1996;6(2):108–111.
70. Schick DM, Meeuwisse WH. Injury rates and profiles among female ice hockey players. *Am J Sports Med* January/February 2003;31(1):47–52.
71. Jorgensen U, Schmidt-Olsen S. The epidemiology of ice hockey injuries. *Br J Sports Med* March 1986;20(1): 7–9.
72. Pinto M, Kuhn JE, Greenfield ML, Hawkins RJ. Prospective analysis of ice hockey injuries at the Junior A level over the course of one season. *Clin J Sport Med* April 1999;9(2):70–74.
73. Tyler T, Zook L, Brittis D, Gleim G. A new pelvic tilt detection device: Roentgenographic validation and application to assessment of hip motion in professional ice hockey players. *J Orthop Sports Phys Ther* November 1996;24(5):303–308.
74. Smith AM, Stuart MJ, Weise-Bjornstal DM, Gannon C. Predictors of injury in ice hockey players. A multvariate, multidisciplinary approach. *Am J Sports Med* July/August 1997;25(4):500–507.
75. Briggs RC, Kolbjornsen PH, Southall RC. Osteitis pubis, Tc-99m MDP, and professional hockey players. *Clin Nucl Med* November 1992;17(11):861–863.
76. Tyler TF, Nicholas SJ, Campell RJ, Donellan S, McHugh MP. The effectiveness of a preseason exercise program to prevent adductor muscle strains in professional ice hockey players. *Am J Sports Med* September/October 2002;30(5):680–683.
77. Bahr R, Reeser JC, Federation Internationale de Volleyball. Injuries among world-class beach volleyball players. The Federation Internationale de Volleyball injury study. *Am J Sports Med* January/February 2003;31(1):119–125.
78. Bartolozzi C, Caramella D, Zampa V, Dal Pozzo G, Tinacci E, Balducci F. The incidence of disk changes in volleyball players. The magnetic resonance findings. *Radiol Med (Torino)* December 1991;82(6): 757–760.
79. Bianco T. Social support and recovery from sport injury: Elite skiers share their experiences. *Res Q Exerc Sport* December 2001;72(4):376–388.
80. Johnson U. Coping strategies among long-term injured athletes. A study of 81 men and women in team and individual sports. *Scand J Med Sci Sports* December 1997;7(6):367–372.
81. Herbert RD, Gabriel M. Effects of stretching before and after exercising on muscle soreness and risk of injury: Systematic review. *BMJ* August 31, 2002; 325(7362):468.
82. Weldon SM, Hill RH. The efficacy of stretching for prevention of exercise-related injury: A systematic review of the literature. *Man Ther* August 2003;8(3):141–150.
83. Connolly DA, Sayers SP, McHugh MP. Treatment and prevention of delayed onset muscle soreness. *J Strength Cond Res* February 2003;17(1):197–208.
84. Nadler SF, Prybicien M, Malanga GA, Sicher D. Complications from therapeutic modalities: Results of a national survey of athletic trainers. *Arch Phys Med Rehabil* June 2003;84(6):849–853.
85. Saal JA, Saal JS. Nonoperative treatment of herniated lumbar intervertebral disc with radiculopathy: An outcome study. *Spine* 1989;14:431–436.
86. Wang JC, Shapiro MS, Hatch JD, Knight J, Dorey FJ, Delamarter RB. The outcome of lumbar discectomy in elite athletes. *Spine* March 15, 1999;24(6):570–573.
87. Mochida J, Nishimura K, Okuma M, Nomura T, Toh E. Percutaneous nucleotomy in elite athletes. *J Spinal Disord* April 2001;14(2):159–164.
88. Watkins RG IV, Williams LA, Watkins RG III. Microscopic lumbar discectomy results from professional and Olympic athletes. *Spine J* March/April 2003;3(2): 100–105.
89. Green JP, Grenier SG, McGill SM. Low-back stiffness is altered with warm-up and bench rest: Implications for athletes. *Med Sci Sports Exerc* July 2002;34(7): 1076–1081.
90. Stone MH. Muscle conditioning and muscle injuries. *Med Sci Sports Exerc* August 1990;22(4):457–462.
91. Ebben WP, Blackard DO. Strength and conditioning practices of National Footbal League strength and conditioning coaches. *J Strength Cond Res* February 2001;15(1):48–58.
92. Kraemer WJ, Ratamess N, Fry AC, et al. Influence of resistance training volume and periodization on physiological and performance adaptations in collegiate women tennis players. *Am J Sports Med* September/October 2000;28(5):626–633.
93. Durell DL, Pujol TJ. A survey of the scientific data and training methods utilized by collegiate strength and conditioning coaches. *J Strength Cond Res* May 2003;17(2):368–373.
94. Greene HS, Cholewicki J, Galloway MT, Nguyen CV, Radebold A. A history of low back injury is a risk factor for recurrent back injuries in varsity athletes. *Am J Sports Med* November/December 2001;29(6):795–800.
95. Nadler SF, Malanga GA, Feinberg JH, Prybicien M, Stitik TP, DePrince M. Relationship between hip muscle imbalance and occurrence of low back pain in collegiate athletes: A prospective study. *Am J Phys Med Rehabil* August 2001;80(8):572–577.
96. Nadler SF, Malanga GA, Feinberg JH, Rubanni M, Moley P, Foye P. Functional performance deficits in athletes with previous lower extremity injury. *Clin J Sport Med* March 2002;12(2):73–78.

97. Nadler SF, Moley P, Malanga GA, Rubanni M, Prybicien M, Feinberg JH. Functional deficits in athletes with a history of low back pain: A pilot study. *Arch Phys Med Rehabil* December 2002;83(12): 1753–1758.
98. Hodges PW. The role of the motor system in spinal pain: Implications for rehabilitation of the athlete following lower back pain. *J Sci Med Sport* September 2000;3(3):243–253.
99. Kreighbaum E, Barthels KM. *Biomechanics—A qualitative approach for studying human movement*, 3rd ed. New York: Macmillan Publishing Company, 1990.
100. Richardson C, Sims K. An inner range holding contraction: An objective measure of stabilizing function of anti-gravity muscle. In: *Proceedings of XI Congress of World Confederation of Physical Therapy.* London, 1991, pp. 829–831.
101. Hoffer J, Andreassen S. Regulation of soleus muscle stiffness in premammillary cats: Intrinsic and reflex components. *J Neurophysiol* February 1981;45(2):267–285.
102. Masamoto N, Larson R, Gates T, Faigenbaum A. Acute effects of plyometric exercise on maximum squat performance in male athletes. *J Strength Cond Res* February 2003;17(1):68–71.
103. Bullock-Saxton J, Janda V, Bullock M. Reflex activation of gluteal muscles in walking. *Spine* 1993;18(6):704–708.
104. Cooke PM, Lutz GE. Internal disc disruption and axial back pain in the athlete. *Phys Med Rehabil Clin N Am* November 2000;11(4):837–865.
105. Morris C. Chiropractic rehabilitation of a patient with S1 radiculopathy associated with a large L-5-S1 disk herniation. *J Manipulative Physiol Ther* January 1999;22(1):38–44.

PART

VI

CLINICAL MANAGEMENT

CHAPTER

31

EVIDENCE-BASED TREATMENT OF BACK PAIN

Nikolai Bogduk

OUTLINE

OBJECTIVES

1. To provide readers with a synopsis of the evidence concerning the treatment of acute and chronic low back pain, highlighting what is and is not effective.
2. To direct readers to the literature that is the source of that evidence.
3. To provide algorithms of how acute and chronic low back pain can be managed in accordance with the available evidence.

INTRODUCTION

Evidence-based medicine has wrought havoc on the management of back pain. Randomized controlled studies and systematic reviews have relentlessly assaulted almost every form of intervention. Few traditional interventions have emerged unscathed.

Most of this research activity has focused on acute low back pain. For this condition, where traditional interventions have been found less than satisfactory they have been replaced by new interventions and paradigm shifts for which there is stronger evidence of efficacy. For chronic low back pain, much of the evidence about current practices is negative, but no proven algorithm for management has emerged.

DEFINITIONS

At present, the International Association for the Study of Pain[1] recognizes a distinction only between acute and chronic pain. Using an arbitrary timescale, it defined *chronic pain* as pain that has been present for longer than 12 weeks, and *acute pain* as pain present for less than this period. Others recognize a further category of acute pain. They restrict the descriptor acute to pain that has been present for less than 5 or 7 weeks, on the grounds that within such a period there is still a good chance that the condition will resolve. Pain that persists beyond this time, but less than 12 weeks, is described as *subacute*.[2] This different term is applied because pain lasting beyond 7 weeks is less likely to resolve spontaneously and threatens to become chronic.

Although these definitions are somewhat arbitrary, they have become relevant and useful. The evidence base for the treatment of each temporal class of pain is different. Interventions that work for acute pain do not necessarily work for chronic pain; interventions for chronic pain may not be appropriate for acute pain; and subacute pain warrants interventions that are somewhat different from those for acute pain.

ACUTE BACK PAIN

What Does Not Work

Bed rest is counterproductive for acute low back pain. There is strong evidence that bed rest does not promote recovery, and that patients who are prescribed or who resort to bed rest are less likely to recover.[3,4] A systematic review found high quality evidence for small but consistent differences in favor of staying active for reduction of pain and improvement in function.[5] It concluded patients should unambiguously be advised to avoid bed rest.

The literature strongly denies any efficacy of particular exercises for acute low back pain. A program of specific exercises offers no attributable benefit, and may be no better than no intervention.[2] Exercise therapy is not more than other treatments with which it has been compared, such as usual care, manual therapy, and nonsteroidal anti-inflammatory drugs.[6] Any benefit of physical activity for acute low back pain is achieved by resuming normal activities of daily living, and does not require specific exercises.

When formally tested, patient education pamphlets provide little or no discernible effect on acute low back pain.[5-7] Such effects that might be attributed to pamphlets are either inconsistent or rapidly extinguished. Although pamphlets can reduce absenteeism, they do not reduce the severity of pain or associated physical problems.[8]

Clinical Pearl: Interventions that work for acute pain do not necessarily work for chronic pain; interventions for chronic pain may not be appropriate for acute pain; and subacute pain warrants interventions that are somewhat different than those for acute pain.

A systematic review identified four low quality studies of back school for acute low back pain and concluded, "there is no evidence that a back school is effective for acute low back pain, because of contradictory results."[2] Two studies, not covered by that review, found no attributable benefit of back school.[9,10]

The older literature on traction related to mixtures of patients with back pain and patients with sciatica. From that literature it is difficult to distill the efficacy of traction explicitly for acute low back pain. Effectively there is no evidence of efficacy of traction for acute low back pain. For subacute back pain, traction has been explicitly shown to provide no therapeutic benefit.[11,12]

An earlier systematic review found that the literature on acupuncture for acute low back pain is limited to studies that reported effects only immediately after treatment.[13] Even under those conditions, the benefits were not statistically superior to those of placebo. A later review, covering more recent studies found that acupuncture offered no greater benefit than either sham acupuncture or treatment with NSAIDs.[16]

The literature on transcutaneous electrical nerve stimulation (TENS) for acute low back pain is limited in volume. One low quality study reported some greater benefit than paracetamol at 6 weeks, but not at 1 or 2 weeks; a better quality study found no benefit over placebo TENS.[2,14]

There is no evidence of efficacy for formal behavioral therapy for acute low back pain.[2] Behavioral counseling confers no added benefit over other measures.[15]

No drug is curative of acute low back pain. At best, analgesics provide some degree of pain relief while recovery occurs naturally with time, or are promoted by other interventions. No studies have explicitly shown that paracetamol (acetominophen) is effective for back pain. Its use is recommended solely on the basis of its generic effects as an analgesic.

Nonsteroidal anti-inflammatory drugs (NSAIDs) are no more effective than placebo for acute low back pain, and no more effective than paracetamol.[20] They do not abolish pain; they offer an average reduction in pain of about only 20 points on a 0–100 scale. For short-term relief, NSAIDs are less effective than heat-wrap therapy.[21] Cox-2 agents are no more effective than COX-1 agents.[22] For short term relief of acute exacerbations of pain, willow bark has proved more effective than placebo, and at least as effective as NSAIDs.[23,24]

Compound analgesics (drugs containing paracetamol and a small amount of codeine) are no more effective than NSAIDs.[14] There is no evidence of efficacy for tricyclic antidepressants.[14]

Clinical Pearl: No drug is curative of acute low back pain. At best, analgesics provide some degree

of pain relief while recovery occurs naturally with time, or are promoted by other interventions.

The efficacy of various muscle relaxants has been studied.[2,14] The data are conflicting for tizanidine and orphenadrine. Diazepam and methocarbamol are not more effective than placebo. Cyclobenzaprine, dantrolene, carisoprodol, and baclofen are each slightly more effective than placebo, but only over periods of 4–10 days. Moreover, the utility of muscle relaxants is limited by a high incidence of central nervous system side effects.

A systematic review and meta-analysis found that manipulative therapy for acute low back pain was not significantly more effective, statistically, than sham therapy.[25] Furthermore, although manipulative therapy was slightly more effective than other therapies, such as exercises, massage, shortwave diathermy, or analgesics, which were judged to be ineffective, the magnitude of difference was clinically questionable.[25] A study published since that review, does not reverse this conclusion.[26]

What Does Work

The literature on manual therapy for acute low back pain is vexatious. Its quality ranges greatly, and the results of systematic reviews seem to change as new reviews are published. In general, it is reasonably evident that manual therapy is somewhat more effective than placebo treatment.[2,14] However, manual therapy is not consistently more effective than other physical interventions, such as exercises, massage, shortwave diathermy, or analgesics.

There is limited evidence that injections of local anaesthetic, with or without a corticosteroid, into tender points in the back are of some short-term benefit to some patients.[16,17] Injections, however, are insufficiently effective to be the single line of therapy, but they may be a useful adjunct to other measures such as manual therapy.[18,19]

Patients who maintain or resume activity are more likely to recover sooner and to have less chronic disability.[4] This activity, however, is nonspecific and global in nature. It does not pertain to undertaking exercises.

For patients who do not improve with simpler measures, more concerted interventions may be required. For those who develop subacute low back pain, a program of stretching exercises, low-impact aerobic exercises, and strengthening exercises, undertaken according to cognitive-behavioral principles, has been shown to reduce both pain and chronic disability.[20] Graded activity programs, consisting of supervised exercises in accordance with the patient's work requirements, are of some benefit for patients with subacute back pain,[21,22] but offer no advantage over simpler interventions for patients with acute low back pain.[23]

Clinical Pearl: Patients who maintain or resume activity are more likely to recover sooner and to have less chronic disability.

Although evidence is lacking that manual therapy, as a sole intervention, is effective for acute low back pain, there is some evidence that manual therapy, combined with exercises, activation, and injections of corticosteroids into tender areas, is both statistically and clinically more effective than physiotherapy.[31,32]

Based on the results of descriptive studies, workplace visits have been recommended on behalf of patients who have not returned to work after an episode of acute low back pain.[24] A workplace visit has been an integral component of some multidimensional programs that have proven successful for patients with subacute low back pain.[21,22] However, the effect of workplace visits cannot be dissected from the effects of other interventions in these studies. One study, however, has shown that adding occupational intervention resulted in reduced absence from work, faster return to work, less disability, less sickness impact, and reduced pain.[25]

Perhaps the most dramatic and enduring results for the treatment of subacute back pain have been those reported by Indahl and colleagues. Through a simple and limited program of intervention they achieved significant improvements in return to work,[26] that persisted at 5-year follow-up.[27] Their intervention consisted of a single consultation, with reinforcement at 3 months and 1 year. It required the physician to explain to the patients the cause of their pain, and to assure patients confidently that light activity would not injure any structure that could be involved in their pain. Patients were encouraged not to be careful, but to maintain light activity and set increasing goals. The physician addressed any fears about back pain that the patient had.

A Synthesis

For the management of acute low back pain, the current literature advocates and supports avoiding passive therapies and monochromatic therapies, i.e., relying on single types of interventions. In contrast, it advocates and supports providing to the patient an explanation of their pain, reassuring them that recovery is likely (without special interventions), maintaining activity, and empowering them to assume responsibility for their own rehabilitation. Adjunctive measures such as manual therapy and analgesics may be used to assist the patient, but the emphasis of therapy lies in addressing the patient's fears about back pain to prevent or reduce disability. If such simple measures prove insufficient, more concerted interventions such as graded exercises in a cognitive-behavioral milieu may need to be added, together with a workplace visit to address occupational impediments to restoration of normal activities.

These interventions can be encapsulated in the acute low back pain algorithm depicted in Figure 31–1. This algorithm is divided into four phases and incorporates a spiral design. The four phases are triage, management, concern, and vigilance. The spiral design involves reviewing the progress of the patient, checking compliance, providing reinforcement, and adding further or more concerted interventions if the patient is not responding.

Triage involves assessing the patient for neurological or red flag conditions that do not constitute simple, acute low back pain. If a serious condition is identified, it is managed appropriately, but outside the context of the algorithm.

Management focuses on the patient's cardinal presenting complaints: "I hurt," "I can't move," "I can't work," and "I'm scared."[29] Each complaint requires enquiry and explanation. Pain relief can be offered by analgesics, manual therapy, or injections. Movement is improved or restored by simple stretching exercises and activation. Return to work is encouraged and assisted as necessary. Fears are addressed and rationalized, and coping strategies are provided.

Clinical Pearl: These interventions can be encapsulated in the algorithm depicted in Figure 31–1. This algorithm is divided into four phases and incorporates a spiral design.

Concern is demonstrated and expressed by reviewing the patient, either to confirm recovery or to recognize failure to improve. In essence, the patient is not abandoned, and treatment is not assumed to have been successful just because the patient did not return.

If recovery is slow, compliance with previous interventions is checked, and if still appropriate these interventions are reinforced. Additional measures may be introduced. If psychosocial factors appear to be paramount, these are addressed in a more concerted manner, up to and including referral for specialist intervention, if required.

At each follow-up a check for red flag conditions is repeated. By this measure the practitioner remains alert to new features that may emerge as a serious condition manifests itself. However, in the absence of new red flag indicators, the practitioner can safely proceed with the algorithm as outlined.

Should a patient not exhibit recovery despite these measures, the possibility of a chronic pain problem developing should be recognized, and action steps taken to implement chronic pain management early in the history. This action is designed to avoid delays in securing appropriate referrals, during which a chronic problem may become more entrenched.

Although this algorithm is based theoretically on the available evidence, it has been field-tested.[30] It has been found to be safe, effective, and cost-effective. Evidence-based practice, according to the algorithm, is modestly better than usual care in terms of symptomatic relief, but is significantly better in terms of less need for continuing care and greater rates of complete recovery. Under this form of management, nearly 80% of patients can expect to be fully recovered by 3 months, and remain that way by 12 months. Moreover, evidence-based care is less expensive. Greater costs incurred by requiring a greater number of consultations to review and monitor patients are offset by savings in reduced use of imaging and expensive drug therapy, less use of referred services, and less use of complementary care and other interventions that patients seek and use.

CHRONIC BACK PAIN

The management of chronic low back pain is far more contentious and controversial than that of acute and subacute low back pain. Although many interventions have been reviewed, and many found wanting, no individual intervention or any program of interventions has been shown to be superlative.

Approaches to chronic low back pain differ in multiple respects. They differ with respect to whether a single practitioner or a team delivers the treatment. They differ with respect to whether special facilities are required. They differ ideologically with respect to whether a diagnosis and specific treatment is pursued *or* the pain and its associated behaviors are treated essentially symptomatically, without regard to specific diagnosis. Figure 31–2 illustrates the polarization and spectrum of strategies.

There is a tension between somatic and behavioral strategies. The somatic strategy assumes that there is a somatic cause for the pain, and seeks to diagnose and/or treat that cause. The behavioral strategy essentially disregards the cause of pain, and seeks instead to treat the secondary manifestations of the pain.

The somatic strategy relies largely on passive interventions that differ with respect to level of invasiveness and technology involved, i.e., level of invasiveness and technology utilized. Within the somatic strategy the "reductionist" approach seeks to identify the cause of pain and treat it specifically. The palliative approach recognizes that there is a somatic cause but that it cannot be identified, but should nevertheless be treated medically, usually with highly technological

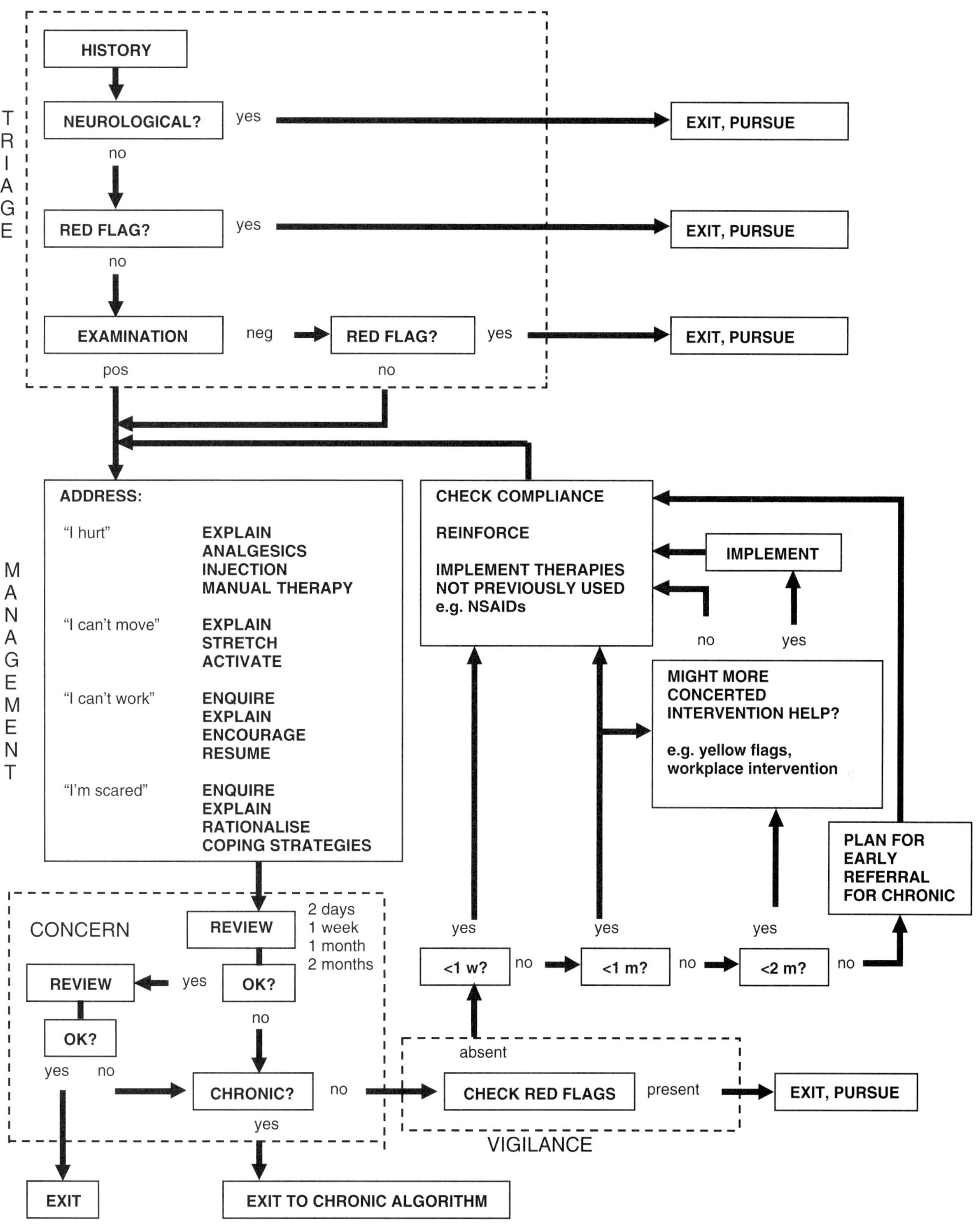

FIGURE 31–1. An algorithm for the management of acute low back pain. (*From Bogduk and McGuirk*[37].)

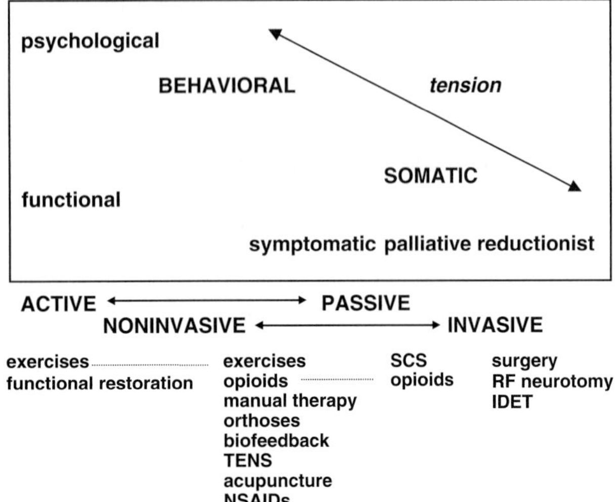

FIGURE 31–2. A schematic summary of the spectrum of strategies and interventions available for chronic low back pain.

interventions. The symptomatic approach assumes a somatic cause and treats it using more traditional interventions.

The behavioral strategy shuns passive interventions and relies instead on active interventions. It disregards any specific cause, and avers pursuit of that cause. Instead, it seeks to reduce the patient's problem by focusing on its behavioral components. Within the behavioral strategy, the psychological approach focuses on what the patients believe, how they feel about their pain, and what they do about it. The functional approach seeks to restore activities of daily living and occupational activities. The functional approach borrows some of the interventions whose roots lie in the symptomatic, somatic approach.

Symptomatic Treatment

The evidence is least favorable for classical, empirical approaches for chronic low back pain. Although NSAIDs are more effective than placebo, there is no evidence of long-term efficacy and every risk of serious side effects with prolonged use.[2,14] Earlier systematic reviews found that antidepressants are not effective. [2,17,40] A more recent review [41] proposed that they are slightly more effective than placebo, but antidepressants have not be tested for longer than 8 weeks. They provide only partial relief, and their utility is limited by their side-effect profile. No muscle relaxant that has been studied for chronic low back pain has been found to be effective.[19] Oral opioids provide only marginal relief of pain, and do not improve disability.[32,33]

For orthoses, transcutaneous electrical nerve stimulation (TENS), and electromyographic biofeedback there is no evidence of efficacy.[2,17,44] Traction is no more effective than sham therapy.[2,4,44] Hydrotherapy is more effective than being put on a waiting list for improving disability, but offers no benefits for pain.[45]

Manual therapy has enjoyed a reputation of being effective for chronic low back pain, but the latest meta-analysis did not support this reputation. Although manipulative therapy is slightly more effective than sham therapy, it is not more effective than other forms of care, including GP care, physiotherapy or exercises, back school, or therapies known to be ineffective.[25] Manipulative therapy was found to be more effective than sham therapies by only 4 points on a 100-point scale.

The efficacy of acupuncture for chronic low back pain remains contentious. An earlier systematic review found insufficient evidence to determine if acupuncture was more than a placebo.[15] A more recent review found acupuncture to be more effective than sham therapy for short-term relief of pain, but the attributable effect was not sustained for longer periods.[16] Furthermore, acupuncture was no more effective than self care education or TENS, and was less effective than manipulation or massage.[16]

Massage is emerging as a viable option for chronic low back pain, although its merits are limited. It is superior to sham therapy, less effective than manipulation, but more effective than corsets, exercises, relaxation, acupuncture, and self-care education.[46]

Of all the traditional, conservative interventions for chronic back pain, exercises are regarded as the most effective. There is an abundant literature reporting that intensive exercises are more effective than usual care, physical modalities, hot packs and rest, behavioral therapy, no exercise, being put on a waiting list, or placebo treatment[2,14]; but no particular type of exercise has been shown to be superior to any other. Exercises, however, do not constitute a cure; they do not eliminate pain. They may or may not reduce pain, but they usually improve functional capacity. In isolation, however, exercises offer only a modest therapeutic benefit, but greater gains have been reported with the use of exercises in the context of multidisciplinary rehabilitation programs.

According to some studies, injection of lignocaine or corticosteroids into tender areas of the back benefits some patients.[44] Those benefits, however, are modest and short-lived.[44] Collectively the studies favor an effect but the pooled outcome data fail to achieve statistical significance.[47]

A particular form of injection therapy is prolotherapy. This involves injecting sclerosing agents into tender sites of ligament attachments. The literature offers mixed results, which vary according to the agents and protocols used.[48] One placebo controlled study provides intriguing results.[49] In that study, some 20% of patients were rendered free of pain by prolotherapy, and a further 20% reduced their pain by half. These results were sustained at 12 months. Intriguingly, statistically equivalent outcomes were achieved by the control treatment, which involved the injection of normal saline. These results strongly suggest that injection, irrespective of the agent used, is the active component of the therapy. Furthermore, no treatment for chronic low back pain has demonstrated relief in such large proportions of patients, sustained for so long. The evidence, therefore, suggests that, of all drugs for chronic low back pain, ironically the most effective is normal saline by injection.[19]

Palliative Treatment

High-tech palliative therapies include spinal cord stimulation and intrathecal opioids. They are interventions performed largely as "salvage" procedures for patients who have exhausted or defied other interventions. Their efficacy, however, has not been assessed in controlled trials, and relies exclusively on descriptive studies.

Spinal cord stimulation has typically been applied to patients with persisting back pain after surgical treatment. On average, about 60% of patients achieve at least 50% relief of their pain, sustained at 12 months. However, only about 30% return to work.[34]

A compilation of the literature on intraspinal opioids[35] reported that success rates vary considerably, and that conditions such as "failed" back tend to be resistant to intraspinal treatment. This form of treatment appears to be distinctly palliative, in that the literature focuses on relief of pain only, and does not report reduction in disability and return to work.

Behavioral Therapy

Purely behavioral therapy is quite clearly more effective than no treatment or being put on a waiting list.[36] In this context it has a moderate positive effect on pain intensity and a small positive effect on general functional status. However, when added to other interventions behavioral therapy confers no long-term or short-term benefit on pain intensity, functional status, or behavioral outcome.[36] Such benefits as might be attributed to behavioral therapy arise when cognitive-behavioral principles have been applied in more physically orientated functional restoration programs.

Functional Restoration

As originally described, functional restoration is a program of management based on sports medicine principles, in which the complaint of pain is essentially disregarded, and management instead focuses on improving the patient's capacity for movement and for tasks specific to his or her occupation. A hallmark of the program is the use of back-testing machines to monitor objectively the changes in range of movement and muscle strength, with regular provision of feedback of gains to the patient. A typical program requires a 3-week live-in period with activities for 57 h/week, involving specific exercises, work simulation, and work hardening, coupled with education and cognitive-behavioral training.[37]

The first studies of functional restoration described an 86% return to work, and a reduction in surgery rates and consumption of health care.[37] A 2-year follow-up confirmed that 86% of patients had remained at work.[38] These results were subsequently replicated by independent investigators,[39,40] and functional restoration has attracted considerable endorsement, at least in the United States.[41] However, each of these studies used a convenience sample as a control group: patients who were denied entry into the treatment program either by their physicians or by their insurance companies. Subsequent studies that used better control groups have not borne out the success rates of the US studies, and have shown no difference to control therapy. A Canadian study[42] compared the functional restoration group with a control group who underwent "usual care," and found an 80% return to work for both groups. There were no significant differences in days lost from work, number of claims, wages lost, or cost of claims. One significant difference was that functional restoration cost more than "usual care."

A Finnish study[43] compared functional restoration with light and unspecific exercises. The males but not the females in the functional restoration group achieved significantly better improvement in flexibility and performance capacity. Their pain and disability, while significantly less from a statistical perspective, was reduced only by a clinically trivial degree. There were no differences in psychological status, sick leave, retirement, use of health care, or endurance.

These studies showed that, when comparable control groups are used, functional restoration is not noticeably superior to other interventions, and that functional restoration appears not to work as well outside the United States. The Finnish investigators[43] concluded that perhaps a difference in social structure bears on the success of functional restoration, or lack thereof. In Finland, patients have the security of a disability pension if they remain with back pain, which is more generous than is available in the United States. Consequently, it may be that in the United States there is a stronger incentive to recover, or conversely, in socialized medical systems there is a disincentive to respond to functional restoration.

Multidisciplinary Treatment Programs

It is not readily evident from the literature exactly how multidisciplinary treatment programs differ from functional restoration programs. Under multidisciplinary treatment some reviewers include some literature that pertains to functional restoration but include other, additional studies.[14,44] The distinction may lie in the extent to which intensive exercises are coupled with behavioral therapy, or the distinction may be artificial or arbitrary. Nevertheless, opinion leaders favor multidisciplinary treatment as the premier approach to managing chronic back pain.[14,45]

Notwithstanding this endorsement, the results of multidisciplinary treatment programs are not uniform or consistent. Compared to control treatment, multidisciplinary treatment does not necessarily achieve better outcomes in terms of pain and disability, and short-term benefits are not necessarily sustained in the long-term.[14] Intensive programs are more effective than less intensive programs with respect reducing pain and improving function,[44] although this distinction relies exclusively on the reported results of one center.[46–49] Some intensive programs report significant improvements in "workreadiness" but others show no benefits in terms of employment status and sick leave.[44] Less intensive programs have not shown improvements in pain, function, or vocational outcomes when compared with non-multidisciplinary outpatient rehabilitation or usual care.[44]

Surgery

Surgery for chronic low back pain is a contentious issue. Reviewers have consistently found no randomized controlled studies of its efficacy. Its reputation rests on observational studies only. A systematic review, now somewhat dated, found that whereas a satisfactory outcome was achieved in an average of 69% of patients, the success rate ranged greatly, from 16% to 95%.[50] More recent reviewers were not persuaded by observational studies, and concluded that there is no acceptable evidence of the efficacy of any form of fusion for degenerative lumbar spondylosis, back pain, or "instability"[51] and no evidence on whether any form of surgery for degenerative lumbar disc disease is effective in returning patients to work.[14]

Two controlled studies have done little to convert this conclusion. In one, surgery was more effective than physical therapy,[69] but the outcomes were modest in both groups. Some 29% of patients felt "much better" after surgery, and 34% felt "better", compared to 15% and 15% of patients treated with physical therapy. However, surgery was not curative. Although mean pain scores for back pain fell from 64 at baseline to 30 at six months, they reverted to 43 by two years. In the other study, the outcomes of surgery were no better than those achieved by counseling and a brief course of supervised exercise, both for pain and for disability.[70]

These aforementioned studies, like most of the literature on fusion, pertain to surgery undertaken without a valid patho-anatomic diagnosis having been made. In effect, surgery was undertaken on the basis of persisting symptoms and imaging findings. Meanwhile, tantalizing results have been reported when surgery has been performed expressly for internal disc disruption (IDD). This condition perhaps best exemplifies the reductionist approach to chronic low back pain.

IDD is a condition characterized by a radial fissure within the affected disc that, somehow, renders it painful. The condition is diagnosed by provocation discography and the demonstration on computed tomography (CT) of a radial fissure.[52] Population studies have shown that radial fissures are not age-related, nor are they related to degeneration, but they correlate strongly with the affected disc being painful.[53] Among patients with chronic low back pain, IDD is the single-most common cause of pain that can be objectively diagnosed, and accounts for at least 40% of cases.[52]

To date, interbody fusion has been the mainstay of treatment for this condition. Many observational studies have reported attractive success rates, based on relief of pain and return to work, as noted in Table 31–1. While such figures remain in the public domain, fusion will continue to be an attractive option for patients with proven IDD who do not benefit from other interventions.

Clinical Pearl: Among patients with chronic low back pain, IDD is the single-most common cause of pain that can be objectively diagnosed, and accounts for at least 40% of cases.

Table 31–1, however, also includes studies with lower success rates. Consequently, it is not evident whether good success rates amount to reporting bias, or are contingent upon patient selection, the skill of the surgeon, or both. How to resolve this issue remains one of the paramount challenges in the treatment of chronic back pain.

Radiofrequency Neurotomy

One of the sources of chronic back pain that can be identified objectively is the lumbar zygapophyseal joint. Pain stemming from these joints can be diagnosed using controlled diagnostic blocks.[61] Among injured workers in the United States with chronic low back pain, the prevalence of lumbar zygapophyseal joint pain is about 15%.[62] In more heterogeneous and older populations the prevalence is about 40%.[63,64] Lumbar zygapophyseal joint pain is, therefore, common and diagnosable. It is also treatable.

Lumbar zygapophyseal joint pain can be relieved using percutaneous lumbar medial branch neurotomy: a procedure also erroneously known as facet denervation or facet rhizotomy. It achieves relief by coagulating the nerves that innervate the painful

TABLE 31–1. **Criteria for Successful Outcome and Success Rates of Observational Studies of Interbody Fusion for Internal Disc Disruption**

	Criteria for Successful Outcome			
Source	>75% Relief of Pain	Return to Work or Normal Activities of Daily Living	No Opioid Medication	Success Rate
Lee et al.[73]	+	+	+	89%
Blumenthal et al.[74]		+	+	74%
Kozak and O'Brien[75]	+	+	+	74%
Gill and Blumenthal[76]	+	+	+	66%
Loguidice et al.[77]		+		61%
Vamvanij et al.[78]	+	+	+	42%
Knox and Champion[79]	+	+		35%

joint or joints. A controlled trial has shown that this procedure is not a placebo.[65] Another study has shown that, in carefully selected patients, pain relief is enduring. Some 60% of patients can expect at least 80% reduction in their pain at 12 months after treatment, and 80% can expect at least 60% relief.[66]

Medial branch neurotomy, however, does not constitute a permanent cure. The coagulated nerves regenerate over a period of 6–12 months, and pain recurs. In that event, repeating the procedure can reinstate pain relief. This need for repeat treatment renders the procedure unattractive in some circles, but no other intervention has been shown to be able to eliminate, let alone relieve, zygapophyseal joint pain.

Clinical Pearl: Medial branch neurotomy does not constitute a permanent cure for zygapophyseal joint pain. The coagulated nerves regenerate over a period of 6–12 months, and pain recurs.

Intradiscal Electrothermal Anuloplasty

Intradiscal electrothermal anuloplasty (IDETA or IDET) is a recent innovation designed explicitly for the treatment of chronic back pain due to IDD. The cardinal attraction of the procedure is that it is a less invasive alternative to surgical fusion.

Observational studies attest to various degrees of success.[90] A placebo-controlled trial showed that the outcomes could not be wholly attributed to a placebo effect.[91] A cohort study with comparison group found that 50% of patients reduced their pain by at least half and returned to work; but moreover, 20% of patients obtained complete relief of pain, and were able to return to work.[92,93] These outcomes were sustained at two years.

Even a modest success rate would make IDET an attractive option to surgical fusion. However, several problems still need to be resolved.

An Algorithm for Chronic Low Back Pain

There is no proven algorithm for the management of chronic low back pain. Moreover, physicians seeking secure help for their patients will be faced with an ideological decision. They will need to decide whether to follow the behavioral or the somatic strategy, and whether to follow a symptomatic or reductionist approach.

Under a behavioral strategy the best option for the patient would be a multidisciplinary treatment program involving intensive exercises coupled with cognitive-behavioral therapy. Under such a program, patients will not necessarily be relieved of their pain, but they stand a reasonable chance of improving function and perhaps being able to return to work.

Under a conservative, somatic strategy, the patient could be treated with exercises or manual therapy, without regard to a specific diagnosis. While such interventions might produce some improvements in pain and function, patients should not be placed under the illusion that these interventions are curative.

Only the reductionist approach offers any prospect of complete or substantial relief of pain. However, it requires establishing a diagnosis first. This will require controlled diagnostic blocks to test for zygapophyseal joint pain, and disc stimulation to test for IDD. Patients with proven zygapophyseal joint pain can be treated with radiofrequency neurotomy. Patients with IDD can be treated with IDET or interbody fusion.

The conundrum that physicians and their patients must confront is where to start: whether to exhaust conservative therapy and multidisciplinary treatment first, in the hope that only a few patients will remain who might require a reductionist strategy; or to follow a reductionist strategy first so as to identify those patients who might benefit from a specific intervention rather than committing all to multidisciplinary treatment and its limited efficacy.

Underlying this conundrum is a fundamental strategic and philosophical issue: Is chronic back pain something that one seeks only to ease or palliate, or does one seek to relieve it completely? In either instance, what is the evidence of success and what is the evidence that patients are really satisfied?

EVIDENCE-BASED MANAGEMENT OF LOW BACK PAIN: A PRACTICAL DEMONSTRATION

Practitioners may have difficulties reconciling the evidence base with what they themselves have been accustomed to doing, and with what they see being done around them. Many of the results of systematic reviews of the literature challenge or refute the efficacy of common practices. This may leave practitioners with the dilemma—what to do.

Ultimately, individual practitioners will need to make a choice. This may entail changing their practices. It may require abandoning certain practices and adopting new ones. This may threaten practitioners' sense of comfort, for they are familiar with what they have been doing, but are not necessarily familiar with new approaches.

Practice guidelines serve to inform practitioners as to what the research literature says is good practice and what is questionable or poor practice. Practitioners then decide if they wish to practice according to the evidence. In making such a decision, however, some practitioners may be at a loss as to how exactly they are supposed to accommodate and incorporate the evidence base. One way of perhaps influencing practitioners is to lead by example, i.e., to provide an account of how someone else deals with this issue. Therefore, the following account describes how the author practically integrates evidence-based principles into the treatment of low back pain.

Clinical Pearl: Practice guidelines serve to inform practitioners as to what the research literature says is good practice and what is questionable or poor practice. Practitioners then decide if they wish to practice according to the evidence.

Acute Low Back Pain

For patients who present with their first episode of back pain, two cardinal responsibilities are assumed. The first is to screen the patients to ensure that they do not have a serious cause for their pain. The second and subsequent responsibility is to promote recovery and to avoid disability. The foremost tool that is exercised in this regard is history. This entails a comprehensive history that records the circumstances of onset and the nature of the pain. How to do this is beyond the province of this chapter, but has been elaborated in detail in previous chapters and elsewhere.[28]

It is also critical to determine that the patients do not have radicular pain (i.e., sciatica). The causes, mechanisms, investigation, and management of radicular pain are distinctly different from that of low back pain.[71] What may be appropriate tests and appropriate treatment for radicular pain are not necessarily appropriate for low back pain, and are usually not appropriate. Failure to understand and to abide by this distinction has been a major problem in the past that has lead to the mismanagement of patients with back pain. Investigations such as electromyography, magnetic resonance imaging (MRI), and CT scanning might be appropriate for radicular pain,[71] but they are not appropriate for low back pain.[28] Interventions such as epidural injections of corticosteroids might be appropriate for radicular pain,[71] but they are not indicated for low back pain.[28] How to make the distinction between radicular pain and low back pain has been elaborated in Chapters 10 and 12, as well as elsewhere.[28,71]

Clinical Pearl: The causes, mechanisms, investigation, and management of radicular pain are distinctly different from that of low back pain.

Having taken a history, and having examined the patient, he or she is then allocated to one of three categories[28]:

Red back pain	In which there is some evidence from history of examination that the patient might have a "red flag" condition, i.e., a fracture, a tumor, or infection.
Yellow back pain	In which the history and examination reveal no suggestion of a serious cause for the pain, but the patient exhibits or expresses a psychosocial "yellow flag," i.e., fears or inappropriate beliefs about the cause of their pain, or that physical, social, or vocational activities will harm them and should be avoided.
Green back pain	In which there is no evidence from history and examination of serious cause of pain, and the patient does not express inordinate fears or misconceptions about their pain, and is potentially able to resume normal activities, and be responsible for their own rehabilitation.

TABLE 31–2. Criteria for Medical Imaging in Patients with Acute Low Back Pain

Severe trauma	Minor trauma in patients:
History of cancer	–over 50 years of age
Unexplained weight loss	–taking corticosteroids
Temperature > 37.8°C	–with osteoporosis
Risk factor for infection	
Neurological signs	
Failure to improve after 1 month	

For the patient with red back pain, one must explain what has raised one's suspicions. The nature and purpose of the investigations that need to be undertaken must be explained. In many cases, this may be no more complicated than obtaining an erythrocyte sedimentation rate, or other blood tests. In most cases it will involve imaging. However, it is important to abide by strict guidelines with respect to imaging.[28] Medical imaging is undertaken only if the patient satisfies one of the criteria listed in Table 31–2. MRI is the modality of choice in this instance. However, imaging is not indicated if the patient does not satisfy the criterion.

For patients with yellow back pain, investigations are not indicated, and they are not required. What is required is a more concerted approach to their fears, misconceptions, and attitudes to their pain.

For patients with green back pain, one can afford to be encouraging and reassuring without reservation, and expect a rapid recovery.

In all instances, however, the author follows a plan of management as outlined by the acute low back pain algorithm depicted in Figure 31–1. Depending on the patients and the nature of their problems, the plan is textured according to their needs. For patients with red back pain, the emphasis will be on relief of pain, until the results of investigations are available. If those results reveal a serious disorder then that disorder is managed as required. That patient no longer is one with simple back pain. He or she is managed for the condition that is diagnosed. If the results of investigations reveal no serious disorder, the patient converts to one with green back pain.

According to the terms of the acute low back pain algorithm, the clinician determines the extent to which the patient's problems lie in "I hurt," "I can't move," "I can't work," and "I'm scared." At the first consultation, the objective is to ensure that the patient does not leave with at least one of these problems having improved to the patient's satisfaction. Remaining or persisting problems can be addressed at subsequent consultations, as required.

For "I hurt," an explanation is primarily provided. Perhaps most critically, patients want to hear that there is not a serious cause for their pain; that they will not get worse; and that there is every chance that they will get better. Irrespective of whether the clinician explains that they have a sprain, or some other simple problem, the objective is to be reassuring. Nor should one feel obliged to stop the pain immediately or pretend to be able to do so. However, natural history is on the clinician's side, and on the patient's side. The odds are that they will progressively recover, even regardless of what treatment is provided. Nevertheless, there are some things that can be done to supplement this recovery. Simple analgesics can be provided, in the form of paracetamol on a time-contingent basis, i.e., at prescribed intervals, not on the basis of "take when desired." The author does not portray other measures, such as manual therapy or injections, as designed to relieve pain. Rather, these might be employed to improve movement.

For "I can't move," again an explanation is provided, not only of why the patient has difficulty moving, but also of what can be done to improve movement. One must emphasize that movement will not be harmful, and explain that the prognosis is worse for patients who rest and who do not make an effort to resume normal activities. For patients with tight or reactive back muscles, one can apply soft tissue mobilization to stretch the muscles in the first instance. However, the critical next step is to empower the patients with means by which they can do this for themselves. For this, they are instructed in simple stretching exercises, and mobilizing maneuvers (like those recommend by McKenzie[72]; see Chapter 22). These are not portrayed as curative, or even as therapeutic. Instead, they are used as a device by which the patient can maintain and increase mobility. They are portrayed as "warm up" exercise before undertaking normal activities of daily living. They are also portrayed as first aid measures: as something to do when the pain starts building up.

For "I can't work," the clinician should explore the circumstances, reasons, and beliefs. In some cases this might be a major problem that cannot be addressed properly at the first consultation, and which will need to be assessed progressively over subsequent consultations. In other instances, reassurance and permission to return to work may be all that is required. If there are legitimate issues concerning work practices and safety, or if the patient requires modified duties, this will need to be negotiated on behalf of the worker. The author undertakes those negotiations if possible. If for logistic reasons this responsibility cannot be assumed, then the assistance of an occupational medicine consultant is required.

"I'm scared" is probably the most unrecognized and most undertreated problem with which patients present. Too often practitioners have assumed that all that they have to do is provide analgesia and some exercises, whereupon the pain, the patient, and their problem will go away. However, fears are the major determinant of disability and failure to recover. Accordingly, it is my responsibility to determine what the patients fear and to do something about it. This requires engaging the patients about their fears, beliefs, and attitudes. Most often, these are simple problems that are dispelled by convincing and confident explanation. More entrenched and resistant fears and beliefs need to be addressed in subsequent consultations.

Clinical Pearl: Too often practitioners have assumed that all that they have to do is provide analgesia and some exercises, whereupon the pain, the patients, and their problem will go away. However, fears are the major determinant of disability and failure to recover.

An important feature of the algorithm for acute low back pain (Fig. 31–1) is to demonstrate concern. This is achieved by scheduling a review. On the one hand, if the patient has recovered or is progressing well, the review consultation establishes that this is the case. Doing so prevents the illusion that "the patient must have recovered because they did not come back." On the other hand, the review allows the clinician continue to help the patient who has not recovered, and shows that he or she has not been abandoned.

If the patient has not recovered, or is progressing only slowly, this presents an excellent opportunity foremost to check compliance. Did the patient understand the interventions that were prescribed, and has he or she used them? If the patient has not, the instruction is repeated to ensure that this time he or she does understand, and can do what is required properly. If he or she has complied, this presents the opportunity to reinforce the explanations and interventions that were offered previously. If necessary, one can then implement interventions not previously used. If paracetamol does not provide sufficient pain relief, one can prescribe an NSAID. If simple exercises and self-mobilization seem to be insufficient, one can consider manipulative therapy with or without injections of local anesthetic into tender areas. If one cannot provide these latter interventions, the clinician can simply coordinate the management of the patient with a colleague who can provide them. In that regard, what the author does not do is refer the patient away, but rather remain pivotal to the patient's management. The clinician can draw upon the services of others, but remains responsible for monitoring the patient's progress.

If psychosocial issues are prominent with the patient, it is important to explore these at the review consultation and subsequent consultations. In most instances, one should be able to make progress with these matters. Only in extreme cases is assistance from behavioral therapists required (see Chapter 19). However, these should preferably be performed early in the evolution of the patient's problem than to wait until they have developed chronic pain.

For patients who have not deteriorated, but who have difficulty successfully assuming responsibility for their own rehabilitation, one might consider enrolling them in a responsible rehabilitation program. In this regard, the author does not accept or rely upon just any rehabilitation provider. It is important to be confident that whoever is used does provide a program *concordant with contemporary evidence-based practice*. The key ingredients of such a program is an exercise program designed to improve function, conducted in a cognitive milieu. That means that the rehabilitation specialists are not relying on passive interventions, or on just an exercise program, but are simultaneously addressing the patient's beliefs and attitudes. Moreover, the therapists need to be convincing, confident, and enthusiastic (if not also charismatic) in order to engender an optimistic environment. The author considers that sending the patient to an outfit that simply does work assessments, and does not express concern and cares about the patient's future welfare, is a waste of expense and effort.

In following this approach, the emphasis has been not on stopping the pain, but on assisting the patient to cope with that pain while he or she recovers naturally. The principal intervention has been behavioral rather than physical; therefore, analgesics or NSAIDs would have been used for pain relief, and simple exercises or manipulative therapy to restore movement. But otherwise, the emphasis has been on how the patient thinks and reacts to the pain. The patient has been provided an explanation. The clinician has been reassuring and encouraging while identifying and addressing any fears and misconceptions. The patient has been encouraged and helped to resume normal activities, including work. The author is encouraged that such an approach is effective by the results of studies that have implemented it.[26,27,30]

Nevertheless, this approach will not be universally successful. A proportion of patients will continue to suffer problems despite the best of measures and intentions. This proportion may be as large as 30%,[26,27,30] although not all of these patients will be seriously or severely disabled. For patients with persisting problems, a new strategy is adopted. Moreover, the author would venture to implement the strategy for chronic pain sooner rather than later: at 2 months rather than waiting for the statutory 3 months, at which time the patient would have officially become "chronic."

Chronic Low Back Pain

The decision whether to follow a palliative or a reductionist approach must be determined. This decision is based on the demeanor of the patients and the nature of their problems. The reductionist approach is suitable for patients without overt, major psychosocial problems—in whom pain and the distress that it causes is the prevailing problem, and who realistically would like something done about it. The palliative approach applies to patients with widespread pain, or those who are considered unable to comply with investigations, or who do not wish to pursue investigations.

Figure 31–3 provides an algorithm for chronic back pain in graphic form. While this chapter briefly explains the evidence-based rationale and reason behind this algorithm, greater detail regarding the overall strategy is presented elsewhere.[37]

All approaches need to be predicated by an assessment of the patient for possible red flag conditions, both by history and by MRI. If a serious cause of pain is recognized or suspected, it should be investigated. If confirmed, the patient exits the algorithm, and the condition is specifically treated. By the same token, patients with more than just back pain should be recognized and separately managed. Widespread pain does not constitute low back pain, and requires a different approach to management.

Another consideration is whether or not the patient has been treated appropriately while their back pain was still in the acute or subacute phase. If the patient has been treated correctly, according to the principles and practices outlined above (see *Acute Low Back Pain* above), there is no point repeating this style of intervention. Since psychosocial problems will already have been addressed, the persistence of pain cannot be attributed to bad treatment or bad attitude. The imperative becomes to locate the source of pain. On the other hand, if the patient has not been managed correctly, the possibility obtains that applying

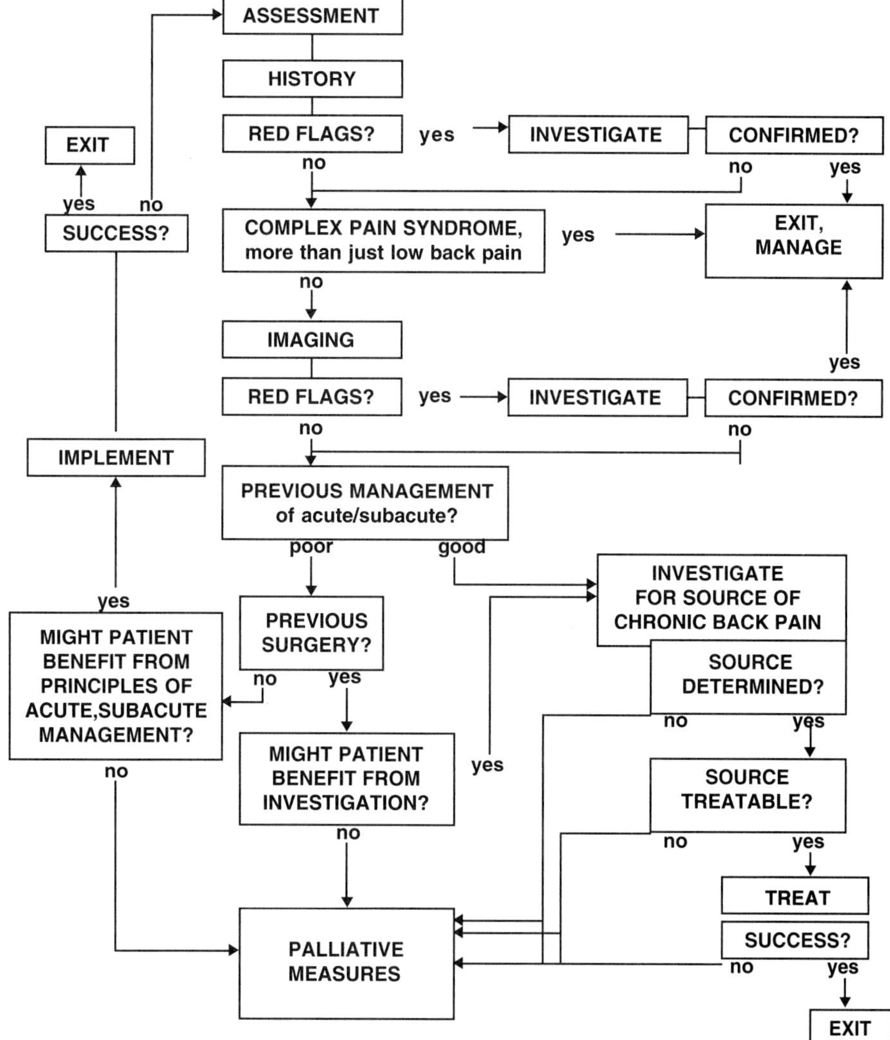

FIGURE 31–3. An algorithm for the management of chronic low back pain. (*From Bogduk and McGuirk*[37].)

the principles of good management of acute low back pain could still benefit the patient. There is no need to rush into investigations, or to adopt palliative measures, if a concerted program of assurance and activation might still help.

As previously noted, an algorithm for the management of chronic low back pain is depicted in Figure 31–1*B*. While this chapter briefly explains the evidence-based rationale and reason behind this algorithm, greater detail regarding the overall strategy is presented elsewhere.[28]

Reductionist Approach

In exercising the reductionist approach, the author starts with an MRI, if one has not already been obtained. On the one hand this test provides clearance—it will show that the patient does not have an occult disorder that has been missed to date, and which requires medical or surgical therapy. On the other hand it provides an assessment of the status of the patient's intervertebral discs.

If the patient has disc disease at multiple levels, the author knows of no specific intervention that is likely to help them. (The author does not believe that three level fusions succeed in relieving pain.) Whereupon the author is reluctant to pursue the reductionist approach further. If the patient has no evidence of disc disease, the author is reluctant to pursue discogenic pain. Although patients might have discogenic pain despite a normal MRI, these patients are few. In patients with a normal MRI, their source of pain is more likely to lie somewhere other than in the discs. For those patients the author pursues investigations of their synovial joints. If, however, the patients have one or two discs that appear to be abnormal whereas their other discs are normal, the author is drawn to investigating them for discogenic pain.

Clinical Pearl: If the patient has no evidence of disc disease, the author is reluctant to pursue discogenic pain. Although patients might have discogenic pain despite a normal MRI, these patients are few.

Synovial Joint Protocol Having decided to pursue source of pain among the synovial joints of the lumbosacral spine, it is important to pay particular attention to the distribution of the pain. If the pain extends above L5, the preference is to investigate for zygapophyseal joint pain. If the pain does not extend above the level of L5, the likelihood of the pain arising from an intervertebral disc or a zygapophyseal joint is low.[73] Accordingly, the likelihood of its source being in the sacroiliac joint is higher than that in the general population. Therefore, sacroiliac joint blocks are undertaken.

If these blocks prove positive, a diagnosis would have been established, and can save the patient from further pursuit of a diagnosis. Unfortunately, there is no sufficiently proven treatment for sacroiliac joint pain. The author is not convinced that arthrodesis works for this condition, and has seen no valid literature to that effect. Nor does the author fall prey to assertions that prolotherapy or radiofrequency denervation works for sacroiliac joint pain. The author does not defer to practitioners who ply these interventions wantonly. The author prepared to enroll patients in studies that conscientiously seek to evaluate any new treatment for sacroiliac joint pain, under ethical approval, but will not refer patients for experimental treatment at the hands of practitioners who are not conducting a proper study. If studies are not available, palliative approach for these patients is pursued.

If sacroiliac joint blocks prove negative, one should be prepared to pursue the possibility of zygapophyseal joint pain, although recognizing that the likelihood of a positive yield is low. Whereas one might prefer simply to pursue a palliative approach for these patients, a screening test for zygapophyseal joint pain is an innocuous investigation that can be undertaken either to rule out zygapophyseal joint pain, or on the remote chance of finding it.

For zygapophyseal joint pain, an appropriate screening test is medial branch blocks at L5, L4, and L3. These blocks can be performed unilaterally for patients with unilateral pain or pain predominantly on one side, or bilaterally in patients with bilateral pain. Screening blocks are undertaken because there are no valid means of implicating a particular joint or a particular level, without performing presumptive blocks. Moreover, lumbar zygapophyseal joint pain is not common. Therefore, the pretest odds are that the patient will not have zygapophyseal joint pain. Therefore, it becomes inefficient to progress by guesswork: testing one joint, then the next, and then another, only to find them all negative. A screening block tests if all the possibly painful joints are negative.

If the screening blocks prove negative, zygapophyseal joint pain would have been ruled out, and investigations cease. If the screening blocks prove positive, investigations can be resumed focusing on particular levels. Under those conditions, the pursuit of further blocks is justified. The screening blocks have indicated that the patient does have zygapophyseal joint pain. Further blocks are required simply to pinpoint which joint or joints are the source of pain. If a diagnosis of zygapophyseal joint pain is established, one can offer the patient treatment by radiofrequency medial branch neurotomy.

Discogenic Pain Protocol For patients in whom the clinician elects to pursue discogenic pain, one should undertake provocation discography and postdiscography CT. If discography proves negative or indeterminate, it is appropriate to cease investigations and follow a palliative approach. If discography proves positive at one or two levels, treatment should be considered.

One option for proven discogenic pain is anterior lumbar interbody fusion. For this treatment, however, a trusted surgeon is required, and on whose technique the clinician has confidence. It is preferable to adopt a palliative approach rather than subject a patient to the risks of poorly performed, major surgery.

Clinical Pearl: For patients in whom the clinician elects to pursue discogenic pain, one should undertake provocation discography and postdiscography CT.

Otherwise, there is the option of offering the patient IDETA. If the clinician does not provide this intervention, then the patient should be referred to a colleague who did, and whose technique is trusted. One should not assume that someone who says that they perform this procedure would necessarily do it properly and well. For this procedure, the patient must satisfy strict indications.[74] Inter alia, they must have preserved disc height, and have a grade III or grade IV fissure in the symptomatic disc, as demonstrated by CT-discography. If the patients satisfy these criteria, they have a 50% chance of reducing their pain by more than half, and a 20% chance of obtaining complete relief. If the patients are not candidates for IDETA, they can exercise the option to undergo anterior fusion, or to resort to palliative measures.

Palliative Approach

Other than medial branch neurotomy, anterior fusion, or IDETA, no other intervention has been shown to be capable of providing substantial and sustained relief from chronic low back pain. Various interventions may provide temporary relief, or partial relief, in some patients, but none is renown as a panacea, and none has been proven to be more than palliative.

For patients for whom reductionist investigations and treatment cannot be offered, a variety of palliative measures are available. In this arena the preference is to use those for which there is some evidence, in order know what the patient can expect.

An intensive, multidisciplinary pain treatment program is one option. One must emphasize on "intensive" because systematic reviews have indicated that only intensive programs are associated with any substantive degree of success.[44] Lesser programs simply do not offer worthwhile outcomes. Even so, the patients must be instructed that they are not undertaking a program that will rid them of their pain. What they can expect is to improve their physical function, and to learn techniques by which they might better be able to cope with their persisting pain.

For patients who have failed back surgery syndrome, the preferred (and only) option is spinal cord stimulation. Although this intervention has not been subjected to controlled trials, the observational data do provide long-term follow-up. One can expect some 50% of patients to obtain 50% or greater reduction of their pain.[34] From personal experience, in an unpublished study by a Master's student, the author can expect 30% of patients to achieve satisfying improvements in pain, mood, and function, and require no need for further treatment. Otherwise, for failed back surgery syndrome there is reason for optimism. Studies not yet published (at the time of this writing) have shown that many of these patients have treatable lesions, provided that they are investigated properly. In particular, some 40% have undiagnosed IDD. Failed back surgery syndrome does not need to be a terminal diagnosis.

For other patients, and for those who fail multidisciplinary treatment, leaves the narrow end of evidence-based management. Few legitimate options apply. Although the controlled trials of opioids for chronic low back pain report less than impressive results, they remain the least contentious option for patients with intractable pain. They are not curative; they do not make the pain go away; but they can constitute some degree of relief for the patient.

The author is less confident about the utility and efficacy of spinal opioids. Although this intervention is suitable for some patients with cancer pain, convincing evidence is lacking of its efficacy for chronic low back pain. Of course, some practitioners provide it, and some patients are drawn to it. However, it does not constitute a "magic" cure for chronic low back pain.

What the author does avoid is treatments known not to work, and which pose a threat to the health of patients because of the attendant risk of complications. These include gratuitous surgery, i.e., surgery performed with no indications other than pain, or surgery performed for conditions known not to be associated with pain, such as spondylosis and spondylolisthesis. The author does not indulge epidural lysis of adhesions, for this intervention has been shown to be no more effective than placebo therapy.[75] For the same reasons the author does not pursue acupuncture, belts, corsets, and traction.

ETHICS

Where the author does have a major concern, as a medical practitioner and on behalf of gullible consumers, is in the ethics of some practices in pain medicine. Too often one encounters and hears of practices that are offered to patients without full and proper disclosure. Interventions are portrayed as a treatment option for low back pain, but those who offer them do not disclose that it is not known if the treatment really works. The practitioner may assert that he or she has found it to work (sometimes) but there is no published evidence as to how well it works, if at all. No studies have shown that the treatment is any more than a glorified (and perhaps expensive) placebo. Worse still are interventions that are portrayed as something that "might" work. In that instance, the provider is simply speculating; they do not even have the experience that it appears to work sometimes.

The ethical insult in these circumstances is that providers do not explain to the patients that the treatment is fundamentally experimental. Instead, the patient is lulled into believing that the practitioner knows what he or she is doing, and because this is a legitimate practitioner the treatment must be legitimate. The facts speak otherwise.

An unproven treatment is fundamentally experimental. By undergoing the treatment, the patient is participating in an experiment but without being told so. The litmus test in these instances is twofold. Would the patients consent to undergo the treatment if they were told of its experimental status, and would their lawyer, if they had one, agree to the treatment? Furthermore, would the insurer pay if it were disclosed that the practitioner was experimenting, and should they pay?

These questions do not preclude trying something new for a patient with an intractable problem, but they ask that the treatment be applied ethically. Practitioners should be able to try new interventions in the interests of their patients, but they should not be allowed to do so covertly, as if it were an accepted treatment. That is what failure to disclose amounts to.

Australia encountered such a problem and dealt with it. When several patients were allegedly injured by injections of epidural steroids, the government commissioned a working party to enquire into the indications, safety, and efficacy of this treatment. The working party found that for the treatment of radicular pain there was insufficient evidence either to proscribe or to recommend epidural steroids.[76] It recommended that since this was an unproven procedure, patients should provide informed consent for the procedure, with that consent being based on a thorough disclosure of the risks and unknown benefits of the procedure. However, the working party also found that there was no evidence to support the use of epidural steroids for back pain as opposed to radicular pain. For back pain, the working party deemed the use of epidural steroids to be experimental, and their use should be restricted to formal research studies. Although the working party issued its report in 1994, no evidence has appeared to justify altering that conclusion.

Similar principles apply to several, if not many, emergent or emerging interventions for low back pain. Usually in the media, instead of peer-reviewed journals, or on the Internet, individuals claim to have a new cure or a new intervention for back pain. These might sound like good ideas, but they have not been tested, let alone proven to work.

An ethical approach would be to declare that this is an unproven intervention, and that volunteers are called for to test it under the aegis of an institutional ethics committee. What is not ethical is to portray the intervention as something that works but only on the basis of the promoter's conviction. Consumers and practitioners alike should be mindful of the distinction between a commercial promotion and a legitimate intervention. Consumers in particular should be mindful that their desperation to find help constitutes a liability. Unscrupulous operators can prey on that desperation simply to achieve financial gain. As protection against being exploited, consumers can ask the following questions:

If it is not proven, why are you charging for this treatment?
What assurances can you give me that I am not being experimented on?
What would my lawyer say if I brought him in?

These same questions can be asked by practitioners, when they offer a treatment, or when they hear of a treatment that has been recommended for their patient.

SUMMARY

1. Few traditional interventions for acute low back pain have emerged as effective following controlled trials and systematic reviews.
2. Addressing the patient's fears and concerns, supporting them to remain active, and avoiding passive interventions, are the hallmarks of evidence-based care for acute low back pain. Studies have vindicated this approach.
3. The evidence does not support traditional passive interventions for chronic low back pain.
4. Current approaches are divided. The reductionist approach seeks to identify the source of pain and then treat it specifically. Although diagnostic tests have been developed to this end, treatment options remain limited. The palliative approach avoids determining the source or cause of pain.

It uses behavioral and multidisciplinary strategies to rehabilitate patients.

5. The evidence supports only multidisciplinary programs centered on intensive exercises.

REFERENCES

1. Merskey H, Bogduk N, eds. *Classification of chronic pain. Descriptions of chronic pain syndromes and definitions of pain terms*, 2nd ed. Seattle: IASP Press, 1994.
2. van Tulder MW, Koes BW, Bouter LM. Conservative treatment of acute and chronic nonspecific low back pain: A systematic review of randomized controlled trials of the most common interventions. *Spine* 1997;22:2128–2156.
3. Koes BW, van den Hoogen HMM. Efficacy of bed rest and orthoses of low back pain. A review of randomized clinical trials. *Eur J Phys Med Rehabil* 1994;4: 96–99.
4. Waddell G, Feder G, Lewis M. Systematic reviews of bed rest and advice to stay active for acute low back pain. *Br J Gen Pract* 1997;47:647–652.
5. Hagen KB, Jamtvedt G, Hilde G, Winnem MF. The updated Cochrane review of bed rest for low back pain and sciatica. *Spine* 2005;30:542–546.
6. van Tulder M, Malmivaara A, Esmail R, Koes B. Exercise therapy for low back pain. A systematic review within the framework of the Cochrane collaboration back review group. *Spine* 2000;25:2784–2796.
7. Gilbert JR, Taylor DW, Hildebrand A, Evans C. Clinical trial of common treatments for low back pain in family practice. *Br Med* 1985;291:791–794.
8. Roland M. Dixon M. Randomized controlled trial of an educational booklet for patients presenting with back pain in general practice. *J Roy Coll Gen Pract* 1989;39:244–246.
9. Cherkin DC, Deyo RA, Street JH, Hunt M, Barlow W. Pitfalls of patient education. Limited success of a program for back pain in primary care. *Spine* 1996;21:345–355.
10. Symonds TL, Burton AK, Tilotson KM, Main CJ. Absence resulting form low back trouble can be reduced by psychosocial intervention at the workplace. *Spine* 1995;20:2738–2745.
11. LeClaire R, Esdaile JM, Suissa S, Rossignol M, Proulx R, Dupuis M. Back school in a first episode of compensated acute low back pain: A clinical trial to assess efficacy and prevent relapse. *Arch Phys Med Rehabil* 1996;77:673–679.
12. Lindequist S, Lundberg B, Wikmark R, Bergstad, Loof G, Ottermark AC. Information and regime at low back pain. *Scand J Rehabil Med* 1984;16:113–116.
13. Beurskens AJ, de Vet HC, Koke AJ, et al. Efficacy of traction for non-specific low back pain: A randomised clinical trial. *Lancet* 1995;346:1596–1600.
14. Beurskens AJ, de Vet HC, Koke AJ, et al. Efficacy of traction for non-specific low back pain: 12-week and 6 month results of a randomized clinical trial. *Spine* 1997;22:2756–2762.
15. Ernst E, White AR. Acupuncture for back pain. A meta-analysis of randomized controlled trials. *Arch Intern Med* 1998;158:2235–2241.
16. Furlan AD, van Tulder M, Cherkin D, Tsukayama H, Lao L, Koes B, Berman B. Acupuncture and dry-needling for low back pain: An updated systematic review within the framework of the Cochrane Collaboration. *Spine* 2005;30:944–963.
17. van Tulder M, Waddell G. Conservative treatment of acute and subacute low back pain. In: Nachemson A, Jonsson E, eds. *Neck and back pain: The scientific evidence of causes, diagnosis, and treatment*. Philadelphia: Lippincott Williams & Wilkins, 2000.
18. Philips HC, Grant L, Berkowitz J. The prevention of chronic pain and disability: A preliminary investigation. *Behav Res Ther* 1991;29:443–450.
19. Bogduk N. Pharmacological alternatives for the alleviation of back pain. *Expert Opin Phamacother* 2004;5:2091–2098.
20. Van Tulder MW, Scholten RJPM, Koes BW, Deyo RA. Nonsteroidal anti-inflammatory drugs for low back pain. A systematic review within the framework of the Cochrane Collaboration Back Review Group. *Spine* 2000;25:2501–2513.
21. Nadler SF, Steiner DJ, Erasala GN, Hengehold DA, Hinkle RT, Goodale MB, Abeln SB, Weingard KW. Continuous low-level heat wrap therapy provides more efficacy than ibuprofen and acetaminophen for acute low back pain. *Spine* 2002;27:1012–1017.
22. Pohjolainen T, Jekunen A, Autio L, Vuorela H. Treatment of acute low back pain with COX-2-selective anti-inflammatory drug nimesulide. Results of a randomised, double-blind comparative trial versus ibuprofen. *Spine* 2000;25:1579–1585.
23. Chrubasik S, Eisenberg E, Balan, Weinberger T, Luzzati R, Conradt C. Treatment of low back pain exacerbations with willow bark extract: a randomised double-blind study. *Am J Med* 2000;109: 9–14.
24. Chrubasik S, Kunzel O, Model A, Conradt C, Black A. Treatment of low back pain with a herbal or synthetic anti-rheumatic: a randomised controlled study. Willow bark extract for low back pain. *Rheumatology* 2001;40:1388–1393.
25. Assendelft WJJ, Morton SC, Yu EI, Suttorp M, Shekelle PG. Spinal manipulative therapy for low back pain. A meta-analysis of effectiveness relative to other therapies. *Ann Int Med* 2003;138:871–881.
26. Grunnesjo MI, Bogfeldt JP, Scardsudd KF, Blomberg SIE. A randomized controlled clinical trial of stay-active care versus manual therapy in addition to stay-active care: functional variables and pain. *J Manipulative Physiol Ther* 2004;27:431–441.
27. Klaber Moffett J, Torgerson D, Bell-Syer S, et al. Randomised controlled trial of exercise for low back pain: Clinical outcomes, costs, and preferences. *Br Med J* 1999;319:279–283.
28. Lindstrom I, Ohlund C, Eck C, Wallin L, Peterson LE, Nachemson A. Mobility, strength, and fitness after a graded activity program for patients with subacute low back pain. A randomized prospective

clinical study with a behavioral therapy approach. *Spine* 1992;17:641–649.

29. Lindstrom I, Ohlund C, Nachemson A. Physical performance, pain, pain behavior and subjective disability in patients with subacute low back pain. *Scand J Rehabil Med* 1995;27:153–160.
30. Sinclair SJ, Hogg-Johnson S, Mondloch MV, Shields SA. The effectiveness of an early active intervention program for workers with soft-tissue injuries. The early claimant cohort study. *Spine* 1997;22:919–931.
31. Blomberg S, Svardsudd K, Mildenberger F. A controlled, multicenter trial of manual therapy in low-back pain: Initial status, sick-leave and pain score during follow-up. *Scand J Prim Health Care* 1992;10:170–178.
32. Blomberg S, Svardsudd K, Tibblin G. Manual therapy with steroid injections in low-back pain: Improvement of quality of life in a controlled trial with four months' follow-up. *Scand J Prim Health Care* 1993;11: 83–90.
33. Frank J, Sinclair S, Hogg-Johnson S, et al. Preventing disability from work-related low-back pain: New evidence gives new hope—if we can just get all the players onside. *Can Med Assoc J* 1998;158:1625–1631.
34. Loisel P, Abenhaim L, Durand P, et al. A population-based, randomized clinical trial on back pain management. *Spine* 1997;22:2911–2918.
35. Indahl A, Velund L, Reikeraas O. Good prognosis for low back pain when left untampered: A randomized clinical trial. *Spine* 1995;20:473–477.
36. Indahl A, Haldorsen EH, Holm S, Reikeras O, Ursin H. Five-year follow-up study of a controlled clinical trial using light mobilization and an informative approach to low back pain. *Spine* 1998;23:2625–2630.
37. Bogduk N, McGuirk B. *Medical management of acute and chronic low back pain. An evidence-based approach.* London: Elsevier, 2002.
38. Watson P. The MSM quartet. *Australas Musculoskeletal Med* 1999;4(2):8–9.
39. McGuirk B, King W, Govind J, Lowry J, Bogduk N. The safety, efficacy, and cost-effectiveness of evidence-based guidelines for the management of acute low back pain in primary care. *Spine*, 2001;26:2615–2622.
40. Turner JA, Denny MC. Do antidepressant medications relieve chronic low back pain? *J Fam Pract* 1993;37:545–553.
41. Salerno S, Browning R, Jackson SL. The effect of antidepressant treatment of chronic back pain. A meta-analysis. *Arch Int Med* 2002;162:19–24.
42. Moulin DE, Lezzi A, Amireth R, Sharpe WKJ, Boyd D, Merskey H. Randomised trial of oral morphine for chronic non-cancer pain. *Lancet* 1996;347:143–147.
43. Jamison RN, Raymond SA, Slawsby EA, Nedelijkov SS, Katz NP. Opioid therapy for chronic noncancer back pain. A randomized prospective study. *Spine* 1998;23:2591–2600.
44. Bogduk N. Management of chronic low back pain. *Med J Aust* 2004;180:79–83.
45. McIlveen B, Robertson V. A randomized controlled study of the outcome of hydrotherapy for subjects with low back or back and leg pain. *Physiotherapy* 1998;84:17–26.
46. Furlan AD, Brosseau L, Imamura M, Irvin E. Massage for low-back pain: a systematic review within the framework of the Cochrane collaboration back review group. *Spine* 2002;27:1896–1910.
47. Nelemans PJ, de Bie RA, Devet HCW, Sturmans F. Injection therapy for subacute and chronic benign low back pain. *Spine* 2001;26:501–515.
48. Yelland MJ, Del Mar C, Pirozzo S, Schoene ML. Prolotherapy injections for chronic low back pain. A systematic review. *Spine* 2004;29:2126–2133.
49. Yelland MJ, Glasziou PP, Bogduk N, Schluter PJ, McKernon M. Prolotherapy injections, saline injections, and exercises for chronic low-back pain: A randomised trial. *Spine* 2004;29:9–16.
50. Turner JA, Loeser JD, Bell KG. Spinal cord stimulation for chronic low back pain: A systematic literature synthesis. *Neurosurgery* 1995;37:1088–1096.
51. Taylor RS, van Buyten JP, Buchsel E. Spinal cord stimulation for chronic back and leg pain and failed back surgery syndrome: A systematic review and analysis of prognostic factors. *Spine* 2004;30:152–160.
52. Dahm P, Nitescu P, Appelgren L, Curelaru I. Efficacy and technical complications of long-term continuous intraspinal infusions of opioid and/or bupivacaine in refractory non-malignant pain: A comparison between the epidural and the intrathecal approach with externalised or implanted catheters and infusion pumps. *Clin J Pain* 1998;14:4–16.
53. van Tulder MW, Ostelo R, Vlaeycn JWS, Linton SJ, Morley SJ, Assendelft WJJ. Behavioral treatment for chronic low back pain. A systematic review within the framework of the Cochrane back review group. *Spine* 2000;25:2688–2699.
54. Mayer TG, Gatchel RJ, Kishino N, et al. Objective assessment of spine function following industrial injury. A prospective study with comparison group and one-year follow-up. *Spine* 1985;10:482–493.
55. Mayer TG, Gatchel RJ, Mayer H, Kishino N, Keeley J, Mooney V. A prospective two-year study of functional restoration in industrial low back injury. *JAMA* 1987;258:1763–1767.
56. Hazard RG, Fenwick JW, Kalisch SM, et al. Functional restoration with behavioural support. A one-year prospective study of patients with chronic low-back pain. *Spine* 1989;14:157–161.
57. Burke SA, Harms-Constas CK, Aden PS. Return to work/work retention outcomes of a functional restoration program: A multi-center, prospective study with a comparison group. *Spine* 1994;19:1880–1886.
58. Hazard RG. Spine update. Functional restoration. *Spine* 1995;20:2345–2348.
59. Mitchell RI, Carmen GM. The functional restoration approach to the treatment of chronic pain in patients with soft tissue and back injuries. *Spine* 1994;19:633–642.
60. Alaranta H, Rytokoski U, Rissanen A, et al. Intensive physical and psychosocial training program for patients with chronic low back pain: A controlled clinical trial. *Spine* 1994;19:1339–1349.

61. Guzman J, Esmail R, Karjalainen K, Malmivaara A, Bombardier C. Multidisciplinary rehabilitation for chronic low back pain: Systematic review. *Br Med J* 2001;322:1511–1516.
62. Waddel G. *The back pain revolution*. Edinburgh: Churchill Livingstone, 1998.
63. Bendix AF, Bendix T, Vaegter K, Lund C, Frolund L, Hom L. Multidisciplinary intensive treatment for chronic low back pain: A randomized, prospective study. *Cleve Clin J Med* 1996;63:62–69.
64. Bendix AF, Bendix T, Ostenfeld S, Bush E, Andersen A. Active treatment programs for patients with chronic low back pain—A prospective, randomized, observer-blinded study. *Eur Spine J* 1995;4:148–152.
65. Bendix AF, Bendix T, Labriola M, Bockgaard P. Functional restoration for chronic low back pain. Two-year follow-up of two randomized clinical trials. *Spine* 1998;23:717–725.
66. Bendix AF, Bendix T, Lund C, Kirkbak S, Ostenfeld S. Comparison of three intensive programs for chronic low back pain patients: A prospective, randomized, observer-blinded study with one-year follow-up. *Scand J Rehabil Med* 1997;29:81–89.
67. Turner JA, Ersek M, Herron L, et al. Patient outcomes after lumbar spinal fusions. *JAMA* 1992;268:907–911.
68. Gibson JNA, Grant IC, Waddell G. The Cochrane review of surgery for lumbar disc prolapse and degenerative lumbar spondylosis. *Spine* 1999;24:1820–1832.
69. Fritzell P, Hagg O, Wessberg P, Nordwall A, Swedish Lumbar Spine Study Group. 2001 Volvo award winner in clinical studies: Lumbar fusion versus nonsurgical treatment for chronic low back pain. A multicenter randomized controlled trial from the Swedish Lumbar Spine Study Group. *Spine* 2001;26:2521–2534.
70. Ivar Brox J, Sorensen R, Friis A, Nygaard O, Indahl A, Keller A, Ingerbrigtsen T, Eriksen HR, Holm I, Koller AK, Riise R, Reikeras O. Randomized clinical trial of lumbar instrumented fusion and cognitive intervention and exercises in patients with chronic low back pain and disc degeneration. *Spine* 2003;28: 1913–1921.
71. Schwarzer AC, Aprill CN, Derby R, Fortin J, Kine G, Bogduk N. The prevalence and clinical features of internal disc disruption in patients with chronic low back pain. *Spine* 1995;20:1878–1883.
72. Moneta GB, Videman T, Kaivanto K, et al. Reported pain during lumbar discography as a function of anular ruptures and disc degeneration. A reanalysis of 833 discograms. *Spine* 1994;17:1968–1974.
73. Lee CK, Vessa P, Lee JK. Chronic disabling low back pain syndrome caused by internal disc derangements. The results of disc excision and posterior lumbar interbody fusion. *Spine* 1995;20:356–361.
74. Blumenthal SL, Baker J, Dossett A, Selby D. The role of anterior lumbar fusion for internal disc disruption. *Spine* 1988;13:566–569.
75. Kozak JA, O'Brien JP. Simultaneous combined anterior and posterior fusion. An independent analysis of a treatment for the disabled low-back pain patient. *Spine* 1990;15:322–328.
76. Gill K, Blumenthal SL. Functional results after anterior lumbar fusion at L5–S1 in patients with normal and abnormal MRI scans. *Spine* 1992;17:940–942.
77. Loguidice VA, Johnson RG, Guyer RD, et al. Anterior lumbar interbody fusion. *Spine* 1988;13:365–369.
78. Vamvanij V, Fredrickson BE, Thorpe JM, Stadnick ME, Yuan HA. Surgical treatment of internal disc disruption: An outcome study of four fusion techniques. *J Spinal Dis* 1998;11:375–382.
79. Knox BD, Chapman TM. Anterior lumbar interbody fusion for discogram concordant pain. *J Spinal Dis* 1993;6:242–244.
80. Carragee EJ, Tanner CM, Khurana S, Hayward C, Welsh J, Date E, Truong T, Rossi M, Hagle C. The rates of false-positive lumbar discography in select patients without low back symptoms. *Spine* 2000;25:1373–1381.
81. International Spine Intervention Society. Lumbar disc stimulation. In: Bogduk N, ed. *Practice Guidelines for spinal diagnostic and treatment procedures.* International Spine Intervention Society, San Francisco, 2004, pp 20–46.
82. Derby R, Lee SH, Kim BJ, Chen Y, Aprill C, Bogduk N. Pressure-controlled lumbar discography in volunteers without low back symptoms. *Pain Med* 2005;6:213–221.
83. Bogduk N. International Spinal Injection Society guidelines for the performance of spinal injection procedures. Part 1. Zygapophysial joint blocks. *Clin J Pain* 1997;13:285–302.
84. Schwarzer AC, Aprill CN, Derby R, Fortin J, Kine G, Bogduk N. Clinical features of patients with pain stemming from the lumbar zygapophysial joints. Is the lumbar facet syndrome a clinical entity? *Spine* 1994;19:1132–1137.
85. Schwarzer AC, Wang S, Bogduk N, McNaught PJ, Laurent R. Prevalence and clinical features of lumbar zygapophysial joint pain: A study in an Australian population with chronic low back pain. *Ann Rheum Dis* 1995;54:100–106.
86. Manchikanti L, Pampati V, Fellows B, Bakhit CE. Prevalence of lumbar facet joint pain in chronic low back pain. *Pain Physician* 1999;2:59–64.
87. van Kleef M, Barendse GAM, Kessels A, Voets HM, Weber WEJ, de Lange S. Randomized trial of radiofrequency lumbar facet denervation for chronic low back pain. *Spine* 1999;24:1937–1942.
88. Dreyfuss P, Halbrook B, Pauza K, Joshi A, McLarty J, Bogduk N. Efficacy and validity of radiofrequency neurotomy for chronic lumbar zygapophysial joint pain. *Spine* 2000;25:1270–1277.
89. Schofferman J, Kine G. Effectiveness of repeated radiofrequency neurotomy for lumbar facet pain. *Spine* 2004;29:2471–2473.
90. Bogduk N, Lau P, Govind J, Karasek M. Intradiscal electrothermal therapy. *Techniques in Regional Anesthesia & Pain Management* 2005;9:25–34.
91. Pauza KJ, Howell S, Dreyfuss P, Peloza JH, Dawson K, Bogduk N. A randomised, placebo-controlled trial of intradiscal electrothermal therapy for the treatment of discogenic low back pain. *The Spine J* 2004;4:27–35.

92. Karasek M, Bogduk N. Twelve-month follow-up of a controlled trial of intradiscal thermal anuloplasty for back pain due to internal disc disruption. *Spine* 2000;25:2601–2607.
93. Bogduk N, Karasek M. Two-year follow-up of a controlled trial of intradiscal electrothermal anuloplasty for chronic low back pain resulting from internal disc disruption. The spine Journal 2002;2:343–350.
94. Bogduk N, Govind J. *Medical management of acute lumbar radicular pain. An evidence-based approach.* Newcastle: Newcastle Bone and Joint Institute, 1997.
95. McKenzie R. *Treat your own back,* 5th ed. Lower Hutt, New Zealand: Spinal Publications, 1997: 42–52.
96. Dreyfuss P, Michaelsen M, Pauza K, McLarty J, Bogduk N. The value of history and physical examination in diagnosing sacroiliac joint pain. *Spine* 1996;21:2594–2602.
97. Karasek M, Bogduk N. Intradiscal electrothermal anuloplasty: Percutaneous treatment of chronic discogenic low back pain. *Tech Reg Anesth Pain Manage* 2001;5:130–135.
98. Waguespack A, Schofferman J, Slosar P, Reynolds J. Etiology of long-term failures of lumbar spine surgery. *Pain Medicine* 2002;3:18–22.
99. Heavner JE, Racz GB, Raj P. Percutaneous epidural neuroplasty: Prospective evaluation of 0.9% NaCl versus 10% NaCl with or without hyaluronidase. *Reg Anaest Pain Med* 1999;24:202–207.
100. Bogduk N, Brazenor G, Christophidis N, et al. *Epidural use of steroids in the management of back pain.* Canberra: National Health and Medical Research Council, 1994.

CHAPTER

32

CLINICAL DECISION MAKING: WHEN TO RECOMMEND BACK SURGERY

Rick Delamarter and Kambiz Hannani

OUTLINE

OBJECTIVES

1. Identification of potential surgical candidates for common surgical procedures.
2. Understanding the indication for various surgeries.
3. Understanding the mechanics and the expected outcomes of various spinal surgery.
4. Strategy for postoperative management.
5. Update on new spinal surgical procedures.
6. Surgical complications and failed back surgery syndrome.

INTRODUCTION

Although most spinal disorders can be managed by nonoperative means, a subset of patients may benefit from surgical intervention. A thorough understanding of the different disorders and the pathophysiology of the disorder are essential in determining the appropriate surgical treatment. This chapter will review the most common spinal disorders associated with low back syndromes and the appropriate surgical treatment when conservative management fails. Because neurocompressive lesions above the level of the lumbar spine can at times cause, complicate, or mimic low back syndromes, several of the more common clinical scenarios and associated surgical solutions will be presented below.

IDENTIFICATION OF POTENTIAL SURGICAL CANDIDATES

A significant number of Americans suffer from low back pain at some point in their lives. Most patients, however, will not require surgical treatment. The key element in identifying a surgical candidate is a thorough history and physical examination with detailed imaging studies. In nonemergency situations, a failed course of multimodal, conservative management has typically been attempted.

Multiple elements in the spine can be responsible for pain. Axial pain is usually secondary to structural or mechanical dysfunction of the disc or facet elements. Peripheral or radicular pain usually originates from neuronal elements.

Pain that has lasted for greater than 6–8 weeks may require further imaging studies as most spinal pain resolve by 6 weeks. Furthermore, deep pain that is present at night can be secondary to infection or tumor, which again require immediate attention.

Factors that exacerbate or relieve pain can help identify the pain generator. Flexion and/or extension may exacerbate spinal pain.

Radicular, peripheral pain following a vertameric distribution is one type of dysesthesia extending to the periphery caused by irritation or compression of the neuronal elements in the spinal column. Nerve root irritation can lead to weakness, numbness, or paresthesias in the extremities. Significant compression of the cauda equina, however, can also present with bowel or bladder dysfunction that can be a surgical emergency. The disc and its syndromes are discussed in great detail in Chapter 6.

Although disc herniations are a common cause of radicular symptoms, canal stenosis as seen in the elderly population can also lead to radicular symptoms. Also known as neurogenic claudication, the degenerative process of aging can lead to a decrease in canal volume, decreasing the space available to the cauda equina. Patients with neurogenic claudication tend to have increasing pain with erect posture and walking; sitting usually resolves their symptoms. If pain does not respond to conservative management and becomes intolerable, surgical intervention may be indicated. Stenotic syndromes are addressed in great detail in Chapter 7.

If the spinal cord is the primary structure being compressed, myelopathic symptoms are commonly seen. Myelopathy can be painless. Cord compression, however, can produce pain. Myelopathy can lead to bowel, bladder, or balance dysfunction. Bilateral weakness and numbness can also be present. With prolonged cord compression, hyperreflexia and spasticity are commonly seen. Severe myelopathy can result in a positive Babinski reflex in which up-going toes are seen with scratching of the outer portion of the foot. Progressive myelopathy and cauda equina syndrome are both absolute indications for surgical intervention in treating spinal pathology.

With a thorough history, the physician formulates a differential diagnosis, which can be refined via the physical examination. During the physical examination, the physician evaluates the spinal range of motion (ROM) and limitations. Gait analysis including toe/heel walking would quickly pinpoint asymmetric loss of motor function or balance. Muscle strength evaluation with a 5-point grading system is essential for evaluating the motor neurons. Distinct nerve root pathology can be identified on the basis of the pattern of weakness noted.

In the lower extremity, straight-leg raising (SLR), which causes radicular symptoms, is commonly seen with disc herniations at the L4/5 and L5/S1 levels. A similar test for disc herniation at the upper levels affecting the femoral nerve is the femoral stretch test. Herniations that irritate the L2 to L4 nerve roots will cause pain when the thigh is extended and knee flexed. These examination procedures are detailed in Chapter 12.

Motor dysfunction and weakness as well as changes in the lower extremity reflexes are commonly seen with radicular symptoms. The L2 nerve root innervates the hip flexors;the L3 and L4 contribute to knee extension; and the L4, L5, and S1 roots innervate inversion/ankle dorsiflexion, extensor hallucis longus, and eversion/plantar flexion, respectively. The patellar reflex is innervated by L4, while the Achilles reflex is innervated by the S1 nerve root. Weakness that is progressive in consecutive examinations with an obvious anatomic cause is considered an indication for surgery.

Clinical Pearl: Absolute indications for surgery include (1) intolerable pain that is not responsive to conservative management, (2) progressive weakness as documented by serial examination, and (3) myelopathic signs/symptoms and/or cauda equina syndrome with bowel and bladder dysfunction.

The physical examination can also help identify patients who are primarily interested in secondary gains from surgical or conservative treatments. Waddell has described multiple nonphysiologic signs, which can identify nonorganic complications. Pain out of proportion to pathology at hand, nonanatomic distribution of radicular symptoms, and severe local tenderness to touch or rolling of the skin are three of the Waddell's criteria. The "twist test" is performed with rotation of the patient's torso, which causes rotation through the knee joint. Lumbar pain with the twist test is a nonanatomic finding. Head compression test with 5 lb causing lumbar pain is a nonanatomic finding. Finally, patients who have a severely positive SLR in the supine position but allow the seated SLR test while being distracted are eliciting a nonorganic finding consistent with Waddell's criteria. Three or more of the above six findings predict a poor response to conservative or surgical treatment of the patient. Waddell's nonorganic tests are discussed and demonstrated in Chapter 14.

In general, by completion of the history and physical examination and the addition of imaging studies, an appropriate treatment plan can be configured. Absolute indications for surgery include the following:

1. Intolerable pain that is not responsive to conservative management.
2. Progressive weakness as documented by serial examination.

3. Myelopathic signs/symptoms and/or cauda equina syndrome with bowel and bladder dysfunction.

SPINAL DISORDERS AND SURGICAL OPTIONS

Although this textbook focuses on low back syndromes, pathologic conditions occur superiorly, which can affect the low back, directly or indirectly, or can present symptoms that may mimic a low back syndrome, leading to a misdiagnosis. Furthermore, these conditions can cause multiple or overlapping conditions, such as myelopathy and local radiculopathy. As such, common surgical procedures for the cervical and thoracic spine will be covered in order to present the reader with a complete overview of this topic.

Cervical Spine Disorders

Cervical Disc Herniation and Spondylosis By age 70, 70% of the population has asymptomatic cervical spondylosis. Fifteen percent of these asymptomatic patients, however, require surgical treatment by 10 years of follow-up.[1] As the natural history of cervical spondylosis is fairly benign, conservative management as well as epidural steroid injections (ESI) are the primary treatment modality.

Cervical spondylosis, however, can progress to cord compression and result in myelopathy. The natural history of cervical myelopathy is not as favorable and is generally considered progressive. When patients present with bowel, bladder, or balance dysfunction, hyperreflexia with progressive weakness, and imaging studies consistent with cord compression, surgical treatment takes priority over conservative management.

Although large central soft disc herniations can cause myelopathy, soft discs tend to be lateral in location and cause radicular pain via compression of exiting roots. Patients may present with some axial complaints but the radicular symptoms are the primary source of discomfort. Conservative management is usually indicated for up to 6 months as long as significant or progressive weakness and myelopathy are not present.

The surgical treatments for soft disc herniation or cervical spondylosis without myelopathy include anterior cervical discectomy and fusion (ACDF), vertebrectomy, and/or posterior laminoforaminotomy.

A single-level discectomy and fusion requires approximately 90 minutes of operative time. The patient is placed under general anesthesia in a supine position with a soft head halter for cervical traction. A transverse incision is placed unilaterally over a neck crease at the appropriate level. The cervical fascia is dissected to identify the interval between the sternocleidomastoid and the medial strap muscles. The carotid sheath and the sternocleidomastoid are retracted laterally, while the esophagus, trachea, and strap muscles are retraced medially. At this point, the appropriate level for discectomy is marked with a needle and identified via x-ray and a discectomy is carried to reach the posterior longitudinal ligament (PLL). The PLL is removed allowing for further removal of bony spurs and extruded disc material that may be narrowing the foramen. The number of hospital day stays depends on the number of levels performed. Usually, the patient stays 1 day or less per level performed. A postoperative cervical collar may be used for 4–8 weeks.

With the placement of bone graft during an anterior cervical fusion, the cervical spine returns to its natural lordotic posture. Furthermore, the graft prevents collapse of the interspace and allows for increased space within the foramina for the exiting nerve roots. Multiple studies have shown ACDF to be very effective in diminishing radicular symptoms; fusion rates of up to 95% for three-level fusion have been reported in the literature.

Clinical Pearl: Horner's syndrome with sympathetic nerve dysfunction can be seen when the sympathetic chain in the area is stretched and is also usually transient.

Complications seen with the anterior approach, although rare, include speech difficulty, donor site morbidity from bone grafting, Horner's syndrome, graft complications, hematoma, neurologic deterioration, and nonunions of the fusion. Speech difficulty is usually seen secondary to stretch of the recurrent laryngeal nerve. The patients tend to have a "hoarse voice" which usually resolves by 1 week. Swallowing difficulty generally resolves by the first postoperative week as the swelling in the area reduces.

Horner's syndrome with sympathetic nerve dysfunction can be seen when the sympathetic chain in the area is stretched and is also usually transient. Hematoma development postoperatively is also uncommon. A drain is usually place intraoperatively to minimize the risk of hematoma development.

Prior to the use of plate fixation anteriorly, graft placement in the interspace was subject to extrusion. Plates are now routinely used and tend to improve fusion rates and decrease graft extrusion without an increase in complication rates.[2]

Soft disc herniations, which are laterally located, can occasionally be removed via a posterior procedure. Through a small 1- to 1.5-in incision, a key hole laminotomy is performed after elevating the paraspinal muscles off of the lamina. The soft disc herniation can be carefully removed below the exiting nerve root.

Cervical Spondylosis with Myelopathy When patients present with multilevel spinal stenosis or myelopathy secondary to stenosis, one may consider a laminectomy, laminoplasty, anterior vertebrectomy, or a combined procedure to help decompress the canal.

Laminoplasty increases the effective volume of the spinal canal while keeping the posterior elements of the cervical spine partially intact.[3,4] The patient is placed in a prone position with a Mayfield head halter holding the neck in a neutral position. The paraspinal muscles are again elevated off of the lamina. The high-speed bur is used to release the lamina partially on one side and completely on the second side. The lamina is subsequently opened similar to a door hinging open on the partially released laminar side. Pulling the lamina away from the cord, which can now fall posteriorly away from any anterior structural compression, significantly increases the available space for the cord.

Clinical Pearl: *Laminoplasty* increases the effective volume of the spinal canal while keeping the posterior elements of the cervical spine partially intact.

Laminoplasty is indicated in multilevel cervical spondylosis (at least three levels). Ossification of the posterior longitudinal ligament (OPLL) is a common entity that results in multilevel cervical stenosis and myelopathy. OPLL is commonly seen in Japan; 80% of the cases are in the cervical spine with 20% divided between thoracic and lumbar spine. The ossified PLL can erode through the dura, which makes an anterior decompression with removal of PLL impossible without significant dural repair. Therefore, posterior decompression is considered ideal for patients with OPLL. A lordotic alignment is required to allow the cord to fall away from anterior compression when the posterior elements are retracted. Laminoplasty, therefore, is contraindicated in kyphotic deformity and in presence of instability.

A *laminectomy* requires a similar surgical approach to a laminoplasty but requires the complete removal of the spinous process and lamina. This can accomplish a similar posterior decompression of a stenotic canal. Laminectomy without a concomitant fusion, however, has an increase incidence of development of kyphotic deformity with progressive axial pain and possible cord compression. Laminoplasty, therefore, has distinct advantages compared to laminectomy without fusion or anterior vertebrectomy with fusion. Laminoplasty retains some motion of the cervical spine and avoids the morbidity of bone grafting compared to fusions.

Anterior corpectomy and fusion is also commonly used for cervical decompression.[5] The surgical approach is similar to ACDF. The high-speed bur is used to remove the vertebrae without injuring the vertebral artery at the lateral border of the uncovertebral joints.[6] After the completion of the vertebrectomy, the PLL is removed for complete decompression of the cord anteriorly. The defect is filled with bone graft (fibular allograft/autograft) or cage placement with autograft bone. A plate can be utilized.[7,8] The authors routinely use a combined anterior and posterior fusion for long segment vertebrectomies. Hospital stay is 3–5 days depending on the number of levels performed. The patient can expect to lose about 10% ROM per level fused.

Corpectomy is indicated in myelopathic patients secondary to anterior compressive disorders (such as OPLL or vertebral tumors), severe multilevel spondylosis, or infections. Corpectomies can also be utilized for revision ACDF.[9] Corpectomy is contraindicated in severe osteoporosis or tracheoesophageal trauma. Results of one-level corpectomy have been similar to two-level discectomies.[10]

Combined anterior corpectomies/discectomies and posterior fusion is used for multilevel corpectomies as described above. Patients with a poor healing potential such as smokers and/or on dialysis/renal failure and patients with a mental handicap that prevents their postoperative cooperation may also benefit from the added posterior stabilization. The combined front and back procedure increases the hospital stay, the postoperative morbidity risks, and the fusion rates but decreases risk of hardware or graft dislodgement and failure.

In summary, cervical spinal disorders can be categorized as those with primarily radicular components versus myelopathy. For radicular pain, soft lateral discs can be addressed posteriorly with a keyhole foraminotomy and discectomy. Central disc herniation or mild to moderate cervical disc spondylosis causing radicular or myelopathic symptoms can be addressed via ACDF with autograft or allograft bone. Plating is optional but tends to improve fusion rates and protect the graft from extrusion. Multisegment disease without myelopathy can be addressed via combined anterior and posterior decompression and fusion for increased fusion rate and avoiding long segment immobilization with plate fixation anteriorly. Finally, myelopathy secondary to multilevel disease and OPLL is best treated with laminoplasty if the patient has a nonkyphotic alignment; corpectomy is used for kyphotic deformities as well as tumor and infections routinely.

Thoracic Spine Disorders

Disc herniations are commonly present in thoracic spine but tend to be asymptomatic. An incidence of 37% asymptomatic thoracic herniations has been reported in the literature.[11] Symptomatic discs are uncommon; thoracic discectomies account for less than 2% of all discectomies performed annually. The most common levels are the T11–T12; 75% of all herniations are present between T8 and T12.

Central disc herniation can produce axial pain and myelopathy. Lateral disc herniations tend to produce radicular symptoms in the chest wall. Disc herniation presentation, however, can be very variable and may mimic lumbar disc herniation or intra-abdominal pathology (such as cholecystitis, aneurysm, or GI tumors). The best imaging study to evaluate thoracic disc herniation is an MRI (magnetic resonance image) or CT (computed tomography) myelogram. As up to 70% of the discs are calcified, CT evaluation can better delineate the calcified anatomy.

Treatment tends to be conservative unless the patient has myelopathic features or has unremitting pain. Manual procedures and active care with bracing and anti-inflammatory medication are commonly started early in the treatment phase. Patients who fail conservative management or have progressive myelopathy may require one of many possible approaches to perform a discectomy with or without fusion. As the thoracic rib cage gives the thoracic spine additional support, fusion is not commonly performed unless a corpectomy is required.[12]

Three surgical approaches are commonly utilized depending on the characteristics of the disc herniation in the thoracic spine. The lateral, extracavetory (costotransversectomy) approach can be used for some paracentral or lateral disc herniations. The approach requires elevation of posterior paraspinal muscle far out over the rib cage. Part of the rib, transverse process, and pedicle are subsequently removed giving the surgeon direct access to the disc space and vertebral body.

The transpedicular approach is also a posterior approach with less muscle dissection. Part of the lamina and medial border of the pedicle are removed to give access to the lateral disc herniation. Central or paracentral discs cannot be addressed via this approach, as the cord would need to be retracted to remove such discs.

The anterior approach is the safest and best suited approach for a central disc herniation as it allows for the best visualization of the disc space.[13] The approach is usually performed by a vascular or thoracic surgeon while an orthopedist performs the discectomy and/or fusion. Thoracoscopic thoracic discectomies are frequently performed with a decrease in morbidity when compared to open anterior discectomies. Up to 83% good to excellent results have been reported in the literature.[14,15]

In summary, thoracic disc herniations tend to be common but are rarely symptomatic. Surgery is reserved for myelopathy or severe radicular pain that cannot be managed conservatively. Surgical decompression can be approached posteriorly or anteriorly; the anterior approach requires entry into the chest cavity but gives excellent visualization and is commonly used for corpectomies for OPLL, tumors, and infections. The posterior extended approach of costotransversectomy allows for good decompression. Finally, for simple lateral disc herniation, a small posterior approach requiring minimal muscle dissection can suffice for discectomy.

Lumbar Spine

Disc Herniations Disc syndromes were addressed in Chapter 6, but will be briefly discussed here also. Although a large portion of the population experience low back pain, only 2% incidence of sciatica is reported in the general population. Multiple factors such as cigarette smoking, age between 30 and 50 years, and stressful occupations with or without heavy lifting contribute to sciatica. Pathophysiology of sciatica or radicular leg symptoms is attributed to the compressive effect of disc herniation upon the nerve root as well as potential inflammatogenic properties of nucleus pulposus.[16]

Clinical Pearl: Although no prospective, randomized study is available, the natural history of disc herniation is considered to be favorable.

Patients tend to present with buttocks and leg pain symptoms; back pain is not the main disabling feature of herniations in most patients. Central herniation, however, can have a significant axial component. Disc herniations can be classified by location or type of herniation. The disc could be central, paracentral, lateral, or far lateral/extraforaminal. Although no prospective, randomized study is available, the natural history of disc herniation is considered to be favorable. Patients with multiple episodes of sciatica, on the other hand, are less likely to be pain-free for prolonged periods.

Weber evaluated 280 patients divided into a surgical and a conservative group. Sixty percent of the conservative group improved within the first 3 months. Within the first 1 year, the surgical group had more satisfied patients.[17,18] The gap between the two groups diminished by the fourth year, however. By the tenth year, the two groups were essentially identical. When patients do not have obvious neurologic compromise with progressive weakness or cauda equina symptoms, one may try conservative management.

Following a failed course conservative management, a microdiscectomy is the surgery of choice for this type of pathology. The surgeon gains access to the disc by elevating the paraspinal muscle and

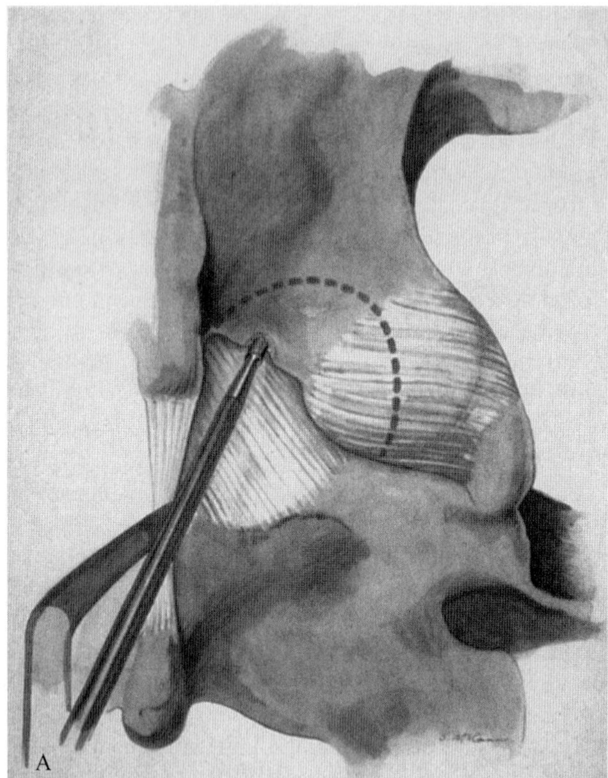

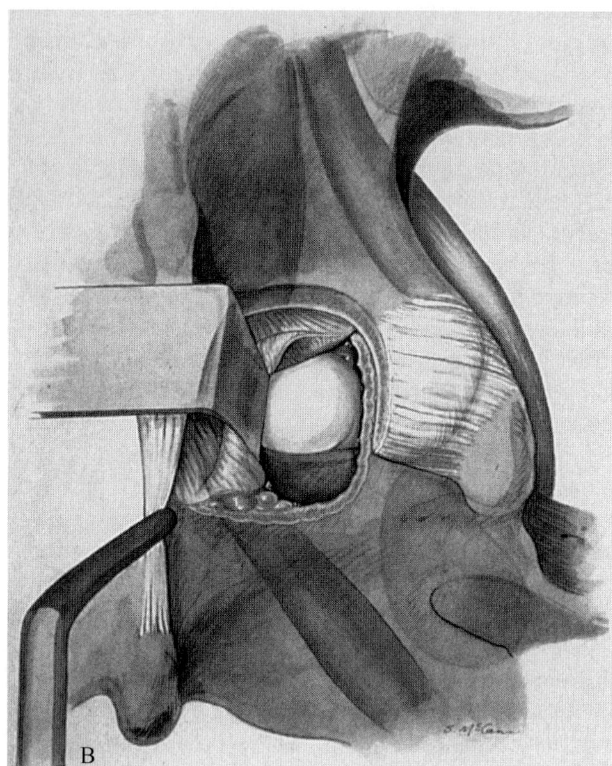

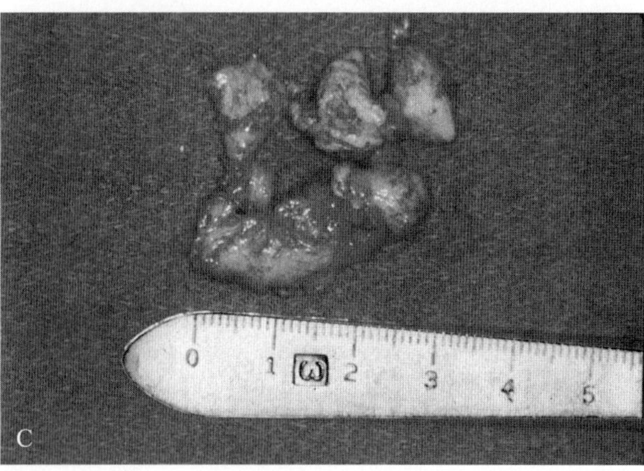

FIGURE 32–1. *A.* Approach used in microdiscectomy: high-speed bur used in the removal of part of the inferior facet to allow visualization of the disc herniation. *B.* Exposure of the disc herniation after the retraction of the nerve roots and cauda equina toward midline. *C.* Disc material removed after microdiscectomy.

removing part of the lamina. When performed with a microscope, a small 1-in incision with minimal soft tissue disruption can be used to complete the discectomy (Fig. 32–1). Percutaneous discectomies have also been performed using arthroscopic equipment.[19,20] In a retrospective study of 307 consecutive patients undergoing a percutaneous discectomy, the authors reported a 90.7% success rate based on the willingness of the patients to undergo the same procedure if faced with the same herniated disc in the future.[20] However, the gold standard at this time is microdiscectomy by using the microscope.

For far lateral discs, a modified approach is used through the paraspinal muscles to reach the intertransverse space. The intertransverse ligament is detached and retracted from the superior border of the inferior transverse process and the lateral aspect of the lamina; at this point, the traversing nerve root is identified and retracted laterally. The herniated disc can easily be removed in addition to any loose fragments noted in the disc space.

Following a microdiscectomy, patients are usually allowed to go home on the first postoperative day. They wear a protective corset for 4–6 weeks to remind the patient to avoid any bending/lifting/or twisting activities. The patients are encouraged to walk by postoperative days 1 or 2 and are able to return to their usual sports by the third postsurgical month.[21]

Clinical Pearl: Following a microdiscectomy, patients are usually allowed to go home on the first postoperative day.

Satisfaction rates postdiscectomies range from 73% to 98% based on the study reviewed. Satisfaction in most studies is based on patient responses to standardized questionnaires and their willingness to undergo the same procedure for similar outcome in the future. Complications from this procedure are uncommon but include continued symptoms, scarring, arachnoiditis, hematoma, infection, or nerve root injury. Early recurrence of symptoms is concerning and needs immediate attention; one needs to rule out an infection, reherniation, and continued lateral recess stenosis. A repeat MRI with contrast is indicated when symptoms have not improved postsurgery at the 2- to 3-week point.

In summary, the lead author's recommended treatment of patients with disc herniation is as follows: patients without obvious progressive neurologic involvement or bowel and bladder dysfunction receive conservative management for up to 3 months postpresentation. If their symptoms are not improved, a microdiscectomy is considered before permanent injury to the nerve root decreases the success of the surgery. The protocol can be modified on the basis of the size, location, and degree of symptomatology experienced by the patient.

Lumbar Stenosis

Unlike disk herniations, which are more common in younger patients, lumbar stenosis is often seen in patients older than 55. The stenotic syndromes were covered in detail in Chapter 7. Nevertheless, a brief review is necessary for the topic at hand. As degenerative processes cause ligamentum hypertrophy and osteophyte formation, the space available to the dural sac gradually decreases. Furthermore, osteophyte formation narrows the foramen for the exiting roots causing radicular symptoms.

Clinical Pearl: Key factors distinguish vascular vs. neurogenic claudication. In vascular claudication, the symptoms are more *distal to proximal* (with mainly calf pain), worse with uphill walking, and improve while lying with the legs extended. In contrast, neurogenic claudication symptoms are *proximal to distal* (with thigh pain), worse with downhill walking (as the spine is extended in this position), and improve with sitting and lying with the hips and knees flexed.

Patients usually present with leg pains and cramping with ambulation. Their symptoms significantly improve with flexion of the spine and sitting. Patients with peripheral vascular disease, however, can also present with worsening leg cramps with walking. Key factors distinguish vascular vs. neurogenic claudication. In vascular claudication, the symptoms are more *distal to proximal* (with mainly calf pain), worse with uphill walking, and improve while lying with the legs extended. In contrast, neurogenic claudication symptoms are proximal to distal (with thigh pain), worse with downhill walking (as the spine is extended in this position), and improve with sitting and lying with the hips and knees flexed.

The natural history of lumbar stenosis is not fully understood. In general, however, 10%–20% of patients with stenosis tend to have progressive symptoms requiring surgical intervention. Prior to surgical intervention, ESIs tend to provide variable length of relief to these patients.

The surgical treatment of stenosis is removal of the lamina and the hypertrophied ligamentum flavum. A midline incision is used to elevate the paraspinal muscles from the lamina bilaterally. Care is taken to avoid injury to the facet capsule, which may destabilize the segment and cause spondylolisthesis requiring future fusion surgery. After removal of all or part of the lamina, the hypertrophied ligamentum is removed from the medial border of the lamina and upper zygapophyseal articulation. The medial portion of the superior articulation of the facet is usually removed (i.e., facetectomy) to decompress the lateral recess area that commonly affects the traversing nerve root. While performing the medial facetectomy, care needs to be exercised to protect at least half of the facet joint in order to avoid instability. If the patient has any preoperative signs of mechanical instability, a laminotomy may be performed in which case only part of the lamina is removed and the spinous process and ligamentous attachment are preserved. Occasionally, a fusion becomes necessary when concern of instability is significant.

Following stenosis decompression, patients are allowed to ambulate and are advanced to a regular diet. Under optimal circumstances, patients typically return to their baseline activities with significant improvement of their claudication by the fourth to fifth week following surgery.

In summary, patients who present with moderate lower extremity symptoms and mild lumbar symptoms and have confirmed spinal stenosis are initially treated with conservative management, including ESI if necessary. A small number of these patients will have progressive neurogenic claudication, which responds favorably to removal of the lamina and ligamentum flavum that cause the stenosis. Extra care needs to be exercised in avoiding destabilization of the surgical levels, as a fusion would then be required in the future.

Lumbar Discogenic Pain

Multiple studies have confirmed the presence of pain fibers at the periphery of the disc anulus. Lumbar disc degeneration increases the above innervation, leading to the diagnosis of internal disc derangement.[22] The presentation, MRI, and discogram findings are the key elements in identifying discogenic pain. As noted in Chapter 17, the gold standard testing for internal disc derangement is discogram followed by postdiscogram CT scan.

Patients with discogenic pain experience symptoms that worsen with activity. Pain can be referred down to the posterior thigh/knee with local tenderness often present. MRI findings are key with loss of T2 high-intensity signal in the disc space (black disc disease). A high-intensity zone on the MRI at the posterior aspect of the anulus has also shown a positive predictive value of 86% for symptomatic discs.[23] Discography, although controversial, can be helpful in determining the symptomatic levels. Forty to sixty percent of patients with discogenic pain tend to improve with conservative management including ESI, therapy, and medications.

A large spectrum of surgical treatment is available. Intradiscal electrothermal therapy (IDET) is a minimally invasive procedure in which a thermal probe is introduced into the disc. It was explained in detail in Chapter 25. Briefly, intradiscal heat is hypothesized to cause shrinkage of the nucleus or sealing of the anulus fibrosus by contraction of collagen fibers. Thermal ablation of sensitive nerve fibers in the outer anulus is achieved with the heating process. Although multiple studies have reported pain improvement in up to 70% of the patients post-IDET treatment, the lead author's experience has not been as encouraging. In evaluating 60 patients 1-year post-IDET procedure, only 40% had less pain and 37% were satisfied; 97% of the patient continued to report pain 1-year postoperatively.

The gold standard surgical treatment for discogenic pain is removal of the pain generator: the offending disc. Interbody fusion can be accomplished via an anterior and/or posterior approach. Alternatively, a fusion can be accomplished by fusing the intertransverse posterolateral gutter region without discectomy. A recent study by Barrick evaluated patients who had obtained a posterolateral fusion without interbody fusion. Twenty patients who continued to have symptoms with the posterolateral fusion had significant improvement in their pain scores after an anterior interbody fusion was performed for the patients.[24] Another study by Lee evaluated 62 patients who underwent posterior interbody fusion for chronic low back pain. Ninety-three percent of the patients returned to work with 89% satisfied with their results at 7-year follow-up.[25]

Posterolateral fusion requires a midline incision with elevation of the paraspinal muscles off of the lamina bilaterally to the transverse processes of the levels to be fused. The transverse processes and lamina are subsequently decorticated and bone graft is placed over the decorticated bone. Bone graft is usually removed for the posterior superior iliac crest regions. New biologic products such as bone morphogenic protein (BMP) is becoming a popular option for use in fusion; BMP will likely improve the fusion rates and minimize bone graft donor site morbidity. The bone graft incorporates into the decorticated bone and effectively prevents any motion from taking place at the interspace between the fused transverse processes. Pedicle screw instrumentation is believed to improve the fusion rate with slight increase in complication rates including nerve root injury via poor placement of the pedicle screws. Nevertheless, most of the literature supports pedicle screw instrumentation in cases where instability is present (such as spondylolisthesis).[26] Although posterolateral fusion does minimize motion posteriorly, the disc may still experience minimal residual motion, which may contribute to continued discogenic postfusion pain. As stated above, discectomy with fusions after successful posterolateral fusions tends to help with pain relief suggesting the importance of performing interbody fusion in discogenic pain patients.

Clinical Pearl: Pedicle screw instrumentation is believed to improve the fusion rate with slight increase in complication rates including nerve root injury via poor placement of the pedicle screws.

Interbody fusion can be accomplished posteriorly or anteriorly. Anterior lumbar interbody fusion (ALIF) requires a retroperitoneal or endoscopic approach to disc removal and placement of graft material.[27–29] The patient is placed in a lateral decubitus position. A flank incision is used with dissection through the external and internal oblique and transversus abdominis muscles. The retroperitoneal space is bluntly dissected to the psoas and the lumbar vertebrae. The ureter should be identified and protected. For the L5–S1 interval, the middle sacral vessels need to be ligated. For the L4–L5 approach, the iliolumbar vein(s) need to be ligated and the vena cava and aorta need to be retracted for access to the disc space. The retroperitoneal approach can also be performed in the supine

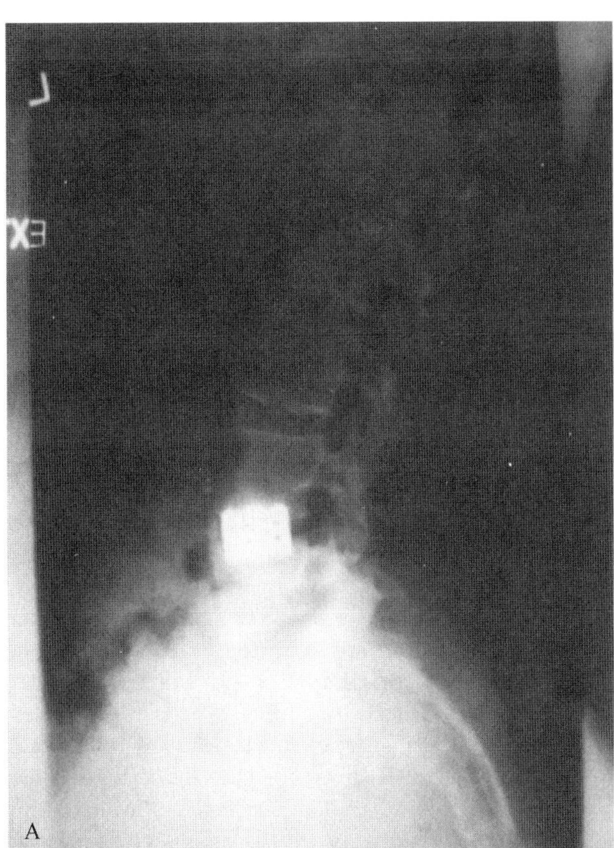

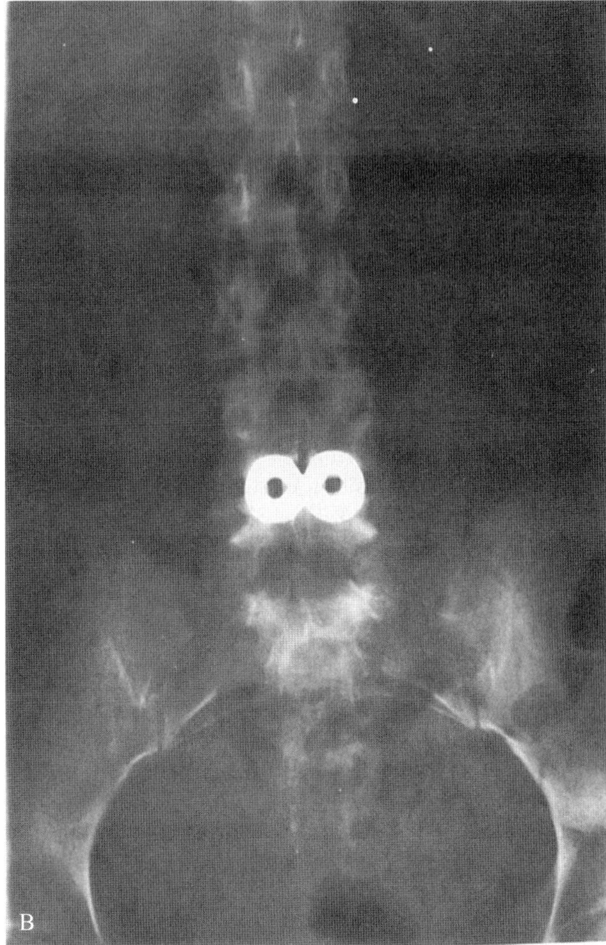

FIGURE 32–2. *A.* Lateral x-ray findings after an anterior interbody fusion using two cylindrical cages. *B.* Anteroposterior view of the cage construct seen in *A.*

position with an intermuscular approach. In this procedure, the rectus is mobilized allowing direct access to the posterior rectus sheath and the arcuate line. The sheath is released allowing for blunt dissection to the retroperitoneum.

The approach is usually performed by a vascular surgeon who places retractors in the retroperitoneum with excellent exposure of the target discs to be excised. After removal of the disc, the interspace can be filled via autograft, allograft, a combination of auto/allograft, or metallic cages filled with graft material. The choice of graft depends on the surgeon's experience and preference. The authors frequently use a femoral ring allograft, which has a cancellous inner portion allowing for faster bony incorporation.

Anterior lumbar interbody fusion (ALIF) can be performed as a stand-alone procedure or combined with posterior instrumentation with or without posterior fusion. Stand-alone anterior fusions are usually utilized in single-level disease with a collapsed interspace. A cage is usually used in this circumstance as bone graft alone has had higher pseudoarthrosis rates (Fig. 32–2). In multilevel disease or single-level disease without disc collapse, a posterior fusion is usually added to the ALIF. After completion of the anterior discectomy, the patient is usually turned to the prone position and the posterolateral fusion technique is used to place bone graft posteriorly with pedicle screw instrumentation.

Clinical Pearl: *Anterior lumbar interbody fusion* (ALIF) can be performed as a stand-alone procedure or combined with posterior instrumentation with or without posterior fusion.

In cases where there is sufficient disc space collapse, a *posterior lumbar interbody fusion* (PLIF) can be used to avoid the anterior retroperitoneal approach. In this procedure, a posterolateral fusion is combined with laminectomy and discectomy. The interspace is subsequently distracted and a bony graft placed posteriorly into the interspace. Disadvantages of PLIF are the need to retract the dural sac during discectomy and the placement of the graft. The authors use the

POLAR (*P*osterior *O*blique *L*umbar *A*rthrodesis) technique in which a cage is introduced after a complete facetectomy from one side in an oblique fashion. With the POLAR technique, the dural sac is retracted minimally to one side only. Furthermore, the cage gives excellent distraction of the interspace.

Clinical Pearl: In cases where there is sufficient disc space collapse, a *posterior lumbar interbody fusion* (PLIF) can be used to avoid the anterior retroperitoneal approach.

Postoperatively, patients with anterior/posterior fusion tend to require hospitalizations of 3–5 days. The patient needs to wear a soft corset for about 3–4 months until a solid fusion is confirmed on x-rays.

A new procedure that is undergoing FDA clinical trials at this time is *prosthetic disc replacement surgery* (PDR). PDR has been used in Europe for several years with promising clinical results. The authors' experience with PDR has also been very positive (Fig. 32–3).

Patients who have discogenic pain with no posterior element pathology such as facet arthropathy or spinal stenosis are excellent candidates for PDR. The advantage of PDR is the removal of a single-level pain-generating disc without the need for a fusion surgery. The continued mobility at the pathologic segment allows for less compromised spinal biomechanics while reducing increased stress on the adjacent disc spaces. Fusion surgery has been shown to increase the junctional, adjacent level discs and facet stresses with increased likelihood of degeneration at the adjacent levels.

The approach for placement of a PDR is the same as the ALIF procedure. After the disc space is clearly exposed, a complete discectomy is performed. Subsequently, equipment specially designed for the insertion of the prosthetic disc is used to distract the interspace and impact the two metallic end plates into position. A polyethylene ball is subsequently placed in between the metallic end plates, which allows for motion at the segment. These patients are allowed to ambulate the first postoperative day. The postoperative stay is usually 2–3 days only.

Potential complications associated with the ALIF are multiple but rare in occurrence. Bone graft collapse and graft extrusion may occur, which results in poor alignment or pseudoarthrosis.

In summary, a large portion of the population has chronic low back pain that can be attributed to discogenic pain. Most of these patients can continue with their daily activities with conservative management. The subset that has failed conservative management may choose surgical intervention. The gold standard surgical treatment is the interbody fusion with or without posterior fusion. The interbody fusion can be accomplished posteriorly or anteriorly. The authors used PLIF in cases with collapsed disc space or patients who have had previous anterior surgery making a revision very difficult and risky. At this time, anterior interbody fusion is recommended in multilevel disc degeneration where the disc space is not significantly collapsed. On the basis of the early results of disc replacement surgery, however, PDR may likely be the surgery of choice for single-level internal disc derangement in the near future.

Spondylolisthesis

Spondylolisthesis is the slippage of one vertebra over another. The most common cause of spondylolisthesis is the occurrence of degenerative changes to the disc and facets allowing for abnormal mobility and slippage of the vertebrae. The degree of slippage was classified by Meyerding into five categories: grade I is less than 25% slippage; grade II is 25%–50% slippage; grade III and IV are 50%–75% and 76%–100% slippage respectively; and spondyloptosis is used to describe grade V, greater then 100% slippage of the vertebrae.

Spondylolisthesis is subcategorized into six types by Wiltse and Newman.[30] Type I is dysplastic or congenital and accounts for 15% spondylolisthesis diagnosed. In this type, facets are dysplastic with orientation that allows for the slippage of one vertebra over another. As there is inherent instability in the structures, this type of slippage tends to be aggressively progressive. High risk of neurologic compromise has been reported requiring surgical decompression and fusion more often than other types of spondylolisthesis.

Clinical Pearl: Spondylolisthesis is subcategorized into six types.

Type II is isthmic spondylolisthesis in which there is a fracture or elongation of the pars interarticularis. This is seen in 5%–7% of the population as a whole and is not commonly symptomatic. Patients present with hamstring tightness and low back pain at an early age (adolescents). The L5/S1 interspace is most commonly affected with L5 nerve root involvement. Pars fractures (spondylolysis) that have not started to slip can be treated via bracing and observation; if the symptoms do not resolve, a repair of the pars defect via the removal of the fibrous nonunion site and bone grafting with wiring has been successful in relieving symptoms.[31,32] Adolescents with grade I slips are observed, whereas those with grade II slippage are encouraged to avoid contact sports. Grade III and higher slippage that is symptomatic require fusion surgery as conservative management fails to inhibit progression at high grades.

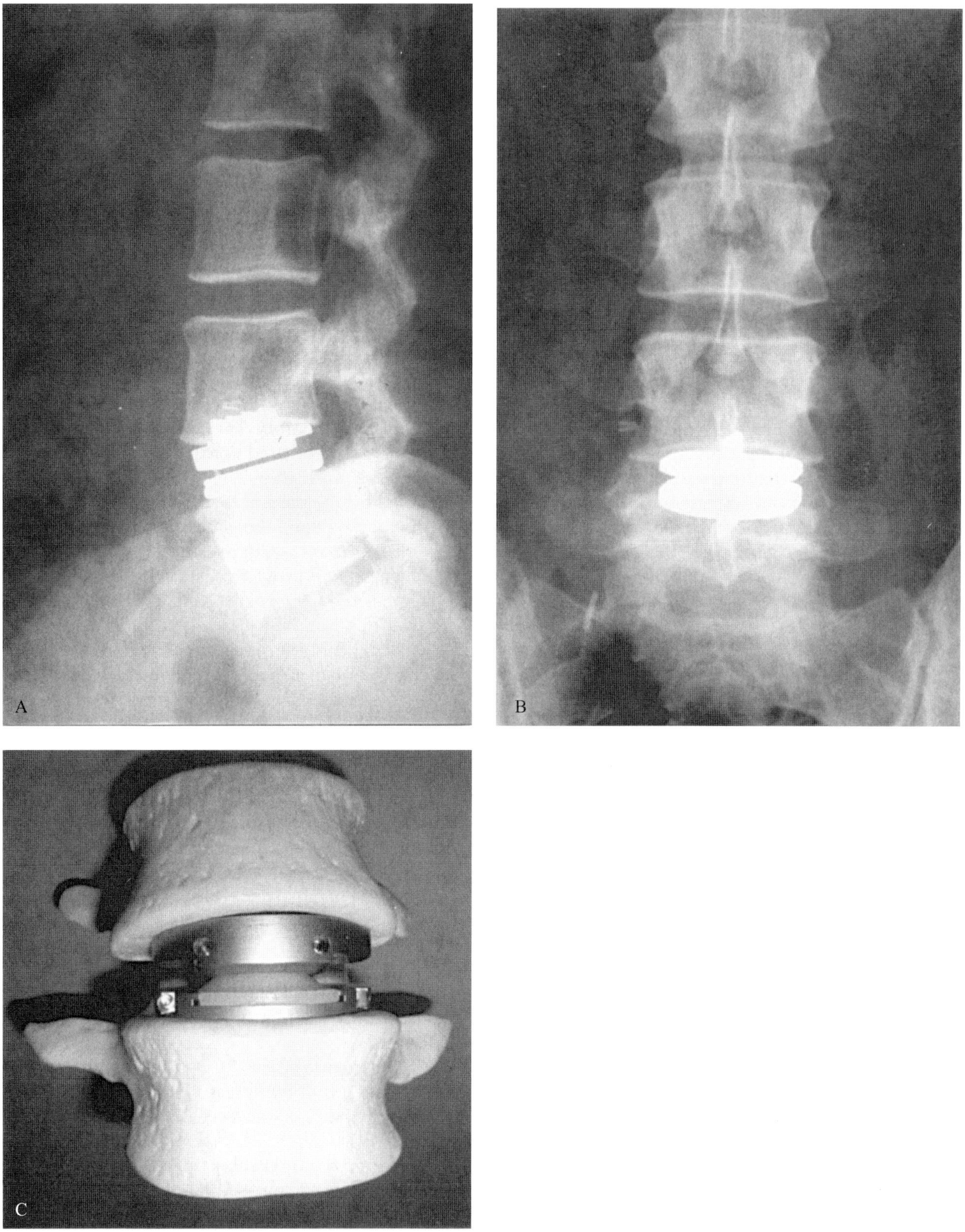

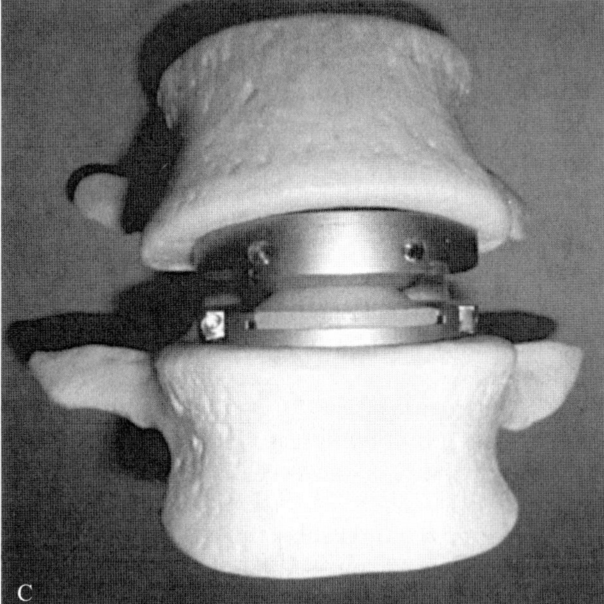

FIGURE 32–3. *A*. Lateral x-ray of the patient undergoing an artificial disc replacement with restoration of the disc height and preservation of lumbar lordosis. *B*. Anteroposterior view of the artificial disc replacement confirming central placement of the device. *C*. Image of the artificial disc replacement.

Type III spondylolisthesis is degenerative. In general, the natural history of degenerative spondylolisthesis is favorable; less than 15% of the patients have clinical deterioration of progressive weakness or incapacitating radicular symptoms.[33] The symptomatic patients usually present with both low back pain and moderate to severe leg symptoms. The low back pain is secondary to the spondylosis and instability experienced by the patients. In degenerative spondylolisthesis, the most common level involved is the L4/L5 interspace with the L5 nerve root radicular pain. The next most common involved level in degenerative spondylolisthesis is the L3/L4 level.

When conservative management has failed, multiple surgical options are available. The goal of surgery is to stabilize the segment via fusion and to decompress the nerve root via foraminotomy and possible distraction of the collapsed segment. Fusions are favored compared to simple decompression because of the high likelihood of progression of the instability after decompression and the continued back symptoms when a fusion is not performed. Herkowitz reviewed 50 patients who underwent decompression with and without fusion and found that patients with fusion had improved low back pain as well as leg symptoms.[34]

The fusion can be performed via a posterolateral technique or a combination of ALIF or PLIF with posterolateral fusion (Fig. 32–4). Interbody fusion can help decompress the foramina by distracting the disc space and increasing the space available for the exiting nerve root within the foramina.[35] In posterolateral fusion, pedicle screw instrumentation has improved fusion rates and decreased the likelihood of progression of the slippage.[36]

The authors recommend interbody fusion in addition to instrumented posterolateral fusion to help with the reduction of the slippage, to gain adequate foraminal height, and to improve the fusion success rate of this surgery. The remaining three types of spondylolisthesis are type IV, V, and VI. Traumatic fractures of the facets are considered a type IV spondylolisthesis and type V and VI are pathologic and iatrogenic spondylolisthesis respectively.

In summary, patients who fail conservative management and present with instability require fusion surgery. This fusion can be performed posteriorly with or without anterior interbody fusion. Fusion rates are improved with instrumentation and addition of interbody grafts. Decompressions with foraminotomies are also crucial in helping with leg symptoms in patients with spondylolisthesis.

Scoliosis

Scoliosis refers to the abnormal curvature of the spine. The deformity is usually in multiple planes including sagittal and coronal planes. A rotational deformity is also usually present. Scoliosis can be subclassified into adult versus pediatric deformity. The most common type of pediatric scoliosis is idiopathic; other types of deformity include neuromuscular, congenital, and syndrome-related. As the idiopathic type is by far the most common, the treatment options for this subtype only will be discussed.[37]

The etiology of idiopathic scoliosis, by definition, is unknown.[38] There, however, is a genetic component to the disorder as seen with increased prevalence within families. Idiopathic scoliosis is usually painless. Deformity accompanied by pain, rapidly progressing scoliosis, or left-sided thoracic scoliosis in the adolescent population needs to be carefully evaluated. A thorough history and physical examination, as well as additional imaging studies such as an MRI, are mandatory. The MRI would help rule out syringomyelia, tethered cord, and Chiari malformations in this population.

Based on the natural history of idiopathic scoliosis in children, guidelines have been developed for treatment options.[39] Curves that are less than 30 degrees tend not to progress, while curves greater than 50 degrees tend to progress approximately 1 degree per year in adulthood. Bracing is commonly used to treat curves between 25 degrees and 40 degrees in skeletally immature patients; bracing needs to be used 24 hours per day. For patients with unrelenting pain and curves over 40 degrees in skeletally immature and 50 degrees in skeletally mature patients, a fusion is usually recommended.

Clinical Pearl: Based on the natural history of idiopathic scoliosis in children, guidelines have been developed for treatment options.

The surgery can be performed as an anterior, posterior, or combined procedure. Anterior release and fusion allows for the fusion of a smaller number of segments with generally improved correction when compared to posterior surgery alone. Combined procedures decrease the risk of pseudoarthrosis and progression of deformity. Fifty percent correction in the deformity is commonly seen with posterior procedures; the correction, however, can be as high as 90% with anterior release.

Although complications are infrequent, spinal cord injury is the feared sequelae of deformity correction. Somatosensory evoked potential (SSEP) monitoring is commonly used to reliably follow changes in cord function in the operating room.

Adult scoliosis presents a very challenging problem. The adult spine is less pliable and has significantly more degenerative changes that cause neural impingement in addition to deformity. Surgical

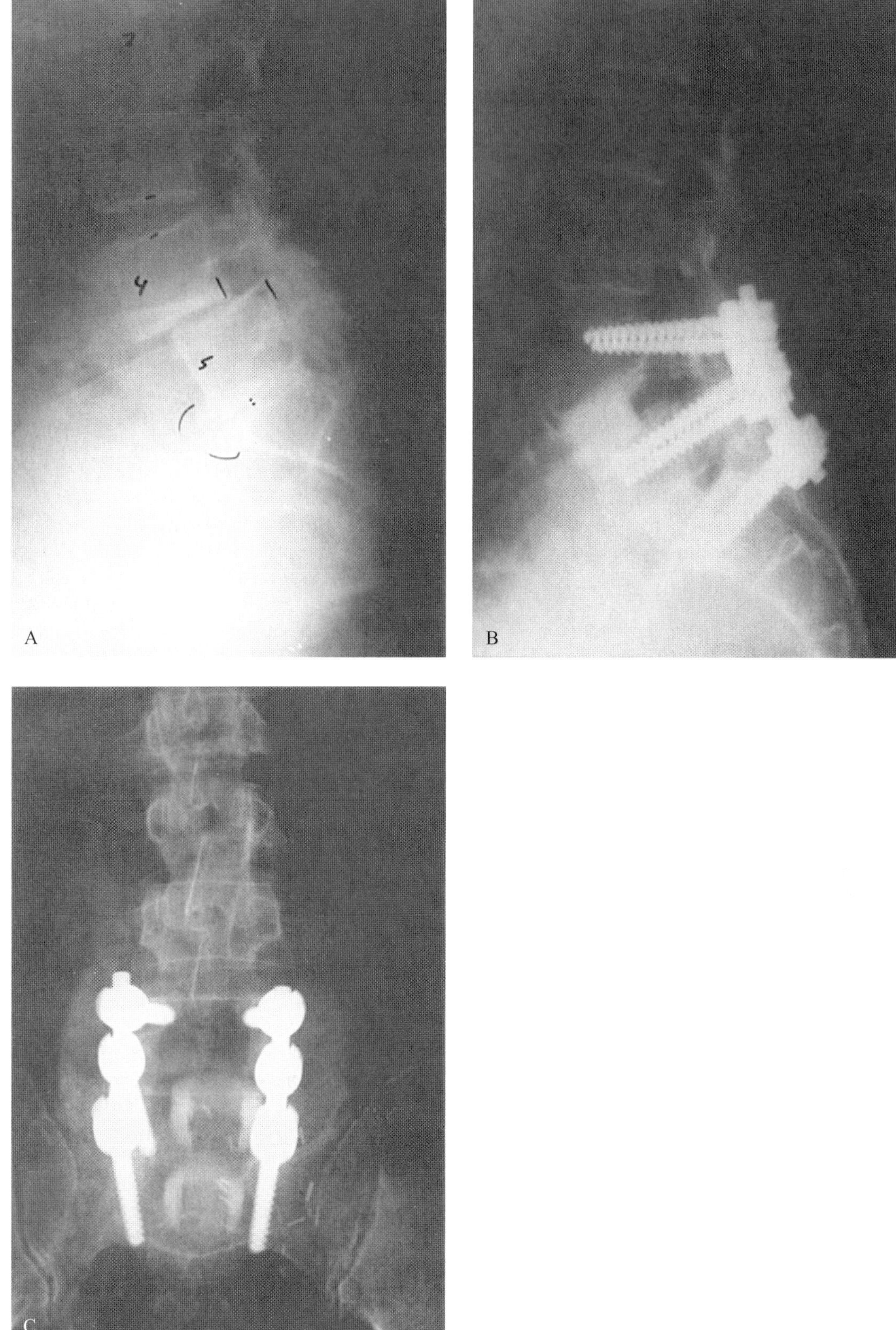

FIGURE 32–4. *A.* Lateral x-ray findings before (demonstrating grade II spondylolisthesis) and *B.* after a combined anterior interbody fusion using allograft femoral bone and posterior stabilization using pedicle screw instrumentation. Note the reduction of spondylolisthesis. *C.* Anteroposterior view of the fusion construct seen in *A.*

decompression is, therefore, important in the adult population. Adult scoliosis can be divided into patients who had idiopathic adolescent deformity versus those who develop degenerative deformity in adulthood. In general, adults with degenerative scoliosis experience greater neurogenic symptoms; patients with previous adolescent idiopathic scoliosis complain more of axial symptoms. In either case, the key factor is determining the source of pain generation. After extensive conservative management fails, surgical decompression versus decompression and fusion are options for these patients. With advancing age, the risk of extensive fusions needed for deformity significantly increases. Generally, patients who have neurogenic claudication and leg symptoms as their major complaint without an extensive curvature are candidates for limited decompression. If extensive scoliosis (greater than 30 degrees) or back pain is also present, a multisegmental fusion extending into the thoracic spine may be necessary. Complications from adult surgery are similar to any other spinal surgery except for the increased frequency and risk in the elderly patients.[40]

Clinical Pearl: Multiple studies have documented accelerated radiographic spondylosis at the adjacent level to fusion levels.

Furthermore, evidence exists that increased intervertebral stress at adjacent motion segments to fusion levels is present.[41] Multiple studies have documented accelerated radiographic spondylosis at the adjacent level to fusion levels.[42,43] Although there is clear accelerated degeneration of the adjacent level, the patients are rarely symptomatic at these levels in long-term follow-ups.[44]

In summary, deformity surgery is used in adolescents who have had curve progression or have curves over 40–50 degrees, depending on their age. Excellent correction can be obtained especially in combined anterior/posterior fusion cases, although subsequent morbidity can occur because of increased loading of the segments immediately above and below the fusion sites. Adult deformity, however, is more difficult to evaluate and treat. Because of the increased medical risk for the elderly, the minimal amount of surgery is preferred. Decompression is usually used in patients with leg symptoms but extensive deformity or back symptoms may require multisegmental fusions to the thoracic spine.

Kyphoplasty

Vertebral compression fracture (VCF) is the most common complication of osteoporosis. Over 700,000 compression fractures are recorded per year in the United States.[45] Fortunately, most compression fractures are benign and are treated conservatively. A few days of bed rest, Calcitonin, and pain medications allow most patients to return to their activities of daily living.

A finite number of patients, however, are left with long-term sequelae from their VCF. The kyphotic deformity commonly seen with multiple thoracic VCF can lead to chronic thoracic and low back pain. The abnormal kyphosis increases the workload of the paraspinal muscles, which may lead to chronic pain and fatigue.

Deformity causes compression of the viscera, which results in early satiety and weight loss in this population. The lung's functional capacity is also significantly reduced, as each VCF causes a 9% loss of forced vital capacity. Patients with multiple VCFs are at significantly increased risk of pneumonia as well.[46,47]

However, a new technique of percutaneous stabilization of vertebral fractures, called "kyphoplasty," allows for restoration of the vertebral body height with injection of cement to stabilize VCFs. The patient is placed in a prone position. Using fluoroscopy, the surgeon introduces a cannula into the vertebral body through the pedicle posteriorly. A balloon is subsequently used to inflate the vertebra to its normal, precompressed height. Subsequently, cement is injected into the void to prevent future collapse.

The procedure is fairly quick and is tolerated very well by the patients. Most patients wake up in the recovery room with their back pain significantly improved.[48] Often, they are able to leave the hospital on the first postoperative day with no further need for medical attention.

SURGICAL COMPLICATIONS AND FAILED BACK SYNDROME

In the process of informed consent, potential complications are communicated with patients. Risks of any type of spinal surgery include infection, nerve injury, paralysis, blood loss, need for reoperation, bone graft donor site morbidity, large vessel injury, and medical complications such as deep venous thrombosis or pulmonary embolism or death.

Risk of nerve injury is increased with the use of pedicle screw fixation. Furthermore, intraoperative monitoring of pedicle screws via electromyography significantly reduces risk of misplaced pedicle screws.[49]

Wound infections have been reported in 1%–6% of spinal surgeries. Instrumented fusions are associated with a higher risk of infection. Deep infections are usually serially irrigated and debrided with acceptable clinical outcome. At 1-year follow-up, 22 patients with deep wound infections who had undergone between 2 and 10 irrigations had no infection recurrence.[50]

Bone grafting is associated with a high risk of complications. Iliac crest bone graft (ICBG) donor site morbidity has been reported in up to 30% of patients, which may last for years.[51] Moreover, allograft bone has the potential for disease transmission and immunologic reaction. The risk of HIV infection, however, has been estimated to be less than 1/1000,000 in properly screened donors.[52]

Although infrequent, certain complications are associated with the ALIF procedures. Bone graft collapse or extrusion and cage malposition or migration can result in poor final alignment or pseudarthrosis. The anterior retroperitoneal approach can be complicated by venous injury requiring repair as well as subsequent thrombosis. Arterial occlusion of internal iliac artery has been reported.[53] Patients who present with ongoing leg pain and weakness in a nondermatomal distribution following ALIF should be evaluated for iliac vessel thrombosis.[54]

Retrograde ejaculation results from injury to the superior hypogastric plexus. This plexus is responsible for bladder neck closure during ejaculation. In a review of 4500 cases, 0.42% of patients experienced retrograde ejaculation.[55] Other rare complications reported in ALIF include pituitary apoplexy, ureteral injury, and pancreatitis.[53,56,57]

Failed back surgery syndrome (FBSS) is characterized by incapacitating symptoms postspinal surgery. The common causes of FBSS include improper patient selection, recurrent or residual disc herniation, arachnoiditis, radiculitis, spinal or spinal neural foraminal stenosis, and failure to correctly identify the structural source(s) of pain.[58] Epidural fibrosis is commonly seen after any type of decompressive surgery; epidural fibrosis, however, has not been associated with increased postoperative symptoms.[59]

Clinical Pearl: The common causes of failed back surgery syndrome include improper patient selection, recurrent or residual disc herniation, arachnoiditis, radiculitis, spinal or spinal neural foraminal stenosis, and failure to correctly identify the structural source(s) of pain.

Treatment for FBSS depends on the cause of the syndrome. Residual or reherniation of disc material and stenosis can be corrected with reoperation. Arachnoiditis, however, does not respond well to surgical intervention. Arachnoiditis can be identified on an MRI by the "empty sac sign"; the nerve roots are matted or "clumped" together with an "empty" thecal sac caused by adhesion of the nerve roots to its walls.[60]

The more common cause of FBSS, however, is poor patient selection. Fusion surgery for degenerative disc disease, for example, has been controversial with a high risk of FBSS. Failure rates of up to 50% have been reported with front and back fusions for chronic low back pain. Unless patients who have undergone at least 6 months of extensive conservative management are carefully selected for surgical intervention, FBSS is not uncommon following spinal fusion for disc degeneration.[61–63]

CONCLUSIONS

This chapter presented a brief overview of common surgical approaches for low back syndromes. A reasonable course of conservative care should be tried and failed in nonemergent cases. Increasing communication and clinical teamwork between conservative care practitioners and surgeons, during both the pre- and postsurgical phases, has become the standard of care. Indeed, the quality of postsurgical care can impact the overall success of the surgery, which was discussed in detail in Chapter 27.

Despite recent advances in technology and new surgical options, the decision to proceed should not be taken lightly. The patient must be provided a reasonable set of options with realistic prognoses, as not all of these cases conclude with great success. The failed back surgery syndrome was discussed, providing a realistic view of those cases that do not fare well. Nevertheless, spinal surgery does provide hope for patients when all other options have been exhausted, and successful cases can dramatically improve the patient's quality and deliver their future back into their own hands.

SUMMARY

General:

1. Surgical intervention is recommended for patients with unremitting pain who have failed conservative management, progressive weakness, or myelopathic symptoms.
2. Cauda equina syndrome is an absolute indication for surgery.

Cervical:

3. Patients with cervical spondylosis or central disc herniation benefit from (ACDF).
4. Allograft bone can be used in ACDF but fusion rates are inferior to autograft bone for two or greater levels of involvement.
5. In ACDF, plate stabilization is used in patients with three or less discs involvement; longer fusion segments require posterior stabilization.
6. Cervical soft lateral disc herniation can be addressed via posterior foraminotomies without a need for fusion.
7. Cervical myelopathy is treated via posterior laminoplasty or laminectomy for three or greater

number of interspaces involved when cervical alignment is not kyphotic.
8. OPLL is a common indication for posterior laminoplasty.
9. Vertebrectomy is used in patients with myelopathy who are kyphotic or have more limited number of levels involved in their pathology.

Thoracic:

10. Thoracic disc disease can cause severe radicular pain or myelopathy.
11. Multiple surgical approaches are available to address thoracic disc herniations.
12. The anterior thoracotomy provides the best exposure to the thoracic disc.

Lumbar:

13. Lumbar stenosis can mimic vascular claudication.
14. Decompressive surgery via removal of lamina and hypertrophied ligamentum flavum has good success for lumbar stenosis.
15. Lumbar disc herniations are commonly seen in younger population with radicular symptoms.
16. Surgical treatment is indicated for lumbar disc herniations if symptoms are not improved by 2–3 months with conservative management.
17. Lumbar discogenic pain is surgically treated by removal of the pain generator, i.e., disc.
18. Discectomy and interbody fusion can be performed anteriorly or posteriorly; posterior approach is utilized in patients with collapsed disc space or previous anterior surgery.
19. Artificial disc replacements are under FDA trials in the United States and are a promising approach to surgical treatment of degenerative disc disease.
20. Spondylolisthesis is treated with posterolateral fusion and instrumentation.
21. Interbody fusion can be added to help with reduction of slippage and improved fusion rates in spondylolisthesis.

Scoliosis:

22. Advanced idiopathic adolescent scoliosis requires surgical fusion via an anterior, posterior, or combined approach.
23. Adult scoliosis is significantly more difficult to assess and treat.
24. Limited decompression is the treatment of choice in elderly patients with degenerative scoliosis.
25. Advanced scoliosis, however, may require extensive fusion with significant potential complications.

REFERENCES

1. Heller JG, Schimandle JH. Operative treatment of degenerative cervical disk disease. *J South Orthop Assoc* 1996;5(3):188–206.
2. Wang J, McDonough P, Kanim L, Endow K, Delamarter R. Increased fusion rates with cervical plating for three-level anterior cervical discectomy and fusion. *Spine* 2001;26(6):643–646; discussion 646–647.
3. Hirabayashi K, Watanabe K, Wakano K, Suzuki N, Satomi K, Ishii Y. Expansive open-door laminoplasty for cervical spinal stenotic myelopathy. *Spine* 1983;8(7): 693–699.
4. Tsuji H. Laminoplasty for patients with compressive myelopathy due to so-called spinal canal stenosis in cervical and thoracic regions. *Spine* 1982;7(1):28–34.
5. Emery SE, Bohlman H, Bolesta M, Jones P. Anterior cervical decompression and arthrodesis for the treatment of cervical spondylotic myelopathy. Two to seventeen-year follow-up. *J Bone Joint Surg Am* 1998; 80(7):941–951.
6. Smith MD, Emery S, Dudley A, Murray K, Leventhal M. Vertebral artery injury during anterior decompression of the cervical spine. A retrospective review of ten patients. *J Bone Joint Surg Br* 1993;75(3):410–415.
7. Suh PB, Kostuik JP, Esses SI. Anterior cervical plate fixation with the titanium hollow screw plate system. A preliminary report. *Spine* 1990;15(10):1079–1081.
8. Vaccaro AR, Falatyn S, Scuderi G, et al. Early failure of long segment anterior cervical plate fixation . *J Spinal Disord* 1998;11(5):410–415.
9. Zdeblick TA, Hughes S, Riew K, Bohlman H. Failed anterior cervical discectomy and arthrodesis. Analysis and treatment of thirty-five patients . *J Bone Joint Surg Am* 1997;79(4):523–532.
10. Wang JC, McDonough P, Endow K, Delamarter R. A comparison of fusion rates between single-level cervical corpectomy and two-level discectomy and fusion. *J Spinal Disord* 2001;14(3):222–225.
11. Wood KB, Blair J, Aepple D, et al. The natural history of asymptomatic thoracic disc herniations. *Spine* 1997;22(5):525–529; discussion 529–530.
12. Albrand OW, and Corkill G. Thoracic disc herniation. Treatment and prognosis. *Spine* 1979;4(1):41–46.
13. Lehman RM, Grunwerg B, Hall T. Anterior approach to the cervicothoracic junction: An anatomic dissection. *J Spinal Disord* 1997;10(1):33–39.
14. Korovessis PG, Stamatakis M, Baikousis A, Vasiliou D. Transthoracic disc excision with interbody fusion. 12 patients with symptomatic disc herniation followed for 2–8 years . *Acta Orthop Scand Suppl* 1997;275:12–16.
15. Bohlman HH, Zdeblick TA. Anterior excision of herniated thoracic discs. *J Bone Joint Surg Am* 1988;70(7): 1038–1047.
16. Olmarker K, Blomquist J, Stromberg J, Nanmark U, Thomsen P, Rydevik B. Inflammatogenic properties of nucleus pulposus. *Spine* 1995;20(6):665–669.
17. Weber H. Lumbar disc herniation. A controlled, prospective study with ten years of observation. *Spine* 1983;8(2):131–140.
18. Weber H. The natural history of disc herniation and the influence of intervention. *Spine* 1994;19(19):2234–2238; discussion 2233.
19. Kambin P. Arthroscopic microdiscectomy. *Arthroscopy* 1992;8(3):287–295.

20. Yeung AT, Tsou PM. Posterolateral endoscopic excision for lumbar disc herniation: Surgical technique, outcome, and complications in 307 consecutive cases. *Spine* 2002;27(7):722–731.
21. Wang JC, Shapiro M, Hatch J, Knight J, Porey F, Delamarter R. The outcome of lumbar discectomy in elite athletes. *Spine* 1999;24(6):570–573.
22. Coppes MH, Marani M, Thomeer R, Groen G. Innervation of "painful" lumbar discs. *Spine* 1997;22(20):2342–2349; discussion 2349–2350.
23. Aprill C, Bogduk N. High-intensity zone: A diagnostic sign of painful lumbar disc on magnetic resonance imaging . *Br J Radiol* 1992;65(773):361–369.
24. Barrick WT, Schofferman J, Reynolds J, et al. Anterior lumbar fusion improves discogenic pain at levels of prior posterolateral fusion. *Spine* 2000;25(7):853–857.
25. Lee CK, Vessa P, Lee JK. Chronic disabling low back pain syndrome caused by internal disc derangements. The results of disc excision and posterior lumbar interbody fusion. *Spine* 1995;20(3):356–361.
26. France JC, Yaszemski M, Lauerman W, et al. A randomized prospective study of posterolateral lumbar fusion. Outcomes with and without pedicle screw instrumentation. *Spine* 1999;24(6):553–560.
27. Boos N, Kalberer F, Schoeb O. Retroperitoneal endoscopically assisted minilaparotomy for anterior lumbar interbody fusion: Technical feasibility and complications. *Spine* 2001;26(2):E1–E6.
28. Mayer HM. A new microsurgical technique for minimally invasive anterior lumbar interbody fusion. *Spine* 1997;22(6):691–699; discussion 700.
29. Zdeblick TA, David SM. A prospective comparison of surgical approach for anterior L4–L5 fusion: Laparoscopic versus mini anterior lumbar interbody fusion. *Spine* 2000;25(20):2682–2687.
30. Wiltse LL, Newman PH, Macnab I. Classification of spondylolysis and spondylolisthesis. *Clin Orthop* 1976;(117):23–29.
31. Gillet P, Petit M. Direct repair of spondylolysis without spondylolisthesis, using a rod-screw construct and bone grafting of the pars defect. *Spine* 1999;24(12):1252–1256.
32. Wu SS, Lee CH, Chen PQ. Operative repair of symptomatic spondylolysis following a positive response to diagnostic pars injection. *J Spinal Disord* 1999;12(1):10–16.
33. Frymoyer JW. Degenerative spondylolisthesis: Diagnosis and treatment. *J Am Acad Orthop Surg* 1994;2(1):9–15.
34. Herkowitz HN, Kurz LT. Degenerative lumbar spondylolisthesis with spinal stenosis. A prospective study comparing decompression with decompression and intertransverse process arthrodesis. *J Bone Joint Surg Am* 1991;73(6):802–808.
35. Blumenthal SL, Baker J, Dossett A, Selby D. The role of anterior lumbar fusion for internal disc disruption. *Spine* 1988;13(5):566–569.
36. Bridwell KH, Sedgewick K, O'Brien M, Lenke L, Baldus C. The role of fusion and instrumentation in the treatment of degenerative spondylolisthesis with spinal stenosis. *J Spinal Disord* 1993;6(6):461–472.
37. Kostuik JP. Operative treatment of idiopathic scoliosis. *J Bone Joint Surg Am* 1990;72(7):1108–1113.
38. Ahn UM, Ahn N, Nallamshetty L, et al. The etiology of adolescent idiopathic scoliosis. *Am J Orthop* 2002; 31(7):387–395.
39. Carr WA, Moe J, Winter R, Lonstein J. Treatment of idiopathic scoliosis in the Milwaukee brace. *J Bone Joint Surg Am* 1980;62(4):599–612.
40. Bradford DS, Tay BK, Hu SS. Adult scoliosis: Surgical indications, operative management, complications, and outcomes. *Spine* 1999;24(24):2617–2629.
41. Lee CK. Accelerated degeneration of the segment adjacent to a lumbar fusion. *Spine* 1988;13(3):375–377.
42. Frymoyer JW, Hanley E, Howe J, Kuhlmann D, Matteri R. Disc excision and spine fusion in the management of lumbar disc disease. A minimum ten-year follow-up. *Spine* Mar 1978;3(1):1–6.
43. Lehmann TR, Spratt K, Tozzi J, et al. Long-term follow-up of lower lumbar fusion patients. *Spine* 1987; 12(2):97–104.
44. Ghiselli G, Wang J, Hsu W, Dawson E. *L5–s1* segment survivorship and clinical outcome analysis after L4–L5 isolated fusion. *Spine* Jun 2003;28(12):1275–1280.
45. Cooper C, Atkinson E, O'Fallon W, Melton L 3rd. Incidence of clinically diagnosed vertebral fractures: A population-based study in Rochester, Minnesota, 1985–1989. *J Bone Miner Res* Feb 1992;7(2):221–227.
46. Lyles KW, Gold D, Shipp K, Pieper C, Martinez S, Mulhausen P. Association of osteoporotic vertebral compression fractures with impaired functional status. *Am J Med* 1993;94(6):595–601.
47. Silverman SL. The clinical consequences of vertebral compression fracture. *Bone* 1992;13(Suppl 2):S27–S31.
48. Lieberman IH, Dudeney S, Reinhardt M, Bell G. Initial outcome and efficacy of "kyphoplasty" in the treatment of painful osteoporotic vertebral compression fractures. *Spine* 2001;26(14):1631–1638.
49. Glassman SD, Dimar J, Puno R, Johnson J, Shields C, Linden R. A prospective analysis of intraoperative electromyographic monitoring of pedicle screw placement with computed tomographic scan confirmation. *Spine* 1995;20(12):1375–1379.
50. Glassman SD, Dimar J, Puno R, Johnson J. Salvage of instrumental lumbar fusions complicated by surgical wound infection. *Spine* Sep 15 1996;21(18):2163–2169.
51. Wimmer C, Kristher M, Gluch H, Ogon M, Stockl B. Autogenic versus allogenic bone grafts in anterior lumbar interbody fusion. *Clin Orthop* Mar 1999;(360):122–126.
52. Buck BE, Malinin TI, Brown MD. Bone transplantation and human immunodeficiency virus. An estimate of risk of acquired immunodeficiency syndrome (AIDS). *Clin Orthop* Mar 1989;(240):129–136.
53. Rajaraman V, Vingan R, Roth P, Heary R, Conklin L, Jacobs G. Visceral and vascular complications resulting from anterior lumbar interbody fusion. *J Neurosurg* 1999;91(Suppl 1):60–64.
54. Hackenberg L, Liljenquist U, Halm H, Winkelmann W. Occlusion of the left common iliac artery and consecutive thromboembolism of the left popliteal artery

following anterior lumbar interbody fusion. *J Spinal Disord* 2001;14(4):365–368.

55. Flynn JC,Price CT. Sexual complications of anterior fusion of the lumbar spine. *Spine* 1984;9(5):489–492.
56. Isiklar ZU, Lindsey RW, Coburn M. Ureteral injury after anterior lumbar interbody fusion. A case report. *Spine* 1996;21(20):2379–2382.
57. Liu JK, Nwagwu C, Pikus H, Couldwell W. Laparoscopic anterior lumbar interbody fusion precipitating pituitary apoplexy. *Acta Neurochir (Wien)* 2001;143(3):303–306; discussion 306–307.
58. Van Goethem JW, Parizel P, van der Hauwe L, De Shepper A. Imaging findings in patients with failed back surgery syndrome. *J Belge Radiol* 1997;80(2):81–84.
59. Cervellini P, Curri D, Bernardi L, Volpin L, Bernardi L, Pinna V, Benedetti A. Computed tomography of epidural fibrosis after discectomy: A comparison between symptomatic and asymptomatic patients. *Neurosurgery* Dec 1988;23(6):710–713.
60. Jinkins JR, Osburn A, Garrett D Jr, Hunt S, Story J. Spinal nerve enhancement with Gd-DTPA: MR correlation with the postoperative lumbosacral spine. *AJNR Am J Neuroradiol* 1993;14(2):383–394.
61. Gertzbein SD, Hollopeter MR, Hall S. Pseudarthrosis of the lumbar spine. Outcome after circumferential fusion. *Spine* 1998;23(21):2352–2356; discussion 2356–2357.
62. Herkowitz HN, Abraham DJ, Albert TJ. Management of degenerative disc disease above an L5–S1 segment requiring arthrodesis. *Spine* 1999;24(12):1268–1270.
63. Herkowitz HN, Sidhu KS. Lumbar spine fusion in the treatment of degenerative conditions: Current indications and recommendations. *J Am Acad Orthop Surg* 1995;3(3):123–135.

CHAPTER

33

PRESURGICAL PSYCHOLOGICAL SCREENING FOR LOW BACK SYNDROMES

Andrew R. Block

OUTLINE

OBJECTIVES

1. Recognize the limitations in effectiveness of spine surgery.
2. Understand psychosocial risk factors for reduced spine surgery outcome.
3. Learn method for combining risk factors in order to determine surgical outcome prognosis.

INTRODUCTION

The outcome of spine surgery is far from uniform. Even when clear surgical indications exist, and the surgery corrects the underlying physical condition, many patients fail to achieve the outcomes they most desire: relief of pain and improvement of functional ability. Turner et al.,[1] reviewing all published research on spinal fusion, found that only about 65%–75% of all patients achieved satisfactory clinical outcomes. In these studies, poorer outcome was associated with a number of factors, including greater numbers of fused levels, and the use of instrumentation. Similarly, Deyo et al.,[2] in a literature review on laminectomy/discectomy, found that the mean success rate of this procedure for relief of spine pain was 67%.

This inconsistency in spine surgery outcome has led researchers and clinicians to examine the factors that affect spine surgery outcome. A growing body of research demonstrates that psychosocial factors are among the most robust predictors of reduced surgical effectiveness. Such issues as a patient's emotional status, social environment, lifestyle, and incentives for improvement appear to exert significant influences upon the extent to which effective spine surgery procedures are accompanied by improvement in symptoms. As will be seen, nonemergent surgery should often be avoided in patients with a high level of psychosocial risk, because even when the surgeon corrects the physical cause of the pain only about 15%–20% of such patients obtain significant pain relief or improvement in functional ability.[3–5] Such results contrast sharply with the excellent outcome obtained by 85%–90% of patients having low levels of psychosocial risk. These findings suggest that for patients with high levels of psychosocial risk, conservative treatment measures, such as chiropractic, physical therapy, or multidisciplinary pain programs, may offer the promise of obtaining the greatest gains in functional ability, while minimizing the potential for iatrogenic effects.

Clinical Pearl: Such issues as a patient's emotional status, social environment, lifestyle, and incentives for improvement appear to exert significant influences upon the extent to which effective spine surgery procedures are accompanied by improvement in symptoms.

The current chapter discusses some of the psychosocial issues that are most strongly associated with diminished spine surgery outcome. Also provided is a guide identifying the most salient issues. A model for presurgical psychological screening is also discussed, with an eye to increasing the awareness of this process to clinicians, both surgeons and nonsurgeons alike. (Much more detailed discussion of these issues can be found in Block et al.[6])

PSYCHOLOGICAL FACTORS ASSOCIATED WITH POOR SURGICAL OUTCOME

Although spine surgery is conducted only on the basis of objectively identifiable pathology, the pain and distress associated with spinal pathology are necessarily subjective. As such, the patient's perception of the injury, the noxious sensations experienced, and the effectiveness of the surgery in improving functioning and lifestyle can be strongly influenced by factors lying far outside the operating room. Many of these factors are psychosocial in nature, including (1) personality conditions and emotional states, (2) cognitive issues, and (3) environmental and historical factors.

Presurgical psychological screening (PPS) identifies such "psychosocial risk factors" through a combination of a diagnostic interview and a psychometric testing. This process allows for objectification and quantification of risk factors for reduced spine surgery outcome. Thus, the psychologist can render a scientifically based determination of the extent to which the clinical outcome of the spine surgery may be negatively compromised.

Clinical Pearl: The psychologist can render a scientifically based determination of the extent to which the clinical outcome of the spine surgery may be negatively compromised.

Personality and Emotional Factors

Personality characteristics are those psychological aspects of a patient that are relatively stable over time. The American Psychiatric Association defines personality as "deeply ingrained patterns of behaviors, which include the way one relates to, perceives, and thinks about the environment and oneself."[7] Such stable characteristics, while exerting strong influences over one's responses to pain, injury, and illness, may be either augmented or diminished by relatively more volatile emotional states. Emotions such as depression, anger, and anxiety may occur as responses to an injury, or in some cases may precede or even be a significant cause of an injury. For example, individuals who are depressed tend to be accident-prone and are therefore likely to suffer injuries that may lead to spine problems.

Long-standing personality traits and more acute and changeable emotional reactions can be objectively assessed through the use of psychometric testing. The most widely used tool for assessing personality traits is the Minnesota Multiphasic Personality Inventory (MMPI), especially in studies of chronic back pain and spinal surgery outcomes, although its use is still considered somewhat controversial.[8] Much of the research on PPS has been conducted using the MMPI, although a growing body of research uses other, more simple instruments.

Pain Sensitivity The single strongest psychosocial risk factor for reduced spine surgery success rates involves "excessive pain sensitivity." This is a relatively stable trait, which is assessed on the MMPI by the Hysteria (Hy) and Hypochondriasis (Hs) scales. These scales are the ones most commonly elevated among patients with heterogeneous chronic pain syndromes and in spine surgery candidates. Patients with elevations on these scales tend to experience pain in excess of that normally expected for a given level of physical pathology. For example, one study[9] found that spine surgery candidates undergoing discography were significantly more likely to report "discordant" pain (i.e., pain upon injection of normal, nondisrupted disc) if they had significant elevations on the MMPI Hy and Hs scales than if their scores on these scales were in the normal range. Both of these scales have been shown to predict poor spine surgery outcome in numerous studies.[3,10–12]

Some studies, in fact, have found the predictive value of these two MMPI scales to exceed the predictive value of medical factors, such as x-rays, computed tomography (CT) scans, and neurological signs. For example, Spengler et al.,[5] examining patients who underwent laminectomy/discectomy, found that MMPI-2 elevations on scales Hs and Hy contributed 26% to a multiple regression equation against clinical outcome (i.e., an equation that mathematically combines all variables to determine which are the strongest outcome predictors), whereas imaging studies contributed only 10% and neurological signs contributed only 3%.

Clinical Pearl: The single strongest psychosocial risk factor for reduced spine surgery results involves "excessive pain sensitivity."

Depression Depression is an emotional condition that can strongly affect spine surgery outcome. Individuals with depression tend to have a low threshold for induced pain,[13] to focus on negative events,[14] and to report significant functional impairment even when direct observation of their behavior proves otherwise.[15] Not surprisingly, higher levels of depression, such as those measured by elevations on the Depression (D) scale of the MMPI, are frequently associated with poor surgical outcome.[12,16,17] Studies using other psychometric tests such as the Beck depression Inventory[18] and a modified version of the Zung depression scale[19] also confirm that depression predicts poor results.

Assessment of depression must evaluate whether this emotional condition is a relatively stable personality trait or a more reactive emotional response to the pain. Some depressive symptoms, such as sleep disturbance, problems with concentration, and weight change, may be a direct result of the experience of continued pain and physical limitations. Perhaps this explains the finding that clinical depression is identified in up to 85% of patients with chronic pain.[20] However, depression is also frequently found in the preinjury history of many patients with back pain. Polatin et al.[21] reported that 39% of the chronic low back pain patients they evaluated displayed symptoms of preexisting depression. For example, in a systematic study of depressed male military veterans with chronic pain, Atkinson et al.[22] found that 58% experienced depression after the pain, whereas 42% of the patients experienced the onset of depression prior to the pain. Finally, Linton,[23] reviewing research on psychosocial risk factors for back pain, found that in 14 of the 16 reviewed studies, depression increased the risk of developing such problems. Depression is a strong risk factor for reduced surgical outcome when it preexists the injury (i.e., when it is a personality trait). When depression exists as an emotional reaction to the injury, it is less of a risk factor, especially if the patient is treated with antidepressant medication.

Clinical Pearl: Depression is a strong risk factor for reduced surgical outcome when it preexists the injury (i.e., when it is a personality trait). When depression exists as an emotional reaction to the injury, it is less of a risk factor, especially if the patient is treated with antidepressant medication.

Anxiety and Stress Most patients being considered for spine surgery experience anxiety, stress, and fear. The pain often causes much of this anxiety, as pain may lead to loss of income, reduction in the quality of marital interaction, and uncertainty about future ability to work. Further, the anticipation of the surgery itself can make patients anxious, as they fear the pain associated with the surgery, and worry about "waking up" afterwards. Unfortunately, a number of studies demonstrate that anxiety and stress can also reduce the outcome of spine surgery.

On the MMPI, the scale that most closely assesses anxiety is the Psychasthenia (Pt) scale. In addition, elevations on this scale are indicative of a tendency toward excessive doubts, fears, obsessions, and compulsions. Elevations on this scale have been found to be associated with poor response to spine surgery.[16,17,24]

Other studies have used scales to more directly assess the role of stress and anxiety in influencing spine surgery results. Trief et al.[19] found that elevated state anxiety scores on the State-Trait Anxiety Inventory (STAI)[25] were significantly associated with lower return to work and less change in reported pain after spine surgery. Kjelby-Wendt et al.,[18] examining discectomy patients, divided subjects into "discontented" and "contented" groups, based in large part on presurgical scores on the STAI. At follow-up 6–12 months postoperative, they found that discontented patients achieved poorer discectomy outcome than did the contented patients, including poorer lumbar range of motion, and greater than twice the duration of postoperative sick leave. Schade et al.[26] studying discectomy results found that "occupational mental stress" had a significant negative correlation with return to work, and had near significant negative correlations with improvement in activities of daily living, as well as reduction in pain. Anxiety appears to reduce surgical effectiveness, regardless of whether it arises from the injury, from environmental conditions, or is a more stable personality trait.

Clinical Pearl: Anxiety appears to reduce surgical effectiveness, regardless of whether it arises from the injury, from environmental conditions, or is a more stable personality trait.

Anger Another major emotion that influences spine surgery outcome is anger. Both clinical experience and research indicate that feelings of anger are prevalent in patients with back pain. For example, Fernandez et al.[27] report on a study in which patients with chronic pain rated the frequency with which they felt six different emotions during the previous 30 days. Fear, guilt, shame, sadness, and envy were all felt commonly, but anger was the most frequently experienced, an average of about 70% of the time.

Anger can be destructive to the spine surgery patient for a number of reasons. Anger can reduce immunosuppression, thereby negatively impacting the postoperative healing process.[28] Further, anger can also adversely influence health-related behaviors, such as smoking, overeating, or alcohol consumption.

Such behaviors can work in opposition to postoperative rehabilitation, a process that requires stamina and dedication to improvement in general health and conditioning.

It may not be surprising, therefore, that research demonstrates a strong negative association of anger with spine surgery outcome. On the MMPI the scale most closely associated with anger is the Psychopathic Deviant (Pd) scale. In addition, patients who score high on the Pd scale tend to be rebellious toward authority figures and aggressive.[29] Pd elevations have been found to be predictive of poor surgical outcome in several studies.[11,12,16]

A more direct test of the influence of anger on spine surgery outcome was conducted by Trief et al.[19] who examined the relationship of spine surgery results to scores on the Cook-Medley Hostility subscale of the MMPI-2. In this study, at 1-year postoperative, patients who had high presurgical hostility scores reported less improvement in daily activities and were significantly less likely to be working compared to patients who had scored low on this scale. As this study measures anger as a trait, it suggests that anger preexisting the pain may correlate with poor results.

Besides its general negative health consequences, anger may also negatively influence spine surgery results because it can alter the patient's priorities, such that vindication or revenge become more important than overcoming the pain. DeGood and Kiernan[30] found that chronic pain patients who are angry and blame their employer for their injury report higher levels of emotional distress and have poorer responses to treatment. For such patients, changes in pain status following surgery may be more closely related to the dynamics of their anger than to changes in the physical pathology.

Clinical Pearl: Research demonstrates a strong negative association of anger with spine surgery outcome. Besides its general negative health consequences, anger may also negatively influence spine surgery results because it can alter the patient's priorities, such that vindication or revenge become more important than overcoming the pain.

Pain-Coping Strategies Since pain is a highly subjective phenomenon, the ways that a patient thinks about the pain, and the patient's behavioral strategies for dealing with the pain, can significantly influence its overall impact. Such pain-coping strategies affect a patient's pain level, in addition to their ability to adjust to and overcome the pain.[31] The term "coping strategies" refers to the specific thoughts and behaviors patients use to manage their pain and their emotional response to that pain.[32] A number of questionnaires have been developed to assess these coping thoughts and behaviors, including the Coping Strategies Questionnaire,[33] the Ways of Coping Checklist,[34] the Vanderbilt Pain Management Inventory,[32] and the Cognitive Coping Strategies Inventory.[35]

The Coping Strategies Questionnaire (CSQ), in particular, has been used in several studies of surgical screening. The CSQ consists of six cognitive and two behavioral coping scales. Cognitive strategies include diverting attention, reinterpreting pain sensations, coping self-statements, ignoring pain sensations, praying or hoping, and catastrophizing (i.e., exaggerated negative self-statements). The two behavioral scales are increasing activity level and increasing pain behavior. In addition, the CSQ contains a measure of the patient's perception of his or her ability to control pain and reduce it.

Block et al.[3] gave the CSQ preoperatively to 204 patients who underwent spine surgery (either laminectomy/discectomy or spinal fusion). A hierarchical regression analysis found that the CSQ Poor Self-Reliance (a combination scale composed of catastrophizing, praying, and reducing activity level) was a significant contributor to the regression equation predicting overall surgical outcome. Gross[36] examined pain intensity, sleep disturbance, and patient-rated surgical outcome in 50 laminectomy patients who were given the CSQ prior to surgery. In this study patients who scored high on a factor termed "Loss of Control" (combining high scores on the catastrophizing scale and low scores on the pain control scale) had greater postoperative pain and reported poorer surgical outcome than did those who scored low on this scale. High scores on the "Self-Reliance" factor (combining high scores on the pain control scale and low scores on the praying/hoping scale) were positively associated with reported surgical outcome and negatively associated with postoperative pain and sleep disturbance. Taken together, these two studies demonstrate that poor pain coping, especially "catastrophizing," can significantly reduce surgical effectiveness.

Clinical Pearl: Poor pain coping, especially "catastrophizing," can significantly reduce surgical effectiveness.

Pathological Distress Thus far, personality and emotional issues have been discussed as if each could be experienced in isolation, e.g., a patient who is depressed is not also angry. However, for many patients the sense of distress is multidimensional, and research demonstrates that patients with broad-ranging, intense distress are particularly vulnerable to obtaining poor clinical outcomes of spine surgery. For example, Riley et al.[37] examined MMPI profiles of 201 spine surgery candidates. The MMPI profiles were then subjected to a cluster analysis and a four-cluster solution was obtained. The outcome of surgery at 6 months postoperative was analyzed by MMPI cluster type. The largest group having all MMPI scales "within normal limits" obtained significant improvement. Similar results were obtained by the second group, which had elevations on scales Hs, D, and Hy (termed the "triad" group). A third cluster, with elevations on scales Hs and Hy only (termed the "V" group), achieved poorer results than did the normal and triad groups. Finally, a "depressed-pathological" group of patients, having elevations on all clinical scales except on scale M–F (the masculine–feminine scale), obtained the worst results.

Additional research[38] has also applied cluster analytic techniques to the MMPI-2 profiles of spine surgery candidates. Examining 222 patients a three-cluster MMPI solution was found. The three clusters obtained include a within-normal-limits group, a triad type profile, and a depressed-pathological profile. As in the Riley et al.[37] study, outcomes varied by MMPI profile type. Twenty-two patients (10% of the total population) fell into the depressed-pathological group, and this group obtained the least improvements in functional ability and pain reduction. The within-normal-limits group, comprising 114 patients, achieved the best surgery results. The remaining patients ($N = 86$), having a triad profile, achieved less pain improvement but similar improvement in functional ability when compared to the within-normal-limits group.

Clinical Pearl: Three primary external factors have been shown to be associated with increased pain behavior: spousal reinforcement, litigation, and workers' compensation and disability payments.

Behavioral and Environmental Factors

Often the factors negatively impacting response to spine surgery lie in the patient's environment—relationships, work, and legal factors. Reactions of significant others, the response of the employer, the legal system, and even actions taken by health-care providers may unwittingly reinforce the patient's pain and disability. One of the major tenets of behavioral psychology is that behaviors increase in frequency when they are followed by rewarding consequences.[39] In some ways, pain behaviors can be considered like any other behaviors in that they occur increasingly when rewarded and decrease in frequency when either ignored or punished.[40] In the research on chronic pain, three primary external factors have been shown to be associated with increased pain behavior: spousal reinforcement, litigation, and workers' compensation and disability payments.

Families and spouses may unknowingly provide rewards for pain behaviors. They may encourage rest, take over the patient's jobs or responsibilities, and provide more attention to the patient when the pain appears greatest, while at the same time, they may ignore the patient when he or she appears to be in less pain because of engaging in alternative "well behaviors," promoting a tendency to avoid such nonreinforced behaviors. A number of studies have demonstrated that such a "solicitous" pattern of spousal response increases the likelihood that patients will report high pain levels,[41] display a high level of pain behaviors,[42] and display less activity during physical exercise.[43]

Another potential source of reinforcement for reduced spine surgery effectiveness is pending legal action. Junge et al.[44] found that spine surgery patients who were applying for disability pension had poorer surgical outcomes than those who were not applying. Several studies have found that a history of having previous medically related lawsuits and other litigation connected with spine injury predicted poor outcome from spine surgery.[4,45] This is not to say that patients with pending litigation are malingering, since they by definition have physical pathology underlying their pain complaints, but rather that financial incentives may make them increasingly pain-sensitive.[46]

Patients who are receiving payments from workers' compensation similarly tend to have poorer responses to spine surgery compared to those who are not receiving such financial compensation.[47–49] However, the explanation for these poorer results does not rest purely on economic considerations. Most patients on workers' compensation, in fact, receive far less in disability payments than they received while working. However, patients with job injuries may exhibit many of the other problems associated with high pain levels and poor treatment outcomes, including job dissatisfaction,[50] heavy physical job demands,[44,49] or directing anger and/or blame toward the employer.[30] All of these problems associated with workers' compensation lead it to be considered as one of the strongest predictors of excessive disability among patients with back injury.[51]

Environmental and Historical Factors

Thus far the focus has been on the patient's current situation—personality, current emotional condition, and factors reinforcing pain in the patient's environment. An examination of the patient's history and background contains much data that can improve the selection process for spine surgery candidates. One factor of particular importance appears to be the existence of mental health problems predating the development of spinal pain. Psychological problems clearly may predispose patients to the development of chronic pain. Bigos et al.,[50] for example, found that employees with high scores on the MMPI Hs and Hy scales were at significant risk of developing occupational back pain complaints over a 4-year period compared to those without such elevations. Moreover, several studies have shown that patients with psychological problems preexisting back injury show reduced spine surgery outcome. Block et al.[3] found that a history of psychological treatment prior to the spine injury contributed significantly to a regression equation of reduced surgical outcome. Keel[52] and Manniche et al.[4] obtained similar results. Such results imply that to the extent that mental health problems are more chronic, intense, and pervasive, they can be expected to have a substantial negative effect on surgical outcome.

Clinical Pearl: Physical and sexual abuse greatly increased the likelihood that individuals would develop chronic pain. Unfortunately, abuse may also predispose patients to have reduced surgical results.

One shocking statistic concerning spine injury is the number of patients who have been abuse victims. Haber and Roos,[53] for example, found that over half of the patients they evaluated for entrance into a multidisciplinary pain program had been victims of physical or sexual abuse, and for over 90% of subjects the abuse occurred during their adult years. Linton,[54] in a general population study, found that physical and sexual abuse greatly increased the likelihood that individuals would develop chronic pain. Unfortunately, abuse may also predispose patients to have reduced surgical results. Schofferman et al.[55] found that spine surgery candidates who reported at least three types of childhood abuse (i.e., sexual, physical, emotional, parental substance abuse, or abandonment) had an 85% clinical failure rate compared to a 5% failure rate among patients who reported no such trauma.

Even marital distress can influence the effectiveness of spine surgery. A number of studies have demonstrated that marital dissatisfaction and problems within a marriage are common in chronic pain patients.[56] Dissatisfied spouses have expectations for outcome that are more negative[57] and tend to attribute the patient's pain to psychological, rather than physical, problems.[58] Schade et al.[26] found that social support by the spouse was significantly associated with greater pain relief in patients undergoing lumbar discectomy. Thus, the quality of the marital relationship should be given consideration, as it may negatively influence treatment outcome.

Clinical Pearl: Abuse of medications and alcohol were associated with a high failure rate among patients undergoing spine surgery.

Finally, patients experiencing chronic pain typically are prescribed narcotic medication to help relieve the pain. However, some spine surgery candidates may become dependent on and addicted to this medication. Two of the studies that looked at the potential role of substance abuse or dependence on spine surgery outcomes found that abuse of medications and alcohol were associated with a high failure rate among patients undergoing spine surgery.[5,59] One must keep in mind, however, that drug addiction and abuse are not defined merely as the taking of large doses of narcotics. Merskey and Moulin[60] state that drug addiction is

> compulsive drug use despite harm, an overwhelming preoccupation with securing a good supply, and the tendency to relapse after withdrawal. Addiction is a behavioral pattern of drug use, in which medication is taken for its psychic effects rather than for its pain-relieving effects (p. 160)

Such a pattern has very strong implications for response to spine surgery.

DETERMINATION OF SURGICAL PROGNOSIS

This brief review presented has shown that there are many identifiable psychological risk factors for poor surgical outcome. A number of studies have attempted to combine such risk factors into a "scorecard" in order to sharpen predictive acumen. The original scorecard study[45] included vague psychosocial factors, such as "gross obesity," "poor psychological background," and "secondary gain." Even so, when combined with some physical and medical predictors, the results were indeed interesting. The results for 280 patients undergoing spine surgery showed that patients who achieved good outcome had higher ratings on the preoperative scorecard than did those who achieved poor outcome, although statistical analyses were not reported. Manniche et al.[4] have confirmed the predictive value of the Finneson and Cooper[45] scorecard, demonstrating that it is a very strong predictor of reduced long-term discectomy results ($p < .00001$). A similar type of scorecard was developed by Spengler et al.[5] and tested on patients undergoing lumbar discectomy. In this study four predictor variables were examined: sciatic root tension signs, radiographic results (CT scan or myelogram), neurological signs (such as atrophy or weakness), and psychological factors (based on MMPI scale elevations). Psychological factors accounted for 24% of the variance in clinical outcome and were much more strongly predictive than were the three medical factors examined, and the scorecard effectively predicted 40% of outcome.

Clinical Pearl: Across many studies, results using "scorecards" demonstrate that about 80%–85% of patients having large number of combined psychosocial risk factors do not achieve good clinical results from spine surgery.

Block et al.[3] investigated the relationship of psychosocial factors to clinical outcome (pain level, improvement in functional ability, and medication use) in 204 patients who underwent laminectomy/discectomy or spinal fusion. In this study, patients were determined to have good outcome at 6 months postoperation if they achieved

1. a pain report of >4 on an 11-point Numeric Pain Rating (NPR) scale;
2. good functional ability (defined as a score of >40/100 on the Owestry Disability Index©[61]);
3. use of either no pain medication or anti-inflammatory medication only.

Patients who achieved two of the above criteria were determined to have fair outcome. Those who achieved 0 or 1 of the criteria were determined to have poor surgery results.

With relatively few factors outcome could be accurately predicted. Outcome was correctly predicted for 83% of cases using a hierarchical regression equation that included psychological factors, especially MMPI elevations on scales D, Hy, Pd, Pt, and Sc, poor pain coping on the CSQ,[33] as well as spousal reinforcement of pain behavior, workers' compensation, pre-injury psychological treatment history, and heavy job requirements. Although a complete description of the PPS scorecard is beyond the scope of this chapter, Figure 33–1 lists the major psychosocial risk factors examined and the relative value they assume in the scorecard. Although the actual PPS model, as used by psychologists, is somewhat complicated, the research by Block et al.[3] suggests that patients whose total psychosocial risk values combine to 10 or greater are generally at high risk for poor outcome of elective spine surgery. Figure 33–2 is a brief overview of the relationship between identified levels of psychosocial risk and recommendations to the surgery arising from PPS.

Psychosocial Risk Factors

Factor Name	Score[a]	Data Source
Job Dissatisfaction	2	Interview
Worker's Comp.	2	Interview
Litigation	2	Interview
Spousal Solicitous.	1	Interview
No spousal support	1	Interview
Abuse & Abandon.	1	Interview
Substance Abuse	2	Interview
Psych. History	2	Interview
Pain Sensitivity	2	TESTING
Depression		
(Chronic)	2	TESTING
(Reactive)	1	
Anger	2	TESTING
Anxiety	2	TESTING
Depressed-Pathological profile	4	TESTING

[a] 1=medium risk, 2=high risk, 4=very high risk
[b] See text for additional references

FIGURE 33–1. Psychosocial risk factors.

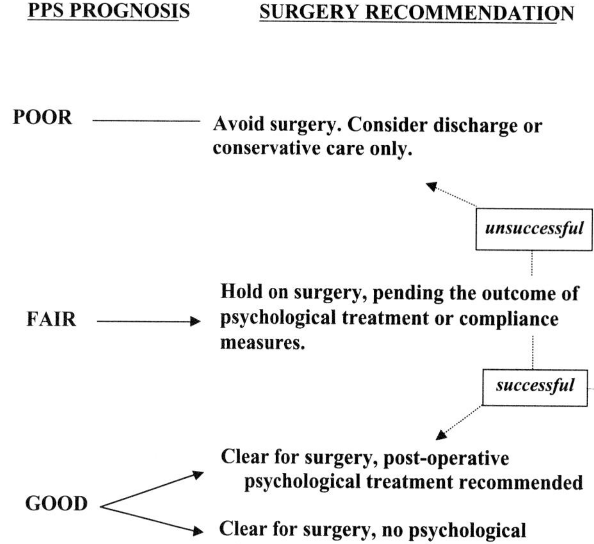

FIGURE 33–2. PPS prognosis and subsequent surgical recommendations.

Clinical Implications

The results reviewed in this chapter provide strong support for the inclusion of PPS in the evaluation of elective spine surgery candidates. Awareness of the psychosocial risk factors described in this chapter can help health-care providers and other physicians involved in the treatment of chronic spine pain patients to make appropriate treatment decisions. Table 33–1 is included in this chapter to help health-care providers recognize when patients may be experiencing emotional and psychosocial difficulties, which could compromise the results of physical treatments. Referral to a psychologist experienced in PPS should be considered when the existence of such difficulties is identified.

This chapter has emphasized the prognostic function of PPS. However, PPS serves a second purpose: it allows the surgeon and other health-care providers to develop individualized treatment plans. Such treatments may be able to facilitate outcome in acceptable surgical candidates, assess and improve motivation in marginal candidates, or stand as surgery alternatives for patients with poor outcome prognoses. For example, for patients with a good PPS prognosis, no psychotherapy is typically needed prior to undergoing

TABLE 33–1. Referral Criteria for Psychological Screening

- Excessive pain behavior
- Symptoms inconsistent with identified pathology
- High levels of depression or anxiety
- Sleep disturbance—insomnia or hypersomnia
- Excessively high or low expectations about treatment outcome
- Marital distress or sexual difficulties
- Negative attitude toward work or employer
- Emotional lability or mood swings
- Inability to work or greatly decreased functional ability (>3 months)
- Excalating or large doses of narcotics or anxiolytics
- Litigation or continuing disability benefits resulting from spine injury

Referral Considerations

0–1 items	Not necessary to refer unless desired by patient
2–3 items	Consider referral
4+ items	Strongly consider referral

surgery. For poor prognosis patients pain relief as a result of spine surgery is unlikely. For such patients an intensive and coordinated treatment intervention, such as that provided by a multidisciplinary pain treatment center, may be effective in providing pain relief even in the absence of correction of underlying pathology. As many poor prognosis patients will not only be unlikely to achieve good surgical outcome, but will go on to be subjected to further surgery, the benefits of avoiding surgery in these patients are multiple. Such a poor prognosis patient who enrolls in an alternative pain management program not only avoids a descent into increasing pain and worsening functional ability, but can also be trained in techniques to achieve self-control over pain, and be helped to accept the limitations imposed by physical and emotional difficulties. In other words, patients can be helped to develop their own means for achieving pain control and improvement in functional ability, rather than relying on the distant hope that surgery will make things better instead of worse.

Many patients examined for PPS have a moderate level of psychosocial risk, so their surgical PPS prognosis is deemed to be "fair." For these patients in the fair prognosis category, treatments may be focused on augmenting the compliance with psychological treatment and/or medical treatment recommendations in order to improve surgical outcome. Such treatments might include required reduction in narcotic medication usage to a predetermined level, smoking cessation prior to surgery, or required weight loss.

Conclusion

Spine surgery is often a patient's last hope for relief from chronic back pain. Unfortunately, many surgical patients do not achieve pain reduction or recovery of function, even though physical pathology has been corrected. Therefore, identification of those patients who are most likely to have a poor surgical outcome is a critical part of the evaluation of spine surgery candidates. The studies reviewed here demonstrate that there are many psychological risk factors that are associated with poor surgical outcome. While many models and "scorecards" exist, it is now clear that examination of such critical risk factors in spine surgery candidates can be an effective means of predicting surgical results. Across many studies, about 80%–85% of high psychosocial risk patients do not have good results from spine surgery. Thus, the inclusion of PPS within the diagnostic regimen of the spine surgery candidate can significantly aid in patient selection and avoid a worsening of problems for high-risk patients.

SUMMARY

1. Psychosocial risk factors predict reduced outcome of spine surgery more strongly than to physical factors.
2. Psychosocial risk factors include emotional, personality, behavioral and historical factors.
3. These risk factors can be quantified and combined to correctly predict the outcome of spine surgery in 83% of cases.
4. Physician should be aware of potential risk factors and refer patients for presurgical psychological screening when such factors are extant in a particular patient's case.

REFERENCES

1. Turner JA, Ersek M, Herron L, et al. Patient outcomes after lumbar spinal fusions. *JAMA* 1992;268(7):907–911.
2. Deyo RA, Diehl A, Rosenthan M. How many days of bedrest for acute low back pain? *NEJM* 1986;315:1064–1070.
3. Block AR, Ohnmeiss DD, Guyer RD, Rashbaum R, Hochschuler SH. The use of presurgical psychological screening to predict the outcome of spine surgery. *Spine J* 2001;1:274–282.
4. Manniche C, Asmussen KH, Vinterberg H, Rose-Hansen EBR, Kramhoft J, Jordan A. Analysis of preoperative prognostic factors in first-time surgery for lumbar disc herniation, including Finneson's and modified Spengler's score systems. *Dan Med Bull* 1994;41:110–115.
5. Spengler DM, Freeman C, Westbrook R, Miller JW. Low-back pain following multiple lumbar spine

procedures: Failure of initial selection? *Spine* 1980;5(4): 356–360.
6. Block AR, Gatchel R, Deardorff WW, Guyer RD. *The psychology of spine surgery*. Washington, DC: American Psychological Association, 2003.
7. American Psychiatric Association. *Diagnostic and statistical manual of mental disorders*, 4th ed. Washington, DC: American Psychiatric Association, 1994.
8. Main CJ, Spanswick CC. Personality assessment and the Minnesota Multiphasic Personality Inventory 50 years on: Do we still need our security blanket? *Pain Forum* 1995;4(2):90–96.
9. Block AR, Vanharanta H, Ohnmeiss DD, Guyer RD. Discographic pain report. Influence of psychological factors. *Spine* 1996;21(3):334–338.
10. Cashion EL, Lynch WJ. Personality factors and results of lumbar disc surgery. *Neurosurgery* 1979;4;141–145.
11. Long C. The relationship between surgical outcome and MMPI profiles in chronic pain patients. *J Clin Psychol* 1981;37:744–749.
12. Herron L, Turner JA, Ersek M, Weiner P. Does the Millon Behavioral Health Inventory (MBHI) predict lumbar laminectomy outcome? A comparison with the Minnesota Multiphasic Personality Inventory (MMPI). *J Spinal Disord* 1992;5(2):188–192.
13. Merskey H. The effect of chronic pain upon the response to noxious stimuli by psychiatric patients. *J Psychosom Res* 1965;9:291–298.
14. Seligman MEP. Learned helplessness and depression in animals and men. In: Spence JT, Carson RC, Thibaut JW, eds. *Behavioral approaches to therapy*. Morristown, N J: General Learning Press, 1976:86–99.
15. Kremer EF, Block AR, Atkinson JJ. Assessment of pain behavior: Factors that distort self-report. In: Melzack R, ed. *Pain management and assessment*. New York: Raven Press, 1983:165–171.
16. Dvorak J, Valach L, Fuhrimann P, Heim E. The outcome of surgery for lumbar disc herniation. II. A 4–17 years' follow-up with emphasis on psychosocial aspects. *Spine* 1988;13(12):1423–1427.
17. Sorenson LV, Mors O. Presentation of a new MMPI scale to predict outcome after first lumbar discectomy. *Pain* 1988;34:191–194.
18. Kjelby-Wendt G, Styf JR, Carlsson SG. The predictive value of psychometric analysis in patients treated by extirpation of lumbar intervertebral disc herniation. *J Spinal Disord* 1999;12:375–379.
19. Trief PM, Grant W, Fredrickson B. A prospective study of psychological predictors of lumbar surgery outcome. *Spine* 2000;25(20):2616–2621.
20. Lindsay P, Wyckoff M. The depression-pain and its response to antidepressants. *Psychosomatics* 1981;22:571–577.
21. Polatin PB, Kinney RK, Gatchel RJ, Lillo E, Mayer TG. Psychiatric illness and chronic low-back pain. The mind and the spine—Which goes first? *Spine* 1993;18(1):66–71.
22. Atkinson JH, Slater MA, Patterson TL, Grant I, Garfin SR. Prevalence, onset and risk of psychiatric disorders in chronic pain patients: A controlled study. *Pain* 1991;45:111–121.
23. Linton SJ. A review of psychological risk factors in back and neck pain. *Spine* 2000;25:1148–1156.
24. Doxey NC, Dzioba RB, Mitson GL. Predictors of outcome in back surgery candidates. *J Clin Psychol* 1988; 44:611–622.
25. Spielberger CD, Gorusch RI, Lushene R. Manual for the State-Trait Anxiety Inventory. Palo Alto: Consulting Psychology Press, 1983.
26. Schade V, Semmer N, Main CJ, Hora J, Boos N. The impact of clinical, morphological, psychosocial and work-related factors on the outcome of lumbar discectomy. *Pain* 1999;80:239–249.
27. Fernandez E, Clark TS, Ruddick-Davis D. A framework for conceptualization and assessment of affective disturbance in pain. In: Block AR, Kremer EF, Fernandez E, eds. *Handbook of pain syndromes: Biopsychosocial perspectives*. Mahwah, NJ: Lawrence Erlbaum Associates, 1999:123–148.
28. Kiecolt-Glaser J, Malarkey W, Chee M, Newton T, Cacioppo J, Mao H, Glaser R. Negative behavior during marital conflict is associated with immunological down-regulation. *Psychosom Med* 1993;55:395–409.
29. Graham JR. *The MMPI-2: Assessing personality and psychopathology*. New York: Oxford University Press, 1990.
30. DeGood DE, Kiernan B. Perception of fault in patients with chronic pain. *Pain* 1996;64:153–159.
31. Turk DC, Rudy TE. Toward an empirically driven taxonomy of chronic pain patients: Integration of psychological assessment data. *J Consult Clin Psychol* 1988;56(2):233–238.
32. Brown GK, Nicassio PM. Development of a questionnaire for the assessment of active and passive coping strategies in chronic pain patients. *Pain* 1987;31: 53–64.
33. Rosensteil AK, Keefe FJ. The use of coping strategies in chronic low back pain patients: Relationship to patient characteristics and current adjustment. *Pain* 1983;17:33–44.
34. Folkman S, Lazarus RS. An analysis of coping in a middle aged community sample. *J Health Soc Behav* 1985;21:219–239.
35. Butler RW, Damarin FL, Bealieu CL, Schewebel AI, Thorn BE. Assessing cognitive coping strategies for acute pain: Psychological assessment. *J Consult Clin Psychol* 1989;1:41–45.
36. Gross AR. The effect of coping strategies on the relief of pain following surgical intervention for lower back pain. *Psychosom Med* 1986;48:229–238.
37. Riley JL, Robinson ME, Geisser ME, Wittmer VT, Smith AG. Relationship between MMPI-2 cluster profiles and surgical outcome in low-back pain patients. *J Spinal Disord* 1995;8(3):213–219.
38. Block AR, Ohnmeiss D. MMPI profiles predict the outcome of spinal surgery. Presented at *North American Spine Society, 15th Annual Meeting*, New Orleans, LA, 2000.
39. Skinner BF. *About behaviorism*. New York: Alfred A. Knopf, 1974.
40. Fordyce WE. *Behavioral methods for chronic pain and illness*. St. Louis, MN: Mosby, 1976.

41. Block AR, Kremer EF, Gaylor M. Behavioral treatment of chronic pain: The spouse as a discriminative cue for pain behavior. *Pain* 1980;9:243–252.
42. Kerns RD, Southwick S, Giller E, Haythornthwaite JA, Jacob MC, Rosenberg R. The relationship between reports of pain-related social interactions and expressions of pain and affective distress. *Behav Ther* 1991;22:101–111.
43. Lousberg R, Schmidt AJ, Groenman NH. The relationship between spouse solicitousness and pain behavior: Searching for more evidence. *Pain* 1992;51: 75–79.
44. Junge A, Dvorak J, Ahrens S. Predictors of bad and good outcomes of lumbar disc surgery: A prospective clinical study with recommendations for screening to avoid bad outcomes. *Spine* 1995;20(4):460–468.
45. Finneson BE, Cooper VR. A lumbar disc surgery predictive score card: A retrospective evaluation. *Spine* 1979;4:141–144.
46. Chapman RC. Pain: The perception of noxious events. In: Sternbach RA, ed. The psychology of pain. New York: Raven Press, 1978:169–202.
47. Haddad GH. Analysis of 2932 workers' compensation back injury cases: The impact of the cost to the system. *Spine* 1987;12(8):765–769.
48. Greenough CG, Fraser RD. The effects of compensation on recovery from low-back injury. *Spine* 1989;14(9):947–955.
49. Davis RA. A long-term outcome analysis of 984 surgically treated herniated lumbar discs. *J Neurosurg* 1994; 80:514–521.
50. Bigos SJ, Battie MC, Spengler DM, et al. A prospective study of work perceptions and psychosocial factors affecting the report of back injury. *Spine* 1991;16(1): 1–6.
51. Frymoyer JW, Cats-Baril WL. An overview of the incidences and cost of low back pain. *Orthop Clin Am* 1987;22:263–271.
52. Keel PJ. Psychosocial criteria for patient selection: Review of studies and concepts for understanding chronic back pain. *Neurosurgery* 1984;15(6):935–941.
53. Haber J, Roos C. Effects of spouse abuse and/or sexual abuse in the development and maintenance of chronic pain in women. *Adv Pain Res Ther* 1985;9:889–895.
54. Linton SJ. A population-based study of the relationship between sexual abuse and back pain: Establishing a link. *Pain* 1997;73:47–53.
55. Schofferman J, Anderson D, Hinds R, Smith G, White A. Childhood psychological trauma correlates with unsuccessful lumbar spine surgery. *Spine* 1992;17(Suppl 6):S1380–S1384.
56. Romano JM, Turner JA, Clancy SL. Sex differences in the relationship of pain patient dysfunction to spouse adjustment. *Pain* 1989;39:289–296.
57. Block AR, Boyer SL, Silbert RV. Spouse's perception of the chronic pain patient: Estimates of exercise tolerance. In: Fields HL, Dubner R, Cervero F, eds. *Advances in pain research and therapy*, Vol. 9. New York: Raven Press, 1985:897–904.
58. Maruta T, Osborne D. Sexual activity in chronic pain patients. *Psychosomatics* 1976;19:531–537.
59. Uomoto JM, Turner JA, Herron LD. Use of the MMPI and MCMI in predicting outcome of lumbar laminectomy. *J Clin Psychol* 1988;44:191–197.
60. Merskey H, Moulin D. Pharmacological treatment in chronic pain. In: Block AR, Kremer EF, Fernandez E, eds. *Handbook of pain syndromes: Biopsychosocial perspectives*. Mahwah, NJ: Lawrence Erlbaum Associates, 1999;149–163.
61. Fairbanks JC, Couper J, Davies JB, O'Brien JP. The Oswestry low back pain disability questionnaire. *Physiotherapy* 1980;66(8):271–273.

CHAPTER

34

MANAGEMENT OF OCCUPATIONAL LOW BACK INJURIES

Alan L. Colledge, Edward B. Holmes, Roger Pack, Hugh I. Johnson, and Scott DeBerard

OUTLINE

OBJECTIVES

1. This chapter will briefly review the history and uniqueness of injuries that occur on the job with the associated mandated entitled benefits.
2. Programs that are in place to assist injured workers to return to their occupation can actually facilitate delayed healing times, increase costs, and create disability.
3. Solutions for health-care providers and employers to prevent and deal with system-induced disability will be discussed extensively under the well-published SPICE model.

INTRODUCTION TO WORKERS' COMPENSATION

The concept of compensating people for injuries received "on the job" has been around for a long time. Even pirates who roamed and plundered in the seventh century had their own elaborate code of "compensation."[1] In the United States "workers' compensation" became a legislated right in the early twentieth century. By 1949, all 50 states had adopted some form of workers' compensation legislation,[2] with each state designing its system to ensure the worker prompt but limited benefits, and to assign to the employer sure and predictable compulsory liability insurance within established parameters. The principal components of these US systems include (1) a statutory program, (2) expeditious resolution of disputed issues, and (3) limited liability without fault. Because workers' compensation is a no-fault insurance program (determining negligence or blame is generally irrelevant), automatic benefits include the following:

(a) Medical treatment coverage including the clinical care, services, and supplies necessary to cure or relieve the effects of an on-the-job injury. This means that the employee does not incur any deductible or out-of-pocket expense for the treatment of a work-related injury or illness.
(b) Indemnity payments replacing wages while the injured employee recovers from an industrial injury and/or reaches clinical stability.[3] All states have varying formulas for the calculation of these indemnity payments, which are often tax-free.
(c) Death benefits, providing weekly payments to the surviving spouse and dependent children of a worker whose work-related injury results in death. Burial and funeral expenses are also paid.
(d) An impairment settlement giving compensation to an injured worker for permanent physical loss from a work-related injury (i.e., scars, disfigurement, amputation, etc.), according to a defined compensation schedule.

As with the other benefits, there are significant differences between the states on the value of settlement amounts and the *methodology used* to calculate permanent partial impairment and disability benefits.[4] The laws of the particular state in which the worker is injured govern the scope and amount of payments for these agreed-upon services.

Notably these systems, adopted to assist injured workers, have become a significant cost to business and paradoxically have been shown to, at times, adversely affect recovery,[5,6] increase disability,[7,8] and decrease the potential to return to work.[9,10] Since their adoption, the cost for administering these programs in the United States has increased exponentially and has now reached 171 billion dollars annually,[11] with the average workers' compensation claim costing $13,182 and each lost time claim averaging $20,000.

Occupational Musculoskeletal Pain

Common musculoskeletal injuries are a particular concern. Most common musculoskeletal ailments are benign and even if they occur at work, most people recover quickly with minimal or no lost time. However, a small number recover much more slowly than expected and generate a considerably greater cost. A 1992 review of 106,961 workers' compensation low back injury cases found that approximately 86% of the costs were incurred by 10% of the injured workers.[13] A similar study of 21,338 work-related musculoskeletal disorders of the upper extremities found that 25% of the claims account for 89% of the costs.[14] Recent statistics from the State of Washington found that 5% of their claims (accounting for 84% of the costs) are not from individuals who have lost limbs or suffered other catastrophic injuries while at work, but rather are from nonverifiable muscle and back complaints.[15]

Clinical Pearl: In the United States, of all work-related injuries, 28% are for soft tissue musculoskeletal strains, which account for approximately 40% of all lost-time injuries.[12]

In the United States, injured workers with skeletal fractures incur an average of 21 days off work and those with amputations incur 18 lost days, while workers with carpal tunnel syndrome complaints average 25 days away from work.[16] Yet a recent study of 3000 randomly selected individuals found carpal tunnel symptoms in 14% of the population.[17] Likewise back pain appears to be a part of living with a recent survey indicating a yearly prevalence in the US population of 15%–20%.[18] Among working-age people surveyed, 50% report back pain symptoms each year.[19,20]

Occupational Back Pain

Throughout the world, occupational low back pain is one of the most commonly encountered conditions in the industrial setting and perhaps best exemplifies the refractory nature of workplace musculoskeletal injuries. Each year approximately 10 million employees in the United States suffer back pain that impairs their work performance and an estimated 1 million employees file workers' compensation claims for back pain.[21] In a survey of 12 states, the US National Safety Council found that occupational back injuries, the most frequently occurring workplace disorder,[22] account for 22% of workplace injuries/illnesses and 32% of workers' compensation costs. In 1986, it was estimated that the total compensable cost of occupational low back cases in the United States was more than 10 billion dollars.[23] Back pain is now the single most expensive category of industrial injury, responsible for 31% of total industrial expenses and is second only to the common cold as a reason for physician office visits in the United States.[24] Back pain results in a loss of 93 million to 250 million workdays per year and is the most common cause of disability in workers under the age of 45.[25] Yet it is important to note that back discomfort appears to be a part of living, with 28% of the adult population reporting some back pain discomfort at any given time and 50% of the population reporting back pain in the previous 6 months.[18,26]

Studies have shown that back pain prevalence rates are comparable for industrialized nations, in particular for the United States and the United Kingdom, but that approaches to treatment vary greatly. Still, the evidence indicates that these variations in treatment have little effect on outcomes.[27]

There is a general lack of consistency in the treatment of back pain in the United States.[28] Increasing awareness of this has led to governmental concern that many patients may be subjected to clinical care that is inappropriate or at least less than optimal.[29,30] As the late Dr. Henry LaRocca stated, "This predicament is not the result of an inadequate fund of available information with which to address the matter. Instead the problem emanates from the lack of a comprehensive and unifying problem-solving strategy."[31]

Many published studies have suggested clinical or rehabilitation tools that can be used to affect this problem; however, the quality of life for disabled individuals and their families, along with significant cost savings for business and industry, depend on identifying and instituting a dynamic, comprehensive system that decreases employee disability, maintains worker productivity, and reduces compensation costs. The SPICE model represents a multifactor system to optimizing clinical and rehabilitation services for injured workers. It represents a philosophical approach to the treatment of injured worker versus a medical treatment guideline. The purpose of this chapter is to outline and summarize the main components of the SPICE model and indicate how this model, if successfully implemented, can be used to reduce work-related disability, reduce compensation cost, and improve patient satisfaction. Generally, statistics from the United States are used to illustrate the concepts of the SPICE model. However, the authors believe the SPICE principles are universally applicable.

SPICE Model for Prevention of Occupational Disability

It is the authors' view that comprehensive application of the SPICE model prevents injuries, facilitates effective treatment, reduces workers' compensation costs, and reduces system-induced disability. Originally published in *The Journal of Occupational Rehabilitation* in 1993,[32] and updated in 2000,[33] the SPICE model continues to be updated and expanded to include clinical and management techniques demonstrated in the literature and in practice to both prevent and manage injuries efficiently and fairly.

SPICE

Over the course of modern warfare and throughout the world, militaries discovered that when soldiers with relatively simple physical complaints were left to heal alone, or received inappropriate treatment for battle-related stress, some became permanently and totally disabled.[34] Placed under combat-induced conditions of anxiety and stress, the soldiers' protective psychological reserves eroded and defense mechanisms began to form. Unchecked, these defenses transformed a relatively simple disorder, such as "fatigue," into an "illness" that was both socially acceptable and serious. Further, once this "illness" was validated by the system, it released the soldier, either consciously or subconsciously, from the unpleasant emotional stress of his or her duties. In response, the militaries evolved a successful treatment model, referred to as "Forward Treatment," to prevent this system-induced disability. Forward treatment is a comprehensive, proactive model developed with over 100 years of experiences of military physicians all over the world to prevent system-induced permanent disability. The model, acronymed SPICE, includes five components, Simplicity, Proximity, Immediacy, Centrality, and Expectancy, and has been adapted for those who deal with injured workers to facilitate return to duty and subsequently reduce claim rates and costs.

During the 1973 Israeli–Arab war, Israeli physicians noted many soldiers had relatively minor physical impairments, yet behaved in a greatly disabled fashion. The best medical care at the time was given to these soldiers, with the shocking result that many of them became permanently disabled and few returning to active duty.[35] Treatment appeared to create iatrogenic (i.e., physician-induced) disability. During the 9 years between the Arab war and the war with Lebanon, Israel had adopted the United States' Forward Treatment concept, as described in this chapter in greater detail. During this Lebanon war, by applying the Forward Treatment philosophy, Israel was able to return 60% of soldiers with injuries similar to the 1973 casualties to full duty within 72 hours.[36]

There are many similarities between military personnel and individuals involved in the disability/workers' compensation environment:

1. Both groups are basically healthy. A certain degree of job-related intelligence has been tested for and is required, and those with preexisting disabilities or serious illnesses have been screened out.
2. Individuals are expected to function in terms of the needs of the "team" rather than the individual.
3. Both groups have legally mandated entitlement programs for "on-the-job" injuries.
4. The number and type of disability complaints are directly related to the intensity of psychosocial stressors to which the subjects are exposed.[37]
5. Psychosocial stressors arise from factors other than the duty that the individual is exposed to. These factors may include personal performance, poor social support, team morale, duty satisfaction, personal belief in supervisors, and economic downturns.[38,39]

While certainly soldiers exposed to battle are highly stressed, many current workers are likewise subjected to unprecedented daily personal stress that carries over into the workplace. Many employees, as they deal with life difficulties, find their life out of control. This includes family relationships, care for elderly parents, reduced job security, and more expectations from employers.

These similarities suggest that the military model of Forward Treatment, validated on the battlefield, provides an extremely useful model for the prevention and treatment of entitled individual's claims and costs.

SIMPLICITY

"Simplicity" comes from the military observation that ominous-sounding diagnostic terminology, complicated tests, and treatment for fairly minor problems (like battle fatigue) only served to strengthen the soldier's rationalization that he or she was indeed seriously ill. Injured workers, like soldiers with stress, at times believe they are suffering from a serious ailment. For example, in one study 60% of patients with back pain believed or had been told they had a "disc prolapse" although only 11% had any evidence of nerve root pain or dysfunction.[40] Another study of 140 patients with mechanical low back pain found 67% were concerned with a serious illness causing their pain. This contrasts with actual statistical experience that only 2% of persons with back pain may require surgery, and less than 1% will have any underlying systemic illness.[41] Regardless of the cause of back pain, approximately 70% of affected people recover in 2–3 weeks and 90% in 6 weeks.[42,43]

Clinical Pearl: This model, given the acronym SPICE, consists of five general components:

***Simplicity*: The concept that simple, benign conditions, treated in a complicated fashion, become complicated.**
***Proximity*: The need to keep the worker associated with the workplace by building morale and support of employees.**
***Immediacy*: The need to deal with industrial claims in a timely manner.**
***Centrality*: All parties involved with workers share a common philosophy and ultimate goal of returning the individual back to gainful employment as quickly as possible.**
***Expectancy*: The concept that individuals often fulfill the expectations placed on them.**

Diagnostic Terminology

"Battle fatigue" has been closely tied with the history of warfare and has been given many names. During the American Civil War it was called "nostalgia"; during World War I, "shell shock"; during World War II, "war neurosis" and "combat exhaustion"; and during the Korean War it was referred to as "combat fatigue." It was discovered that the more ominous-sounding the "diagnosis," the worse the soldier responded. Many times it appeared that the diagnosis given to stressed soldiers became a self-fulfilling prophecy with the prognosis directly related to the initial diagnostic label given to the individual soldier.)

Concerns about diagnostic "labeling" (which refers to the unintended, and usually adverse, consequences of simply assigning a diagnostic label to an anxious individual) have long been recognized. Researchers have shown that simply informing a person who feels that he or she has a "disease" (such as asymptomatic hypertension) can cause an increase in "sick behavior."[44] For this reason, the military abandoned ominous-sounding labels such as "shell shock" or "war neurosis" and replaced them with more benign names, such as "battle fatigue" or "combat reaction."

The problem of back pain terminology is well recognized. A recent review of over 7000 low back pain medical articles revealed a pronounced lack of uniformity in diagnostic terminology. This lack of common terminology has been identified as a major barrier to research and a key challenge to defining methods of treatment.[45] One study showed 20 current diagnostic terms ranging from the mundane "lumbar strain" to the exotic "metameric cellulotenoperiostomyalgic syndrome."[46] In reality, only 10%–20% of patients can be given a precise pathoanatomical diagnosis.[47]

Health-care providers should apply concepts of simplicity by (a) providing an explanation of the most likely pain mechanisms; (b) reassuring the patient that serious disease is absent and that only benign conditions exist; and (c) providing information about the favorable prognosis of the natural history of the condition. Business and disability claim managers should reemphasize the simplicity of the diagnosis and discuss the likelihood of return to regular duty in the time frames given by the treating practitioner. Return-to-work programs should emphasize the clinician's findings and allow light-duty and other return-to-work activities that specifically follow the natural healing process of the injury.

Clinical Pearl: Unjustified diagnoses must be replaced with clear, nonthreatening terms such as "simple strain."

Testing

Sophisticated testing procedures can at times reinforce severity of the illness to the injured worker. Clinicians should limit the use of expensive diagnostic tests unless it is strongly suspected that the results of such tests would significantly change the course of treatment. Health care practitioners must remember that many of the imaging "findings" will have nothing to do with the patient's current symptoms and are more likely the result of the natural aging process. A recent study of spinal MRIs in 98 asymptomatic subjects revealed that while 36% of the subjects had normal disks at all levels, 52% had at least one bulge involving at least one level, 27% had a protrusion, 1% an extrusion, and 38% had abnormalities involving more than one intervertebral disk. Not surprisingly, physical findings increased with the age of the subject. The conclusion is that many asymptomatic people have disk bulges or protrusions and the discovery of disk bulges or protrusions in people with back pain may often be merely coincidence.[48] In general, current image findings correlate poorly with back pain[49–52] and are performed more frequently on workers' compensation patients than on comparative group health patients.[53] In addition to the psychological impact of expensive testing and the results thereof, one must consider the impact on physical health. It is estimated that, depending on technique, a 5-view LS spine x-ray series exposes the patient to the same amount of gonadal radiation as nearly 200 chest x-rays. The impact on the health and well-being of the patient and his or her reproductive potential may be significant, especially in those undergoing multiple back x-rays, CT scans, and other radiological procedures. Because specific diagnoses are rare, and sophisticated testing procedures can have an adverse effect on the patient's illness behavior, adequate reassurance and education is often more effective in the long-term treatment of the compensated patient and is no more time-consuming.

Clinical Pearl: Overemphasizing the potential seriousness of a patient's symptoms can lead to the injured employee overreacting to his or her illness and subsequently negatively affecting recovery.

Psychosocial Sensitivity

Health-care providers and managers dealing with claimants should be sensitive to the psychosocial impact on the somatic components of the claim with their associated clinical impacts on the long-term outcome of the case. Clinicians must keep in mind the increasing volume of valid studies demonstrating the role of pain and illness behavior in certain patients. Behavioral signs of distress should not be immediately interpreted as physical disorders. The behavior component of a patient's condition can often be more important than the underlying presumed physical problem. The *Performance APGAR*, discussed later in this chapter, provides an effective tool for practitioners to use to help quantify patient motivation and sincerity of effort.[54] With this information, the practitioner can more readily quantify other subjective reports and findings of the examination.

Treatment

During World War II, the military used such exotic and complex-sounding treatments as "narcosynthesis" or "electroconvulsive therapy."[55] The use of these treatment modalities often strengthened the soldier's rationalization that he or she was significantly physically or mentally ill, or as Barsky suggests, "Attention to a symptom amplifies it, whereas distractions diminish it."[56]

Current treatments for musculoskeletal pain often fare no better than the exotic "cures" applied during World War II and, like those cures, today's medical care has the potential to prolong disability by reinforcing illness behavior. Recent studies have shown that some providers are using expensive, time-consuming treatment modalities, with little attention to the efficacy of the treatments used.[57,58] A recent review of workers' compensation cases in eight states for claims that had incurred over 7 days lost time for the same type injury found the cost could vary as much as 200%. As described previously, in third world countries, where expensive diagnostic and treatment modalities are not available, there is little evidence of back disability being a problem.[59–61] This inconsistency among providers for the same condition creates a high degree of unnecessary variability among providers, increased costs, controversy over billings, increasing administrative time and worker frustration, litigation, and subsequent payer costs.

Currently, those treating patients must remember that of all that is done in routine medical practice, only about 10%–20% has a basis in published scientific research.[62] This means that 80% of current treatment is subjective, based upon expert opinion or consensus, or simply not substantiated by current evidence. This partially explains the significant practice variations that exist for treatment of some conditions throughout the United States.[63–65] One needs to be cognizant of the fact that various studies use different end points as measures of success. Some studies measure the ability to return to gainful employment whereas others measure subjective pain relief. Outcomes, such as reporting those injured workers who are able to return to an occupational role, have been considered by some to be a "harsh" or "inappropriate" measure of success.[66] One study reported that 52% of injured workers undergoing spinal cord stimulation for pain obtained good to very good relief; however, less than 5% returned to any kind of work.[67]

Clinical Pearl: From the practical point of view, returning an injured/disabled worker back to productive employment should be the ultimate measure of successful worker rehabilitation.

Medication

Relief of pain and improvement in function is a major goal of workers presenting with low back pain. Several classes of medications (and combinations thereof) are commonly used, including nonsteroidal anti-inflammatory drugs (NSAIDs), acetaminophen, muscle relaxers, and narcotics analgesic. These medications provide temporary pain relief until the body's natural healing process is able to provide more longer-lasting relief.

It appears that the most effective medications for reducing mechanical low back pain are acetaminophen and NSAIDs, such as ibuprofen and aspirin, which are generally safe and relatively inexpensive.[68,69] NSAIDs have been demonstrated to be effective in treating low back pain. Specific choice of the nonsteroidal, however, is less likely to be important as there is no particular NSAID that has been demonstrated to be superior to the others. However, if one NSAID is not working, one may be considered from another class of NSAIDs before abandoning the class or adding on other medications. For the elderly chronic steroid users, or those with upper gastrointestinal (GI) symptoms, one may consider beginning with COX-2 inhibitors or Tylenol. NSAIDs are less clearly effective for neurogenic back pain. Acetaminophen may also be just as effective as NSAIDS. In the elderly, pregnant, renally impaired, or those with upper GI disease, it should be considered as first-line therapy. Newer, longer-acting preparations may make its use more practical.

Muscle relaxers, although also effective for the treatment of low back pain, should be used for more severe symptoms. They should be considered before narcotics for symptoms beyond NSAIDs and acetaminophen. Bensodiazepines, despite sometimes being used as a muscle relaxer, have been shown to be addictive in treating low back pain. Narcotics have been shown to provide pain relief, but with more risk of addition. In addition to reduced efficacy, narcotic medications have significant side effects including tolerance, addiction, depression and repression of endorphins.[71] When controlled substances are prescribed, it should be for a fixed time interval, before reevaluation.

Clinical Pearl: Caution must be taken with patients taking daily or high doses of NSAIDs. Studies have reported up to 31% of patients developing endoscopic confirmed gastric duodenal ulcers with chronic use.[70]

Treatment of neurogenic low back pain with oral steroids is somewhat controversial. There are no well-designed placebo controlled studies that demonstrate a clear benefit. Potential determents such as hyperglycemia, steroid psychosis, and avascular necrosis should limit their potential use to those with severe neurogenic acute back pain.

Injections and Other Invasive Techniques

A number of studies have looked at the use of injection procedures for the treatment of low back pain.[46,72,73] Infiltration of trigger points has not been shown to be particularly effective. Epidural injections of cortisone and local anesthetics have been the topic of a number of clinical studies, with variable results, and their use remains controversial.[74] Facet joint injections are also a common injection therapy. However, like trigger point injections, no significant studies are available which verify their effectiveness. Selective nerve root injections have, however, been proven effective in identifying the site of the origin of the pain. Radio frequency lesioning for the treatment of back pain has likewise shown limited success.[75]

Bed Rest

Overemphasis of pain and discomfort alone and over-prescription of rest may indeed be a major factor of iatrogenic disability. The rationale for bed rest is the observation that intradiscal pressure is lowest in the lying position and many patients actually feel better with bed rest. However, protracted bed rest leads to a catabolic state with general malaise, bone demineralization, and loss of muscle strength.[76,77] There is also evidence that rest and inactivity actually inhibit healing and lead to increased psychological distress and depression, loss of work habit, and progressive loss of job opportunity.[78] Feeling better in the short term and getting better in the long term can often be two entirely different outcomes. Return to normal activities (including work) should be the objective of all treatment and management efforts.

Treatment Guidelines

Over the past decade aggressive and coordinated attempts have been undertaken to facilitate improvement, reduce variation, and standardize care in the provider and payer systems. These have mostly been done through the development of comprehensive treatment guidelines. Unfortunately, these guidelines appear to have done little to modify treatment patterns and have come under severe criticism.[79] These guidelines have been developed by systematically reviewing the current available medical literature, and where there are deficiencies, experts have developed consensus on interpretation.[80] Most often, these reviews of the literature generally find the available evidence to be "sparse and of poor quality,"[81,82] necessitating the guidelines or recommendations to be published largely on the consensus of members of the given task force.[46] Naturally, the major criticism of guidelines is selection bias of the panel members based upon the criteria of what literature was reviewed. Therefore, the composition of the reviewing panel and the sponsoring organization often interjects bias that can influence the final guideline recommendations. Another criticism of guidelines is that they seem only to focus on utilization issues often without addressing the role of psychosocial distress. Therefore it is the authors' opinions that rather than providers argue from a bias selection of the literature to substantiate their treatment plan, the providers should be able to readily demonstrate their treatment's value by objectifying and quantifying improvement in their patient's function.

Physical Medicine Modalities

Currently there is a marked increase in the use of physical medicine for injured workers, now accounting for nearly 40% of the medical dollars billed in some states.[83] Yet, passive modalities, such as traction, electrical stimulation, ultrasound, thermal agents, acupuncture, and diathermy are controversial as to their value in healing tissues.[27,29,46,81,82] Although these modalities may provide some measure of temporary symptom relief, they are expensive with minimal evidence of long-term efficacy. Unfortunately, passive modalities can create dependency and can distract patients from more responsible and effective treatment.[85] An example of a passive modality illustrating this point is hot/cold packs. For over a decade, the medical literature is explicit that there is insufficient value to justify the cost of these modalities. Yet according to the 1996 report of the California Workers' Compensation Institute, 35 million dollars were spent on the passive modalities of electrical stimulation, hot or cold packs, massage, and ultrasound, with 15 million being spent on manipulation and 18 million being spent on active conditioning.[86] Likewise a recent review of physical medicine charges for a major insurer of group health care found that 62% of physical therapy and 82% chiropractic charges were for these same passive modalities, with the remaining percent of billing for active treatment.* This has provoked some to observe that, irrespective of what we know from the medical literature, as long as a procedure is reimbursed, that procedure will continue to be performed and billed.[87] This continues to be true for the use of other physical modalities including diathermy, massage, ultrasound, cutaneous laser treatment, massage and electrical stimulation. Although they may provide some measure of temporary symptom relief, the Agency of Health Care Research, almost a decade ago, stated that their "use is of insufficiently proven benefit to justify their cost."[85]

Ergonomics

Although originally promising, prospective studies utilizing ergonomics and education have failed to demonstrate significant reduction in claims.[88] Ergonomic interventions apparently reach a point of diminishing returns. The 50-year quest to eliminate offending biomechanical stresses from the workplace has not had any positive impact on back pain or back pain claims in the workplace.[89]

Conditioning

The key to musculoskeletal symptom control is balancing mechanical stress against the more debilitating effect of inactivity on the protective musculature. Aerobic exercise, physical conditioning, and psychosocial support appear to be very beneficial for the worker with a soft tissue injury.[90,91] Recovery is inevitably dependent on conditioning of the protective and supportive musculature to compensate for any structural deficit caused by the injury. If strength is sufficient, a patient may return to full function, not because the back is "cured," but because there is sufficient muscular compensation to tolerate the discomfort of activity.

Surgery

Since the first article describing surgical decompression for disc herniation causing sciatica appeared in 1934,[92] the number of spinal surgeries performed in the United States has increased exponentially.

* Authors data collection of 2002 billings of physical medicine services comparing trends of active to passive treatment.

According to the National Hospital Discharge Survey, spinal fusion rates increased 200% from 1979 to 1987.[93] This increase in surgery appears to parallel an increase in related disability.[94] Too often, surgery is performed on patients who encourage it, expecting it to be a cure. Some patients, consciously or subconsciously, desire surgery to validate their disability, or even to assuage guilt.[95,96] The natural history of a "herniated disc" is to stabilize itself. Failure to operate very seldom produces serious adverse effects, even in patients with discogenic paresis.[97,98] Long-term outcomes demonstrate that nonoperative treatment of a disc herniation is often as effective as surgical intervention and much more cost-effective.[99] In fact, Weber has demonstrated that surgery in the working age group is a "luxury for speeding recovery when there are very strong pre-operative indications."[100] Likewise, the outcomes for spinal fusion in compensated low back surgery patients appear less than optimal.

Comparative studies of surgery rates in the United States and the United Kingdom show the disparity between treatment patterns. With comparable prevalence of back injuries in the two countries, approximately 20% of those in the United States who see an orthopedic surgeon will have back surgery, whereas only 3% of those in the United Kingdom who see a surgeon will have back surgery.[27]

Clinical Pearl: A number of studies[101] have shown that between 30% and 60% of compensated patients show evidence of poor outcomes following lumbar fusion.

Outcomes and Common Goals of Providers, Payors, and Patients

While relieving pain is certainly desirable, pain is very subjective, its measurement is unreliable, and pain does not always correlate with function. In treating injured workers the primary focus of treatment for health care providers should not be reducing pain but improving function, with an emphasis on return to gainful employment. Achieving this goal requires a coordinated commitment that measures and records objective improvement. In the United States, The Labor Commission of the State of Utah has developed an instrument that performs this function. Called the "Restorative Services Agreement" (or RSA), the instrument requires a provider who bills for restorative services to benchmark and then demonstrate improvements in three objective areas. Those areas are (1) functional ability as it relates to the essential job functions, (2) hours the injured worker is able to work each day, and (3) the patient's own report of pain reduction with a pain scale. Regarding function, the provider is to obtain at least three measurable and objective essential physical job functions (i.e., lifting, carrying, range of motion, sitting, tolerance, etc.) necessary for the injured worker to return to work. The injured worker's capacity is then tested and benchmarked to these essential functions as part of the initial evaluation. Every sixth visit, the capacity is extrapolated from the job-specific conditioning, and authorization for continued treatment is granted depending on the patient's functional improvement. Increased function and reduced cost have validated the use of the RSA.[102]

Summary

Application of Simplicity in treating and managing a disability claimant allows an approach to recovery that parallels the natural history of the injury. Intervention is provided to improve function, and continued only as long as the worker is able to demonstrate objective improvement. As the patient receives more efficacious treatment, there is a concomitant reduction in disability, in patient impairment, and in costs for employers.

PROXIMITY

"Proximity" deals with the need to evolve a work family both by developing worker morale and, when a claim occurs, by keeping the injured individual as closely involved and associated with the workplace as possible.

Prior to 1917, the British army routinely removed "battle-stressed" casualties from its duty stations, sending them home to England. It was assumed that returning the soldier to a more comfortable, stable environment would relieve the "battle stress" symptoms. Unfortunately, the reverse was found to be true. Many of those who returned to England for "battle stress" became refractory to treatment. After World War II, one seventh of all military discharges were due to mental conditions. Of the 200,000 soldiers on England's pension list, one fifth had a permanent diagnosis of "war neurosis."

Later, in World War II, British and French physicians noted that soldiers with battle stress improved more rapidly when treated in permanent hospitals near the battlefront. The recovery rate was better still for those simply treated in casualty-clearing stations near the front line. The most successful recovery was found when encouragement, rest, persuasion, and suggestion (Simplicity) were given within the combat organization itself, close to battle lines (Proximity).

The Israeli Defense Forces (IDF) validated the concept of proximity during the 1973 Arab-Israeli War and the 1982 war with Lebanon. In the 1973 conflict, all psychiatric casualties were evacuated to the rear of the battlefront. None of these casualties were returned to combat duty during the war, and many became chronically disabled.[103]

Sobered by the incidence of these psychiatric casualties, and the failure of the Israeli medical system to successfully rehabilitate any of them, the Israeli military adopted the doctrine of Forward Treatment, i.e., brief treatment (physical replenishment—water, food, sleep, and the opportunity to recount battle experiences) near the front, with a rapid return to combat duty. To implement this new approach, the IDF deployed mental health specialists with each medical battalion, operating from 2 to 5 km from the front. With this system in place, 60% of combat reaction cases were returned to combat duty within 72 hours.[36,103]

The second element of Proximity is the concept of developing and maintaining soldier morale. The military found that in addition to battle intensity and battle stress, a variety of personal and unit factors influence whether an injured soldier performs well or becomes a psychiatric casualty. In 1973, IDF soldiers from units with good leadership, good unit cohesion, and who had stable personal and family lives were less likely to become psychiatric casualties[39] and more likely to perform well and to be decorated for heroism.[104,105] In 1982, good personal and unit morale also protected IDF soldiers from psychiatric breakdown.[36]

Often the unhappy and disappointing aspects of a worker's home life can be mitigated at work. Work creates status and builds self-esteem. Work defines identity, breeds self-reliance, provides personal security, and offers an opportunity for personal advancement. Through work we gain skills and develop personal efficacy.[106] Being away from work, especially as the result of a disability, encourages introspection and maladaptive behavior that can lead to increased illness behavior. Many workers, once injured, feel abandoned by their employers and coworkers. That feeling leads to erosion of the personal benefits of work. One major United States review of 8500 injured workers in six states who were losing work time found that only 48% of employers had taken the trouble to call them during their recovery time with only 33% of employers offering a return-to-work program.[107]

Clinical Pearl: All those involved with managing entitlement claims must remember that working is one of the most potent modalities in preventing iatrogenic disability.

Proximity for the industrial worker is not limited to simply maintaining geographical closeness. Proximity includes all elements identified as generally improving the physical, mental, and social work environment. Perceptive employers agree with W. Edward Demming that the individual worker is the company's most important asset and that respect for individuals is paramount for business success.[108] Today, employees are under unprecedented stress with marked increases in single parenting, divorce, teenage pregnancy, caring for grandchildren, and suicide. Consider the following demographic changes in the United States during the last 30 years:

- Illegitimate birth rates have increased by more than 400%.[109]
- The percentage of families headed by a single parent has more than tripled.[110]
- The divorce rate has more than doubled.[111] Many project that about half of all new marriages will end in divorce.
- Teenage suicide has increased by almost 300%.[112]
- Scholastic Aptitude Test scores among all students have dropped 73 points.[113]
- Every year, four million women are beaten by their partners.[114]
- One fourth of all adolescents contract a sexually transmitted disease before they graduate from high school.[111]

The challenge for employers is finding a means of developing a "work family" and assisting their employees in being able to come to work ready to give 100%, managing their life's stresses, and fulfilling their individual goals and purposes in life. Figure 34–1 represents a comprehensive overview of occupational services that an employer can implement to help select a healthy employee population, what they can do to keep them healthy, and programs to incorporate when an injury occurs to prevent delayed recovery from occurring. Indicators of the erosion of an individual's or employee's psychosocial reserves and an attendant potential for an injury claim can be indirectly measured by levels of tardiness, use of health insurance, quality of work, employee turnover, reduced productivity, accident and illness rates, property damage, grievances filed, and percentage of employees using employee assistance programs.

Human Resources

Personnel policies that are clear and evenly enforced can prevent undue employee frustration, and help to maintain a productive attitude among employees.[115,116] Occasionally employees will have an unrealistic idea about the financial benefits associated with being disabled. All employees should be educated about their rights as employees and what to expect, medically as well as financially, if a work-related accident occurs. A major review of injured workers found that one half of injured workers had received

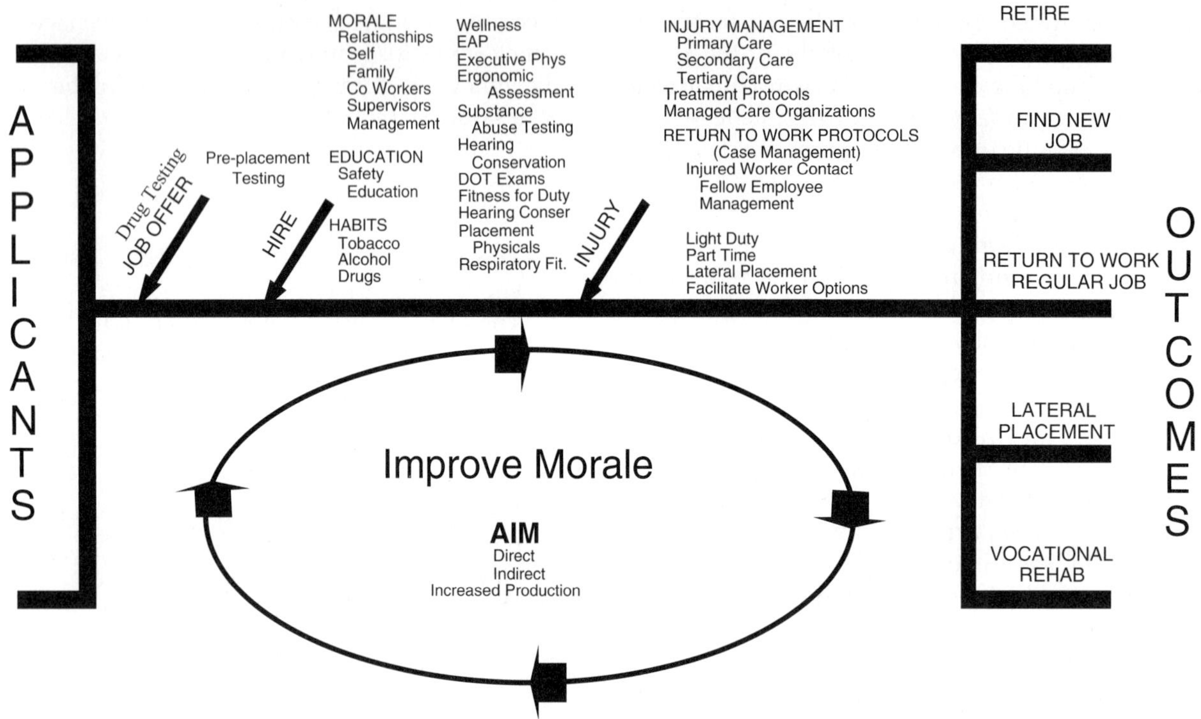

FIGURE 34–1. Comprehensive employer services.

no information from their employer regarding what procedure to follow to get appropriate treatment.[107]

Qualified human resources staff should also provide channels for communication and dispute resolution. The majority of compensation-related litigation is directly related to the frustration, ignorance, unrealistic expectations, and/or fear level of the injured workers.[117] Human resource policies that educate, accommodate return-to-work programs, and reduce anxiety in the worker also reduce litigation.[107,117]

In one study involving a Canadian geriatric hospital[118] it was found that 46% of nursing aids initiated low back industrial claims, with an 82% recurrence rate. The hospital, in an effort to control these workers' compensation losses, implemented a program of back school training, with individual education on injury prevention and careful follow-up of reported injuries. They found that there was essentially no change in the injury and recurrence rates among their employees.

However, when this same hospital began a *personnel policy* of immediate contact following an injury and regular 10-day follow-up contacts, coupled with evaluation of retraining and early return-to-work possibilities, they found they were three times more effective in reducing time loss and recurrence rates for low back injuries. In another study of 31,200 Boeing employees,[37] a strong correlation was found between the incidence of lost-time soft tissue injuries and a poor supervisor relationship. This was manifest through a poor appraisal rating performed within the 6 months preceding an injury. A similar recent major study has been completed with urban transit operators.[119] These studies demonstrate that an employer's policies can often be more successful in returning employees to work in a timely manner and in reducing the number of claims, than clinicians can be by treating injuries.

Clinical Pearl: The lesson to be learned here is that making employees feel that they are valued in the workplace can have a significant impact on the employer's bottom line.

Safety

A major review of injured workers in the United States found that only 44% had received special training or information on how to prevent injuries.[107] Companies utilizing safety teams, videotaped safety meetings, incentives for worker participation, safety audits, safety management review of all accidents, placement of safety coordinators, and fatigue prevention programs have demonstrated a 30%–90% reduction in claims.[120] Management commitment to safety should focus on identifying and reducing hazards, not injuries.

Drug Testing Program

In 1990 the United States Navy found that 41% of sailors under the age of 25 tested positive for some drug use. Now with 10 years of random drug testing the current rate has been cut to 2%.[121] Of 4375 US Postal Service employees, nationwide, that underwent pre-employment drug tests, 8.4% tested positive.[122,123] The group testing positive had 41% higher absenteeism, 1.5 times more involuntary turnover, and 1.7 times greater likelihood of quitting than the group that had negative drug tests. A major study of 1500 of the state of Louisiana's largest workers' compensation policyholders performed a 1-year study of implementing preemployment, postincident, and random drug screening and demonstrated 50% reduction in workplace accidents with a cost savings of 22%.[124]

Unions

Many employers have found that rather than fight a union's involvement in their workplace, they can benefit from involving union officials in the development of safety and disability prevention programs. Unions should assist with lateral placement for injured employees, and establishment and enforcement of light-duty or alternative duty programs, as mandated under the Americans with Disability Act.[125] Such participation by Union representatives gives ownership and support that will help ensure the program's success.

Wellness

The general health of an individual worker contributes to any incident that may occur, as well as contributing to the worker's response to that incident. A US study of 1652 firefighters tested several areas of general fitness including endurance, isometric strength, spine flexibility, blood pressure, and postexercise heart rate. Participants were divided into three groups, highest fitness, middle fitness, and lowest fitness, based on the results of the testing. The subsequent workers' compensation back injuries and costs for these firefighters were then analyzed in relation to their prior fitness results. The frequency of subsequent injury for the lowest fitness firefighters was 10 times higher than that of the highest fitness group. The cost per claim for the lowest fitness group was 13% higher than for the middle fitness group. The highest fitness group had too few claims to make an accurate estimation of future costs per claim.[126]

Employers can contribute to a higher level of health and wellness by providing a work-site culture, which encourages healthy lifestyles. Travelers Insurance, with 36,000 employees, introduced the Taking Care Program in 1986. Based on 4 years of experience, Travelers now reports an estimated return of approximately $3.40 for every dollar invested in health promotion.[127]

Clinical Pearl: Successful employee wellness programs include convenience, supportive corporate culture, management support, and employee involvement in decision making, clear goals, and comprehensive, long-range planning.

Injury Response

When injuries do occur, the safety program should enforce the management's concern for the injured worker and the impact of the injury on other workers. Work-site injuries should be investigated, but not in an atmosphere of distrust. Investigations should focus on clarification of how the injury occurred, both to assist the injured worker and to take steps to prevent similar accidents from occurring in the future. This does not reduce the need to monitor all disability claims for potential fraud. However, an immediate positive response, while investigating facts of the claim, greatly increases trust and confidence in the system. With that trust established fraud is more readily identified since the desire to "get back at the company" is greatly reduced.

Return to Work

Resumption of work has also been shown to be a significant part of the treatment for an injury or illness, even benefiting patients suffering from chronic pain.[128] Studies have shown that workers who return to their original employer are usually better off financially than workers who choose other options, such as alternative vocational rehabilitation plans that include retraining or new job placement.[129,130] Conversely, prolonged time away from work makes recovery and eventually returning to work progressively less likely. The longer an injured worker is kept away from the work site, the less likely it becomes that he or she will ever return to productive employment.[131,132] A recent Canadian study revealed that promptly offering modified duty reduced lost time by 30%–50%.[133] Unfortunately, clinicians, management, and labor all too often encourage disability by prolonging the injured worker's separation from the workplace. This is particularly true when the employer requires "100% recovery" prior to any work release. A "100% recovery" policy may prove more costly to the employer than any modified duty expense. Effective accomplishment of returning impaired individuals to work requires the combined efforts, of the individual, health-care provider, and employer, to carefully evaluate the patient's ability and then, if necessary, consider efforts to provide reasonable accommodations.

Utilizing the concepts of Proximity in the treatment of disability and occupational injury claims can significantly affect a company's profitability and employee morale, along with creating a very real reduction in human suffering.

IMMEDIACY

The need for immediate treatment was one of the first principles identified in dealing with soldiers suffering from "battle fatigue." Often, when there was a large influx of casualties, soldiers suffering from "war neurosis" were not treated immediately. Instead, attention was focused on more life-threatening injuries. Left to their own devices, these same soldiers were found to be more refractory to treatment when it was eventually offered, and more likely to need further rearward evacuation. The soldier's time away weakened his bonds with the unit and allowed him to solidify and rationalize the severity of his symptoms. In other words, a soldier near to his unit in space (proximity) and time (immediacy) can generally expect to return to it. This expectation decreases with distance, in space and/or time.

A vivid illustration of the effectiveness of applying "Immediacy" was recounted in a Wall Street Journal article describing the aftermath of a 1985 airline crash at the Dallas/Fort Worth (United States) airport. On August 2, 1985, wind shear slammed a Delta L-1011 to the ground, short of the runway. The accident severely injured many, and killed 137 people. In the immediate aftermath of the accident Delta Airlines' management sought for ways to comfort the bereaved. Within hours of the crash, the airline had dispatched employees to be with the family of every casualty. These Delta representatives provided clothing, financial aid, assistance in locating lost articles, and in general made themselves available to provide whatever was necessary at this most critical period in these families' lives.

As a result of the bonds created by this early intervention, many crash victims and their families found it difficult to sue Delta, whom they had come to see as a friend instead of an adversary. Of a possible 152 passenger claims in the crash, only 65 suits were filed, and about 50 of these suits have been settled, most without litigation. This is impressive when compared with the 1982 US Pan Am crash in New Orleans, Louisiana. In this incident Pan Am did not employ "early bonding" tactics and at least three fourths of the 146 passenger deaths resulted in litigation.[134]

Critical Time Periods

If, however, the absence from work is prolonged, permanent disability may be reinforced, and the chance to return to that job diminishes significantly.[131,132]

Clinical Pearl: Many clinical studies have validated the concept that timely treatment and return to work facilitates return to productivity.

Within these studies of return-to-work parameters, several critical time periods have been identified.[135] All musculoskeletal soft tissue injuries should show some objective improvement within 2 weeks regardless of the treatment imposed. Delay of expected time periods alerts the management team to potential recovery delays, triggering movement to a more aggressive treatment mode.[29] If pain persists beyond 3 months, treatment should expand to concentrate on psychosocial factors associated with pain that might be complicating the clinical problem.

CENTRALITY

"Centrality" refers to the military's practice of making certain that all combat medical decisions, treatments, and evacuations are funneled through a central screening process. This ensures that only skilled personnel, trained in the Forward Treatment philosophy, are in contact with the soldiers at this critical period. This aspect of Centrality prevents the anxious soldiers from being exposed to confusing terminology, diagnostics, and treatments, thereby reducing iatrogenic disorders.

Too often in today's health-care system a patient encounters a confusing maze of conflicting diagnosis and treatments. Specialists will sometimes recommend tests that have already been performed and often it is perceived that no one is directing care. With no one to take full responsibility for the direction of treatment, other members of the management team (the patient and employer) are often confused as to what to expect and when to expect it.

To prevent this from occurring, health-care providers must become more professionally coordinated, using the concepts of immediacy and expectancy in approaching the full spectrum of the patient's biological, psychological, and social needs. Often, at this point, like the soldier left to his own devices or subjected to inappropriate and poorly coordinated care, the will or ability to work has been lost, disability is well established, and irretrievable harm has come to the patient and his or her family. To prevent such adverse outcomes the concept of centrality is embodied in the case manager. Many workers' compensation insurance carriers as well as provider networks employ case mangers to act as a central point of contact for the clinician, employer, and injured worker. Studies have shown the effectiveness of case manager involvement in workers' compensation cases. Efforts, such as case management, that improve centrality will

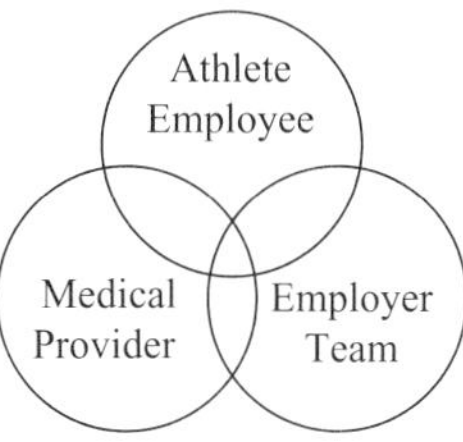

FIGURE 34–2. Athletic and employer model.

help minimize adverse outcomes and improve return-to-work potential.

The Athletic Model

The team concept is not unique to the military. Athletic teams consistently rely on the collective energy and abilities of each member to attain success. It is well recognized that athletes recover from injuries very quickly. This efficient recovery is the result of a treatment model wherein common recovery goals are shared by a "team," including the clinician, the coach, team members, and the injured athlete. The result of this "team" approach is that an athlete, highly motivated and well supported, is able to return quickly to full function. If any supportive team element is missing or if all does not share the same goal, return to activity can be delayed (see Fig. 34–2).

Team Approach. This model approaches treatment by sharing accountability equally among all involved entities with a return to productivity as the common goal (see *Expectancy*). Just as with the injured athlete, the entitled (compensated) worker needs a structured, comprehensive approach to recovery. When the athletic model is applied, the worker becomes the "athlete" and the employer takes the role of "coach" and fellow workers the "team." The success of this model is dependent on three components: (1) motivation and physical capability of the injured worker (the "athlete"), (2) appropriate treatment, (3) the desire of the employer (the "coach") and coworkers (the "fellow athletes") to have the injured worker return to work, manifested by the employer's willingness to support and accommodate the worker. Together, these components provide a structured and comprehensive approach to optimize recovery outcomes for the compensated worker. These include increased employee/employer communication, reduction in lost time and associated indirect costs, disability management, avoidance of litigation, and the reduction of unnecessary medical costs. This approach ensures that all the patient's issues, including sociological and psychological concerns, are addressed and obstacles to recovery are removed. Injured or disabled employees usually seek legal assistance because of misinterpretation and miscommunication. A multidisciplinary, centralized team approach could potentially avert such cases by resolving communication issues before they require litigation.[139]

Employee Motivation

Most compensated injuries are minor and heal uneventfully with little or no disability. However, in some injured workers, recovery can take longer than can be explained by physical symptoms alone, indicating the presence of nonbiological issues that serve to prolong the disability. A review of the available literature demonstrates that compensation benefits alone can significantly affect motivation toward recovery.[137,138]

The principal difference in recovery rates between compensated and noncompensated patients appears to lie in motivation—motivation of the injured employee, the employer, the insurance carrier, government, and providers. All parties involved in the recovery of a compensated patient are required to recognize the unique set of expectations, critical periods, and specific needs that must be met to attain return-to-work status.

Current research has shown conclusively that in cases of delayed recovery, nonphysical factors are often present directly impacting the injured employee's motivation.[139–141] There might be a single factor or a combination of factors present, i.e., social, emotional, neurotic, economic, and even sometimes-vindictive motives. Beneath this lies the original physical complaint that maintains the disability compensation payment.

Epidemiological studies reveal distinct characteristics in the occupational and psychological profiles of people disabled by soft tissue injuries, particularly low back pain.[142,143] For example, job dissatisfaction, monotony, and stress are common characteristics. Persons facing these problems are more likely to suffer from depression, anxiety, hypochondriasis, and hysteria.

These nonbiological factors have an even greater impact on motivation when the entitled patient retains an attorney and becomes a legal claimant.[136,139] Once this happens the patient is obligated to prove and preserve injury or illness. To improve physically jeopardizes the ability to prevail in a suit. Additionally, the worker's own credibility is placed at risk. Hence, the disability continues throughout the litigation process, even in the absence of any objective clinical basis for the disability. Because legal counsel is usually sought only after a patient feels abandoned or "wronged" by the employer, personnel policies that prevent such adversarial relationships can have a significant financial impact on the company, as they may prevent costly litigation. Simple personnel policies can provide positive reinforcement for an injured worker, and also allow the employer to maintain control of an industrial claim.

Measuring Employee Motivation and Sincerity of Effort: The Performance APGAR

Making an objective determination of the amount of effort an individual expends to recover from injury or illness is an essential component in making stability and capability statements. Individuals whose effort and motivation are less than optimal may overuse treatment, have increased medical costs, more disability payments, and a prolonged recovery.

Clinical Pearl: The Performance APGAR (*A*cceptance, *P*ain, *G*ut, *A*cting, and *R*eimbursement) is a new standardized reporting methodology, which is a comprehensive summary of current methods used to measure the amount of personal commitment and effort the injured worker is currently expending or has expended to improve their condition.

In order to simplify and justify assessments of motivation, effort, and credibility, the authors have developed the *Performance APGAR*. Originally developed by Virginia Apgar in 1951, to measure a newborn's health, others in the literature have built on this model as a basis for other types of measures.[144–147] Most APGAR models are rated on a scale of 0–10, with 10 representing normal. As with others, this Performance APGAR score is scaled from 0 to 10 and can be used to quantify effort at the initial visit, as a summary of progress at subsequent visits, or on the final determination of capability.

Motivation and effort can conceivably be plotted along a continuum with the physiologic bone ligament complex responses to loading conditions[148,149] and with psychosocial factors determining how one performs in relationship to these physiological limits. Elite athletes perform much closer to their physiological limits than most persons.

Currently, a number of procedures are promoted for a clinician to objectively assess motivation, including Waddell's nonorganic signs,[150] dynometric grip strength variation,[151] bell-shaped force curves,[152] Rey 15-Item Test for Malingering,[153] and rapid exchange grip.[154] Other evaluations include the correlation between musculoskeletal evaluation and functional capacity evaluation,[155] documentation of pain behaviors and symptom magnification,[156,157] and the ratio of heart rate to pain intensity.[158] The Social Security Administration uses an assessment of the credibility of allegations in their overall disability evaluation process. Table 34–1 provides an example of a tabular assessment of credibility for use within the Performance APGAR.

Like the infant APGAR, which is given at birth, the Performance APGAR is a composite summary of methods used to determine patient motivation level and is rated on a scale of 1–10. A score of 7–10 is consistent with what is optimally expected from a motivated patient, a score of 4–6 indicates concern about motivation, and a score of 0–3 suggests poor patient motivation to improve their functional abilities. The Performance APGAR scores can be used for many different types of impairments. These scores can be given at each visit or over a series of visits and provide the reader with an indication of the motivation a patient is currently expending to improve their condition.

A work sheet for the comprehensive Performance APGAR score is shown in Table 34–2 along with descriptors for each variable. Each of the five categories of the APGAR can be given a value of up to 2, making the maximum composite score of 10, consistent with acceptable motivation and effort. The five components of the APGAR are described. Each section of the APGAR has multiple possible measures that can be scored. When scoring, the single best method under each letter is chosen which is most appropriate for a particular patient. Alternatively, if there are several items under a specific letter (A, P, G, A, or R) that have been tested, these may be averaged to estimate a mean score for that letter. The Performance APGAR provides an easy mnemonic by which to remember a method to quantify patient motivation, credibility, and effort.[159]

Treating the Total Patient—The Health-Care Provider

Such clinicians must be sensitive not only to the biological pathology, but also to psychosocial issues, which may limit motivation for return to work. In sports medicine, the provider must have an understanding of the game, and knowledge of how the team interacts. The same principles apply in the occupational medicine arena.

Clinical Pearl: Clinicians whose treatment regimens have demonstrated the ability to effectively return the employee to work should treat injured workers.

Clinicians who treat the injured worker should be comfortable with the type of work required for an injured worker to perform his or her job and determine the capability of the patient. Health care providers providing regular care to certain employers or plants should tour the facilities and review the job descriptions to become familiar with the jobs performed by their patients. These ability decisions carry

TABLE 34–1. **APGAR Creditability Assessment**

	Not Consistent with the Objective Evidence and/or Expected Outcome/Severity (0 Points)	Partially Consistent with the Objective Evidence and/or Expected Outcome/Severity (1 Point)	Fully Consistent with the Objective Evidence and/or Expected Outcome/Severity (2 Points)
Impact of symptoms or condition on ADLs			
Type, dosage, effectiveness, and side effects of medications			
Treatment sought and received			
Opinions about function given by other treating and examining sources in the file			
Inconsistencies or conflicts in the allegations, statements, or medical evidence in the file			
		Total credibility score = ___ (0–10)	
Credibility determination: Total credibility score of 0–3 = Not credible Total credibility score of 4–7 = Partially credible Total credibility score of 8–10 = Fully credible			Result of credibility determination to be used in the APGAR table

Note: Each of the five areas should be scored 0, 1 or 2 points. The five area scores are then totaled for an overall credibility score of *x*/10. This score is then used in the credibility section of table 1 (not, partially, or fully credible).

heavy legal and ethical responsibilities as fitness for duty decisions are often directly related to the individual's earning capacity and/or disability benefits. The clinician should also be well informed on workplace parameters such as the availability of modified duty.

Employer's Responsibility

Applying the concept of centrality, employers have two main responsibilities: (1) to prevent injuries from occurring and (2) creating a favorable return-to-work environment for the injured employee. To accomplish this the employer must understand and support the concept that timely work integration is critical to the rehabilitation of the injured employee.

Clinical Pearl: Clinicians should very seldom remove the injured employees from work. They should make clinical determinations of physical capability, with the administrative decisions of accommodations being left to the employer.[125]

Employers should evaluate work restrictions given by the clinician and make an administrative decision, in consultation with the provider, about when and in what capacity the injured worker may return to the work site, whether in the same job or a modified position. Employers must be willing to accommodate early return to work during the rehabilitation phase, prior to the worker's full recovery.

Limited Residual Physical Capacity

Many essential job functions require a significant amount of physical capability to perform. All individuals are at points in their lives, irrespective of motivation, health care, or employment concerns, where they may not be able to physically do what they would like. Just as injured athletes all reach a time where a change in careers is inevitable, so workers doing significant physical work will need to have serious discussion regarding accommodation of the labor-intensive essential functions of their work. Employers would do well to identify those jobs in which it is unlikely that anyone could continue till retirement and develop plans for engineering changes that will accommodate physical limits or, if necessary, shifting aging workers to less physically demanding work.

TABLE 34–2. **Work Sheet for the Performance APGAR**

			Scoring Options			Score up to 2 points
			0	1	2	
A	Acceptance (choose best test or average)	If this just does not get any better, what will you do?	I can't live like this	I am going to have some problems	I will live with it	A =___
		Are you satisfied with your job?	Not satisfied	Partially satisfied	Satisfied	
P	Pain (choose best test or average)	Pain drawing	Nonphysiologic	Some of it physiologic	Physiologic	P =___
		Pain behaviors score (AMA Guides Table 18-5)	Exaggerated or nonphysiologic	Mixed or ambiguous	Appropriate and confirm clinical findings	
G	Gut (intuition) (choose best test or average)	Credibility tool (see Table 2)	Not credible	Partially credible	Credible	G =___
		Intuition of effort	Poor effort	Partial effort	Excellent effort	
		Duration	Much longer than expected	Longer than expected	As expected	
A	Acting (choose best test or average)	Consistency with distractions	Poor consistency	Partial consistency	Excellent consistency	A =___
		Waddell signs	More than 2 Waddell signs	2 Waddell signs	0 to 1 Waddell sign	
		Grip strength testing	Unreliable grip strength (high variance, etc.)	Partial validity	Reliable grip strength	
R	Reimbursement	Compensation/ litigation	Someone else liable WC, PI, disability application Attorney representing	Someone else liable WC, PI, disability application	No one liable	R =___

Total Performance APGAR Score = ___
(Add A, P, G, A, R sections for a maximum of 10)

EXPECTANCY

"Expectancy," the final component of the SPICE model, reflects the fact that injured workers often fulfill the clinical and labeling expectations placed on them.

Again, the military system provides a startling illustration of the role Expectancy plays in the recovery of compensated individuals.

To fully understand why Expectancy plays such a vital role in human performance, it is necessary to recognize that belief or expectation can significantly affect the clinical outcomes.[160] Some authors suggest that the patient's expectations may influence outcomes more strongly than any clinical therapy.[161] Often referred to as the nonspecific effect of healing, or placebo, these effects have been reported to be strongest when the patient is anxious, the health care provider is perceived as having great expertise, the patient and clinician believe the treatment is powerful, and the treatment is considered both impressive and expensive. The clinician's friendliness, warmth, interest, sympathy, prestige, empathy, positive attitude toward the patient, and positive attitude toward the treatment have all been found to significantly influence positively the outcomes.[162,163] All health-care providers should understand the significant role played by the placebo effect in the healing of their patients.

A review of treatments for angina pectoris, originally believed efficacious but later found to be ineffective or no better than placebo, have demonstrated 63%–100% objective improvements,[164,165] far better than the usual 30% usually explained by placebo. Other studies have reproduced these findings.[166] A review of 2504 discectomies for lumbar disk disease that report negative surgical exploration found that 37% of the patients reported complete relief from sciatica and 43% complete relief from back pain,[167] results similar to those reporting improvement with surgery.

Goals

The setting of a personal goal higher than would be assigned by another can lead to increased success. Because there is little difference in effectiveness between assigned goals and self-set goals,[168,169] the clinician is able to exert a healthy influence on patients' goals and expectations without prejudicing the clinical outcome.

Cathlove and Cohen used a "Directive Return to Work" approach in a multimodality rehabilitation program for workers' compensation patients.[170] Patients were divided into two groups, one directed in return to work, the other left to routine treatment, with no specific return-to-work goals identified. In the directed group, patients were informed at program entry that they would need to resume work within 1–2 months. This return-to-work understanding was part of the initial "treatment contract." The staff continually reinforced this concept by actively initiating return-to-work discussions and by guiding patients in setting work goals commensurate with their abilities. Sixty percent of patients in the directed group became gainfully employed. This is striking when compared to the nondirected group, where only 25% returned to gainful employment. Nine months later, 90% of the directed patients who had resumed work were still working. In contrast, only 75% of the nondirected group who had returned to work remained employed.

The Clinician's Role in Treatment and Patient Expectation

Often patients unrealistically expect to be made completely well from a disorder or illness that will likely leave the patient with residual symptoms. The lay press, family members, and other care providers often facilitate such unrealistic expectations. Left with symptoms, frustration with the conventional health care, and with encouragement from peers and family, many desperate workers have resorted to aggressive surgeries or alternative health-care therapies.[171] As with anyone being left with a personal loss, these workers will go through the five stages of grief outlined by Kubler Ross: denial, anger, bargaining, depression, and then finally acceptance[172] (see Fig. 34–3). Comprehensive programs have demonstrated that those patients who receive encouragement to engage in normal activities return to work sooner than those who receive more conventional treatment.[163]

Clinical Pearl: The practitioner's goal must be to provide the worker with realistic expectations of a disorder. This includes reviewing with the patient the risk and benefits of intervention as it compares to the natural history of the disorder and facilitating acceptance and independence.

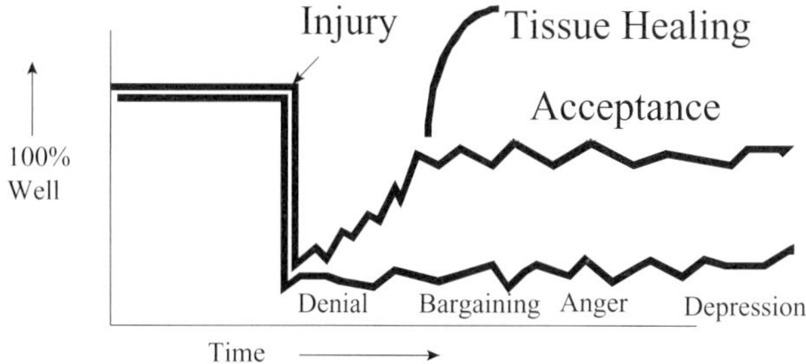

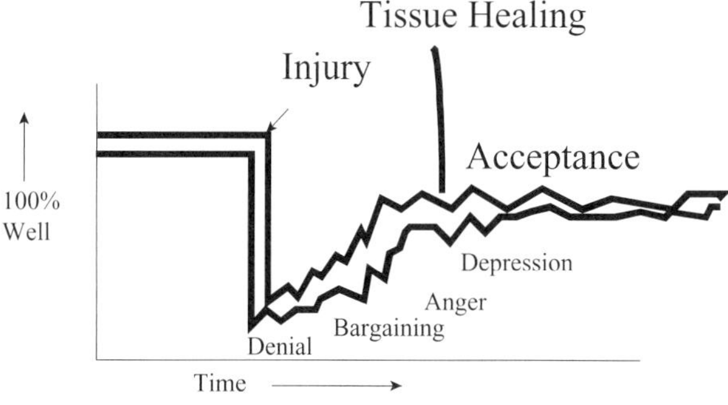

FIGURE 34–3. Recovery curves: Psychological acceptance over time should parallel tissue healing.

Expected Administrative Issues Needing to be Completed with Occupational Back Pain

Reporting Information on Injured Workers The unique needs of those responsible for injured workers require that practitioner reports are complete, objective, and defensible. The attending clinician is the person most knowledgeable regarding the condition, progress, and final status of the injured employee. Therefore, it is imperative that this provider renders the final disposition on the care of the worker.

The Clinician's Report at Stability Administrative rules and regulations for occupational health care vary between countries and, indeed, between regions within those countries. This is especially true in the United States, where workers' compensation systems can be quite disparate. The following generic overview of the reporting strategy and process is provided here as a model for the reader to understand the process. Specific reporting rules and regulations must be learned on an individual basis.

The clinical report at stability is a comprehensive report prepared after the injured worker is medically stable, sometimes referred to as maximum medical improvement (MMI), or fixed state of recovery. Other common terms include maximum therapeutic benefit (MTB) and permanent and stationary (P and S). As this is an administrative document, the final disposition of the examiner should include the following information:

1. *Diagnosis*: The examiner needs to clearly state the diagnosis as substantiated from the medical record. The examiner should also define, as clearly as possible, the relationship of the diagnosis to the industrial event. It is recognized that, in many cases, specific pathological diagnoses are not clearly evident. The examiner has the responsibility to provide a diagnostic impression that is as closely correlated to the clinical findings as possible.
2. *Stability*: Medical stability, MMI, or fixed state of recovery, refers to a date on which the period of healing has ended and the condition of the worker is not expected to materially improve or deteriorate by more than 3% Whole Person in the ensuing year.[173,174] It is important to note that medical stability may not be used to terminate necessary medical care. The date of medical stability and the date on which the worker qualifies for an impairment rating can be two separate dates.
3. *Calculation of Impairment*: Using appropriate rating criteria for the jurisdiction within which he or she works, the examiner should calculate the residual impairment, based on clinical findings established during the medical examination and information found in the medical records. Those states that use the *American Medical Association* (AMA) Guides to the evaluation of permanent impairment (Guides) must try to be consistent with their rating methodology and be careful to prevent controversy and unnecessary litigation. Unfortunately this lack of consistency inherent within the guides is a concern and has provoked calls for serious revisions to address this issue.[175,176] A number of studies have demonstrated poor reliability of the AMA Guides' spinal range of motion model to estimate impairment in patients with chronic low back pain.[177,178] As a solution to this troublesome area, some states have adopted their own methodology to calculate impairment ratings and likewise demonstrated their reliability.[184,185]

   Clinical Pearl: Further studies have shown that spinal range of motion is unreliable and dependent on the age and sex of the patient,[179,180] osteoarthritis,[181] and the time of the day the measurements were taken,[182] and have no relationship to disability.[183]

4. *Apportionment*: The examiner must identify and list any factors, occupational and nonoccupational, which add to, or are a part of, the impairment, but are not directly resultant from the injury.
5. *Capabilities Assessment*: If requested, the clinician should make a statement as to the current functional capacity of the patient. It is his or her responsibility to determine whether the impairment results in functional limitations and to inform the employer about an individual's ability and limitations. It is the employer's responsibility to identify and determine whether reasonable accommodations are possible to enable the individual's performance of the essential job activities.[186] Not only does this clearly establish physical abilities, but also facilitates the patient/employer relationship for return to work. The Workplace Functional Ability Medical Guidelines,[187,188] is an excellent, comprehensive system review and report form. Functional ability evaluations should be performed or requested only if the carrier or self-insured employer makes a specific request for this service.
6. *Future Medical Treatment*: If requested, the examiner should be specific in identifying what treatment may be required in the future as a direct result of the industrial accident.
7. *Utah Performance APGAR*: Because impairment ratings outcomes are often contingent upon the effort an individual has made to improve his or condition, it is recommended that each impairment rating should include a Performance APGAR score as described above.[189,190]

CONCLUSION

Comprehensive problem-solving solutions are now mandatory to prevent the creation of costly disability. Health-care providers, disability managers, and business managers must coordinate the redirection of treatment to the whole person, recognizing all the factors that influence successful return to work. Claude Bernard once wrote, "The greatest error in the advancement of medical science has been the search for a single cause for a single disease."[191] Or, as Aristotle (384–322 BC) said, "Treatment of the part should never be attempted without treatment of the whole. That is the error of our day, separation of the body from the soul."

SUMMARY

1. The SPICE model, as outlined above, combined with the Performance APGAR and the other methods proposed in this chapter, provides the much-needed structure for a comprehensive problem-solving strategy.
2. The authors feel this strategy will help in preventing work-related claims.

3. When work-related claims do occur this strategy provides for management in an efficient, fair, and timely manner, thereby preventing iatrogenic disability.

REFERENCES

1. *J Am Insur* 2nd Quarter, 1986.
2. US Chamber of Commerce. 1997 Analysis of Workers' Compensation Laws, 1997.
3. *The guides to the evaluation of permanent impairment*, 5th ed. Chicago: American Medical Association, 2000:2.
4. Swezey, CL. Workers' compensation law. In: Ladou J, ed. *Occupational medicine*. East Norwalk, CT: Appleton & Lange, 1990:17.
5. Hunter SJ, Shaha S, Flint DF, et al. Predicting return to work, A long-term follow-up study of railroad workers after low back injuries. *Spine* 1998;23(21):2319–2328.
6. Rainville J, Sobel JB, Hartigan C, Wright A. The effect of compensation involvement on the reporting of pain and disability by patients referred for rehabilitation of chronic low back pain. *Spine* September 1, 1997;22(17):2016–2024.
7. Guest GH, Drummond PD. Effect of compensation on emotional state and disability in chronic back pain. *Pain* 1992;48:125–130.
8. Milhous RL, Haugh LD, Frymoyer JW, et al. Determinants of vocational disability in patients with low back pain. *Arch Phys Med Rehabil* 1989;70:589–593.
9. Fredrickson BE, Trief PM, Van Beveren P, Yuan HA, Baum G. Rehabilitation of the patients with chronic back pain: A search for outcome predictors. *Spine* 1988;3:351–353.
10. Guck TP, Meilman PW, Skultery FK, Dowd ET. Prediction of long-term outcome of multidisciplinary pain treatment. *Arch Phys Med Rehabil* 1986;7:233–236.
11. Leigh JP, Markowitz SB, Fahs M, Shin C, Landrigan P. Occupational injury and illness in the United States. *Arch Intern Med* July 28, 1997;157(14):1557–1568.
12. National Safety Council. *Accident facts*, 1998 edition. Itasca, IL: National Safety Council, 1998.
13. Hashemi L. Length of disability and cost of workers' compensation low back pain claims. *JOEM* October 1997;39(10):937–945.
14. Hashemi L, Webster BS, Clancy EA, Courtney TK. Length of disability and cost of work-related musculoskeletal disorders of the upper extremity. *J Occup Environ Med* March 1998;40(3):261–269.
15. State of Washington, Department of Labor and Industries. *Attending doctor's handbook.* Olympia, WA: Washington State Department of Labor and Industries, 1996:4.
16. US Dept of Labor Statistics, April 22, 1999. http://www.bls.gov/oes/oes_con.htm.
17. Atroshi I, Gummesson C, Johnsson R, Ornstein E, Ranstam J, Rosen I. Prevalence of carpal tunnel syndrome in a general population. *JAMA* July 14, 1999;282(2):153–158.
18. Andersson GB. The epidemiology of spinal disorders. In: Frymoyer JW, ed. The adult spine: Principles and practice. New York: Raven Press, Ltd., 1991:107–146.
19. Vällfors B. Acute, subacute and chronic low back pain: Clinical symptoms, absenteeism and working environment. *Scand J Rehabil Med Suppl* 1985;11:1–98.
20. Sternbach RA. Survey of pain in the United States: The Nuprin pain report. *Clin J Pain* 1986;2(1): 49–53.
21. *Back injuries: Costs, causes, cases and prevention*. Washington, DC: Bureau of National Affairs, 1988:80.
22. National Safety Council. *Accident facts.* Chicago: National Safety Council, 1990:38.
23. Webster B, Snook S. The cost of compensable low back pain. *J Occup Med* 1990;32:13–15.
24. Lemrow N, Adams D, Coffey R, et al. The 50 most frequent diagnosis-related groups (DRGs), diagnosis, and procedures: Statistics by hospital size and locations. In: *Hospital studies program research note 13.* Rockville, MD: Agency for Health Care Policy and Research, Public Health Services, September 1990. DHHS Publication No. (PHS) 90-3465.
25. Bigos S, Bowyer O, Braen G, et al. Acute low back problems in adults. In: *Clinical practice guideline*, Quick reference guide number 14. Rockville, MD: US Department of Health and Human Services, Public Health Service, Agency for Health Care Policy and Research, December 1994. AHCPR Publication No. 95-0643.
26. Cassidy JD, Carroll LJ, Cote P. The Saskatchewan Health and Back Pain Survey. The prevalence of low back pain and related disability in saskatchewan adults.
27. Waddell G. Low back pain: A twentieth century health care enigma. *Spine* 1996;21:2820–2825.
28. *Darthmouth Atlas of musculoskeletal health care.* American Hospital Association Press, 2000. http://www.dartmouthatlas.org/.
29. *Acute low back problems in adults: Assessment and treatment*. AGHCPR Guidelines No. 14. Rockville, MD: AGHCPR, December 1994.
30. Tacci JA, Webster BS, Hashemi L, Christiani DC. Clinical practices in the management of new onset, uncomplicated, low back workers' compensation disability claims. *J Occ Environ Med* 1999;41(5):397–404.
31. LaRocca H. Scientific approach to the assessment and management of activity-related spinal disorders [Editorial]. *Spine* 1987;12(7S):S8 (European edition).
32. Colledge AL, Johnson HI. SPICE—A model for the prevention iatrogenic low back pain within the current workers compensation system. *J Occup Rehabil* September 1993;3(3):172–178.
33. Colledge AL, Johnson HI. SPICE—A model for reducing the incidence and costs of occupationally entitled claims. *Occup Med: State Art Rev* October–December 2000;15(4):723–739.
34. Belenky GL. Psychiatric casualties: The Israeli experience. *Psychiatr Ann* August 1987;17(8):528.
35. Belenky GL. Psychiatric casualties: The Israeli experience. *Psychiatr Ann* August 1987;17(8):530.

36. Belenky GL, Noy S, Solomon Z. Battle stress: The Israeli experience. *Mil Rev* 1985;65:28–37.
37. Bigos S, Nachemson AL. Work for all: For those with low back pain as well. *Clin Orthop* 1983;179:77–85
38. Nachemson AL. Newest knowledge of low back pain. A critical look. *Clin Orthop* 1992;279:8–20
39. Noy S. Stress and personality as factors in the causation of combat reaction. In: Belenky GL, ed. *Contemporary studies in combat psychiatry*. Westport, CT: Greenwood Press, 1987.
40. Waddell G. An approach to backache. *Br J Hosp Med* September 1982;28(3):187, 190–191, 193–194.
41. Deyo RA, Diehl AK. Cancer as a cause of back pain: Frequency and diagnostic strategies. *Clin Res* 1987; 35:738A.
42. Andersson GBJ, Svensson H-O, Oden A. The intensity of work recovery in low back pain. *Spine* 1983;8: 880–884.
43. Nachemson AL. The natural course of low back pain. In: White AA, Gordon SL, eds. *Idiopathic low back pain*. St Louis: C.V. Mosby, 1982.
44. Haynes RB, Sackett DL, Taylor DW, et al. Increased absenteeism from work after detection and labeling of hypertensive patients. *New Engl J Med* 1978;299:741.
45. LeBlanc FE, et al. Scientific approach to the assessment and management of activity-related spinal disorders. 3. Dx of the problem. *Spine* 1987;12(7S) [Supp 1]:S16 (European edition).
46. Nachemson A. Scientific approach to the assessment and management of activity related spinal disorders. A monograph for clinicians. Report of the Quebec Task Force on spinal disorders. *Spine* 1987; 12(75)[Suppl 1]:S1–S59.
47. Bigos SJ, Battie M. Overdiagnosis and over prescription of low back pain: Acute care to prevent back disability. *Clin Orthop* 1987;221:121–130, 304.
48. Jensen MC, Brant-Zawadzki M, Obuchowski N, et al. Magnetic resonance imaging of the lumbar spine in people without back pain. *NEJM* July 14, 1994; 331(2).
49. Bigos SJ, Hansson T, Castillo RN, Beecher PJ, Wortley MD. The value of preemployment roentgenographs for predicting acute back injury claims and chronic back disability. *Clin Orthop Rel Pes* October 1992;283: 124–129.
50. LaRocca H, Macnab I. Value of pre-employment radiographic assessment of the lumbar spine. *Ind Med* June 1970;39(6):253–258.
51. Marora A, Schwartz A. Relation between the low back pain syndrome and x-ray findings. 1. Degenerative osteoarthritis. *Scand J Rehabil Med* 1976;8:115–125.
52. Paajanen H, Erkintalo M, Dahlstrom S, Kuusela T, Svedstrom E, Kormano M. Disc degeneration and lumbar instability. Magnetic resonance examination of 16 patients. *Acta Orthop Scand* August 1989;60(4): 375–358.
53. Oleinick A, Gluck JV, Guire KE. Diagnostic and management procedures for compensable back injuries without serious associated injuries. Modeling of the 1991 injury cohort from a major Michigan compensation insurer. *Spine* January 1998;23(1):93–110.
54. Colledge AL, Holmes E, et al. APGAR, Determining patient compliance and motivation. *Disabil Med* September–December 2001;1(2):5–19.
55. Jones FD, Hales RE. Military combat psychiatry: A historical review. *Psychiatr Ann* August 1987;17(8):526.
56. Barsky AJ. Amplification, somatization, and the somatoform disorders. *Psychosomatics* 1992;33:28–34.
57. Koes BW, Bouter LM, van Mameron H, et al. A randomized clinical trial of manual therapy and physiotherapy for persistent back and neck complaints: Subgroup analysis and relationship between outcome measures. *J Manip Physiol Ther* May 1993;16(4): 211–219.
58. Hadler NM. Diagnosis and treatment of backache. In: *Medical management of the regional musculoskeletal disease*. Hadler NM ed. Orlando: Gurne & Stratton, 1984:3–52.
59. Anderson RT. Orthopaedic ethnography in rural Nepal. *Med Anthropol* 1984;8:46–59.
60. Waddell G. A new clinical model for the treatment of low back pain. 1987 Volvo Award in Clinical Sciences. *Spine* 1987;12:632–644.
61. World Health Organization. *Epidemiology of work-related diseases and accidents*. Organization technical report series 777. Copenhagen, Denmark: WHO, 1986.
62. Williamson JW, Braswell HR, Horn SD. Validity of medical staff judgments in establishing quality assurance priorities. *Med Care* April 1979;17(4):331–346.
63. Deyo RA, Cherkin D, Conrad D, Volinn E. Cost, controversy, crisis: Low back pain and the health of the public. *Annu Rev Public Health* 1991;12:141–156.
64. Keller RB, Soule DN, Wennberg JE, Hanley DF. Dealing with geographic variations in the use of hospitals: The experience of the Maine medical assessment foundation orthopaedic study group. *J Bone Joint Surg* October 1990;72A(9):1286–1293.
65. Volinn E, Mayer J, Diehr P, Van Koevering D, Connell FA, Loeser JD. Small area analysis of surgery for low-back pain. *Spine* 1992;17(5):575–581.
66. Fishbain DA, Rosomoff HL, Goldberg M, et al. The prediction of return to the workplace after multidisciplinary pain center treatment. *Clin J Pain* 1993;9: 3–15.
67. Kupers RC, Van den Oever R, Van H Oudenhove B, et al. Spinal cord stimulation in Belgium. *Pain* 1994; 56:211–216.
68. Deyo RA. Conservative therapy for low back pain: Distinguishing useful from useless therapy. *JAMA* 1983;250:1057–1062.
69. Cherkin DC. Medication use for low back pain in primary care. *Spine* March 1, 1998;23:607–614.
70. Miller DR. Treatment of nonsteroidal anti-inflammatory drug-induced grastropathy. *Clin Pharm* August 1992;11(8):690–704.
71. Ohnmeiss P, Stith W, Gilbert P, Rashbaum R. Treatment of acute back pain in lumbar disc disease. *Spine State Art Rev* 1989;3:69.

72. Nachemson AL. *Low back pain, causes, diagnosis and treatment* (in Swedish). Stockholm: The Swedish Council of Technology Assessment in Health Care, 1991.
73. Jackson RP. The facet syndrome—Myth or reality? *Clin Orthop* 1992;279:110.
74. Carette S, Leclaire R, Marcoux S, et al. Epidural corticosteroid injections for sciatica due to herniated nucleus pulposus. *N Engl J Med* June 5, 1997; 336(23):1634–1640.
75. Leclaire R, Fortin L, Lambert R, Bergeron TM, Rossignol M. Radiofrequency facet joint denervation in the treatment of low back pain a placebo-controlled clinical trial to assess efficacy. *Spine* 2001;26(13)1411–1417.
76. Deyo RA, Diehl AK, Rosenthal M. How many days of bedrest for acute low back pain? A randomized clinical trial. *N Engl J Med* 1986;315:1064–1070.
77. Hrudey WP. Overdiagnosis and overtreatment of low back pain: Long term effects. *J Occup Rehabil* 1991;1(4):308.
78. Bortz WM. The disuse syndrome. *West J Med* 1984; 141:691–694.
79. Richardsen W, Berwick D, Bisgard J, et al. *Crossing the chasm: A New Health System for the 21st Century*. Institute of Medicine, US Committee on Quality Health in America. Washington, DC: National Academy Press, 2001.
80. Cassidy D. The QTF on whiplash-associated disorders—Impact and update. *AAPM&R 61st Annual Assembly and 13th World Congress of the International Federation of Physical Medicine and Rehabilitation*, November 1999.
81. Update Quebec Task Force guidelines for the management of whiplash-associated disorders technical report, January 2001 Motor Accidents Authority Level 22580 George Street, Sydney NSW, 2000.
82. Scientific monograph of the QTF on whiplash-associated disorders, Redefining "whiplash" and its management. *Spine* 1995;20(85, Suppl).
83. California Workers' Compensation Institute, Bulletin October 16, 1997.
84. Philadelphia panel evidence-based clinical practice guidelines on selected rehabilitation interventions for low back pain. *Phys Ther* October 2001;81(10):1641–1674.
85. Feine JS, Lund JP. An assessment of the efficacy of physical therapy and physical modalities for the control of chronic musculoskeletal pain. *Pain* 1997;71: 5–23.
86. California Workers' Compensation Institute Bulletin. Research abstract: Billing under the California official medical fee schedule, August 1997.
87. *Mooney v Back Letter*, 122 November 2001.
88. Daltroy LH. A controlled trial of an educational program to prevent low back injuries. *N Engl J Med* 1997;37:322–328.
89. Hadler NM. Workers with disabling back pain. *New Engl J Med* 1997;337:341–343.
90. Bouchard C. Discussion: Heredity, fitness and health. In: Bouchard C, Shephard R, Stephens T, Sutton J, McPherson B, eds. *Exercise, fitness and health.* Human Kinetics, Champaigne, IL 1990:147–153.
91. Estlander AM, et al. Effects and follow-up of a multimodal treatment program including intensive physical training for low back pain patients. *Scand J Rehabil Med* 1992;23:97–102.
92. Mixter WJ, Barr JS. Rupture of the intervertebral disc with involvement of the spinal canal. *N Engl J Med* 1934;211:210.
93. *The back letter: A digest of current information and literature.* (Bulletin), Vol. 7, No. 6. Hagerstown, MD: Lippincott, Williams and Wilkins, p. I, 1992.
94. Antonakes JA. Claims costs of back pain. *Best's Rev* 1981;9:36.
95. Goodwin PA. Prolonged disability for job-related injury. *Am Fam Physician.* November 1988;38(5):165–170.
96. Engel GL. Psychogenic pain and the pain-prone patient. *Am J Med* 1959;26:899–918.
97. Delauche-Cavallier MC, et al. Lumbar disc herniation—Computed tomography scan changes after conservative treatment of nerve root compression. *Spine* 1992;17(8).
98. Dubourg G, Rozenberg S, Fautrel B. A pilot study on the recovery from paresis after lumbar disc herniation. *Spine* 2002;27(13):1426–1432.
99. Saal JA, Saal JS. Nonoperative treatment of herniated lumbar intervertebral disc with radiculopathy—An outcome study. *Spine* 1989;14(4).
100. Weber H. Lumbar disc herniation—A controlled, prospective study with ten years of observation. *Spine* 1983;8:131–140.
101. DeBerard MS, Masters KS, Colledge AC, Schleusener RL, Schlegel JD. Outcomes of posterolateral lumbar fusion in Utah patients receiving workers' compensation: A retrospective cohort study. *Spine* 2001;26(7):738–747.
102. Colledge A, Sewell J, Crohm G. Controlling physical therapy and chiropractic utilization within the workers' compensation system—a retrospective review. A three-year analysis of 63,000 workers' compensation claims. IAIABC Journal 2004 (Fall);41(1):110–125.
103. Noy S, Levy R, Solomon Z. Mental health care in the Lebanon war. *Isr J Med Sci* 1984;20:360–365.
104. Gal R. Courage under stress. In: Breznitz S, ed. *Stress in Israel.* New York: Van Nostrand Reinhold Co., 1983.
105. Gal R. Combat stress—An opportunity for heroism. In: Belenky GL, ed. *Contemporary studies in combat psychiatry.* Westport, CT: Greenwood Press, 1987.
106. Panzarella JP. The nature of work, job loss, and the diagnostic complexities of the psychologically injured worker. *Psychiatr Ann* 1991:21:10–15.
107. Out of site, but not out of mind, injured/ill workers and their experiences with workers' compensation system. A review of 8,592 injured workers in 6 states. Study commissioned by Intracorp. 1996.
108. Walton M. *Thc Demming management method.* New York: Putnam, 1986.

109. US Department of Health and Human Services, National Center for Health Statistics. *Mon Vital Stat Rep* June 24, 1996;44(11S). http://www.os.dhhs/gov/
110. US Bureau of the Census, as published in the *Statistical Abstracts of the US*, October 1996:99.
111. US Bureau of the Census. Current Population Reports, pp. 23–180, and National Center for Health Statistics, Advance Data from Vital and Health Statistics, no. 194, 1996.
112. National Center for Health Statistics, Mortality Statistic Branch. Vital Statistics of the U.S. 1975–1990;2.
113. US Department of Education. *The condition of education*. The Office of Educational Research and Improvement, 1996.
114. Nahser EB, Mehrtens SE. *What's really going on?* Chicago: Corporantes, 1993:12.
115. Fitzler SL, Berger RA. Attitudinal change: The Chelsea back program. *Occup Health Saf* 1982;51:24–26.
116. Battie MC. Minimizing the impact of back pain: Workplace strategies. *Sem Spine Surg* March 1992;4(1):20–28.
117. California Workers' Compensation Institute (Bulletin). Report to the governor and legislature, July 1985.
118. Wood DJ. Design and evaluation of a back injury prevention program within a geriatric hospital. *Spine* 1987;12(2).
119. Krause N. Psychosocial job factors, physical workload, and incidence of work related spinal injury: A 5 yr prospective study of urban transit operators. *Spine* 23(23):2507–2516.
120. *Workers' Compensation Monitor*, (bulletin) July 1998:10.
121. Burt M, Biegel Y, Farley EC. *Worldwide highlights from the worldwide survey of non-medical drug use and alcohol use among military personnel.* Bethesda, MD: Burt Associates, 1980.
122. Normand J. Relationship between drug test results and job performance indicators. Presented at the *97th American Psychological Association Meeting*, New Orleans, LA, 1989.
123. Zwerling C, Ryan J, Orav EJ. The efficacy of preemployment drug screening for marijuana and cocaine in predicting employment outcome. *JAMA* 1990;264(2):639–643.
124. *Creating a drug free workplace: How to design and implement an effective program.* Louisiana Workers' Compensation Corp., 2002. http://www.lwcc/resourse orderform.cfm
125. *Americans with Disabilities Act* 42 USC § 12101 (1991).
126. Lee D, Cady MD. Strength and fitness and subsequent back injuries in firefighters. *J Occup Med* April 1979;21(4):86–91.
127. Lynch WD, Golaszewski TJ, Clearie AF, Snow D, Vickery DM. Impact of a facility-based corporate fitness program on the number of absences from work due to illness. *J Occup Med* January 1990;32(1):9–12.
128. Mayer TG, Gatchel RJ, Kishono N, et al. Objective assessment of spine function following industrial injury: A prospective study with comparison group and one year follow up. *Spine* 1985;10:483–493.
129. Gice J, Tomokins K. Cutting costs with return to work programs. *Risk Manage* 1988;35:62–65.
130. Taylor T. Working around workers' injuries. *Nations Bus* 1988;76:39–40.
131. Dworkin RH, Handlin DS, Richlin DM, Brand L, Vannucci C. Unraveling the effects of compensation, litigation, and employment on treatment response in chronic pain. *Pain* 1985;23:49–59.
132. Stung JP. The chronic disability syndrome. In: Aronoff GM, ed. *Evaluation and treatment of chronic pain.* Baltimore, MD: Urban & Schwarzenberg, 1985.
133. Yassi A, Tate R, Cooper JE, Snow C, Vallentyne S, Khokhar JB. Early intervention for back-injured nurses at a large Canadian tertiary care hospital: An evaluation of the effectiveness and cost benefits of a two-year pilot project. *Occup Med (Lond)* August 1995; 45(4):209–214.
134. Bean E. Damage control after 137 people died in its Texas jet crash, Delta helped families. *Wall Street J* November 7, 1988.
135. Nachemson A, et al. Management guidelines. *Spine* September 1987;12(7S) [Supp 1] (European edition).
136. Litigation and workers' compensation: A report to industry. Report to the governor and California legislature, July 1979.
137. Cotton P. Symptoms may return after carpal tunnel surgery. *JAMA* April 17, 1991;265(15).
138. Worral JD, Appel D. The impact of workers' compensation benefits on low back claims. In: Hadler NM, ed. *Clinical concepts in regional musculoskeletal illness.* Orlando; Grune and Stratton, 1987:281–297.
139. Hunter S. Predicting return to work, A long-term follow-up study of railroad workers after low back injuries. *Spine*. 1998;32(21):2319–2328.
140. Bigos SJ, Andary MT. The practitioner's guide to the industrial back problem. Part I. Helping the patient with the symptoms and pathology. *Sem Spine Surg* March 1992;4(1):42–54.
141. Brodsky CM. Psychological factors contributing to somatoform disease attributed to the workplace. The case of intoxication. *J Occup Med* 1983;25:459–464.
142. Bigos SJ, Battie MC, Spengler DM. A prospective study of work perceptions and psychosocial factors affecting the report of back injury. *Spine* January 1991; 16(1):1–6. Erratum in: Spine June 1991; 16(6):688.
143. Craufurd DI, Creed F, Jayson MI. Life events and psychological disturbances in patients with low back pain. *Spine* 1990;15(6):490–494.
144. Jepson H, Talashek M, Tichy A. The APGAR score: Evolution, limitations, and scoring guidelines. *Birth* June 1991;18:83–92.
145. Norwood S. The social support APGAR: Instrument development and testing. *Res Nurs Health* 1996; 19:143–152.
146. Smilkstein G, Ashworth C, Montano M. Validity and reliability of the family APGAR as a test of family function. *J Fam Pract*, 1982;15(2):303–311.
147. Gwyther R, Bentz E, Drossman D, Berolzheimer N. Validity of the family APGAR in patients with irritable bowel syndrome. *Clin Res Methods* 1993;25(1):21–25.

148. Woo SLY, An KN, Arnoczky SP, Wayne JS, Fithian DC, Myers BS. Anatomy, biology, and biomechanics of tendons, ligament, and meniscus. In: Simon SR, ed. *Orthopedic basic science*. Rosemont, IL: American Academy of Orthopedic Surgeons, 1994:45–87.
149. Woo SL, Vogrin TM, Abramowitch SD. Healing and repair of ligament injuries in the knee. *J Am Acad Orthop Surg* 2000;8:364–372.
150. Waddell G, McCulloch JA, Kummel E, Venner RM. Nonorganic physical signs in low-back pain. *Spine* 1980;5:117–125.
151. Portney LG, Watkins MP. *Foundations of clinical research: Applications to practice*. East Norwalk, CT: Appleton & Lange, 1993:680.
152. Stokes HM. The seriously uninjured hand: Weakness of grip. *J Occup Med* 1983;25:683–684.
153. Simon MJ. Use of Rey Memory Test to assess malingering in criminal defendents. *J Clin Psychol.* November 1994;50(6):913–917.
154. Lister G. *The hand: Diagnosis and Indications*, 4th ed. New York: Churchill Livingstone, 2002:162–163.
155. Isernhagen SJ. *Isernhagen Work Systems functional capacity evaluation*. Duluth, MN: Isernhagen Work Systems, 1996:52a–52b, 83.
156. Matheson LN. Use of the BTE Work Simulator to screen for symptom magnification syndrome. *Ind Rehabil Q* 1989;2(2):5–31.
157. Solomon PE. Measurement of pain behavior. *Physiother Can* 1996;48:52–58.
158. Borg G, Holmgren A, Lindblad I. Quantitative evaluation of chest pain. *Acta Med Scand Suppl* 1981;644: 43–45.
159. Johns R, Colledge A, Holmes E. Fitness for duty evaluations. *Disability Evaluation*, 2nd ed. Chicago, IL, Mosby, AMA Publication 2003.
160. Hall H, Iceton JA. Back school: An overview with specific reference to the Canadian back education units. *Clin Orthop* 1983;179:10–17.
161. Repko GR, Cooper R. A study of the average workers' compensation case. *J Clin Psych*, 1983;39:287–295.
162. Turner JA, Deyo RA, Loeser JD, Von Korff M, Fordyce WE. The importance of placebo effects in pain treatment and research. *JAMA* May 1994;271(20): 1609–1614.
163. Hagen EM, Eriksen HR, Ersin H. Does early intervention with a light mobilization program reduce long-term sick leave for low back pain? *Spine* 2000;25:1973–1976.
164. Diamond EG. Comparison of internal mammary ligation and sham operation for angina pectoris. *Am J Caridol* 1960;5:483–486.
165. Cobb LA. An evaluation of internal mammary artery ligation by a double blind technique. *N Engl J Med* 1959;260:1115–1118.
166. Goodman P. Response of patients with myofascial pain dysfunction syndrome to mock equilibration. *J Am Dent Assoc* 1976;93:755–758.
167. Spangfort EV. The lumbar disc herniation: A computer aided analysis of 2504 operation. *Acta Othorp Scand* 1972:142(Suppl):1–95.
168. Ashworth DN. An experimental study of the effects of three participative goal setting strategies on perception of goal difficulty, goal acceptance, satisfaction and task performance. *Diss Abstr Int* 1980;40(12): 63–64.
169. Alexy B. Goal setting and health risk reduction. *Nurs Res* 1985;34(5):283–288.
170. Catchlove R, Cohen K. Effects of a directive return to work approach in the treatment of workmans' compensation patients with chronic pain. *Pain* 1982;14: 181–191.
171. Astin JA. Why patients use alternative medicine: Results of a national study. *JAMA* May 1998; 279(19):1548–1553.
172. Noyes R Jr, Clancy J. The dying role: Its relevance to improved patient care. *Psychiatry* February 1977; 40(1):41–47.
173. *Guides to the Evaluation of Permanent Impairment*, 5th ed. Chicago American Medical Association, 2001:19.
174. *Guides to the Evaluation of Permanent Impairment*, 5th ed. Chicago, IL. American Medical Association, 2001:315.
175. Impairment ratings trends in the Texas workers' compensation system. *Tex Monit* Fall 1999;4(3):7–9.
176. Spieler EA, Barth PS, Burton JF Jr, Himmelstein J, Rudolph L. Recommendations to guide revision of the Guides to the Evaluation of Permanent Impairment. *JAMA* 2000;283:519–523.
177. Nitschke JE, Nattrass CL, Disler PB, Chou R, Ooi KT. Reliability of the American Medical Association Guides' model for measuring spinal range of motion. Its implication for whole-person impairment rating. *Spine* February 1, 1999;24(3):262–268.
178. Madson TJ, Youdas JW, Suman VJ. Reproducibility of lumbar spine range of motion measurements using the back range of motion device. *J Orthop Sports Phys Ther* August 1999;29(8):470–477.
179. Nilsson N, Hartvigsen J, Christensen HW. Normal ranges of passive cervical motion for women and men 20–60 years old. *J Manipulative Phys Ther* June 1996; 19(5):306–309.
180. Russell P, Pearcy MJ, Unsworth A. Measurement of the range and coupled movements observed in the lumbar spine. *Br J Rheumatol* June 1993;32(6):490–497.
181. Weiner DK, Distell B, Studenski S, Martinez S, Lumansky L, Bangiorni D. Does radiographic osteoarthritis correlate with flexibility of the lumbar spine? *Am Geriatr Soc* March 1994;42(3):257–263.
182. Ensink FB, Saur PM, Frese K, Seeger D, Hildebrandt J. Lumbar range of motion: Influence of time of day and individual factors on measurements. *Spine* June 1, 1996;21(11):1339–1343.
183. Poitras S, Loisel P, Prince F, Lemaire J. Disability measurement in persons with back pain: A validity study of spinal range of motion and velocity. *Arch Phys Med Rehabil* October 2000;81(10):1394–1400.

184. Colledge AL. *Utah Labor Commission's impairment rating guide*. Salt Lake City, UT: Utah Labor Commission, 2002.
185. Colledge AL. Methodology to reduce variation for impairment ratings in workers' compensation. *Disabil Med* February 2001:38–42.
186. *The guides to the evaluation of permanent impairment*, 5th ed. Chicago: American Medical Association, 2001:15.
187. Colledge AL, Johns RE Jr. *Unified fitness.* Report for the workplace. Occ Med October–December 2000; 15(4):723–737.
188. Colledge AL, Johns RE Jr, Thomas MH. Functional abilities assessment: Guidelines for the workplace. *JOEM* March 1999;41(3):172–180.
189. Demeter S. Fitness for duty, disability evaluation. In: Demeter S, Andersson G, Smith G, eds. *Disability evaluation*. Chicago: AMA and Mosby. 1996.
190. Colledge AL, Holmes E. Utah Performance APGAR. *Disability* Fall, 2002.
191. Bernard C. *An introduction to the study of experimental medicine.* In: Green HC, trans. New York: Dover, 1957.

CHAPTER

35

CLINICAL MANAGEMENT OF CHRONIC, DISABLING LOW BACK SYNDROMES

Vert Mooney, Joe L. Verna, and Craig E. Morris

OUTLINE

OBJECTIVES

1. To discuss clinical strategies to clinicians in the challenging field of chronic disabling low back disorders.
2. Discuss practical assessment strategies for chronic disabling low back disorders.
3. Demonstrate multidisciplinary clinical strategies to chronic, disabling back disorders.
4. Demonstrate exercise strategies for chronic disabling low back disorders.
5. Demonstrate standardized treatment protocols for chronic disabling low back disorders.
6. To emphasize the importance of the multidisciplinary team concept in the management of chronic, disabling low back disorders.

BACKGROUND

Low back pain is currently one of the leading causes of disability in the United States, with disability rates for low back pain climbing at 14 times the rate of the population growth.[1] The costs of these soft tissue injuries to the industrial society are immense and the scope of the problem continues to grow.[2–8] Low back pain is the leading cause of disability between ages of 19 and 45 years, and accounts for approximately 41% of workers' compensation expenses ($20–50 billion, annually).[9] Furthermore, low back pain effects 60%–80% of the general population at some point during their lifetime and 28%–30% are suffering from low back pain at any given time.[10] In addition, military low back injury and disability rates are comparable to, and in some cases exceed, those of the civilian populations.[11]

Attaching specific diagnoses to low back pain is difficult and, as previously discussed, elusive, as there is often no identifiable source of pain or injury. Typically, low back pain episodes are characterized by the context of their course and have been described as acute, subacute, chronic, or recurrent. Some controversy exists regarding the definition of these terms. Frymoyer has defined acute low back pain as pain that exist from 0 to 6 weeks after onset of symptoms, subacute as 6 to 12 weeks, and chronic as greater than 12 weeks.[12] Frymoyer's classification of low back pain falls within the time frame of natural history and definition of acute back problems outlined in the Clinical Practice Guidelines published by the US Department of Health of Human Services' Agency for Health Care Policy and Research (AHCPR).[13]

The natural history of low back pain suggests that approximately 90% of patients suffering from a first episode of acute low back will be asymptomatic within 3 months.[14] Therefore, the natural history of low back pain may serve as a reference point for treatment and recovery expectations. However, there is a very high recurrence rate (40%–60%) among those suffering first time low back pain.[15] In addition, there are apparent morphological changes in the lumbar extensors muscles, namely atrophy and asymmetry, which exist long after the resolution of pain.[16] It is also important to note that the majority of medical and disability expenses are attributed to a small minority of low back pain cases. It is estimated that 15% of all spinal disorders that are not resolved within 6 months become chronic and that this chronic pain population accounts for 85% of all costs.[3–9]

The traditional approach in physical medicine for the rehabilitation of acute, subacute, and chronic low back pain, has been, and unfortunately often continues to be, the use of passive modalities, such as ultrasound and hot packs. Although modalities have continued to change with time, the therapeutic results have remained mostly disappointing. In many states, such as California for example, the workers' compensation system's fee schedule is based on providing procedures in combination with modalities without any justification for efficacy or therapeutic rational. The combination of modalities with exercise may certainly be justified if the modalities used enhance the patient's compliance by temporally reducing symptomatology or increasing range of motion to enable the patient to perform at a higher level while exercising and thus enhance the quality of their performance.

In 1994, the AHCPR published *Acute Low Back Pain Problems in Adults: A Clinical Practice Guidelines*.[13] These guidelines were systematically developed to assist practitioners and patients with the decision-making process for appropriate health care. An independent multidisciplinary panel of private sector clinicians and other experts commissioned by the AHCPR developed the guidelines based on published scientific literature regarding acute low back pain. Peer review and field reviews were combined to evaluate the validity, reliability, and utility of the guidelines for acute low back pain in clinical practice. The AHCPR guidelines represented one of the most extensive literature searches, critical reviews, and syntheses of empirical evidence related to low back pain.

Some adjustments should be made to reflect new findings regarding back schools, bed rest, lumbar corsets, and epidural injections. It is likely that minor updates will be needed in a timely manner, but no specific mechanism to achieve this was presented.[17,18]

Clinical Pearl: The most recent review by Shekelle et al[17] indicates that the AHCPR Guidelines are largely still valid and a reasonably accurate interpretation of the scientific literature.

The AHCPR guidelines define acute low back pain as activity intolerance or limitation related to back pain symptoms of less than 3 months' duration. In the absence of contraindications, the AHCPR recommendations for the treatment of acute low back pain include

- NSAIDS (nonsteroidal anti-inflammatory drugs) or acetaminophen.
- Spinal manipulation.
- Two to four days of bed rest with gradual return to normal activities for patients with severe low back pain. The bed rest recommendation has been removed because of the now well-accepted deconditioning effect.[19–21]
- Aerobic activities that minimally stress the back (e.g., walking, biking, and swimming).
- Gradual increase conditioning exercises for back extensor muscles, especially if low back pain persists.

Moreover, the AHCPR panel found no evidence of benefit from passive physical agents in some modalities such as ice, heat, massage, traction, ultrasound, and transcutaneous electrical nerve stimulation. In addition, the panel reported that there was no evidence to support the use of trigger point, ligaments, and facet joint injections, needle acupuncture, and dry needling for acute low back pain. The use of oral steroids, calcium, and antidepressant medications was also not recommended. Furthermore, the panel found that prolonged bed rest (for more than 4 days) was not appropriate in the treatment for acute low back problems because it could lead to debilitation and deconditioning. An independent panel in the State of Florida reconfirmed these guidelines.[22] To further confirm the negative impact of bed rest, a recent review of randomized studies on bed rest by Haen et al.[19] showed that bed rest had no positive effects and some slightly harmful effects. Because of apparent economic pressures, passive modalities, such as ultrasound and electrical stimulation, continue to be used in spite the lack of evidence necessary to support their use. A review of 10 randomized controlled trials found that 8 demonstrated no benefit for the use of passive modalities, and only 2 demonstrated a possible benefit.[20] These modalities are inexpensive to apply by assistants and aids in therapy centers. In most states, such as California, maximum reimbursement for physical medicine can only be achieved if they are included in treatment.[23] This fact demonstrates the power of political lobbying in the face of negative support on a scientific basis.

Recent research has identified histochemical pathologies, deconditioning effects, morphological changes, and functional abnormalities in the lumbar extensor musculature of patients with low back pain.[24] Furthermore, a low level of trunk muscle endurance has been implicated as a primary risk factor for low back injury with an inverse relationship existing between back extension endurance (Biering–Sorensen test) and the likelihood of future low back pain episodes.[25] However, this relationship has not been clearly shown to exist with trunk extension strength.[26,27] In addition, the reduction of painful symptoms following lumbar extensor strength training has not been shown to be well correlated with increases in lumbar extension strength.[28] Because of these findings, it has been suggested that exercise programs for low back pain should emphasize endurance movements (longer duration, lower intensity) rather than strength (shorter duration, higher intensity).[29] Specifically, progressive resistance exercises (particularly for the lumbar extensors) have been frequently prescribed and have been shown to be effective for the treatment of low back pain.[28,29,35,36] The US Department of Health and Human Services currently recommends gradually increasing conditioning exercises for back extensors for the treatment of acute back pain.[13]

Clinical Pearl: By the mid-1980s, evidence began to appear suggesting that aggressive "sports medicine" approaches were more effective than traditional methods in treating low back pain.[30–34]

Acute low back pain has been described as "activity intolerance" and it is recommended that an initial assessment consist of a focused clinical history and physical examination. The AHCPR guidelines denote that the initial assessment provides an opportunity for the clinician to establish a rapport with the patient and to become aware of the impact of the symptoms on their activity.[13]

THE CHRONIC BACK SYNDROME

The following discussion will be focused on the care of people with chronic recurrent back problems. The majority of these have failed previous treatments of various types. Some of them have had surgical care. It is assumed that this population had their problem for at least 6 months—most of them far longer. They have typically been screened for an alternative source of back pain such as infection or tumor, and although they may have been declared a candidate for surgery, a trial of nonoperative care has been authorized. Indeed, many of the patients, though considered good surgical candidates by their physicians, are fearful of surgery and wish to find an alternative approach to control their pain.

Pain is generally the patient's major presenting symptom. Some also have weakness, paresthesia, and/or stiffness. What generally drives them to seek further attention, however, is their pain. Most of them, when initially seen, are taking one or more medications such as narcotics, anti-inflammatories, and muscle relaxants. Some are seemingly, hopelessly habituated, adding to the clinical complexity of their case.

The lead authors of this chapter oversee several multidisciplinary clinic dedicated to complex musculoskeletal injuries, including surgical interventions and rehabilitation. This discussion will be an outgrowth of this experience and the somewhat eclectic model that has subsequently evolved from such experience. It must be recognized that there are many approaches to chronic low back pain. Some of them are well represented, perhaps more individually, in other chapters in this textbook.

This phrase would imply that one would expect the patient to develop some enthusiasm for taking responsibility in his or her own care. This may not always be possible. The authors will discuss our approach to that challenging group of people.

Clinical Pearl: The underlying philosophy of this treatment program is centered on the somewhat rhetorical question: "Do you just want to feel better, or get better?"

JUSTIFICATION FOR TREATMENT

Chronic recurrent back pain is essentially based on two interrelated factors. The first factor, more clearly understood at least by clinicians trained in the care of musculoskeletal disease, is structural abnormalities. The second, no doubt of equal importance, is the nonstructural factor. This factor can further be subdivided into psychosocial, psychiatric, and socioeconomic subcategories. Both structural and nonstructural issues are important and must be addressed.

This has been documented by several other studies.[34,37] Why should this be true?

In the case of chronic recurrent low back pain, it certainly is appropriate to expect that there has been some tissue deterioration or some "weak link" that has developed. The authors have evidence that in the case of disc injury, which may result in painful deterioration, there is a buildup of abnormal chemicals within the disc such as nitric oxide, phospholipase, and various metalloproteases.[38] Furthermore, degenerated and symptomatic discs, determined by discography, have an increased level of acidity as reflected by lower pH.[39] It is important to note that non-painful, degenerative discs are not acidic, but rather have a neutral pH. This would seem to indicate, for reasons not yet clear, that there is some sort of stagnation of metabolic events within the painful disc and perhaps in other soft tissues. Therefore, in order to improve metabolism of poorly vascularized tissues such as the intervertebral disc, increased physical activity may be quite useful. Enhanced fluid exchange by such physical activity would certainly seem to be a reasonable therapeutic strategy.

Clinical Pearl: In regards to the structural factors, it has been the authors' experience that the medical diagnosis does not seem to influence the expected outcome or variation in treatment.[30]

There are other important changes that occur when there is a homeostatic imbalance associated with degeneration and injury. In a fascinating series of studies of both patients with back pain and normal subjects at the Physiotherapy Department at the University of Queensland in Brisbane, some important insight as to new muscular changes has been achieved. The researchers' tools for analysis were real-time cross-sectional ultrasound measurements of the spinal musculature and fine wire electrode electromyographic (EMG) analysis of specific muscles. With the aid of ultrasound visualization, one could place the fine wire electrodes and insure their position in the appropriate muscles. Even the very thin transversalis (AKA-abdominis transversus) muscle—the deepest of the abdominal muscles—could be monitored with this method. At various levels, the multifidus muscle could also be monitored by such a method.

In one of the Australian studies, patients complaining of initial-onset back pain were analyzed for their muscle mass.[24] These patients demonstrated a relative decrease in mass of the multifidus on the painful side compared to the non-painful side. In contrast, the control group, with no history of back pain and matched by age and sex, displayed bilaterally equal and normal mass of the multifidus musculature. The most startling discovery, however, was that the atrophy occurred quite early, sometimes only 2 weeks after the onset of back pain. Another surprising finding, with important nonsurgical spinal implications, was the persistence of the demonstrated atrophy. Numerous patients from this study were evaluated several months later, following the resolution of their back pain. In spite of a total resolution of pain, the multifidus atrophy persisted. Obviously, continued inhibition of muscle activity in some manner existed interfering with a return of normal mass with daily activity.[40] It is also notable that the patients who exercised their low back extensors in this subacute population demonstrated only a 30% recurrence rate at 1-year follow-up, while those who did not exercise their lumbar extensors had an 80% recurrence rate.[24]

The importance of inhibition and facilitation of muscle activity was also demonstrated by more studies from this Australian group.[41,42] Using the fine wire electrode technology for myoelectric analysis, they could instantaneously monitor muscle activity as the subject was performing normal functional activities. It was apparent that whenever the upper extremities were moved or the position of the torso changed, the abdominis transversus musculature, in concert with the multifidi, was active several milliseconds before the arm or torso activity was initiated to accompany myoelectric activity of the governing muscles for the activity. These muscles, the transversalis and multifidus, partnered with the pelvic floor and diaphragm, work as torso stabilizers. Under conditions of movement, these muscles increase intra-abdominal pressure (the "pressurized canister"), and normally contract *prior to* the activation of muscles that would, for example, initiate extremity motion. This physiological apparatus, a system whereby intrinsic trunk muscles, mediated via the central nervous system, contract prior to target peripheral muscles, has been called the "feedforward mechanism." However, with the onset of back pain, this function is compromised and the myoelectric activity of the multifidus and transversalis is delayed, hindering torso stabilization. This probably has implications concerning recurrence, and indeed, treatment.

Do these studies have relevance for chronic recurrent back problems? Studies by the authors, using magnetic resonance imaging (MRI) and surface electrode myography, demonstrated similar findings.[43] In this study, all patients with chronic back pain had significant fatty infiltration into the multifidus musculature. This was specific in that other torso musculature and the iliopsoas seen in the axial MRI slices did not demonstrate similar fatty infiltration typical of muscle atrophy (Fig. 35–1*A* and 35–1*B*). When tested, the subjects in this series averaged about 45% below expected normal strength. However, muscle strength was returned to normal in all the patients with back pain in this study after 16 training sessions (8 weeks). Of

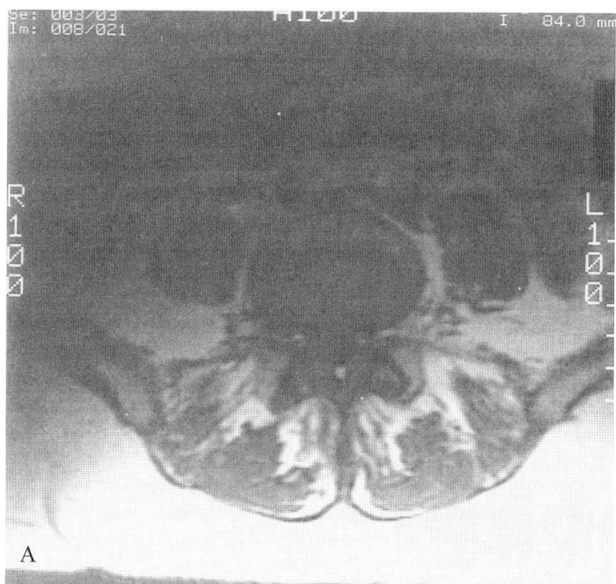

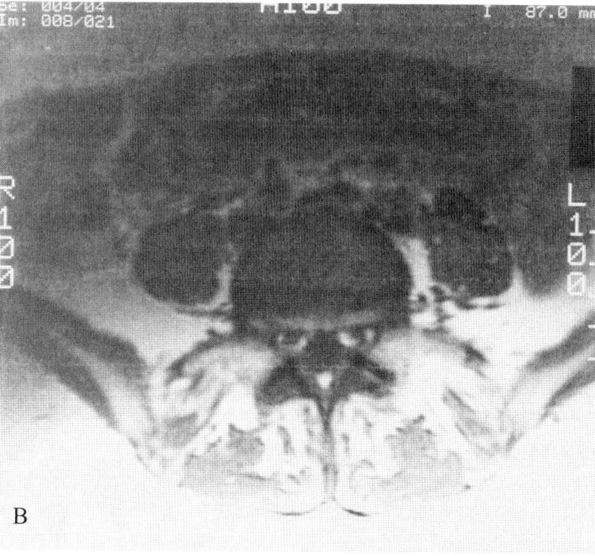

FIGURE 35–1. *A.* MRI axial view of the multifidus at L4–L5 in a normal individual. *B.* MRI axial view of L4–L5 of an individual with chronic back pain. Note the extreme amount of fatty infiltration and associated atrophy of especially the multifidus muscles.

interest was the fact that there was no consistent correlation between increased muscle mass and improved strength (Fig. 35–2*A* and 35–2*B*). There was not much change in muscle mass and fatty infiltration seen in the MRI 8 weeks after initiation of training. Thus, this study demonstrates that there truly is an inhibition of normal muscle function after back injury associated with pain and degeneration. The effects of this inhibition can therefore be corrected with physical training.

These observations are not unique to one group. Parkkola et al. noted that fatty infiltration in the lumbar extensors of patients with chronic low back pain was higher than in healthy individuals. Interestingly, the fatty infiltration was localized to the lumbar extensors in these chronic patients, whose other skeletal muscle demonstrated far lower fat levels.[44] Alaranta et al. noted similar findings using computed tomography scanning: the more severe the back pain, the greater the atrophy noted in the lumbar extensor muscles only.[45] Using the same technology, Mayer et al. noted a significant amount of muscle atrophy in postoperative patients.[46] Other studies using EMG technology demonstrated similar findings to the authors'.[47,48] They demonstrated that the amplitude of myoelectric signals in extensors is considerably diminished whereas lumbar flexors function normally. This variation in EMG activity supports the concept that the lumbar flexors function normally in patients with low back pain, whereas lumbar extensors do not.[49] Also, the evidence is clear that back pain or surgery causes atrophy and muscle inhibition and, hence, atrophy of the lumbar extensors, especially the multifidus. Is there a rationale why the small lumbar extensors should be so at risk on the occasion of chronic recurrent back pain?

Historical and Morphological Perspectives

A reasonable theory takes account of the relatively new function of the multifidi as postural muscles in human primates. This requires, of course, the multifidus to reflexively maintain this relatively new functional position. Because this reflex activity is not as deeply imbedded in the nervous system, these phylogenetically reflexes can be more easily troubled by injury and/or pain. Interestingly, a similar phenomenon seems to occur in the knee. It is well recognized that knee injury, especially the anterior cruciate ligament, will cause rapid atrophy of the quadriceps, especially the vastus medialis. Again, the human is the only primate that stands with a fully extended knee at 180 degree. The patella is least constrained, or stabilized, by anatomic features (i.e., ligaments and fascia) when the knee is fully extended. Thus, the unique function of the vastus medialis occurs in the human primates in that it has the phylogenetically "new" job of restraining the patella. Like the multifidus mentioned above, the vastus medialis also atrophies rapidly after injury. The progressive exercise programs for the injured knee routinely achieve reversal of the inhibition and atrophy. That certainly is the current standard of care for the knee. Should lumbar extensor strengthening be the standard of care following back injury?

Clinical Pearl: Phylogenetically speaking, human postural reflexes for the upper and lower extremities are buried deep within the subconscious

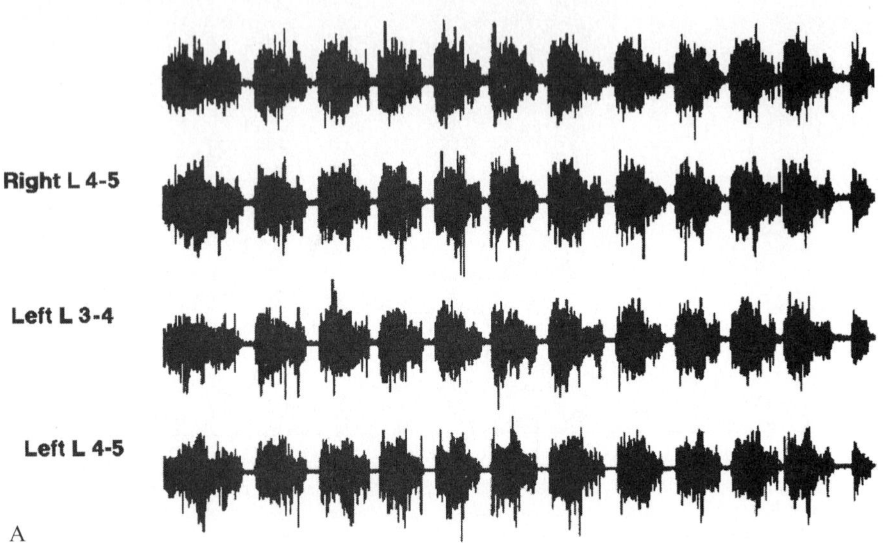

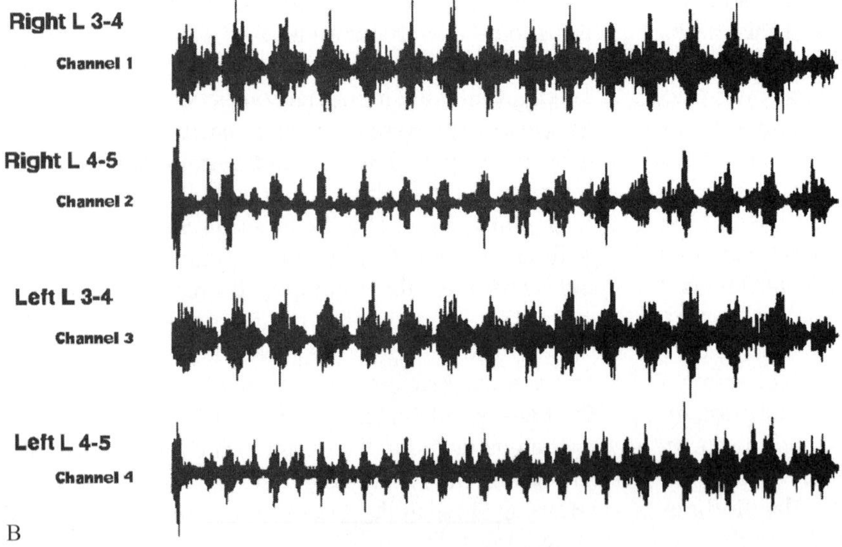

FIGURE 35–2. *A.* Example of myoelectric findings of an individual carrying out lumbar flexion extension exercises on MedX equipment at the beginning of their training program. *B.* Myoelectric findings from the same individual after completing the 8-week program using the same resistance as was present at the beginning of treatment. Note the diminished amplitude of the myoelectric signal demonstrating the training effect, creating a more efficient motor control. Each peak represents maximum multifidus activity at the extreme of extension.

nervous system based on thousands or perhaps millions of years of evolution. Only the human, among primates, stands with a lordosed lumbar spine in the upright posture.

Actually, the current state of spine rehabilitation bares some resemblance to the status of cardiac rehabilitation in the late 1960s. At that time rehabilitation for post cardiac infarct patients was quite varied. There certainly was a lack of knowledge of what cardiac patients could tolerate. At that point exercise was not thought to be beneficial. The first real data emerged in 1969 when Robert Bruce first published studies regarding graded exercise testing on a treadmill.[50] Measurement tools, of course, were essential to confirm safety and efficacy. Electronic monitoring with the Holter monitor allowed cardiac monitoring while exercise was progressing. But it was not until the early 1980s that the "Bruce protocol" became standardized for cardiac assessment in this country. Thus, it took more than a decade to gain acceptance.[51]

It was not until 1986 that treatment protocols for chronic low back pain based on measurement of function were established.[52] It was not until the 1990s that standard test protocols for soft tissue injuries to the back were published.[51,53] A credible report on a significant number of patient using functional restorations in a measured manner was not reported until 1987.[34] This was a very intense and expensive program. A program using standardized exercise protocols was later developed and was first published in 1995.[28] Although initially there was considerable enthusiasm for this equipment, which could basically perform only spinal testing, it was not especially useful for physical training. Therefore, it gradually fell out of favor, probably because there was an insufficient cost–benefit ratio.[54] Many of the computerized systems for functional testing of back problems failed to gain support from the medical and scientific community because of a lack of credibility following critical and influential articles.[27,55] These articles point out that the computerized equipment failed to provide standardized test protocols and derived variables of questionable reliability and scientific standard such as power, work, and agonist/antagonist ratios. In other words, if the measurement becomes too sophisticated and does not offer sufficient insight as to the measurable benefit, it may not be worth the effort. However, the lead authors perceive the critical report by Newton and Waddell,[55] to be biased in that it did not evaluate one brand of equipment (MedX, Ocala, FL) that had established normative values for spinal strength by standardized protocols. In addition to its assessment capability, the lead authors have found it to function as an excellent exercise tool. The authors have therefore continued to use this equipment routinely during treatment protocols (Fig. 35–3). *(The authors feel it appropriate to state that there is no financial relationship with the manufacturer.)*

The value of a defined protocol is the methodology from which an effective exercise prescription can be determined. In order to provide a defined protocol, it is necessary to have a measurement tool from which objective data may be derived. Without the use of some measurement, it is very difficult to determine a meaningful measure of progress. Without measurement of dose of an activity, it is difficult to determine efficacy of the activity. Actually, there were similar cost arguments concerning objective measurement tools for knee rehabilitation in its early stages, but they are no longer present. The use of exercise equipment for knee rehabilitation is now well accepted. Unfortunately, the back is more complex than the knee, and exactly how and what to measure has not yet reached the level of consensus accepted for the knee.

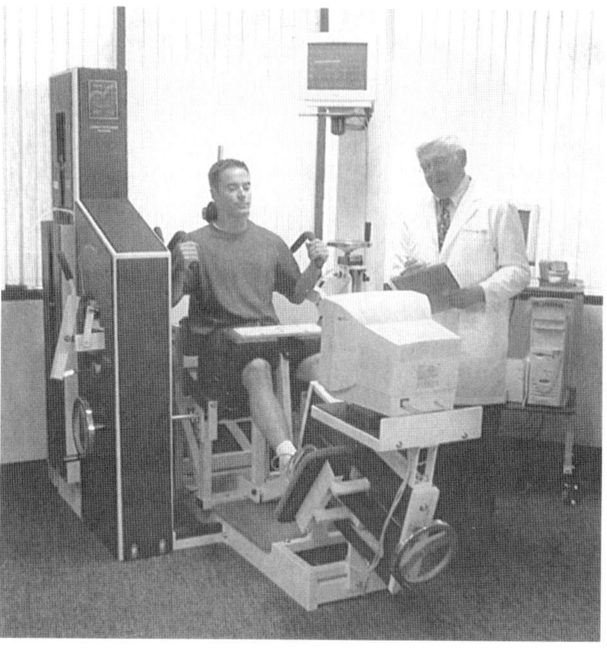

FIGURE 35–3. Subject carrying out a MedX training program with feedback from the VCR screen.

In order to determine the importance of isolating the low back extensors during strength training, Mayer et al. performed a comparative study of this region.[56] In this article, isometric back extension strength was measured with and without pelvic stabilization (restraint) at various points of back extension on a lumbar extension dynamometer in 33 healthy subjects. In this study, lumbar extensor torque values were similar for the stabilized and unstabilized tests at 5 of the 7 angles tested. The unstabilized tests produced higher torque values than the stabilized test only at the two most extended angles. Recent work by this group demonstrated that training on a dynamometer without stabilization results in strength gains that are similar to those visualized with stabilized training.[57] These studies concluded that pelvic stabilization, as measured by dynamometry, is not necessary to increase lumbar extension strength, and that training without pelvic stabilization is quite practical. Furthermore, training without stabilization may be more closely related to typical spinal functional activities.

One important aspect of computerized dynamometry is the counterbalanced design with regard to the individual's torso while seated. Because of the counterbalance, minimal physical effort is needed to create motion. Thus, resistance exercise at a very low level can be accomplished. This is important for patients with back pain, where deconditioning often leads to painful exacerbations with relatively minor loading of the lumbopelvic musculature. One of the problems with a standard gym extensor training device known as a Roman chair is that the demand on back strength is so severe at the starting positions, either at 45 degrees or 0 degree. To resolve this problem, a back extension machine has been recently developed to allow the performance of progressive resistance exercises at a starting point where controlled, minimal loading of the lumbopelvic region occurs. This lumbar extension machine is a variable angle Roman chair which can be adjusted from 75 degrees relative to horizontal (i.e., almost vertical) to 0 degree relative to horizontal (i.e., horizontal), in 15-degree increments (Fig. 35–4). As the angle from horizontal decreases on the variable angle Roman chair, the load applied in the low back muscles increases, which has been verified by EMG testing.[58] Moreover, by varying the location of the subject's hands and arms, farther away from the axis of rotation at the lumbosacral spine, increases in the loading, and hence the degree of resistance has been measured.[58] Thus, this device has been incorporated into the authors' treatment programs.

As noted above, the use of standardized equipment is vital in achieving standardized protocols for progressive resistance exercises. With the availability of such tools, improvements in mobility, strength, and endurance can be measured. These are necessary components to document that an individual is improving, an important issue for the patient, clinician, and payer of care. Once accepted measures for improvement are in place, a plethora of treatment strategies can be implemented to determine the most efficacious means available. The feedback of improving performance is an important component of an active rehabilitation program.

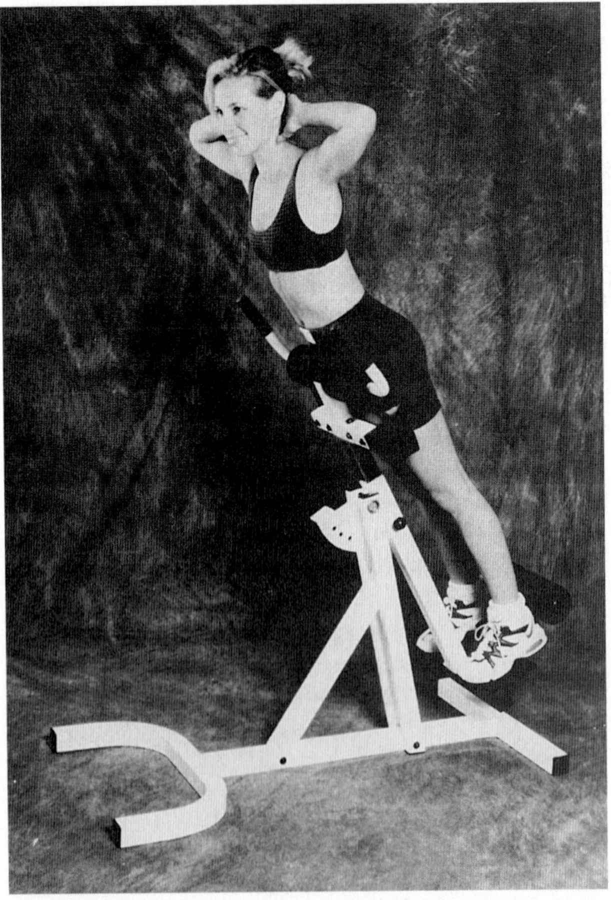

FIGURE 35–4. The variable angle Roman chair. The angle at which the subject performs exercises can be adjusted to go as far as horizontal, allowing for measurable functional gains.

NONSTRUCTURAL FACTORS

It is no surprise to any clinician involved with care of chronic low back pain that there are frequently psychological, social, and organizational factors that contribute to the chronic pain problem. Although this topic is addressed in detail in Chapter 19, these factors will be briefly addressed here for the benefit of the reader. These factors are summarized by what is called the "biopsychosocial model for chronic conditions." Melzack and Wall established this model with what is known as the "gate control theory of pain."[59] This theory points out that the pain message from injured tissue passes through multiple neurological gates. These gates can be opened or closed, or left partially opened, by psychological and motivational factors.

First there is the underlying personality, which involves one's coping strategies. In the centers treating severely chronic problems, personality disorders have been found to be as high as 59% of the patient population.[60] In this context, a personality disorder is indicative of long-standing maladaptive and inflexible behavior patterns that do not readily respond to attempts at intervention. When tested, these disorders are labeled hypochondriasis, depression, and hysteria. The interface of fear, pain, and anxiety with these personality disorders were demonstrated by an interesting study from Barnes et al.[61] In this study, the Minnesota Multiphasic Personality Inventory (MMPI) measure was administered to patients with chronic pain at the beginning of a rehabilitation program and then 6 months later. Prior to treatment, the elevated levels of the personality disorders were significant. Following 6 months of rehabilitation, most of these patients returned to work and their follow-up scores were brought to normal levels. Thus, even though an individual may have underlying personality disorder, in the appropriate context, that individual is treatable and may return to a normal life.

Clinical Pearl: Pain perception is modulated by one's thoughts and emotional experience, such as depression, anger, and anxiety. A clinician dealing with chronic back pain has to be aware of these factors.

The extreme deviation of personality disorders, labeled psychiatric disorders, are identified by various tests, organized and labeled with roman numerals. This system of classification is known as the *Diagnostic and Statistical Manual of Mental Disorders*.[62] To demonstrate how significant a factor these disorders might be, Polatin et al. evaluated patients at a multimodel nonoperative interdisciplinary treatment program for patients with chronic back pain.[60] In this study it was found that 77% of the patients in their lifetime could be diagnosed as having a psychiatric disorder, and 59% currently had a psychiatric disorder. The most significant findings from the study, however, were that 95% of those with previous histories of anxiety disorders experienced these symptoms *before* the onset of their back pain. Also, 54% of patients diagnosed with depression experienced their depression prior to their back pain. Of course, these statistics apply to individuals with the most severe chronicity and resistance to improvement. This paints a very complex picture of chronic pain disorders, leading one to wonder which condition, structural or emotional, precedes the other. A multidimensional program would be required to provide appropriate treatment for such complex cases.

Stress is certainly a factor in chronic pain complaints. In a recent study, Lampe et al. studied patients with chronic back pain whose pain had a clear organic etiology and also patients with back pain of unknown origin (nonorganic group).[63] Not surprisingly, significantly more members of the nonorganic group had at least one highly stressful event preceding the most recent episode of back pain. Also, these patients reported more exhaustion and difficulty in coping than their counterparts in the organic group. Stress seems to be associated with overload. *Overload* can be defined as a level of demand exceeding one's coping capacity, or ability to "deal with it." Increasing structure and predictability, improving one's ability to organize the present and anticipate the future, has been recognized as a mechanism for addressing stress. Such a method would appear to be logical as structure and predictability form the basis of establishing better control over one's life. These are factors important in an organized protocol-driven treatment program.

While this chapter is not designed to deeply delve into these issues, the authors cannot overemphasize their importance. Furthermore, the authors feel that ignoring or avoiding these issues for the patient with chronic back pain may interfere with a more complete or rapid recovery. Chronic back pain certainly results in significant personal stress, but also stress in the patient's family. This is related to financial concerns as well. In these situations the family can either reinforce disability and create dependent behaviors, or be too supportive and encourage positive behaviors. Family members' presence on the occasion of a treatment program may indeed be helpful.[64]

Clinical Pearl: Other factors related to, and somewhat intertwined with, personality and stress, of course, are the socioeconomic factors. These factors are represented by their place in society, family, and the workplace.

Occupational issues are certainly another important nonstructural factor for chronic back syndromes. The authors have found that a simple question on the intake questionnaire is one of the best predictors as to successful completion of a rehabilitation program. That question is simply "Do you like your job?" Those who say "no" may not respond to active treatment. Another predictor question is "Do you expect to be back at your job in 6 months?" A positive answer here is highly predictable of success. A third question may be "What is good and bad about your job?" This response may assist in exposing and resolving difficulties that were previously undetected or ignored. Certainly, job satisfaction is an important reason to resolve pain problems. Intertwined with that, however, is the entire compensation system. Compensation appears to effect frequency of reported injuries. Studies have shown that an increase in benefits results with an increase in number of claims and duration of claims.[65]

Interestingly, the physical demands of one's job are not typically the cause of an injury. In a study of patients with low back pain, Gatchel et al. isolated several potential etiological factors and discussed their influence on the development and predictability of chronic disability.[66] This study evaluated a large cohort of patients with acute low back pain within 6 weeks of acute back pain onset. They were then followed for 1 year and evaluated for various psychosocial variables to differentiate between those who returned to work and those did not. As expected, there was a high self-report of pain and disability and elevated hysteria scores on the MMPI for those who did not return to work. Also of interest, the diagnosis and its severity were found to be very poor predictors of chronicity, as were the physical demands of the job. In this study, the authors tested the strength of a healthy group of shipyard workers and followed them for 2 years. The authors found that even though this workplace registered in with high levels of physical stress, this was not ultimately a predictor of chronicity.[67] Of those who made claims of back pain in the 2-year follow-up, all demonstrated normal back strength at the time of initial testing. In fact, 10 of the 12 workers with back pain showed slightly stronger than average strength at initial testing.

The above discussion, however, brings up the important question of how to cope with significant issues of the biopsychosocial model. Some programs in the

United States have accepted this challenge, aggressively using a multidisciplinary approach.[68] These programs, while using the "sports medicine" model for the physical treatment, also intensely integrate psychological/psychiatric support. The patient/client is there all day—perhaps 5 ½ days per week, and the program typically lasts 3–4 weeks. Also, there is an intense preadmission indoctrination and postadmission follow-up program. Because of the high staff-to-patient ratio, they are necessarily expensive (over $25,000). But, as the PRIDE program in Dallas, TX, has demonstrated, it can successfully return high numbers of employees with disability back to work and effectively maintain their work status and productivity once they return.

For patients with chronic pain with significant emotional involvement, an even more comprehensive and intensive program is needed. Ideally, this should be an inpatient program with considerable psychosocial expertise among the members of the treating team. Such programs are known as tertiary treatment program centers.

Even the tertiary programs had significant dropout rates. In the original report from the intense PRIDE program, only about 55% of the original treatment group completed the program.[34] In the authors' experiences, with a less intense but more prolonged program involving less psychosocially impaired individuals, about a quarter of the 1025 patients in the study group dropped out. Causes included insufficient motivation to complete the program, as well as health insurance factors and travel problems.[30]

Clinical Pearl: The mechanism to identify appropriate patients for treatment in a tertiary treatment program involves determination of their motivation and willingness to participate in a program using active exercises.

It is difficult to derive an accurate comparison between these two types of programs—the intense program, all day long on a daily basis, versus the more typical program, an hour and a half two to three times a week program. The efficacy of these programs has to be measured, not only by the dropout rate, but also by other parameters of benefit. Return to work may not be the most critical parameter of evaluation owing to several interweaving factors, including job availability, age, vocational rehabilitation, work status prior to injury, etc., all of which can confound the reliability of this measure. Probably the most reliable measure is the rate of reutilization of the health-care system for the same complaint. *Reutilization* is defined as the percentage of individuals who resume treatment for the same condition. In the study of Mayer et al.[34] there was a 30% reutilization rate at 1 year. In the authors' center study, there was an 11% 1-year reutilization rate.[30] By contrast, a very careful study in North Carolina analyzed 269 individuals who reported persistent back pain with recurrence rate of 2.5 occasions during a 1-year period. This amounted to a reutilization rate of 73%, with 10% undergoing subsequent surgery.[69]

Indeed, this type of treatment program, which the lead authors use for chronic back pain, has demonstrated effectiveness in the only prospective randomized study comparing specific exercises with a non-treatment group.[70] In this study, 54 patients with chronic low back pain were randomly assigned to a 10-week exercise program similar to our program or were placed on a waiting list. They all underwent psychological testing as well. In this study, the exercise program was carried out twice weekly for 4 weeks and then once weekly for 6 weeks. The exercise program was successful in relieving back pain, while the control group was not. In follow-up, the psychological testing improved in those who were in the exercise group, but deteriorated in those who were not. This study demonstrated not only the efficacy of exercise, but also the positive psychological impact of an exercise program. The participants in this program were significantly disabled with back pain of 85 months' duration, and were out of work for 24 months on average.

What are the mechanisms for predicting successful outcomes among potential participants in an active exercise program? Even more important, how does one predict those who will return to gainful activity?

FUNCTIONAL CAPACITY AND MOTIVATIONAL TESTING

A small percentage of patients willfully mislead the examiner for secondary gain. Such cases are usually apparent on initial evaluation in that the claimant demonstrates an inability to carryout any significant activity. The authors have found that this false behavior can be documented on MedX equipment by varying the feedback to the patient. The amount resistance can be changed, but its feedback on the screen that the patient is watching appears to be the same. Those who are truly dishonest will attempt to recreate their outcomes with each attempt, thus confirming their lack of honesty because their outcomes should vary as the resistance levels vary.[71] Such dishonesty is unusual, and the need to carry out this type of measuring is usually to document increased patient performance and ultimately substantiate the appropriate discharge of the patient.

A much more important reason for testing is to assess the individual's perception of disability-associated abnormal illness behavior, such as anxiety and fear. These problems are frequently treatable in an active rehabilitation setting. A standardized evaluation scheme was developed, initially identified as the CAL-FCP, to determine abnormal illness behavior cases.[72] The CAL-FCP is in the process of being converted into a computer-based test known as the Multidimensional Task Ability Profile. (MTAP)

The unique feature of the CAL-FCP is that the patient is allowed to state their believed physical capacity. This is done by a series of comparable photographs of individuals carrying out normal daily activities and also during specific physical testing maneuvers. The pictures are graded by the patient on a scale of 1 to 5, with the numbers corresponding to whether they can perform the activity or not, or do not know. The pictures also display activities with varying degrees of physical demand[73] (Fig. 35–5). Scoring of the pictures can be translated to the five levels of physical demand known as the Physical Demand Characteristics, which is currently used by many states as a disability measure.[74]

In addition to this pen and paper test is the CAL-FCP test, a measure that contains a health questionnaire and a job demand questionnaire. The purpose of this questionnaire is to provide information about the evaluee's perception of job demands against which the performance of later tests can be compared. In addition, this questionnaire extends the time of the evaluee's seated activity in order to evaluate their tolerance level. The questionnaire phase of the test should take about an hour to complete, which is an excellent measure to evaluate sitting capacity.

Lateral pinch test and power grip tests are done with appropriate dynamometers. A standing range of motion is then evaluated in the Cal-FCP test. The lift capacity test is carried out by a system known as the EPIC Lift Capacity test (ELC).[75] In this test, blinded weights are lifted in a standardized manner to heights relative to the height of the individual (Fig. 35–6). Heart rate is monitored during this test to assure cardiac safety standards. Next, a carrying test is accomplished, where the individual carries varying weights (blinded) over a 100-ft course. The evaluee performs a stair-climbing test carrying a blinded weight while stepping up and down on an 8-in step for 15 repetitions.

The combination of all these tests results in an effort rating. The series of 50 pictures (Spinal Function Sort) have several pictures displaying the same physical effort, but portrayed in a different manner. This can help to determine inconsistency in the patient's perceived abilities to perform work. Then, the relationship between perceived physical capacities, determined by the Spinal Function Sort, can be compared to the actual achievement in the ELC test. Normally, these two tests should have a similar rating. The ELC test should demonstrate an increase in heart rate commensurate with the physical demands. If the heart rate does not elevate, one can assume no serious effort is being made. For the pinch and grip test where the achievement is likewise blinded, consistency of outcomes is also evaluated. After all of these evaluations are completed, the clinician/technician then assigns a three-level effort rating to the patient: reliable effort, questionable effort, or unreliable effort.

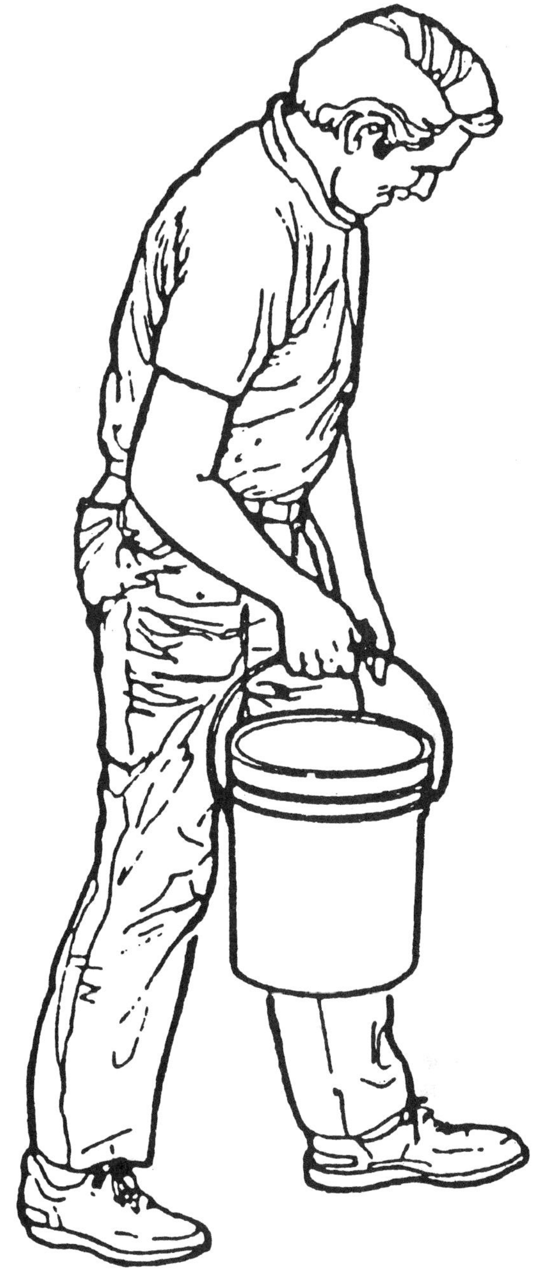

FIGURE 35–5. A drawing on the Spinal Function Sort demonstrating physical activity.

As noted above, the role of functional capacity testing is not only to identify an individual's reliability and willingness to participate in an active exercise

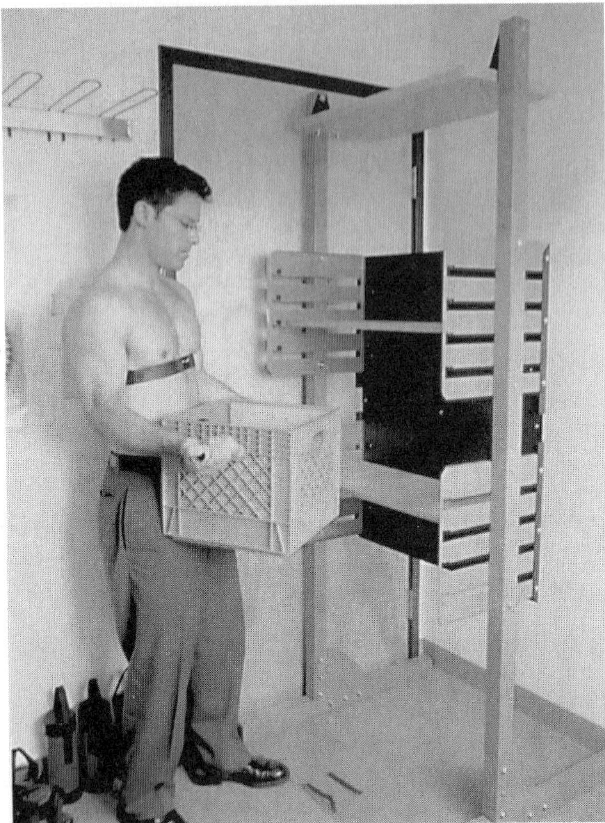

FIGURE 35–6. The EPIC Lift Capacity test demonstrating the subject lifting blinded weights to heights that are adjusted according to the individual's height. Note that the heart rate is monitored.

program, but also to establish a level of work capacity and level of impairment/disability following the completion of a rehabilitation program. Most of the patients being treated are involved with return-to-work issues or questions regarding permanent disability. The benefit of the CAL-FCP test is that it does address disability issues. Disability, as opposed to impairment, refers to the capacity to carry out work activity, social activity including sports, and self-care. Impairment merely implies the physical limitation without implication of how that deters the individual from normal human activity. Thus, the CAL-FCP also evaluates the degree of pain in terms of severe, moderate, slight, and minimal, while pain frequency is defined as constant, frequent, intermittent, and occasional. These are the specific adjectives required for rating in California, but can be generalized to adapt to other systems as well. Certainly a reasonable goal for any rehabilitation program, especially as applied to the injured worker, would be to return to work in as high a degree of function as possible.

Clinical Pearl: By actually testing lifting capacity, as well as carrying capacity, a clear statement can be made as to an individual's job status when compared to the description of the job to which they intend to return.

PROTOCOL FOR TREATMENT OF CHRONIC RECURRENT BACK PAIN

The underlying philosophy of treatment is that physical restoration is the goal. As noted above, there is good evidence that chronic recurrent problems create functional deficits such as weakness and associated stiffness, and tissue incompetence.[30,34,37] Also, there is no doubt that, in most cases, significant psychological aspects interweave with the chronic pain problem.

The lead authors expect that because their multidisciplinary approach is based on a physical training program, at least 6–8 weeks will be required to achieve the training effect. In explaining this model to both payers and patients, the following analogous scenario is presented: High-caliber athletes prepare to play for professional sports by attending "training camp" at least 6 weeks before their particular season begins. Part of the training is conditioning, even for these gifted and extraordinarily well-conditioned individuals.

It is important to communicate to both the patient and the payer that the "sports medicine" model necessitates the utilization of exercise equipment. The authors point out that if the patient were an injured professional athlete, he or she would be referred to the team's athletic trainer. Indeed, the athlete would be supervised using specialized exercise equipment. They would not simply be placed on a home program alone. They would not just receive passive care in the form of ultrasound, massage, or even manipulation. The treatment they would receive is called physical training, not physical therapy. If there were a more efficient way to treat these valuable athletes, who are essentially injured workers who have suffered an on-the-job trauma, the team owners would certainly use such an approach. The same attitude should be applied to the industrial athlete: injured workers.

The equipment and tools mentioned above allow the authors to identify a patient's baseline deficits and to monitor progress. One of the most important psychological benefits of equipment is the unbiased nature of feedback to the patient. Their performance is objectively measured and cannot be hidden or falsified. Thus, all involved, including therapists, physicians, payers, and certainly the patient, are aware of their progress, or lack thereof. Certainly for the chronic recurrent condition, sudden resolution of pain is not to be expected. Nonetheless, there is the appreciation that the exercise therapy program is improving function without increasing pain, which can be a very positive motivator for the patient. In this manner, the tentative, anxious patient can be encouraged to continue the program.

Clinical Pearl: Another important aspect of utilizing exercise equipment is the feedback of improved performance in spite of continued discomfort. This can be a powerful approach to combat illness behavior, as the patient learns to focus primarily on function rather than pain.

Another aspect of a training program is the avoidance of overtraining. True resistance exercise requires rest periods of at least 1 day between each strenuous exercise event. Consequently, the training schedule is two to three times a week. The patient should also return to some modified duty at work as quickly as possible to avoid habituation to disability and minimize deconditioning.

One final aspect of a progressive training program carried out by knowledgeable clinicians is the positive perception of exercise itself. Certainly there is nothing mystical about a graded exercise program. Exercise is medicinal for mental, cardiovascular, metabolic, and musculoskeletal conditions. This perception of the benefits of exercise is an important aspect in successful treatment.

Recently, an interesting paper comparing the efficacy of acupuncture to that of massage was published.[76] In this study, these two passive modes of care were provided to 135 patients in a random manner. The patients were also queried as to their expectation of efficacy from either acupuncture or massage. Although it is no surprise, this paper documented patients who had a positive attitude toward either acupuncture or massage prior to treatment fared much better with either form of treatment than those who had a negative view. This study provides an excellent example of the *placebo* and *nocebo* phenomena. Thus, a treatment program should be provided with the expectation, by both the therapist and the patient, that it will be successful. A positive attitude by all involved is extremely important in determining the ultimate success of that program. Patients with a persistently negative attitude may even have to be sequestered in their treatment programs in order to avoid negatively affecting other patients undergoing simultaneous treatment.

Clinical Pearl: Placebo represents the well-known "Pavlovian"conditioned responses activated by positive anticipation of healing. Nocebo is the lesser known opposite effect, creating negative expectations about symptoms that can have a devastating effect on patient recovery.[77,78]

STANDARDIZED TREATMENT PROTOCOLS

Measurement Driven Rehabilitation Systems, Inc. (MDRS) has developed a multidisciplinary, common sense treatment approach for musculoskeletal injuries. The MDRS approach consists of four phases of treatment, a model that mimics the standardized model used in cardiac rehabilitation by cardiologists worldwide. All phases of care center on an active approach to the treatment of spinal and extremity injuries, which is guided by focusing on function rather than pain, inactivity, and/or intolerance. These phases are intended to provide general treatment guidelines, including goal criteria and time lines in order to assure efficient progression of all treatment programs.

MDRS Phase I Rehabilitation: Acute Nonmovement Directional Treatment

Phase I is intended for the acute/subacute injury. The goals of the treatment techniques are to reduce pain and inflammation, promote movement, increase patient knowledge, and allow for further evaluation. Phase I patients typically do not benefit from a specific movement pattern (e.g., do not centralize, but may peripheralize according to McKenzie principles explained in Chapters 15 and 22), which decreases symptoms and improves function. Thus, Phase I mainly is a hands-on/palliative approach, which uses therapeutic modalities, soft tissue and joint mobilization/manipulation, further evaluation of movement patterns, home exercise programs, patient education, and/or low intensity lumbar stabilization exercises. These lumbar stabilization exercises are designed to activate the multifidus, transverse abdominis, and quadratus lumborum muscles in a low-grade manner as per the protocols described by Hides et al.[16] If a clear improvement is attained within 2 weeks of Phase I care, the patient is progressed to Phase II. If no clear improvement is demonstrated after 2 weeks of palliative care in Phase I, the patient is progressed to Phase III.

To summarize, Phase I includes the following clinical tools:

1. Therapeutic modalities
2. Soft tissue mobilization and manipulation
3. Further evaluation and movement pattern exploration according to McKenzie principles (discussed in Chapters 15 and 22)
4. Low-intensity lumbar stabilization exercises
5. Patient education
6. Home exercise program

MDRS Phase II Rehabilitation: Movement-Directed Treatment

When a specific movement pattern is found to decrease symptoms and/or improve function, the patient progresses to Phase II. In Phase II, a clear beneficial movement pattern is established, allowing movement-specific treatment for the patient. The treatment principles of Phase II involve movement-directed progression of range of movement force. Thus, the goal of Phase II is to promote symptom and functional improvement through well-directed, specific movement patterns. This rehabilitation includes utilization of McKenzie end-range loading movement patterns, activation of the intrinsic lumbar muscles, and/or joint-specific manipulation (Fig. 35–7). If the patient remains symptomatic following 6 weeks of combined Phase I and II treatment, the patient is progressed to Phase III.

To summarize, Phase II includes the following clinical tools:

- Progressive resistive exercises
- Progressive aerobic exercises
- Lumbar stabilization exercises
- Manipulation
- Patient education
- Home exercise programs

MDRS Phase III Rehabilitation: Isolated Strength and Functional Restoration

Phase III activities promote increased isolated strength and general conditioning, along with a gradual progression of functional ability. This phase is essential if the medical history indicates a significant pattern of recurrence, if symptoms persist for greater than 6 weeks from injury, or a significant loss of strength or function has been noted. The target at this phase involves the gradual correction of the weak link. By the end of this phase, treatment should emphasize activities that promote achievement of functional goals. Throughout this phase, objective data regarding strength and function are collected periodically to provide justification for continuation or discontinuation of treatment. Documentation of both objective progression and reliable patient effort must be evident in order to justify the progression of treatment. Phase III treatment principles mainly involve movement-directed progressive increases in range of motion (ROM) and force production (FORCE) of functional movements. Gradual endurance conditioning of trunk musculature, isolated progressive resistive exercise, aerobic exercises, patient education, and home exercise are also included. Phase III is complete when a patient reaches a plateau in functional improvement demonstrated by the objective tests, such as isometric lumbar extension strength, functional capacity evaluation, and trunk extension endurance (Biering–Sorensen test). In addition, if a patient demonstrates an unreliable effort or noncompliance during objective tests, the program is discontinued and the patient is discharged from care.

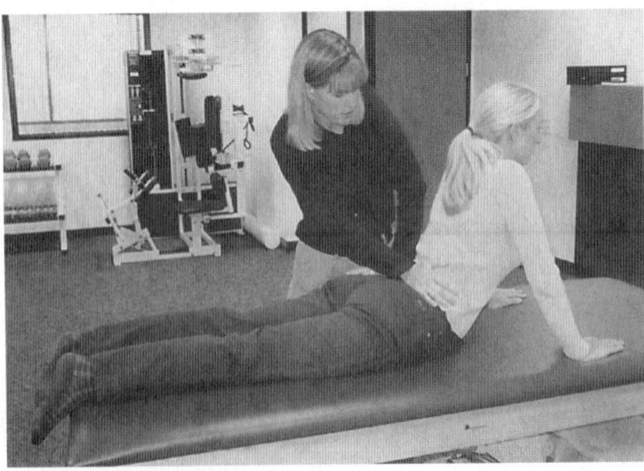

FIGURE 35–7. Clinician carrying out McKenzie training for treatment of the low back.

To summarize, Phase III includes the following clinical tools:

1. Isolated strengthening and endurance exercises for the lumbar extensors
2. Restoration of functional movements
3. Movement-directed progression ROM and FORCE
4. Clinic-simulated or on-site activities of daily living
5. Progressive resistive exercise
6. Progressive aerobic exercise
7. Lumbopelvic stabilization exercises
8. Patient education
9. Home exercise program

MDRS Phase IV: Maintenance and On-Site Programs

The final MDRS phase for each case can vary greatly, depending on the patient's needs, goals, functional capacity, and resources. The chief goal of this phase is to reinforce the patient's independence and provide a safe and reliable return to function. Achieving independence shows more permanent improvement in the patient's function and a positive change in overall lifestyle. This phase may include work-site visits, maintenance programs at local fitness clubs, home, or sport-specific exercise program. Phase IV is typically not performed in the clinic, but rather in a gym, at a work site, home, or athletic field environment.

Patient Education

MDRS provides a large educational component in all phases of the treatment programs. It is crucial that all patients understand the etiology of their problem and also what would be required to maintain the benefits of the program. It is the responsibility of each clinical staff member to ensure that patients are educated properly regarding their condition and treatment program. In many clinical cases, educational videotapes are available to reinforce patient knowledge. The first section of the tape discusses back conditions specifically in terms of anatomy and physiology. The second section focuses on rehabilitation, the pain cycle, stress management, or any lifestyle factors that the patient may want to incorporate into his or her program. The third section examines proper posture and body mechanics. The fourth and final section discusses specific exercise the patient should be responsible for completing during and after rehabilitation to ensure a rapid recovery while minimizing risk of recurrence.

It should be emphasized that the patient is treated in the clinic for approximately 2%–3% of their total week. This is simply not a sufficient period of time to enable a complete recovery of chronic back syndrome. Patients are therefore expected to be involved in a home exercise program that is progressively increased with each visit. This home exercise program should begin to develop during the first week of treatment. By the third week, the therapist should commence discussing home or alternative exercise facilities that would allow a continuation of conditioning following discharge from treatment. By the time the therapy is reduced to a frequency of once per week, the patient should have established an alternative means to sustain the general conditioning program that was initiated in the clinic. These exercises can be performed at home, in a private health facility, or through MDRS clinic base maintenance programs. Any of these options may be effective, but the best choice for each patient depends on individual needs, time, and resources.

The Team Concept

The lead authors use a multiprofessional model in which patients with spine-related diagnoses are evaluated by physical therapists, chiropractors, and exercise physiologists. Since this team-based evaluation and treatment approach differs from traditional clinics, it is imperative to provide a clear explanation of the strategy to the patient. Dialog with the patient should include an explanation of how a team approach provides a multifaceted degree of expertise on each case. This explanation includes the credentials and clinical roles of each patient care team member. The patient care team supervisor (a licensed provider) is identified and the patient is informed that the supervisor will decide whose expertise on the team is most appropriate to guide the patient through the different phases of their treatment program. These evaluations are standardized, using McKenzie evaluation, diagnosis, and management for the cervical, thoracic, and lumbar spine. McKenzie protocol forms, specific to each spinal region, are used to document the results of the mechanical evaluation. These forms provide a degree of inter-examiner standardization and communication between the disciplines employed at MDRS.

CONCLUSION

Chronic, disabling low back pain is an epidemic of the industrialized world. While there are many intervening factors summarized by the term "psychosocial" (implying that not all back pain is structural), structural abnormalities must still be treated in a rationale manner. The most effective approaches can only be demonstrated by measuring the dose of accepted treatment options and the ensuing effect on symptoms and function. In the model prepared here, active exercise, which is easily definable and quantifiable, is the centerpiece of physical rehabilitation.

SUMMARY

1. This chapter presented a multimodal model for the treatment of chronic back syndromes.
2. After appropriate assessment and functional outcomes measures are obtained, treatment can proceed with numerous available options. In short, these include manual procedures, medications, counseling, and exercises.
3. One of the most commonly used manual procedures is spinal manipulative therapy (SMT), a subject that is discussed at length in three other chapters of this textbook. Clinicians typically explain to the patient that SMT is designed to assist and restore normal spinal biomechanics while simultaneously reducing pain. Because it is a passive procedure, SMT should be a part of a program that also includes remedial exercises.
4. Another passive clinical tool is medication. Utilization guidelines for medication are covered in another chapter, but a remedial exercise program must be integrated into this approach also. The risks associated with prolonged utilization of medication, such as morbidity and mortality, must always be taken into consideration.
5. In conjunction with the passive strategies to reduce pain such as manipulation and medication, active care must also be integrated in the form of supervised and independent exercise.
6. Home active programs that explore "end-ranging" and promote independent exercise will be prescribed long-term.
7. From the initial visit the doctor must educate the patient regarding function, emphasizing independent active care rather than symptomatic relief. The locus of control must be placed on the patient by empowering them with activity-based

treatment strategies and tools to help them achieve independence.

8. Continued education regarding best self-care and independence from treatment needs to be encouraged throughout the patient's care and exercise program.
9. The overall goal of treatment is improved function as well as pain reduction.
10. Inherent in this program is the establishment of a baseline level of spinal function (e.g., range of motion, strength, endurance, sitting tolerance, Spinal Function Sort), periodic reevaluations of this function to monitor progress, and a final assessment at the conclusion of treatment to demonstrate improvement.

REFERENCES

1. Statistics NCfH. *Prevalence of selected impairments.* Hyattsville, MD: National Center for Health Statistics, 1981.
2. Pope M, Frymoyer J, Andersson G. *Occupational low back pain.* New York: Praegar Scientific, 1984.
3. Mooney V, Cairns D. Management in the patient with clinical low back pain. *Orthop Clin North Am* 1978;9:543–547.
4. LeBlanc F. Quebec Task Force on Spinal Disorders: Scientific approach to the assessment and management of activity related spinal disorders. A monograph for physicians. *Spine* 1987;12(Suppl):1–59.
5. Nachemson A. Work for all: For those with low back pain as well. *Clin Orthop* 1983;179–182.
6. Nachemson A. The lumbar spine: An orthopedic challenge. *Spine* 1976;2:59–72.
7. Nachemson A. The newest knowledge of low back pain: A critical look. *Clin Orthop* 1992;270:8–20.
8. Nachemson A, Bigos S. *The low back. Adult orthopedics.* New York: Churchill Livingstone, 1984:843–937.
9. Spengler D, Bigos S, Martin N, She J, Fisher L. Back injury in industry: A restrospective study. *Spine* 1986; 11(3):241–245.
10. Kirkaldy-Willis W, Burton C, Cassidy J. *Managing low back pain*, 2nd ed. New York: Churchill Livingstone, 1988.
11. Rohrer M, Santos-Eggimann B, Paccaud F, Haller-Maslov E. Epidemiologic study of low back pain in 1,398 swiss conscripts between 1985 and 1992. *Eur Spine J* 1998;3(1):2–7.
12. Frymoyer J. Back pain and sciatica. *NEJM* 1988;318: 291–300.
13. Bigos S, Bowyer O, Braen G, et al. Acure low back pain problems in adults: Assessment and treatment. *Clinical Practice Guideline, Quick Reference Guide*, Vol. 14. Rockville, MD: US Department of Health and Human Services, Public Health Service; Agency for Health Care Policy and Research, 1994.
14. Andersson G, Svensson H, Od'en A. The intensity of work recovery in low back pain. *Spine* 1983;8(8, Nov–Dec):880–884.
15. Croft P, McFarlane G, Papegeorgiou A, Thomas E, Silman A. Outcome of low back pain in general practice: A prospective study. *BMJ* 1998;316:1356–1359.
16. Hides J, Richardson C, Jull G, Hodges P. *Therapeutic exercise for spinal segmental stabilization in low back pain: Scientific basis and clinical approach*,1st ed. United Kingdom: Churchill Livingstone, 1999.
17. Shekelle P, et al. Validation of the Agency for Health Care Policy and Research guidelines: How quickly do guidelines become outdated? *JAMA* 2002;286(12): 1461–1467.
18. Browman G. Development and aftercare of clinical guidelines: The balance between rigor and pragmatism. *JAMA* 2001;286(12):1509–1511.
19. Haen K, Hilde G, Jantveldt G, Winnen M. The Cochrane review of bed rest for acute low back pain and sciatica. *Spine* 2000;25(22):2932–2939.
20. Robertson V, Baker K. A review of therapeutic ultrasound: Effectiveness studies. *Phys Ther* 2001;81:339–350.
21. Saltin B, Blomqvist G, Mitchell J, Johnson R, Wildenthal K, Chapman C. Response to exercise after bed rest and after training. *Circulation* 1968;38(Suppl):1–78.
22. State of Florida AfHCA, University of Florida. Patients with low back pain or injury: Medical practive guidelines. *J Back Musculoskeletal Rehabil* 1999;12(1):35–65.
23. California Worker's Compensation Official Medical Fee Schedule. Division of Workers' Compensation, Division of Industrial Relations. State of California, 1999.
24. Hides J, Stakes M, Saide M, Jull G, Cooper D. Evidence of lumbar multifidus muscle wasting ipislateral to symptoms in patients with acute/subacute low back pain. *Spine* 1994;19(2):165–172.
25. Biering-Soresnen F. Physical measurements as risk indicators for low back trouble over a one-year period. *Spine* 1984;9(2):106–119.
26. Battie M, Bogos S, Fisher L. Isometric lifting strength as a predictor of industrial back pain reports. *Spine* 1989;14:851–856.
27. Newton M, Thow M, Somerville D, Henderson I, Waddell G. Trunk strength testing with iso-machines. Part 2. Experimental evaluation of the Cybex II back testing system in normal subjects and patients with chronic low back pain. *Spine* 1993;18(7):812–824.
28. Nelson B, O'Reilly E, Miller M, Hogan M, Wagner J, Kelly C. The clinical effects of intensive, specific exercise on chronic low back pain: A controlled study of 895 consecutive patients with 1-year follow-up. *Orthopedics* 1995;18(10):971–981.
29. McGill S. Evidence for improving exercise regimens. *Phys Ther* 1998;78:754–765.
30. Leggett S, Mooney V, Nelson B, Dreisinger T, Van Zytveld J, Vie L. Restorative exercise for clinical low back pain: A prospective two-center study with 1 year follow-up. *Spine* 1999;24(9):889–898.
31. Mooney V, Gulick J, Pearlman M, et al. Relationships between myoelectric activity, strength and MRI of lumbar extensor muscles in back pain patients and normal subjects. *J Spine Disord* 1997;10(4):348–356.
32. Mayer T. Orthopedic conservative care: The functional restoration approach. *Spine* 1986;10(4):348–356.

33. Mayer T, Gatchel R, Kishino N, et al. Objective assessment of spine function following industrial injury: A prospective study with comparison group and one-year follow-up. *Spine* 1985;10(6):1762–1769.
34. Mayer T, Gatchel R, Mayer H, Kishino N, Keeley J, Mooney V. A prospective two-year study of functional restoration in industrial low back injury: An objective assessment procedure. *JAMA* 1987;258(13):1763–1768.
35. Mitchell R, Carmen G. The functional restoration approach to the treatment of chronic pain in patients with soft tissue and back injuries. *Spine* 1994;19:623–644.
36. Manniche C, Christensen I, Benmtzen L, Hesselhoe G. Intensive dynamic exercises for chronic low back pain clinical trial. *Pain* 1991;47:53–63.
37. Hazard R, Fenwick J, Kalish S, et al. Functional restoration with behavioral support: A one-year perspective study of chronic low back pain patients. *Spine* 1989;14:157–165.
38. Mooney V, Saal J, Saal J. Clinical symposia—Evaluation and treatment of low back pain. *CIBA* 1996;48(4):1–36.
39. Kitano T, Zerwekh J, Usui Y, Edwards M, Flicker P, Mooney V. Biochemical changes associated with the symptomatic human intervertebral disc. *Clin Orthop Rel Res* 1993;293:372–377.
40. Hides J, Richardson C, Jull G. Multifidus muscle recovery is not automatic following resolution of acute first episode low back pain. *Spine* 1996;21:2763–2769.
41. Hodges P, Richardson C. Relationship between limb movement speed and associated contraction of trunk muscles. *Ergonomics* 1997;40:1220–1230.
42. Hodges P, Richardson C. Delayed postural contraction of transversus abdominis in low back pain associated with movement of the lower limbs. *J Spinal Disord* 1998; 11:46–56.
43. McKenzie R. *Treat your own back*. Waikaniae, New Zealand: Spinal Publications, 1980.
44. Parkkola R, Rytokoski R, Korman O. Magnetic resonance imaging of the disc and trunk muscles in patients with chronic low back pain and healthy subjects. *Spine* 1993;18:830–836.
45. Alaranta H, Tallroth K, Soukka A, Heliovaara M. Fat content in lumbar extensor muscles and low back disability: A radiographic and clinical comparison. *J Spinal Disord* 1993;6:137–140.
46. Mayer T, Vanharanto H, Gatchal R. A comparison of CT muscle measurements and isokinetic strength in post-operative patients. *Spine* 14(1):33–36.
47. Robinson M, Cassisi J, O'Connor P, McMillan N. Lumbar EMG during isotonic exercise: Chronic low back pain patients versus controls. *J Spinal Disord* 1992;5: 8–15.
48. Robinson M, Cassisi J, O'Connor P. Reliability of lumbar isometric torque in patients with chronic low back pain. *Phys Ther* 1992;72:186–190.
49. Ross E, Parianpour M. The effect of resistance level on muscle coordination patterns and movement profiled during trunk extension. *Spine* 1993;18:1829–1838.
50. Bruce R, McDonough J. Stress testing in screening for cardiovascular disease. *Acad Med (U.S.)* 1969;45:1288–1305.
51. Graves J, Webb D, Pollick M, et al. Pelvic stabilization during resistance training: Its effect on the development of lumbar extension strength. *Arch Phys Med Rehabil* 1994;75(2):210–215.
52. Mayer T, Gatchel R, Kishino N, et al. A prospective short-term study of chronic low back pain patients utlizing novel objective functional measurement. *Pain* 1986;25:53–68.
53. Graves J, Pollock M, Carpenter D, et al. Quantitative assessment of full range of motion isometric lumbar extension strength. *Spine* 1990;15:289–294.
54. Mooney V. Physical measurements of the lumbar spine. *Phys Med Rehab Clin North Am* 1998;9(2):391–410.
55. Newton M, Waddell G. Trunk strength testing with iso-machines. Part 1. Review of a decade of scientific evidence. *Spine* 1993;18(7):801–811.
56. Mayer J, Graves J, Li Y, Udermann B, Ploutz-Snyder L. Specificity of training and isolated lumbar extension strength. *Med Sci Sports Exer Suppl* 1998;30(5):206S.
57. Mayer J, Graves J, Udermann B, Ploutz-Snyder L. Development of lumbar extension strength: Effect of pelvic stabilization during resistance training. *J Back Musculoskel Rehab* 2002;16(1):25–31.
58. Mayer J, Graves J, Robertson V, Verna J, Pierra E, Ploutz-Snyder L. Electromyographic activity of the lumbar extensor muscles: The effect of angle and hand position during roman chair exercise. *Arch Phys Med Rehabil* 1999;80(7):751–755.
59. Melzack R, Wall P. Pain mechanisms: A new theory. *Science* 1965;150:971–979.
60. Polatin P, Kinney R, Gatchel R, Lillo E, Mayer T. Psychiatric illness and chronic low back pain. *Spine* 1993;18:66–71.
61. Barnes D, Gatchel R, Mayer T, Barnett J. Changes in the MMPI profile levels of chronic low back pain patients following successful rehabilitation. *J Spinal Disord* 1990;3:353–355.
62. American Psychiatric Association. *Diagnostic and statistical manual of mental disorders (DSM-III-R)*. Washington, DC: American Psychiatric Association, 1987.
63. Lampe A, Sollner W, Krismer M, et al. The impact of stressful life events on exacerbation of chronic low back pain. *J Psychosom Res* 1998;44:555–563.
64. Turk D, Flor H, Rudy T. Pain and families. 1. Etiology, maintenance, and psychosocial impact. *Pain* 1987;30:3–27.
65. Worrall J, Appel D. The impact of workers' compensation benefits on low back claims. In: Hadler N, ed. *Clinical concepts in regional musculoskeletal illness.* New York: Grun and Stratton, 1987:281–297.
66. Gatchel R, Polatin P, Mayer T. The dominant role of psychosocial risk factors in the development of chronic low back pain disability. *Spine* 1995;20:2702–2709.
67. Mooney V, Kenney D, Leggett S, Holmes B. Relationship of lumbar strength in shipyard workers to workplace injury claims. *Spine* 1996;21(17):2001–2005.
68. Mayer T, Polatin P. Tertiary nonoperative interdisciplinary programs. The functional restoration variant of the outpatient chronic pain management program. In: Mayer, TG, Gatchal R., ed. *Occupational musculoskeletal disorders*. Philadelphia: Lippincott Williams & Wilkins, 2000:Chapt. 36, 639–649.

69. Carey T, Evans A, Hadler N, et al. Care seeking among individuals with chronic low back pain. *Spine* 1995;20:312–317.
70. Risch S, Norvell N, Pollock M, et al. Lumbar strengthening in chronic low back pain patients: Physiologic and psychological benefits. *Spine* 1993;18:232–238.
71. Mooney V, Leggett S, Holmes B, Negri S. Strength testing can identify malingering. *J Workers Compens* 1992; 2(1):55–64.
72. Matheson L, Mooney V, Grant J, Leggett S, Kenny K. Stadardized evaluation of work capacity. *J Back Musculoskeletal Rehabil* 1996;6:249–265.
73. Matheson L, Matheson M, Grant J. Development of a measure of perceived functional ability. *J Occup Rehabil* 1993;3(1):15–30.
74. World Health Organization. *International classification of impairments, disabilities and handicaps*. Geneva: World Health Organization, 1980.
75. Matheson L. Effects of age, gender and body mass on lift capacity. *J Occup Rehabil* 1996;6(4):26–30.
76. Kalauokalani D, Cherkin D, Sherman K, Koepsell T, Deyo R. Lessons from a trial of acupuncture and massage for low back pain: Patient expectations and treatment effects. *Spine* 2001;26(13):1418–1424.
77. Kasdan ML, Lewis K, Bruner A, Johnson AL. The nocebo effect: Do no harm. *J S Orthop Assoc* Summer 1999; 8(2):108–113.
78. Barsky AJ, Saintfort R, Rogers MP, Borus JF. Nonspecific medication side effects and the nocebo phenomenon. *JAMA* February 6, 2002;287(5):622–627.

CHAPTER

36

RISK MANAGEMENT FOR LOW BACK SYNDROMES

James Kutz, David Chapman-Smith, and Craig E. Morris

OUTLINE

OBJECTIVES

1. Describe the professional risk involved in clinical practice.
2. Describe strategies to minimize the risks as part of an overall management program.
3. Explain the issues associated with mal practice.
4. Explain the issues associated with sexual misconduct.
5. Explain the importance of informed consent and provide examples to implement this into clinical practice.

INTRODUCTION

A 45-year-old legal secretary was receiving physical therapy at a hospital for low back pain. After the therapy was completed, she was told she could leave. Getting off the table, the woman fell. According to her, the therapist was negligent for leaving a cord over her legs, for not lowering the table, and for not assisting her off the table. The therapist denied that there was a cord over the secretary's legs and did not believe that the grown woman required assistance from the table. Although the jury found the therapist to be 30% negligent, the defendant's portion of the verdict returned by the jury was $555,534.00![1] Five seconds, or even less, of additional time simply assisting the patient off of the table would probably have avoided that verdict.

The term "risk management" is common among North American clinicians. Far too often, however, the concept is relegated to a second-tier consideration, presumably addressed by securing errors and omissions insurance, also known as professional liability or malpractice insurance. Unfortunately, as important as risk management has been in the past, it is of even greater significance today. This is true internationally, with claims rates and litigation proliferating for chiropractors and all health professionals in Europe, Australia, and Asia. A decade ago it was almost unheard of for a clinician to be sued for malpractice in Japan or Latin America—but not today.

Health-care providers around the world should be aware that this is a reflection of an evolving change in social attitudes as to the respective rights of health professionals and patients. An era of paternalism, reflected in the expression "the physician knows best," has been supplanted by an era that places emphasis on patient and consumer rights. Many countries have recently passed into law a patient bill of rights dealing with areas such as rights to information on alternative treatment options, informed consent, confidentiality and privacy, appropriate and skilled treatment, and respect for the dignity of patients and their family, cultural, and religious concerns as these have an impact on healing and health care. For example, a March 1994 meeting of the World Health Organization Regional Office for Europe, held in Amsterdam and hosted by the Netherlands, was attended by representatives of 36 European countries and produced a detailed Declaration on the Promotion of Patients' Rights in Europe which covered all the above-mentioned rights in detail.[2]

Therefore, although the primary focus of this chapter is the practitioner's need to minimize the risk from claims of wrongful conduct (i.e., malpractice), risk management today encompasses other important considerations that deserve at least a brief discussion. In addition, although this publication deals primarily with the conservative management of low back syndromes, the risk management factors discussed here are essentially universal in their application—that is, they apply to all conditions managed and all treatment methods utilized.

Finally, there is a positive side to risk management. This is that it leads to improved standards of care and enhances patient satisfaction and one's reputation in practice. Satisfying the requirements of informed consent means that, for example, in the event that a patient suffers vertebral artery dissection, stroke, and permanent paralysis following manual treatment, a rare event but one experienced by a number of manual care clinicians giving perfectly competent care, the clinician will find some solace in knowing the patient was informed and aware of this remote risk.

WHAT ARE THE RISKS THAT NEED TO BE MANAGED?

Any practitioner treating patients needs to address a number of different risks. For example, practitioners face the risk of licensure sanctions from their regulatory board. They run the risk of performing valuable, expensive services, only to be denied reimbursement by some third-party payer. Practitioners run the risk of losing eligibility to participate in managed care organizations or to serve as participating providers. Every day there is the risk of being subject to criminal and other sanctions imposed by those who regulate the health-care industry, including government investigators whose special job is to ensure that there has been no irregularity in, for example, billing practices. Unless they practice alone (without any supporting staff), practitioners run the risk of being held liable for the neglectful and/or improper acts of their professional corporations, the acts of their partners, and the acts of staff or auxiliary personnel. Practitioners also run the risk of losing their esteemed professional reputations when they become the subject of some investigation, licensure charge, expulsion from managed care programs, or even worse, publicity associated with unproven allegations of professional malpractice.

The practitioner must zealously address each of these issues in order to minimize claims of professional malpractice. Indeed practitioners who lose their professional licenses to their regulatory board or find themselves subject to criminal sanction for fraud billing need not worry about professional malpractice. This is for the simple reason that they will find themselves precluded from practicing their chosen profession by reason of that conviction or regulatory discipline. Thus, the remainder of this chapter will focus upon the more commonly recognized and discussed risk for those in the health-care professions—protecting one's self to the greatest extent possible from claims of professional malpractice and being vigilant with respect to these other sources of risk, any one of which can have serious impact on one's practice.

PROFESSIONAL MALPRACTICE—WHAT IS IT?

Although there are many variations and nuances concerning what constitutes professional malpractice across North America and around the world, what constitutes negligence for violation of the informed consent doctrine, and what subjects the health-care provider to claims of professional wrongdoing, certain basic principles remain applicable wherever one practices. Almost every jurisdiction within the United States defines professional malpractice as containing three components. For success in such a claim a patient needs to prove the following:

1. An act or omission by the practitioner that falls below the reasonable and *acceptable standard of care*;
2. That this act or omission by the health-care provider is the *proximate cause* (or substantial

factor and therefore one of the proximate causes) of the patient's injuries; and

3. That the patient, by reason of that act or omission, has suffered damages.[3]

Each of these three components is relatively simple and straightforward but is reviewed below in further detail. However, first a comment on the term "professional malpractice" is necessary. Don't be confused by this—it is really nothing more than another name for a lawsuit premised upon common law principles of "negligence." Everyone knows what negligence is: it exists when the driver of an automobile hits a pedestrian because the driver is traveling too fast; it exists when the department store owner allows water to collect upon his exterior sidewalks when a reasonable person would know that freezing temperatures may cause that water to turn to ice causing passers-by to slip and injure themselves; it exists when the tavern owner continues to sell alcohol to the knowingly intoxicated patron; and it exists when the electrician wires the home in an unacceptable manner, with the result that the home burns to the ground. In reality, the negligence claim against a health-care professional is no different.

The Acceptable Standard of Care

As a threshold point, no malpractice claim exists unless the doctor's standard of care has fallen below an acceptable standard. Thus, the question becomes what is or is not an acceptable standard of care? In those cases dealing with slippery sidewalks and speeding vehicles, the standard is known as the "reasonable man" standard.* When a jury determines whether or not the department store owner was negligent, it simply assesses whether a reasonable store owner under like circumstances would have allowed the water to puddle and freeze or, viewed from the alternate end, whether it is unreasonable to impose upon that department store owner the duty to keep the sidewalk continuously free from water that might freeze and expose passers-by to danger. When we look at the electrician, the situation may seem different but it comes back to the same question—"What is the acceptable standard of care for that particular type of individual?" In other words, the electrician who wired the home will be adjudged by the jury on the basis of whether his or her conduct, as an electrician, fell below the standard of performance of the "objective" reasonable electrician. To amplify, the electrician is not adjudged by the standard of "Joe Homeowner," who may have wired the home that way, but rather the standard of a professional electrician. This brings us to doctors. Like electricians, their liability for negligence and malpractice will be adjudged by whether or not the standard of care of any one of them fell below the standard of care expected from the objective reasonable doctor.

The "reasonable doctor" concept, simple as it may sound on its face, becomes a little more complex, depending on the jurisdiction wherein the doctor practices. For example, simply because another professional practices differently, or employs another school of thought, does not mean that the accused doctor's conduct fell below an acceptable standard of care. Indeed, there are a number of different ways to treat an ailment, and the key legal question becomes whether this doctor's conduct fell below a standard established by that which is generally recognized within the profession.[4] At the same time, one of the critical defenses available to any doctor is the "two schools of thought defense."[5] Although this defense may vary somewhat from jurisdiction to jurisdiction, it stands for the proposition that so long as your care was at a standard that is recognized by "an appreciable number of like practitioners," you are entitled to seek a jury instruction that liability should not be imposed simply because *doctors of the same profession but of another school of thought* would have done something differently.**

How is the Standard of Care Determined? Standard of care can be determined through common sense, learned treatises, expert testimony, and sometimes by the state of technology. Most commonly, a malpractice standard of care must be established through expert testimony. The reason for this, in the eyes of the judicial system, is simple. What constitutes an acceptable standard of care from a member of a particular health profession or specialty is a matter of opinion that is beyond the comprehension and experience of the lay juror and, therefore, expert testimony is required to establish the purported standard of care. This predictably creates the "battle of the experts" in malpractice cases, where the injured plaintiff

*The use of the word "man" is not intended to be sexist and derives from a centuries-old legal precept that was forged long before women ever had the right to vote.

**For example, the worker who injures his lower back can seek treatment from a medical doctor (ex family practitioner), a doctor of chiropractic, a physical therapist, or a physiatrist. The medical doctor may order bed rest and medication to reduce inflammation and soreness. Conversely, if that injured worker presents to the doctor of chiropractic, he will likely receive some modalities of physical therapy and possibly manipulation. However, he will not receive a prescription for pain medication. The physical therapist may treat with physical modalities but not engage in manipulation. And, lastly, the physiatrist may do any or all of these procedures. This does not mean that any one of the practitioners has fallen below an acceptable standard of care inasmuch as an appreciable number of health-care providers practice each of these approaches in terms of treating the injured worker. However, the validity of these defenses, as usual, is decided by juries.

retains one or more experts who opine that the standard has been breached and the defendant doctor presents other experts who opine that the standard has been met. The defendant doctor's standard of care, they respond, was fully consistent with that of reasonable fellow practitioners. The end result of this is that the question of whether a standard or duty of care has been violated is usually a matter of disputed expert evidence that is decided by the jury.

There are some malpractice situations that do not require expert testimony. For example, in most jurisdictions, it would not be necessary to produce an expert for the purpose of opining that a surgical sponge left in the abdomen of a patient who has had her appendix removed constitutes neglect. In this same vein, most jurisdictions would not require expert testimony for the purpose of rendering an opinion that a standard of care is violated when a defendant doctor amputates the patient's left leg when it was the right leg that should have been amputated.* However, whether a practitioner has fallen below the standard of care in failing to *use certain diagnostic* methods or in delivering a particular form of treatment for a specific patient, and is therefore negligent and liable for malpractice, are matters of fact to be determined on the basis of expert evidence.

Learned Treatises and Clinical Guidelines The learned treatise doctrine is simple. It recognizes the fact that publications in the field of health care or medicine are often relied upon by those who practice in that area. Therefore, the doctrine permits most practitioners to rely upon those treatises or journals for the purpose of assisting them in establishing protocols or standards of care when interacting with patients.[6] For example, a textbook that is widely used in medical, osteopathic, chiropractic, or physical therapy schools and that deals with where and when a practitioner should secure diagnostic testing can indeed provide important evidence as to what the appropriate standard of care in that area of practice should be. However, in order to qualify as a learned treatise, the publication must broadly be adopted and recognized within the applicable health-care community. It remains subject, of course, to a challenge from the other side that the treatise is not the prevailing point of view or, as noted above, that another substantial school of thought disagrees with the principles set forth in that treatise. The bottom line consideration for the practitioner, however, is that he or she is better protected when his or her standard of care aligns with the standards of care established in generally recognized learned treatises.

A very significant development in many countries since the early 1990s has been the development of more authoritative professional and governmental guidelines for the clinical management of patients. Practicing in conformity with these will often represent compelling evidence of practice in accordance with the reasonable and legal standard of care.

To illustrate this, one can look at an example of chiropractic clinical guidelines, the Mercy Center Guidelines in the United States.[7] These are evidence-based clinical guidelines developed by a representative committee of 35 research and clinical experts using accepted consensus methods. In Chapter 12 of the guide, titled *Contraindications and Complications*, there are specific recommendations on absolute and relative contraindications for chiropractic care. Under Articular Derangement, there are, for example, the following two recommendations:

1. Degenerative joint disease, osteoarthritis, degenerative discopathy, and spondyloarthrosis are *not contraindications* to high-velocity thrust procedures to the area of pathology but treatment modification may be warranted during active inflammatory phases.
2. In patients with spondylolysis and spondylolisthesis, caution is warranted when high-velocity thrust procedures are used. These conditions are *not contraindications*, but with progressive slippage they may represent a *relative contraindication*.

Imagine a case in which a patient is claiming damages for malpractice supported by a chiropractic expert witness offering the opinion that the defendant chiropractor fell below the standard of care because he used high-velocity adjustment that, in the opinion of this expert, was contraindicated because of the presence of degenerative joint disease (DJD). Recommendation 1 above from the Mercy Center Guidelines represents a persuasive combination of expert testimony (the consensus clinical judgment of an expert panel of 35 doctors of chiropractic) and learned treatise that DJD is not a contraindication to such adjustive care and is likely to be preferred by the court over the opinion of the patient's chiropractic expert witness. One can imagine a similar factual situation involving spondylolisthesis and Recommendation 2.

Clinical guidelines from individuals or trade organizations from within a profession do not guarantee of course. Much depends on their quality. But they can be of value if they have appropriate quality and authority, and address directly the issues of negligence raised in the particular case.

*A legal principle known generally as *res ipsa loquitur* or exclusive control (depending on the jurisdiction) creates a situation where there is a presumption of negligence and it is the defendant rather than the plaintiff who has the burden of disproving the presumption. The quintessential example of this doctrine is demonstrated in the surgical sponge situation where the patient would not be put to the burden of proving why a surgical sponge was left in her stomach. *Ales v Ryan*, 8 Cal2d 82, 64 P2d 409 (Cal 1936) (sponge left in abdomen).

Professional licensing boards in North America and around the world now commonly give guidelines and statements of policy defining acceptable standards of care. Practice in accordance with these is compelling evidence of meeting acceptable standards of care because of the governmental authority of these agencies. It is important to be aware of such standards or guidelines or practice parameters. In the same way that practice in accordance with these is a major step toward protecting yourself against malpractice claims, practice in conflict with these represents a problem.

Although practitioners are not required to follow the standards of a nongovernmental trade organization, the plaintiff's attorney will test both the practitioner and his or her experts to test the extent to which the practitioner's conduct is at odds with any standards or guidelines that have been established.

Technology and Specialty Status The clinicians must be concerned with clinical technologies and understand their significance in this context. Many years ago, a provider could not be accused of having failed to secure the results of MRI testing for example, for the simple reason that there was no such available technology. However, in the United States today everyone who treats a patient with a low back complaint without MRI screening runs the risk of being accused of having injured or exacerbated the lumbosacral area because of the failure to secure an MRI prior to commencing conservative treatment. Putting to one side the question whether the standard of care within the health-care community dictates the early utilization of MRIs for expected disk-related problems, the point to be made here is that, as technology evolves, the practitioners standard of care needs to keep pace with that of technology and the doctor needs to be wary of predictable claims from patients whose attorneys and experts will challenge any treatment unless it is preceded by a battery of diagnostic testing.

With regard to specialization, a standard of care can be imposed at a higher level if the practitioner is a "specialist." As a general rule, though once again the principle of law varies according to state and jurisdiction, if the practitioner is one who holds special postdoctoral status, he or she may be held to a higher standard of care than the general practitioner.[8] By way of example, the family doctor practicing in a heavily rural community may be held to a lesser standard of care than the neurosurgeon who practices at the Mayo Clinic. The theory behind this is that the enhanced status and/or location (i.e., access to advanced technology) compels that higher standard.

The final, catchall consideration deals with one's professional peers. In short, if one practices in the same manner as his or her peers, the risk against claims alleging that one's practice protocols do not meet an acceptable standard of care. Obviously, the "peer" consideration combines virtually every other consideration discussed above but it should not be overlooked. Remember also that-plaintiff attorneys are daily attempting to "establish" or "create" new standards of care under case law as determined in the courtroom, and frequently they are successful. Indeed, as long as a question of fact exists, there will be some uncertainty because lay jurors will ultimately decide your fate. Their decisions, regrettably, frequently depend upon issues wholly unrelated to the merits of any charge of malpractice.*

Proximate Cause or Substantial Factor

The second element of a successful professional malpractice claim is proof that the doctor's conduct was the "proximate cause" of the injuries for which the patient seeks recovery. What is a proximate cause? Strictly understood it is that act which was the necessary, immediate cause for someone suffering an injury, but most courts have expanded that definition to the benefit of the plaintiff patient, simply requiring him or her to prove that the doctor's conduct was a "substantial factor" which brought about the harm or that the doctor engaged in conduct which "increased the likelihood" that injury would follow. This second component of a negligence claim is important and frequently becomes the focus of the defense attorney representing the doctor. Specifically, even though the doctor's conduct may be proven to have fallen below an acceptable standard of care, this is insufficient by itself for the plaintiff to win the case. The malpractice must be proven to have caused the injury and loss. Conversely, even if the patient proves proximate cause, he or she nevertheless loses unless he or she can also prove a breach of some standard of care.

By way of example, assume a provider performs cervical manipulation, which is subsequently followed by evidence of vertebral artery dissection and stroke. If the stroke occurs while the patient is in the office, it will be difficult to argue that the treatment was not a substantial factor in bringing about harm to the

*Although we read everyday in the newspapers that major lawsuits have been dismissed prior to trial by defense motions, take little comfort in those anecdotal rulings. A malpractice claim, unlike commercial or business litigation, is not subject to dispositive motions, unless the patient cannot make out a *prima facie* case. Unfortunately for the doctor, making out a *prima facie* case is a relatively simple task in the area of malpractice, and so long as some expert, somewhere, is willing to render an opinion that your conduct fell below an acceptable standard of care and that said conduct was a substantial factor in bringing about some harm to your patient, the case goes, *ipso facto*, to a jury. It matters not that the opinion is weak or fraught with holes. Rather, so long as the expert meets the relaxed standard of being an expert, and so long as that expert's report opines on both the standard of care and causation, a jury question exists such that your fate will not be determined by a judge, but rather gets placed in the hands of a jury.

patient. However, that gets the patient only half way home. There is the second question as to whether performance of the manipulation fell below an acceptable standard of care. If the plaintiff is unable to convince a jury that the cervical manipulation was contraindicated, or that it was performed in an unacceptable manner, there is no recovery regardless of the injury. In this scenario, the doctor's defense focuses on the first prong or criterion for a successful case—breach of standard of care.

There is a second scenario that must be addressed. Under this second hypothetical situation, the doctor is accused of having herniated a disk in the lumbar region because of a spinal manipulative procedure. Once again the doctor can argue that the manipulation was appropriate, not contraindicated, and within the standard of care. He or she can further argue, however, that the manipulation played no substantial role (i.e., was not a proximate cause) in the herniation. Even if the doctor performed manipulations over a period of months without imaging or reassessment, suggesting a breach of standard of care, nevertheless, the plaintiff is not entitled to a recovery unless the second element of the case is proved—namely that the negligent care was a substantial factor in bringing about the injury of which the plaintiff complains. The usual defense to this type of case is expert testimony from the defendant doctor that the herniated disk preexisted treatment and this was the cause of the low back pain to begin with, and that the manipulation had nothing to do with the increased pain the patient subsequently experienced. Therefore, the doctor's conduct, even if it failed to meet some standard of care, was not a proximate cause of the disc herniation and pain.

Damages

The third element a patient must prove in a professional malpractice claim is that he or she suffered injury and loss requiring compensation in the form of "damages." A treatise in itself could be written on this subject. As a bottom line, a doctor found liable for damages will be held responsible for the injured patient's lost time away from work, all future work loss potential, medical expenses, and pain and suffering. Whereas work loss and medical expenses are identifiable and ascertainable, the doctor is at the mercy of the jury on the extent and value of "pain and suffering."*

*There is frequent discussion of punitive damages in the area of professional malpractice. Within the scope of this chapter, simply bear in mind that punitive damages can be awarded if the doctor's conduct reaches the point of gross negligence, reckless disregard, or intentional wrongdoing. See generally for a collection of cases, Allowance of Punitive Damages in Medical Malpractice Action, 35 ALR 5th 145.

INFORMED CONSENT

The doctrine of informed consent is well known but frequently misunderstood by members of the legal and health-care professions. Its origin and its focus vary depending upon the state, region, or country. In most cases, this doctrine is based upon a patient's right "to intelligently reject or accept treatment."[9] In those jurisdictions where it is based upon this concept, a duty is imposed on the doctor to make a reasonable disclosure of all material facts relevant to the decision the patient is required to make.** What is "material" is generally understood as any risk that is pertinent and appropriate for disclosure as part of the decision to undergo the treatment. Predictably, that which is or is not "material" frequently becomes the subject of litigation.

Clinicians are called upon every day to help alleviate severe low back pain and its syndromes, which interfere with a patient's work and enjoyment of life. Should conservative care providers inform the patient that the treatment protocols they are recommending might exacerbate the existing condition? Should the provider advise the patient that a side posture lumbar manipulation might result in disk injury or increased symptomatology? Is this a "material risk" that needs to be disclosed? In some jurisdictions it may be, in others perhaps not. (This may be compared with the risk of vertebral artery injury or stroke after manipulation, which, although rare, is a much clearer material risk because of the potential for severe harm.) Although there is no hard and fast answer, the doctor is better protected against all claims of lack of informed consent when there has been a disclosure of any risk of significant harm that could, in fact, occur.

Courts have defined two different standards for determining what is a material risk. Courts in most countries hold that a risk is material if a "reasonable patient would want to know about the risk." Another school of thought, found in many jurisdictions in the

**It should be noted that a minority of jurisdictions have refused to extend the doctrine of informed consent beyond principles grounded in battery to theories premised on the general negligence of health-care providers for failing to advise the patient of risks associated with a course of treatment, whatever that treatment may be. For example, the Pennsylvania Supreme Court has held repeatedly that the doctrine of informed consent is premised on principles of battery only. See, e.g., *Morgan v MacPhail*, 550 Pa202, 704 A2d 617 (1997). Indeed, the court has stated that the informed consent doctrine derives from the very fact that surgical or operative procedures, if not consented to, amount to a battery, *Id.* Because of this rationale, the Court has refused to apply the doctrine of informed consent to nonsurgical or operative procedures. Therefore, under Pennsylvania law, the chiropractor, physiatrist, or osteopath who performs a manipulation is under no obligation to advise his or her patient of the risks associated with the same. See *Matukonis v Trainer*, 441 Pa Super 570, 657 A2d 1314 (1995).

United States, stands for the proposition that a risk is material only if a "reasonable doctor" would inform his patients. The "reasonable patient" approach is growing, and is consistent with the increase in patient rights generally. Regardless of what standard applies where a provider practices, jury members are lay people who will probably end up asking, "Is that something that I would have wanted to know before the treatment was provided?" They may very well disregard the strict legal test they should be following.

Two major practical issues with respect to informed consent are first how to prove that it has been given, and second the process of obtaining informed consent. On the first, many jurisdictions now require a written informed consent signed by the patient, rather than simply a verbal consent noted in the file by the doctor. In an era of increased patient rights, the trend toward written consents will likely increase with time. Written consent forms, and increasingly the use of videotapes, audiotapes, or pamphlets, even when not strictly required by law, are valuable means of documenting that consent was obtained and of ensuring uniform disclosure in relation to common treatment procedures. It is a question of fact in each case whether the patient gave an informed consent, and when facts are disputed objective evidence is invaluable. To perhaps restate this concept more philosophically, *the palest ink is superior to the sharpest memory.**

Practitioners, educators, and lawyers will likely disagree into the future on the question of just how detailed an informed consent document should be and, for that matter, whether informed consent should be an oral process as opposed to a written process as opposed to some combination thereof. Continuing with the theme that the patient's signature on a physical document is more difficult for that patient to "run from" when the malpractice claim is filed, the question then becomes just how detailed that form should be. One strong school of thought adheres to the concept that the informed consent document cannot be too comprehensive or too detailed. That school of thought ascribes to the belief that all reasonable risks should be listed; any physical touching of the body should be acknowledged as a component of the treatment; and the document should expressly note that the patient has the right to decline assessment or treatment. Further, the document should be clear that the practitioner cannot assume responsibility for harm from treatment, if the patient consents to treatment, or the consequences of lack of treatment if the patient chooses to decline treatment after having discussed and read the potential risks inherent in the medical procedures at issue. Appendix 1 provides a summary of the key aspects that should be covered in the body of an informed consent form. Appendix 2 provides an example of a second form, to be completed by the clinician during the initial history, covering the patient's mental or emotional status at the time of signing the form.

Another approach is to use a more concise consent form describing only the material risk or risks of the treatment to be given. The benefits and risks of alternative treatments or no treatment are dealt with verbally. Appendix 3 provides a generic sample, developed by one of the authors (D.C.S.) for use in Canada. This covers some typical aspects of conservative treatment, including manual procedures of the lumbar and cervical spine.

Information must be disclosed in a clear manner that can be understood by the patient. Consent forms couched in general language and lacking detailed risk/benefit information will not be accepted as evidence of informed consent. The risk of vertebral artery injury causing stroke that exists with cervical manipulation can be used as an example. This is a remote but foreseeable and material risk that may have serious consequences. It should, in general, be disclosed if there is to be a valid informed consent from the patient. If a clinician who performs spinal manipulation in practice were to use a written consent form that simply referred to a risk of "vertebral artery injury" and omitted any reference to stroke, production of this written form signed by the patient would, probably, not be accepted as evidence of valid disclosure and informed consent. The first question the defendant will be asked in cross-examination will be "Why did you choose not to mention the risk of stroke on the consent form?" Everyone knows the answer, and the patient will be believed when, in evidence, he or she denies knowing what "injury to the vertebral artery" is and explains that no form would have been signed or acceptable if the word "stroke" had been used.

Now moving to the second major practical issue, the process of obtained informed consent—this is as important as the contents of the consent. This is because a valid informed consent requires not only disclosure of information but also evidence that the patient understood the disclosed facts. Signature of a consent form with clear information creates a presumption that the patient understood what was signed. However, a defendant clinician is in a stronger position legally if the injured patient now claiming damages, and having the sympathy of the court, had a clear opportunity to discuss the risks disclosed. The strongest position of all is created by the clinician talking to the patient before treatment, referring to the consent form, asking if it has been understood, receiving a positive answer, and noting this in the file.

Readers are reminded once more that they should consult with a local attorney on both the form of

*Check your jurisdiction. There may be a statutory or regulatory requirement compelling the doctor to secure written consent.

consent and process of obtaining consent to ensure compliance with applicable laws in their state or jurisdiction. Some states provide that a written consent form meeting statutory requirements shall, if signed by a patient, create a presumption that informed consent was given. (See Florida Medical Consent Law, which stipulates informed consent requirements for specified health-care professionals in Florida.[10]) Even in these jurisdictions, however, the key question remaining is whether the form itself provided adequate information.[11]

SEXUAL MISCONDUCT: THE ERA OF ZERO TOLERANCE

Few areas of risk management in health-care practice have undergone greater change in the past generation than that of professional misconduct for sexual impropriety. Many changes in society, including changes in patient rights, women's rights, cultural and sexual mores, and multiculturalism, have produced an era of "zero tolerance." Issues relating to sexual boundaries are no longer gray; they are black and white. All practitioners, especially those who have been in practice for 15 years or more, must understand and respect these changes. The days of telling a joke with a sexual innuendo to a patient, for example, are over.

Because of the hands-on nature of their work, practitioners using manual methods of examination and treatment are at special risk of allegations of sexual impropriety or misconduct. This is particularly the case in the management of low back syndromes, where patients must disrobe to varying degrees and the body regions of the sacrum, hips, pelvis, and torso will often require examination and treatment. The situation is further complicated by the fact that patients in many health-care practices come from a variety of ethnic and cultural backgrounds, with very different attitudes toward personal relationships and physical contact. Social mores vary considerably from country to country, and in different regions of the same country. Many patients have unresolved psychological or even psychiatric conditions that may not be apparent to a clinician until behavior triggered by the unconscious crossing of a line of perceived impropriety. Few issues are more traumatic for a patient than a perceived invasion of physical or sexual propriety. Few things are as traumatic for a clinician as allegations of sexual impropriety or abuse, whether or not they are true or proven in disciplinary proceedings or other litigation.

On the other hand, failure to properly examine a patient, for any reason, and this includes concern about claims of sexual impropriety, is negligent clinical behavior. When clinicians accept the responsibility of managing a patient, they accept the responsibility of performing a thorough and professional examination to assess the basis of any presenting conditions. This requires inspection of the body region in question, and perhaps other regions that may be clinically/functionally associated with the patient's complaint. Disrobing, observation, and palpation will frequently be necessary for appropriate assessment of the patient.

A complete commentary on issues of sexual misconduct would require a chapter in itself, but the following comments may provide a helpful framework for clinicians to follow. Clinicians should also be familiar with relevant laws and professional guidelines in their community or jurisdiction.

1. Always be sensitive to the fact that all patients have differing needs and comfort levels. A golden rule to follow is that "people don't like surprises." The clinician must anticipate any scenario in which patients may feel uncomfortable and forewarn them, using common language to explain in detail what procedures will be used and are deemed necessary.
2. If the clinician feel any hesitation from a patient, then it is better to avoid the planned procedure and present an alternative approach. If one proceeds when a patient is clearly uncomfortable about an examination or treatment exceeding his or her comfort zone, then the clinician is in error. The only question is to what degree.
3. A third person, an assistant, generally a female, should always be available to be in the room whenever the clinician or patient so requests, and the patient should always be aware of the opportunity to have this chaperone present. The decision to request a chaperone or to refuse a procedure is of course the patient's right.
4. The clinician's feelings are equally important, of course, and the clinician must feel comfortable and confident to proceed with optimal treatment. If this feeling is compromised, for any reason, then the patient should be referred to another clinician.
5. Entering any level of sexual relationship with a patient is clearly inappropriate and represents professional misconduct. Whenever adults come in contact with one another, romance is a possibility. It is not uncommon for clinicians to be married to former patients. How does this occur in an ethical manner, without risk and without professional misconduct? At the first sign of any change in the relationship from professional to personal, the clinician must explain to the patient that, for a personal or potentially romantic relationship to begin, the professional relationship must end. As such

the patient should then be referred to another clinician, preferably one outside the clinician's current office or clinic. This development should be duly documented and signed by the clinician and the patient, and the patient's clinical records should then be forwarded to the new treating clinician at no charge to the patient or new clinician.

6. Historically, the greatest danger of a sexual misconduct case arises where there is a male clinician and a female patient. However, claims of sexual misconduct by female and male patients against female or male clinicians are now being made, and clinicians who believe that they have some sort of gender immunity from an allegation of sexual impropriety from any patient are placing themselves at increased risk. For example, even an office policy that a disrobed female be given a gown, but not necessarily a male, may be seen by some male patients as prejudicial and inappropriate, and expose the clinician to risk of complaint. Women and men should be given equally dignified procedures protecting their privacy.
7. One thing to consider that will help patients better anticipate what will occur during their initial examination is that part of the informed consent form or other intake documentation outline what type of procedures are to be performed and what these entail. The form should explain that the clinician's protocols routinely include examination procedures such as looking at (inspection) and touching (palpation—testing the tone and range of motion of soft tissues and joints) of all body parts or regions that may be clinically associated with the patient's complaints. This form should also explain the right of a patient to request a chaperone in the examination/treatment room at any time and the right to refuse any procedure or treatment.
8. If the clinician, does not feel comfortable with a particular patient at any time, yet feels that further examination or one or more regions of the body are necessary for appropriate and professional care, these clinician's concerns should be prudently respected. Call an assistant, of the same sex as the patient, into the room. For example, the low back should often be examined in the event of leg pain to rule out sciatica. Failure to properly examine is negligent clinical behavior, even if the clinician feels concerns about the risk of a claim of sexual impropriety from the patient in question. In such an

Again, if in doubt, think—"Will my conduct be deemed acceptable in the eyes of 12 jurors?" If the answer is "no," think again!

STRATEGIES TO PROTECT AGAINST CLAIMS OF MALPRACTICE OR VIOLATIONS OF THE INFORMED CONSENT DOCTRINE

Risk management really is a misnomer, in that "risk minimization" probably states more accurately the goal of the doctor. This may seem a trivial difference in wording, but it represents a significant difference of attitude and clinical strategizing that will be addressed. A brief summary of strategies that must be enacted are first covered.

First, beyond question, be certain you have professional errors and omissions insurance coverage in place, whether mandatory or not!

Second, ensure that the coverage is adequate to cover one's needs. The amounts vary in different regions. In the United States, for example, there are few professional malpractice claims where the demanded damages are less than $100,000 and claims are often for damages of $1–2 million. Be farsighted and spend a little more money on premiums in order to ensure adequate protection. The goal is to "sleep at night," to be protected against the large claim that may take one's home and future.

Third, in a practice with partners, ensure that there is adequate coverage for their conduct also, as partners are generally mutual beneficiaries of successes and jointly responsible for liabilities.

Fourth, if the clinic is structured as a professional corporation, ensure that there is a rider on any policy that protects the professional corporation and all of its employees as well as the clinician(s). Many insurance carriers refuse to insure professional fictional entities, unless the health-care professional has taken affirmative steps to make the professional corporation a "named insured" on policies. Importantly, there is an increasing number of lawsuits against professional corporations premised upon claims that ordinarily would not exist against sole practitioners. For example, if the clinician, as a single practicing doctor, injure a patient, the only legitimate claim that can be advanced against that clinician is the traditional malpractice claim itself. Not so for the clinician who practices in the professional corporation. Indeed, the professional corporation can be sued for having failed to properly train, supervise, and/or monitor those who practice within the professional corporation that is a very different and distinct tort from the malpractice claim. For this reason, ensure that coverage exists for the acts or conduct of all of those who work with you, whether they are fellow physicians, assistants, employees, or independent contractors.

Fifth, remember that it is no defense to a malpractice claim against a clinician for injuries caused by a doctor hired and placed within the facility because he or she is categorized in some agreement as an "independent contractor," rather than as an employee. Quite simply, so long as the treating patient is led to believe that the doctor who treated him or her is within the clinician's sphere of control, he or she will be held liable under principles of vicarious liability without regard to the fact that the other doctor is described as an independent contractor in a contract. In this regard, regardless of whether it is the clinic owner or the independent contractor who brings up the topic, be sure to address insurance issues with one another. For example, consider having the independent contractor name the owner as an "additional insured" on his or her errors and omissions policy and require that independent contractor to produce for you, on an annual basis, evidence that he or she has, in good standing, such insurance.

Sixth, be sure to have coverage that protects against all events, past, present, and future. Some carriers write insurance based upon when the claim is made and some policies provide coverage based upon the occurrence of the wrongdoing. Seek advice if necessary but be certain that there is coverage for all acts and conduct. Whether identified as "tail" or "head" coverage, bear in mind that these are terms of art and reference to them may not necessarily mean that you are fully protected. In this day and age of physician mobility, mergers of practice, termination of affiliations and its like, one of the fundamental pitfalls that can befall a practitioner is to "lose" coverage for the malpractice claim that has yet to be asserted.

Seventh, even beyond the professional liability insurance consideration, be sure to have comprehensive liability insurance. What happens if one of the clinical assistants assaults a young patient in one of the treatment rooms? The professional liability carrier may very well argue that because the conduct was criminal or involved sexual intimacy, there are express exclusions, thus entitling the carrier to decline a defense or refuse to indemnify you in litigation. It may very well be that the general comprehensive liability carrier would argue the same but, at a minimum, to the extent claims were directed against the owner/clinician for failing to properly monitor and supervise employees, the owner/clinician would more likely be protected under his or her general liability policy, even if the professional liability carrier were to deny coverage. In any event, one must protect one's self to the greatest extent possible, which leads to the next critical point.

Eighth, have established protocols in your office. Have written procedures as to how you go about hiring professional and support staff. Do reasonable, background checks. Secure references and keep them in the personnel file.

Ninth, have written procedures as to how staff members should interact with patients; how risks are discussed with patients; how referrals are to be made in order to ensure against, inter alia, claims that you failed to properly refer for alternative treatment or diagnostic testing. Every day patients bring lawsuits claiming that serious medical conditions went undetected in circumstances where the doctor had recommended that the patient seek out other health-care providers or diagnostic testing services to determine whether there was any other physiological problem affecting the patient. There is no better rebuttal to a claim of failure to diagnose than a detailed, in-writing note confirming that the patient was directed to see specialists "x" but refused to do so. Whereas, the doctor may be required to "lead the horse to water," but his or her duty usually ends at that point where the patient "refuses to drink."

Tenth, have protocols that prohibit personal relationships between staff and patients. Nearly every jurisdiction is creating regulations that hold that sexual boundary violations are subject to severe sanction. The topic of sexual boundaries with respect to patients has been dealt with previously in this chapter.

Eleventh, while on the issue of personal relationships, have protocols that prohibit such relationships between and among the staff. One employee's interest in another employee adds significant additional risk to the employer because of potential lawsuits regarding employee harassment and hostile work environment.

Twelfth, be sure your clinical records are thorough, legible, and supportable. If you are not proud of your clinical files, rethink how you create them!

Finally, one of the most important considerations of them all must not be forgotten—the clinician's relationship with his or her patients. Patients are much more likely to take legal action against a health professional they do not like or respect or against someone who has not treated them fairly or pleasantly. Equally, they will either not take action or are more likely to limit their claims if they know the doctor is a conscientious person placing their best interests and welfare above his or her own. There are numerous examples of this.

A striking example in Canada in the 1990s involved a young professional woman who suffered a stroke and quadriplegia after cervical manipulation. She had a large claim of several millions because of a very high loss of future earning potential. She and other members of her family had a history of successful treatment from the clinician involved, respected his character and professional skills, and knew he was married with a young family. Although he was liable for damages because he had not mentioned the risk of stroke and obtained an informed consent, the plaintiff settled her claim at the level of his insurance coverage rather than see him and his family lose their home and security. It was necessary to get a special court approval for the settlement, because it was so far below the plaintiff's full entitlement to damages.

The Insurance Issue A doctor's "records" are not simply his or her clinical records. They also include any insurance-related records of the patient, which may become significant in a malpractice claim, and are therefore relevant to risk management. The smart plaintiff lawyer always requests the insurance records because those records, almost without exception, contain diagnostic codes identifying what treatment was provided and what the doctor believed to be the diagnosis. In this regard, when the doctor is accused of having performed certain procedures or having reached a certain diagnosis that was inaccurate, his or her position can be tested by both the clinical records as well as the records submitted to the insurance company for reimbursement. In short, be certain that the insurance records are consistent with the clinical records; otherwise, the inconsistency, although arguably irrelevant to the injury, may become a critical issue in a subsequent malpractice claim.

In addition, be careful not to govern treatment by "that which the insurance company will pay for." Although the doctor is not required to work without fair reward, once the doctor/patient relationship becomes established it remains in place until lawfully terminated. During that time, treatment of the patient should be governed by the standards previously discussed in detail. Reassessments should be performed based upon standards, not insurance coverage. Diagnostic testing should be based upon standards, not insurance coverage. And, most importantly, insurance reimbursement requests should be based upon the actual diagnosis and the actual services provided rather than utilizing those codes that provide for maximum reimbursement.

A similar problem occurs in the managed care arena, a uniquely structured and controlled medical management model that has gained acceptance in various forms in several industrialized countries. Suppose the clinician is given permission to treat an HMO (health maintenance organization) patient six times, but no more, without the consent of the gatekeeper. On visit number six, that patient remains in extreme pain; it is the clinician's opinion that he or she needs additional conservative low back therapy, and yet, the patient's HMO will not approve additional care. What should be done? Simply stated, when the clinician agrees to treat a patient, the doctor/patient relationship is created and it continues until lawfully terminated by either the patient or you. Termination by the patient is easy. Terminations by the doctor, on the other hand, are far more difficult and may involve considerations such as abandonment and breaches of standard of care for which the doctor will be held liable. Again, a useful test is to ask the following question: "If I terminate treatment or refuse to provide treatment in this case now, how will this look if I am subsequently accused of professional malpractice?" Simply stated, each clinician must govern his or her standards of practice by professional standards. Recent appellate decisions at the US federal and state court level suggest that HMOs, a unique type of insurance and provider consortium, can be held liable under claims of professional malpractice and their like for failing to permit reimbursement for needed medical care. The clinician must diligently protect himself or herself from being a co-defendent in the name of reimbursement.

The Clinical Records

Various treatises, publications, and government standards provide basic requirements for the doctor's clinical file. Some insurance companies will deny reimbursement unless certain forms are completed. From the malpractice perspective, this entire, complex issue of recordkeeping can be summarized with the following question: "If the provider's clinical records are the subject of a two foot by three foot blowup in a medical malpractice case, will that provider feel comfortable defending those records?" If your answer is yes, then the records are probably adequate. If the answer is "no," is the provider managing the level of practice risk intelligently?

The Altered Record

"Dr. A" treated a patient Mr. Smith for 3 months a year ago. Now Dr. A receives in the mail a release of medical information form with a request from a lawyer that the file be photocopied and turned over to the lawyer. Dr. A reviews the records; Dr. A know that Mr. Smith had complications subsequent to his treatment and notes that the records are less than stellar. Dr. A want very much to supplement the existing clinical file before it is turned over to the attorney. What does Dr. A do?

Although the better school of thought is to refrain from modifying the records in any manner, if Dr. A feel absolutely compelled to do so, be sure that any additions or supplements to the records are initialed and accurately dated. Although this creates a "red flag" and a point of concern, this is far better than alteration of records in such a manner as to suggest that the "additions" were made on a date other than when they were made. Indeed, such alterations can create major problems. They may subject the clinician to claims of fraud and will likely puncture a large hole in a malpractice case against the provider that otherwise would have been wholly defensible. Every day malpractice cases are decided or settled under unfavorable terms because a doctor who, with hindsight, believed that his or her records should look better and thus has altered the clinical file.

In addition, have protocols in place to ensure that no set of clinical records is provided to an attorney or discharged patient without the doctor being aware of the request. Despite a busy schedule, the provider should personally review that clinical file before it is provided to the lawyer or the discharged patient, and under no circumstance, should an original record be turned over without the clinician retaining a full and complete set of those records.

CONCLUSION

Although chiropractic, medical, osteopathic, or physical therapy schools may teach students that which *they* need to know from a *clinical* perspective, the formal education setting does little to assist the doctor in how his or her office should function operationally, staff-wise, insurance-wise, and document-wise. There is perhaps no more fundamental rule to be followed by a health-care provider than "document, document, document"! Lawyers say that "if it is not in writing, it does not exist," and there is no reason why the health-care profession should not be governed by this wise adage.

The more comprehensive and legible the clinical file, the more assured one can be of a legitimate defense to any claim of wrongdoing or malpractice. Remember *in particular* that the provider's duty to a patient is governed by common law or regulatory standards that govern your profession generally. The day the clinician allow insurance coverage and insurance considerations to dictate the means by which his or her practice is the day that the exposure to potential claims of malpractice is enhanced.

Be sure to discuss the clinical findings and proposed treatment plan with the patient. Whether or not a written informed consent form is used, be certain that the patient is given a reasonable opportunity to discuss material risks associated with treatment and other options for care. Where there is no written consent form, have the patient initial the chart reflecting that these discussions have taken place. Whenever possible, have the patient fill out information in his or her own handwriting. Every day lawyers representing patients take the position that the doctor wrote self-serving information concerning the patient's complaints of pain and other information provided by the patient. One of the easiest ways to eliminate this attack is to have the patients, in their own hand, explaining what they were doing when they became injured, where they did it, and why they are coming for treatment. As the doctor/patient encounter continues, continue to ask this question: "If this patient ever sues me for malpractice, will I be confident in my clinical records and the treatment regimen I provided? If the answer to that question in the affirmative, effective risk minimization or management is probably in place and this is of great importance to the interests of all parties involved—the patient, the malpractice insurer, and any third-party payer involved, but finally and very importantly, that health care provider.

SUMMARY

1. Risk management comprises a multitude of strategies that protect both the clinician and patient.
2. Risk management was previously necessary in only a few select countries, but increasing pressures for patient protection and more organized legal and health care systems globally now require the implementation of this strategy everywhere.
3. Clinicians must be proactive in establishing organized risk "minimalization" policies for their clinics. This includes employee training and written policy statements.
4. Informed consent is a keystone of risk management, allowing the patient, or potential patient, to clearly understand the reasonable risks of assessment and treatment in advance.
5. Proper informed consent can make the difference regarding the filing of a malpractice action, if the patient was duly informed of the risk of an untimely event that later occurred.
6. Because of the intimate nature of the doctor-patient relationship, all efforts to guard against the appearance of sexual impropriety must be employed. This can at times be difficult when issues of patient modesty conflicts with the need to clinically assess and provide treatment.
7. Ultimately, good risk management means good communication between healthcare provider and patient. This translates into good healthcare practices and a more appreciative patient who is aware that appropriate time and care was taken.

APPENDIX 1: CHECKLIST FOR TOPICS THAT SHOULD BE COVERED IN AN INFORMED CONSENT FORM

1. Opening statement, expressed in the first person (e.g., I .... understand ....), that the patient or legal guardian understands that he or she is requesting and consenting to assessment and/or treatment from the clinician(s) and staff of the clinic.
2. The patient understands and agrees to undergo the components of assessment in order for the clinic staff to arrive at a diagnosis. Specific examples of common assessment methods, such as inspection and palpation of involved body regions, should be included.
3. The patient understands and agrees that he or she has the right to refuse assessment procedures, but that the staff has the right to discontinue the assessment or treatment because of the absence of assessment information necessary for optimal care.
4. The patient is informed, as specifically as is practical, of the various treatment options provided at the clinic and of the known risks involved. Specific examples of some of the more common procedures performed at the clinic and of their risks are important.
5. The patient understands that the staff will answer questions regarding procedures and risks, in addition to explaining other treatment options, but that the patient must accept the responsibility to ask enough questions so that he or she can decide whether or not to proceed with treatment.
6. The patient has read the entire document and consents to initiate assessment and/or treatment at the clinic.
7. The patient has had, and continues to have, the opportunity to ask any and all questions and to decline assessment or treatment procedures.
8. The patient understands that he or she, or the clinician, can request a second staff member in the room at any time during assessment and/or treatment.
9. The patient understands that the clinicians and staff are there for the benefit of the patient and that the optimal communication between patient and staff is in the patient's best interest. Therefore, the patient is invited to inquire about any aspect of his or her condition at any time before, during, or after the visit to the clinic.

There should be lines at the bottom of the form allowing for printed names and signatures of the patient, a guardian where appropriate, a witness, and a translator.

A short line and space at the beginning of each topic, to be initialed by the patient to confirm specific agreement of each topic, is recommended.

APPENDIX 2: PATIENT STATUS AT TIME OF INFORMED CONSENT PROCESS

Based on my personal observations of the patient's medical history and direct conversation with the patient, I conclude that throughout the consent process the patient was:

- ☐ Of legal age
- ☐ Well-oriented
- ☐ Disoriented as to ----------------------------
- ☐ Coherent and lucid
- ☐ On prescription/OTC medication but unimpaired
- ☐ Proficient in understanding the English language
- ☐ Assisted in understanding by an interpreter. (Interpreter's name: ----------------------------)
- ☐ Resolute in denying the use of alcohol and/or recreational drugs prior to consent
- ☐ Unable to give legal consent
- ☐ Consent given thru legal guardian

____

Name Relationship

Patient's questions (if any) and information supplied are as follows:

____

____

____

Comments:

____

____

I certify that the above accurately describes the above named patient's status during the informed consent process on

____

Date Signature of Doctor

(Reprinted withpermission by Charles W. Theisler, from his Form and Sample Letter Book.)

*APPENDIX 3: INFORMED CONSENT TO TREATMENT

Please read this consent form, discuss it with your clinician if you would like to, and then sign where indicated at the bottom. Clinicians who use spinal manual therapy techniques, such as for example joint adjustment or manipulation or mobilization, are advised to inform patients that there are or may be some risks associated with such treatment. In particular:

(a) While rare, some patients have experienced muscle soreness, ligament sprains or strains, or rib fractures following spinal adjustments.
(b) There have been reported cases of injury to a vertebral artery following neck adjustment, manipulation, and/or mobilization. Such vertebral artery injuries may on rare occasion cause stroke, which may result in serious neurological injury and/or physical impairment. This form of complication is an extremely rare event, occurring about 1 time per 1 million to 2 million treatments.
(c) There have been reported cases of disc injuries following spinal manual therapy, although no scientific study has ever demonstrated that such injuries are caused, or may be caused, by adjustment or manipulative techniques and such cases are also very rare.

Treatment provided at this clinic, including spinal adjustment or manipulation, has been the subject of much research conducted over many years and has been demonstrated to be an appropriate and effective treatment for many common forms of spinal pain, pain in the shoulders/arms/legs, headaches, and other similar symptoms. Treatment provided at this clinic may also contribute to your overall well-being. The risk of injury or complication from manual treatment is substantially lower than the risk associated with many medications, other treatments and procedures frequently given as alternative treatments for the same forms of musculoskeletal pain and other associated syndromes.

Your clinician will evaluate your individual case, provide an explanation of care and a suggested treatment plan, or alternatively a referral for consultation and/or further evaluation if deemed necessary.

Acknowledgment: I acknowledge I have discussed, or have been given the opportunity to discuss, with my clinician the nature of the treatment in general and my treatment in particular as well as the contents of this consent.

Consent: I consent to the treatment(s) offered or recommended to me by my clinician, including joint adjustment or manipulation to the joints of my spine (neck and back), pelvis, and extremities (shoulder, upper limbs, and lower limbs). I intend this consent to apply to all my present and future treatment at this clinic.

Dated this ____ day of ______, 20___.

____________________	________________________________
Patient Signature (Legal Guardian)	Signature of Guardian (when applicable)
Name:____________________	Name: ____________________________
(Please print name of patient)	(Please print name of guardian)
Name: ____________________	____________________________
(Please print name of witness/translator)	Signature of Witness/Translator

* This is a sample form and is not intended as a final product. Each clinician should utilize informed consent forms that satisfy the requirements of his or her community, in addition to his or her unique practice standards.

REFERENCES

1. *Source*: 1996 Verdictum Juris, Tri-Service Reference No. 92-22-02.
2. World Health Organization. *Promotion of the rights of patients in Europe*. The Hague: Kluwer Law International, 1995.
3. See, e.g., *Hanson v Grode*, 76 Cal App 4th 601, 606 90 Cal Rptr 2d 396, 400 (1999). (In any medical malpractice action, the plaintiff must establish "(1) the duty of the professional to use such skill, prudence, and diligence as other members of his profession commonly possess and exercise; (2) a breach of that duty; (3) a proximate causal connection between the negligent conduct and the resulting injury; and (4) actual loss or damage resulting from the professional's negligence.") (citations and internal quotations omitted); *Monahan v Weichert*, 82 AD2d 102, 105 442 NYS2d 295, 297 (1981). (Court opining that it is incumbent upon plaintiff to prove the following: "(1) the duty to possess the requisite skill and knowledge as is possessed by the average member of the medical profession in the community in which he practices; (2) the duty to exercise ordinary and reasonable care in the application of that professional knowledge and skill; or (3) the duty to use his best judgment in the application of his knowledge and skill.") (citation omitted); *Hamil v Bashline*, 481 Pa256, 392 A2d 1280 (1978).
4. See, e.g., *Flowers v Torrance Memorial Hospital Medical Center*, 884 P2d 142, 145 (Cal 1994). ("...the standard for professionals is articulated in terms of exercising 'the knowledge, skill and care ordinarily possessed and employed by members of the profession in good standing...' "); *Bardessono v Michels*, 3 Cal3d 780, 788, 478 P2d 480, 484 (Cal 1971). ("The courts require only that physicians and surgeons exercise in diagnosis and treatment that reasonable degree of skill, knowledge, and care ordinarily possessed and exercised by members of the medical profession under similar circumstances.") (citation omitted).
5. See, e.g., *Brannan v Lankenau Hospital*, 490 Pa588, 597, 417 A2d 196, 200 (1980). ("...where competent medical authority is divided, a physician will not be held responsible if in the exercise of his judgment he followed a course of treatment advocated by a considerable number of his brethren in good standing in his community.") (citation omitted).
6. See, e.g., *Ohligschlager v Proctor Community Hospital*, 55 Ill2d 411 (1973) and *Mulder v. Parke Davis & Co.*, 288 Minn 332, 181 NW2d 882 (1970) (accepting the PDR as evidence of a physician's standard of care).
7. Haldeman S, Chapman-Smith D, Petersen, DM, eds. Guidelines for chiropractic quality assurance and practice parameters. In: *Proceedings of the Mercy Center Consensus Conference*. Gaithersburg, MD: Aspen Publishers, 1997.
8. See *Jordan v Bogner*, 844 P2d 664 (Colo 1993) (collecting an array of cases discussing the applicable standards of care for specialists and nonspecialists); *Fales v Books*, 570 NW2d 841 (Neb 1997); *Didato v Strehler*, 554 SE2d 42 (Va 2001).
9. See, e.g., *Cobbs v Grant*, 8 Cal3d 229, 104 Cal Rptr 505, 502 P2d 1 (1972); *Arato v Vedon*, 5 Cal 4th 1172, 858 P2d 598 (1993).
10. Fla Stat Ann §766.103 (West 1992).
11. *Parikh v Cunningham*, 493 So2d 999 (Fla 1986).

CHAPTER

37

LOW BACK SYNDROMES: A FINAL PERSPECTIVE

Craig E. Morris

OUTLINE

OBJECTIVE

1. Provide commentary regarding the current status and future direction of the management of low back syndromes.

INTRODUCTION

The chapters of this textbook have encapsulated the current state of clinical affairs regarding low back syndromes (LBS). While volumes can be written on this topic, the information herein presents the reader with a comprehensive overview of this daunting subject at the beginning of the twenty-first century. This chapter will now provide a brief commentary on factors governing the evolution of management of LBS, for today and the foreseeable future. Whereas the first chapter of this textbook presented an overwhelming scenario of disabling LBS, this chapter is designed to provide a more optimistic future.

Indeed, the current standards of clinical practice are based upon a staggering array of scientific information, fine tuned by meta-analyses and "best-practice" guidelines. While such progress is impressive, it is important to be able to place it in some sort of perspective. A historical perspective is presented here. Viewed from the past, the current understanding and management of LBS would be remarkable. Conversely, future generations will probably have a different perspective. What will future historians think about today's concepts regarding the management of LBS? It is the perspective of a future generation that perhaps might allow us to properly appraise our current perspective regarding LBS. Therefore, presumptuous as it is and unrealistic as it may be, a brief, futuristic, retrospective commentary will be given regarding today's management of LBS.

FUTURE RETROSPECTIVE VIEW

Perhaps future historians will look at the current understanding of LBS as a transitional period between the information age and the *knowledge age*, defined as the era when truths within the information are isolated, distilled and acknowledged by spinal specialists. Once these truths become evident, then the knowledge age would transition to the *wisdom age*, defined as a period when knowledge is properly applied. If this transition were to occur, what would be the stepping-stones leading to such wisdom, and how would they apply to LBS? Key topics might include the following.

Overcoming Information Overload

This issue was discussed in the first chapter, describing the advent of reams of scientific information of varying quality that was far beyond what one clinician could possibly review or assimilate. One solution to information overload occurred with introduction of *treatment guidelines*, first started in the late twentieth century. While initially simplistic in their recommendations because of a dearth of quality research, this new model provided a means for moving mountains of clinical research forward into a synthesized, contemporary, manageable document from which clinicians could derive a clear clinical direction. Initial problems occurred because of overreliance on these guidelines, blocking treatment for those who were in need of methods before supporting research of acceptable quality became available. However, this was overcome with time, as atypical cases gradually became better understood and managed.

In retrospect, one of the most important occurrences in the evolution of the guideline process took place in Great Britain when the 1994 CSAG document[1] was superseded biannually by updated guidelines. These versions, known as the Royal College of General Physicians[2] (RCGP) Guidelines, allowed for structured guideline growth as technologies and methodologies continued to evolve and the number of quality research papers expanded. Also, this ongoing process allowed guidelines developers the opportunity to mature in this new clinical craft.

The "Low Back Guidelines" model continued to evolve and became quite popular by the dawn of the twenty-first century. No less than 11 countries had established such monograms to provide direction for their respective constituencies.[3] Although there were some consistent recommendations among all of them, significant variations in treatment also occurred, perhaps because of regional preferences, panel makeup, and panelist bias. Because the acute phase of research for LBS was more plentiful than for the chronic phase, only one of the sets of the initial 11 national guidelines even addressed the chronic stage (the Danish Guidelines).[4]

The evolution of the guideline process reached a new milestone in the year 2005 with the advent of the *European Guidelines for Low Back Pain Problems*. Mandated by the European Union in order to attempt to gain better insights and a more organized, strategic approach to the epidemic of disabling LBS, these guidelines comprised the first evidence-based, multinational documents for this topic. These guidelines included a group of four subsets: acute, subacute, chronic nonspecific back pain, and the pelvic girdle.[3,5–7]

Multidisciplinary Organizations

As specialty groups divided the practice of medicine in the twentieth century, barriers were established in the various emerging schools of thought regarding the evaluation and treatment of LBS. Additional clinical disciplines, including chiropractic, osteopathy, and physical therapy added to that complexity. The scenario became more intricate as international perspectives, including linguistic barriers and idiomatic expressions, magnified the challenges of organized and structured progress.

One answer to overcoming this diversity was established with the formation of the World Health Organization (WHO).[8] Based in Switzerland, the WHO was designed to bring disparate health-care groups from around the world together for the common good of humanity. In addition, the Council for International Organizations of Medical Sciences (CIOMS),[9] founded by the WHO and the United Nations Education, Scientific and Cultural Organization (UNESCO)[10] in 1949, gradually provided entry to qualified science-based disciplines (i.e., medicine, osteopathy, dentistry, chiropractic, and physical therapy). The WHO and CIOMS have both provided groundbreaking forums for international, interprofessional, and interspecialty dialogue in health care.

The general strategy of the WHO was later integrated into a nongovernmental, transcultural society for specialists dedicated to LBS. The International Society for the Study of the Lumbar Spine (ISSLS)[11] was established in 1974, which brought together leading authorities from around the world to share their experiences and research. By the turn of the twenty-first century, ISSLS set the standard in international, interprofessional low back research. Instead of being based upon degree, specialty, or pedigree, members earned entry on the basis of their respective clinical academic excellence. True to its international nature, the ISSLS meeting is held at a different location around the world annually. This esteemed body provides attendees with the latest in LBS research and a forum to discuss and debate this rapidly evolving field.

In North America, the American Back Society (ABS)[12] was established in the 1980s utilizing the same basic principles of interprofessional sharing of ideas and camaraderie as previously noted. ABS meets annually for several days and includes scientific presentations, grand rounds among a variety of specialists, and breakout sessions for various specialties.

Finally, the new century brought another global strategy to confront the problem of musculoskeletal pain, including a heavy influence on LBS. The "Bone and Joint Decade"[13,14] was initiated in the year 2000 and involves a 10-year plan among governmental and nongovernmental organizations from around the world to work together in order to reduce human suffering by

- raising awareness of the growing burden of musculoskeletal disorders on society,
- empowering patients to participate in their own care,
- promoting cost-effective prevention and treatment, and
- advancing understanding of musculoskeletal disorders through research to improve prevention and treatment.

These organizations provide prime examples of principles that set the gold standard for interdisciplinary collaboration at the beginning of the twenty-first century and allowed for a more unified and organized global elevation in clinical standards for LBS.

Diagnostic Division of Nonspecific Back Pain

By the year 2000, there were essentially three evidence-based classifications of LBS[3]:

1. Serious or "red flag" conditions
2. Nerve root/radicular conditions
3. Nonspecific back pain

As stated in the initial chapter, the first two classifications comprise less than 15% of all low back problems,[15] leaving the remainder to be placed in the generic nonspecific back pain classification. There are a number of conditions that fall under the umbrella of nonspecific back pain that have received varying degrees of clinical acceptance, some of which were described in earlier chapters. These include the following:

1. Posterior joint pain stemming from the zygapophyseal (the so-called facet syndrome) and/or the sacroiliac joints
2. Internal disc derangement
3. Posterior joint syndromes
4. McKenzie syndromes
5. Myofascial pain
6. Joint dysfunction
7. Combinations of the above diagnoses

The lack of a universally accepted classification system that subdivides nonspecific back pain remained one of the key barrier to gaining control of disabling LBS. Without having such a system upon which to base diagnoses, research designed to determine the efficacy for each of the various classifications was stymied.

Bouter et al. exposed this issue in 1998, stating, "There clearly is a need for an evidence-based classification system for low back pain. Because tenable theoretical framework is lacking, it is difficult to know which determinants of low back pain should be quantified."[16]

Once established, a universally accepted, evidence-based classification system for LBS paved the way for evidence-based treatments according to those diagnoses, indeed a major move forward.

Overcoming "Terminological Chaos"

Janda stated in 1990 that one of the great remaining challenges in health care was that of "terminological chaos."[17] He coined this term to highlight the problem of imprecise and vague clinical descriptors that created barriers to communication and, hence, progress. There are a number of such terms involving the spine that are commonly used today by clinicians, nonclinicians, or both. For example, terms such as sciatica, radiculopathy, radiculitis, instability, stabilization, and spasm can vary greatly in their definitions. Is pain extending from the back to the buttock considered sciatica? Are sciatica and radiculopathy synonymous terms? Do surgeons and rehabilitation specialists define "instability" in the same manner? Why is the term *degenerative disc disease* used, when painless degenerative discs are so commonplace? Terms describing the intervertebral disc vary greatly, leading to confusion as to what is actually being stated.

A pivotal paper was published in 2001 that provided key insights into the solution for terminological chaos. Fardon et al. presented a paper designed to clarify nomenclature regarding lumbar disc pathology.[18] Although this had been previously attempted by others, the unique part of this paper was that its authors were composed of a combined task force from the North American Spine Society (NASS), the American Society of Neuroradiology (ASN), and the American Society of Spine Radiology (ASSR). This paper became known as the NASS Guidelines for disc nomenclature, and helped to clarify confusing terminology that was typically conflicting or diverging. For example, the paper distinguishes between focal (i.e., less than 25% of the circumference) and broad-based (i.e., greater than 25% of the circumference) disc protrusions. This paper also resolved the issue of degenerative disc disease by stating, "Causal connections between degenerative changes and symptoms are often difficult clinical distinctions. The term (i.e., degenerative disc disease) carries implications of illness that may not be appropriate if the only manifestations are from imaging. The preferred term for description of imaging manifestations alone, or imaging manifestations of uncertain relationship to symptoms, is degenerated disc rather than degenerative disc disease."

The NASS Guidelines for disc nomenclature provided an excellent example of a proactive approach to solving one of the many problems confronting spine specialists. While earlier attempts to clarify disc terminology resulted in limited change, this paper received much broader multiprofessional and multispecialty support. With such acceptance at the upper levels of professional organizations, changes in standards of nomenclature then become integrated within other associations and teaching institutions, gradually filtering down to the individual clinician. This is indeed progress in action.

Obesity, Deconditioning, and LBS

The initial chapter of this textbook discussed the societal aspects of the industrial evolution of many countries around the world during the nineteenth and twentieth centuries. With increasing prosperity came increases in quality of life such as an increased availability of food, a reduction in laborious work, and increased leisure time. This reversal of fortune led to the advent of a new scenario in which a reduction of physical demands and an abundance of available nutrients led to positive caloric imbalances. Ergo, a new type of malnutrition, overweight and obesity, was introduced to the masses.[19] This combination of increased levels of human adiposity and physical deconditioning later expanded from industrialized nations to the populations of countries that were becoming industrialized.[8] It has been estimated that two thirds of the world's burden of diseases will be attributable to chronic noncommunicable diseases by 2020, most of these strongly associated with diet.[8] Unfortunately, there remains a widespread opinion that obesity is generally a cosmetic issue rather than the disease that it is now accepted to be.[20]

The incidence of overweight and obese humans at the beginning of this century has been estimated between 1.0 billion[14] and 1.7 billion people,[21] comprising between one sixth and one fourth of the global population. This rate affects far more than just the industrialized countries, as the emerging countries are heavily involved in what has also been called an obesity epidemic by the WHO.[19,22] Ironically, the two groups of humanity who have the lowest levels of obesity are those of the lowest socioeconomic group of the poorest countries, protected by limited access to food, and those of the highest socioeconomic status of the wealthiest countries, presumably with reduced risk due to education and other means (structured diet programs, medical strategies, structured exercise programs, etc.) to avoid the problem.[23]

The international rate of obesity has steadily climbed over the past several decades.[8,13] As this problem has gained increasing attention, it has gradually become associated with a variety of conditions, including diabetes, asthma, cardiovascular conditions, psychological sequelae,[20] and musculoskeletal pain including LBS.[24–26]

There is evidence that the problem of obesity often becomes established during childhood and adolescence.[27] This pattern has been associated with increasing levels of sedentary activities, which may vary among ethnic groups and genders.[28,29] In an era of increased computer games, video, and television, it appears as though humans often will forego physical activities, such as sports and playground games, as long as they remain mentally engrossed with passive activities.[30,31] This, when combined with the availability of food, results in a caloric imbalance in which the intake outpaces that which is being expended. These behaviors, learned early on in life, become exceedingly difficult to change in later years.[32]

Because deconditioning and obesity have been associated with increased risk of chronic LBS,[33] this relatively recent new complication represents yet another challenge that must be confronted and resolved. Fortunately, there is evidence of increasing organization in this battle. The International Obesity Task Force (IOTF)[34] was established in 1994 by the International Association for the Study of Obesity.[35] Its purpose is to collaborate with the WHO and to inform the world about the urgency of what they call the "millennium disease" and to persuade governments that the time to act is now. It is this type of focused international and multidisciplinary attention that is necessary to overcome this disease that threatens to present countries with unmanageable costs and provides a significant complication regarding LBS. The IOTF was instrumental in establishing the body mass index (BMI) as a key measure of obesity.[35]

Unfortunately, there is little available literature regarding clinical management of LBS complicated by obesity. Milissas et al. demonstrated a complete resolution of presurgical back pain among 19 of 29 morbidly obese patients who lost weight 2 years following vertical banded gastroplasty, while the remaining 10 symptomatic cases noted less pain and reduced doses of pain medication.[36] Clearly, more research is necessary to determine a greater understanding of the etiology and management of obesity and its association with LBS.

Flag Expansion

The establishment of the term "red flags" was one of the most successful strategies in the history of LBS, bringing forward universal acceptance of new and important clinical concept. Introduced in the US acute low back pain guidelines in 1994,[37] "red flags" became a rapidly accepted term to define potentially serious conditions at times associated with LBS. This topic was explained in detail in Chapter 10.

On the basis of the successful establishment of red flags, the term of "yellow flags" was later introduced to address important psychosocial factors that tend to create barriers to recovery.[38] Like its crimson predecessor, the yellow warning system found great success in its universal acceptance.

The early twenty-first century brought the establishment of two additional flags, which were given the blue and black color designations.[39] These "third generation" flags were explained in detail in Chapter 11. Because they actually describe subsets of psychosocial factors of chronicity, they should be considered subcategories of the yellow flags. The black and blue flags involve aspects of chronicity and disability associated specifically with the workplace. Because of its importance, the "black flags" emphasize sociooccupational aspects of work (e.g., job satisfaction, health benefits and insurance, work conditions, etc.), whereas the "blue flags" focus on one's work status. While the most recent flags received less widespread attention to date, the importance of highlighting these crucial barriers to recovery was a welcome addition to the flag strategy for LBS.

Research Evolution

The first chapter of this textbook briefly described the formation of the Cochrane Collaboration, an international body designed to bring organization and structure to the subject matter of health-care research. This represented a major step forward in the entire health-care field and the topic of LBS has been no less affected.

The integration of new technologies and refined methodologies continues to emerge as the research evolution continues to advance. Such progression includes those who publish the scientific literature and also those who systematically review the literature. The Cochrane Collaboration Back Task Force for Spinal Disorders established guidelines for systematic literature reviews in 1997.[40] In order to keep pace with emerging trends in research, these methods were updated in 2003.[41]

In 1998, Jadad et al. compared Cochrane systematic reviews and meta-analyses with those of paper-based publications and found the Cochrane reviews to have greater methodological rigor and be more frequently updated.[42] However, Shea et al. compared Cochrane systematic reviews (which is an electronically published format whose studies may later be published in paper-based journals) with systematic reviews in paper-based publications.[43] Using multi-item checkoff assessment tools, the overall quality of both the Cochrane and paper-based reviews was found to be surprisingly low. The authors stated, "This represents a serious situation because clinicians, health policy makers, and consumers are often told that systematic reviews represent the best available evidence." Fortunately, the authors also noted that the Cochrane Collaboration took immediate steps to rectify these faults between the time the research results were completed and the time the paper was accepted for publication. This provides an excellent example of adaptability to problem areas in one's scientific method once recognized, while reminding all to avoid the pitfall of overreliance on the summaries of any group or entity, regardless of their stature.

Other issues regarding the advancement of systematic reviews continue to move forward. For example, the question of language bias was raised in order to determine whether randomized trials published in non-English journals should be included in the systematic review process. Moher et al. found that the quality of *complementary and alternative medicine* (CAM) studies were higher than the *conventional medicine* (CM) intervention studies of non-English publications.[44] As such, they concluded that language restrictions do not appear to bias the CM studies because their quality was less than optimal, while there was substantial bias in the CAM systematic reviews. As international research standards increase, it stands to reason that language barriers will logically continue to be breached, leading to increasingly high and homogenous standards. This in turn would lead to greater levels of quality as larger and more diverse research subject pools are tapped.

Finally, the latter part of the twentieth century brought forward a topic of critical importance in the advancement of research and the guidelines upon which they rely. This involves ethical aspects of research, specifically the issue of conflict of interest among researchers and publications. This is not a new issue. For example, Klein noted concerns regarding sources of research funding and conflicts of interest in his 1979 article involving the relatively new phenomenon of the controlled clinical trial.[45] Three years later, Bean warned about the increasingly controversial relationship between universities and the free enterprise system.[46] Five years after that, Hoppin noted that industry support for university-based research increased 38% between 1980 and 1985 and discussed concerns about issues including conflict of interest (COI) and fulfillment of expectations (FOE).[47]

COI are not simply confined to North America or Western Europe. Recent concerns arising from Central European countries during their transition from socialist-era health care and research suggest the problem is widespread.[48,49]

Of course, industry bringing additional revenues to the field of research in any field of science is not in itself a bad thing. Indeed, much quality research and numerous emerging technologies have been brought forward using this strategy. The question is therefore not whether private sector financial support for emerging technologies and research should be continued or omitted, but rather how these important resources can be utilized in a manner that ethically allows for unbiased studies.

COI issues persisted in the research world into the 1990s. In 1993, members of the influential *International Committee of Medical Journal Editors* (ICMJE) convened in London and drafted a *conflict of interest statement*.[50] They stated that COI for a given manuscript exists when a participant in the peer review and publication process—author, reviewer, and/or editor—has ties to activities that *could* inappropriately influence his or her judgment, regardless of whether that judgment is, in fact, affected. Financial relationships with industry (for example, employment, consultancies, stock ownership, honoraria, expert testimony), either directly or through immediate family members, are usually considered the most important COI. However, conflicts can occur for other reasons, such as personal relationships, academic competition, and intellectual passion. The committee recommended that authors, reviewers, and editorial staff disclose any potential conflicts that might bias their work. Any reviewer or editorial staff with an acknowledged conflict may then require disqualification from the project.

Because of continued COI in health-care research "being taken more seriously by doctors and by society at large," a 1998 editorial in the *British Medical Journal* stressed the importance of transparency among those involved in the research.[51] The editors of this publication then outlined additional measures to further ensure unbiased research in their pages.

Unfortunately, recent papers show that conflicts and compromises remain a problem. For example, Buchkowsky and Jewesson recently reviewed 500 articles randomly chosen from five influential journals over a 20-year period. They found that industry-sponsored and mixed-funding clinical trials are common and have continued to increase in frequency.[52] Earlier that year, Friedman and Richter used three different measures and concluded with each that COI is widespread among the authors of published manuscripts and that those authors are more likely to present positive findings (i.e., supportive of the entity with which they are or were associated).[53]

In September 2004, an editorial statement by the ICMJE provided a new strategy to combat another aspect of COI.[54] This involved researchers and publishers who failed to publish their studies because they failed to demonstrate a significant effect of a given treatment (i.e., a positive trial) or equivalence of two treatment methods (i.e., noninferiority trial). Instead, trials that demonstrated a given treatment was less effective than the standard treatment (i.e., inferiority trial) or those that failed to clearly determine either a positive or negative result (i.e., inconclusive trial) were simply not published. The ICMJE considered all results to be of value and took a stand against the selective reporting of research. They therefore established a strategy that requires researchers of prospective trials to register their trials in a public repository in advance if they wish for their results to be published in the 11 ICMJE-member journals.

These examples demonstrate the importance of clinicians remaining vigilant as independent critical reviewers of the literature and of emerging guidelines. Each clinician must realize that today's research or guidelines are not final products, but rather the latest in an ongoing production. In order for clinicians to provide the optimal treatment for their specific patient's needs, a dynamic balance between clinical experience, clinical research, and clinical guidelines must be continually re-established.

Education

"Other reforms are remedial; education is preventative."—Horace Mann.

One must remember that the word "doctor" stems from the Latin word for "teacher." And so it is that those associated with resolving the epidemic of disabling LBS must hold education as their preeminent modality. Such education can be directed at clinicians and laypersons.

Education of the clinician occurs in many ways. This can include attending post-professional meetings, where the latest in research and professional approaches are demonstrated. Education also occurs by reviewing publications such as periodicals, Internet-based instructional courses, and textbooks such as this.

As noted in Chapter 1, there is growing evidence of variations in health-care provisions based upon racial and ethnic differences.[55–57] Therefore, additional emphases must be placed on the education of clinicians regarding this vital topic. Because of its importance, this commentary recommends the establishment of a new clinical flag, a so-called *rainbow flag*, to assist health-care providers and educational institutions in emphasizing this subject. Educational strategies must include a better understanding of how pain and disability is perceived among different ethnic groups and how clinicians can integrate this information into providing the fair, respectful, and responsible management of members of such groups. Betancourt and Maina[58] recently presented "the first detailed systematic examination of racial/ethnic disparities in health care" and provided specific recommendations for academic health centers to ameliorate this problem. Even more recent research has further helped to highlight the importance of this topic.[59,60,61]

A second new clinical flag designation is recommended for this chapter, one that may be uncomfortable for some health providers. This is the establishment of clinical *"Green Flags"*, designed to place an emphasis on another risk factor of chronicity, *the clinician*. This color is designated because green is a color that is analogous to nature, health and life, This presents a new model in that the focus is established on the other side of the doctor-patient relationship. As such, a variety of issues that can, but should not, influence clinical standards of practice may be brought to light and isolated. From the clinician's personal and professional biases, understanding of current clinical standards, and even prejudices, topics can be brought forward for additional consideration in the hopes of elevating the provider's clinical excellence.

Clinicians must understand and respect their potential impact on their patients, not only their treatment, but also their patient education. For example, how a clinician explains questionably significant disc findings on MRI can either empower the patient to increasing confidence and self-sufficiency, or stigmatize him or her and begin the nightmare of fear avoidance behavior, deconditioning, a plethora of treatment, deconditioning and short or long disability. Green Flags education can assist in overcoming these issues.

This text has demonstrated that there remain a wide variety of clinical options and schools of thought regarding the healthcare subset of LBS, and it will be a long time before universal agreement on these topics arrives. Nevertheless, strategies that promote patient independence and exercises with little or no consequences should be emphasized, while those that promote clinician dependence and deconditioning with unacceptable benefit should be avoided. Once these topics are brought forward, it is hoped that clinicians will welcome the opportunity to learn about themselves and subsequently appreciate how changes in their own personal green flags will help their patients and, hopefully, improve their own professional outcomes.

Layperson instruction can be provided in a variety of ways, from in-office patient consultation to various educational materials and public presentations to mass media programming designed to reach large populations. Each opportunity is important, as it may establish a key cornerstone for greater individual or group understanding that may result in one's increased self-dependence and quality of life.

Given the plethora of available information regarding LBS, the clinician must ultimately decide what approach to take in disseminating information to his or her patient. In addition to the amount of information provided, an ethical decision must be made about how this information should be presented. After all, the clinician can choose to provide information that magnifies or trivializes the severity of the patient's condition, a decision that can be based on many factors. In addition, these choices can also be utilized to influence a patient in the direction the clinician feels will best assist that patient. While each patient's circumstances are unique, each clinician must strive to establish the strongest clinical and ethical foundation possible upon which to base the management of that particular case.

One of the key topics for patient education involves the psychosocial complication of "illness behavior", a topic that was discussed in several chapters of this textbook. It has become clear to me that the greatest restrictions in life are often self-imposed. This is particularly true of the potential emotional and physical devastation caused by fearful avoidance of any painful activities, which is a type of illness behavior that leads to physical deconditioning. This barrier to recovery is common because it combines the instinctive reactions to avoid pain-provoking activities with long-held beliefs regarding pain, many of which are cultural. However, as was discussed in the first chapter, the health-care community facilitated fear-avoidance behavior for nearly a century by directing its patients with LBS to bed rest, reinforcing the notion that activity would "re-injure" their healing tissues.

Ralph Waldo Emerson stated, "The antidote for fear is knowledge." This truth forms the basis of overcoming fear avoidance, and it is incumbent on the clinician to observe his or her patient's unique concerns with the issues of illness behavior in order to educate the patient in a manner that the patient can tolerate and absorb. As with determining the proper dosages of medications or manual treatment methods, the ability to determine the type and amount of patient education is individually unique and involves the art of health care. After all, this science-based approach nevertheless requires human factors such as empathy, compassion, sensitivity, respect, patience, and the ability to be a good listener, a commodity that many patients feel is in short supply among clinicians. Healthcare providers who strive to improve in their human relations skills effectively establish greater opportunities to educate their patients.

Large-scale preventative education regarding LBS is a strategy that has met with some recent success. Buchbinder et al. performed an Australian population-based public education campaign and research across the state of Victoria using television commercials, which resulted in a decline in the number of reported back claims, rates of days compensated, and medical payments for back-related claims.[62]

Interestingly, these commercials also appeared to have a positive effect on clinicians who treat LBS. A follow-up study by these authors indicated that beliefs about back pain remained more positive 3 years later.[63] In short, the population had learned and this translated into long-term changed attitudes, behaviors, and results.

This type of mass media education appears to have significant merit in teaching populations about the psychosocial factors of LBS. Because habits and beliefs are most effectively instilled early in life, it certainly makes sense to target educational programs to youths in order to better prepare them for future life challenges, as is likely to occur with LBS.

Evidence-Based Health Care

One of the problems of western health care in the later 20th century was the costly over utilization of inappropriate procedures and the under utilization of appropriate and efficacious procedures. Evidence-based health care was designed to be a partial solution to this conundrum.

In terms of history, this paradigm developed rapidly, perhaps too rapidly. Its strength appeared to be in its reasonableness, basing treatment on quality research that demonstrated efficacy. Unfortunately, there were early problems because of inherent inequities in this strategy. These problems, which can be called *evidence-based barriers*, require explanation.

First, there was simply an insufficient volume of high-quality trials available to provide comprehensive, evidence-based guidelines at the beginning of the twenty-first century. In the absence of such research, many procedures were either allowed or disallowed by health-care systems consensus based upon the vote of a selected panel of clinicians. Typically composed of leading specialists, panel decisions affected patients and clinicians alike. However, this method at times left inadequate provisions to address issues of bias among panelists. Therefore, such documents could not be considered strictly evidence-based, but rather partially evidence-based, consensus documents.

Second, evidence-based health care (EBHC) provided the opportunity for those whose methods were validated, perhaps because their model was relatively simple to prove or had stronger backing (i.e., financial, political, etc.), to flourish in the established health-care systems. This was an excellent approach to block diagnostic and therapeutic methods that would later fall by the wayside because of their proven lack of efficacy. Unfortunately, other more complex or inadequately supported, yet effective approaches encountered hurdles (administrative, financial, political, and/or professional) that slowed their progress. Because these methods were later proven to be valid, many patients who would have previously benefited were instead blocked access. For EBHC to be effective, it must be able to subclassify assessment and treatment methods into at least three categories: methods whose efficacy is either proven, unproven, and disproven. At the beginning of the twenty-first century, there were really only two divisions because methods that were unproven were synonymous with disproven. As the volume of quality research increased, the division of unproven versus disproven methods became clarified, allowing each group to be addressed individually.

One example of an evidence-based barrier is that of specific exercises for LBS. At the turn of the twenty-first century, there was insufficient evidence to prove that specific exercises were more effective than generic exercise for nonspecific back pain. Of course, without the benefit of accepted diagnostic subdivisions (as discussed earlier), proving the efficacy of specific exercises remains a major challenge. Nevertheless, there is some evidence that this obstacle is gradually being overcome. Following up on prior studies with similar results, Long et al. recently demonstrated strong support for the benefits of specific exercises consistent with specific mechanical diagnoses among acute, subacute, and chronic patients.[64] Conversely, exercises inconsistent with the mechanical diagnoses were far less effective.

With time, the evidence-based barriers and evidence-based biases that hampered the progress of EBHC became clarified and overcome. Perhaps if the health-care world had been a little more careful in organizing this model, the inappropriate barriers and biases would have been lessened.

Additional Responsibilities

With increasing understanding of disabling LBS, it becomes clear that resolving this epidemic requires a *societal* approach. From governmental agencies to teaching institutions, from health-care provider associations to the companies who finance health care and health-related pensions, from attorneys protecting their injured patient's rights to their legal counterparts who provide the defensive strategies, from the clinician to the patient, a greater level of responsibility is necessary. This responsibility requires the practical integration of incoming information, the knowledge of its proper application, and ultimately, the wisdom of optimal management.

This type of responsibility requires that the practice of health care integrates with, yet supersedes, the business and politics of health care. The clinician, like the parent of a child, must accept that the ultimate goal is to return the individual to the highest level of self-dependence possible, which entails directing the patient away from deleterious behavior of clinical dependencies such as unnecessary recurrent office visits, medications, and clinical procedures. The patient must understand that they are ultimately responsible for their own health and subsequently organize a lifestyle that reflects this responsibility.

SUMMARY

And so it is that the topic of disabling LBS, defined as a societogenic condition in the initial chapter, will continue to be problematic for the foreseeable future because of a variety of complex and recalcitrant barriers encumbering progress. Many of these barriers have been spotted, while others are only now coming to light. Still, there may be a few that remain elusive. The speed of which the disabling LBS epidemic will resolve may indeed be commensurate with the society's capacity to adapt, which is by definition, complex and cumbersome.

Assessment and treatment of LBS is, for the most part, under the control of the clinician. Management of disabling LBS is less so, because of a variety of outside factors.

Nevertheless, there is no doubt that multifaceted progress continues. Key organizational strategies are being established to overcome the menace of disabling LBS to governments, institutions, and families. The fact that these devastating effects but will be resolved is certain, because it is human nature to overcome challenges once they become delineated. In the end, the issue is not whether this problem will become controlled, but rather when this will occur. The irony of this is that both the solutions and the barriers are in our hands. It is only a matter of time.

REFERENCES

1. CSAG–(Clinical Standards Advisory Group). Clinical Standards Advisory Group Report on Back Pain. London: HMSO, 1994.
2. RCGP–(Royal College of General Practitioners). *Clinical guidelines for the management of acute low back pain.* London: RCGP, 1996.
3. European Commission, Research Directorate General, Department of Policy, Co-ordination and Strategy. *European guidelines for the management of chronic nonspecific low back pain*. COST ACTION B13. Brussels: European Commission, 2004.
4. Danish Institute for Health Technology Assessment. *Low back pain. Frequency, management and prevention from an HTA perspective*. Danish Health Technology Assessment, 1999.
5. European Commission, Research Directorate General, Department of Policy, Co-ordination and Strategy. *European guidelines for the management of acute nonspecific low back pain in primary care*. COST ACTION B13. Brussels: European Commission, 2004.
6. European Commission, Research Directorate General, Department of Policy, Co-ordination and Strategy. *European guidelines on the diagnosis and treatment of pelvic girdle pain*. COST ACTION B13. Brussels: European Commission, 2004.
7. European Commission, Research Directorate General, Department of Policy, Co-ordination and Strategy. *European guidelines for prevention in low back pain*. COST ACTION B13. Brussels: European Commission, 2004.
8. www.who.int
9. "http://www.cioms.ch"
10. "http://www.unesco.org"
11. www.issls.org
12. americanbacksoc.org
13. "http://www.boneandjointdecade.org"
14. Lidgren L. The Bone and Joint Decade 2000–2010 (www.boneandjointdecade.org). *Bull World Health Organ* September 2003;81(9): 629.
15. Nachemson AL, Waddell G, Norlund AI. Epidemiology of neck and low back pain. In: Nachemson AL, Jonsson E, eds. *Neck and back pain: The scientific evidence of causes, diagnosis and treatment*. Philadelphia: Lippincott Williams & Wilkins, 2000:165–188.
16. Bouter L, van Tulder M, Koes B. Methodologic issues in low back pain research in primary care. *Spine* September 15, 1998;23(18):2014–2020.
17. Janda V. Differential diagnosis of muscle tone in respect of inhibitory techniques. In: Paterson JK, Burn L, eds. *Back pain, an international review.* Dordrecht, The Netherlands: Kluwer Academic Press, 1990:196–199.
18. Fardon D, Milette P, Appel B, et al. Nomenclature and classification of lumbar disc pathology. *Spine* 2001; 26(5):E93–E113.
19. World Health Organization. *Obesity and overweight*, 2003. www.who.int/dietphysicalactivity/publications/facts/obesity/en/
20. Reilly J, Methven E, McDowell Z, et al. Health consequences of obesity. *Arch Dis Child* 2003;88:748–752.
21. Deitel M. Overweight and obesity worldwide now estimated to involve 1.7 billion people. *Obes Surg* June 2003;13(3):329–330.
22. Montiero C, Conde W, Lu B, Popkin B. Obesity and inequities in health in the developing world. *Int J Obes Relat Metab Disord* September 2004;28(9):1181–1186.
23. Zhang Q, Wang Y. Socioeconomic inequality of obesity in the United States: Do gender, age, and ethnicity matter? *Soc Sci Med* March 2004;58(6):1171–1180.
24. Bener A, Alwash R, Gaber T, Lovasz G. Obesity and low back pain. *Coll Antropol* June 2003;27(1):95–104.
25. Andersen R, Crespo C, Bartlett S, Bathon J, Fontaine K. Relationship between body weight gain and significant knee, hip, and back pain in older Americans. *Obes Res* 2003;11:1159–1162.
26. Leboeuf-Yde C. Body weight and low back pain. A systematic literature review of 56 journal articles reporting on 65 epidemiologic studies. *Spine* January 15, 2000;25(2):226–237.

27. Sjolie A. Persistence and change in nonspecific back pain among adolescents: 3-year prospective study. *Spine* November 1, 2004;29(1):2452–2457.
28. Gordon-Lawson P, Adair L, Popkin B. Ethnic differences in physical activity and inactivity patterns and overweight status. *Obes Res* March 2002;10(3): 141–149.
29. Flodmark C, Lissau I, Moreno L, Pietrobelli A, Widhalm K. New insights into the field of children and adolescents' obesity: The European perspective. *Int J Obes Relat Metab Disord* October 2004;28(10):1189–1196.
30. Andersen R, Crespo C, Bartlett S, Cheskin L, Pratt M. Relationship of physical activity and television watching with body weight and level of fatness among children. *J Am Med Assoc* 1998;279:938–942.
31. Balague F, Nordin M, Skovron M, Dutoit G, Yee A, Waldburger M. Non-specific low-back pain among school children: a field survey with analysis of some associated factors. *J Spine Disord* 1994;7:374–379.
32. Barnekow-Bergkvist M, Hedburg G, Janlert U, Jansonn E. Physical activity pattern in men and women at the ages of 16 and 34 and development of physical activity from adolescence to adulthood. *Scand J Med Sci Sport* 1996;6:359–370.
33. Verbundt J, Seelen H, Vlayen J, et al. Disuse and deconditioning in chronic low back pain: Concepts and hypotheses on contributing mechanisms. *Eur J Pain* 2003;7(1):9–21.
34. www.iotf.org
35. Dietz W, Bellizzi M. Introduction: The use of body mass index to assess obesity in children. *Am Soc Clin Nutr* July 1999;70(1):123S–125S.
36. Melissas J, Volakakis E, Hadjipavlou A. Low-back pain in morbidly obese patients and the effect of weight loss following surgery. *Obes Surg* June 2003;13(3):389–393.
37. Bigos S, Bowyer O, Braen G, et al. *Acute low back problems in adults.* Clinical Practice Guideline No. 14. AHCPR Publication No. 95-0642. Rockville, MD: Agency for Health Care Policy and Research, Public Health Service, US Department of Health and Human Services, December 1994.
38. Kendall NAS, Linton SJ, Main CJ. *Guide to assessing psychosocial yellow flags in acute low back pain: Risk factors for long term disability and work loss.* Wellington, NZ: Accident Rehabilitation and Compensation Insurance Corporation of New Zealand and the National Health Committee, 1997.
39. Main CJ, Spanswick CC, eds. *Pain management: An interdisciplinary approach.* Edinburgh: Churchill Livingstone, 2000.
40. van Tulder M, Assendelft W, Koes B, Bouter L. Method guidelines for systematic reviews in the Cochrane Collaboration Back Review Group for Spinal Disorders. *Spine* October 15, 1997;22(20):2323–2330.
41. van Tulder M, Furlan A, Bombardier C, Bouter L. Updated method guidelines for systematic reviews in the Cochrane Collaboration Back Review Group. *Spine* June 15, 2003;28(12):1290–1299.
42. Jadad A, Cook D, Jones A, et al. Methodology and reports of systematic reviews and meta-analyses: A comparison of Cochrane reviews with articles published in paper-based journals. *JAMA* July 15, 1998;280(3):278–280.
43. Shea B, Moher D, Graham I, Pham B, Tugwell P. A comparison of the quality of Cochrane reviews and systematic reviews published in paper-based journals. *Eval Health Prof* March 2002;25(1):116–129.
44. Moher D, Pham B, Lawson M, Klassen T. The inclusion of reports of randomised trials published in languages other than English in systematic reviews. *Health Technol Assess* 2003;7(41):1–90.
45. Klein J. Medical ethics and controlled clinical trials. *Ann Otol Rhinol Laryngol Suppl* September/October 1979;88(5 Pt 2, Suppl 60):99–106.
46. Bean L. Entrepreneurial science and the university. *Hastings Cent Rep* October 1982;12(5):5–9.
47. Hoppin M. A university perspective on pharmaceutical and industry support of research. *Am J Clin Nutr* July 1987;46(Suppl 1):226–228.
48. Tikk A. Conflict of interest in medical research in Estonia. *Sci Eng Ethics* July 2002;8(3):317–318.
49. Nersesyan A. Conflicts of interest in science in Armenia. *Sci Eng Ethics* July 2002;8(3):291–293.
50. Angell M, Clever L, Colaiani L, et al. Conflict of interest. International Committee of Medical Journal Editors. *Ann Intern Med* April 15, 1993;118(8):646–647.
51. Editorial. Beyond conflict of interest. *BMJ* 1998;317: 291–292.
52. Buchkowsky S, Jewesson P. Industry sponsorship and authorship of clinical trials over 20 years. *Arch Pharmacother* April 2004;38(4):57–85.
53. Friedman L, Richter E. Relationship between conflicts of interest and research results. *J Gen Intern Med* January 2004;19(1):51–56.
54. Editorial. A statement from the International Committtee of Medical Journal Editors. *MJA* 2004;181(6):293–294.
55. Tait R, Chibnall J, Andresen E, Hadler N. Management of occupational back injuries: Differences among African Americans and Caucations. *Pain* December 2004;112(3):389–396.
56. Chibnall J, Tait R. Confirmatory factor analysis of the Pain Catastrophizing Scale in African American and Caucasian Workers' Compensation claimants with low back injuries. *Pain* February 2005;113(3):369–375.
57. Green C, Anderson K, Baker T, et al. The unequal burden of pain: Confronting racial and ethnic disparities in pain. *Pain Med* September 2003;4(3):277–294.
58. Betancourt J, Maina A. The Institute of Medicine report "Unequal Treatment": Implications for academic health centers. *Mt Sinai J Med* October 2004;71(5):314–321.
59. Vaccarino U, Rathore S, Wenger N, et al. Sex and racial differences in the management of acute myocardial infarction, 1994 through 2002. *N Engl J Med* Aug 18, 2005;353(7):671–682.
60. Jha A, Fisher E, Li Z, Orav E, Epstein A. Racial trends

in the use of major procedures among the elderly. *N Engl J Med* Aug 18, 2005;353(7):683–691.

61. Trivedi A, Zaslavsky A, Schneider E, Ayanian J. Trends in the quality of care and racial disparities in medicare managed care. *N Engl J Med* Aug 18, 2005;353(7):692–700.
62. Buchbinder R, Jolley D, Wyatt M. Population based intervention to change back pain beliefs and disability: Three part evaluation. *BMJ* 2001;322:1516–1520.
63. Buchbinder R, Jolley D. Population based intervention to change back pain beliefs: Three year follow up population survey. *BMJ* February 7, 2004;328:321–322.
64. Long A, Donelson R, Fung T. Does it matter which exercise? A randomized control trial of exercise for low back pain. *Spine* December 1, 2004;29(23):2593–2602.

Index

Note: page references with an f or a t indicate a figure or table on designated page.

B

C

F

G

N

O

Q

T

W

X